D1605090

LATE-LIFE MOOD DISORDERS

LATE-LIFE
MOOD DISORDERS

Edited By

Helen Lavretsky, MD
DEPARTMENT OF PSYCHIATRY BIOBEHAVIORAL SCIENCES
SEMEL INSTITUTE FOR NEUROSCIENCE HUMAN BEHAVIOR
DAVID GEFFEN SCHOOL OF MEDICINE AT UCLA
LOS ANGELES, CA

Martha Sajatovic, MD
DEPARTMENTS OF PSYCHIATRY AND NEUROLOGY; AND
NEUROLOGICAL OUTCOMES CENTER
UNIVERSITY HOSPITALS CASE MEDICAL CENTER
CLEVELAND, OH

Charles F. Reynolds III, MD
WESTERN PSYCHIATRIC INSTITUTE AND CLINIC
UNIVERSITY OF PITTSBURGH SCHOOL OF MEDICINE
PITTSBURGH, PA

OXFORD
UNIVERSITY PRESS

OXFORD
UNIVERSITY PRESS

Oxford University Press is a department of the University of Oxford.
It furthers the University's objective of excellence in research, scholarship,
and education by publishing worldwide.

Oxford   New York
Auckland   Cape Town   Dar es Salaam   Hong Kong   Karachi
Kuala Lumpur   Madrid   Melbourne   Mexico City   Nairobi
New Delhi   Shanghai   Taipei   Toronto

With offices in
Argentina   Austria   Brazil   Chile   Czech Republic   France   Greece
Guatemala   Hungary   Italy   Japan   Poland   Portugal   Singapore
South Korea   Switzerland   Thailand   Turkey   Ukraine   Vietnam

Oxford is a registered trademark of Oxford University Press
in the UK and certain other countries.

Published in the United States of America by
Oxford University Press
198 Madison Avenue, New York, NY 10016

Library of Congress Cataloging-in-Publication Data
Late-life mood disorders / edited by Helen Lavretsky, Martha Sajatovic, Charles F. Reynolds III.
p. ; cm.
Includes bibliographical references and index.
ISBN 978–0–19–979681–6 (alk. paper)
I. Lavretsky, Helen.   II. Sajatovic, Martha.   III. Reynolds, Charles F., 1947–
[DNLM: 1. Mood Disorders.   2. Aged. WM 171]
616.85'27—dc23
2012031575

1 3 5 7 9 8 6 4 2
Printed in the United States of America
on acid-free paper

To our teachers, students, and patients

CONTENTS

Contributors   xi
Preface   xix

SECTION 1: INTRODUCTION TO
LATE-LIFE MOOD DISORDERS

1 A National Institute of Mental Health
   Perspective on Geriatric Mood Disorder
   Research   3
   Jovier D. Evans and George Niederehe

2 Research Priorities in Late-Life
   Mood Disorders: An International
   Perspective   17
   Briony Dow, Xiaoping Lin, Jean Tinney,
   Betty Harambous, and David Ames

3 Epidemiology of Late-Life Mood
   Disorders: Rates, Measures, and
   Populations   32
   Patricia Marino and Jo Anne Sirey

4 Public Health Burden of Late-Life Mood
   Disorders   42
   Mijung Park and Jürgen Unützer

5 Late-Onset Mood Disorders: *ICDs* and
   DSMs   61
   Roger Peele

SECTION 2: DIAGNOSIS AND
COMORBID CONDITIONS

6 The Diagnosis and Treatment of Unipolar
   Depression in Late Life   79
   John Snowdon and Osvaldo P. Almeida

7 Bipolar Disorder   104
   Robert C. Young and Nahla A. Mahgoub

8 Non-Major Depression   129
   Ipsit V. Vahia, Ganesh Kulkarni,
   Thomas W. Meeks, and Dilip V. Jeste

9 Anxious Depression: Application of a
Unified Model of Emotional Disorders
to Older Adults 144
*Andrew J. Petkus, Eric J. Lenze, and
Julie Loebach Wetherell*

10 The Social Determinants of Depression
in Older Adulthood 164
*Stephen E. Gilman, Hannah Carliner, and
Alex Cohen*

11 Depression in Dementia 177
*Christopher M. Marano, Paul B. Rosenberg, and
Constantine G. Lyketsos*

12 The Challenge of Suicide Prevention in
Later Life 206
Yeates Conwell and Alisa O'Riley

13 Bereavement and Complicated Grief in
Older Adults 220
*M. Katherine Shear, Angela Ghesquiere, and
Michael Katzke*

14 Current Issues in Informal Caregiving
Research: Prevalence, Health Effects,
and Intervention Strategies 236
Richard Schulz

15 Post-Stroke Depression and Vascular
Depression 254
Sarah Volk and David C. Steffens

16 Depression and Medical Illness in Late
Life: Race, Resources, and Stress 270
Briana Mezuk and Joseph J. Gallo

17 Comorbid Neurological Illness 295
Dylan Wint and Jeffrey Cummings

18 Substance Abuse Comorbidity 315
David W. Oslin and Amy Helstrom

19 Comorbid Pain Disorders 329
Jordan F. Karp and Jonathan McGovern

20 Bidirectional Relationships Between
Sleep, Insomnia, and Depression 347
*Chiara Baglioni, Mathias Berger, and
Dieter Riemann*

SECTION 3: TREATMENT AND
PREVENTION

21 Use of Adjunctive Therapy in Older
Depressed Adults Who Are Resistant to
Antidepressant Treatment 363
J. Craig Nelson

22 Psychotherapy 390
Patricia A. Areán

23 Electroconvulsive Therapy and
Neuromodulation in the Treatment of
Late-Life Mood Disorders 406
William M. McDonald and Arshya Vahabzadeh

24 Complementary and Alternative
Medicine Approaches for Treatment
and Prevention in Late-Life Mood
Disorders 432
*David Merrill, Martha Payne, and
Helen Lavretsky*

25 Prevention of Depression in Later Life:
A Developmental Perspective 448
Aartjan T. F. Beekman, Pim Cuijpers, and Filip Smit

26 Depression Medication Treatment
Adherence in Later Life 457
*Kara Zivin, Janet Kavanagh, Susan Maixner,
Jo Anne Sirey, and Helen C. Kales*

SECTION 4: CARE DELIVERY SYSTEMS

27 Depression in Long-Term Care 477
Christina Hui and David L. Sultzer

28 Late-Life Depression in the Primary
Care Setting: Toward a Patient-Centered
Future 500
*Marsha Wittink, Paul Duberstein, and
Jeffrey M. Lyness*

29 Depression in Older Adults Receiving
Hospice Care 516
*Abhilash K. Desai, Daphne Lo, and
George T. Grossberg*

30 Late-Life Mood Disorders
and Home-Based Services and
Interventions 532
*Kisha N. Bazelais, Yolonda R. Pickett, and
Martha L. Bruce*

31 Novel Platforms for Care Delivery: Internet-Based Interventions and Telepsychiatry   546
Pim Cuijpers, Heleen Riper, and Aartjan T. F. Beekman

SECTION 5: NEUROBIOLOGY AND BIOMARKERS

32 Structural Neuroimaging in Late-Life Mood Disorders   559
Sean J. Colloby and John T. O'Brien

33 Molecular Neuroimaging in Late-Life Depression   572
Anand Kumar, Olusola Ajilore, Brent Forester, Jaime Deseda, Matthew Woodward, and Emma Rhodes

34 Functional Neuroimaging in Late-Life Mood Disorders   586
Meenal J. Patel, Howard J. Aizenstein, and Gwenn S. Smith

35 Cognitive Biomarkers in Depression   606
Oliver J. Robinson and Barbara J. Sahakian

36 Neuropathological Markers in Late-Life Depression   627
José Javier Miguel-Hidalgo and Grazyna Rajkowska

37 Pharmacogenetics of Late-Life Depression   643
Greer M. Murphy, Jr.

38 Pharmacokinetics and Pharmacodynamics in Late Life   655
Kristin L. Bigos, Robert R. Bies, and Bruce G. Pollock

39 Psychoneuroimmunology of Depressive Disorders: Implications for Older Adults and Late-Life Depression   675
Michael R. Irwin

40 The HPA Axis and Late-Life Depression   689
Keith Sudheimer, John Flournoy, Anda Gershon, Bevin Demuth, Alan Schatzberg, and Ruth O'Hara

41 Clinical Prediction Models   704
Wesley K. Thompson, Ji-in Choi, and Stewart Anderson

42 Integration of Biological, Clinical, and Psychosocial Predictors of Treatment Response Variability in Late-Life Depression   714
Linda Garand, Ellen M. Whyte, Meryl A. Butters, Elizabeth R. Skidmore, Jordan F. Karp, and Mary Amanda Dew

43 Conclusion   742
Helen Lavretsky, Martha Sajatovic, and Charles F. Reynolds III

Index   747

CONTRIBUTORS

Howard J. Aizenstein, MD, PhD
Department of Psychiatry and Clinical and
    Translational Sciences
University of Pittsburgh School of
    Medicine; and
Department of Bioengineering
University of Pittsburgh
Pittsburgh, PA

Olusola Ajilore, MD, PhD
Department of Psychiatry
University of Illinois-Chicago
Chicago, IL

Osvaldo P. Almeida, PhD
Centre for Medical Research
The University of Western Australia
Crawley, WA, Australia

David Ames, BA, MD, FRCPsych, FRANZCP
National Ageing Research Institute
Royal Melbourne Hospital
Department of Psychiatry
University of Melbourne
Parkville, Victoria, Australia

Stewart Anderson, PhD
Department of Biostatistics
University of Pittsburgh
Pittsburgh, PA

Patricia A. Areán, PhD
Department of Psychiatry
University of California, San Francisco
San Francisco, CA

Chiara Baglioni, PhD
Department of Psychiatry and Psychotherapy
Freiburg University Medical Center
Germany

Kisha N. Bazelais, PhD
Department of Psychiatry
Weill Cornell Medical College
White Plains, NY

Aartjan T. F. Beekman, MD
Department of Psychiatry; and
EMGO Institute for Care and Health Research
VU University Medical Centre
Amsterdam, The Netherlands

Mathias Berger, MD
Department of Psychiatry and
  Psychotherapy
Freiburg University Medical Center
Germany

Robert R. Bies, PharmD, PhD
School of Pharmacy
University of Pittsburgh
Pittsburgh, PA

Kristin L. Bigos, PhD
Lieber Institute for Brain Development
Johns Hopkins Medical Campus
Baltimore, MD

Martha L. Bruce, PhD, MPH
Department of Psychiatry
Weill Cornell Medical College
White Plains, NY

Meryl A. Butters, PhD
Department of Psychiatry
University of Pittsburgh School of Medicine
Pittsburgh, PA

Hannah Carliner, MPH
Department of Society, Human Development
  and Health
Harvard School of Public Health
Boston, MA

Ji-in Choi
Department of Biostatistics
University of Pittsburgh
Pittsburgh, PA

Alex Cohen, PhD
Faculty of Epidemiology and
  Population Health
London School of Hygiene and Tropical
  Medicine
London, UK

Sean J. Colloby, PhD
Institute for Ageing and Health
Newcastle University
Campus for Ageing and Vitality
Newcastle Upon Tyne, UK

Yeates Conwell, MD
Department of Psychiatry
University of Rochester School of Medicine and
  Dentistry; and
Center for the Study of the Prevention of Suicide
Rochester, NY

Pim Cuijpers, PhD
Department of Clinical Psychology; and
EMGO Institute for Care and Health Research
VU University and VU University Medical Center
Amsterdam, The Netherlands

Jeffrey Cummings, MD
Cleveland Clinic Lou Ruvo Center for Brain Health
Las Vegas, NV

Bevin Demuth, MSW
Department of Psychiatry and Behavioral Sciences
Stanford University School of Medicine
Stanford, CA; and
Sierra-Pacific Mental Illness Research and
  Education Center
Department of Veterans Affairs
Palo Alto, CA

Abhilash K. Desai, MD
Department of Geriatric Psychiatry
Sheppard Pratt Hospital
Baltimore, MD

Jaime Deseda
Department of Psychiatry
Harvard Medical School
McLean Hospital
Belmont, MA

Mary Amanda Dew, PhD
Departments of Psychiatry, Psychology,
  Epidemiology, Biostatistics, and
Clinical and Translational Science
University of Pittsburgh School of Medicine
Pittsburgh, PA

Briony Dow, PhD
National Ageing Research Institute
Royal Melbourne Hospital
University of Melbourne
Departments of Psychiatry and Social Work
Parkville, Victoria, Australia

Paul Duberstein, PhD
Department of Psychiatry
University of Rochester Medical Center
Rochester, NY

Jovier D. Evans, PhD
Geriatrics Research Branch
National Institute of Mental Health, NIH
Bethesda, MD

John Flournoy
Department of Psychiatry and
   Behavioral Sciences
Stanford University School of Medicine
Stanford, CA; and
Sierra-Pacific Mental Illness Research and
   Education Center
Department of Veterans Affairs
Palo Alto, CA

Brent Forester, MD
Department of Psychiatry
Harvard Medical School
McLean Hospital
Belmont, MA

Joseph J. Gallo, MD, MPH
Department of Mental Health
Johns Hopkins Bloomberg School of
   Public Health
Baltimore, MD

Linda Garand, PhD
Department of Health and
   Community Systems
University of Pittsburgh School of Nursing
Pittsburgh, PA

Anda Gershon, PhD
Department of Psychiatry and Behavioral Sciences
Stanford University School of Medicine
Stanford, CA; and
Sierra-Pacific Mental Illness Research and
   Education Center
Department of Veterans Affairs
Palo Alto, CA

Angela Ghesquiere, PhD
Department of Psychiatry
Weill Cornell Medical College
White Plains, NY

Stephen E. Gilman, ScD
Departments of Society, Human Development
   and Health and Epidemiology
Harvard School of Public Health; and
Department of Psychiatry
Massachusetts General Hospital
Boston, MA

George T. Grossberg, MD
Departments of Neurology and Psychiatry, Anatomy
   and Neurobiology,and Internal Medicine
Saint Louis University School of Medicine
St. Louis, MO

Betty Harambous, MSW
National Ageing Research Institute
Royal Melbourne Hospital
Parkville, Victoria, Australia

Amy Helstrom, PhD
Department of Psychiatry
Philadelphia VA Medical Center; and
Mental Illness Research, Education, and
   Clinical Center (MIRECC)
Philadelphia, PA

Christina Hui, MD
Department of Psychiatry and Biobehavioral
   Sciences
David Geffen School of Medicine at UCLA; and
VA Greater Los Angeles Healthcare System
Los Angeles, CA

Michael R. Irwin, MD
Cousins Center for Psychoneuroimmunology
Semel Institute for Neuroscience
University of California, Los Angeles
Los Angeles, CA

Dilip V. Jeste, MD
Department of Psychiatry; and
Sam and Rose Stein Institute for Research on
   Aging
University of California, San Diego, CA

Helen C. Kales, MD
National VA Serious Mental Illness Treatment
   Resource & Evaluation Center (SMITREC); and
Department of Psychiatry
University of Michigan Health System
Ann Arbor, MI

Jordan F. Karp, MD
Departments of Psychiatry, Anesthesiology, and
Clinical and Translational Science
Western Psychiatric Institute and Clinic
University of Pittsburgh School of Medicine
Pittsburgh, PA

Michael Katzke, JD
Columbia University School of Social Work
New York, NY

Janet Kavanagh
Department of Psychiatry
University of Michigan Health System
Ann Arbor, MI

Anand Kumar, MD
Department of Psychiatry
University of Illinois-Chicago
Chicago, IL

Ganesh Kulkarni, MBBS
San Diego State University
San Diego, CA

Helen Lavretsky, MD
Department of Psychiatry and Biobehavioral
  Sciences
Semel Institute for Neuroscience and Human
  Behavior
David Geffen School of Medicine at UCLA
Los Angeles, CA

Eric J. Lenze, MD
Department of Psychiatry
Washington University School of Medicine
St. Louis, MO

Xiaoping Lin
National Ageing Research Institute
Royal Melbourne Hospital
Parkville, Victoria, Australia

Daphne Lo, MD
Department of Internal Medicine
University of Colorado, Denver
Aurora, CO

Constantine G. Lyketsos, MD, MHS
Department of Psychiatry and Behavioral Sciences
Johns Hopkins Bayview Medical Center
Baltimore, MD

Jeffrey M. Lyness, MD
Department of Psychiatry
University of Rochester Medical Center
Rochester, NY

Nahla A. Mahgoub, MD
Department of Psychiatry
Weill Cornell Medical College
White Plains, NY

Susan Maixner, MD
Department of Psychiatry
University of Michigan Health System
Ann Arbor, MI

Christopher M. Marano, MD
Department of Psychiatry and Behavioral Sciences
Johns Hopkins Bayview Medical Center
Baltimore, MD

Patricia Marino, PhD
Department of Psychiatry
Weill Cornell Medical College
White Plains, NY

William M. McDonald, MD
Department of Psychiatry and
  Behavioral Sciences
Emory University School of Medicine
Atlanta, GA

Jonathan McGovern
Western Psychiatric Institute and Clinic
University of Pittsburgh School of Medicine
Pittsburgh, PA

Thomas W. Meeks
Department of Psychiatry
University of California, San Diego, CA

David Merrill, MD, PhD
Department of Psychiatry and Biobehavioral
  Sciences
Semel Institute for Neuroscience and Human
  Behavior
David Geffen School of Medicine at UCLA
Los Angeles, CA

Briana Mezuk, PhD
Department of Epidemiology and Community
  Health
Virginia Commonwealth University
Richmond, VA

José Javier Miguel-Hidalgo, PhD
Department of Psychiatry and Human Behavior
University of Mississippi Medical Center
Jackson, MS

Greer M. Murphy, Jr., MD, PhD
Department of Psychiatry and Behavioral Sciences
Stanford University School of Medicine
Stanford, CA

J. Craig Nelson, MD
Department of Psychiatry
University of California, San Francisco
San Francisco, CA

George Niederehe, PhD
Geriatrics Research BranchNational Institute
    of Mental HealthNational Institutes of
    HealthBethesda, Maryland

John T. O'Brien, DM
Institute for Ageing and Health
Newcastle University
Campus for Ageing and Vitality
Newcastle Upon Tyne, UK

Ruth O'Hara, PhD
Department of Psychiatry and Behavioral Sciences
Stanford University School of Medicine
Stanford, CA; and
Sierra-Pacific Mental Illness Research and
    Education Center
Department of Veterans Affairs
Palo Alto, CA

Alisa O'Riley, PhD
Department of Psychiatry
University of Rochester School of Medicine and
    Dentistry; and
Center for the Study of the Prevention of Suicide
Rochester, NY

David W. Oslin, MD
Department of Psychiatry
Philadelphia VA Medical Center; and
Mental Illness Research, Education, and Clinical
    Center (MIRECC)
Philadelphia, PA

Mijung Park, PhD, MPH RN
Department of Health and Community Systems
University of Pittsburgh School of Nursing
Pittsburgh, PA

Meenal J. Patel
Department of Bioengineering
University of Pittsburgh
Pittsburgh, PA

Martha Payne, PhD, RD, MPH
Department of Psychiatry and Behavioral Sciences
Neuropsychiatric Imaging Research Laboratory
Duke University School of Medicine
Durham, NC

Roger Peele, MD, DLFAPA
Behavioral Health and Crisis Center
    Montgomery County
Rockville, MD

Andrew J. Petkus, MA
SDSU/UCSD Joint Doctoral Program in Clinical
    Psychology
San Diego, CA

Yolonda R. Pickett, MD
Department of Psychiatry
Weill Cornell Medical College
White Plains, NY

Bruce G. Pollock, MD, PhD
Campbell Family Mental Health Research Institute
Centre for Addiction and Mental Health
Departments of Psychiatry and Pharmacology
University of Toronto, CA

Grazyna Rajkowska, PhD
Department of Psychiatry and Human Behavior
University of Mississippi Medical Center
Jackson, MS

Charles F. Reynolds III, MD
Western Psychiatric Institute and Clinic
University of Pittsburgh School of Medicine
Pittsburgh, PA

Dieter Riemann, PhD
Department of Psychiatry and Psychotherapy
Freiburg University Medical Center
Freiburg, Germany

Heleen Riper, PhD
Departments of Clinical Psychology and
    Psychiatry; and
EMGO Institute for Care and Health Research
VU University Medical Centre
Amsterdam, The Netherlands

Emma Rhodes
Department of Psychiatry
University of Illinois-Chicago
Chicago, IL

Oliver J. Robinson, PhD
National Institute of Mental Health
Bethesda, MD

Paul B. Rosenberg, MD
Department of Psychiatry and
    Behavioral Sciences
Johns Hopkins Bayview Medical Center
Baltimore, MD

Barbara J. Sahakian, PhD
Department of Psychiatry
University of Cambridge; and
MRC/Wellcome Trust Behavioural and Clinical
    Neuroscience Institute
Cambridge, UK

Martha Sajatovic, MD
Departments of Psychiatry and
    Neurology; and
Neurological Outcomes Center
University Hospitals Case Medical Center
Cleveland, OH

Alan Schatzberg, MD
Department of Psychiatry and Behavioral Sciences
Stanford University School of Medicine
Stanford, CA

Richard Schulz, PhD
Departments of Psychiatry, Epidemiology,
    Sociology, Psychology, Community Health, &
    Health and Rehabilitation Sciences
University Center for Social and Urban
    Research; and
Aging Institute of UPMC Senior Services
University of Pittsburgh, PA

M. Katherine Shear, MD
Center for Complicated Grief, Columbia
    University School of Social Work and Columbia
    University College of Physicians and Surgeons
New York, NY

Jo Anne Sirey, PhD
Department of Psychiatry
Weill Cornell Medical College
White Plains, NY

Elizabeth R. Skidmore, PhD
Department of Occupational Therapy
University of Pittsburgh School of Health &
    Rehabilitation Sciences
Pittsburgh, PA

Filip Smit, PhD
Department of Epidemiology and
    Biostatistics
EMGO Institute for Care and Health Research
VU University Medical Centre
Amsterdam, The Netherlands

Gwenn S. Smith, PhD
Department of Psychiatry and
    Behavioral Sciences
John Hopkins University School of Medicine
Baltimore, MD

John Snowdon, FRCPsych, FRANZCP, MD
Department of Psychological Medicine
Concord Clinical School
The University of Sydney
Sydney, Australia

David C. Steffens, MD
Department of Psychiatry
University of Connecticut Health Center
Farmington, CT

Keith Sudheimer, PhD
Department of Psychiatry and
    Behavioral Sciences
Stanford University School of Medicine
Stanford, CA

David L. Sultzer, MD
Department of Psychiatry and Biobehavioral
    Sciences
David Geffen School of Medicine at
    UCLA; and
VA Greater Los Angeles Healthcare System
Los Angeles, CA

Wesley K. Thompson, PhD
Department of Psychiatry
University of California, San Diego
San Diego, CA

Jean Tinney, PhD
National Ageing Research Institute
Royal Melbourne Hospital
Parkville, Victoria, Australia

Jürgen Unützer, MD, MPH, MA
Department of Psychiatry and
  Behavioral Sciences
University of Washington School of Medicine
Seattle, WA

Arshya Vahabzadeh, MD
Department of Psychiatry and Behavioral Sciences
Emory University School of Medicine
Atlanta, GA

Ipsit V. Vahia, MD
Department of Psychiatry; and
Sam and Rose Stein Institute for Research on
  Aging
University of California,
San Diego, CA

Sarah Volk, MD
Department of Psychiatry
University of North Carolina School of Medicine
Chapel Hill, NC

Julie Loebach Wetherell, PhD
VA San Diego Healthcare System
Department of Psychiatry
University of California,
San Diego, CA

Ellen M. Whyte, MD
Departments of Psychiatry and Physical Medicine
  and Rehabilitation
University of Pittsburgh School of Medicine
Pittsburgh, PA

Dylan Wint, MD
Cleveland Clinic Lou Ruvo Center for Brain Health
Las Vegas, NV

Marsha Wittink, MD, MBE
Department of Psychiatry and Department of
  Family Medicine and Community Health
University of Rochester Medical Center
Rochester, NY

Matthew Woodward
Department of Psychiatry
Harvard Medical School
McLean Hospital
Belmont, MA

Robert C. Young, MD
Department of Psychiatry
Weill Cornell Medical College
White Plains, NY

Kara Zivin, PhD
National VA Serious Mental Illness Treatment
  Resource & Evaluation Center (SMITREC)
University of Michigan Health System
Ann Arbor, MI

PREFACE

WITH THE global population aging, a greater number of older adults will experience mood disorders in later life. Over the next four decades the number of individuals aged 60 years and older will nearly triple, increasing from 672 million in 2005 to almost 1.9 billion by 2050 (http://www.un.org). By mid-century projected life expectancy in developed countries will be 82 years, and there will be two elderly persons for every child (http://www.un.org). Late-life mood disorders carry additional risk for suicide, medical comorbidity, disability, and family caregiver burden. More clinicians and researchers involved in care of older adults will have to deal with late-life mood disorders as primary or coexisting problems. More clinicians and caregivers will need guidance in finding successful treatments for older adults with depressive or bipolar disorders. More researchers will face the issue of inadequate treatment response in the presence of medical and neurological comorbid disorders and psychosocial issues like bereavement and caregiver stress, or social isolation and loneliness that perpetuate the chronic course of depression and determine poor treatment outcomes. This urgent need generated the impetus for a book that will address inquiries from the geriatric mental health practitioners and researchers, as well as the interested lay public, and will cover broad aspects of the up-to-date information about neurobiology, diagnosis, and care for older adults with mood disorders.

Our unique book represents a comprehensive compendium of knowledge about the course, prognosis, treatment, and prevention of late-life mood disorders. Detailed review of recent research advances in understanding neurobiology and psychosocial origins of geriatric mood disorders in the first decade of the 21st century is provided by the international group of 110 leading experts in the field, who carefully review the latest developments and "gold standards" of care or methodologies but also project the anticipated future directions of research and translation into clinical practice. These most prominent experts in their respective fields deliver key messages in a way that is user friendly, relevant, and influential for future clinical and research trends.

This volume is intended to target a broad audience of clinical researchers and clinicians. The content of the book will increase clinicians' and researchers' competency in recent research findings and broaden their diagnostic and therapeutic perspectives and power of observation that will prepare them to deal with the challenges of finding appropriate effective treatments for older adults with mood disorders. The discussion of the data is presented in a textbook format and can be used for training of students of geriatric mental health. Individual chapters can be used as references on a particular topic for interested clinicians and researchers who are dedicated to the treatment and study of mood disorders in older people might consider this volume an essential part of their library.

Section 1 (Introduction to Late-Life Mood Disorders) addresses clinical phenomenology and diagnosis of late-life mood disorders, and it provides new information on the latest edition of the diagnostic classification systems of mental disorders: *The Diagnostic Statistical Manual*, fifth edition (*DSM-5*), and the *International Classification of Disorders*, 11th edition (*ICD-11*), as well as the recent epidemiological studies of late-life mood disorders. Section 2 (Diagnosis and Comorbid Conditions) provides new information on emerging new trends in diagnosing major neuropsychiatric disorders comorbid with other medical and cognitive disorders, and in the context of psychosocial stress. Much of the new research is related to the neurobiology of coexisting cognitive, vascular, pain, and sleep disorders. These chapters will also provide an update on the available treatment options for the disorders. Section 3 (Treatment and Prevention) provides an overview and an update of the main principles of treatment

and new trends in prevention of late-life mood disorders. Section 4 (Care Delivery Systems) provides an update on the state of the established health care systems (e.g., nursing homes, medical settings); evolving research in the palliative care and hospice setting, home health, Internet, and telemedicine; and the third-world countries' approach to care for elderly depressed. Finally, Section 5 (Neurobiology and Biomarkers) focuses on the use of biomarkers in research and clinical practice with a preview of potential use for developing individualized treatments for older adults with mood disorders. Future directions for research and translation into clinical practice are summarized in Chapter 43.

This volume differs from other publications because it covers a wide variety of diagnostic and treatment approaches to primary and secondary geriatric depressive and bipolar disorders in older adults. It also brings an international perspective to the diagnostic classification, as well as the latest understanding of the psychosocial origins and neurobiological mechanisms of late-life mood disorders, treatment, and preventive strategies in this vulnerable and growing population of older adults. Many chapters bridge science and policy, identifying future directions of therapeutics and models of treatment development with direct relevance for reimbursement for quality and evidence-based interventions. It is our hope that this book will increase professional and public awareness of the complexity of late-life mood disorders and will help disseminate the current knowledge and identify areas for future research. Ultimately, we hope it will help improve treatment outcomes and quality of life of those suffering from late-life mood disorders and their families.

The Editors

SECTION 1

INTRODUCTION TO LATE-LIFE MOOD DISORDERS

1

A NATIONAL INSTITUTE OF MENTAL HEALTH PERSPECTIVE ON GERIATRIC MOOD DISORDER RESEARCH

Jovier D. Evans and George Niederehe

THE NATIONAL Institute of Mental Health (NIMH) is the lead federal agency in the United States responsible for supporting research on mental and behavioral disorders. The mission of the NIMH is to transform the understanding and treatment of mental illnesses through basic and clinical research, paving the way for prevention, recovery, and cure. With an annual budget of roughly $1.4 billion (http://www.nimh.nih.gov/about/budget/fy-2012-budget-congressional-justification.shtml, accessed April 29, 2012), NIMH funds research by scientists across the country as well as in an intramural research program on the National Institutes of Health (NIH) campus. Through its extramural program, NIMH supports more than 2,000 research grants and contracts at universities and other institutions across the country and overseas. Investigators propose projects through grant applications that are evaluated by peer reviewers and must apply for renewals at intervals in order to receive continued funding.

Approximately 500 scientists work in the NIMH intramural research program. Intramural scientists range from molecular biologists working in laboratories to clinical researchers working with patients at the NIH Clinical Center. Because it involves basic science as well as clinical trials, the program is structured to facilitate interdisciplinary studies.

To accomplish this mission, the Institute is interested in supporting basic and clinical science that will lead to new discoveries regarding major public health problems such as late-life mood and anxiety disorders, as well as translational research efforts to speed the movement of scientific findings into clinical applications for and broad dissemination to those suffering with these disorders. To move this work forward, the Institute endeavors to foster innovative thinking and ensure that a full array of research approaches is used to further discovery and translation in the evolving science of brain, behavior, and experience. From the NIMH perspective, there are particular needs for research aimed at deepening our mechanistic understanding of mood and anxiety disorders and at expanding science-based approaches to intervening in their course.

The United States today has more aged adults than at any other time in its history, and this number is rapidly increasing. As of May 2010, the US Bureau of the Census estimated that 40.2 million Americans are 65 years or older, comprising 13% of the population. By 2050, this age segment will have more than doubled to over 88.5 million older adults (Vincent & Velkoff, 2010). Along with this rapid growth in numbers, the proportion of older adults with mood and anxiety disorders is also expected to increase. Much of this increase may be due to the fact that as people in general live longer, they may experience more chronic, age-related diseases that may predispose them to develop concomitant mental disorders, as well as to changing characteristics of the older adult cohort (e.g., baby boomers may have more prior psychiatric and substance abuse histories, relative to their pre–World War II parents; Hybels & Blazer 2003; Jeste et al., 1999). Current estimates suggest that by 2020, depression will be second only to heart disease in its contributions to the global burden of disease (Chapman & Perry, 2008). This rapid increase in our aging adult cohorts creates an increased need to understand and reduce the public health burden of mood and anxiety disorders on older Americans.

Mood and anxiety disorders in late life are very common and often comorbid with other mental and physical illnesses (Alexopoulos, Schultz, & Lebowitz, 2005; Kessler et al., 2010). Within a 12-month period, anxiety disorders affect 7%–12% and depressive disorders 2.6%–5% of adults over 65 (Byers, Yaffe, Covinsky, Friedman, & Bruce, 2010; Gum, King-Kallimanis, & Kohn, 2009; Kessler et al., 2005). Late-life major depressive disorder (MDD) frequently manifests as physical symptoms and is often underrecognized, misdiagnosed, and undertreated. It tends to be more recurrent and chronic than depression in younger patients. Generalized anxiety disorder (GAD), characterized by pervasive, excessive, and uncontrollable worry about everyday situations, has a prevalence rate of 7% among older adults and frequently manifests itself in later years (Gum et al., 2009; Lenze & Wetherell, 2009). In addition, these forms of disorder often occur together in the elderly, though in general the anxiety features remain relatively understudied in this population (Gum et al., 2009; King-Kallimanis, Gum, & Kohn, 2009).

Among older adults, mood and anxiety disorders are associated with physical illness and cognitive impairment, and they result in reduced quality of life and increased functional disability and suicide risk (Alexopoulos, 2005; Lenze & Wetherell, 2009; Steffens, 2009). Of particular note, a significant risk associated with late-life depression is that of excess mortality (Alexopoulos, 2005; Schoevers et al., 2009; Thomas & O'Brien, 2009). Depression has been shown to predict less successful outcomes of treatment for other physical conditions, particularly cardiovascular and cerebrovascular disease, and to increase death rates among the elderly (Thomas & O'Brien, 2006). The significant toll that GAD takes on daily functioning, quality of life, and morbidity/mortality parallels that seen in MDD (Brenes et al., 2007, 2008). There is a pressing need to understand the pathways whereby mood and anxiety disorders contribute to these negative consequences and to develop more effective treatments to alleviate their symptoms among the elderly.

To improve our understanding of late-life mood and anxiety disorders and our capacity to treat and prevent them, as spelled out in its Strategic Plan (National Institute of Mental Health, 2008; Insel, 2009), NIMH will advance research and promote research training to fulfill the following four objectives: (1) promote discovery in the brain and behavioral sciences to fuel research on the causes of mental disorders; (2) chart mental illness trajectories to determine when, where, and how to intervene; (3) develop new and better interventions that incorporate the diverse needs and circumstances of people with mental illness; and (4) strengthen the public health impact of NIMH-supported research. This chapter highlights opportunities for research on late-life mood and anxiety disorders across the translational spectrum from bench to bedside and from bedside to the community.

DIMENSIONAL ASPECTS OF PSYCHOPATHOLOGY AND BEHAVIOR

One specific subobjective of the Strategic Plan that may be relevant to geriatric mental health concerns the Research Domain Criteria (RDoC) project. Strategy 1.4 of the NIMH Strategic Plan calls for the development, for research purposes, of new ways of classifying psychopathology based on dimensions of observable behavior and neurobiological measures. The RDoC project has been launched by NIMH to implement this strategy. The goal is to create a framework for research classifications that reflect functional dimensions stemming from translational research on genes, circuits, and behavior (Cuthbert & Insel, 2010). An NIMH project group has been established to define basic dimensions of functioning (such as fear circuitry or working memory) to be studied across multiple levels of analysis, from genes to neural circuits to behaviors, cutting across disorders as traditionally defined.

One of the most fundamental implications of this approach will be alterations in how clinical samples are composed for research. Under the RDoC framework, study participants might be screened, characterized, and grouped primarily on the basis of a gene polymorphism, a response to an imaging task, or their performance on an executive functioning task, independent of a traditional *Diagnostic and Statistical Manual of Mental Disorders* (DSM) psychiatric diagnosis. The goal is to advance the study of basic mechanisms of mental disorder by fully outlining and developing evidence for crosscutting features of psychopathology at multiple levels of analysis, ranging from the behavioral to the molecular and cellular, with particular emphasis on neurocircuitry (Cuthbert & Insel, 2010; Insel & Cuthbert, 2009; Insel et al., 2010).

Such a dimensional approach to the phenotypic characterization of mood disorder may be particularly useful in geriatric research where most older adults have comorbid diagnoses that do not fit neatly into specific DSM categories, and it may open up numerous questions for investigation that do not fit well into a categorical diagnostic framework. For example, what is the neurobiological significance of subsyndromal depression in old age? What mechanisms underlie the relationship of depression and anxiety among older adults? Are there similar or different neurobiological circuits involved in the expression of particular illness behaviors in younger versus older adults? Such questions are ripe targets for future clinical neuroscience research among older adults.

INTEGRATING NEUROBIOLOGY AND BASIC NEUROSCIENCE INTO THE STUDY OF LATE-LIFE MOOD AND ANXIETY DISORDERS

Genomic Research

As a field, geriatric mental health research needs to capitalize on recent findings and methodological

advances in the fields of genomics, neuroscience, and the biology of aging and integrate these findings and approaches into the study of late-life mood and anxiety disorders. The failure of genome-wide association studies to identify clear-cut genetic causes for psychiatric disorders has underlined the multigenetic complexity of these disorders and certainly suggests that research focused on single nucleotide polymorphisms is unlikely to provide comprehensive explanations for the pathophysiology of mood disorders (Moskvina et al., 2009). More work is needed to examine complex patterns of genetic influence on or risk for the expression of psychopathology in later life, utilizing broad arrays of genetic factors and their interactions, including interactions with environmental influences (Psychiatric GWAS Consortium Steering Committee, 2009).

Such research regarding the genetic regulation of late-life disorders will require not only the examination of comprehensive gene expression profiles but a focus on integrating such factors as the basic biology of normal aging, the molecular pathways of CNS aging, and the genetics of longevity. A wide variety of genes that have been linked with molecular brain aging, such as BDNF, sirtuins, and other genetic polymorphisms, may play a role in the development of neuropsychiatric disorders (Glorioso & Sibille, 2011). In their review of this topic, these authors discuss several techniques for investigating these potential research avenues, most notably the use of postmortem brain microarray studies to identify possible genetic markers of molecular brain aging.

A recent gene by environment interaction study by Kohli and colleagues (2011) that has been heralded as pointing to a new way to understand how complex neurobiological systems may interact and impact psychiatric disorder (Tost & Meyer-Lindenberg, 2011) also provides an example of the importance of taking the aging process into account. In this research, genome-wide association (GWAS) methods initially identified a risk variant for MDD (rs 1545843) on chromosome 12q21.31 in a German sample (N = 353 index cases and 366 healthy controls). This risk variant finding was replicated in a meta-analysis of data from six other independent samples of German, Dutch, United Kingdom, and African American origin, thereby basing the overall finding on data accumulated from over 15,089 unrelated individuals. Furthermore, the investigators used human gene expression studies and high-resolution magnetic resonance imaging (MRI) and magnetic resonance spectroscopy

(MRS) neuroimaging studies to examine the functional relevance of the identified genetic locus in humans, and they established a role for it in environmental interactions by examining its hippocampal expression in a mouse model of chronic stress. The findings across these various methodologies converged on suggesting the SLC6A15 neuronal transporter gene as a susceptibility factor for depression.

However, Kohli et al. also discovered that this finding did not replicate in the Rotterdam study (Hofman et al., 2007), where the average age of 72 years for those experiencing an incident depressive episode was significantly older than that seen in any of the other samples used, either the German discovery sample (average age, 50.4 years) or the other replication samples (age range, 39.3 to 48.7). In addition, in the other samples, rs1545843 was significantly associated with depression only among individuals younger than 55 years and not in the older age subgroups, leading the investigators to suggest that late-life depression may be pathophysiologically distinct from MDD and more closely related to vascular disease and the future expression of cognitive impairment. These striking findings illustrate the critical importance of evaluating aging as a major variable in genetic and other neurobiological research on mood disorders, and they pose a fundamental question for future research: With late-life disorders, are we talking about the same set of illnesses that occur among younger adults with mood and anxiety disorders?

Neuroimaging Research to Understand Pathophysiology

Neuroimaging research on geriatric mood and anxiety disorders has used a variety of approaches to delineate the pathophysiology and associated mechanisms of illness. Much of the work done with midlife and older adult samples has documented both structural and functional abnormalities in depressed patients (for a more complete review, see Gunning & Smith, 2011; Smith et al., 2007). Many of the studies have documented structural changes in the frontal, limbic, and subcortical structures thought to be involved in the affective and cognitive abnormalities of depression (Benjamin & Steffens, 2011). Functional neuroimaging studies have found both hypo- and hyperactivation of these networks, with the patterns varying according to aspects of depression severity, age, and comorbid

conditions (Aizenstein et al., 2009; Andreescu et al., 2009; Gunning & Smith, 2011). The findings of increased white matter changes among older adults with MDD and the use of novel techniques such as diffusion tensor imaging have led to network-based theories of cerebrovascular changes consistent with the vascular depression hypothesis (Alexopoulos, 2006). Advances in technology are now allowing investigators to take more mechanistic approaches to the study of pathophysiology of depression and its relationship to clinical outcomes and treatment response. It will be useful to examine neuroimaging markers in future studies of clinical efficacy and treatment response in order to expand understanding of both disease mechanisms and treatment effects.

Inflammation

As systemic inflammatory processes have been related in the literature both to a myriad of physical and neuropsychiatric illnesses (Miller, Maletic, & Raison 2009) and to aspects of biological aging (Brinkley et al., 2009), the study of inflammatory pathways is apt to be a ripe area for research on the pathophysiology of age-related depression. The "cytokine hypothesis of depression" assumes that inflammatory mediators play a role in the pathophysiology of depression (Maes, 1995; Maes et al., 1994, 2009). In both cross-sectional and longitudinal studies, investigators have noted that inflammatory mechanisms are indeed elevated among older adults with depression; although the evidence suggests a potential causal role in the development of disorder, the exact mechanisms remain unclear (Bremmer et al., 2008; Lotrich, El-Gabalawy, Guenther, & Ware, 2011; Milaneschi et al., 2009). In one review, it has been noted that systemic inflammation as well as recurring life stressors contribute to the negative outcomes seen in both physical and mental health conditions among older adults (Rosano, Marsland, & Gianaros, 2011).

Biomarkers of Aging

We view it as important that investigators of biological mechanisms in late-life mood and anxiety disorders incorporate measures of the biological aging process into their studies, so as to advance investigation of how the pathways leading to aging and to disease may interact. A peripheral marker of cellular aging that may hold promise for integrating the biological aging process into geriatric mood and anxiety disorder research comes from the study of telomeres and telomerase activity (Blackburn et al., 1989; Harley, Futcher, & Greider, 1990). Wolkowitz and colleagues (2010) have posited that depression is associated with premature aging of certain cells both in the peripheral bloodstream and in the central nervous system, that this is traceable to specific biochemical mediators, and that this may account for some of the disability associated with depression. According to this theory of the aging process, chronic stress leads to changes in glucocorticoids, which drive changes in various gene expression patterns and cytokine functions, that lead to changes in telomere length and function, which in turn prompt cellular senescence. More research is needed to determine whether peripheral markers of this aging process have counterparts in the central nervous system and reflect biological changes of significance in depression. In a preliminary study, Wolkowitz, Mellon, and colleagues (2011) have found that telomere length was inversely correlated with oxidative stress in both depressed patients and controls, and with inflammation among depressed subjects. They also noted that although there were no group differences, overall telomere length was inversely related to lifetime depression exposure, such that patients who were above the median (>9.2 years of cumulative duration of depression) had significantly shorter telomere length. It should be noted that findings linking this marker with depression exposure or pathophysiology may not be specific to depression, as other studies have suggested similar manifestations of accelerated aging in bipolar disorder (Yatham et al., 2009) and in schizophrenia (Kirkpatrick, Messias, Harvey, Fernandez-Egea, & Bowie, 2008).

Other meaningful indices of biological aging to consider for incorporation into mood and anxiety disorder research include markers of allostatic load, which represents the degree of "wear and tear" on the body in response to stressful situations. This model proposes that chronic stressors impact the homeostatic mechanisms responsible for neuroendocrine, sympathetic, and cellular functions that may contribute to senescence and alter trajectories of disease across the life span (for a review, see Juster, McEwen, & Lupien, 2010). Research into the relationships between allostatic load and mood and anxiety disorders among older people may be especially meaningful for identifying protective or "resilience" factors as well as pathways of risk that can guide

efforts to develop preventive interventions for these disorders.

DEVELOPMENTAL TRAJECTORIES AND LATE-LIFE MOOD DISORDERS

Those who take the viewpoint that many of the major mental disorders are neurodevelopmental in nature often concentrate only on the early developmental periods of life, and the time window within which the neurodevelopmental process has been examined has ranged primarily from prenatal exposures to late adolescence or early adulthood. There is a gap in the research literature regarding key periods of risk or vulnerability for manifesting mood and anxiety disorder in the later developmental course. Research is needed that examines developmental changes throughout the life span to determine whether there are particularly sensitive periods or other transitions relevant to late-life mood disorders.

Efforts to understand the neurobiological trajectories leading to late-onset disorders would be aided by assuring that more biological information gathered from older adults gets added to ongoing repository efforts in psychiatry. Specifically, studying older adults with late-onset mood and anxiety disorder and either establishing brain banks for these samples or adding their tissue into existing banks would significantly increase the available evidence around the neuropathological mechanisms responsible for the development of these disorders in late life and potentially identify new trajectory-altering targets to be studied in younger patients. It is equally important to bank tissue samples from those with early-onset and recurrent mood and anxiety disorders throughout their life cycle so as to clarify the neurobiological trajectories characteristic of aging with chronic disorder.

Novel methodologies for studying long-range patterns of change, such as accelerated longitudinal designs (Thompson, Hallmayer, & O'Hara, 2011), offer the possibility of examining aging-related trajectories in an efficient manner by tracking multiple age cohorts over relatively brief periods. Similarly, extension of current studies of middle-aged participants to include comparisons with older samples may help to accelerate research on trajectories and advance our understanding of the key antecedents for both positive and negative outcomes in later life. In summary, trajectory-related studies examining different developmental periods of risk have the potential to lead to the discovery of new targets for intervention and preemption of disease.

Menopause as a Critical Period

One meaningful transition for study may come with menopause, as a natural midlife developmental period during which major, aging-related biological changes occur. Emerging findings from the scientific study of estrogen effects on the aging brain may help inform translational work in areas of cognition and mood, most specifically in relation to the development of hormonal therapies for brain disorders (Morrison, Brinton, Schmidt, & Gore, 2006). As a context for research, menopause offers opportunities for many potential "natural experiment" studies on the effects of developmental changes in estrogen levels and dynamics. Although one role for menopause-related research has traditionally been in helping to account for group-level sex differences in the incidence and expression of mental disorder, another may be in tracking changes at the individual level.

Prior research findings regarding the influence of menopause on the risk of developing depression have been mixed and controversial. In a longitudinal investigation of women who were premenopausal when they entered the large, NIH-supported Study of Women's Health Across the Nation, investigators determined that women were at two to four times increased risk of experiencing a major depressive episode during menopause or shortly thereafter, as compared to when they were premenopausal. While history of major depression was also a strong predictor of depressive episodes throughout the study, the menopause effect was independent of women's depression history and a number of other potential precipitants, such as stressful life events, psychotropic medication use, and measured changes in reproductive hormone levels (Bromberger et al., 2011). Longitudinal research on hormonal factors and other gender-related neural differences with aging may help elucidate risk or protective mechanisms operating along general pathophysiological pathways to depression. If such mechanisms can be identified through longitudinal trajectory research, they may then be made targets for the development of preventive strategies that can be broadly useful for younger as well as older individuals (Hindi, Dew, Albert, Lotrich, & Reynolds, 2011; Reynolds, 2009).

Effects of Earlier Exposures and Experiences

Likewise, early life and other premenopausal exposures may increase risk or be protective for the development of mood and anxiety disorders in old age. Clinical investigators have increasingly come to suspect that vulnerability to late-life mental disorder may build up over considerable periods of time and be influenced by developmental processes occurring much earlier in the life cycle. Recent work has highlighted the influence of early life stressors on the development of depression among older adults (Ritchie et al., 2009; Salum, Polanczyk, Miguel, & Rohde, 2010).

Research into risk or protective early life factors influencing older adults requires exploration of larger models of aging and disease and how these may interact with the expression of psychiatric disturbances into later life; it also includes the use of data or samples linking together broader spans of the life cycle than has been typical in mood and anxiety disorder research. For example, studies of vascular disease as a process that may lead to depression and other comorbid illness in late life need to be done in middle-aged or young adults (Hannestad et al., 2006; Taylor et al., 2007). An examination of white matter disease earlier in life may identify other targets for prevention that could be addressed.

Epigenetics appears to offer one promising approach to understanding how earlier experiences and environments may eventuate in the later occurrence of disease. For example, the study of epigenetic mechanisms for the development of neurological disorders has pointed to some interesting avenues for research around both synaptic plasticity and cognitive deterioration (Zeng et al., 2011). There are difficulties, however, in developing a uniform way to examine the influence of aging itself in a systematic enough fashion so as to capture environmental influences on gene expression and regulation over time (Kahn & Fraga, 2009, Lotrich, 2011). Other opportunities might include more research on how epigenetic mechanisms identified in younger adults may be altered as a function of chronicity of disease or age.

Mechanisms of Excess Mortality

Furthermore, studies that examine mood and anxiety disorder trajectories as they relate to other clinical outcomes in late life are needed to deepen understanding of the underlying neurobiological processes at work. In particular, research examining mechanisms of increased morbidity and mortality among patients with mood and anxiety disorder should be an important area of focus. Such mechanistic studies may potentially identify modifiable intervening factors and pathways, such as markers of cardiovascular illness that could be treated to preempt the adverse impact of mood disorders on health and longevity. Different avenues of comorbidity research have included studies examining the interaction of mood disorders with cerebrovascular or cardiovascular disease (Alexopoulos 2003); metabolic illness, such as diabetes (Ajilore et al., 2007); and cognitive decline or dementia (Butters et al., 2008; Steffens et al., 2006). A future challenge will be translating findings regarding such interactions into novel clinical targets to be integrated into treatment of mood and anxiety disorders.

CLINICAL INNOVATION AND THE TRANSLATION OF RESEARCH FINDINGS TO BENEFIT PUBLIC HEALTH

Treatment Development Research

While a range of effective interventions are available for mood and anxiety disorders, there remains a considerable need for developing innovative approaches that overcome the shortcomings of these interventions when applied to geriatric mental health care. According to a Cochrane Database review, current psychopharmacological approaches to the treatment of late-life mood disorder have been shown to be effective for alleviating symptoms in about two thirds of those receiving treatment (Mottram, Wilson, & Strobl, 2006). A recent meta-analysis has shown that most second-generation antidepressant medications were beneficial compared to placebo in alleviating symptoms, but that full remission with these agents was difficult to achieve for a significant proportion of patients (Nelson, Delucchi, & Schneider, 2008). Another Cochrane review of treatment regimens noted that medications were effective in treating late-life depression, and combination therapies (medications and psychotherapy) were effective as well. However, a large proportion of patients still do not fully recover and can remain disabled and at risk for other negative outcomes (Wilson, Mottram, & Vassilas, 2008). Moreover, older adults' response to treatment often occurs somewhat more slowly and/ or proves to be less sustained over time than that of younger adults. Although such treatment shortcomings are not unique to older adults, they may pose more acute problems for geriatric patients.

Advances in delineating the pathophysiology of mood and anxiety disorders have opened pathways for developing novel interventions that, for example, might target different or additional neurotransmitter systems to those addressed by current antidepressant medications or that might utilize varied techniques (e.g., pharmacological, behavioral, cognitive, device driven) to modulate the activity of brain circuits that have been identified as hyper- or hypoactive in depression and anxiety. NIMH is committed to supporting research to develop new drugs and other interventions that will target, demonstrably engage, and modify putative mechanisms underlying mood disorder as well as having significant impact on symptomatic and functional outcomes. While relatively little of such intervention development work may focus on strategies uniquely for older adults, it is critical that the research examine a broad age range rather than excluding older adults, and that there be early identification of the interventions for which age differences do moderate the feasibility or outcomes.

A related need is for studies aimed at improving the safety of pharmacotherapy for mood and anxiety disorders among older adults. Numerous reports have documented health- and mortality-related risks associated with the use of antidepressant medications by older adults (e.g., Ciechanowski et al., 2004; Smoller et al., 2009), as well as with other psychotropic medications frequently used adjunctively in the treatment of mood and anxiety disorders (e.g., antipsychotic medications, benzodiazepines). While the iatrogenic risks of these treatments must be weighed against those associated with untreated mood disorders themselves, clearly an expanded treatment armamentarium offering clinicians and patients more options would aid in maximizing treatment safety. A research agenda that prioritizes safety will include the development of novel alternative interventions (both new medications and nonpharmacological strategies) designed to avoid or reduce the risk of triggering treatment-related serious adverse events in older patients.

Personalizing Interventions

A recent National Advisory Mental Health Council Workgroup report, *From Discovery to Cure* (National

Advisory Mental Health Council, 2010), lays forth a charge to the research community to move beyond large efficacy and effectiveness trials that examine merely average levels of response and instead to begin testing questions critical for the development of novel personalized and/or preemptive interventions. The report defines the interventions that are needed for matching treatments to patients as follows: "Personalized interventions refer to aspects of the individual that differentially predict response to a treatment. Preemptive means that the disease process will be arrested before illness occurs or early in the course, so that more negative consequences do not happen."

To pursue this agenda in geriatric mental health, more research needs to be done examining predictors and/or moderators of treatment outcomes. Predictors are defined as baseline variables that have a main effect on treatment outcomes but do not necessarily interact with the difference between treatment conditions when specific interventions are compared. In contrast, moderators are baseline factors that are associated with a between-treatment groups effect (i.e., an interaction) and thus are predictive of the outcomes attributable to a particular intervention. According to a recent review of the extant literature, commonly studied predictors of poorer treatment outcome have included age, baseline severity of depression, baseline anxiety, comorbid personality disorder, poorer perceived or self-rated health, baseline stress, and signs of endogenous depression (Kiosses, Leon, & Arean, 2011). Meanwhile, age, severity of baseline depression and anxiety, and cognitive dysfunction are the main variables that have been studied in comparative treatment designs as potential moderators of depression and/or disability outcomes. In the field of geriatric mental health, the moderating influence of various forms and degrees of cognitive impairment deserves a great deal more investigation, particularly as to predicting which older adults will or will not benefit from cognitively oriented intervention strategies. Other key clinical factors to examine as potential moderator variables include comorbidity and functional status.

Other lines of neurobiological research are providing additional biomarkers that should be included in intervention studies as measures that might help improve personalization and lead to more efficient treatment delivery. For example, incorporating neuroimaging methods into examination of treatment response may point to useful predictors of

treatment response (Gunning & Smith, 2011; Smith et al., 2007). The integration of genomic characteristics into treatment studies may also prove beneficial (Andreescu & Reynolds, 2011; Kiosses et al., 2011). In addition, it may be that differing sorts of predictors will prove critical for the personalization of different treatment modalities. Panels combining genetic, neuroimaging, and clinical predictors may be necessary to personalize effective interventions for difficult-to-treat older adults.

Another line of research to be pursued relative to making personalized care available might be termed the development of "personalizable" interventions. As opposed to using predictive indices to assist with choices between treatment options, the notion here is to enhance the tailored delivery of a particular intervention approach by making it more inherently flexible and responsive to the individual's needs, preferences, and circumstances. For example, several promising modular, multimodal interventions for anxiety in older adults have been piloted where only those modules need to be administered that are directly applicable to the particular patient and presenting problems (Paukert et al., 2010; Wetherell et al., 2009).

EFFICACY TO EFFECTIVENESS AND IMPLEMENTATION RESEARCH

The NIMH has made efforts to support research on interventions and assessment methods that can be disseminated efficiently into improved care approaches, with effectiveness sufficient to produce a public health impact in real-world clinical practice. Specifically, during the last decade the Institute supported comparative effectiveness trials examining the relative outcomes of empirically supported interventions, and it has recently been launching strong efforts in the area of implementation and dissemination research (Chambers, Wang, & Insel, 2010). Given the myriad of health and comorbidity concerns that are dealt with in geriatric health care, health services research in the area of late-life mood and anxiety disorders is well positioned to be a leading force in the development of real-world approaches to complex care.

According to a schema outlined by Alexopoulos and Bruce (2009), existing interventions for late-life depression fill differing roles in helping depressed older adults and have been studied to varying degrees along the continuum that runs from establishing an intervention's efficacy to demonstrating its effectiveness under real-world conditions to determining how to best implement and disseminate it across diverse practice settings and communities. While there is no complete consensus on which existing interventions are supported by convincing evidence of efficacy or effectiveness, clearly a substantial evidence base has been accumulating for various approaches. In one recent review of psychotherapies that have been studied for the treatment of late-life MDD, although none fully met the criteria specified for having established efficacy in the acute treatment of the disorder, the reviewers found sufficient evidence for viewing three psychosocial interventions as promising, pending more replication research: problem-solving therapy, cognitive-behavioral therapy, and treatment initiation and participation program (Kiosses et al., 2011).

Another review focused on community interventions that have a solid evidence base was conducted by an expert panel convened by the Centers for Disease Control and Prevention (CDC) through the Prevention Research Centers' Health Aging Network (PRC-HAN). The panel highlighted depression care management (DCM) as having been shown to be an effective treatment delivery system, and it recommended DCM, as well as individual cognitive-behavioral therapy, as effective community-based treatments for depression in older adults (Frederick et al., 2007; Snowden, Steinman, & Frederick, 2008; Steinman et al., 2007). DCM models exist for providing depression care, particularly in primary care settings (Improving Mood-Promoting Access to Collaborative Treatment, or IMPACT; Unützer et al., 2002) but also as applied to home settings (Program to Encourage Active and Rewarding Lives for Seniors, or PEARLS; Ciechanowski et al., 2004). Existing evidence on efficacy was found to be insufficient to recommend any other forms of psychosocial intervention at that time, including skills training programs, exercise, group psychotherapy, and psychotherapies without a cognitive-behavioral focus (Steinman et al., 2007).

A recent report published by the Substance Abuse and Mental Health Services Administration (SAMHSA) outlined evidence-based practices for the treatment of depression among older adults (Substance Abuse and Mental Health Services Administration, 2011). For the purpose of this report, evidence-based practice was defined as the integration of the best research evidence with clinical expertise and patient values, as defined by the Institute of Medicine (2001). The report noted that

effective treatments include psychotherapy interventions, antidepressant medications, outreach services, and collaborative and integrated mental and physical health care, with variable degrees of scientific evidence for the use of these evidence-based practices. This report suggested that there is currently a need to develop further implementation studies to improve both generalizability and uptake of these practices.

While there clearly is room for more effectiveness research, given that a number of interventions have been shown to be reasonably effective for use with depressed and anxious older adults, we tend to agree that perhaps the more pressing public health needs are for studies of how to tailor treatments to be more capable of reaching people in their local communities, to take account of the social and environmental constraints with which many older adults may have to contend, and to "scale up" these interventions for broader implementation and dissemination. A significant focus is therefore needed on studying how to deliver effective interventions in real-world settings, such as board and care facilities, Meals on Wheels programs, and primary care clinics, and on how to train, deploy, and supervise personnel capable of carrying out this work.

The greatest barriers to implementation of empirically established psychotherapies for late-life mood and anxiety disorders concern the general lack of availability of mental health care providers trained to provide these interventions, and the typical separation of mental health and physical health services. Accordingly, considerable attention will be needed in the research on personnel and organizational issues. These matters, coupled with a general lack of recognition of emotional concerns among older adults, contribute to the underutilization of mental health services for seniors in community settings. At a systems research level, there is scant research on organizational features and financing methods that are optimal for building and sustaining mental health programs that serve the needs of older adults with mood and anxiety disorders both well and in a cost-effective manner.

Research is needed on major challenges and barriers to moving effective interventions into real-world clinical practice in various settings, so as to identify strategies for accomplishing this goal effectively and successfully. With respect to the PEARLS program, implementation barriers have included inadequate funding, inadequate program management, the need to ensure fidelity to established program protocols, accessibility problems, competition between depression intervention steps and case managers' other job demands, failure of many older clients to expect benefit from depression treatment, issues in dealing with medical comorbidity, and lack of intervention packages diversified for non-English speakers (Snowden et al., 2008). For the IMPACT program, major barriers have included difficulties convincing primary care physicians to institute systematic screening for depression efforts (though these providers are capable of following treatment guidelines for depression, few offices actually screen for it) and lack of sufficient third-party reimbursement for the intervention, which has limited the broad dissemination of the model.

All of these areas point to a need for more research in implementation science, particularly for studies that can advance the real-world translation of best practices to communities that have been traditionally underserved. In a review of implementation research, Unutzer (2008) has noted that if we want to see widespread adoption of evidence-based treatments and quality improvement efforts, more work will need to be done to change the settings and approaches for training, examine economic theories around the demand for evidence-based care, and push policy makers and insurance companies to improve incentives around providing evidence-based care.

Disclosures

Neither Jovier Evans nor George Niederehe have any financial disclosures to note.

REFERENCES

Aizenstein, H. J., Butters, M. A., Wu, M., Mazurkewicz, L. M., Stenger, V. A., Gianaros, P. J., ... Carter, C. S. (2009). Altered functioning of the executive control circuit in late-life depression: Episodic and persistent phenomena. *American Journal of Geriatric Psychiatry, 17*(1), 30–42.

Ajilore, O., Haroon, E., Kumaran, S., Darwin, C., Binesh, N., Mintz, J., & Kumar, A. (2007). Measurement of brain metabolites in patients with type 2 diabetes and major depression using proton magnetic resonance spectroscopy. *Neuropsychopharmacology, 32*(6), 1224–1231.

Alexopoulos, G. S. (2003). Vascular disease, depression, and dementia. *Journal of the American Geriatrics Society, 51*(8), 1178–1180.

Alexopoulos, G. S. (2005). Depression in the elderly. *Lancet, 365*(9475), 1961–1970.

Alexopoulos, G. S. (2006). The vascular depression hypothesis: 10 years later. *Biological Psychiatry, 60*(12), 1304–1305.

Alexopoulos, G. S., & Bruce, M. L. (2009). A model for intervention research in late-life depression. *International Journal of Geriatric Psychiatry, 24*(12), 1325–1334.

Alexopoulos, G. S., Schultz, S. K., & Lebowitz, B. D. (2005). Late-life depression: A model for medical classification. *Biological Psychiatry, 58*(4), 283–289.

Andreescu, C., Butters, M., Lenze, E. J., Venkatraman, V. K., Nable, M., Reynolds, C. F., III, & Aizenstein, H. J. (2009). fMRI activation in late-life anxious depression: A potential biomarker. *International Journal of Geriatric Psychiatry, 24*(8), 820–828.

Andreescu, C., & Reynolds, C. F., III. 2011. Late-life depression: Evidence-based treatment and promising new directions for research and clinical practice. *Psychiatric Clinics of North America, 34*(2), 335–355.

Benjamin, S., & Steffens, D. C. (2011). Structural neuroimaging of geriatric depression. *Psychiatric Clinics of North America, 34*(2), 423–435.

Blackburn, E. H., Greider, C. W., Henderson, E., Lee, M. S., Shampay, J., & Shippen-Lentz, D. (1989). Recognition and elongation of telomeres by telomerase. *Genome/National Research Council Canada, 31*(2), 553–560.

Bremmer, M. A., Beekman, A. T. F., Deeg, D. J. H., Penninx, B. W. J. H., Dik, M. G., Hack, C. E., & Hoogendijk, W. J. G. (2008). Inflammatory markers in late-life depression: Results from a population-based study. *Journal of Affective Disorders, 106*(3), 249–255.

Brenes, G. A., Kritchevsky, S. B., Mehta, K. M., Yaffe, K., Simonsick, E. M., Ayonayon, H. N., ... Penninx, B. W. (2007). Scared to death: Results from the Health, Aging, and Body Composition study. *American Journal of Geriatric Psychiatry, 15*(3), 262–265.

Brenes, G. A., Penninx, B. W. J. H., Judd, P. H., Rockwell, E., Sewell, D. D., & Wetherell, J. L. (2008). Anxiety, depression and disability across the lifespan. *Aging and Mental Health, 12*(1), 158–163.

Brinkley, T. E., Leng, X., Miller, M. E., Kitzman, D. W., Pahor, M., Berry, M. J., ... Nicklas, B. J. (2009). Chronic inflammation is associated with low physical function in older adults across multiple comorbidities. *Journal of Gerontology Series A: Biological Sciences Medical Sciences, 64*(4), 455–461.

Bromberger, J. T., Kravitz, H. M., Chang, Y. F., Cyranowski, J. M., Brown, C., & Matthews, K. A. (2011). Major depression during and after the menopausal transition: Study of Women's Health Across the Nation (SWAN). *Psychological Medicine, 41*(9), 1879–1888.

Butters, M. A., Young, J. B., Lopez, O., Aizenstein, H. J., Mulsant, B. H., Reynolds, C. F., III, ... Becker, J. T. (2008). Pathways linking late-life depression to persistent cognitive impairment and dementia. *Dialogues in Clinical Neuroscience, 10*(3), 345–357.

Byers, A. L., Yaffe, K., Covinsky, K. E., Friedman, M. B., & Bruce, M. L. (2010). High occurrence of mood and anxiety disorders among older adults: The National Comorbidity Survey Replication. *Archives of General Psychiatry, 67*(5), 489–496.

Chambers, D. A., Wang, P. S., & Insel, T. R. (2010). Maximizing efficiency and impact in effectiveness and services research. *General Hospital Psychiatry, 32*(5), 453–455.

Chapman, D. P., & Perry, G. S. (2008). Depression as a major component of public health for older adults. *Preventing Chronic Disease, 5*(1), A22.

Ciechanowski, P., Wagner, E., Schmaling, K., Schwartz, S., Williams, B.,Diehr, P., ... LoGerfo, J. (2004). Community-integrated home-based depression treatment in older adults: A randomized controlled trial. *Journal of the American Medical Association, 291*(13), 1569–1577.

Cuthbert, B. N., & Insel, T. R. (2010). Toward new approaches to psychotic disorders: The NIMH Research Domain Criteria project. *Schizophrenia Bulletin, 36*(6), 1061–102.

Frederick, J. T., Steinman, L. E., Prohaska, T., Satariano, W. A., Bruce, M., Bryant, L., ... Snowden, M., Late Life Depression Special Interest Project Panelists (2007). Community-based treatment of late life depression an expert panel-informed literature review. *American Journal of Preventive Medicine, 33*(3), 222–249.

Glorioso, C., & Sibille, E. (2011). Between destiny and disease: Genetics and molecular pathways of human central nervous system aging. *Progress in Neurobiology, 93*(2), 165–181.

Gum, A. M., King-Kallimanis, B., & Kohn, R. (2009). Prevalence of mood, anxiety, and substance-abuse disorders for older americans in the National Comorbidity Survey-Replication. *American Journal of Geriatric Psychiatry, 17*(9), 769–781.

Gunning, F. M., & Smith, G. S. (2011). Functional neuroimaging in geriatric depression. *Psychiatric Clinics of North America, 34*(2), 403–422.

Hannestad, J., Taylor, W. D., McQuoid, D. R., Payne, M. E., Krishnan, K. R., Steffens, D. C., & Macfall, J. R. (2006). White matter lesion volumes and caudate volumes in late-life depression. *International Journal of Geriatric Psychiatry, 21*(12), 1193–1198.

Harley, C. B., Futcher, A. B., & Greider, C. W. (1990). Telomeres shorten during ageing of human fibroblasts. *Nature, 345*(6274), 458–460.

Hindi, F., Dew, M. A., Albert, S. M., Lotrich, F. E., & Reynolds, C. F., III. (2011). Preventing depression in later life: State of the art and science circa 2011. *Psychiatric Clinics of North America, 34*(1), 67–78.

Hofman, A., Breteler, M. M., Van Duijn, C. M., Krestin, G. P., Pols, H. A., Stricker, B. H., ... Witteman, J. C. (2007). The Rotterdam study: Objectives and design update. *European Journal of Epidemiology, 22*, 819–829.

Hybels, C. F., & Blazer, D. G. (2003). Epidemiology of late-life mental disorders. *Clinics in Geriatric Medicine, 19*(4), 663–696.

Insel, T. R. (2009). Translating scientific opportunity into public health impact: a strategic plan for research on mental illness. *Archives of General Psychiatry, 66*(2), 128–133.

Insel, T. R., & Cuthbert, B. N. (2009). Endophenotypes: Bridging genomic complexity and disorder heterogeneity. *Biological Psychiatry, 66*(11), 988–989.

Insel, T. R., Cuthbert, B., Garvey, M., Heinssen, R., Pine, D. S., Quinn, K., ... Wang, P. (2010). Research domain criteria (RDOC): Toward a new classification framework for research on mental disorders. *Americn Journal of Psychiatry. 167*(7), 748–751.

Institute of Medicine. (2001). *Crossing the quality chasm: A new health system for the 21st century*. Washington, DC: Institute of Medicine.

Jeste, D. V., Alexopoulos, G. S., Bartels, S. J., Cummings, J. L., Gallo, J. J., Gottlieb, G. L., ... Lebowitz, B. D. (1999). Consensus statement on the upcoming crisis in geriatric mental health: Research agenda for the next 2 decades. *Archives of General Psychiatry, 56*(9), 848–853.

Juster, R. P., McEwen, B. S., & Lupien, S. J. (2010). Allostatic load biomarkers of chronic stress and impact on health and cognition. *Neuroscience and Biobehavioral Reviews, 35*(1), 2–16.

Kahn, A., & Fraga, M. F. (2009). Epigenetics and aging: Status, challenges, and needs for the future. *The Journal of Gerontology. Series A, Biologocial Sciences and Medical Sciences, 64*(2), 195–198.

Kessler, R. C., Birnbaum, H., Bromet, E., Hwang, I., Sampson, N., & Shahly, V. (2010). Age differences in major depression: Results from the National Comorbidity Survey Replication (NCS-R). *Psychological Medicine, 40*(2), 225–237.

Kessler, R. C., Chiu, W. T., Demler, O., Merikangas, K. R., & Walters, E. E. (2005). Prevalence, severity, and comorbidity of 12-month DSM-IV disorders in the National Comorbidity Survey Replication. *Archives of General Psychiatry, 62*(6), 617–627.

King-Kallimanis, B., Gum, A. M., & Kohn, R. (2009). Comorbidity of depressive and anxiety disorders for older americans in the National Comorbidity Survey-Replication. *American Journal of Geriatric Psychiatry, 17*(9), 782–792.

Kiosses, D. N., Leon, A. C., & Arean, P. A. (2011). Psychosocial interventions for late-life major depression: Evidence-based treatments, predictors of treatment outcomes, and moderators of treatment effects. *Psychiatric Clinics of North America, 34*(2), 377–401, viii.

Kirkpatrick, B., Messias, E., Harvey, P. D., Fernandez-Egea, E., & Bowie, C. R. (2008). Is schizophrenia a syndrome of accelerated aging? *Schizophrenia Bulletin, 34*(6), 1024–1032.

Kohli, M. A., Lucae, S., Saemann, P. G., Schmidt, M. V., Demirkan, A., Hek, K., ... Binder, E. B. (2011). The neuronal transporter gene SLC6A15 confers risk to major depression. *Neuron, 70*(2), 252–265.

Lenze, E. J., & Wetherell, J. L. (2009). Bringing the bedside to the bench, and then to the community: A prospectus for intervention research in late-life anxiety disorders. *International Journal of Geriatric Psychiatry, 24*(1), 1–14.

Lotrich, F. E. (2011). Gene-environment interactions in geriatric depression. *Psychiatric Clinics of North America, 34*(2), 357–376.

Lotrich, F. E., El-Gabalawy, H., Guenther, L. C., & Ware, C. F. (2011). The role of inflammation in the pathophysiology of depression: Different treatments and their effects. *Journal of Rheumatology, 88*, 48–54.

Maes, M. (1995). Evidence for an immune response in major depression: A review and hypothesis. *Progress in Neuro-Psychopharmacology and Biological Psychiatry, 19*(1), 11–38.

Maes, M., Scharpe, S., Meltzer, H. Y., Okayli, G., Bosmans, E., D'Hondt, P., ... Cosyns, P. (1994). Increased neopterin and interferon-gamma secretion and lower availability of l-tryptophan in major depression: Further evidence for an immune response. *Psychiatry Research, 54*(2), 143–160.

Maes, M., Yirmyia, R., Noraberg, J., Brene, S., Hibbeln, J., Perini, G., ... Maj, M. (2009). The inflammatory & neurodegenerative (I&ND) hypothesis of depression: Leads for future research and new drug developments in depression. *Metabolic Brain Disease, 24*(1), 27–53.

Milaneschi, Y., Corsi, A. M., Penninx, B. W., Bandinelli, S., Guralnik, J. M., & Ferrucci, L. (2009). Interleukin-1 receptor antagonist and incident depressive symptoms over 6 years in older persons: The inchianti study. *Biological Psychiatry, 65*(11), 973–978.

Miller, A. H., Maletic, V., & Raison, C. L. (2009). Inflammation and its discontents: The role of cytokines in the pathophysiology of major depression. *Biological Psychiatry, 65*(9), 732–741.

Morrison, J. H., Brinton, R. D., Schmidt, P. J., & Gore, A. C. (2006). Estrogen, menopause, and the aging brain: How basic neuroscience can inform hormone therapy in women. *Journal of Neuroscience, 26*(41), 10332–10348.

Moskvina, V., Craddock, N., Holmans, P., Nikolov, I., Pahwa, J. S., Green, E., ... O'Donovan, M. C. (2009). Gene-wide analyses of genome-wide association data sets: Evidence for multiple common risk alleles for schizophrenia and bipolar disorder and for overlap in genetic risk. *Molecular Psychiatry, 14*(3), 252–360.

Mottram, P., Wilson, K., & Strobl, J. (2006). Antidepressants for depressed elderly. *Cochrane Database of Systematic Reviews*, (1), CD003491.

National Advisory Mental Health Council. (2010). *From discovery to cure: Accelerating the development of new and personalized interventions for mental illnesses.* Report of the National Advisory Mental Health Council's Workgroup, August 2010. Rockville, MD: US Department of Health and Human Services, National Institutes of Health, National Institute of Mental Health.

National Institute of Mental Health. (2008). *National Institute of Mental Health strategic plan.* (US Department of Health and Human Services, National Institutes of Health, Ed.). Bethesda, MD: NIH Publication.

Nelson, J. C., Delucchi, K., & Schneider, L. S. (2008). Efficacy of second generation antidepressants in late-life depression: A meta-analysis of the evidence. *American Journal of Geriatric Psychiatry, 16*(7), 558–567.

Paukert, A. L., Calleo, J., Kraus-Schuman, C., Snow, L., Wilson, N., Petersen, N. J., ... Stanley, M. A. (2010). Peaceful mind: An open trial of cognitive-behavioral therapy for anxiety in persons with dementia. *International Psychogeriatrics/IPA, 22*(6), 1012–1021.

Psychiatric GWAS Consortium Steering Committee. (2009). A framework for interpreting genome-wide association studies of psychiatric disorders. *Molecular Psychiatry, 14*(1), 10–17.

Reynolds, C. F., III. (2009). Prevention of depressive disorders: A brave new world. *Depression and Anxiety, 26*(12), 1062–1065.

Ritchie, K., Jaussent, I., Stewart, R., Dupuy, A. M., Courtet, P., Ancelin, M. L., & Malafosse, A. (2009). Association of adverse childhood environment and 5-HTTLPR genotype with late-life depression. *Journal of Clinical Psychiatry, 70*(9), 1281–1288.

Rosano, C., Marsland, A. L., & Gianaros, P. J. (2011). Maintaining brain health by monitoring inflammatory processes: A mechanims to promote successful aging. *Aging and Disease, 2*(5), 1–18.

Salum, G. A., Polanczyk, G. V., Miguel, E. C., & Rohde, L. A. (2010). Effects of childhood development on late-life mental disorders. *Current Opinion in Psychiatry, 23*(6), 498–503.

Schoevers, R. A., Geerlings, M. I., Deeg, D. J., Holwerda, T. J., Jonker, C., & Beekman, A. T. (2009). Depression and excess mortality: Evidence for a dose response relation in community living elderly. *International Journal of Geriatric Psychiatry, 24*(2), 169–176.

Smith, G. S., Gunning-Dixon, F. M., Lotrich, F. E., Taylor, W. D., & Evans, J. D. (2007). Translational research in late-life mood disorders: Implications for future intervention and prevention research. *Neuropsychopharmacology, 32*(9), 1857–1875.

Smoller, J. W., Allison, M., Cochrane, B. B., Curb, J. D., Perlis, R. H., Robinson, J. G.,...Wassertheil-Smoller, S. (2009). Antidepressant use and risk of incident cardiovascular morbidity and mortality among postmenopausal women in the Women's Health Initiative study. *Archives of Internal Medicine, 169*(22), 2128–2139.

Snowden, M., Steinman, L., & Frederick, J. (2008). Treating depression in older adults: Challenges to implementing the recommendations of an expert panel. *Preventing Chronic Disease, 5*(1), A26.

Steffens, D. C. (2009). A multiplicity of approaches to characterize geriatric depression and its outcomes. *Current Opinion in Psychiatry, 22*(6), 522–526.

Steffens, D. C., Otey, E., Alexopoulos, G. S., Butters, M. A., Cuthbert, B., Ganguli, M.,...Yesavage, J. (2006). Perspectives on depression, mild cognitive impairment, and cognitive decline. *Archives of General Psychiatry, 63*(2), 130–138.

Steinman, L. E., Frederick, J. T., Prohaska, T., Satariano, W. A., Dornberg-Lee, S., Fisher, R.,...Snowden, M., Late Life Depression Special Interest Project Panelists (2007).

Recommendations for treating depression in community-based older adults. *American Journal of Preventive Medicine, 33*(3), 175–181.

Substance Abuse and Mental Health Services Administration. (2011). *The treatment of depression in older adults: Selecting evidence-based practices for treatment of depression in older adults*. HHS Pub. No. SMA-11–4631. Rockville, MD: Center for Mental Health Services, Substance Abuse and Mental Health Services Administration, US Department of Health and Human Services.

Taylor, W. D., Bae, J. N., MacFall, J. R., Payne, M. E., Provenzale, J. M., Steffens, D. C., & Krishnan, K. R. (2007). Widespread effects of hyperintense lesions on cerebral white matter structure. *American Journal of Roentgenology, 188*(6), 1695–1704.

Thomas, A. J., & O'Brien, J. T. (2006). Mood disorders in the elderly. *Psychiatry, 5*(4), 127–130.

Thomas, A. J., & O'Brien, J. T. (2009). Mood disorders in the elderly. *Psychiatry, 8*(2), 56–60.

Thompson, W. K., Hallmayer, J., & O'Hara, R. (2011). Design considerations for characterizing psychiatric trajectories across the lifespan: Application to effects of APOE-{varepsilon}4 on cerebral cortical thickness in alzheimer's disease. *American Journal of Psychiatry, 168*(9), 894–903.

Tost, H., & Meyer-Lindenberg, A. (2011). A new, blue gene highlights glutamate and hippocampus in depression. *Neuron, 70*(2), 171–172.

Unützer, J. (2008). Evidence-based treatments for anxiety and depression: Lost in translation? *Depression and Anxiety, 25*(9), 726–729.

Unützer, J., Katon, W., Callahan, C. M., Williams, J. W., Jr., Hunkeler, E., Harpole, L.,...Langston, C. (2002). Collaborative care management of late-life depression in the primary care setting: A randomized controlled trial. *Journal of the American Medical Association, 288*(22), 2836–2845.

Vincent, G. K., & Velkoff, V. A. (2010). *The next four decades, the older population in the United States: 2010–2050*. Current population reports, P25–1138. Washington, DC: US Census Bureau.

Wetherell, J. L., Ayers, C. R., Sorrell, J. T., Thorp, S. R., Nuevo, R., Belding, W.,...Patterson, T. L. (2009). Modular psychotherapy for anxiety in older primary care patients. *American Journal of Geriatric Psychiatry, 17*(6), 483–492.

Wilson, K. C., Mottram, P. G., & Vassilas, C. A. (2008). Psychotherapeutic treatments for older depressed people. *Cochrane Database of Systematic Reviews* (1), CD004853.

Wolkowitz, O. M., Epel, E. S., Reus, V. I., & Mellon, S. H. (2010). Depression gets old fast: Do stress and depression accelerate cell aging? *Depression and Anxiety, 27*(4), 327–338.

Wolkowitz, O. M., Mellon, S. H., Epel, E. S., Lin, J., Dhabhar, F. S., Su, Y.,...Blackburn, E. H. (2011). Leukocyte telomere length in major depression: Correlations with chronicity, inflammation and oxidative stress—preliminary findings. *PLoS ONE, 6*(3), e17837.

Yatham, L. N., Kapczinski, F., Andreazza, A. C., Trevor Young, L., Lam, R.

W., & Kauer-Sant'anna, M. (2009). Accelerated age-related decrease in brain-derived neurotrophic factor levels in bipolar disorder. *International Journal of Neuropsychopharmacology, 12*(1), 137–139.

Zeng, Y., Tan, M., Kohyama, J., Sneddon, M., Watson, J. B., Sun, Y. E., & Xie, C. W. (2011). Epigenetic enhancement of BDNF signaling rescues synaptic plasticity in aging. *Journal of Neuroscience, 31*(49), 17800–17810.

2

RESEARCH PRIORITIES IN LATE-LIFE MOOD DISORDERS

AN INTERNATIONAL PERSPECTIVE

Briony Dow, Xiaoping Lin, Jean Tinney, Betty Harambous, and David Ames

MOOD DISORDERS are common in late life. Against the background of population aging, a burgeoning research literature about this group of disorders has emerged (Banerjee et al., 2011; Cooper et al., 2011; Hindi, Dew, Albert, Lotrich, & Reynolds, 2011). This chapter presents a summary of research priorities in this area in the next 5–10 years for international researchers. It starts with a brief discussion of important issues that underlie future research in late-life mood disorders, including sociodemographic changes and advances in technology. It then presents a bird's eye view of current research in late-life mood disorders and identifies important gaps in this research. The chapter concludes with recommendations on research priority areas that are likely to create the most exciting opportunities for the late-life mood disorder field in the next 5–10 years.

IMPORTANT ISSUES UNDERLYING FUTURE RESEARCH

Before the discussion of priority areas for future research on late-life mood disorders, it is important to highlight some important social and economic factors, including sociodemographic changes, health care provision for older people, and advances in technology (see Table 2.1), that influence and have profound implications for future research in this area.

Current and future research on late-life mood disorders takes place against a background of inexorable population aging. In addition to this trend, the populations of many countries are also becoming racially and ethnically more diverse due to the influences of globalization and migration. There are also significant minority indigenous populations in many countries, including but not limited to Australia, Brazil, Canada, Taiwan, and the United States. Within this context, more cultural studies will be needed to improve our understanding of how cultural diversity, interactions between cultures, and the evolution of cultures affect the experience of late-life mood disorders. Other important sociodemographic changes that have implications for future research include high divorce and remarriage rates in many developed countries, increasing workforce

Table 2.1 Important Issues That Affect Future Research in Late-Life Mood Disorders

Sociodemographic changes	Population aging
	Increasing cultural diversity in many populations
	Significant minority populations in some countries
	Higher divorce and remarriage rates
	Increasing workforce participation among women
	Characteristics of baby boomers
Health care for older people with mood disorders	Increasing number of older people with mood disorders
	Strained health resources
	Shortage of care staff for the aged
Advances in technology	Advances in neuroimaging
	Advances in information technology
	Advances in communication technology

participation among women, and the characteristics of the younger cohort of the baby boomer generation, who will be entering their 60s and 70s over the next 20 years. For example, in a society with high divorce and remarriage rates, falling fertility rates (partly due to delayed age of childbearing), and smaller family size, it is important to investigate the impact of changed family structures on family care for older people with mood disorders.

Consistent with the trend of population aging, there will be an increasing number of older people diagnosed with mood disorders who require professional help. However, health care resources are strained in many countries (Snowdon, 2007, 2010a; Walsh, Currier, Shah, Lyness, & Friedman, 2008) and the persistent adverse economic conditions will exacerbate this problem. Against this background, the issues of program evaluation and cost effectiveness will be very important research topics in future studies. Furthermore, there is a shortage of aged care staff working with older people, which could be explained by a reluctance among health students to work with older people (Koder & Helmes, 2006; Lee, Volans, & Gregory, 2003; Lovell, 2006). These studies suggest that workforce issues, and in particular how to increase students' interest in working with older people, will need to be further investigated in future research.

Technological developments have had a profound influence on society in the last 100 years. Advances in neuroimaging and information technology have made important contributions to

research on late-life mood disorders in the past decade. Studies in neuroimaging have helped us to gain a better understanding of the anatomy, functional circuitry, and biochemistry of major mood disorders in older people (Kumar & Ajilore, 2009; Smith & Alexopoulos, 2009). New developments in information technology have helped to improve the assessment and management of late-life mood disorders, in particular, among people living in rural and remote areas. With exciting and cutting-edge developments in these areas, there is no doubt that they will continue to contribute to future research in late-life mood disorders, but it is important that we use these tools to accumulate useful knowledge and to provide meaningful benefit to older people with mood disorders, rather than succumbing to the ever-present temptation to use them as little more than high-tech toys.

DEPRESSION

Depression, both major and minor, is the late-life mood disorder that is best understood, but it nevertheless presents a wide range of unanswered questions and challenges for urgent future research. There is general acknowledgement that late-life depression is a complex, multifactorial disorder or group of disorders, highly prevalent, often undetected, untreated, or undertreated, and strongly correlated with a range of physical comorbidities and psychological and life adversity factors.

This section gives an overview of current research activity and knowledge about depression in older people, identifying gaps in this knowledge, and makes recommendations for future research directions.

Summary of Current Knowledge

Recent research articles fall into the major categories of detection/diagnosis, prevalence, prevention, and treatment/interventions.

The term *depression* can refer to both depressive disorders and depressive symptoms. In modern research and clinical practice, diagnoses of depressive disorders are made most often using either the criteria of the World Health Organization's *International Classification of Diseases*, tenth revision (*ICD-10*) (World Health Organization, 1992) or the American Psychiatric Association's *Diagnostic and Statistical Manual of Mental Disorders*, fourth edition (*DSM-IV*) (American Psychiatric Association, 1994; Dow, Lin, Tinney, Haralambous, & Ames, 2011), though these venerable diagnostic systems will be replaced by newly revised criteria in the next year or two.

DETECTION/DIAGNOSIS

The growing interest in research on geriatric depression could focus on earlier diagnosis to help doctors better detect depression at the primary care level (Kua & Ho, 2008). One important step will be improvement in diagnostic tools, for example, integration of late-life issues into the *DSM-5* (Kupfer, Kuhl, & Regier, 2009).

Current research on diagnosis has raised a number of key themes. The application of biomarkers to clinical practice may be on the horizon if further research is able to refine their sensitivity and specificity (Blumberger, Daskalakis, & Mulsant, 2008).

Neuroimaging is becoming increasingly important in proposed clinical trials and longitudinal studies (Ajilore & Smith, 2011). Hoptman et al. (2006) argue that structural neuroimaging is central for the conceptual advancement of the field of geriatric depression. The early characterization of brain changes associated with the presence of cardiovascular diseases holds promise for clinical applications in psychiatry, providing new perspectives for the prevention of old-age psychiatric disorders (de Toledo Ferraz Alves, Ferreira, & Busatto, 2010).

Another associated issue is vascular depression and the links between depression and stroke (Almeida, 2008; Baldwin, 2005). There is a strong argument that older patients presenting with the problems of cognitive decline and depression should have vascular risk assessed and treated, although further research is required to determine whether the management of these vascular risk factors actually decreases the risk of depression and cognitive decline (Flicker, 2008). In accordance with the vascular depression hypothesis, apparent differences in the morphological changes between younger and older patients may suggest a differing pathological basis in major depressive disorders (Khundakar & Thomas, 2009). The vascular depression hypothesis has considerable utility and potential to help us understand the relationship between depressive and vascular disorders, but the extent to which depression contributes to vascular disease remains controversial and further prospective studies are needed (Culang-Reinlieb, Johnert, Brickman, & Steffens, 2011).

PREVALENCE

There is a need for more studies targeted to where knowledge is lacking regarding prevalence, risk factors, adequate diagnosis, adequate representation/inclusion in clinical trials, and culturally relevant assessment tools in ethnically diverse older people (Faison & Mintzer, 2005). For example, ethnic minorities in the United States and the United Kingdom and other developed countries are understudied in terms of prevalence and development of culturally appropriate interventions, as well as delayed diagnosis and treatment (Akincigil et al., 2012; Cañive & Escobar, 2009), and too little is known about depression in developing countries.

We agree with Djernes (2006) that high prevalence of depression and low rates of treatment represent a challenge that requires a greater involvement of the primary care sector and greater collaboration between primary care practitioners and old-age psychiatrists.

Limited research addresses the association between cognitive impairment and depression (Huang, Wang, Li, Xie, & Liu, 2011; Kumar, Aizenstein, & Ballmaier, 2008). A recent well-conducted study reported disappointing findings from antidepressant treatment of depression in dementia (Banerjee et al., 2011). It would be of great value to know to what extent this condition is treatable, and, if so, how best to treat it.

Findings from studies in developing countries suggest that key areas for future research will be the epidemiology of mental disorders in rural areas, the direct and indirect costs of psychogeriatric conditions, the evaluation of the cost-effectiveness, and the financial sustainability of early detection programs, and treatment and rehabilitation models (Chiu, Tsoh, & Lam, 2007).

PREVENTION

The current evidence base for primary prevention of depression in older people is weak, and further trials are warranted (Forsman, Schierenbeck, & Wahlbeck, 2011). Interventions that are reported to work in preventing late-life depression include antidepressant medications in standard doses and problem-solving treatment (Baldwin, 2010). Prevention is feasible, particularly when integrated into a care model, such as collaborative care (Baldwin, 2010).

Social support is an important factor in preventing onset and progression of depression (Meeks, Vahia, Lavretsky, Kulkarni, & Jeste, 2011); effective social interventions can be initiated by social/health care workers and family and friends (Blazer, 2005). Other protective factors cited are good health and the maintenance of cognitive function (Blazer, 2005).

Some of the challenges for further research into the prevention of depression include the need for more efficacy in trials in specific target groups, better pathophysiological models to inform the choice of interventions, and further investigation of the cost-effectiveness of depression prevention (Reynolds, 2009).

TREATMENT AND INTERVENTIONS

Treatment

According to Frazer, Christensen, and Griffiths (2005), treatments with the best evidence of effectiveness are antidepressants, electroconvulsive therapy (ECT), cognitive-behavioral therapy, reminiscence therapy, problem-solving treatment, bibliotherapy (for mild to moderate depression), and exercise. For an overview on current research on psychotherapy, see Chapter 22 in this book.

There is limited evidence to support the effectiveness of transcranial magnetic stimulation, dialectical behavior therapy, interpersonal therapy, light therapy (for people in nursing homes or hospitals),

St John's wort, and folate in reducing depressive symptoms (Frazer et al., 2005).

Kasckow and Zisook (2008) argue that more research is needed to refine our treatment approaches toward older people with depression. Pharmacological agents in combination with psychosocial interventions appear to be useful treatments for depressive symptoms in this group of older patients (Felmet, Zisook, & Kasckow, 2011).

Despite the aforementioned reference to the effectiveness of ECT, its use remains controversial (Dombrovski & Mulsant, 2007; Frazer et al., 2005; Ganguli, 2007; Greenberg & Kellner, 2005) with only a few studies assessing its efficacy in older subjects specifically (van Schaik et al., 2012). Greenberg and Kellner (2005) highlighted the need for prospective studies to clarify specific indications, efficacy, and side effects of ECT in patients with dementia in particular. Chapter 23 in this book summarizes current research and knowledge on ECT and neuromodulation for late-life mood disorders. Despite some evidence of success in limiting the relapse rate in patients with combined ECT and pharmacological treatment, questions remain about how often and for how long ECT should be continued. On the other hand, there is increasing evidence that transcranial magnetic stimulation may be an effective noninvasive treatment for some forms of depression (refer to Chapter 23 in this book).

There appears to be no significant difference between the effectiveness of psychotherapy for younger and older adults (Cuijpers, van Straten, Smit, & Andersson, 2009). Group cognitive-behavioral therapy is effective in older adults with depression. However, conclusions that can be drawn are limited (Krishna et al., 2011). Psychological treatments are effective in the treatment of depression in older adults (the effect is comparable to the effect of pharmacological treatments), and further dissemination of these treatments is justified (Cuijpers, van Straten, & Smit, 2006). In many countries small numbers of practitioners with competence in the delivery of psychological treatments to older people, and a willingness to work with older patients, markedly limit the availability of such therapies.

Alexopoulos et al. (2008) argue that indices of anterior cingulate cortex dysfunction may be used to identify subgroups of depressed elderly patients with distinct illness course and treatment needs, and it may serve as the theoretical background for novel treatment development.

Some studies have identified the benefits of combined treatments and others discuss the use of augmenting agents to traditional antidepressant maintenance therapies (Andreescu & Reynolds, 2011; Dew et al., 2007; Reynolds et al., 2006). Reynolds et al. (2011) found that in recurrent major depression, both nortriptyline and interpersonal therapy were superior to placebo in preventing or delaying recurrence. A review by Carvalho et al. (2007) concluded that the augmentation therapy with the best evidence was the lithium-antidepressant combination, especially in patients not responding to tricyclic agents. Another large double-blind randomized clinical trial found that combination pharmacotherapy (olanzapine plus sertraline) was efficacious for the treatment of major depression with psychotic features, suggesting it provided physicians an alternative to the use of ECT (Meyers et al., 2009). Gaps in this research will be discussed in the next section.

Interventions

Interventions found effective in the treatment of depression in community-dwelling older people include multidisciplinary, collaborative depression care management (Frederick et al., 2007), particularly personalized interventions at the individual level (Alexopoulos & Bruce, 2009). Other effective models are interventions that combine case management with problem-solving treatment (Areán & Alexopoulos, 2007). Interventions potentially helpful but requiring further evidence include psychotherapy for mental illness in late life (Areán & Alexopoulos, 2007) and reminiscence interventions in a psychiatric context (Coleman, 2005). In a recent randomized controlled trial, Banerjee et al. (2011) found that antidepressant treatments for depression in dementia were no more effective than placebo, although they carried increased risk of adverse events. They recommend reconsideration of the use of antidepressants as a first-line treatment of depression in Alzheimer's disease (Banerjee et al., 2011). One encouraging finding from this study was that the severity of depression in dementia tended to diminish over time, even when placebo treatment was used.

Physical activity interventions obtain clinically relevant outcomes in the treatment of depressive symptoms. However, further research is needed to establish medium- to long-term effects and cost-effectiveness (Blake, Mo, Malik, & Thomas, 2009). Effectiveness of psychosocial interventions has been demonstrated.

Issues/Gaps

There are a number of important gaps in current knowledge about late-life depression. These fall into the major categories of detection/diagnosis, prevalence, prevention, and treatment/interventions. There is also a lack of rollout into practice of research findings, for example, on the benefits of multifaceted personalized studies and the translation of research findings into large populations.

DETECTION/DIAGNOSIS

There is an absence of information or knowledge about neuroimaging, biomarkers, integration of psychiatry with primary care, and sleep disturbances. Ancoli-Israel and Alessi (2005) argue that a better understanding of sleep disturbance to assist in day-to-day management of psychiatric illness is needed. In relation to neuroimaging, further work is required on integrating research neuroimaging methods with clinical trials or longitudinal studies (Ajilore & Smith, 2011). In terms of diagnostic tools, there are gaps in the existing *DSM-IV* and ongoing debate about the proposed *DSM-5* and the importance of integrating late-life issues.

PREVALENCE

There are gaps in knowledge of prevalence of depression in ethnically diverse older people. This includes prevalence, risk factors, adequate diagnosis, adequate representation/inclusion in clinical trials, and culturally relevant assessment tools (Bell & McBride, 2011; Faison & Mintzer, 2005).

Primary care practitioners face challenges in addressing the high prevalence and low rates of treatment of depression in older people. Further knowledge is required regarding the links between depression and cognitive impairment (Bhalla & Butters, 2011).

PREVENTION

Little is known about effective means of preventing depression in older people. Specific areas of concern are people living in rural areas and/or developing countries, people with dementia, suicide prevention, and links between depression and conditions as diverse as vascular disease and schizophrenia (Felmet et al., 2011). Collaborative care models of prevention are underdeveloped (Baldwin, 2010).

TREATMENT AND INTERVENTIONS

At a practitioner level, further knowledge is required on how to help doctors treat depression in both community-dwelling older people and those in residential care. In most countries there is a need to better integrate psychiatry with primary care services for older people (Kennedy, 2005).

Many treatment studies involve younger populations, and there is increasing but still imperfect knowledge about antidepressant tolerability in older people that may vary markedly between individuals according to their state of health. In addition, even though depression is a remitting, relapsing disorder, there is far less evidence in relation to effective prophylaxis against relapse in relation to treatment of future episodes and how long to continue such treatment. The data on the effectiveness of transcranial magnetic stimulation, interpersonal therapy, light therapy (for people in nursing homes or hospitals), and St John's wort and folate in reducing depressive symptoms indicate that these areas all require further investigation. There is debate about the effective use of ECT in older people, and prospective studies are needed to "clarify specific indications, efficacy and side effects of ECT in patients with dementia" (Greenberg & Kellner, 2005, p. 276). Questions also remain about optimal frequency and continuation of treatments, and the possibilities offered by combined treatments (see Chapter 23 in this book).

Directions for Future Research

Several important directions for future research focusing on older adults with serious depressive illness are suggested. Controlled clinical trials using real-world populations of vulnerable older people are required. For example, investigations of predictors of suicidality that eliminate patients at risk are unlikely to investigate the most effective treatment for those at greatest risk (see Chapter 6 in this book). People aged 75 and over are clearly underrepresented in the clinical trials of potential antidepressants; the inclusion of at least 25% of subjects aged 75 and over is recommended for future trials (Giron, Fastbom, & Winblad, 2005). The exclusion from trials of those most likely to need treatment means that, although the data obtained may be scientifically credible, "they do not reflect the clinical environment in which the product will be prescribed" (Yastrubetskaya, Chiu, & O'Connell, 1997).

There is a need for agreed diagnostic criteria and validation of the tools for detection of depression in older people, especially those with other comorbid psychiatric disorders. Other directions for research include multifactorial interventions, individually tailored interventions, and integrated approaches to treatment that reflect most recent research evidence. This could mean psychological therapies as first-line therapies, combination of pharmacological and psychosocial interventions, or other therapies such as exercise.

More studies are needed on new pharmacological treatments and on research on existing drug options. This includes side effects of antidepressants, tolerability in older people, and optimal duration of treatment (Kok, Heeren, & Nolen, 2011; Mottram, Wilson, & Strobl, 2006).

Content areas for clinical trials should include combined interventions concerning depression and comorbidities such as pain, dementia, cardiovascular disease (Snowdon, 2010b), Parkinson's disease, anxiety, diabetes, and chronic obstructive pulmonary disease.

Further clinical research should include trials on mechanisms underlying psychiatric disorders and subsyndromal (Bruce, 2010) and minor depression, and rigorous studies to test whether older adults with minor depression or dysthymia receive greater benefits from psychotherapy than from medication. More controlled studies that randomly assign older depressed patients to pharmacotherapy, psychotherapy, and control groups are needed.

Studies seeking to define the subtype population need to include comprehensive neuropsychological and neuroimaging evaluations to examine the relative value and contribution of functional outcomes and the underlying pathophysiology burden (Sneed & Culang-Reinlieb, 2011). Also the longitudinal course needs to be characterized.

Future research into biomarkers of depression should include homocysteine, cytokines, and endothelial dysfunction (Teper & O'Brien, 2008). Outcome domains focusing on the predictive, moderating, and mediating roles of a wide range of psychopathological, medical, functional, and psychosocial factors will also complement interventions and biomarker research approaches (Alexopoulos & Morimoto, 2011; Almeida, 2011).

Further understanding of the onset, course, and outcomes of psychiatric disorders gained from epidemiologic studies will be critical in the future (Hybels & Pieper, 2009). Studies with older people should include thorough cognitive and mood assessments, including measures of depression and anxiety.

There are potential ways to close the gap between knowledge and clinical practice. Suggestions include building cross-disciplinary research teams, partnerships with the community, improving communication in long-term care, raising awareness and training clinicians in the new technologies, and focusing on more holistic and person-centered approaches to care. There is a need to encourage psychotherapists to engage with older adults. There is growing evidence that social interventions can make a difference in patients' lives.

In summary, research approaches to late-life depression need to be flexible and multidirectional, clinical and psychosocial, focusing on both community and residential care populations. Our ultimate goal should be a combined treatment and prevention model like that which has so successfully reduced cardiovascular morbidity and mortality over the past few decades. Although we have made progress in treatment science in older adults, we have done much less in indicated and selective prevention, despite the evidence that such approaches have the potential to reduce the incidence of major and minor episodes by as much as 25% (Cuijpers, Beekman, & Reynolds, 2012).

BIPOLAR DISORDER

Bipolar disorder (BPD) occurs in approximately 0.5%–1% of the world population (Sajatovic & Chen, 2011). Onset is most common in younger age groups with only approximately 0.1% prevalence in older people (Vasudev & Thomas, 2010), implying that many people with BPD do not survive into late life. However prevalence is much higher in care homes and some hospitals (up to 10%) (Vasudev & Thomas, 2010). BPD in old age is a complex and heterogeneous condition. It may be associated with cognitive impairment (Depp & Jeste, 2004), cerebrovascular disease, and diabetes (McIntyre et al., 2006; Tsai et al., 2009).

Late-onset BPD patients tend to have a milder illness (less manic severity), but higher medical and neurological burden (cerebrovascular disease and cognitive decline). They are also less likely to have a family history of BPD compared with early-onset BPD patients. There is also some evidence of increased white matter changes as seen in increased white matter hypersensitivities on neuroimaging (Vasudev & Thomas, 2010). Furthermore, there appear to be differences in health service usage among younger and older onset BPD patients with younger patients more likely to use inpatient services and older BPD patients using more case management and outpatient care (Young, 2005).

Drug treatments are the main management strategy for older BPD patients (Young, 2005). A major difficulty for clinicians, older patients, and their families is managing the side effects of these drugs. Older patients with BPD may be prone to specific drug-related side effects, such as renal impairment or extrapyramidal symptoms and, when side effects occur, the sequelae may lead to marked disability (e.g., fall leading to hip fracture). Clinicians also need to be alert to the possibility of age-related reduced ability to metabolize and clear psychotropic drugs, treatment adherence, and the development of medication intolerance over time (Sajatovic, Herrman, & Shulman, 2009). Mood stabilizers, such as lithium, may also interact with other commonly prescribed drugs for older people, such as diuretics (Shulman, 2010).

There has been some research into the short-term and longer term consequences of lithium treatment (Shulman, 2010) and how it compares with the currently available alternatives (Sajatovic et al., 2009). Shulman (2010) argues that, as the best understood of the range of alternatives available, lithium should continue to be prescribed but cautions that dosage and serum lithium levels should be closely monitored in older adults. He also points out that clinicians also need to balance the quality-of-life risks of bipolar relapse and suicide against the risk of renal impairment. There is also some evidence that lithium may exert a protective effect against cognitive decline (Shulman, 2010; Young, 2011).

Some of the challenges in conducting research with older BPD patients are the lack of an agreed cutoff age and the limited sample size within a clinical setting as well as the complexity of comorbidities, drug sensitivities, and interactions (Young & Shulman, 2009).

Treatment of late-life BPD is currently based on evidence drawn from studies of younger BPD patients. There is limited evidence to support specific biologic or psychosocial interventions for either acute or long-term care of older adults with BPD.

There is general agreement in the literature that we need to know much more about BPD in older age, and to do this we need collaborative, multicenter studies to get adequate numbers, as much research to date has addressed relatively small numbers in single centers. Research needs to include further investigation of lithium treatment for older adults. Specific research questions are the efficacy of lithium as both an acute and maintenance treatment for late-life BPD; whether lithium (and other mood stabilizers) are effective in suicide prevention; whether lithium is protective for dementia; and the long-term effect of lithium on renal function in people of advanced years. Promising recent research on the therapeutic use of lithium reported evidence of good antisuicidal properties and potential antimanic effects, as well as reduced prevalence of Alzheimer's disease in patients with BPD, suggesting that lithium treatment may indeed be protective for dementia (Young, 2011). Other research directions for older age BPD include better understanding of the relationship between BPD and shared or overlapping contributors, such as cognitive decline and medical comorbidity (Lala & Sajatovic, 2012). More research is needed to understand illness trajectory, relationship to cognitive status, and treatments that optimize all levels of health and functioning. We need to better understand subtypes of BPD by age of onset.

We also need specific treatment guidelines for older adults that may differ from recommendations in current treatment guidelines. These may include recommendations about multifactorial treatments, including drug, psychoeducation for patients and families, and optimal care environments. We would benefit from multimethod studies that include clinical and behavioral measures as well as structural and functional neuroimaging in order to identify the characteristics that can help to identify older BPD subtypes that may have different prognoses, require different use of existing treatments, or respond to novel treatments.

More research is needed to refine neuroimaging findings, especially white matter hyperintensities, with a view to improving understanding of the pathogenesis of mania. More research is needed to better understand the patterns and extent of health care usage among older people with BPD.

Finally, BPD often has a significant effect on friendships and family relationships. With late-life BPD, family members may have been affected over many years by the consequences of this disorder. There is a lack of research about how to support families and friends so they can continue to interact with and assist the older person with BPD.

In summary, we need better to understand the pathogenesis and trajectory of BPD, how best to treat BPD in older people, including better understanding of the place of lithium in an effective treatment regime, and how service systems can best respond to older people with BPD and their families, taking into account their likely medical and cognitive comorbidities.

ANXIETY DISORDERS

Anxiety is more common than depression in older people (Wetherell, Maser, & van Balkom, 2005), but it has been studied far less (Bryant, Jackson, & Ames, 2008). Like depression, anxiety symptoms are more prevalent than anxiety disorders (however defined) with up to 24% of older people experiencing some symptoms of anxiety (Bryant et al., 2008) compared with approximately 5.6% when DSM-IV-TR criteria are used (Grenier et al., 2011). Anxiety is also more prevalent in clinical than community settings (Bryant et al., 2008). Particular at-risk groups for anxiety are women, people with neurodegenerative disorders and associated dementias, those in institutional care, and caregivers (Bryant et al., 2008), with up to 25% of caregivers of people with dementia experiencing clinically significant anxiety (Cooper, Balamurali, & Livingston, 2007). Anxiety can also have serious adverse consequences for older people, including reduced life satisfaction, poorer quality of life, greater health care utilization, increased onset of disability, mortality for suicide, and increased cardiovascular disease, with older men at particular risk (Bryant et al., 2008; Porensky et al., 2009).

At present if an older person presents to his or her primary care practitioner with anxiety, it is unlikely to be detected or treated and, if detected, most likely to be treated with benzodiazepines, which can have adverse consequences for older people, such as increased risk of falling, or antidepressant monotherapy (Lenze & Wetherell, 2011). Benzodiazepine treatment rates are falling, but their prescription is still common, although it has long been established that these drugs have numerous harmful side effects. There is a need for more public awareness of older age anxiety as well as education for primary care practitioners about detection and treatment of anxiety in older age (Lenze & Wetherell, 2011).

Anxiety in late life is still underresearched compared with depression, but there has been a substantial increase in research on older age anxiety in recent years (Flint, 2009). Some of the questions being asked include whether current diagnostic criteria for anxiety are appropriate for older adults (Bryant, 2010); what is the nature of anxiety in older people and how is it different from depression (Flint, 2005, 2009); what is the relationship between anxiety and cognitive decline (Bryant, 2010); and how can we best prevent, detect, and treat anxiety in older adults (Beekman, 2008; Lenze & Wetherell, 2009).

Diagnostic Criteria for Anxiety in Older Age

The current *DSM-IV* criteria for diagnosing anxiety disorders may not be appropriate for diagnosing anxiety in older people. For example, the criteria for social phobia include experiencing a marked and persistent fear of social situations and significant interference with social activities. Older people may be experiencing both of these but may have other reasons that are seen as acceptable in later life (such as avoidance of night driving) to account for these symptoms. The current *DSM-IV-TR* criteria for generalized anxiety disorder require that the person experiences his or her worry as "excessive," but older people may be less likely to describe their symptoms as excessive due to stoicism and/or stigma associated with mental health problems that are characteristic of their generation (Bryant, 2010; Flint, 2005). The problem with this is that older people who may have debilitating symptoms of anxiety (subthreshold anxiety) (Grenier et al., 2011) may not receive a diagnosis or treatment.

Nature of Older Age Anxiety

Another difficulty in diagnosing older age anxiety is differentiating the symptoms from depression, cognitive decline, and physical morbidity. For example, the symptoms of insomnia may mirror those of anxiety, and older people may worry excessively about their memory decline, which may be a symptom of anxiety, depression, or cognitive decline. There seem to be two approaches to this difficulty in the literature. Some question the benefit of studying older age depression and anxiety as separate disorders, suggesting that "an approach that embraces the continuities and similarities of late-life generalized anxiety and depression may well be richer, more informative and more clinically meaningful than an approach that continues to treat generalized anxiety disorder as a discrete categorical entity" (Flint, 2009, p. 443). Others suggest that there needs to be more

focus on specific presentations of anxiety in older people, such as avoidance or hyperarousal, in order to tease out how anxiety is experienced and therefore should be treated (Böttche, Kuwert, & Knaevelsrud, 2012; Flint, 2005). Grenier et al. (2011) suggests that perhaps older age anxiety should be seen as "a continuum in terms of the number of symptoms, frequency, impairment or severity" rather than an "all-or-nothing phenomena" (p. 325).

Relationship Between Anxiety and Cognitive Decline

There appears to be a two-way relationship between anxiety and cognitive decline (Beaudreau & O'Hara, 2008). There is some evidence that severe anxiety and generalized anxiety disorder affect cognitive performance, but mild anxiety can have the opposite effect (Beaudreau & O'Hara, 2008). Similarly, clinically significant anxiety may predict accelerated cognitive decline (Beaudreau & O'Hara, 2008). Hippocampal neurodegeneration in Alzheimer's disease may also reduce the brain's ability to manage anxiety states, accounting for the high levels of anxiety (70%) in patients with Alzheimer's disease (Beaudreau & O'Hara, 2008).

Prevention, Detection, and Treatment of Anxiety

Little is known about how to prevent anxiety in older adults. To date, there are no published studies that focus on prevention (Lenze & Wetherell, 2009). As stated earlier, there is a need for much greater awareness among the general public and clinicians working with older people about the prevalence and consequences of anxiety. This lack of awareness, together with the problems of diagnosis, also touched on earlier, makes detection difficult.

A review of 32 studies of anxiety in older adults (n = 2,484) found that there were greater improvements when patients were treated with pharmacotherapy than behavioral interventions and concluded that pharmacotherapy, specifically benzodiazepines and selective serotonin reuptake inhibitors, should be the treatment of choice for older adults who do not have medical conditions that preclude this form of treatment (Pinquart & Duberstein, 2007). However, the authors called for more randomized controlled trials that directly compare behavioral and pharmacological interventions with similar inclusion criteria, as direct comparison could not be made between these treatment types and it was not always possible to work out whether those enrolled in pharmacological treatments were also receiving behavioral interventions and vice versa (Pinquart & Duberstein, 2007). Furthermore, for many older people, there are both immediate and long-term adverse effects from pharmacotherapy treatments (McClive-Reed & Gellis, 2011). The main behavioral treatment that has been trialed on older subjects is cognitive-behavioral therapy. This has been found to be of some benefit to older people (Hendriks, Voshaar, Keijsers, Hoogduin, & vanBalkom, 2008; Pinquart & Duberstein, 2007), but it is unclear whether relaxation alone, which is often a component of cognitive-behavioral therapy is just as effective as combined cognitive-behavioral therapy and relaxation (Cooper, Balamurali, Selwood, & Livingston, 2007). A review of non-pharmacological approaches to treatment of anxiety in people with dementia found that behavioral and cognitive-behavioral approaches, music therapies, animal-assisted therapies, exercise, and touch therapies showed clinical promise, but the evidence base was not strong (McClive-Reed & Gellis, 2011).

Directions for Future Research

There is a need for consensus about how anxiety, including subthreshold anxiety, in older age should be defined. This consensus should include the views of older people and their caregivers, as clinicians rely on patient and informant reports to identify symptoms, so these symptoms have to have validity for those reporting them. The diagnostic criteria should be sensitive and appropriate for older people and should be accompanied by valid measures (Beekman, 2008; Mohlman et al., 2012). In particular, measures of anxiety in older people with cognitive impairment need further development (Beekman, 2008).

There is a need for research into prevention of anxiety in older age, but this again requires an understanding of what triggers anxiety from the point of view of the older person. This might include interventions to strengthen cognition, coping strategies (Cooper, Balamurali, Selwood et al., 2007), resilience, prophylactic behavioral interventions, and/or public awareness campaigns about safety and security for older people.

Society also requires more cross-disciplinary research, including psychosocial, behavioral, and

biological approaches (Lenze & Wetherell, 2009; O'Hara, 2006). There is an opportunity to increase our understanding of the neurological aspects of anxiety through advances in neuroimaging (Lenze & Wetherell, 2009). There is also a need for more well-designed studies that focus on anxiety specifically (rather than as a subset of depression) that clearly identify the inclusion criteria for participants, the symptoms or disorders that are targeted, and the interventions used (Böttche et al., 2012; Bryant et al., 2008; Cooper, Balamurali, Selwood et al., 2007; Flint, 2007; Grenier et al., 2011; Hendriks et al., 2008).

While perhaps not a research direction as such, researchers should contribute to awareness raising and education about older age anxiety through translational research activities.

Finally, there is a need for translational research that evaluates the effectiveness, cost, and feasibility of treatments for anxiety in a range of settings but particularly primary health settings as there is currently little takeup of the interventions known to be of benefit (Lenze & Wetherell, 2011; McClive-Reed & Gellis, 2011).

CONCLUSION

Despite increased awareness of older age mood disorders in recent decades, there are still a number of questions that remain unanswered. New technologies and an aging population provide an opportunity for us to address these questions and increase our understanding of these conditions. Better understanding should encompass better methods of assessment, more appropriate treatment options for older people and their families, and public education about these conditions. Future research should not only provide answers to academic questions but seek to implement findings in the real world, enabling older people to benefit from the knowledge gained through better access to assessment and treatment that improves their quality of life. As most of us will live to be old, many of us will experience older age mood disorders and will be grateful for research that has the potential to improve the well-being of older people.

Disclosures

Professor David Ames is director of the National Ageing Research Institute and holds grants from Australia's National Health and Medical Research

Council. He is clinical leader of the Australian Imaging Biomarkers and Lifestyle study of aging, whose chief funding sources since 2006 have been Australia's Commonwealth Science and Industry Research Organisation and the Science Industry Endowment Fund, but the study has received some funds from Pfizer, Astra Zeneca, GE, and Merck. Professor Ames has served on advisory boards for Eli Lilly, Janssen, Novartis, and Pfizer, but all but the Eli Lilly board are dormant at present. He has received support to attend conferences from each of these entities, but none of this support has been received within the last 18 months. He has received money for giving talks sponsored by these entities and also for giving talks sponsored by Lundbeck. Only Pfizer has paid him for talks in the past 12 months. He has given unpaid advice to the pharmaceutical company Prana and has undertaken drug trials for Pfizer, Prana, Lundbeck, and Eli Lilly within the last 2 years. He is a member of the International Psychogeriatric Association and edited their journal *International Psychogeriatrics* from 2003 to 2011. He has been chief medical advisor to Alzheimer's Australia for the last year. Professor Ames is salaried by the University of Melbourne and derives some income from private practice as a psychiatrist and from public sector work as a consultant psychiatrist for Melbourne Health and St Vincent's Health. In no year has his income from services to pharmaceutical companies ever exceeded 10% of his total income from all sources.

Dr. Briony Dow has no conflicts to disclose. She is funded by the National Ageing Research Institute and is in receipt of a National Health and Medical Research Council (Australia) project grant.

Dr. Jean Tinney has no conflicts to disclose. She is funded by the National Ageing Research Institute.

Ms. Betty Haralambous has no conflicts to disclose. She is funded by the National Ageing Research Institute.

Ms. Xiaoping Lin. has no conflicts to disclose. She is funded by the National Ageing Research Institute and is in receipt of an Australian Postgraduate Award Scholarship, funded by the Australian Federal Government.

REFERENCES

Ajilore, O., & Smith, G. (2011). Neuroimaging in geriatric psychiatry: Integrative research as the next frontier. *American Journal of Geriatric Psychiatry, 19*(1), 1–3.

Akincigil, A., Olfson, M., Siegel, M., Zurlo, K. A., Walkup, J. T., & Crystal, S. (2012). Racial and ethnic disparities in depression care in community-dwelling elderly in the United States. *American Journal of Public Health, 102*(2), 319–328.

Alexopoulos, G. S., & Bruce, M. L. (2009). A model for intervention research in late-life depression. *International Journal of Geriatric Psychiatry, 24*(12), 1325–1334.

Alexopoulos, G. S., Gunning-Dixon, F. M., Latoussakis, V., Kanellopoulos, D., & Murphy, C. F. (2008). Anterior cingulate dysfunction in geriatric depression. *International Journal of Geriatric Psychiatry, 23*(4), 347–355.

Alexopoulos, G. S., & Morimoto, S. S. (2011). The inflammation hypothesis in geriatric depression. *International Journal of Geriatric Psychiatry, 26*, 1109–1118.

Almeida, O. P. (2008). Vascular depression: Myth or reality? *International Psychogeriatrics, 20*(4), 645–652.

Almeida, O. P. (2011). Guest Editorial: Evolution, depression and the interplay between chance and choices. *International Psychogeriatrics, 23*(7), 1021–1025.

American Psychiatric Association. (1994). *Diagnostic and statistical manual of mental disorders* (4th ed.). Washington, DC: Author.

Ancoli-Israel, S., & Alessi, C. (2005). Sleep and aging. *American Journal of Geriatric Psychiatry, 13*(5), 341–343.

Andreescu, C., & Reynolds, C. F. (2011). Late-life depression: Evidence-based treatment and promising new directions for research and clinical practice. *Psychiatric Clinics of North America, 34*, 335–355.

Areán, P. A., & Alexopoulos, G. (2007). Psychosocial interventions for mental illness in late-life. *International Journal of Geriatric Psychiatry, 22*(2), 99–100.

Baldwin, R. C. (2005). Is vascular depression a distinct sub-type of depressive disorder? A review of causal evidence. *International Journal of Geriatric Psychiatry, 20*(1), 1–11.

Baldwin, R. C. (2010). Preventing late-life depression: A clinical update. *International Psychogeriatrics, 22*(Special Issue 8), 1216–1224.

Banerjee, S., Hellier, J., Dewey, M. E., Romeo, R., Ballard, C., Baldwin, R.,...Burns, A. (2011). Sertraline or mirtazapine for depression in dementia (HTA-SADD): A randomised, multicentre, double-blind, placebo-controlled trial. *Lancet, 378*, 403–411.

Beaudreau, S., & O'Hara, R. (2008). Late-life anxiety and cognitive impairment: A review. *American Journal of Geriatric Psychiatry, 16*(10), 790–803.

Beekman, A. (2008). Anxiety in aging: A newly chartered territory. *American Journal of Geriatric Psychiatry, 16*(10), 787–789.

Bell, C. C., & McBride, D. F. (2011). A commentary for furthering cultural sensitivity within research in geriatric psychiatry. *American Journal of Geriatric Psychiatry, 19*(5), 397–402.

Bhalla, R. K., & Butters, M. A. (2011). Cognitive functioning in late-life depression. *British Columbia Medical Journal, 53*(7), 357–360.

Blake, H., Mo, P., Malik, S., & Thomas, S. (2009). How effective are physical activity interventions for alleviating depressive symptoms in older people? A systematic review. *Clinical Rehabilitation, 23*(10), 873–887.

Blazer, D. G. (2005). Depression and social support in late life: A clear but not obvious relationship. *Aging and Mental Health, 9*(6), 497–499.

Blumberger, D. M., Daskalakis, Z. J., & Mulsant, B. H. (2008). Biomarkers in geriatric psychiatry: Searching for the holy grail? *Current Opinion in Psychiatry, 21*(6), 533–539.

Böttche, M., Kuwert, P., & Knaevelsrud, C. (2012). Posttraumatic stress disorder in older adults: An overview of characteristics and treatment approaches. *International Journal of Geriatric Psychiatry, 27*(3), 230–239.

Bruce, M. (2010). Subsyndromal depression and services delivery: At a crossroad? *American Journal of Geriatric Psychiatry, 18*(3), 189–192.

Bryant, C. (2010). Anxiety and depression in old age: Challenges in recognition and diagnosis. *International Psychogeriatrics, 22*(4), 511–513.

Bryant, C., Jackson, H., & Ames, D. (2008). The prevalence of anxiety in older adults: Methodological issues and a review of the literature. *Journal of Affective Disorders, 109*(3), 233–250.

Cañive, J., & Escobar, J. (2009). New research on aging minority groups is timely and incorporates state of the art methodologies. *American Journal of Geriatric Psychiatry, 17*(11), 913–915.

Carvalho, A. F., Cavalcante, J. L., Castelo, M. S., & Lima, M. C. O. (2007). Augmentation strategies for treatment-resistant depression: A literature review. *Journal of Clinical Pharmacy and Therapeutics, 32*, 415–428.

Chiu, H. F-K., Tsoh, J., & Lam, L. C-W. (2007). Studies from emerging countries: An encouraging development. *Current Opinion in Psychiatry, 20*(6), 544–550.

Coleman, P. G. (2005). Uses of reminiscence: Functions and benefits. *Aging and Mental Health, 9*(4), 291–294.

Cooper, C., Balamurali, T. B. S., & Livingston, G. (2007). A systematic review of the prevalence and covariates of anxiety in caregivers of people with dementia. *International Psychogeriatrics, 19*(02), 175–195.

Cooper, C., Balamurali, T. B. S., Selwood, A., & Livingston, G. (2007). A systematic review of intervention studies about anxiety in caregivers of people with dementia. *International Journal of Geriatric Psychiatry, 22*(3), 181–188.

Cooper, C., Katona, C., Lyketos, K., Blazer, D. G., Brodaty, H., Rabins, P. V., ... Livingston, G. (2011). A systematic review of treatments for refractory depression in older people. *American Journal of Psychiatry, 168*(7), 681–688.

Cuijpers, P., Beekman, A. T. F., & Reynolds, C. F. (2012). Preventing depression: A global priority. *Journal of the American Medical Association, 307*(10), 1033–1034.

Cuijpers, P., van Straten, A., & Smit, F. (2006). Psychological treatment of late-life depression: A meta-analysis of randomized controlled trials. *International Journal of Geriatric Psychiatry, 21*(12), 1139–1149.

Cuijpers, P., van Straten, A., Smit, F., & Andersson, G. (2009). Is psychotherapy for depression equally effective in younger and older adults? A meta-regression analysis. *International Psychogeriatrics, 21*(01), 16–24.

Culang-Reinlieb, M. E., Johnert, L. C., Brickman, A. M., & Steffens, D. C. (2011). MRI-defined vascular depression: A review of the construct. *International Journal of Geriatric Psychiatry, 26*, 1101–1108.

de Toledo Ferraz Alves, T. C., Ferreira, L. K., & Busatto, G. F. (2010). Vascular diseases and old age mental disorders: An update of neuroimaging findings. *Current Opinion in Psychiatry, 23*(6), 491–497.

Depp, C., & Jeste, D. V. (2004). Bipolar disorder in older adults: a critical review. *Bipolar Disorder, 6*, 343–367.

Dew, M. A., Whyte, E. M., Lenze, E. J., Houck, P. R., Mulsant, B. H., Pollock, B. G., ... Reynolds, C. F., III. (2007). Recovery from major depression in older adults receiving augmentation of antidepressant pharmacotherapy. *American Journal of Psychiatry, 164*(6), 892–899.

Djernes, J. K. (2006). Prevalence and predictors of depression in populations of elderly: A review. *Acta Psychiatrica Scandinavica, 113*, 372–387.

Dombrovski, A. Y., & Mulsant, B. H. (2007). ECT: The preferred treatment for severe depression in late life. *International Psychogeriatrics, 19*(01), 10–14.

Dow, B., Lin, X., Tinney, J., Haralambous, B., & Ames, D. (2011). Guest Editorial: Depression in residential care homes for older people. *International Psychogeriatrics, 23*(5), 681–699.

Faison, W. E., & Mintzer, J. E. (2005). The growing, ethnically diverse aging population: Is our field advancing with it? *American Journal of Geriatric Psychiatry, 13*(7), 541–544.

Felmet, K., Zisook, S., & Kasckow, J. W. (2011). Elderly patients with schizophrenia and depression: Diagnosis and treatment. *Clinical Schizophrenia and Related Psychoses, 4*(4), 239–250.

Flicker, L. (2008). Vascular factors in geriatric psychiatry: Time to take a serious look. *Current Opinion in Psychiatry, 21*(6), 551–554.

Flint, A. (2005). Anxiety and its disorders in late life: Moving the field forward. *American Journal of Geriatric Psychiatry, 13*(1), 3–6.

Flint, A. (2007). Anxiety disorders in later life: From epidemiology to treatment. *American Journal of Geriatric Psychiatry, 15*(8), 635–638.

Flint, A. (2009). Late-life generalized anxiety: The constraint of categorization. *American Journal of Geriatric Psychiatry, 17*(6), 441–444.

Forsman, A. K., Schierenbeck, I., & Wahlbeck, K. (2011). Psychosocial interventions for the prevention of depression in older adults: Systematic review and meta-analysis. *Journal of Aging and Health, 23*(3), 387–416.

Frazer, C. J., Christensen, H., & Griffiths, K. M. (2005). Effectiveness of treatments for depression in older people. *Medical Journal of Australia, 182*(12), 627–632.

Frederick, J. T., Steinman, L. E., Prohaska, T., Satariano, W. A., Bruce, M., Bryant, L., ... Snowden, M. (2007). Community-based treatment of late life depression: An expert panel-informed literature review. *American Journal of Preventive Medicine, 33*(3), 222–249.

Ganguli, M. (2007). For debate: The evidence for electroconvulsive therapy (ECT) in the treatment of severe late-life depression. *International Psychogeriatrics, 19*(1), 9–10.

Giron, M. S. T., Fastbom, J., & Winblad, B. (2005). Clinical trials of potential antidepressants: to what extent are the elderly represented: A review. *International Journal of Geriatric Psychiatry, 20*(3), 201–217.

Greenberg, R. M., & Kellner, C. H. (2005). Electroconvulsive therapy: A selected review. *American Journal of Geriatric Psychiatry, 13*(4), 268–281.

Grenier, S., Préville, M., Boyer, R., O'Connor, K., Béland, S., Potvin, O., ... Scientific Committee of the ESA Study. (2011). The impact of DSM-IV symptom and clinical significance criteria on the prevalence estimates of subthreshold and threshold anxiety in the older adult population. *American Journal of Geriatric Psychiatry, 19*(4), 316–326.

Hendriks, G. J., Voshaar, R. C. O., Keijsers, G. P. J., Hoogduin, C. A. L., & vanBalkom, A. J. L. M. (2008). Cognitive-behavioural therapy for late-life anxiety disorders: A systematic review and meta-analysis. *Acta Psychiatrica Scandinavica, 117*, 403–411.

Hindi, F., Dew, M. A., Albert, S. M., Lotrich, F. E., & Reynolds, C. F. (2011). Preventing depression in later life: State of the art and science circa 2011. *Psychiatric Clinics of North America, 34*(1), 67–78.

Hoptman, M. J., Gunning-Dixon, F. M., Murphy, C. F., Lim, K. O., & Alexopoulos, G. S. (2006). Structural neuroimaging research methods in geriatric depression. *American Journal of Geriatric Psychiatry, 14*(10), 812–822.

Huang, C-Q., Wang, Z-R., Li, Y-H., Xie, Y-Z., & Liu, Q-X. (2011). Cognitive function and risk for depression in old age: A meta-analysis of published literature. *International Psychogeriatrics, 23*(4), 516–525.

Hybels, C., & Pieper, C. (2009). Epidemiology and geriatric psychiatry. *American Journal of Geriatric Psychiatry, 17*(8), 627–631.

Kasckow, J. W., & Zisook, S. (2008). Co-occurring depressive symptoms in the older patient with schizophrenia. *Drugs and Aging, 25*(8), 631–647.

Kennedy, G. J. (2005). Should primary care be the primary site of geriatric mental health care? *American Journal of Geriatric Psychiatry, 13*(9), 745–747.

Khundakar, A. A., & Thomas, A. J. (2009). Morphometric changes in early- and late-life major depressive disorder: Evidence from postmortem studies. *International Psychogeriatrics, 21*(05), 844–854.

Koder, D. A., & Helmes, E. (2006). Clinical psychologists in aged care in Australia: A question of attitude or training? *Australian Psychologist, 41*, 179–185.

Kok, R., Heeren, T., & Nolen, W. (2011). Continuing treatment of depression in the elderly: A systematic review and meta-analysis of double-blinded randomized controlled trials with antidepressants. *American Journal of Geriatric Psychiatry, 19*(3), 249–255.

Krishna, M., Jauhari, A., Lepping, P., Turner, J., Crossley, D., & Krishnamoorthy, A. (2011). Is group psychotherapy effective in older adults with depression? A systematic review. *International Journal of Geriatric Psychiatry, 26*(4), 331–340.

Kua, H. E., & Ho, R. (2008). The many faces of geriatric depression. *Current Opinion in Psychiatry, 21*(6), 540–545.

Kumar, A., Aizenstein, H., & Ballmaier, M. (2008). Multimodal neuroimaging in late-life mental disorders: Entering a more mature phase of clinical neuroscience research. *American Journal of Geriatric Psychiatry, 16*(4), 251–254.

Kumar, A., & Ajilore, O. (2009). Neuroimaging and geriatric psychiatry: The story of an interdisciplinary science and mental illness in the elderly. *American Journal of Geriatric Psychiatry, 17*(1), 1–3.

Kupfer, D., Kuhl, E., & Regier, D. (2009). Research for improving diagnostic systems: consideration of factors related to later life development. *American Journal of Geriatric Psychiatry, 17*(5), 355–358.

Lala, S. V., & Sajatovic, M. (2012). Medical and psychiatric comorbidities among elderly individuals with bipolar disorder: A literature review. *Journal of Geriatric Psychiatry and Neurology, 25*(1), 20–25.

Lee, K., Volans, P. J., & Gregory, N. (2003). Trainee clinical psychologists' views on recruitment to work with older people. *Aging and Society, 23*, 83–97.

Lenze, E. J., & Wetherell, J. L. (2009). Bringing the bedside to the bench, and then to the community: A prospectus for intervention research in late-life anxiety disorders. *International Journal of Geriatric Psychiatry, 24*(1), 1–14.

Lenze, E. J., & Wetherell, J. L. (2011). Anxiety disorders: New developments in old age. *American Journal of Geriatric Psychiatry, 19*(4), 330–339.

Lovell, M. (2006). Caring for the elderly: Changing perceptions and attitudes. *Journal Of Vascular Nursing, 24*, 22–26.

McClive-Reed, K. P., & Gellis, Z. D. (2011). Anxiety and related symptoms in older persons with dementia: Directions for practice. *Journal of Gerontological Social Work, 54*(1), 6–28.

McIntyre, R., Konarski, J., Soczynska, J., Wilkins, K., Panjwani, G., Bouffard, B.,…Kennedy, S. H. (2006). Medical comorbidity in bipolar disorder: Implications for functional outcomes and health service utilization. *Psychiatric Services, 57*(8), 1140–1144.

Meeks, T. W., Vahia, I. V., Lavretsky, H., Kulkarni, G., & Jeste, D. V. (2011). A tune in "a minor" can "b major": A review of epidemiology, illness course, and public health implications of subthreshold depression in older adults. *Journal of Affective Disorders, 129*(1–3), 126–142.

Meyers, B. S., Flint, A. J., Rothschild, A. J., Mulsant, B. H., Whyte, E. M., Peasley-Miklus, C.,…STOP-OP Group. (2009). A double-blind randomized controlled trial of olanzapine plus sertraline vs olanzapine plus placebo for psychotic depression. *Archives of General Psychiatry, 66*(8), 838–847.

Mohlman, J., Bryant, C., Lenze, E. J., Stanley, M. A., Gum, A., Flint, A.,…Craske, M. G. (2012). Improving recognition of late life anxiety disorders in Diagnostic and Statistical Manual of Mental Disorders, Fifth Edition: Observations and recommendations of the Advisory Committee to the Lifespan Disorders Work Group. *International Journal of Geriatric Psychiatry, 27*, 549–556.

Mottram, P. G., Wilson, K., & Strobl, J. J. (2006). Antidepressants for depressed elderly. *Cochrane Database of Systematic Reviews, 1*, CD003491.

O'Hara, R. (2006). Stress, aging, and mental health. *American Journal of Geriatric Psychiatry, 14*(4), 295–298.

Pinquart, M., & Duberstein, P. (2007). Treatment of anxiety disorders in older adults: A meta-analytic comparison of behavioral and pharmacological interventions. *American Journal of Geriatric Psychiatry, 15*(8), 639–651.

Porensky, E., Dew, M., Karp, J., Skidmore, E., Rollman, B., Shear, M., & Lenze, E. J. (2009). The burden of late life generalized anxiety disorder: Effects on disability, health related quality of life and health care utilization. *American Journal of Geriatric Psychiatry, 17*, 473–482.

Reynolds, C. F. (2009). Prevention of depressive disorders: A brave new world. *Depression and Anxiety, 26*(12), 1062–1065.

Reynolds, C. F., Butters, M. A., Lopez, O., Pollock, B. G., Dew, M. A., Mulsant, B. H., et al. (2011). Maintenance treatment of depression in old age: A randomized, double-blind, placebo-controlled evaluation of the efficacy and safety of donepezil combined with antidepressant pharmacotherapy. *Archives of General Psychiatry, 68*(1), 51–60.

Reynolds, C. F., Dew, M. A., Pollock, B. G., Mulsant, B. H., Frank, E., Miller, M. D.,…DeKosky, S. T. (2006). Maintenance treatment of major depression in old age. *New England Journal of Medicine, 354*(11), 1130–1138.

Sajatovic, M., & Chen, P. (2011). Geriatric bipolar disorder. *Psychiatric Clinics of North America, 34*(2), 319–333.

Sajatovic, M., Herrman, N., & Shulman, K. I. (2009). Acute mania and bipolar affective disorder. In M. Abou-Saleh, C. Katona, & A. Kuma (Eds.), *Principles and practice of geriatric psychiatry* (3rd ed.). Chichester: John Wiley and Sons Ltd.

Shulman, K. I. (2010). Lithium for older adults with bipolar disorder: Should it still be considered a first-line agent? *Drugs Aging, 27*(8), 607–615.

Smith, G. S., & Alexopoulos, G. S. (2009). Neuroimaging in geriatric psychiatry. *International Journal of Geriatric Psychiatry, 24*(8), 783–787.

Sneed, J., & Culang-Reinlieb, M. (2011). The vascular depression hypothesis: An update. *American Journal of Geriatric Psychiatry, 19*(2), 99–103.

Snowdon, J. (2007). Psychogeriatric services in the community and in long-term care facilities: Needs and developments. *Current Opinion in Psychiatry, 20*(6), 533–538.

Snowdon, J. (2010a). Mental health service delivery in long-term care homes. *International Psychogeriatrics, 22*(Special Issue 7), 1063–1071.

Snowdon, J. (2010b). Protection from late life depression. *International Psychogeriatrics, 22*(5), 844–845.

Teper, E., & O'Brien, J. T. (2008). Vascular factors and depression. *International Journal of Geriatric Psychiatry, 23*(10), 993–1000.

Tsai, S., Kuo, C., Chung, K., Huang, Y., Lee, H., & Chen, C. (2009). Cognitive dysfunction and medical co-morbidity in elderly outpatients with bipolar disorder. *American Journal of Geriatric Psychiatry, 17*(12), 1004–1011.

van Schaik, A. M., Comijs, H. C., Sonnenberg, C. M., Beekman, A. T., Sienaert, P., & Stek, M. L. (2012). Efficacy and safety of continuation and maintenance electroconvulsive therapy in depressed elderly patients: A systematic review. *American Journal of Geriatric Psychiatry, 20*(1), 5–17.

Vasudev, A., & Thomas, A. (2010). Bipolar disorder' in the elderly: What's in a name? *Maturitas, 66*(3), 231–235.

Walsh, P., Currier, G., Shah, M., Lyness, J., & Friedman, B. (2008). Psychiatric emergency services for the U.S. elderly: 2008 and beyond. *American Journal of Geriatric Psychiatry, 16*(9), 706–717.

Wetherell, J. L., Maser, J. D., & van Balkom, A. (2005). Anxiety disorders in the elderly: Outdated beliefs and a research agenda. *Acta Psychiatrica Scandinavica, 111,* 401–402.

World Health Organization. (1992). *International statistical classification of diseases and related health problems* (10th ed., text rev.). Geneva, Switzerland: Author.

Yastrubetskaya, O., Chiu, E., & O'Connell, S. (1997). Is good clinical research practice for clinical trials good clinical practice? *International Journal of Geriatric Psychiatry, 12*(2), 227–231.

Young, A. H. (2011). More good news about the magic ion: Lithium may prevent dementia. *British Journal of Psychiatry, 198,* 336–337.

Young, R., & Shulman, K. (2009). Bipolar disorders in late life: Early days, gradual progress. *American Journal of Geriatric Psychiatry, 17*(12), 1001–1003.

Young, R. C. (2005). Bipolar disorder in older persons: Perspectives and new findings. *American Journal of Geriatric Psychiatry, 13*(4), 265–267.

3

EPIDEMIOLOGY OF LATE-LIFE MOOD DISORDERS

RATES, MEASURES, AND POPULATIONS

Patricia Marino and Jo Anne Sirey

AS THE largest generation in American history enters older adulthood, we prepare ourselves for the mental health needs of a heterogeneous population of individuals ranging from 60 to 100 years old. Adults reaching age 65 have an average life expectancy of an additional 18.6 years (19.9 for females and 17.2 for males) (US Department of Health and Human Services, 2011). At the present, there are an estimated 39.6 million adults aged 65+ in 2009 comprising 13% of the population. This is expected to grow to 55 million by the year 2020. The group of oldest older adults, age 85 plus, now estimated at 5.7 million, will grow to 6.6 million by 2020. The older adult population represents a wide range of functional levels, medical burden, and psychiatric needs. In this chapter we describe the rates of late-life mood disorders, taking into account the range of individuals in this population. Steffens notes that estimates of prevalence are affected by person-related factors such as settings, inclusion/exclusion factors, and methodological factors such as assessment type, attribution of symptoms that overlap with medical

symptoms, and the degree of representativeness (Steffens, Fisher, Langa, Potter, & Plassman, 2009). To capture the heterogeneity in the population, the rates we present include the assessments used and the settings where the sample is collected. We review the reported rates of unipolar and bipolar disorders without a systematic review of the gender and race/ethnic variation that is emerging.

The rates of late-life mood disorders vary across studies with a number of factors that contribute to the identification and documentation of late-life mood disorders. Factors include variability in the definition of mood disorders, measures used to evaluate depression, and settings from which data are collected. In addition, when later life is defined as age 60 years or older, we are characterizing a population that spans 40 years. These factors contribute to the heterogeneity that is the hallmark of late-life mood disorders (Alexopoulos, 2005; Lebowitz et al., 1997). As we review the rates of reported later life mood disorders, particular attention will be paid to the assessment methods used and the populations sampled. This focus represents the increasing move out into the "community" and the increased efforts to detect the prevalence of later life mood disorders in settings that support older persons. In this volume, other chapters will describe in great detail the diagnostic nomenclature, the personal and public costs, the treatments, and the outcomes. In the medical settings we will only review the rates of late-life mood disorders, with more in-depth discussion provided in Chapters 28–31, where mood disorders in nursing home settings, palliative care, primary care, and home care settings are reviewed. Additionally, the prevalence conditions comorbid with depression, including anxiety (Chapter 9), medical conditions (Chapter 16), and cognitive impairment (Chapter 17), will also be discussed in depth in later chapters.

To organize our review of late-life mood disorders, we will discuss the rates of unipolar depression, bipolar disorder, and nonmajor depression using the framework of settings and populations that are sampled within those settings. At the simplest level the selected settings can be divided into research data on rates of mood disorders drawn from (1) representative community samples, (2) medical settings, and (3) community service settings. Finally, we will define older adults as those individuals who are aged 60 or older. While age 65 is frequently thought of as the beginning of later life due to its association with retirement age, we will use 60 to include those studies that are conducted in aging service settings where eligibility for Elderly Nutrition Programs, authorized under Title III, Grants for State and Community Programs on Aging, and Title VI, Grants for Native Americans, under the Older Americans Act services begins at age 60.

ASSESSMENT OF DEPRESSION

Research assessment of unipolar depression and nonmajor depression is traditionally done using diagnostic assessments by trained evaluators using such standardized interview instruments as the Structured Clinical Interview for the *DSM-IV* (Spitzer et al., 1995). However, the increase in awareness of the public health importance of depression has led to expanded detection of depression to settings beyond traditional mental health or research settings. This increase in awareness and detection has expanded the use of assessment tools that can be quickly and effectively used in community settings, often with only minimal training.

Several screening tools, rating scales, and diagnostic interviews for depression have been developed and are frequently used in assessing depression and depressive symptoms in older adults. The Patient Health Questionnaire (PHQ-9), the Geriatric Depression Scale (GDS), and the Center of Epidemiologic Studies Depression Scale (CES-D) are screening tools most commonly used in community-based setting to identify the presence of depression or symptoms of depression. The PHQ-9 is a nine-question survey in which the patient or subject gives a self-report of the depressive symptoms he or she has been experiencing over the last 2 weeks. (Kroenke, Spitzer, & Williams, 2001; Kroenke et al., 2002) The PHQ-2 is a two-item survey and is a quick and valid measure for the assessment of depression in the community. The PHQ-2 consists of the first two items of the full nine-item PHQ-9 that evaluate the gateway symptoms of depression, including depressed mood and anhedonia (lack of interest/enjoyment in activities). The GDS asks similar questions to the PHQ-9; however, it is a 15-question survey and is focused on depressive symptoms experienced over the last week (Yesavage et al, 1983). The CES-D is a survey comprised of 20 questions also used to examine depressive symptoms in the last 7 days (Radloff, 1977).

The most commonly used diagnostic interviews for diagnosing major depression or minor depression and subsyndromal depression are the Composite International Diagnostic Interview (CIDI) and the Structured Clinical Interview for *DSM* Disorders (SCID). The CIDI is a diagnostic interview based on the *DSM-IV* and *ICD-10* criteria for mood disorders. It is generally used in large epidemiological studies and assesses both the presence and severity of several mood disorders (such as major depression, generalized anxiety disorder, and panic disorder). The SCID is a diagnostic interview based on the *DSM-IV* criteria for mood (SCID-I) and is used to diagnose a mood disorder. These measure assess depression and symptoms of depression based on the diagnostic criteria set forth in the *DSM-IV-TR*.

UNIPOLAR DEPRESSION

Types of Unipolar Depression

The category of unipolar disorder includes major depressive disorder (major depression), dysthymic disorder, and minor or subsyndromal depression. Dysthymic disorder is defined by the *DSM-IV-TR* as depression defined by any two depressive symptoms on the SCID lasting 2 or more years in length. Prevalence of dysthymic disorder varies among studies from 0.7% to 8.1%. This may be due to the assessment and diagnosis of dysthymia. In some studies dysthymic disorder has been included in the category of subsyndromal depression (Grabovich, Lu, Tang, Tu, Lyness, 2010; Lyness, Chapman, McGriff, Drayer, & Duberstein, 2009) and the individual prevalence of each diagnosis was not reported. Minor depression is defined by the *DSM-IV-TR* as having only two to four symptoms rather than the five or more needed for major depression. Subsyndromal is defined as an indication of depression defined by any two depressive symptoms on the SCID (Grabovich et al., 2010).

Population Representative Samples

The traditional method to identify prevalence of mental health need uses random identification of a representative sample of older adults. These studies use a multiple-frame approach to estimation and inference to characterize the general population. In these samples individuals with a range of functional abilities and medical burden who are community dwelling are surveyed using standardized surveys and claims databases. These studies have traditionally documented low rates of mental health needs among older adults when compared to younger adult samples.

In 2003, data were published from the 1997–1998 Healthcare for Communities (HCC) Household Telephone Survey on rates of unipolar depression and use of mental health services among adults aged 18 years and older. Telephone interviews of 9,585 adults were conducted using the CIDI to determine mental health need followed by questions about mental health use. Among the older adults (N = 1,538), 5.74% met criteria for depression (either major depression or dysthymia) as compared to 12.84% in the younger group (ages 18–29) and 11.52% in the middle group (ages 30–64) (Klap, Unroe, & Unützer, 2003). The National Comorbidity Study-Replication (NCS-R) gathered face-to-face data on a nationally representative sample of 9,282 adults age 18 and older (Kessler et al., 2004; Kessler & Merikangas, 2004). To identify the rates of unipolar depression, two analyses have been completed. Gum and colleagues found a 12–month prevalence of major depression using the CIDI of 2.3% for older adults with an additional

0.5% meeting CIDI criteria for dysthymia (Gum, King-Kallimanis, & Kohn, 2009). In a further analysis the prevalence for older adults was analyzed to examine age groups within the older adult subgroup. The rate was highest among adults between the ages of 65 and 74 at 3.1% with a decline for years 75–84 (1.1%) and 85 years and older (1.8%) (Byers, Yaffe, Covinsky, Friedman, & Bruce, 2010). There were no differences noted between race/ethnic groups.

The Behavioral Risk Surveillance System (BRFSS) is used by the Centers for Disease Control and Prevention to help states identify health issues and behaviors (Byers, Arean, & Yaffe, 2012). In 2006, a state-based, random-digit dialed-telephone survey of noninstitutionalized adults to collect data on health and health risks was conducted. Using the PHQ-8, surveyors found that 5.0% of older adults endorsed significant depressive symptoms (State of Mental Health and Aging in America; http://apps.nccd.cdc.gov/MAHA/MahaHome.aspx). In a follow-up report, based on data collected in 2006 and 2008, the rate was increased to 6.8% of adults aged 65 and older who were suffering from any depression on the PHQ-8 (Morbidity and Mortality Weekly Report, October 1, 2010/59(38); 1229–1235).

Medicare is the largest insurer of adults aged 65 and older with 93.5% of older adults covered (A Profile of Older Adults: 2010, Administration on Aging, http://www.aoa.gov/aoaroot/aging_statistics/Profile/2010/15.aspx). Combining Medicare claims with interviews with enrolled adults conducted through the Medicare Current Beneficiary Survey (MCBS) rates of depression were estimated for those insured. Among 20,966 persons with observations from 1992 to 1998, the rates of depression diagnosed and treated increased significantly. The proportion of individuals aged 65 and older with any depression jumped from 2.8% in 1992 to 5.8% in 1998 (Crystal, Sambamoorthi, Walkup, & Ankicigil, 2003). Looking specifically at the rates of depression diagnosis over a 13-year span, Akincigil and colleagues found that major depression diagnosis rates almost doubled from 2.3% in 1992 to 6.3% in 2005 (Akincigil et al., 2011). The greatest increase in depression diagnosis was with the category of adults aged 85 and older (7.1% in 2005). Within those rates almost a quarter had the diagnosis of major depression (23.1%) with the other diagnoses in the nonmajor depression diagnostic category. Other notable trends included a gap in depression diagnoses between older adults that were White and those that were African American and Hispanic. These findings document a disparity that has been noted in community treatment setting samples (Cooper-Patrick, et al. 1999; Sirey et al., 1999; Kales et al., 2005).

Health and Retirement study reported by AOA HHS shows that from 1998 to 2006, 10% to 12% of men over 65 had clinically relevant depressive symptoms as did 17% to 19% of women using the CES-D. To examine the rates of depression among older adults with varying levels of cognitive functioning, Steffens and colleagues examined the ADAMS sample of the Health and Retirement Study (HRS). The ADAMS sample is proxy measures that were collected on the participant's health and mental health status to supplement self-report data. In a sample of 851 for which the CIDI short form was used to measure depression over the age of 70, 11.19% of individuals had major depression (Steffens et al., 2009).

Medical Settings

The medical settings that serve older adults include primary care settings, home health care, long-term care, and hospital settings. These settings vary in the presentation of older adults who utilize their services. The transitional state of the medical setting as well as the overall severity of disability and chronic illness among the older adults that present in this setting may be factors in the assessment and presentation of depression. A growing body of research has found that depression is often associated with greater health care utilization, making medical settings an important venue for the identification of depressive symptoms.

In a primary care setting it was found that 6.9% of the population endorsed minor depression, 37.6% met criteria for subsyndromal depression (Grabovich et al., 2010), 1% met criteria for dysthymia (Lyness, King, Cox, Yoediono, & Caine, 1999), and 4.8% met criteria for major depression (Lyness et al., 2009). Lyness and colleagues pioneered research in late-life subsyndromal depression in primary care settings (Lyness et al., 1999, 2007, 2009). Their work indicates a higher rate of subsyndromal depression compared to minor or major depression among older adults in a primary care setting. The subsyndormal group was also found to have a greater rate of functional disability (Lyness et al., 2007). Approximately 8%–10% of older adults with subthreshold depression developed major depression per year (Meeks, Vahia, Lavretsky, Kulkarni, & Jeste,

2011). In additional primary care studies a 10% per year conversion rate for subthreshold depression to major depression was reported compared to 2% per year major depression incidence among nondepressed peers (Lyness et al., 2002).

Hospital-based settings including emergency departments (EDs) serve a population of older adults with either chronic or acute medical illness. Older adults in the United States frequent EDs with 15 million ED visits in 2000 (Shah et al., 2011; Shah et al., 2011). Screening for depression in ED settings identified a 15% rate of depression among older adults presenting with acute exacerbation of medical symptoms (Shah et al., 2011; Shah et al., 2011). At 2-week follow-up 28% of those individuals who initially screened positive for depression continued to endorse symptoms of depression. Reasons for this variability may reflect changes in clinical state confounding for medical conditions. Among older adults in a hospital-based setting 21.6% were found to meet criteria for major depression and 27.9% with minor depression (Koenig, 1997). When compared with patients without depression, those patients with major depression were more likely to report overall greater severity of medical illness and symptoms of pain or other somatic symptoms (Koenig, 1997). Research on longitudinal risk of major depression among this population is limited. Individuals with medical illnesses, including coronary heart disease and postmyocardial infarctions, have been found to have a higher rate (14%–42%) of conversion from minor depression to major depression (Hance, Carney, Freedland, & Skala, 1996; Schleifer et al., 1989).

Home health care programs are designed to provide short-term home care services, including skilled nursing, nurse's aide, and social services, to individuals who are too medically or functionally compromised to visit a physician or clinic without help. A prevalence rate of 13.5% of major depression is found for Medicare home health care patients (Bruce et al., 2002; Raue et al., 2003) with meaningful rates of suicidal ideation (Raue, Meyers, Rowe, Heo, & Bruce, 2007). When minor or other subsyndromal depressions are included in the calculations, the rates of depression increase to approximately one-third of all geriatric home health care patients (Bruce et al., 2002; Ell, Unützer, Aranda, Sanchez, & Lee, 2005).

With increasing age of the US population, especially among those aged 85 and above, there is a greater number of older adults requiring long-term care services. It is estimated that 4% to 5% of persons 65 years and older reside in a nursing home (US Board of the Census, 1993; Sirrocco, 1994) and that as many as 50% of older adults will enter nursing home at some point in their lives (Cohen, Tell, & Wallack, 1986; Murtaugh, Kemper, & Spillman, 1990). The prevalence of depression in nursing homes varies, depending on the method of assessment and time frame. Estimates of prevalence of clinical depression among the elderly nursing home residents range from 9% to 30% (Gruber-Baldini, Zimmerman et al., 2005; Parmelee, Katz, & Lawton, 1989; Payne et al., 2002; Rovner, 1993), with rates of any depressive symptoms ranging from 25% to 66% (Gruber-Baldini, Zimmerman et al., 2005; McCurren, Dowe, Rattle, & Looney, 1999; Ryden et al., 1999). Many studies have determined that depression is underdetected and undertreated in nursing homes (Brown, Lapane, & Luisi, 2002; Gruber-Baldini, Zimmerman et al., 2005; Ryden et al., 1999; Webber et al., 2005), especially among older adults with dementia (Brown et al., 2002). Symptoms of depression are often present in individuals with dementia. The prevalence of major depression in patients with Alzheimer's disease is approximately 17% and even higher in those with subcortical dementias (Alexopoulos, 2005). Research of the conversion of minor depression or subsyndromal depression to major depression is limited in this population. Research has reported up to a 23% conversion rate in a long-term care setting (Parmelee, Katz, & Lawton, 1992).

In conclusion, the research supports the higher prevalence of major depression in medical treatment settings: 5% to 10% in primary care (Hybels & Blazer, 2003), 14% in home health care (Bruce, 2002), and 24% in long-term care (Hyer, 2005) in comparison to community-dwelling older adults. The relationship of depression and disability is bidirectional with empirical evidence suggesting that late-life depression promotes disability, and likewise, disability increases the risk of depression (Wilkins, Kiosses, & Ravdin, 2010). Overall the greater the medical burden, the higher the risk of depression (Alexopoulos, 2005).

Community Service Settings

With the increase in awareness of the personal, social, and economic costs of depression among older adults, depression screening has become more widely integrated in community-based settings that service nutritional and social needs of older adults. These settings offer the opportunity for detection of depression in the context of providing other services. In some cases, the depression screening can be integrated into a "whole person approach" or offered as an additional routine assessment. These community subsamples include large numbers of individuals who benefit from the aging-related services provided through the State Departments of Aging through Area on Aging Agencies funded by federal monies through the Older Americans Act. These older persons include those who have impairments in activities of daily living and need nutritional support (e.g., home meal service, congregate meals), special crisis intervention (e.g., elderly crime victims services), or seek support. In an early review of community-based studies, higher rates of depression were found in the oldest old and those with physical disability and cognitive impairment (Blazer, 2003).

Depression screening in these settings is often conducted as part of a partnership that may bridge the typical siloed approach to services. Sirey and colleagues formed a partnership with the local Area on Aging Agency to integrate screening into all routine meals provided to homebound older adults. In this sample of 403 meal recipients, 12.2% of older adults reported moderate or clinically significant depression on the PHQ-9 with an additional 15% reporting mild symptoms (Sirey et al., 2008). Using this screening tool, a large number of older adults (13%) reported thoughts of death and dying or hurting themselves (PHQ-9 item 9). Among those adults with clinically significant depression, only one third were in mental health care. In other settings that serve ambulatory older adults within the aging service network, rates of depression are high. In a sample of 313 older adults attending meal programs at nutritional centers, 17% of study participants met criteria for major or minor depression using the SCID diagnostic interview (Bruce & Sirey 2006). These data are consistent with the review of community studies finding the prevalence of subsyndromal depression to range from 4% to 22.9% in community-dwelling older adults (Meeks et al., 2011). Though research is limited, in a sample of older adult community residents who were identified as endorsing symptoms of minor depression at 1-year follow-up had converted to major depression (Parmelee et al., 1992).

Recently, a more in-depth exploration of depression among aging services found that 31% had clinically significant depressive symptoms and 27% met criteria for a current major depressive episode on the SCID. Among those individuals with depression, a higher percentage of individuals were in mental health care with 61% being treated with medication. This reflects both the high rates of depression and the growing numbers of older adults who are both suffering from unipolar depression and prescribed a medication (Richardson et al., 2012). These data are consistent with the more recent 30% depression rates reported by the Nutrition, Aging, and Memory in Elders (NAME) Study, which sampled older adults receiving home care throughout the Boston, Massachusetts, area and administered the CES-D (Mwamburi et al., 2011). In the NAME study, of the 976 older adults screened, 34% screened positive for depression using the CES-D cutoff of 16 and above.

Research on the relapse or recurrence rate of major, minor, or subsyndromal depression in older adults is limited to clinical trials. Recurrence rates in late-life depression have been found to range from 50% to 90% in a period of 2 to 3 years (Zis, Grof, Webster, & Goodwin, 1980). Data from a meta-analysis conducted both in primary care and in community secondary care settings showed that after 2 years, 21% of older depressed patients had died and among the survivors, approximately 50% remained depressed (Cole, Bellavance, & Monsour, 1999). Relapse rate in late life has been found to be greater than in midlife depression (Mitchell & Subramaniam, 2005). The median time to recurrence has also been found to be significantly different among age groups, with the older group (age 65–79) experiencing a more rapid time to recurrence then younger old age group (51–64) (Mueller et al., 2004).

Factors such as anxiety and lack of social networks and support have been found to impede remission from depression among older adults (Wallace et al., 2012). The comorbidity of anxiety and depression ranges from 1.8% to 8.4% in community settings (Lenze et al., 2000). Co-occurrence of anxiety and depression is frequently associated with increased severity and poorer response to treatment among older adults. On the other hand, social support has been identified to have a positive and protective effect in an older adult population. There is a large body of evidence that documents the benefits of social support in patient recovery of both minor and major depression (Alexopoulos et al., 1996; Hybels, Blazer, & Steffens, 2005; Lyness et al., 2006; Nasser & Overholser, 2005).

BIPOLAR DEPRESSION

Bipolar disorder is a serious and chronic mental disorder characterized by periods of mania, hypomania, mixed episodes, and depressive episodes. Despite the chronic and serious nature of the diagnosis, there is a lack of knowledge about bipolar disorder in the elderly (Cassano, McElroy, Brady, Nolen, & Placidi, 2000; Depp & Jeste, 2004). Depressive symptoms are particularly disabling for individuals with bipolar disorder and occur over a great proportion of an individual's life compared to manic symptoms (Sajatovic et al., 2011). There is little information available regarding standardized ratings of depressive symptoms in geriatric bipolar disorder (Young et al., 2007). Furthermore, the clarification of depressive symptoms in bipolar disorder is confounded by the presence of depressive symptoms in depressive, manic, hypomanic, and mixed episodes. Research has found rates of moderate to severe depressive symptoms as high as 11% in a sample of geriatric bipolar patients with a diagnosis of type I bipolar disorder, mania, mixed-manic of hypomanic episodes (Sajatovic et al., 2011). The mixture of manic and depressive symptoms has also been found to be more severe with increased irritability, agitation, anxiety, and psychotic features (Akiskal et al., 1998; Cassidy, Yatham, Berk, & Grof, 2008).

Most bipolar studies and reported prevalence rates are based on samples of older adults diagnosed with bipolar disorder with varying mood states. Community- and population-based studies indicate a marked decline in the prevalence of bipolar disorder in late life (Depp & Jeste, 2004). In community samples the prevalence of bipolar disorder in late life has been found to range from 0.1% to 0.5% (Hirschfeld et al., 2003; Weissman et al., 1988). Inpatient psychiatry samples report a range from 4.7% to 18.5% (Moak, 1990). There are limitations to the reported prevalence rates as several studies reported only individuals in the manic state (Depp & Jeste, 2004). The prevalence of older adults diagnosed with bipolar disorder receiving services in outpatient clinics and community-based mental health services ranges from 2% (Speer, 1992) to 8% (Molinari & Rosenberg, 1983).

CONCLUSION

In sum, there appear to be no change in the prevalence rates of depression reported among older adults sampled in large-scale epidemiologic population studies.

However, as we look more closely at subpopulations of older adults, where there is greater medical burden, disability, and social service needs, the depression rates are much higher. Evidence from comorbidity studies has demonstrated that time to remission may be longer and rates of remission may be lower when medical comorbidity is present (Mitchell & Subramaniam, 2005). It is these populations where depression may also take its greatest toll.

Disclosures

Dr. Marino has no conflicts to disclose. She is supported by individual grants from the National Institute for Mental Health (R01 MH087557, U01MH062518), van Amerigen Foundation, and the Weill Cornell ACISR (P30 MH086943).

Dr. Sirey has no conflicts to disclose. She is supported by individual grants from the National Institute for Mental Health (R01 MH087557, R01 MH079265) and the Weill Cornell ACISR (P30 MH086943).

REFERENCES

Akincigil, A., Olfson, M., Walkup, J. T., Siegel, M. J., Kalay, E., Amin, S., ... Crystal, S. (2011). Diagnosis and treatment of depression in older community-dwelling adults: 1992–2005. *Journal of the American Geriatrics Society*, 59(6), 1042–1051.

Akiskal, H. S., Hantouche, E. G., Bourgeois, M. L., Azorin, J. M., Sechter, D., Allilaire, J. F., ... Châtenet-Duchêne, L. (1998). Gender, temperment, and teh clinical picture in dysphoric mixed mania; findings from a French national study (EPIMEN). *Journal of Affective Disorders*, 50, 175–186.

Alexopoulos, G. S. (2005). Depression in the elderly. *Lancet*, 365(9475), 1961–1970.

Alexopoulos, G. S., Meyers, B. S., Young, R. C., Kakuma, T., Feder, M., Einhorn, A., & Rosendahl, E. (1996). Recovery in geriatric depression. *Archives of General Psychiatry* 53(4), 305–312.

Blazer, D. G. (2003). Depression in late life: Review and commentary. *Journal of Gerontology A: Biological Sciences Medical Sciences*, 58(3), 249–265.

Brown, M., Lapane, K., & Luisi, A. F. (2002). The management of depression in older nursing home residents. *Journal of the American Geriatrics Society*, 50(1), 69–76.

Bruce, M., & Sirey, J. (2006). Depression and Medicare Part D enrollment in vulnerable elders. In M. L. Bruce & J. A. Sirey (Es.), *NIMH Biennial Research Conference on the Economics of Mental Health*, September 25–29, 2006, Bethesda.

Bruce, M. L. (2002). Psychosocial risk factors for depressive disorders in late life. *Biological Psychiatry*, 52(3), 175–184.

Bruce, M. L., McAvay, G. J., Raue, P. J., Brown, E. L., Meyers, B. S., Keohane, D. J., ... Weber, C.. (2002). Major depression in elderly home health care patients. *American Journal of Psychiatry*, 159(8), 1367–1374.

Byers, A. L., Arean, P. A., & Yaffe, K. (2012). Low use of mental health services among older americans with mood and anxiety disorders. *Psychiatric Services*, 63(1), 66–72.

Byers, A. L., Yaffe, K., Covinsky, K. E., Friedman, M. B., & Bruce, M. L. (2010). High occurrence of mood and anxiety disorders among older adults: The National Comorbidity Survey Replication. *Archives of General Psychiatry*, 67(5), 489–496.

Cassano, G., McElroy, S., Brady, K., Nolen, W. A., & Placidi, G. F. (2000). Current issues in the identification and management of bipolar spectrum disorders in "special populations." *Journal of Affective Disorders*, 59(Suppl 1), S69–S79).

Cassidy, F., Yatham, L., Berk, M., & Grof, P. (2008). Pure and mixed manic subtypes: A review of diagnostic classification and validation. *Bipolar Disorder*, 6, 343–367.

Cohen, M., Tell, E., & Wallack, S. S. (1986). The lifetime risks and costs of nursing home use among the elderly. *Medical Care*, 24(12), 1161–1172.

Cole, M. G., Bellavance, F., & Mansour, A. (1999). Prognosis of depression in elderly community and primary care populations: A systematic review and meta-analysis. *American Journal of Psychiatry*, 156, 1182–1189.

Cooper-Patrick, L. G. J., Gonzales, J. J., Vu, H. T., Powe, N. R., Nelson, C., & Ford, D. E. (1999). Race, gender, and partnership in the patient-physician relationship. *Journal of the American Medical Association*, 282(6), 583–589.

Crystal, S., Sambamoorthi, U., Walkup, J. T., & Ankicigil, A. (2003). Diagnosis and treatment of depression in the elderly medicare population: Predictors, disparities, and trends. *Journal of the American Geriatrics Society*, 51(12), 1718–1728.

Depp, C. A., & Jeste, D. V. (2004). Bipolar disorder in older adults: A critical review. *Bipolar Disorder*, 6, 343–367.

Ell, K., Unützer, J., Aranda, M., Sanchez, K., & Lee, P. J. (2005). Routine PHQ-9 depression screening in home health care: Depression, prevalence, clinical and treatment characteristics and screening implementation. *Home Health Care Service Quarterly*, 24(4), 1–19.

Grabovich, A., Lu, N., Tang, W., Tu, X., Lyness, J. M. (2010). Outcomes of subsyndromal depression in older primary care patients. *American Journal of Geriatr Psychiatry, 18*(3), 227–235.

Gruber-Baldini, A. L., Zimmerman, S., Boustani, M., Watson, L. C., Williams, C. S., & Reed, P. S. (2005). Characteristics associated with depression in long-term care residents with dementia. *Gerontologist, 45 Special No. 1*(1), 50–55.

Gum, A. M., King-Kallimanis, B., & Kohn, R. (2009). Prevalence of mood, anxiety, and substance-abuse disorders for older Americans in the national comorbidity survey-replication. *American Journal of Geriatr Psychiatry, 17*(9), 769–781.

Hance, M., Carney, R., Freedland, K. E., & Skala, J. (1996). Depression in patients with coronary heart disease. A 12-month follow-up. *Gerneral Hospital Psychiatry, 18*, 61–65.

Hirschfeld, R. M., Calabrese, J. R., Weissman, M. M., Reed, M., Davies, M. A., Frye, M. A.,...Wagner, K. D. (2003). Screening for bipolar disorder in community. *Journal of Clinical Psychiatry, 64*, 53–59.

Hybels, C. F., & Blazer, D. G. (2003). Epidemiology of late-life mental disorders. *Clinics in Geriatric Medicine, 19*, 663–696.

Hybels, C., Blazer, D. G., & Steffens, D. C. (2005). Predictors of partial remission in older patients treated for major depression: The role of comorbid dysthymia. *American Journal of Geriatric Psychiatry, 13*(8), 713–721.

Hyer, L. (2005). Depression in long-term care. *Clinical Psychology: Science and Practice, 12*(3), 280–299.

Kales, H. C., Neighbors, H. W., Valenstein, M., Blow, F. C., McCarthy, J. F., Ignacio, R. V.,...Mellow, A. M. (2005). Effect of race and sex on primary care physicians' diagnosis and treatment of late-life depression. *Journal of the American Geriatrics Society 53*(5), 777–784.

Kessler, R. C., Berglund, P., Chiu, W. T., Demler, O., Heeringa, S., Hiripi, E.,...Zheng, H. (2004). The US National Comorbidity Survey Replication (NCS-R), design and field procedures. *International Journal of Methods in Psychiatric Research, 13*(2), 69–92.

Kessler, R. C., & Merikangas, K. R. (2004). The National Comorbidity Survey Replication (NCS-R), background and aims. *International Journal of Methods in Psychiatric Research, 13*(2), 60–68.

Klap, R., Unroe, K. T., & Unützer, J. (2003). Caring for mental illness in the United States: A focus on older adults. *American Journal of Geriatric Psychiatry, 11*(5), 517–524.

Koenig, H. (1997). Differences in psychosocial and health correlates of major and minor depression in medically ill older adults. *Journal of American Geriatrics Society, 45*(12), 1487–1495.

Kroenke, K., Spitzer, R. L., & Williams, J. B. (2001). The PHQ-9: Validity of a brief depression severity measure. *Journal of General Internal Medicine, 16*(9), 606–613.

Kroenke, K., & Spitzer, R. L. (2002). The PHQ-9: A new depression diagnostic and severity measure. *Psychiatric Annals, 32*, 509–515.

Lebowitz, B. D., Pearson, J. L., Schneider, L. S., Reynolds, C. F., 3rd, Alexopoulos, G. S., Bruce, M. L.,...Parmelee, P. (1997). Diagnosis and treatment of depression in late life. Consensus statement update. *Journal of the American Medical Association, 278*(14), 1186–1190.

Lenze, E., Mulsant, B., Shear, M. K., Alexopoulos, G. S., Frank, E., & Reynolds, C. F., 3rd. (2000). Comorbidity of depression and anxiety disorders in late life. *Depression and Anxiety, 14*, 86–93.

Lyness, J., Heo, M., Datto, C. J., Ten Have, T. R., Katz, I. R., Drayer, R.,...Bruce, M. L. (2006). Outcomes of minor and subsyndromal depression among elderly patient in primary care settings. *Annals of Internal Medicine, 144*(7), 496–505.

Lyness, J. M., Caine, E. D., King, D. A., Conwell, Y., Duberstein, P. R., & Cox, C. (2002). Depressive disorders and symptoms in older primary care patients: One-year outcomes. *American Journal of Geriatric Psychiatry, 10*, 275–282.

Lyness, J. M., Chapman, B. P., McGriff, J., Drayer, R., & Duberstein, P. R. (2009). One-year outcomes of minor and subsyndromal depression in older primary care patients. *International Psychogeriatrics, 21*, 60–68.

Lyness, J. M., King, D. A., Cox, C., Yoediono, Z., & Caine, E. D. (1999). The importance of subsyndromal depression in older primary care patients: Prevalence and associated functional disability. *Journal of the American Geriatrics Society, 47*, 647–652.

McCurren, C., Dowe, D., Rattle, D., & Looney, S. (1999). Depression among nusing home elders: Testing an intervention strategy. *Applied Nursing Research, 12*(4), 185–195.

Meeks, T. W., Vahia, I. V., Lavretsky, H., Kulkarni, G., & Jeste, D. V. (2011). A tune in a minor can b major: A review of epidemiology, illness course, and public health implications of subthreshold depression in older adults. *Journal of Affective Disorders, 129*(1–3), 126–142.

Mitchell, A. J., & Subramaniam, H. (2005). Prognosis of depression in old age compared to middle age: A system review of comparative studies. *American Journal of Psychiatry, 162*, 1588–1601.

Moak, G. (1990). Characteristics of demented and non-demented geriatric admissions to a state hospital. *Hospital and Community Psychiatry, 41,* 799–801.

Molinari, V., & S. Rosenberg (1983). Bipolar disorder in the elderly. *Journal of Psychiatric Treatment and Evaluation, 5,* 325–330.

Mueller, T. I., Kohn, R., Leventhal, N., Leon, A. C., Solomon, D., Coryell, W., Endicott, J., ... Keller, M. B. (2004). The course of depression in elderly patients. *American Journal of Geriatric Psychiatry, 12*(1), 22–29.

Murtaugh, C., Kemper, P., & Spillman, B. C. (1990). The risk of nursing home use in later life. *Medical Care, 28*(10), 952–962.

Mwamburi, D. M., Liebson, E., Folstein, M, Bungay, K., Tucker, K. L., & Qiu, W. Q. (2011). Depression and glycemic intake in the homebound elderly. *Journal of Affective Disorders 132*(1–2), 94–98.

Nasser, E., & Overholser, J. (2005). Recovery from major depression: The role of support from family, friends, and spiritual beliefs. *Acta Psychiatrica Scandanavica, 111,* 125–132.

Parmelee, P., Katz, I. R., & Lawton, M. P. (1989). Depression among institutionalized aged: Assessment and prevalence estimation. *Journal of Gerontology, 44*(1), M22–M29.

Parmelee, P., Katz, I. R., & Lawton, M. P. (1992). Incidence of depression in long-term care settings. *Journal of Gerontology, 47,* M189–M196.

Payne, J., Sheppard, J., Steinberg, M., Warren, A., Baker, A., Steele, C., ... Lyketsos, C. G. (2002). Incidence, prevalence, and outcomes of depression in residents of a long-term care facility with dementia. *International Journal of Geriatric Psychiatry, 17*(3), 247–253.

Radloff, A. (1977). The CES-D Scale: A self-report depression scale for research in the general population. *Applied Psychological Measurement, 1,* 385–401.

Raue, P. J., Meyers, B. S., McAvay, G. J., Brown, E. L., Keohane, D., & Bruce, M. L. (2003). One-month stability of depression among elderly home-care patients. *American Journal of Geriatric Psychiatry, 11*(5), 543–550.

Raue, P. J., Meyers, B. S., Rowe, J. L., Heo, M., & Bruce, M. L. (2007). Suicidal ideation among elderly homecare patients. *International Journal of Geriatric Psychiatry 22*(1), 32–37.

Richardson, T. M., Friedman, B., Podgorski, C., Knox, K., Fisher, S., He, H., & Conwell, Y. (2012). Depression and its correlates among older adults accessing aging services. *American Journal of Geriatric Psychiatry, 20*(4), 346–354.

Rovner, B. (1993). Depression and increased risk of mortality in the nursing home patient. *American Journal of Medicine, 94*(5A), 19S–22S.

Ryden, M., Pearson, V., Kaas, M. J., Hanscom, J., Lee, H., Krichbaum, K., ... Snyder, M. (1999). Nursing interventions for dperssion in newly admitted nursing home residents. *Journal of Gerontological Nursing, 25*(3), 20–29.

Sajatovic, M., Jurdi, R. A, Gildengers, A., Greenberg, R. L., Tenhave, T., Bruce, M. L., ... Young, R. C. (2011). Depression symptom rating in geriatric patients with bipolar mania. *International Journal of Geriatric Psychiatry, 26*(11), 1201–1208.

Schleifer, S., Macari-Hinson, M., Coyle, D. A., Slater, W. R., Kahn, M., Gorlin, R., & Zucker, H. D. (1989). The nature and course of depression following myocardial infarction. *Archives of Internal Medicine, 149,* 1785–1789.

Shah, M. N., Jones, C. M., Richardson, T. M., Conwell, Y., Katz, P., & Schneider, S. M. (2011). Prevalence of depression and cognitive impairment in older adult emergency medical services patients. *Prehospital Emergency Care, 15*(1), 4–11.

Shah, M. N., Richardson, T. M., Jones, C. M., Swanson, P. A., Schneider, S. M., Katz, P., & Conwell, Y. (2011). Depression and cognitive impairment in older adult emergency department patients: Changes over 2 weeks. *Journal of the American Geriatric Society, 59*(2), 321–326.

Sirey, J. A., Bruce, M. L., Carpenter, M., Booker, D., Reid, M. C., Newell, K. A., & Alexopoulos, G. S. (2008). Depressive symptoms and suicidal ideation among older adults receiving home delivered meals. *International Journal of Geriatric Psychiatry, 23*(12), 1306–1311.

Sirey, J. A., Meyers, B. S., Bruce, M. L., Alexopoulos, G. S., Perlick, D. A., & Raue, P. (1999). Predictors of antidepressant prescription and early use among depressed outpatients. *American Journal of Psychiatry, 156*(5), 690–696.

Sirrocco, A. (1994). *Nursing homes and board and care homes. Advanced data from vital and health statistics.* Hyattsville, MD: National Center for Health Statistics.

Speer, D. (1992). Differences in social resources and treatment history among diagnostic groups of older adults. *Hospital and Community Psychiatry, 43,* 270–274.

Spitzer, R., Gibbon, M., & Williams, J. B. (1995). *Structured Clinical Interview for Axis I DSM-IV Disorders (SCID).* Washington, DC: American Psychiatric Association Press.

Steffens, D. C., Fisher, G. G., Langa, K. M., Potter, G. G., & Plassman, B. L. (2009). Prevalence of depression among older Americans: The Aging, Demographics and Memory Study. *International Psychogeriatrics, 21*(5), 879–888.

US Board of the Census. (1993). *Nursing home population:1990.* Washington, DC: Government Printing Office.

US Department of Health and Human Services. (2011). Adminstration on aging, profile of older Americans: 2010. Washington, DC: Author.

Wallace, M., Dombrovski, A., Morse, J. Q., Houck, P. R., Frank, E., Alexopoulos, G. S., ... Schulz, R. (2012). Coping with health stresses and remission from late-life depression in primary care: A two-year prospective study. *International Journal of Geriatric Psychiatry 27,* 178–186.

Webber, A., Martin, J., Harker, J. O., Josephson, K. R., Rubenstein, L. Z., & Alessi, C. A. (2005). Depression in older patients admitted for postacute nursing home rehabiliation. *Journal of American Geriatrics Society, 53*(6), 1017–1022.

Weissman, M., Leaf, P., Tischler, G. L., Blazer, D. G., Karno, M., Bruce, M. L., & Florio, L. P. (1988). Affective disorders in five US communities. *Psychological Medicine, 18,* 141–153.

Wilkins, V. M., Kiosses, D., & Ravdin, L. D. (2010). Late-life depression with comorbid cognitive impairment and disability: Nonpharmacological interventions. *Clinical Interventions in Aging, 5,* 232–331.

Yesavage, J. A., Brink, T. L., Rose, T. L., Lum, O., Huang, V., Adey, M., & Leirer, V. (1983). Development and validation of a geriatric depression screening scale: A preliminary report. *Journal of Psychiatric Research, 17,* 37–49.

Young, R. C., Peasley-Miklus, C., & Schulberg, H. C. (2007). Mood rating scales and the psychopathology of mania in old age. In M. Sajatovic & F. C. Blow (Eds.), *Bipolar Disorder in Later Life* (pp. 17–26). Baltimore, MD: The John Hopkins University Press.

Zis, A. P., Grof, P., Webster, M., & Goodwin, F. K. (1980). Predictors of relapse in recurrent affective disorders. *Psychopharmacology Bulletin, 16,* 47–49.

4

PUBLIC HEALTH BURDEN OF LATE-LIFE MOOD DISORDERS

Mijung Park and Jürgen Unützer

THE WORLD Health Organization (WHO) has identified mood disorders as leading causes of disability worldwide (Murray & Lopez, 1997; World Health Organization, 2001). Depressive and bipolar disorder together cause more lost quality of life, lost productivity, and chronic impairment than ischemic heart disease and cerebrovascular disease. Depression is among the most common mood disorders in older adults, whereas bipolar disorder, although less frequent, can be more burdensome to the older adults, their family members, and caregivers. Understanding the burden of late-life mood disorders is particularly important because the proportion of older adults will increase from 17% to 26% of the total adult population over the next 20 years. It is projected that the number of people older than 65 with psychiatric disorders will reach 15 million by 2030 (Jeste et al., 1999), with the majority suffering from mood disorders. In this chapter, we review the public health burden of mood disorders in late life.

BURDEN OF ILLNESS

We define "burden of illness" as the value of resources that are expended or foregone as a result of a health problem, in this case late-life mood disorders. This includes the costs and the pain and suffering of affected individuals, their families, and society. This definition encompasses the full societal cost of illness, including quantifiable elements as well as subjective elements that can be harder to quantify (McGuire et al., 2002). Traditionally, the term "burden of illness" has been used interchangeably with "cost of illness." Most studies have distinguished between direct costs and indirect costs of illness. Direct costs refer to the resources used to treat an illness such as medical expenditures. Indirect costs refer to the lost productivity, the effects of the illness on the ability of either patients or their caregivers to work (e.g., lost income) or engage in other activities (e.g., cleaning the house).

BURDEN OF LATE-LIFE MOOD DISORDERS

Burden Associated With Increased Mortality

Individuals with mood disorders die younger than individuals without those disorders. Analyses of a 17-year follow-up of a nationally representative US sample (Druss, Zhao, Von Esenwein, Morrato, & Marcus, 2011) show that the mean age of death was 63.4 years for persons with affective disorders compared to 74.4 years for their counterparts without reported mental disorders, a difference of 11 years. A recent review (Depp, Ojeda, Mastin, Unützer, & Gilmer, 2008) concluded that the people with mood disorders experience elevated mortality rates up to four-fold greater than those without mood disorders. Standardized mortality ratios (SMRs) among those with mood disorders were found to be 1.64 for males and 1.59 for females (Angst, Stassen, Clayton, & Angst, 2002).

LATE-LIFE DEPRESSION AND MORTALITY

The evidence for the association between late-life depression and mortality is mixed (Murphy, Smith, Lindesay, & Slattery, 1988; Wulsin, Vaillant, & Wells, 1999). Although most published studies have reported late-life depression as an independent risk factor for mortality, other studies have not found this association. For example, Schulz et al (2000) examined the association between baseline depressive symptoms and 6-year all-cause mortality among a community sample of 5,201 community-living adults age 65 and older. After controlling for sociodemographic characteristics, severity of comorbid medical conditions, and health risk factors, higher baseline depressive symptoms were associated with a 24% higher risk of death. On the contrary, Callahan et al. (1998) analyzed data from 3,767 adults aged 60 years and older in primary care settings and found no association between baseline depressive symptoms and 5-year all-cause mortality. These inconsistent findings may be due to variations in research methods such as measures of depression used, how depression is operationalized, samples used, the length of observation period for ascertaining mortality, and the choice of covariates. Additionally, most published studies in this area are secondary analyses of observational studies in which the primary research question was not the relationship of late-life depression and mortality. As a result, the literature on this topic may be limited by publication bias and by unmeasured risk factors contributing to mortality that are missed in observational analyses.

Several authors have reported gender variations in mortality rates associated with late-life mood disorders (Mallon, Broman, & Hetta, 2000; Ryan et al., 2008). The prevalence of late-life depression is higher among women than men, but older women are less likely than men to die when depressed. One study showed that depressed older men experienced three-fold greater odds for death compared to older women (Barry, Allore, Guo, Bruce, & Gill, 2008). Another study showed that depressed Swedish older men experienced approximately 1.9 times higher adjusted total death rates than nondepressed counterparts. Such associations were not statistically significant among older women (Mallon et al., 2000). Ryan et al. (2008) examined whether gender modifies the association between depression, treatment, and mortality among 7,363 community-dwelling older adults in France. They found higher rates of death in men with depression and men using antidepressants. In women, depression also increased the risk of mortality, but women with severe depression who took antidepressant medications did not have an increased risk of death.

LATE-LIFE BIPOLAR DISORDER AND MORTALITY

Robust evidence exists for the association between bipolar disorder and mortality. Roshanaei-Moghaddam and Katon (2009) reviewed 17 studies involving aggregated 331,000 persons with bipolar spectrum disorders. They found 35% to two-fold higher mortality from natural causes among patients with bipolar spectrum disorders than the comparison group. A 22-year longitudinal, population-based study (Ösby, Brandt, Correia, Ekbom, & Sparén, 2001) found that Standardized Mortality Ratios of people with bipolar disorder for all natural causes were 1.9 for males and 2.1 for females.

Few studies have examined the mortality associated with late-life bipolar disorders. This may be reflective of the shorter life expectancy among individuals with bipolar disorders. Nonetheless, the available evidence suggests that late-life bipolar disorder is associated with increased mortality.

Compared to persons never hospitalized, SMRs of late-life bipolar disorder range between 1.4 and 1.7 for men and between 1.3 and 1.9 for women (Laursen et al., 2007). Compared to unipolar depression, bipolar disorders increase the risk for death by two-fold (Gildengers et al., 2008).

LATE-LIFE MOOD DISORDERS AND SUICIDE

Older Americans have the highest rate of suicide of any other population group in the United States (Centers for Disease Control and Prevention, 2009). Suicide rates increase with age, and men outnumber women suicide completers by a substantial percentage, especially in the elderly (Conwell et al., 1998). The majority of deaths by suicide among the elderly are closely associated with an episode of an affective disorder (Charney et al., 2003; Manthorpe & Iliffe, 2010). Late-life depression is a powerful predictor of suicide among older adults (Conwell, 2001; Conwell, Duberstein, & Caine, 2002; Heisel & Duberstein., 2005). Data showed that between 71% and 95% of suicide victims aged 65 years and over had a major psychiatric disorder at the time of death, and major depressive disorder is present in up to 75% of all older suicide victims (Waern, Runeson et al., 2002). Although the rates of completed suicide are higher in later life, studies show that older adults are less likely to endorse suicidal ideation or attempt suicide than younger subjects (Conwell & Thompson, 2008). Older adults who have history of attempted suicide have a high mortality rate from later completed suicide and death from other causes (Hepple & Quinton, 1997). These risks remain heightened many years after an attempt (Jenkins, 2002). Suicide associated with late-life mood disorders is described in more detail in Chapter 11 of this volume.

Burden Associated With Increased Morbidity

Mood disorders are associated with increased morbidity, delayed recovery and negative prognosis among those with medical illness, elevated premature mortality associated with comorbid medical illness, increased functional impairment, and treatment costs (Alexopoulos et al., 2002; Barry, Allore, Bruce, & Gill, 2009; Bermudes, Keck, & Welge, 2006; Ciechanowski, Katon, & Russo, 2000; Enger, Weatherby, Reynolds, Glasser, & Walker, 2004;

Evans et al., 2005; Harris & Barraclough, 1998; Lin et al., 2004). Comorbid mental-physical disorders are associated with greater disability than mental or physical disorders alone (Kessler, Ormel, Demler, & Stang, 2003).

Medical burdens associated with mood disorders are particularly relevant to older adults among whom multimorbidity is common (Charney et al., 2003). Eighty-eight percent of older adults have one or more chronic illnesses, with one quarter of this group having four or more conditions (Wolff, Starfield, & Anderson, 2002). In the following section, we will review the current understanding on medical burdens of late-life mood disorders and underlying mechanisms for such burdens.

MEDICAL BURDEN OF LATE-LIFE DEPRESSION

The interaction between depression and chronic medical illness is complex and bidirectional (Katon, 2003). Strong evidence shows that depression or depressive symptoms increase morbidity and mortality associated with medical illnesses such as cardiovascular disease (Lesperance, Frasure-Smith, Talajic, & Bourassa, 2002; van Melle et al., 2004), diabetes (Anderson, Freedland, Clouse, & Lustman, 2001; Li, Ford, Strine, & Mokdad, 2008), cerebrovascular disease (Kales, Maixner, & Mellow, 2005), HIV/AIDS (Himelhoch & Medoff, 2005; Mayne, Vittinghoff, Chesney, Barrett, & Coates, 1996), chronic pain (Bair, Robinson, Katon, & Kroenke, 2003; Bonnewyn et al., 2009; Geerlings, Twisk, Beekman, Deeg, & van Tilburg, 2002), obesity (Blaine, 2008), osteoporosis (Cizza, Ravn, Chrousos, & Gold, 2001; Yirmiya & Bab, 2009), cancer (Fann et al., 2008; Pinquart & Duberstein, 2010), and dementia (Katon, Lyles, Parker, Karter, Huang, & Whitmer 2012).

A meta-analysis (Van der Kooy et al., 2007) found that depressed mood increased the risk for cardiovascular diseases by 43%–63%. Among those who have depression, older adults age 65 and older experienced up to 2.5-fold increased risk for stroke relative to young adults age between 18 and 29. Older adults with a history of depression experience 1.5-fold increased risk for stroke compared to those without history of depression (Larson, Owens, Ford, & Eaton, 2001). Furthermore, post–myocardial infarction depression is associated with 2.36-fold increase in all-cause mortality (Frasure-Smith, Lesperance, & Talajic, 1995; van Melle et al., 2004).

Evidence suggests a dose–response relationship between the severity of depression and risk for negative cardiac outcomes (Lesperance et al., 2002). Another study found that being diagnosed with depression increased the risk of new-onset coronary heart disease by 2.69, whereas having depressive symptoms increased risk of coronary disease by 1.64 (Barth, Schumacher, & Herrmann-Lingen, 2004; Van der Kooy et al., 2007).

Recent meta-analyses have shown that depression and depressive symptoms increase the risk for developing type 2 diabetes (Knol et al., 2006; Mezuk, Eaton, Albrecht, & Golden, 2009) and for negative diabetes outcome such as complications and death (de Groot, Anderson, Freedland, Clouse, & Lustman, 2001; Kilbourne et al., 2005; Lin et al., 2009). Among older adults, depression or depressive symptoms are associated with up to 150% increased risk for developing type 2 diabetes (Arroyo et al., 2004; Carnethon et al., 2007; Golden et al., 2004). A longitudinal study (Demakakos, Pierce, & Hardy, 2010) found that those with depressive symptoms had approximately a 62% increased risk for developing type 2 diabetes. Having major depression elevated all-cause mortality of those with diabetes by 1.52-fold (Lin et al., 2009). Having comorbid depression and diabetes seems to have a synergetic effect on morbidity and mortality (Black, Markides, & Ray, 2003; Oslin et al., 2002). Patients with major depression and diabetes were 1.5- to 2-fold more likely to have three or more cardiovascular risk factors as patients with diabetes without depression (Katon et al., 2004).

Late-life depression increases the odds of painful physical symptoms compared to those without depression by 2.06-fold (Bonnewyn et al., 2009) and is associated with poor cancer prognosis (Fann, Fan, & Unützer, 2009).

MEDICAL BURDEN OF LATE-LIFE BIPOLAR DISORDER

Older adults with bipolar disorder have high rates of medical illnesses such as stroke, diabetes, or adverse drug reactions (Evans, 2000; Fenn et al., 2005). In their study of hospitalized older adults age 50 and older, Regenold et al. (2002) found that individuals with bipolar disorders experienced two-fold greater rates of type 2 diabetes than expected for an age-, race-, and gender-matched group in the general US population.

MECHANISMS OF INCREASED MEDICAL BURDENS OF LATE-LIFE MOOD DISORDERS

A growing body of evidence has demonstrated that the interaction between mood disorders and medical illnesses is complex and bidirectional (Katon, 2003) (Fig. 4.1). Various mechanisms for how mood disorders increase the burden of medical illness have been suggested and include physiological, behavioral, cognitive, and social factors.

Biological Mechanisms

Multiple biological links have been suggested as potential mediators for the adverse effects of comorbid mood disorders on diabetes- and cardiovascular-related mortality. Depression has been associated with vascular pathology, which in turn, is strongly correlated with ischemic heart disease and cerebrovascular disease. Elevated levels of proinflammatory cytokines, which can contribute to the development and progression of atheroscerosis, also occur in patients with depression (Monteleone, 2010). Depression is linked to increased platelet activation and hypercoagulability (Joynt, Whellan, & O'Connor, 2004; von Känel, Mills, Fainman, & Dimsdale, 2001). Depression-related alteration in neurohormonal mechanisms, such as hypothalamic-pituitary-adrenal axis hyperactivity and increases in plasma control, may be associated with increased congestive heart failure risk (Grippo & Johnson, 2002). On the other hand, some medications prescribed for the treatment of mental illness, particularly second-generation or atypical antipsychotic medications, are known to cause metabolic and cardiovascular side effects (American Diabetes Association, 2004; Newcomer & Hennekens, 2007).

Behavioral Mechanisms

Late-life mood disorders are associated with unhealthy lifestyles, poor adherence to treatment, poor health services usage, and receiving poor quality of care. And having chronic disease may increase functional impairment, which increases the risk of depression. Studies have found strong associations between late-life mood disorders and unhealthy lifestyles such as inactivity, smoking, alcohol use, and poor diet (Lasser et al., 2000; van Gool et al., 2003). For example, a 6-year longitudinal, prospective cohort study of 1,280 Dutch older adults (van Gool et al., 2003) showed that individuals who had

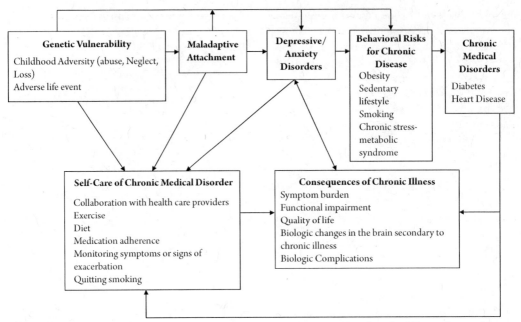

FIGURE 4.1 A conceptual model of interaction between major depression and medical illness. (From Katon, W. J. (2003). Clinical and health services relationships between major depression, depressive symptoms, and general medical illness. *Biological Psychiatry*, 54(3), 216–226. Used with permission from Elsevier.)

persistent depression experienced an increase in cigarette consumption. Furthermore, individuals who are newly diagnosed with depression experienced large decreases in minutes of physical activity and a higher risk of changing to sedentary lifestyles. Another study (Katon et al., 2004) concluded that patients with diabetes without cardiovascular disease who met criteria for major depression were significantly more likely to be smokers, to be obese, to lead a more sedentary lifestyle, and to have poor diabetes control compared to nondepressed patients with diabetes without heart disease.

Older adults with mood disorder have difficulties in adhering to treatment such as medications, dietary changes, or rehabilitation (Kilbourne et al., 2005; Kreyenbuhl et al., 2008; Lin et al., 2004). Because most medical illnesses require active self-management behavior to optimize treatment outcomes (Wagner, 1998; Wagner et al., 2001), improving depression can increase patients' ability to successfully manage their illness and improve health outcomes.

Older adults with mood disorders are also more likely to delay seeking care (Kim et al., 2007), less likely to receive preventative services such as smoking cessation (Currie et al., 2008; Desai, Rosenheck, Druss, & Perlin, 2002; Druss, Rosenheck, Desai, & Perlin, 2002; Prochaska, Schane, Leek, Hall, & Hall, 2008), and are more likely to receive poor quality of care for their psychiatric and medical conditions (Desai et al., 2002; Druss et al., 2002; Wells, Schoenbaum, Unützer, Lagomasino, & Rubenstein, 1999).

Psychological/Cognitive Mechanisms

Decreased self-efficacy and negative outlook on the future are typical symptoms of mood disorders. These symptoms can have a negative effect on older adults' ability to successfully manage their chronic illness. Patients with low self-efficacy were more likely to have depression following major surgery, and poorer functional status (Kurlowicz, 1998), ineffective disease management (Arnstein, 2000; Marks & Allegrante, 2005), and decreased help-seeking behaviors (Cohen & Williamson, 1991). Clark and Dodge (2001) concluded that baseline self-efficacy was a predictor of several disease management behavior at both 4 months and 12 months, including using medicine as prescribed, getting adequate exercise, managing stress, and following a recommended diet. Perceived stigma, minimization of the need for care, hopelessness related to depression, or poor judgment related to the manic symptoms associated with bipolar disorder may hinder older adults from seeking effective care for their mood or medical disorders (Sirey et al., 2001).

Social Mechanisms

Mood disorders interfere with normative social roles such as parent, marital partner, and colleagues. Social network members may avoid interaction with persons with severe depression or the affective instability associated with bipolar disorder (Joiner, Alfano, & Metalsky, 1993). Patients with the intense emotional distress common with mood disorders often require continued support, and they may fatigue and deteriorate their social network. Social support improves physical health by promoting positive health practices, positive views of the world, and providing resources for facing and avoiding stressful life events (Cohen & Wills, 1985). Hence, interference with these network functions can increase the risk for adverse mental and physical health outcomes. Social pressures from network members may also influence the use of health services, either promoting or discouraging seeking help in the face of symptom reports.

Burdens Associated With Disability and Quality of Life

Abundant evidence demonstrates a strong cross-sectional association between mood disorders and decrements in self-reported functional status or quality of life. Late-life mood disorders are associated with a significant level of disability and losses in quality of life (Katz, 1996; Lenze et al., 2001).

DISABILITY

Disability is defined as restriction in or lack of ability to perform an activity due to impairment (WHO, 1980). Such activities include interpersonal relationships, work or school, or physical activities. Physical activities include activities of daily living (ADLs) such as feeding, dressing, bathing, and toileting, or instrumental activities of daily living (IADLs) such as cleaning, paying bills, and preparing food. For older adults, physical disability is often a more prominent issue than role disability. In 1997, persons age 65 and older accounted for 54% of all physical disability in the United States (Lenze et al., 2001).

Impaired functioning associated with depressive symptoms has been shown to be comparable or worse than functional losses associated with several major chronic medical conditions (Alexopoulos et al., 2002). There are strong associations between late-life depression and disability (Bruce, 2001; Stuck et al., 1999). A recent meta-analysis (Schillerstrom, Royall, & Palmer, 2008) concluded that adjusted odds ratios measuring the longitudinal association between depression and disability ranged from 1.16 to 5.47 among community-dwelling older adults. Oslin and colleagues (2002) found that functional decline associated with medical illnesses was related to increased depressive symptoms among older adults.

With bipolar disorder, social, family, and occupational disabilities are the rule rather than the exception (Bauer, 2001). Without adequate treatment, a person with bipolar disorder at age 25 can expect to lose 14 years of effective major activity (e.g., work, school, family role function) and 9 years of life (Department of Health, Education, and Welfare, 1979). Fifteen percent of persons with bipolar disorder are unemployed for at least 5 consecutive years, and over 25% of those under age 65 receive disability payments (Klerman, Olfson, Leon, & Weismann, 1992). Although there are less published data in older adults, we estimate that for affected individuals, the functional losses associated with late-life bipolar disorder are at least as great as those reported for late-life depression.

QUALITY OF LIFE

Late-life mood disorders diminish quality of life (QOL) of older adults and their loved ones (Doraiswamy, Khan, Donahue, & Richard, 2002). Depressed patients in primary care settings have been shown to have worse QOL than general medical patients within the same clinics with common diseases such as hypertension, arthritis, diabetes, and heart disease (Ormel et al., 1993). The degree of decrement in QOL is proportional to the severity of depressive symptoms (Jaffe, Froom, & Galambos, 1994; Pyne et al., 1997). Unützer et al. (1996) found that older adults with depressive symptoms at baseline had 0.23 fewer quality adjusted life years (QALYs) over the 4 years than those without depressive symptoms. In this study of 2,558 older adults, depression was associated with greater losses in QALYs than most chronic medical disorders, including diabetes and cancer.

LOSS OF PRODUCTIVITY

Numerous studies have demonstrated an association between mood disorders and lost work productivity via either unemployment or time missed from work because of illness. In 2000, the economic impact of depression was estimated at $51.5 billion of lost productivity and $18 billion in lost earnings (Greenberg et al., 2003). Depression was associated with a 2.5-fold increase in probability of missing work because of illness and a 50% increase in time lost from work (Kessler et al., 1999). Research with bipolar patients demonstrated that patients with bipolar disorder had a seven-fold increase in likelihood of missing work because of illness (Olfson et al., 1997) and a 40% reduction in likelihood of paid employment (Zwerling et al., 2002).

Traditionally, loss of productivity has been less emphasized when considering burdens of late-life mood disorders. However, as more older adults are working full time or part time, the burdens of mood disorder on labor market and work productivity are expected to grow. By 2016, workers age 65 and over are expected to account for 6.1% of the total labor force, up sharply from their 2006 share of 3.6% (US Bureau of Labor Statistics, 2008).

Depression can force people to retire early, limiting their ability to sustain income. Doshi and colleagues (2008) found that depressed older men had 60% increased odds for retiring compared to men without depression. On the other hand, depressed women had 38% higher odds of retiring in the presence of active depression. Given that catastrophic medical events are relatively common at this older age (French & Jones, 2004), a substantial amount of the individual's retirement savings may be required to pay for health care expenditures.

Burden on Formal Care

The use of health care resources among older adults with mood disorders may be substantial compared to those without mood disorders and even to those with other serious mental disorders (Sajatovic, 2002). Older adults with mood disorders use more inpatients and partial hospitalization, case management, and skills training. Medicare beneficiaries age 65 and older spent an average of $2,430, or 19% of their average annual income, for out-of-pocket health care costs in 1999. This excludes the costs of home care and long-term nursing services. The direct and indirect costs of depression have been estimated at $43 billion each year, not including pain and suffering and diminished quality of life. In their study with patients with diabetes and comorbid depression, Desai and colleagues (2002) found that the total primary and ambulatory costs were higher among patients with the highest severity of depression symptoms.

Late-life depression is particularly costly because of the excess disability it causes and its deleterious interaction with physical health. Studies have shown health care costs are significantly higher among elderly patients with depressed symptoms compared to those without depression (Himelhoch, Weller, Wu, Anderson, & Cooper, 2004). Unützer et al. (1997) found that elderly patients with significant depressive symptoms had total health care costs 50% higher per year than those without symptoms. Katon et al. (2003) examined large HMO administrative data and similarly found 43% to 52% higher health care cost among depressed elderly patients compared with their nondepressed counterparts, after adjustment for chronic medical illness. This increase was seen in every component of health care costs, with only a small percentage due to mental health treatment. For elderly individuals with at least one chronic medical condition, the presence of a depressive symptom increased the odds of acute medical service use (Himelhoch et al., 2004). Elderly Medicare beneficiaries with depressive symptoms were at least twice as likely to use emergency department services and medical inpatient hospital services, as compared with those without depression. Comorbidity can also confound the evaluation of the impact of depression on outcomes in outpatients (Luber et al., 2001). The strong association between depression and increased use of health services is seen at all levels of medical comorbidity, and the relationship seems to be multiplicative (Simon, 2003).

Treating elderly persons with depression is more expensive than treating their younger counterparts. Elderly patients were treated in general hospitals in Maryland for major depression at nearly the same rate as nonelderly patients. The average cost of treating the elderly patients was, however, 2.3 times higher and the average length of stay nearly 8 days longer than those of the nonelderly patients (Brown, 2001).

Bipolar disorder is also an extremely costly problem for the nation's health care systems. Simon and Unützer (1999) found that the direct costs shouldered by patients treated for bipolar disorder exceed that of patients treated for depression, diabetes, and general medical conditions. Approximately 5% of bipolar patients accounted for 95% of the total costs of inpatient treatment in the population. Wyatt and Henter (1995) estimated that, as of 1991, affective disorders account for approximately 21% of the direct costs of all mental illnesses, with the total economic burden of bipolar disorder alone estimated at $45 billion per year. Direct costs totaling $7 billion consist of expenditures for inpatient and outpatient care, which are treatment related, as well as non-treatment-related expenditures such as those for the criminal justice system used by individuals with manic-depressive illness. Indirect costs, which were $38 billion, include the lost productivity of both wage earners ($17 billion) and homemakers ($3 billion), suicides among institutionalized individuals ($8 billion), and family caregivers of bipolar disorder ($6 billion).

Although the overall percentage of older adults with bipolar disorder is relatively small, these individuals have a disproportionate impact on the health care system. While bipolar disorder is more prevalent in younger populations, elderly patients with bipolar disorder account for the same proportion of diagnoses in psychiatric emergency room visits (Shulman, 1997; Wingerson, Russo, Ries, Dagadakis, & Roy-Byrne, 2001) and inpatient psychiatric hospitals (Brown, 2001) as younger patients. Older adults with bipolar disorder were hospitalized at the similar rate as those with schizophrenia, although their length of stay was shorter (Depp & Jeste, 2004; Sajatovic, 2002). Elderly patients and veterans with bipolar disorder have longer hospital stays than younger patients and are more likely to use outpatient services (Sajatovic, Blow, Ignacio, & Kales, 2005). The average cost for treating elderly patients with bipolar disorder was almost twice as large as their younger counterparts and similar to their depressed counterparts (Brown, 2001).

Burden of Late-Life Mood Disorders on Family and Informal Care

The impacts of mood disorders in later life are felt across a broad spectrum of family life: work, leisure, income, children, family health, and relationships with extended family, friends, and neighbors (Maurin & Boyd, 1990). Late-life depression can cause impoverishment of older adult's household via income losses and medical expenses that trigger a spiral of asset depletion and indebtedness (Wagstaff, 2002).

According to a national survey (National Alliance for Caregiving/AARP, 2004), 44.4 million Americans provide care to their family members. Thirteen percent of them were over 65 years of age. Studies have shown that the burden from caregiving can compromise immune, cardiovascular, and endocrine functioning and increase the risk for morbidity and mortality (Talley & Crews, 2007). Over 24 months, after adjusting for marital status, intervention status, and number of medical comorbidities, those reporting any caregiving burden had over 30 more days with depression compared to those with no caregiving burden (Thompson, Fan, Unützer, & Katon, 2008). Another study showed that minor depressive symptoms were common in caregivers (Russo, Vitaliano, Brewer, Katon, & Becker, 1995).

National data indicate that depressive symptoms in older adults will require additional hours of assistance from their family members, with associated costs reaching approximately $9 billion (Langa et al., 2004). Family members of depressed older adults experience moderate to high levels of caregiver burden, similar to family caregivers of older adults with Alzheimer's disease (van Wijngaarden, Schene, & Koeter, 2004). Caregivers who feel burdened by patients' depressive symptoms may be less able to be supportive with regard to the setbacks that patients encounter during treatment, such as treatment side effects and the difficulty of adhering to prescribed treatment (Perlick et al., 2004).

Bipolar patients and their caregivers must contend with the high rates of chronicity and recurrent illness associated with the disorder (Otto, Reilly-Harrington, & Sachs, 2003). These multiple recurrent episodes are disruptive to family, social, and vocational functioning (Miklowitz, 2008). A study showed that families with a member with bipolar disorder, compared with matched families, made approximately three times more outpatient physician visits, inpatient hospital stays, and received prescription medications (Chatterton, Ke, Lewis, Rajagopalan, & Lazarus, 2008). Their total annual health care costs were more than three-fold higher for bipolar families compared with matched families.

Caregiving can impact work; it increases exit from the workforce and missed work time (absenteeism), and it decreases productivity while at work (presenteeism) (Pitsenberger, 2006). Individuals engaged heavily in caregiving are more likely to have left a job or retired early than matched noncaregivers (Lilly, Laporte, & Coyte, 2007). Minorities (Covinsky et al., 2001), low-income caregivers (Kneipp, Castleman, & Gailor, 2004), and women (Carmichael & Charles, 2003; Johnson & Lo Sasso, 2006) are more likely to leave the workforce because of their caregiving role. Caregivers who remain in the workforce are more likely to miss work than noncaregiver employees (Lilly et al., 2007), with lower income, minority, and female caregivers being most likely to miss time from work (Neal & Wagner, 2001). The impact of caregiving on work productivity increases as the intensity of caregiving increases; for example, assisting with a greater number of tasks, caring for an individual with cognitive limitations, or providing more hours of caregiving (Covinsky et al., 2001). In addition to absenteeism, caregiving may impede productivity while at work through negative health effects (Burton, Chen, Conti, Pransky, & Edington, 2004; Pinquart & Sorensen, 2005) or decreased ability to concentrate on work activities (Stephens, Franks, & Atienza, 1997).

SPECIAL CONSIDERATIONS FOR BURDEN OF LATE-LIFE DEPRESSION

Certain segments of the population experience particular burdens of late-life mood disorders. These groups include older adults with lower socioeconomic status (SES) or less education and those from ethnic/racial minority groups. Poverty and poor health are intertwined. Poor people have worse health outcomes than better-off people. This association reflects causality running in both directions: Poverty breeds ill health, and ill health keeps poor people poor (Wagstaff, 2002). Lower SES is also associated with less favorable depression treatment outcome (Cohen et al., 2006). Compared to older adults residing in a low-income neighborhood, middle-income Census tracts were more likely to respond to antidepressant treatment and less likely to report suicidal ideation. In a recent meta-analysis, compared with old people with more education, those with less education had a 1.49-fold higher risk for depression (Yong-Hong et al., 2010). Older men from ethnic minority groups are particularly unlikely to receive depression treatment in primary care (Hinton, Zweifach, Oishi, Tang, & Unützer, 2006; Klap, Unroe, & Unützer, 2003; Unützer et al., 2003).

STRATEGIES FOR ADDRESSING PUBLIC HEALTH BURDENS

Considering the significant societal burdens associated with late-life mood disorders, it is imperative to reduce such burdens. Depression is one of the most common health problems in older adults, but it is often undetected, undiagnosed, untreated, or undertreated (Unützer, 2002; Wells et al., 2002).

Prevention and Early Detection

Given the risks for deleterious effects of late-life mood disorders on individual and family health, improving access to care, prevention and early detection, and quality of depression treatment will reduce the burden of late-life depression (Charney et al., 2003; Whyte & Rovner, 2006). Undetected and untreated mood disorders at a young age can increase disability and burdens of illness in later life. Depressive symptoms independently predict the development of persistent limitations in ADLs and mobility as middle-aged persons advance into later life. Middle-aged persons with depressive symptoms may be at greater risk for losing their functional independence as they age (Covinsky et al., 2010).

Unfortunately, prevention and early detection of late-life mood disorders remain problematic. A recent meta-analysis showed that primary care providers detected only 40%–50% of depression among older adults and they were less successful detecting depression among older adults than among younger adults (Mitchell, Rao, & Vaze, 2010). Only about one in five older adults with depression receives effective treatment for depression in primary care (Unützer, 2002). Approximately 31% of National Depressive and Manic-Depressive Association members waited more than 10 years from the time they first exhibited signs of their illness to seeking professional guidance or treatment. After the first encounter with a professional, a majority of the members waited more than 5 years to be correctly diagnosed (Lish, Dime-Meenan, Whybrow, Price, & Hirschfeld, 1994).

Literature on prevention strategies of late-life depression is limited but growing. For late-life depression, directing prevention efforts toward selected high-risk groups could help reduce the incidence or recurrence of depression and is likely to be more cost-effective than universal prevention approaches (Schoevers et al., 2006; Smit, Ederveen, Cuijpers, Deeg, & Beekman, 2006;

Willemse, Smit, Cuijpers, & Tiemens, 2004). In a recent meta-analysis on short-term psychotherapeutic interventions aimed at people with subsyndromal depressive symptoms, these were found to reduce the incidence of depression by 30% (Cuijpers et al., 2005). A randomized clinical trial (Veer-Tazelaar et al., 2009) concluded that stepped-care approaches are effective in reducing the risk of late-life depression and anxiety disorders. Short-term problem-solving treatments in primary care seemed to prevent depression among elderly patients with age-related macular degeneration in primary care (Rovner, Casten, Hegel, Leiby, & Tasman, 2007). The authors recommend booster or rescue treatments to sustain problem-solving treatment's preventative effect. Another study (Robinson et al., 2008) has demonstrated the effectiveness of escitalopram and problem-solving therapy for the prevention of poststroke depression. Prevention of late-life depression is discussed in Chapter 25.

Treatment

Effective educational and organizational interventions for late-life mood disorders can lead to reduction of societal burden of illness via decreasing mortality and morbidity (Gallo et al., 2007), reducing long-term health care cost (Unützer et al., 2008), decreasing disability, and increasing productivity (Schoenbaum et al., 2001). Currently, one of the most effective approaches to treating late-life depression is collaborative care programs such as IMPACT (Improving Mood: Promoting Access to Collaborative Treatment for Late-life Depression; Unützer et al., 2008), PROSPECT (Prevention of Suicide in Primary Care Elderly: Collaborative Trials; Bruce et al., 2004), and TEAM care (Katon et al., 2010). Such collaborative care programs, in which primary care providers collaborate closely with mental health providers to offer evidence-based pharmacological and psychotherapy treatments, can double the effectiveness of usual care for depression (Gilbody, Bower, Fletcher, Richards, & Sutton, 2006; Unützer, Schoenbaum, Druss, & Katon, 2006). The largest study of collaborative care to date also showed that treating depression reduced functional impairment from chronic pain (Lin et al., 2003). Collaborative care approaches can also increase the use of evidence-based depression treatments and improve health outcomes in older minorities and poor older Americans (Arean

et al., 2005; Ayalon, Arean, Linkins, Lynch, & Estes, 2007; Miranda, Azocar, et al., 2003; Miranda, Duan, et al., 2003; Yeung et al., 2010). On the contrary, treating depression alone does not seem to improve outcomes of comorbid diabetes and coronary heart disease, although it improves patients' self-management and adherence to treatment (Katon et al., 2006; Lin et al., 2003, 2004; Williams, et al., 2004). In a recent study called TEAM care, Katon and colleagues (2010) extended collaborative care to focus on depression, diabetes, and heart disease and found that this approach was associated with better adherence to treatment and better outcome in both depression and comorbid diabetes and coronary health disease than care as usual. Addressing late-life depression may also have spillover benefits to family. For example, Martire et al. (2010) concluded that treatment of late-life depression has benefits that extend to family caregivers. Caregiver education and support may strengthen these effects.

Disclosures

Dr. Unützer receives grant and contract funding from the National Institute of Mental Health, the John A. Hartford Foundation, the Alaska Mental Health Trust Authority, the George Foundation, the Hogg Foundation for Mental Health, and the Henry M. Jackson Foundation/Department of Defense. He provides technical assistance and /or consultation to the Community Health Plan of Washington, Public Health of Seattle & King County, AARP Services Incorporated, and the National Council of Community Behavioral Health Care. He also serves as an advisor to the Carter Center Mental Health Program, the Institute for Clinical Systems Improvement, and the World Health Organization.

Dr. Park has no conflicts to disclose. She is funded by Geriatric Mental Health Services Research Fellowship by the National Institutes of Health (2 T32 MH 73553–6)

REFERENCES

Alexopoulos, G. S., Buckwalter, K., Olin, J., Martinez, R., Wainscott, C., & Krishnan, K. R. (2002). Comorbidity of late life depression: An opportunity for research on mechanisms and treatment. *Biological Psychiatry, 52*(6), 543–558.

American Diabetes Association. (2004). Consensus Development Conference on Antipsychotic Drugs and Obesity and Diabetes. *Diabetes Care, 27*(2), 596–601.

Anderson R. J., Freedland K. E., Clouse R. E., & Lustman P. J. (2001). The prevalence of comorbid depression in adults with diabetes. *Diabetes Care, 24*(6), 1069–1078.

Angst, F., Stassen, H. H., Clayton, P. J., & Angst, J. (2002). Mortality of patients with mood disorders: Follow-up over 34–38 years. *Journal of Affective Disorders, 68*(2–3), 167–181.

Arean, P. A., Ayalon, L., Hunkeler, E., Lin, E. H., Tang, L., Harpole, L., ... IMPACT Investigators. (2005). Improving depression care for older, minority patients in primary care. *Medical Care, 43*(4), 381–90.

Arnstein, P. (2000). The mediation of disability by self efficacy in different samples of chronic pain patients. *Disability and Rehabilitation, 22*(17), 794–801.

Arroyo, C., Hu, F. B., Ryan, L. M., Kawachi, I., Colditz, G. A., Speizer, F. E., & Manson, J. (2004). Depressive symptoms and risk of type 2 diabetes in women. *Diabetes Care, 27*(1), 129–133.

Ayalon, L., Arean, P. A., Linkins, K., Lynch, M., & Estes, C. L. (2007). Integration of mental health services into primary care overcomes ethnic disparities in access to mental health services between black and white elderly. *American Journal of Geriatric Psychiatry, 15*(10), 906–912.

Bair, M. J., Robinson, R. L., Katon, W., & Kroenke, K. (2003). Depression and pain comorbidity: A literature review. *Archives of Internal Medicine, 163*(20), 2433–2445.

Barnow, S., & Linden, M. (2000). Epidemiology and psychiatric morbidity of suicidal ideation among the elderly. *Crisis: The Journal of Crisis Intervention and Suicide Prevention, 21*(4), 171–180.

Barry, L. C., Allore, H. G., Bruce, M. L., & Gill, T. M. (2009). Longitudinal association between depressive symptoms and disability burden among older persons. *Journals of Gerontology Series A: Biological Sciences and Medical Sciences, 64A*(12), 1325–1332.

Barry, L. C., Allore, H. G., Guo, Z., Bruce, M. L., & Gill, T. M. (2008). Higher burden of depression among older women: The effect of onset, persistence, and mortality over time. *Archives of General Psychiatry, 65*(2), 172–178.

Barth, J., Schumacher, M., & Herrmann-Lingen, C. (2004). Depression as a risk factor for mortality in patients with coronary heart disease: A meta-analysis. *Psychosomatic Medicine, 66*(6), 802–813.

Bauer, M. S. (2001). The collaborative practice model for bipolar disorder: Design and implementation in a multi-site randomized controlled trial. *Bipolar Disorders, 3*(5), 233–244.

Bermudes, R. A., Keck, P. E., Jr., & Welge, J. A. (2006). The prevalence of the metabolic syndrome in psychiatric inpatients with primary psychotic and mood disorders. *Psychosomatics, 47*(6), 491–497.

Black, S. A., Markides, K. S., & Ray, L. A. (2003). Depression predicts increased incidence of adverse health outcomes in older Mexican Americans with type 2 diabetes. *Diabetes Care, 26*(10), 2822–2828.

Blaine, B. (2008). Does depression cause obesity? *Journal of Health Psychology, 13*(8), 1190–1197.

Blazer, D. (1983). Impact of late-life depression on the social network. *American Journal of Psychiatry, 140*(2), 162–166.

Bonnewyn, A., Katona, C., Bruffaerts, R., Haro, J. M., de Graaf, R., Alonso, J., & Demyttenaere, K. (2009). Pain and depression in older people: Comorbidity and patterns of help seeking. *Journal of Affective Disorders, 117*(3), 193–196.

Brown, S. L. (2001). Variations in utilization and cost of inpatient psychiatric services among adults in Maryland. *Psychiatric Services, 52*(6), 841–843.

Bruce, M. L. (2001). Depression and disability in late life: Directions for future research. *American Journal of Geriatric Psychiatry, 9*(2), 102–112.

Bruce, M. L., Ten Have, T. R., Reynolds, C. F., III, Katz, I. I., Schulberg, H. C., Mulsant, B. H., ... Alexopoulos, G. S. (2004). Reducing suicidal ideation and depressive symptoms in depressed older primary care patients: A randomized controlled trial. *Journal of the American Medical Association, 291*(9), 1081–1091.

Burton, W. N., Chen, C-Y., Conti, D. J., Pransky, G., & Edington, D. W. (2004). Caregiving for ill dependents and its association with employee health risks and productivity. *Journal of Occupational and Environmental Medicine, 46*(10), 1048–1056.

Callahan, C. M., Wolinsky, F. D., Stump, T. E., Nienaber, N. A., Hui, S. L., & Tierney, W. M. (1998). Mortality, symptoms, and functional impairment in late-life depression. *Journal of General Internal Medicine, 13*(11), 746–752.

Carmichael, F., & S. Charles (2003). The opportunity costs of informal care: does gender matter? *Journal of Health Economics, 22*(5), 781–803.

Carnethon, M. R., Biggs, M. L., Barzilay, J. I., Smith, N. L., Vaccarino, V., Bertoni, A. G., ... Siscovick, D. (2007). Longitudinal association between depressive symptoms and incident type 2 diabetes mellitus in older adults: The cardiovascular health study. *Archives of Internal Medicine, 167*(8), 802–807.

Centers for Disease Control and Prevention (CDC). (2009). National suicide statistics at a glance:

Suicide rates* among persons ages 65 years and older, by race/ethnicity and sex, United States, 2002–2006. http://www.cdc.gov/violenceprevention/suicide/statistics/rates05.html Retrived on Octorber 30, 2012.

Change-Quan, H., Zheng-Rong, W., Yong-Hong, L., Yi-Zhou, X, & Qing-Xiu, L. (2010). Education and risk for late life depression: A meta-analysis of published literature. *International Journal of Psychiatry in Medicine*, 40(1), 109–124.

Charney, D. S., Reynolds, C. F., III, Lewis, L., Lebowitz, B. D., Sunderland, T., Alexopoulos, G. S, ... Depression and Bipolar Support Alliance. (2003). Depression and bipolar support alliance consensus statement on the unmet needs in diagnosis and treatment of mood disorders in late life. *Archives of General Psychiatry*, 60(7), 664–672.

Chatterton, M., Ke, X., Lewis, B. E., Rajagopalan, K., & Lazarus, A. (2008). Impact of bipolar disorder on the family: Utilization and cost of health care resources. *Pharmacy & Therapeutics*, 33(1), 15–34.

Ciechanowski, P. S., Katon, W. J., & Russo, J. E. (2000). Depression and diabetes: Impact of depressive symptoms on adherence, function, and costs. *Archives of Internal Medicine*, 160(21), 3278–3285.

Cizza, G., Ravn, P., Chrousos, G. P., & Gold, P. W. (2001). Depression: A major, unrecognized risk factor for osteoporosis? *Trends in Endocrinology and Metabolism*, 12(5), 198–203.

Clark, L. (2001). La Familia: Methodological issues in the assessment of perinatal social support for Mexicanas living in the United States. *Social Science and Medicine*, 53(10), 1303–1320.

Cohen, A., Houck, P. R., Szanto, K., Dew, M. A., Gilman, S. E., & Reynolds, C. F., III. (2006). Social inequalities in response to antidepressant treatment in older adults. *Archives of General Psychiatry*, 63(1), 50–56.

Cohen, S., & Williamson, G. M. (1991). Stress and infectious disease in humans. *Psychological Bulletin*, 109(1), 5–24.

Cohen, S., & Wills, T. A. (1985). Stress, social support, and the buffering hypothesis. *Psychological Bulletin*, 98(2), 310–357.

Conwell, Y. (2001). Suicide in later life: A review and recommendations for prevention. *Suicide and Life-Threatening Behavior*, 31, 32–47.

Conwell, Y., & Brent, D. (1995). Suicide and aging I: Patterns of psychiatric diagnosis. *International Psychogeriatrics*, 7(02), 149–164.

Conwell, Y., Duberstein, P. R., & Caine, E. D. (2002). Risk factors for suicide in later life. *Biological Psychiatry*, 52(3), 193–204.

Conwell, Y., Duberstein, P. R., Cox, C., Herrmann, J. H., Forbes, N. T., Caine, E. D. (1996). Relationships of age and axis I diagnoses in victims of completed suicide: A psychological autopsy study. *American Journal of Psychiatry*, 153(8), 1001–1008.

Conwell, Y., Duberstein, P., Cox, C., Herrmann, J., Forbes, N., & Caine, E. D. (1998). Age differences in behaviors leading to completed suicide. *American Journal of Geriatric Psychiatry*, 6, 122.

Conwell, Y., & Thompson, C. (2008). Suicidal behavior in elders. *Psychiatric Clinics of North America*, 31(2), 333–356.

Covinsky, K. E., Eng, C., Lui, L. Y., Sands, L. P., Sehgal, A. R., Walter, L. C., ... Yaffe, K. (2001). Reduced employment in caregivers of frail elders. *Journals of Gerontology Series A: Biological Sciences and Medical Sciences* 56(11), M707–M713.

Covinsky, K. E., Yaffe, K., Lindquist, K., Cherkasova, E., Yelin, E., & Blazer, D. G. (2010). Depressive symptoms in middle age and the development of later-life functional limitations: The long-term effect of depressive symptoms. *Journal of the American Geriatrics Society*, 58(3), 551–556.

Coyne, J. C. (1976). Depression and the response of others. *Journal of Abnormal Psychology*, 85(2), 186–193.

Cuijpers, P., Van Straten, A., & Smit, F. (2005). Preventing the incidence of new cases of mental disorders: A meta-analytic review. *Journal of Nervous and Mental Disease*, 193(2), 119–125.

Currie, S. R., Karltyn, J., Lussier, D., de Denus, E., Brown, D., & El-Guebaly, N. (2008). Outcome from a community-based smoking cessation program for persons with serious mental illness. *Community Mental Health Journal*, 44(3), 187–194.

de Groot, M., Anderson, R., Freedland, K. E., Clouse, R. E., & Lustman, P. J. (2001). Association of depression and diabetes complications: A meta-analysis. *Psychosomatic Medicine*, 63(4), 619–630.

Demakakos, P., Pierce, M. B., & Hardy, R. (2010). Depressive symptoms and risk of type 2 diabetes in a national sample of middle-aged and older adults. *Diabetes Care*, 33(4), 792–797.

Department of Health Education and Welfare. (1979). Department of Health, Education and Welfare Medical Practice Project. A state-of-the-science report for the Office of the Assistant Secretary for the US Department of Health, Education, and Welfare. Baltimore, MD: Policy Research.

Depp, C. A., & Jeste, D. V. (2004). Bipolar disorder in older adults: A critical review. *Bipolar Disorders*, 6(5), 343–367.

Depp, C., Ojeda, V. D., Mastin, W., Unützer, J., & Gilmer, T. P. (2008). Trends in use of antipsychotics and mood stabilizers among Medicaid beneficiaries with bipolar disorder, 2001–2004. *Psychiatric Services, 59*(10), 1169–1174.

Desai, M. M., Rosenheck, R. A., Druss, B. G., & Perlin, J. B. (2002). Mental disorders and quality of diabetes care in the Veterans Health Administration. *American Journal of Psychiatry, 159*(9), 1584–1590.

Doraiswamy, P. M., Khan, Z. M., Donahue, R. M., & Richard, N. E. (2002). The spectrum of quality-of-life impairments in recurrent geriatric depression. *Journals of Gerontology Series A: Biological Sciences and Medical Sciences, 57*(2), M134-M137.

Doshi, J. A., Cen, L., & Polsky, D. (2008). Depression and retirement in late middle-aged U.S. workers. *Health Services Research, 43*(2), 693–713.

Druss, B. G., Rosenheck, R. A., Desai, M. M., & Perlin, J. B. (2002). Quality of preventive medical care for patients with mental disorders. *Medical Care, 40*(2), 129–136.

Druss, B. G., Zhao, L., Von Esenwein, S., Morrato, E. H., & Marcus, S. C. (2011). Understanding excess mortality in persons with mental illness 17-year follow up of a nationally representative US survey. *Medical Care, 49*(6), 599–604.

Enger, C., Weatherby, L., Reynolds, R. F., Glasser, D. B., & Walker, A. M. (2004). Serious cardiovascular events and mortality among patients with schizophrenia. *Journal of Nervous and Mental Disease, 192*(1), 19–27.

Evans, D. L. (2000). Bipolar disorder: Diagnostic challenges and treatment considerations. *Journal of Clinical Psychiatry, 61*(Suppl 13), 26–31.

Evans, D. L., Charney, D. S., Lewis, L., Golden, R. N., Gorman, J. M., Krishnan, K. R., ... Valvo, W. J. (2005). Mood disorders in the medically ill: Scientific review and recommendations. *Biological Psychiatry, 58*(3), 175–189.

Fann, J. R., Fan, M. Y., & Unützer, J. (2009). Improving primary care for older adults with cancer and depression. *Journal of General Internal Medicine, 24*(Suppl 2), S417–S424.

Fann, J. R., Thomas-Rich, A. M., Katon, W. J., Cowley, D., Pepping, M., McGregor, B. A., & Gralow, J. (2008). Major depression after breast cancer: A review of epidemiology and treatment. *General Hospital Psychiatry, 30*(2), 112–126.

Fenn, H. H., Bauer, M. S., Altshuler, L., Evans, D. R., Williford, W. O., Kilbourne, A. M., ... VA Cooperative Study #430 Team. (2005). Medical comorbidity and health-related quality of life in bipolar disorder across the adult age span. *Journal of Affective Disorders, 86*(1), 47–60.

Frasure-Smith, N., Lesperance, F., & Talajic, M. (1995). Depression and 18-month prognosis after myocardial infarction. *Circulation, 91*(4), 999–1005.

French, E., & Jones, J. B. (2004). On the distribution and dynamics of health care costs. *Journal of Applied Econometrics, 19*(6), 705–721.

Gallo, J. J., Bogner, H. R., Morales, K. H., Post, E. P., Lin, J. Y., & Bruce, M. L. (2007). The effect of a primary care practice-based depression intervention on mortality in older adults. *Annals of Internal Medicine, 146*(10), 689–698.

Geerlings, S. W., Twisk, J. W. R., Beekman, A. T., Deeg, D. J., & van Tilburg, W. (2002). Longitudinal relationship between pain and depression in older adults: Sex, age and physical disability. *Social Psychiatry and Psychiatric Epidemiology, 37*(1), 23–30.

Gilbody, S., Bower, P., Fletcher, J., Richards, D., & Sutton, A. J. (2006). Collaborative care for depression: A cumulative meta-analysis and review of longer-term outcomes. *Archives of Internal Medicine, 166*(21), 2314–2321.

Gildengers, A. G., Whyte, E. M., Drayer, R. A., Soreca, I., Fagiolini, A., Kilbourne, A. M., ... Mulsant, B. H. (2008). Medical burden in late-life bipolar and major depressive disorders. *American Journal of Geriatric Psychiatry, 16*(3), 194–200

Golden, S. H., Williams, J. E., Ford, D. E., Yeh, H. C., Paton Sanford, C., Nieto, F. J., & Brancati, F. L. (2004). Depressive symptoms and the risk of type 2 diabetes. *Diabetes Care, 27*(2), 429–435.

Greenberg, P. E., Kessler, R. C., Birnbaum, H. G., Leong, S. A., Lowe, S. W., Berglund, P. A., & Corey-Lisle, P. K. (2003). The economic burden of depression in the United States: How did it change between 1990 and 2000? *Journal of Clinical Psychiatry, 64*(12), 1465–1475.

Grippo, A. J., & Johnson, A. K. (2002). Biological mechanisms in the relationship between depression and heart disease. *Neuroscience and Biobehavioral Reviews, 26*(8), 941–962.

Harris, E., & Barraclough, B. (1998). Mortality risk from mental disorders: A meta-analysis. *British Journal of Psychiatry, 173*, 11–53.

Heisel, M. J., & Duberstein, P. R. (2005). Suicide prevention in older adults. *Clinical Psychology: Science and Practice, 12*(3), 242–259.

Hepple, J., & Quinton, C. (1997). One hundred cases of attempted suicide in the elderly. *British Journal of Psychiatry, 171*(1), 42–46.

Himelhoch, S., & Medoff, D. R. (2005). Efficacy of antidepressant medication among HIV-positive individuals with depression: A systematic review and meta-analysis. *AIDS Patient Care and STDs*, *19*(12), 813–822.

Himelhoch, S., Weller, W. E., Wu, A. W., Anderson, G. F., & Cooper, L. A. (2004). Chronic medical illness, depression, and use of acute medical services among medicare beneficiaries. *Medical Care*, *42*(6), 512–521.

Hinton, L., Zweifach, M., Oishi, S., Tang, L., & Unützer, J. (2006). Gender disparities in the treatment of late-life depression: Qualitative and quantitative findings from the IMPACT trial. *American Journal of Geriatric Psychiatry*, *14*(10), 884–892.

Jaffe, A., Froom, J., & Galambos, N. (1994). Minor depression and functional impairment. *Archives of Family Medicine* *3*(12), 1081–1086.

Jenkins, R. (2002). Addressing suicide as a public-health problem. *Lancet*, *359*(9309), 813–814.

Jeste, D. V., Alexopoulos, G. S., Bartels, S. J., Cummings, J. L., Gallo, J. J., Gottlieb, G. L., ... Lebowitz, B. D. (1999). Consensus statement on the upcoming crisis in geriatric mental health: Research agenda for the next 2 decades. *Archives of General Psychiatry*, *56*(9), 848–853.

Johnson, R. W., & Lo Sasso, A. T. (2006). The impact of elder care on women's labor supply. *Inquiry*, *43*(3), 195–210.

Joiner, T. E., Alfano, M. S., & Metalsky, G. I. (1993). Caught in the crossfire: Depression, self-consistency, self-enhancement, and the response of others. *Journal of Social and Clinical Psychology*, *12*(2), 113–134.

Joynt, K. E., Whellan, D. J., & O'Connor, C. M. (2004). Why is depression bad for the failing heart? A review of the mechanistic relationship between depression and heart failure. *Journal of Cardiac Failure*, *10*(3), 258–271.

Kales, H. C., Maixner, D. F., & Mellow, A. M. (2005). Cerebrovascular disease and late-life depression. *American Journal of Geriatric Psychiatry*, *13*(2), 88–98.

Katon, W., Lin, E. H. B., Von Korff, M., Ciechanowski, P., Ludman, E., Young, B., ... McGregor, M. (2010). Integrating depression and chronic disease care among patients with diabetes and/or coronary heart disease: The design of the TEAMcare study. *Contemporary Clinical Trials*, *31*(4), 312–322.

Katon, W., Lyles, C. R., Parker, M. M., Karter, A. J., Huang, E. S., & Whitmer, R. A. (2012). Association of depression with increased risk of dementia in patients with type 2 diabetes: The diabetes and aging study. *Archives of General Psychiatry*, *69*(4), 410–417.

Katon, W., Unützer, J., Fan, M. Y., Williams, J. W. Jr., Schoenbaum, M., Lin, E. H., & Hunkeler, E. M. (2006). Cost-effectiveness and net benefit of enhanced treatment of depression for older adults with diabetes and depression. *Diabetes Care*, *29*(2), 265–270.

Katon, W. J. (2003). Clinical and health services relationships between major depression, depressive symptoms, and general medical illness. *Biological Psychiatry*, *54*(3), 216–226.

Katon, W. J., Lin, E., Russo, J., & Unützer, J. (2003). Increased medical costs of a population-based sample of depressed elderly patients. *Archives of General Psychiatry*, *60*(9), 897–903.

Katon, W. J., Lin, E. H. B., Russo, J., Von Korff, M., Ciechanowski, P., Simon, G., ... Young, B. (2004). Cardiac risk factors in patients with diabetes mellitus and major depression. *Journal of General Internal Medicine*, *19*(12), 1192–1199.

Katz, I. R. (1996). On the inseparability of mental and physical health in aged persons lessons from depression and medical comorbidity. *American Journal of Geriatric Psychiatry*, *4*(1), 1–16.

Kessler, R. C., Barber, C., Birnbaum, H. G., Frank, R. G., Greenberg, P. E., Rose, R. M., ... Wang, P. (1999). Depression in the workplace: Effects on short-term disability. *Health Affairs*, *18*(5), 163–171.

Kessler, R. C., Ormel, J., Demler, O., & Stang, P. E. (2003). Comorbid mental disorders account for the role impairment of commonly occurring chronic physical disorders: Results from the National Comorbidity Survey. *Journal of Occupational and Environmental Medicine*, *45*(12), 1257–1266.

Kilbourne, A. M., Reynolds, C. F., III, Good, C. B., Sereika, S. M., Justice, A. C., & Fine, M. J. (2005). How does depression influence diabetes medication adherence in older patients? *American Journal of Geriatric Psychiatry*, *13*(3), 202–210.

Kim, M. M., Swanson, J. W., Swartz, M. S., Bradford, D. W., Mustillo, S. A., & Elbogen, E. B. (2007). Healthcare barriers among severely mentally ill homeless adults: Evidence from the Five-site Health and Risk Study. *Administration and Policy in Mental Health and Mental Health Services Research*, *34*(4), 363–375.

Klap, R., Unroe, K. T., & Unützer, J. (2003). Caring for mental illness in the United States: A focus on older adults. *American Journal of Geriatric Psychiatry*, *11*(5), 517–524.

Klerman, G. L., Olfson, M., Leon, A. C., & Weismann, M. M (1992). Measuring the need for mental health care. *Health Affairs*, *11*(3), 23–33.

Kneipp, S. M., Castleman, J. B., & Gailor, N. (2004). Informal caregiving burden: An overlooked aspect of the lives and health of women transitioning from welfare to employment? *Public Health Nursing, 21*(1), 24–31.

Knol, M., Twisk, J., Beekman, A. T., Heine, R. J., Snoek, F. J., & Pouwer, F. (2006). Depression as a risk factor for the onset of type 2 diabetes mellitus. A meta-analysis. *Diabetologia, 49*(5), 837–845.

Kreyenbuhl, J., Dixon, L. B., McCarthy, J. F., Soliman, S., Ignacio, R. V., & Valenstein, M. (2008). Does adherence to medications for type 2 diabetes differ between individuals with vs without schizophrenia? *Schizophrenia Bulletin, 36*, 428–435.

Kurlowicz, L. H. (1998). Perceived self-efficacy, functional ability, and depressive symptoms in older elective surgery patients. *Nursing Research, 47*(4), 219–226.

Langa, K. M., Valenstein, M. A., Fendrick, A. M., Kabeto, M. U., & Vijan, S. (2004). Extent and cost of informal caregiving for older americans with symptoms of depression. *American Journal of Psychiatry, 161*(5), 857–863.

Larson, S. L., Owens, P. L., Ford, D., & Eaton, W. (2001). Depressive disorder, dysthymia, and risk of stroke: Thirteen-year follow-up from the Baltimore Epidemiologic Catchment Area Study. *Stroke, 32*(9), 1979–1983.

Lasser, K., Boyd, J. W., Woolhandler, S., Himmelstein, D. U., McCormick, D., & Bor, D. H. (2000). Smoking and mental illness: A population-based prevalence study. *Journal of the American Medical Association, 284*(20), 2606–2610.

Lenze, E. J., Rogers, J. C., Martire, L. M., Mulsant, B. H., Rollman, B. L., Dew, M. A., ... Reynolds, C. F., III. (2001). The association of late-life depression and anxiety with physical disability: A review of the literature and prospectus for future research. *American Journal of Geriatric Psychiatry, 9*(2), 113–135.

Lesperance, F., Frasure-Smith, N., Talajic, M., & Bourassa, M. G. (2002). Five-year risk of cardiac mortality in relation to initial severity and one-year changes in depression symptoms after myocardial infarction. *Circulation, 105*(9), 1049–1053.

Lilly, M. B., Laporte, A., & Coyte, P. C. (2007). Labor market work and home care's unpaid caregivers: A systematic review of labor force participation rates, predictors of labor market withdrawal, and hours of work. *Milbank Quarterly, 85*(4), 641–690.

Lin, E. H., Katon, W., Von Korff, M., Tang, L., Williams, J. W., Jr., Kroenke, K., ... Unützer, J. (2003). Effect of improving depression care on pain and functional outcomes among older adults with arthritis: A randomized controlled trial. *Journal of the American Medical Association, 290*(18), 2428–2429.

Lin, E. H. B., Heckbert, S. R., Rutter, C. M., Katon, W. J., Ciechanowski, P., Ludman, E. J., ... Von Korff, M. (2009). Depression and increased mortality in diabetes: Unexpected causes of death. *Annals of Family Medicine, 7*(5), 414–421.

Lin, E. H. B., Katon, W., Von Korff, M., Rutter, C., Simon, G. E., Oliver, M., ... Young, B. (2004). Relationship of depression and diabetes self-care, medication adherence, and preventive care. *Diabetes Care, 27*(9), 2154–2160.

Lish, J. D., Dime-Meenan, S., Whybrow, P. C., Price, R. A., & Hirschfeld, R. M. (1994). The National Depressive and Manic-depressive Association (DMDA) survey of bipolar members. *Journal of Affective Disorders, 31*(4), 281–294.

Luber, M. P., Meyers, B. S., Williams-Russo, P. G., Hollenberg, J. P., DiDomenico, T. N., Charlson, M. E., & Alexopoulos, G. S. (2001). Depression and service utilization in elderly primary care patients. *American Journal of Geriatric Psychiatry, 9*(2), 169–176.

Mallon, L., Broman, J-E., & Hetta, J. (2000). Relationship between insomnia, depression, and mortality: A 12-year follow-up of older adults in the community. *International Psychogeriatrics, 12*(03), 295–306.

Manthorpe, J., & Iliffe, S. (2010). Suicide in later life: Public health and practitioner perspectives. *International Journal of Geriatric Psychiatry, 25*(12), 1230–1238.

Marks, R., & Allegrante, J. P. (2005). A review and synthesis of research evidence for self-efficacy-enhancing interventions for reducing chronic disability: Implications for health education practice (Part II). *Health Promotion Practice, 6*(2), 148–156.

Martire, L. M., Schulz, R., Reynolds, C.F., III, Karp, J. F., Gildengers, A. G., & Whyte, E. M. (2010). Treatment of late-life depression alleviates caregiver burden. *Journal of the American Geriatrics Society, 58*(1), 23–29.

Maurin, T. M., & Boyd, B. C. (1990). Burden of mental illness on the family: A critical review. *Archives of Psychiatric Nursing, 6*, 99–107.

Mayne, T. J., Vittinghoff, E., Chesney, M. A., Barrett, D. C., & Coates, T. J. (1996). Depressive affect and survival among gay and bisexual men infected with HIV. *Archives of Internal Medicine 156*(19), 2233–2238.

McGuire, T., Wells, K. B., Bruce, M. L., Miranda, J., Scheffler, R., Durham, M., ... Lewis, L. (2002). Burden of illness. *Mental Health Services Research, 4*(4), 179–185.

Mezuk, B., Eaton, W. W., Albrecht, S., & Golden, S. H. (2009). Depression and type 2 diabetes over the lifespan: A meta-analysis. *Diabetes Care, 32*(5), e57.

Miklowitz, D. J. (2008). *Bipolar disorder: A famiy-focused treatment approach*. New York: Guilford Press.

Miranda, J., Azocar, F., Organista, K. C., Dwyer, E., & Areane, F.. (2003). Treatment of depression among impoverished primary care patients from ethnic minority groups. *Psychiatric Services, 54*(2), 219–225.

Miranda, J., Duan, N., Sherbourne, C., Schoenbaum, M., Lagomasino, I., Jackson-Triche, M., & Wells, K. B. (2003). Improving care for minorities: Can quality improvement interventions improve care and outcomes for depressed minorities? Results of a randomized, controlled trial. *Health Services Research, 38*(2), 613–630.

Mitchell, A. J., Rao, S., & Vaze, A. (2010). Do primary care physicians have particular difficulty identifying late-life depression? A meta-analysis stratified by age. *Psychotherapy and Psychosomatics, 79*(5), 285–294.

Monteleone, P. (2010). The association between depression and heart disease: The role of biological mechanisms. In *Depression and heart disease* (pp. 39–56). New York: Wiley.

Murphy, E., Smith, R., Lindesay, J., & Slattery, J. (1988). Increased mortality rates in late-life depression. *British Journal of Psychiatry, 152*(3), 347–353.

Murray, C., & Lopez, A. (1997). Alternative projections of mortality by cause 1990–2020: Global Burden of Disease Study. *Lancet, 349*, 1498–1504.

National Alliance for Caregiving/AARP. (2004). *Caregiving in the US*. Washington, DC: Author

Neal, M., & Wagner, D. (2001). *Working caregivers: Issues, challenges and opportunities for the aging network* (National Family Caregivers Support Program Selected Issue Brief). Washington, DC: Administration on Aging.

Newcomer, J. W., & Hennekens, C. H. (2007). Severe mental illness and risk of cardiovascular disease. *Journal of the American Medical Association, 298*(15), 1794–1796.

Olfson, M., Fireman, B., Weissman, M. M., Leon, A. C., Sheehan, D. V., Kathol, R. G., ... Farber, L. (1997). Mental disorders and disability among patients in a primary care group practice. *American Journal of Psychiatry, 154*(12), 1734–1740.

Ormel, J., Von Korff, M., Van den Brink, W., Katon, W., Brilman, E., & Oldehinkel, T. (1993). Depression, anxiety, and social disability show synchrony of change in primary care patients. *American Journal of Public Health, 83*(3), 385–390.

Ösby, U., Brandt, L., Correia, N., Ekbom, A., & Sparén, P. (2001). Excess mortality in bipolar and unipolar disorder in Sweden. *Archives of General Psychiatry, 58*(9), 844–850.

Oslin, D. W., Datto, C. J., Kallan, M. J., Katz, I. R., Edell, W. S., & Ten Have, T. (2002). Association between medical comorbidity and treatment outcomes in late-life depression. *Journal of the American Geriatrics Society, 50*(5), 823–828.

Otto, M. W., Reilly-Harrington, N., & Sachs, G. S. (2003). Psychoeducational and cognitive-behavioral strategies in the management of bipolar disorder. *Journal of Affective Disorders, 73*(1–2), 171–181.

Perlick, D. A., Rosenheck, R. A., Clarkin, J. F., Maciejewski, P. K., Sirey, J., Struening, E., & Link, B. G. (2004). Impact of family burden and affective response on clinical outcome among patients with bipolar disorder. *Psychiatric Services, 55*(9), 1029–1035.

Pinquart, M., & Duberstein, P. R. (2010). Depression and cancer mortality: A meta-analysis. *Psychological Medicine, 40*(11), 1797–1810.

Pinquart, M., & Sorensen, S. (2005). Ethnic differences in stressors, resources, and psychological outcomes of family caregiving: A meta-analysis. *Gerontologist, 45*(1), 90–106.

Pitsenberger, D. (2006). Juggling work and elder caregiving: Work-life balance for aging American workers. *American Association of Occupational Health Nurses Journal, 54*(4), 181–5.

Prochaska, J. J., Schane, R., Leek, D., Hall, S. E., & Hall, S. M. (2008). Investigation into the cause of death of a 56-year-old man with serious mental illness. *American Journal of Psychiatry, 165*(4), 453–456.

Pyne, J. M., Patterson, T. L., Kaplan, R. M., Ho, S., Gillin, J. C., Golshan, S., & Grant, I. (1997). Preliminary longitudinal assessment of quality of life in patients with major depression. *Psychopharmacology Bulletin, 33*(1), 23–29.

Regenold, W. T., Thapar, R. K., Marano, C., Gavirneni, S., & Kondapavuluru, P. V. (2002). Increased prevalence of type 2 diabetes mellitus among psychiatric inpatients with bipolar I affective and schizoaffective disorders independent of psychotropic drug use. *Journal of Affective Disorders, 70*(1), 19–26.

Robinson, R. G., Jorge, R. E., Moser, D. J., Acion, L., Solodkin, A., Small, S. L., ... Arndt, S. (2008). Escitalopram and problem-solving therapy for prevention of poststroke depression. *Journal of the American Medical Association, 299*(20), 2391–2400.

Roshanaei-Moghaddam, B., & Katon, W. (2009). Premature mortality from general medical illnesses among persons with bipolar disorder: A review. *Psychiatric Services, 60*(2), 147–156.

Rovner, B. W., Casten, R. J., Hegel, M. T., Leiby, B. E., & Tasman, W. S. (2007). Preventing depression in age-related macular degeneration. *Archives of General Psychiatry, 64*(8), 886–892.

Russo, J., Vitaliano, P. P., Brewer, D. D., Katon, W., & Becker, J. (1995). Psychiatric disorders in spouse caregivers of care recipients with Alzheimer's disease and matched controls: A diathesis-stress model of psychopathology. *Journal of Abnormal Psychology, 104*(1), 197–204.

Ryan, J., Carriere, I., Ritchie, K., Stewart, R., Toulemonde, G., Dartigues, J. F., ... Ancelin, M. L. (2008). Late-life depression and mortality: Influence of gender and antidepressant use. *British Journal of Psychiatry, 192*(1), 12–18.

Sajatovic, M. (2002). Aging-related issues in bipolar disorder: A health services perspective. *Journal of Geriatric Psychiatry and Neurology, 15*(3), 128–133.

Sajatovic, M., Blow, F. C., Ignacio, R. V., & Kales, H. C. (2005). New-onset bipolar disorder in later life. *American Journal of Geriatric Psychiatry, 13*(4), 282–289.

Schillerstrom, J. E., Royall, D. R., & Palmer, R. E. (2008). Depression, disability and intermediate pathways: A review of longitudinal studies in elders. *Journal of Geriatric Psychiatry and Neurology, 21*(3), 183–197.

Schoenbaum, M., Unützer, J., Sherbourne, C., Duan, N., Rubenstein, L. V., Miranda, J., ... Wells, K. (2001). Cost-effectiveness of practice-initiated quality improvement for depression: Results of a randomized controlled trial. *Journal of the American Medical Association, 286*(11), 1325–1330.

Schoevers, R., Smit, F., Deeg, D. J., Cuijpers, P., Dekker, J., van Tilburg, W., & Beekman, A. T. (2006). Prevention of late-life depression in primary care: Do we know where to begin? *American Journal of Psychiatry, 163*, 1611–1621.

Schulz, R., Beach, S. R., Ives, D. G., Martire, L. M., Ariyo, A. A., & Kop, W. J. (2000). Association between depression and mortality in older adults: The cardiovascular health study. *Archives of Internal Medicine, 160*(12), 1761–1768.

Shulman, K. I. (1997). Disinhibition syndromes, secondary mania and bipolar disorder in old age. *Journal of Affective Disorders, 46*(3), 175–182.

Simon, G. (2003). Social and economic burden of mood disorders. *Biological Psychiatry, 54*, 208–15.

Simon, G. E., & Unützer, J. (1999). Health care utilization and costs among patients treated for bipolar disorder in an insured population. *Psychiatric Services, 50*(10), 1303–1308.

Sirey, J. A., Bruce, M. L., Alexopoulos, G. S., Perlick, D. A., Friedman, S. J., & Meyers, B. S. (2001). Stigma as a barrier to recovery: Perceived stigma and patient-rated severity of illness as predictors of antidepressant drug adherence. *Psychiatric Services, 52*(12), 1615–1620.

Smit, F., Ederveen, A., Cuijpers, P., Deeg, D., & Beekman, A. (2006). Opportunities for cost-effective prevention of late-life depression: An epidemiological approach. *Archives of General Psychiatry, 63*(3), 290–296.

Stephens, M. A. P., Franks, M. M., & Atienza, A. A. (1997). Where two roles intersect: Spillover between parent care and employment. *Psychology and Aging, 12*(1), 30–37.

Stuck, A. E., Walthert, J. M., Nikolaus, T., Büla, C. J., Hohmann, C., & Beck, J. C. (1999). Risk factors for functional status decline in community-living elderly people: A systematic literature review. *Social Science and Medicine, 48*(4), 445–469.

Talley, R. C., & Crews, J. E. (2007). Framing the public health of caregiving. *American Journal of Public Health, 97*(2), 224–228.

Thompson, A., Fan, M. Y., Unützer, J., & Katon, W. (2008). One extra month of depression: The effects of caregiving on depression outcomes in the IMPACT trial. *International Journal of Geriatric Psychiatry, 23*(5), 511–516.

US Bureau of Labor Statistics (2008). *BLS spotlight on statistics older workers.*

Unützer, J. (1996). *Depressive symptoms, quality of life, and the use of health services in HMO patients age 65 and over: A four-year prospective study.* Seattle: University of Washington.

Unützer, J. (2002). Diagnosis and treatment of older adults with depression in primary care. *Biological Psychiatry, 52*(3), 285–92.

Unützer, J., Katon, W., Callahan, C. M., Williams, J. W., Jr., Hunkeler, E., Harpole, L., ... Oishi, S. (2003). Depression treatment in a sample of 1801 depressed older adults in primary care. *Journal of the American Geriatrics Society, 51*(4), 505–514.

Unützer, J., Katon, W. J., Fan, M. Y., Schoenbaum, M. C., Lin, E. H., Della Penna, R. D., & Powers, D. (2008). Long-term cost effects of collaborative care for late-life depression. *American Journal of Managed Care, 14*(2), 95–100.

Unützer, J., Patrick, D. L., Simon, G., Grembowski, D., Walker, E., Rutter, C., & Katon, W. (1997). Depressive symptoms and the cost of health services in HMO patients aged 65 years and older. A 4-year prospective study. *Journal of the American Medical Association, 277*(20), 1618–1623.

Unützer, J., Schoenbaum, M., Druss, B. G., & Katon, W. J. (2006). Transforming mental health care at the interface with general medicine: Report for the Presidents Commission. *Psychiatric Services, 57*(1), 37–47.

Van der Kooy, K., van Hout, H., Marwijk, H., Marten, H., Stehouwer, C., & Beekman, A. (2007). Depression and the risk for cardiovascular diseases: systematic review and meta analysis. *International Journal of Geriatric Psychiatry, 22*(7), 613–626.

van Gool, C. H., Kempen, G. I., Penninx, B. W., Deeg, D. J., Beekman, A. T., & van Eijk, J. T. (2003). Relationship between changes in depressive symptoms and unhealthy lifestyles in late middle aged and older persons: Results from the Longitudinal Aging Study Amsterdam. *Age and Ageing, 32*(1), 81–87.

van Melle, J. P., de Jonge, P., Spijkerman, T. A., Tijssen, J. G., Ormel, J., van Veldhuisen, D. J., ... van den Berg, M. P. (2004). Prognostic association of depression following myocardial infarction with mortality and cardiovascular events: A meta-analysis. *Psychosomatic Medicine, 66*(6), 814–822.

van Wijngaarden, B., Schene, A. H., & Koeter, M. W. (2004). Family caregiving in depression: Impact on caregivers' daily life, distress, and help seeking. *Journal of Affective Disorders, 81*(3), 211–222.

von Känel, R., Mills, P. J., Fainman, C., & Dimsdale, J. E. (2001). Effects of psychological stress and psychiatric disorders on blood coagulation and fibrinolysis: A biobehavioral pathway to coronary artery disease? *Psychosomatic Medicine, 63*(4), 531–544.

Veer-Tazelaar, P. J., van Marwijk, H. W. J., van Oppen, P., van Hout, H. P., van der Horst, H. E., Cuijpers, P., ... Beekman, A. T. (2009). Stepped-care prevention of anxiety and depression in late life: A randomized controlled trial. *Archives of General Psychiatry, 66*(3), 297–304.

Waern, M., Runeson, B. S., Allebeck, P., Beskow, J., Rubenowitz, E., Skoog, I., & Wilhelmsson, K. (2002). Mental disorder in elderly suicides: A case-control study. *American Journal of Psychiatry, 159*(3), 450–455.

Wagner, E. (1998). Chronic disease management: What will it take to improve care for chronic illness? *Effective Clinical Practice, 1,* 2–4.

Wagner, E., Glasgow, R., Davis, C., Bonomi, A. E., Provost, L., McCulloch, D., ... Sixta, C. (2001). Quality improvement in chronic illness care: A collaborative approach. *Joint Commission Journal on Quality Improvement, 27,* 63–80.

Wagstaff, A. (2002). Poverty and health sector inequalities. *Bulletin of the World Health Organization, 80,* 97–105.

Wells, K. B., Miranda, J., Bauer, M. S., Bruce, M. L., Durham, M., Escobar, J., ... Unützer, J. (2002). Overcoming barriers to reducing the burden of affective disorders. *Biological Psychiatry, 52*(6), 655–675.

Wells, K. B., Schoenbaum, M., Unützer, J., Lagomasino, I. T., & Rubenstein, L. V. (1999). Quality of care for primary care patients with depression in managed care. *Archives of Family Medicine, 8*(6), 529–536.

Whyte, E. M., & Rovner, B. (2006). Depression in late-life: Shifting the paradigm from treatment to prevention. *International Journal of Geriatric Psychiatry, 21*(8), 746–751.

Willemse, G. R. W. M., Smit, F., Cuijpers, P., & Tiemens, B. G. (2004). Minimal-contact psychotherapy for sub-threshold depression in primary care: Randomised trial. *British Journal of Psychiatry 185*(5), 416–421.

Williams, J. W., Jr., Katon, W., Lin, E. H., Nöel, P. H., Worchel, J., Cornell, J., ... Unützer, J. (2004). The effectiveness of depression care management on diabetes-related outcomes in older patients. *Annals of Internal Medicine, 140*(12), 1015–1024.

Wingerson, D., Russo, J., Ries, R., Dagadakis, C., & Roy-Byrne, P. (2001). Use of psychiatric emergency services and enrollment status in a public managed mental health care plan. *Psychiatric Services, 52*(11), 1494–1501.

Wolff, J. L., Starfield, B., & Anderson, G. (2002). Prevalence, expenditures, and complications of multiple chronic conditions in the elderly. *Archives of Internal Medicine, 162*(20), 2269–2276.

World Health Organization. (1980). *International classification of impairments, disabilities and handicaps: A manual of classification relating to the consequences of disease.* Geneva, Switzerland: Author.

World Health Organization. (2001). Burden of mental and behavioural disorders. In *The World Health Report 2001- Mental health: New understanding, new hope* (pp. 19–45). Geneva, Switzerland: Author.

Wulsin, L. R., & Singal, B. M. (2003). Do depressive symptoms increase the risk for the onset of coronary disease? A systematic quantitative review. *Psychosomatic Medicine, 65*(2), 201–210.

Wulsin, L. R., Vaillant, G. E., & Wells, V. E. (1999). A systematic review of the mortality of depression. *Psychosomatic Medicine, 61*(1), 6–17.

Wyatt, R. J., & Henter, I. (1995). An economic evaluation of manic-depressive illness-1991. *Social*

Psychiatry and Psychiatric Epidemiology, 30(5), 213–219.

Yeung, A., Shyu, I., Fisher, L., Wu, S., Yang, H., & Fava, M. (2010). Culturally sensitive collaborative treatment for depressed Chinese Americans in primary care. *American Journal of Public Health, 100*(12), 2397–2402.

Yirmiya, R., & Bab, I. (2009). Major depression is a risk factor for low bone mineral density:

A meta-analysis. *Biological Psychiatry, 66*(5), 423–432.

Zwerling, C., Whitten, P. S., Sprince, N. L., Davis, C. S., Wallace, R. B., Blanck, P. D., & Heeringa, S. G. (2002). Workforce participation by persons with disabilities: The National Health Interview Survey Disability Supplement, 1994 to 1995. *Journal of Occupational and Environmental Medicine, 44*(4), 358–364.

5

LATE-ONSET MOOD DISORDERS

*ICD*s AND *DSM*s

Roger Peele

AS SUGGESTED in other chapters of this volume, patient care, research, and clinical education might improve if there were greater recognition of late onset in mood disorders. One way recognition would be enhanced is if the diagnostic system used in medicine recognized this designation.

Recognition is dependent on two classification systems, *The International Classification of Diseases* (*ICD*) and the *Diagnostic and Statistical Manual of Mental Disorders* (*DSM*). We will review the histories of the *ICD*s and *DSM*s, the present status of depressive disorders in these two classifications, and, specifically, the lack of a status "late onset." Lastly, we will review the ways we might increase this recognition in future *ICD*s and *DSM*s.

THE INTERNATIONAL CLASSIFICATION OF DISEASES

In Europe during the late 1800s, there developed the wish to have an international classification of diseases. After some conferences, one was published in 1900. As shown in Table 5.1, an edition was developed about every 10 years for the first half of the 20th century. The development of later editions has been at a slower pace, due to the need to attain ratification of the World Health members, now numbering 193 members (International Advisory Group for the Revision of *ICD-10* Mental and Behavioral Disorders).

The earlier editions of *The International Classification of Diseases* (*ICD*) focused on mortality, so there was no classification of psychiatric diseases in the first five editions except for those closely identified with neurology, such as paresis. The latest *ICD*s are much broader, wanting "to enable the assessment and monitoring of mortality, morbidity, and other relevant parameters related to health" (International Advisory Group for the Revision of *ICD-10* Mental and Behavioral Disorders).

Nations are allowed to expand on the *ICD*s to meet that particular nation's needs. The United States' expansion is titled "Clinical Modification"

Table 5.1 International Classification of Diseases

ICD-1	1900
ICD-2	1910
ICD-3	1921
ICD-4	1930
ICD-5	1939
ICD-6	1949 (first to contain psychiatric disorders)
ICD-7	1958
ICD-8A	1968 ("A" = "Adapted for use in the United States")
ICD-9	CM 1979 ("CM" = "Clinical Modification" for use in the United States)
ICD-10	1992 (not yet used in the US except for international reporting of deaths)
ICD-10	CM is scheduled for October 1, 2013
ICD-11	Scheduled for 2015

(CM), for example, "ICD-9-CM." In Canada, it is ICD-9-CA. In general, the modifications are reflected in additional digits to the ICD codes.

In the United States, the ICD-CM is promulgated by a federal agency within the Department of Health and Human Services, the National Center for Health Statistics (NCHS). Each winter, the NCHS receives suggestions for clinical modifications. The Center holds hearings in the spring and announces its decisions in August. The decisions are effective on the next October 1 throughout the United States, for both the private and public sectors. For example, the Center received suggested additions to the 2009 version of ICD-9-CM in the winter of 2009–2010, held hearings in the spring of 2010, and announced the Center's decisions in August 2010, which were effective October 1, 2010. (The US federal government's annual cycle begins October 1, not January 1.)

The Center's decisions are public, not copyrighted, and can be downloaded for free. The total document runs over a thousand pages, with many pages having three columns. Even though free, attractive editions of ICD-9-CM are bought in the United States for about $80, in September, soon after the NCMS decisions are public—in time for government agencies, hospitals, clinics, and others to implement the changes by October 1.

The ICD-9-CM consists of two main parts:

1. An alphabetical listing of medical disorders, for example, "depression, major, recurrent episode, 296.3." The alphabetical part of ICD-9-CM is unsatisfactory in two ways:
   a. Some major entities cannot be found, such as "bipolar."

   b. On finding an entity in the listing, it may not include the CM distinction. For example, "depression, major, recurrent episode, 296.3" is unsatisfactory in that the clinician also often needs to specify the fifth digit for the electronic record systems (including billing systems) to accept the code the code. To be useful, the alphabetical system should have the 0 to 6 fifth digit spelled out, 0 = unspecified, 1 = mild, and so on, for those codes under ICD-9-CM's recurrent major depression.

2. A numerical ("tabular") listing, for example, "296.52 Bipolar I disorder, most recent episode depressed, moderate." The tabular entries include synonyms and exclusions. For 296.52, for example, includes "manic-depressive psychosis, circular type but currently depressed" and excludes "brief compensatory or rebound mood swings" and refers the reader to another code, "296.99," for that disorder. In general, the numerical part of ICD-9-CM is problem free.

For clinicians who electronically search for codes or names, the process is within easy reach. For example, if a clinician has finished an examination of a patient and concluded that the patient has dysthymic disorder, the clinician can search "dysthymic disorder" and "ICD-9-CM," and "300.4" pops up. Same with "dysthymic disorder" and "ICD-10-CM" and up pops "F34.1." Or if one only has the code and wants to know the name, one types in "300.4" and "ICD-9-CM" and "dysthymic disorder" pops up. While search engines can freely provide the clinician with the names and codes of disorders, the DSMs will remain of considerable value to clinicians because the *DSMs* will define the terms as well as provide valuable general information about each disorder. Moreover, if the American Psychiatric Association is able to keep their Practice Guidelines current, a *DSM* tied electronically to the Practice Guidelines would be very valuable. For example, the clinician determines that the patient has borderline personality disorder and the electronic version of *DSM* has a tie to the Borderline Personality Disorder Practice Guideline.

As noted in Table 5.1, *ICD-10* was published in 1994, yet *ICD-10-CM* is not yet implemented in the United States. Why? Most of the codes in *ICD-9* begin with a number. *ICD-10* codes begin with a letter. For computer systems of government agencies and private companies, there are huge costs associated with switching from codes that begin with a number to codes that begin with a letter. So pleas to postpone implementing *ICD-10-CM* were granted by NCHS year after year. Eventually, NCHS decided it could no longer postpone implementation and had set a deadline of October 1, 2013, for implementation throughout American medicine, but strong objections led to a postponement until October 1, 2014. It is not clear that NCHS can stick with that date if the American Medical Association and others object.

Table 5.2 shows the outline of *ICD-10*. Most of the diagnoses used by mental health specialists are in Chapter V, where all the codes begin with an "F." Some codes in Chapter VI, XVIII, XIX, XX, and XXI will also be used by mental health clinicians. Those interested in seeing late-onset depression into the *ICD-10-CM* will probably be focused on Chapter V, but the other targets deserve consideration.

Even though not yet in use, NCHS has been making changes in *ICD-10-CM* periodically. For example, in 1999, NCHS had Michael First, MD, editor of *DSM-IV* and *DSM-IV-TR*, change Chapter V of *ICD-10-CM* to coincide with *DSM-IV-TR* nomenclature. Thus, any sticker-shock for clinicians first exposed to *ICD-10-CM* of Chapter V should be limited only to the codes, as the names of the disorders in Chapter V are very similar to *DSM-IV-TR*'s.

Table 5.3 outlines the sections of Chapter V.

Table 5.4 outlines the diagnoses of the mood disorders within Chapter V.

ICD-11

Since the work of *ICD-10* was completed in the early 1990s, the World Health Organization (WHO) has been developing *ICD-11*. A draft of *ICD-11* is to be completed in 2014. It is hoped that the draft will be approved by the WHO Assembly in 2015. Four questions the writers of *ICD-11* have tentatively been resolved:

1. What is a mental illness? *ICD-11*'s answer is likely to be the same as *ICD-10*'s: "A clinically recognizable set of symptoms or behaviors associated in most cases with distress and with interference with personal functions." *DSM-III, IIIR*, and *IV-TR* have definitions of mental disorders that are far more complex and will likely not be used by *ICD-11*. Obviously, advocating for the distinction "late-onset depression" will fit within *ICD*'s definition focused on distress and interference with personal functions.

2. Who will use *ICD-11*? *ICD-11* is being developed with the belief that there are a very board range of users. A major consideration in the development of *ICD-11* is that nearly half of the people in the world live in countries where there is less than 1 psychiatrist per 100,000 people. Thus, psychiatrists cannot be the sole professional constituency. In developing *ICD-11*, many professions as well as laypersons are regarded as important users, whose needs must be considered (International Advisory Group for the Revision of *ICD-10* Mental and Behavioral Disorders). Given the broad use of the *ICD*s, many distinctions within a major category may not be welcomed, but late-onset depression should not be too challenging for *ICD-11*'s broad number of users.

3. Are mental disorders to be conceptualized as universal or culture bound? Universality of specific categories of mental disorders is an inherent assumption in *ICD-10*. While the *ICD-11* draft is not yet set, it appears that the *ICD-10*'s tilt toward universality will continue in *ICD-11* (International Advisory Group for the Revision of *ICD-10* Mental and Behavioral Disorders). Since "late-onset depression" is universal, this proviso is not a barrier to including "late-onset depression" in *ICD-11*.

4. What is the primary orienting principle: clinical, research, education, or public health? The guiding question is, "How can a diagnosis and classification manual assist in increasing coverage and enhancing mental health care across the world?" (International Advisory Group for the Revision of *ICD-10* Mental and Behavioral Disorders). In part, this question would suggest a focus on epidemiology and statistics, but information without practice will not reduce disease burden. To do this, it is even more important that the classification provide a basis for identifying

Table 5.2 Chapters of *ICD-10*

CHAPTER	BLOCKS	TITLE
I	A00-B99	Certain infectious and parasitic diseases
II	C00-D48	Neoplasms
III	D50-D89	Diseases of the blood and blood-forming organs and certain disorders involving the immune mechanism
IV	E00-E90	Endocrine, nutritional, and metabolic diseases
V	F00-F99	Mental and behavioral disorders
VI	G00-G99	Diseases of the nervous system
VII	H00-H59	Diseases of the eye and adnexa
VIII	H60-H95	Diseases of the ear and mastoid process
IX	I00-I99	Diseases of the circulatory system
X	J00-J99	Diseases of the respiratory system
XI	K00-K93	Diseases of the digestive system
XII	L00-L99	Diseases of the skin and subcutaneous tissue
XIII	M00-M99	Diseases of the musculoskeletal system and connective tissue
XIV	N00-N99	Diseases of the genitourinary system
XV	O00-O99	Pregnancy, childbirth, and the puerperium
XVI	P00-P96	Certain conditions originating in the perinatal period
XVII	Q00-Q99	Congenital malformations, deformations and chromosomal abnormalities
XVIII	R00-R99	Symptoms, signs, and abnormal clinical and laboratory findings, not elsewhere classified
XIX	S00-T98	Injury, poisoning, and certain other consequences of external causes
XX	V01-Y98	External causes of morbidity and mortality
XXI	Z00-Z99	Factors influencing health status and contact with health services
XXII	U00-U99	Codes for special purposes

people with the greatest mental health needs when they come into contact with health care systems, and ensuring that they have access to appropriate and cost-effective forms of treatment. The classification must lend itself to use in countries and settings with limited resources, especially primary care settings, and be usable by a range of mental health professionals, nonspecialty health professionals, and even lay health care workers (International Advisory Group for the Revision of *ICD-10* Mental and Behavioral Disorders). The concept of "late-onset depression" should be very usable.

In addition to the broad mandates of *ICD*, another wish of those developing Chapter V, the Mental and Behavioral Health chapter, is harmonization with the *DSMs*. As of November 2010, the outline of Chapter V (with more details shown for Mood Disorders) (Hyman, 2010):

Neurodevelopmental Cluster
F–0: Neurodevelopmental Disorders
F–1: Primary Psychotic Disorders
Emotional Cluster
F–2: Bipolar and related diagnoses
F–3: Mood Disorders
Distress Disorders, examples: Major Depression; Dysthymia
Anxious Depression, example: Mixed anxiety-depression
F–4: Anxiety Disorders
F–5: Disorders related to an environmental stressor

Table 5.3 *ICD-10-CM*'s Chapter V, Mental and Behavior Disorders Outline

F00-F09	Organic, including symptomatic, mental disorders
F10-F19	Mental and behavioral disorders due to psychoactive substance use
F20-F29	Schizophrenia, schizotypal and delusional disorders
F30-F39	Mood (affective) disorders
F40-F48	Neurotic, stress-related and somatoform disorders
F50-F59	Behavioral syndromes associated with physiological disturbances and physical factors
F60-F69	Disorders of adult personality and behavior
F70-F79	Mental retardation
F80-F89	Disorders of psychological development
F90-F98	Behavioral and emotional disorders with onset usually occurring in childhood and adolescence
F99	Unspecified mental disorder

Table 5.4 *ICD-10-CM* Mood Disorders

F30 Manic episodes
F30.1 Manic episode without psychotic symptoms
F30.10 Manic episode without psychotic symptoms, unspecified
F30.11 Manic episode without psychotic symptoms, mild
F30.12 Manic episode without psychotic symptoms, moderate
F30.13 Manic episode, severe, without psychotic symptoms
F30.2 Manic episode, severe with psychotic symptoms
F30.3 Manic episode in partial remission
F30.4 Manic episode in full remission
F30.8 Other manic episodes
Hypomania
F30.9 Manic episode, unspecified
Mania NOS
F31 Bipolar disorders
F31.0 Bipolar disorder, current episode hypomanic
F31.1 Bipolar disorder, current episode manic without psychotic features
F31.10 Bipolar disorder, current episode manic without psychotic features, unspecified
F31.11 Bipolar disorder, current episode manic without psychotic features, mild
F31.12 Bipolar disorder, current episode manic without psychotic features, moderate
F31.13 Bipolar disorder, current episode manic without psychotic features, severe
F31.2 Bipolar disorder, current episode manic severe with psychotic features
Bipolar disorder, current episode manic with mood-congruent psychotic symptoms
Bipolar disorder, current episode manic with mood-incongruent psychotic symptoms
F31.3 Bipolar disorder, current episode depressed, mild or moderate severity
F31.30 Bipolar disorder, current episode depressed, mild or moderate severity, unspecified
F31.31 Bipolar disorder, current episode depressed, mild
F31.32 Bipolar disorder, current episode depressed, moderate
F31.4 Bipolar disorder, current episode depressed, severe, without psychotic features
F31.5 Bipolar disorder, current episode depressed, severe, with psychotic features

(Continued)

Table 5.4 *(Continued)*

Bipolar disorder, current episode depressed with mood-incongruent psychotic symptoms

Bipolar disorder, current episode depressed with mood-congruent psychotic symptoms

F31.6 Bipolar disorder, current episode mixed

F31.60 Bipolar disorder, current episode mixed, unspecified

F31.61 Bipolar disorder, current episode mixed, mild

F31.62 Bipolar disorder, current episode mixed, moderate

F31.63 Bipolar disorder, current episode mixed, severe, without psychotic features

F31.64 Bipolar disorder, current episode mixed, severe, with psychotic features

Bipolar disorder, current episode mixed with mood-congruent psychotic symptoms

Bipolar disorder, current episode mixed with mood-incongruent psychotic symptoms

F31.7 Bipolar disorder, currently in remission

F31.70 Bipolar disorder, currently in remission, most recent episode unspecified

F31.71 Bipolar disorder, in partial remission, most recent episode hypomanic

F31.72 Bipolar disorder, in full remission, most recent episode hypomanic

F31.73 Bipolar disorder, in partial remission, most recent episode manic

F31.74 Bipolar disorder, in full remission, most recent episode manic

F31.75 Bipolar disorder, in partial remission, most recent episode depressed

F31.76 Bipolar disorder, in full remission, most recent episode depressed

F31.77 Bipolar disorder, in partial remission, most recent episode mixed

F31.78 Bipolar disorder, in full remission, most recent episode mixed

F31.8 Other bipolar disorders

F31.81 Bipolar II disorder

F31.89 Other bipolar disorder

Recurrent manic episodes NOS

F31.9 Bipolar disorder, unspecified

F32 Major depressive disorder, single episode

F32.0 Major depressive disorder, single episode, mild

F32.1 Major depressive disorder, single episode, moderate

F32.2 Major depressive disorder, single episode, severe without psychotic features

F32.3 Major depressive disorder, single episode, severe with psychotic features

Single episode of major depression with mood-congruent psychotic symptoms

Single episode of major depression with mood-incongruent psychotic symptoms

Single episode of major depression with psychotic symptoms

ingle episode of psychogenic depressive psychosis

Single episode of psychotic depression

Single episode of reactive depressive psychosis

F32.4 Major depressive disorder, single episode, in partial remission

F32.5 Major depressive disorder, single episode, in full remission

F32.8 Other depressive episodes

Atypical depression

Post-schizophrenic depression

F32.9 Major depressive disorder, single episode, unspecified

Depression NOS

Depressive disorder NOS

(Continued)

Table 5.4 *(Continued)*

Major depression NOS

F33 Major depressive disorder, recurrent

F33.0 Major depressive disorder, recurrent, mild

F33.1 Major depressive disorder, recurrent, moderate

F33.2 Major depressive disorder, recurrent severe without psychotic features

F33.3 Major depressive disorder, recurrent, severe with psychotic symptoms

Endogenous depression with psychotic symptoms

Recurrent severe episodes of major depression with mood-congruent psychotic symptoms

Recurrent severe episodes of major depression with mood-incongruent psychotic symptoms

Recurrent severe episodes of major depression with psychotic symptoms

Recurrent severe episodes of psychogenic depressive psychosis

Recurrent severe episodes of psychotic depression

Recurrent severe episodes of reactive depressive psychosis

F33.4 Major depressive disorder, recurrent, in remission

F33.40 Major depressive disorder, recurrent, in remission, unspecified

F33.41 Major depressive disorder, recurrent, in partial remission

F33.42 Major depressive disorder, recurrent, in full remission

F33.8 Other recurrent depressive disorders

Recurrent brief depressive episodes

F33.9 Major depressive disorder, recurrent, unspecified

Monopolar depression NOS

F34 Persistent mood (affective) disorders

F34.0 Cyclothymic disorder

Affective personality disorder

Cycloid personality

Cyclothymia

Cyclothymic personality

F34.1 Dysthymic disorder

Depressive neurosis

Depressive personality disorder

Dysthymia

Neurotic depression

Persistent anxiety depression

F39 Unspecified mood (affective) disorder

Includes: affective psychosis NOS

F–6: Obsessive-compulsive spectrum and Stereotypic behavioral disorders

   Somatic meta-cluster

   F–7: Somatic symptom disorders

   F–8: Feeding and eating disorders

   F–9: Sleep disorders

   F–10: Disorder of Sexual Function

   Externalizing meta-cluster

   F–11: Antisocial and Disruptive Disorders

F–12: Substance-related and Addictive Disorders

Neurocognitive meta-cluster

   F–13: Neurocognitive Disorders (non-developmental)

   Disorders Not Yet Assigned

   F–15 Other Disorders (paraphilias; factitious disorders)

No suggestion of "Late-Onset Depression" in this draft.

A point as to the order of the codes: Because of the interest in harmonizing and because of the logic of this *ICD-11* proposal, we may see *DSM-5* organized as suggested by the *ICD-11*'s organization. *DSM-5* authors can shuffle the numbers of *ICDs* anyway they want—just as *DSM-III, IIIR,* and *IV* authors paid little attention to *ICD*'s organization of the codes. In summary, *DSM-5* must adhere to *ICD-9-CM* codes and want to be ready for *ICD-10-CM* codes, but they can ignore the organization of the codes of the *ICDs*.

THE DIAGNOSTIC AND STATISTICAL MANUAL OF MENTAL DISORDERS

Soon after its founding in 1844, the American Psychiatric Association (APA) developed diagnostic systems to classify the psychiatrically ill, with an emphasis during the APA's first hundred years on those patients in hospitals. During World War II, the classification systems were found to be insufficient in classifying men who physicians decided were too mentally unfit to be enlisted and insufficient in classifying psychiatric combat casualties. The APA decided to develop a new classification of mental disorders based on the experiences during World War II. To increase the consistency in the way terms were used, definitions of each term were included (see Table 5.5).

World War II mental casualties were conceptualized as a reaction to combat, and the authors of *DSM-I* used "reaction" rather than "disorder," "disease," or "illness." Two examples (American Psychiatric Association, 1952):

Manic depressive reactions: "*These groups comprise the psychotic reactions which fundamentally are marked by severe mood swings, and a tendency to remission and recurrence. Various accessory symptoms such as illusions, delusions, and hallucinations may be added to the fundamental affective alteration.*"

Schizophrenic Reactions, defined as "*It represents a group of psychotic disorders characterized by fundamental disturbances in reality relationships and concept formations, with affective, behavioral, and intellectual disturbances in varying degrees and mixtures. The disorders are marked by strong tendency to retreat from reality, by emotional disharmony, unpredictable disturbances in stream of thought, regressive behavior, and in some, a tendency to 'deterioration.'*"

Table 5.5 Editions of the *Diagnostic and Statistical Manual of Mental Disorders* (DSM)

DSM–I, 1952
    Chair: George Raines, MD
DSM–II, 1968
    Chair: Ernest M. Gruenberg, MD
DSM–III, 1980
    Chair: Robert L. Spitzer, MD
DSM–IIIR, 1987
    Chair: Robert L. Spitzer, MD
    Text Editor; Janet B. W. Williams, DSW
DSM–IV, 1994
    Chair: Allen Frances, MD
    Vice-Chair: Harold Alan Pincus, MD
    Editor: Michael B. First, MD
DSM–IV–TR, 2000
    Michael B. First, Editor, Text and Criteria
DSM–5, 2013
    Chair: David J. Kupfer, MD
    Vice-Chair: Darrel A. Regier, MD, MPH

In the early 1960s, the United States signed an international treaty that said that it would use the *International Classification of Diseases. DSM-I* was not consistent with the *ICD* as to names or codes, so the APA developed *DSM-II* (1968), which was consistent as to names and codes of *ICD-8* (1966). This resulted in the loss of "reaction" in the titles of diseases, for example, "Manic Depressive Illness" and "Schizophrenia." The *DSM-I*-like definitions of disorders remained.

The *DSMs* have to use the *ICD* codes. Because there are more *DSM* entities than available codes, many codes are used more than once. For example, the code for other Drug-Induced Disorders, 292.89, is used with 24 different *DSM-IV* disorders. The *ICD-10* switch to the first code being a letter rather than a number vastly increases the codes that are available. When *DSM-5* promulgates its entities in *ICD-10-CM*, almost all entities will have a unique code if *DSM-5* does not markedly expand the number of entities. If NCHS agreed to add "Late-Onset Depression" to all of the depression diagnoses, it appears they could all have a unique code. .

All *DSMs* have had severity dimensions, but, unless the dimension was coded, it is fair to say they have been infrequently used. Unlike the other

DSMs, DSM-II had severity dimensions coded for all disorders—mild, moderate, severe, and so on. Only mood disorders and mental retardation have retained coded dimensions in subsequent DSMs, although dimensions that were uncoded were championed in the text of all DSMs. Some of those working on DSM-5 want to see all mental disorders have a severity code, like DSM-II. To add coded dimensions to the classification of medical conditions in the United States, it will be necessary to have those codes in ICD-10-CM. At the moment, as to mental disorders, ICD-10-CM only has severity codes for mood disorders and mental retardation.

DSM-III (1980) brought huge changes to the DSMs. The following sections were added, a vast increase in background information about each disorder.

- Diagnostic features
- Associated features
- Cultural and gender features
- Prevalence
- Course
- Familiar patterns
- Differential Dx
- Decision trees
- Glossary

Diagnostic Criteria (a substitute for DSM-I and DSM-II definitions)

Five axes were expected to be addressed when providing the DSM-III diagnosis:

I. Psychiatric Disorders
II. Personality Disorders, Mental Retardation, and Traits
III. Other Medical Conditions
IV. Psychosocial Problems
V. Level of Functioning

The DSM-III's Diagnostic Criteria replaced DSM-I's and DSM-II's prototype definitions to increase reliability. Moreover, the expansion of information in DSM-III made the manual not only a diagnostic manual but also a book on psychopathology. Eventually, the DSM-III became not just a US-focused publication but the international text on psychopathology. Within this text, the importance of age of onset as age impacts the associated signs or impacts the course could be described briefly.

DSM-III-R (1987) and DSM-IV's (1994) presentation of mood disorders was quite similar to

DSM-III's. DSM-IV introduced two new ways of organizing the entities. First, all substance-related disorders are presented twice. They are listed in the substance-related section as well as listed in the clinical manifestation section, for example, cocaine mood disorder is listed in the substance-related section and in mood disorders. The second new way of organizing entities related to organic disorders. The term "organic" was discontinued and replaced with listing the medical condition with the symptomatology, for example, "Mood Disorder due to Multiple Sclerosis." Authors of DSM-IV wanted to increase the chances that clinicians would keep substance abuse and somatic conditions in the differential when diagnosing mood disorders.

DSM-IV-TR (2000) made no significant changes in the Diagnostic Criteria sets, but it greatly improved the other parts of text, for example, greater accuracy regarding laboratory findings.

Beginning in 1999, the staff at the American Psychiatric Association, under the direction of Darrel Regier, began the preparations for DSM-5 (initially "DSM-V," but changed to Arabic numbers because those numbers are easier to use for updates, e.g., "DSM-5.1.") Regier's office sponsored a number of publications, eight stepping stones so to speak, as to what should be in DSM-5. Some highlights as to mood disorders:

1. *A Research Agenda for DSM-V* (Kupfer, First, & Regier, 2002). This volume reviews the scientific developments of the prior decade that might impact DSM-5. This volume notes considerable interest in dimensions, and it does so without any reference to the experience with dimensions in prior DSMs. The latest DSM-5 proposals include severity scales for almost all disorders, consistent with the theme of this 2002 volume.

2. *Advancing DSM: Dilemmas in Psychiatric Diagnosing*. This book's foreword begins with a challenge from a past NIMH director, Steve Hyman (Hyman, 2003, p. xii):

- "Despite these successes (of the DSMs), there are clear problems and unresolved controversies related to DSM-IV-TR, the most recent version of DSM. If a relative strength of DSM is its focus on reliability, a fundamental weakness lies in the problems related to validity. Not only persisting but looming larger is the question of whether DSM-IV-TR truly carves nature at the joints—that is, whether the entities described in the manual are truly 'natural kinds' and not arbitrary chimeras."

- "In reifying *DSM-IV-TR* diagnoses, one increases the risk that science will get stuck, and the very studies that are needed to better define phenotypes are held back."

1. A recent brilliant summary of Hyman's thinking: "The most important goal is to help the APA get out of the *DSM-III-R-R-R* rut without blowing up clinical practice" (Hyman, personal communication, March 14, 2011),

2. In various ways, authors of chapters in this book address possible major redirections that *DSM-5* might take, none specific to mood disorders, other than the suggestion that *DSM-5* might want to include subclinical mood disorders, disorders that lack the clinically significant distress or disability expected of disorders to be included in the *DSM*. It would be difficult to claim that any of the suggestions of this book led directly to any of the present *DSM-5* proposal. Hyman's challenge still remains unmet.

3. *Dimensional Models of Personality Disorders* (Widiger, Simonsen, Sirovatka, & Regier, 2006). This book's main reflection that could impact depression is the suggestion that *DSM-5* be reorganized into internalizing and externalizing spectra, and that depressive signs and symptoms, that is, depressive personality, would fall under internalizing spectra. At the time of this writing, however, "Depressive Personality" is not proposed for *DSM-5* (www.dsm5.org, as of June 30, 2011).

4. *Relational Processes and DSM-V: Neuroscience, Assessment, Prevention, and Treatment* (Beach et al., 2006). It has been appealing to many clinicians to diagnosis not just illnesses but problematic relationships, because of the potential gains in clinical results when those relationships are addressed. In *DSM-IV*'s development, there was considerable interest in enhancing a relationship-based diagnostic system, but studies led to the conclusion that there was insufficient evidence to justify such (Frances, Clarkin, & Ross: Family/relational problems in *DSM-IV* Sourcebook, Vol 3. Edited by Widiger TA, Frances AJ, Pincus HA, et al. Washington, DC, American Psychiatric Association, 1997, pp. 521–530). Even so, in the *DSM-IV-TR* Appendix B, under entities "Provided for Further Study," there is a Global Assessment of Relational Functioning

Scale (GARF) (*DSM-IV-TR*, pp. 814–816). The GARF offers the potential of indicating family difficulties brought on by late-onset depression, but the GARF has not been frequently used. This 2006 book states the importance of relationships, dismisses the GARF, but it does not arrive at any substantial suggestions that have found their way into proposals for *DSM-5* as promulgated at www.dsm5.org (as of June 30, 2011). Part of the challenge is to attain any agreement on classifying pathological relationships within a medical system that is focused on diseases of individuals. It appears that interests in noting the impact of late-onset depression in relationships is to look for *ICD-10-CM* Z-Codes that might be applicable. If not yet in Z-Codes, they could be proposed to NCHS.

5. *Age and Gender Considerations* (Narrow, First, Sorpvatka, & Regier, 2007). Five chapters of this book are of special interest as to late-onset depression:

a) "Aging-Related Diagnostic Variations." This chapter points to the lack of recognition of depression in the elderly, but in the case of major depressive disorder, "there is not much evidence in favor of major age-associated differences in pathognomonic features when co-morbidity is taken into account" (p. 274). More important, the author suggests, is a need for a full consideration of both depression and the other somatic illnesses.

b) "Late-Life Depression: A Model for Medical Classification." This chapter provides a broad research approach to uncovering a classification of late-life depression, reaching biopsychosocial contributions to the person's suffering that in turn could become the basis of a medical classification. This chapter does not propose a classification system for *DSM-5*, instead focusing on what is needed before we can justify making recommendations as to late-life depression.

c) "Challenges of Diagnosing Psychiatric Disorders in Medically Ill Patients." This chapter raises questions as to whether context-dependent factors should be part of the diagnostic system, for example, the patient is dying. Even before terminal states, an *ICD-9-CM* diagnosis might apply, "Failure to thrive in adults," with signs much like those of major depressive disorder. The authors propose that a separate axis containing factors that contribute to adverse outcomes of somatic illnesses would be useful to those managing somatic illnesses. More generally, the authors wonder whether classification of the dying and of patients with frailty would be improved if the classification proposals came from studies of patients with those conditions. The authors ask, would that population be better served to have a classification that evolved from studies of them rather than to apply a classification system based on people who are not dying and do not have frailty?

d) "Use of Biomarkers in the Elderly." Ideal biomarkers, the authors suggest, are "a fundamental feature of the underlying pathophysiology of a disease and distinguish that illness from other conditions with an acceptable positive and negative predictive value. The biomarker should be reliable, relatively noninvasive, simple to perform, and inexpensive" (Narrow et al., p. 317). The authors focus on Alzheimer's and conclude an acceptable biomarker is not yet available.

e) "Impact of Psychosocial Factors on Late-Life Depression." The authors review the importance of psychosocial factors and stress the need for improved psychosocial assessment. (Comment: Not addressed by the authors is the potential of *ICD-9-CM*'s V-codes and *ICD-10-CM*'s Z-codes to name and code the relevant physical, psychological, and social stresses on patients. Those working on *DSM-5* may want to identify any factors related to late-onset mood disorders that are clinically important and propose to NCHS that the factors be added to the V-codes of *ICD-9-CM* and the Z-codes of *ICD-10-CM*.)

6. *Dimensional Approaches in Diagnostic Classification* (Helzer, Kraemer, Krueger, & Wittchen, 2008). This book reviews the PHQ-9 as a dimensional approach to major depressive disorder, notes a few problems, and concludes favorably that it "would facilitate recognition, guide treatment, and be acceptable to consumers, providers, and funders" (p. 49). Of course, dimensions have been part of all *DSM*'s mood disorders since *DSM-II*, but could we attain a greater reliability by being more specific as to scoring the dimensions? At present, the *DSM-5* Work Group on Mood Disorders points to three alternatives without taking sides: PHQ-9, CGI, and a third eight-point scale of 0= not assessed, 1 = normal, 2 = borderline mentally ill, 3 = mildly ill, 4 =

moderately ill, 5 = markedly ill, 6 = severely ill, and 7 = among the most extremely ill patients.

(Comment: Without more information, it is difficult to say how the third option increases reliability over the recent *DSM*'s mild, moderate, severe without psychotic features, with psychotic features, in partial remission, in full remission, and unspecified. Many clinicians might prefer the more longitudinal specifiers of recent *DSM*s. The APA's Practice Guidelines for Major Depressive Disorder uses the *DSM-IV-TR* breakdown. Additionally, other factors being equal, the more a scale is differentiated, the more likely reliability decreases.)

7. *Somatic Presentations of Mental Disorders* (Dimsdale, Xin, Kleinman, & Patel, 2009). This book notes the close relationship between depression and somatoform disorders and makes no recommendations that *DSM-5*'s handling of depression be different than *DSM-IV-TR*'s.

8. *The Conceptual Evolution of DSM-5* (Regier, Narrow, & Kuhl, 2011). The major focus on this book is on dimensions. "Late-onset" is defined as ">60 years," and even though that designation is defined, the authors do not champion it as a classification distinction, writing that "the fundamental phenomenology of depressive illness is essentially the same in terms of diagnostic criteria, involving relatively cohesive core symptoms regardless of age at onset" (Regier et al., 2011, p. 329). While not impacting the basic classification, *DSM-5* will address age-related issues in the text of each entity. Furthermore, criteria sets of depression might address age-related topics, such as "role-function thresholds for persons who are retired" (Regier et al., 2011, p. 331). As to age-related subtypes of depression, a case is made for such in children, but not for late life. However, what might deserve consideration, the authors suggest, is a lower threshold of symptoms in the late-onset population. Any initiatives wishing to add "late-onset" as a code in future *ICDs/DSMs* will want to be aware of this book's opposing arguments.

THE *DSM-5* TASK FORCE

In 2006, the APA formed the *DSM-5* Task Force and selected *DSM*-experienced psychiatrists as chair (David Kupfer) and vice-chair (Darrel A. Regier). Over two dozen others were appointed to the Task Force, several being quite pertinent to the subject of this book: The Mood Disorders Work Group is chaired by Jan A. Fawcett, MD, and one of the editors of this book chairs The Sleep-Wake Disorders Work Group, Charles F. Reynolds, III, MD. The *DSM-5* effort differs from past *DSM* efforts in the following ways:

1. In addition to work groups for a subset of disorders, there are also study groups for:
    a. Diagnostic spectra
    b. Life span developmental approaches
    c. Gender and cross-cultural issues
    d. Psychiatric/general medical interface
    e. Impairment assessment
    f. Diagnostic assessment instruments
2. The appointment process of members of the Task Force and members of the Work Groups has been closely monitored as to potential conflicts of interests. Furthermore, there is a $10,000/year upper limit on any earnings related to subjects that Task Force members might be working on. The limits on *DSM-5* advisors is less stringent, but it is understood that they can only advise and that they have no vote in the decisions that are made. Past *DSM*s have involved about a thousand advisors, and it is anticipated that *DSM-5* will eventually approach the same number.
3. There is a Web site that has the current *DSM-5* proposals, www.dsm5.org, and periodically, there is an opportunity for comment by all, both professionals and the public. Each comment is reviewed by at least one member of the relevant Work Group.
4. There is a Scientific Review Board that reflects on all proposed changes (more infra).
5. There is a Clinical and Public Health committee to reflect on controversial issues and to address entities that might be a consideration for *DSM-5* even if it was not scientifically mature enough to pass the Scientific Review Board but seen as a needed addition to *DSM-5*.
6. While *DSM* thinking had been presented at APA Annual meetings with *DSM-III*, *DSM-III-R*, and *DSM-IV*, the presentations have been far more extensive with *DSM-5* with half a dozen presentations not unusual at Annual meetings. Also, in recent years, the *American Journal of Psychiatry* has often had editorials on *DSM-5*.
7. The plans are for the Task Force to make final decisions in 2012, then present a *DSM-5* draft to the APA governance (Assembly and Board of Trustees) for approval in 2012, and to publish in time for the APA annual meeting, May 2013. *DSM-5* will have both *ICD-9-CM* and *ICD-10-CM* codes.

Mood Disorders Work Group Proposals for *DSM-5* Disorders for Depression

    1. Disruptive Mood Dysregulation Disorder (proposed as a childhood disorder)
    2. Major Depressive Disorder, Single Episode
    3. Major Depressive Disorder, Recurrent
    4. Chronic Depressive Disorder (Dysthymia)
    5. Premenstrual Dysphoric Disorder
    6. Mixed Anxiety/Depression
    7. Substance-Induced Depressive Disorder
    8. Depressive Disorder Associated With a Known General Medical Condition
    9. Other Specified Depressive Disorder
    10. Unspecified Depressive Disorder

The major changes from *DSM-IV-TR* are the addition of Disruptive Mood Dysregulation Disorder, Premenstrual Dysphoric Disorder, Mixed Anxiety/Depression, and Other Specified Disorder. Of special interest to those focused on late-onset depression are (1) Mixed Anxiety/Depression and (2) Other Specified Depressive Disorder (Mood Disorders Work Group, n.d.).

Mixed Anxiety/Depression *DSM-5* Proposal

Those interested in late-onset depression will want to ascertain whether this entity, now in *DSM-IV-TR*'s listing of disorders for further study (*DSM-IV-TR*, pp. 780–781), meets a need. The *DSM-5* proposed criteria of this disorder includes the following (Mood Disorders Work Group, n.d.):
"The patient has *three or four* of the symptoms of major depression which must include depressed mood and/or anhedonia), and they are accompanied by anxious distress. The symptoms must have lasted at least 2 weeks, and no other *DSM* diagnosis of anxiety or depression must be present, and they are both occurring at the same time.

"Anxious distress is defined as having two or more of the following symptoms: *irrational worry, preoccupation with unpleasant worries, having trouble relaxing, motor tension, fear that something awful may happen.*"

The Mood Disorder Work Group rationale for establishing this Disorder (Mood Disorders Work Group, n.d.):
"This diagnosis has been in the Appendix of *DSM-IV*, and is in the *ICD-10*. It has not

previously been defined *precisely*. (The *ICD* definition states that symptoms of both anxiety and depression are both present, but neither set of symptoms, considered separately is sufficient to justify a diagnosis.)

"The advantages of this proposal are that it ensures that symptoms of *both* disorders are indeed present and distressing (*DSM-IV*), and the ambiguity of the *ICD-10* criteria are also avoided."

"The Mood Workgroup is considering a simple method by which a clinician is able to rate anxiety severity on a single dimension, useful for both mixed anxiety depression and major depression accompanied by anxiety:

"Anxious Symptoms:

b. describes (irrational) worries

c. feeling uneasy

d. feeling nervous

e. motor tension

f. feels something awful may happen" (Mood Disorders Work Group, n.d.)

Advocates of late-onset depression will want ascertain whether this addition reaches the late-onset depression symptomatology.

Other Specified Depressive Disorders

DSM-5 will likely not use "Not Otherwise Specified" as used in *DSM-IV-TR* but, instead, use two categories, Other Specified Depressive Disorder and Unspecified Depressive Disorder. Thus, Late-Onset Depression Syndrome could be identified and described in *DSM-5* as one of the Other Depressive Disorders. While the codes would not be unique, being described in Other Depressive Disorders does alert clinicians that there is a specific syndrome, which is a much more useful communication than *DSM-IV's* "Depression, NOS." Should proponents of Late-Onset Depression believe they can justify a syndrome that differs some from other depressive disorders, they could propose to the *DSM-5* Task Force that they have a paragraph in *DSM-5's* sections on Other Depressive Disorders, provide the preferred name and a paragraph describing it. Proponents might want to propose two: There are two coding options in *ICD-9-CM*. Proponents would need to decide whether "episodic" is wanted.

296.99 Other Episodic Mood Disorder or Late Onset Type

311 Depressive disorder, Not Elsewhere Classified, Late Onset Type

As to *ICD-10-CM*, there are three options:

F32.8 Other Single Episode Depressive, Late Onset Type

F33.9 Other Recurrent Depressive Disorder, Late Onset Type

F343.8 Other Persistent Mood Disorder, Late-Onset Type

DSM-5 PROPOSALS FOR BIPOLAR DISORDERS

The *DSM-5* proposal for bipolar disorders looks very similar to *DSM-IV-TR* (Mood Disorders Work Group, n.d.), as follows:

Bipolar I Disorder

Bipolar II Disorder

Cyclothymic Disorder

Substance-Induced Bipolar Disorder

Bipolar Disorder Associated With a Known General Medical Condition

Other Specified Bipolar Disorder

Unspecified Bipolar Disorder.

In looking at this list, one sees two changes: (1) There is no Mixed Type; (2) *DSM-IV-TR's* Not Otherwise Specified (NOS), like the depressive disorders, is divided into Other and Unspecified. Thus, as said earlier for Depressive Disorders, one could consider having a Late-Onset name and paragraph with Bipolar disorders.

In place of the Mixed Type, it is proposed that a Mixed Feature Specifier be available for Manic, for Hypomanic, and for Bipolar Depressed Episodes. The criteria are as follows (Mood Disorders Work Group, n.d.):

"A. If predominantly Manic or Hypomanic, full criteria are met for a Manic Episode (see Criteria for **Manic Episode**) or Hypomanic Episode (see **Criteria for Hypomanic Episode**), and at least three of the following symptoms are present nearly every day during the episode:

1. Prominent dysphoria or depressed mood as indicated by either subjective report (e.g., feels sad or empty) or observation made by others (e.g., appears tearful).

2. Diminished interest or pleasure in all, or almost all, activities (as indicated by either subjective account or observation made by others).

3. Psychomotor retardation nearly every day (observable by others, not merely subjective feelings of being slowed down).
4. Fatigue or loss of energy.
5. Feelings of worthlessness or excessive or inappropriate guilt (not merely self-reproach or guilt about being sick).
6. Recurrent thoughts of death (not just fear of dying), recurrent suicidal ideation without a specific plan, or a suicide attempt or a specific plan for committing suicide.

B. If predominantly Depressed, full criteria are met for a Major Depressive Episode (see Criteria for Major Depressive Episode), and at least three of the following symptoms are present nearly every day during the episode.
• Elevated, expansive mood
• Inflated self-esteem or grandiosity
• More talkative than usual or pressure to keep talking
• Flight of ideas or subjective experience that thoughts are racing
• Increase in energy or goal-directed activity (either socially, at work or school, or sexually)
• Increased or excessive involvement in activities that have a high potential for painful consequences (e.g., engaging in unrestrained buying sprees, sexual indiscretions, or foolish business investments).
• Decreased need for sleep (feeling rested despite sleeping less than usual (to be contrasted from insomnia)

C. Mixed symptoms are observable by others and represent a change from the person's usual behavior.

D. For those who meet full episode criteria for both Mania and Depression simultaneously, they should be labeled as having a Manic Episode, with mixed features, due to the marked impairment and clinical severity of full mania.

E. The mixed symptom specifier can apply to depressive episodes experienced in Major Depressive Disorder, Bipolar I disorders, Bipolar II disorders, and Bipolar Disorder Not Elsewhere Classified.

F. The mixed symptoms are not due to the direct physiological effects of a substance (e.g., a drug of abuse, a medication, or other treatment)."

While DSM-5 would have this mixed type specifier, there could be complications as to coding as, at present, Mixed type is part of ICD-9-CM and the mixed specifier is not.

RELATIONSHIP BETWEEN *ICD*S AND *DSM*S

The DSMs and ICDs have an interlocking relationship in which they both provide some leadership to the other. The DSMs have to live within the ICDs, but only as to the first three digits. The APA can suggest to the NCHS changes every year as to the fourth and fifth codes with the corresponding name changes, leading to the ICD-CMs being more advanced than the ICDs. When the ICDs are constructed, they look toward the DSMs for ideas on how to improve the psychiatric part of the ICD. Because the World Health Organization is composed of nearly 200 countries, the approval process is slow. Despite the challenges, both ICD and DSM authors have attempted to achieve consistency, "harmonization," between the two. Helpful is having some members be part of both groups. As to the development of ICD-11 and DSM-5, again, the two teams are working to keeping the other informed, there is some overlap of membership, and harmonization is the wish of both.

WAYS THAT "LATE ONSET" MIGHT BECOME PART OF *DSM-5*

Before reviewing ways that "late onset" can become part of DSM-5, we should note a minor problem. DSM-IV-TR defines "late onset" with one mood disorder, dysthymia, and the definition, unfortunately, is older than 21. Since the typical clinician and researcher ignores this distinction, it does not provide any substantial hurdle for those of us championing "late onset" other than to see this older wording remove.

Proposals for change could be directed to NCHS or to the DSM-5 Task Force. If a proposal goes to NCHS that an entity be added to ICD-9-CM/ICD10-CM is successful, that could lead to adoption by DSM-5, as the APA always wants the DSMs to be consistent with the ICDs.

Both of these bodies are open to suggestions from many sources. To obtain recognition of late-onset depression, advocacy would be made to NCHS in order that it has a code in ICD-9-CM/ICD-10-CM, the only way to achieve a recognized medical code in the United States. This would involve making the recommendation late in a calendar year to NCHS and presenting the rationale at the NCHS hearing several months later. By late summer, one would know the results. If successful, the code would be applicable that October 1. Traditionally, the APA changes its *DSM* text to be consistent with *ICDs* in the next printing of the book, not waiting for a new *DSM*. Thus, if a submission of a "Late-Onset" code specifier was made to NCHS in 2013 and accepted by NCHS in 2014, it could be in the next printing of *DSM-5*. NCHS's revision process is annual and exact information as to timing and documentation can be obtained at http://www.cdc.gov/nchs/. To repeat: When thinking of adding an entity to *ICD-9-CM/ICD-10-CM*, remember that regardless of when the next *DSM* is published, the APA will feel pressed to recognize mental disorders accepted by NCHS and make the changes in the next printing of the *DSM*. While not guaranteed, if one is successful in NCHS accepting Late-Onset Depression as a coded specifier, it could begin appearing in *DSM-5* soon after NCHS acceptance—not have to wait for a subsequent edition of *DSM*. *DSM-IV-TR* recognized changes in the printing of *DSM-IV-TR*. No waiting for *DSM-5*. There is a proposal that the *DSM* be published yearly, but that idea will probably not be accepted for several years.

There are signs and symptoms of late-onset depression that a clinician might want to emphasize as an additional code beyond the depression diagnosis. Some possibilities available in *ICD-9-CM* coding:

Agitation or Restlessness: In *ICD-9-CM*, 799.29. In *ICD-10-CM*: R45

Anosognosia: In *ICD-9-CM*, 780.00. In *ICD-10-CM*: R41.89

Mild Cognitive Impairment: *ICD-9-CM*, 331.83. *ICD-10-CM*, G31.84

Suicidal ideation:*ICD-9-CM*, V62.84. *ICD-10-CM*, R45.481. *DSM-5* may have a Suicide Risk Severity scale to help monitor that aspect of the patient's illnesses.

An opportunity to classify patients with depression, obviously including late-onset conditions, which are related to another medical condition, is part of *ICD-9-CM* and *ICD-10-CM*. In *ICD-9-CM*, the choices include 293.83, Mood Disorder Due To (indicate the somatic condition).

In *ICD-10-CM*, the following three choices:

F06.31 Mood disorder due to known physiological condition with depressive features

F06.32 Mood disorder due to known physiological condition with major depressive-like episode

F06.34 Mood disorder due to known physiological condition with mixed features.

CONCLUSION

There are several routes to increasing the recognition of late-onset depression in *DSMs* and *ICDs*. Because of efforts to harmonize the two, recognition in either is likely to lead to recognition in both. In addition to the *ICD-10-CM* chapter on mental disorders, advocates can consider targeting other chapters, such as *ICD-10-CM*'s Z-codes for a place in the classification system. A less prominent option is noncoded recognition in the *DSMs* under the "Other" categories. Pending progress in getting late-onset depression recognized in *ICD* and *DSM* classification systems, clinicians can consider documenting specific signs of late-depression that are already in the nomenclature and coding of *ICD-9-CM* and *ICD-10-CM*.

Disclosure

Dr. Peele has no conflict of interests to disclose. He is fully funded by the Montgomery County, Maryland, government.

REFERENCES

American Psychiatric Association. (1952). *Diagnostic and statistical manual of mental disorders*. Washington, DC: Author.

American Psychiatric Association, DSM-5 Scientific Review Committee. (2011, February 1). Introductory comments for "The structure of the requested memos outlining evidence for change ."

Beach, S. R. H., Wamboldt, M. Z., Kaslow, N. J., Heyman, R. J., First, M. B., Underwood, L. G., & Reiss, D. (Eds.). (2006). *Relational process and DSM-V: Neuroscience, assessment, prevention, and treatment*. Washington, DC: American Psychiatric Association.

Dimsdale, J. E., Xin, Y., Kleinman, A., & Patel, V. (Eds.). 2009. *Somatic presentations on mental disorders*. Washington, DC: American Psychiatric Association.

Helzer, J. E., Kraemer, H. C., Krueger, R. F., & Wittchen, H-U. (2008). *Dimensional approaches in diagnostic classification*. Washington, DC: American Psychiatric Association.

Hyman, S. (2003). Forward. In K. A. Phillips, M. B. First, & H. A. Pincus (Eds.), *Advancing*

DSM: Dilemmas in psychiatric diagnosis (pp. xx–xx). Washington, DC: American Psychiatric Association.

Hyman, S. (2010, December 11–12). *Metastructure.* Presentation to the Board of Trustees Meeting.

International Advisory Group for the Revision of ICD-10 Mental and Behavioural Disorders. (2011). A conceptual framework for the revision of the ICD-10 classification of mental and behavioural disorders. *World Psychiatry 10,* 86–92.

Kupfer, D. J., First, M. B., & Regier, D. A. (Eds.). (2002). *A research agenda for DSM-V.* Washington, DC: American Psychiatric Association.

Mood Disorders Work Group, DSM-5 Task Force. (n.d.). *Depressive disorders.* Retrieved June 30, 2011 from the American Psychiatric Association Web site, http://www.dsm5.org/proposedrevision/Pages/DepressiveDisorders.aspx

Narrow, W. E., First, M. B., Sorpvatka, P. J., & Regier, D. A. (2007). *Age and gender considerations in psychiatric diagnosing.* Washington, DC: American Psychiatric Association.

Regier, D. A., Narrow, W. E., & Kuhl, E. A. (Eds.). (2011). *The conceptual evolution of DSM-5.* Washington, DC: American Psychiatric Association.

Widiger, T. A., Simonsen, E., Sirovatka, P. J., & Regier, D. A. (Eds.). (2006). *Dimesional models of personality disorders.* Washington, DC: American Psychiatric Association.

SECTION 2

DIAGNOSIS AND COMORBID CONDITIONS

6

THE DIAGNOSIS AND TREATMENT OF UNIPOLAR DEPRESSION IN LATE LIFE

John Snowdon and Osvaldo P. Almeida

IN GENERAL parlance, depression means a state of dejection—a lowering of spirits that is commonly related to real or perceived loss. Such depression may be transient or prolonged. Temporarily depressed mood and depression that last only a few hours or days (even if associated with disturbed sleep and appetite) do not usually require clinical interventions. If they persist longer, with various physical and emotional manifestations, and prolonged interference with ability to function (physically, socially, emotionally, and/or cognitively), they are called depressive disorders. How a distressing situation affects an individual (*and whether a clinically significant depression develops*) will depend on a complexity of factors, including genetic vulnerability, previous experience of loss or stress, and the perceived meaning of the situation for the individual. For example, awareness that a serious illness is causing or will lead to physical limitations might be much more depressing for one person than another. If self-esteem, sense of self-worth, and control over one's life are detrimentally affected by a medical condition, depression may develop. The pattern of factors associated with late-life depression tends to be different from that associated with depression earlier in life, and depression tends to present differently in old age.

This chapter focuses on unipolar depression in late life. The *Diagnostic and Statistical Manual of Mental Disorders*, fourth edition (*DSM-IV*; American Psychiatric Association, 1994) divides Mood Disorders into "the Depressive Disorders ('unipolar depression'), the Bipolar Disorders, and two disorders based on etiology—Mood Disorder Due to a General Medical Condition and Substance-Induced Mood Disorder." It distinguishes the depressive from bipolar disorders by the fact that the latter are associated with one or more past episodes of mania, hypomania, or mixed affect. A small proportion of bipolar disorder cases do not declare themselves as bipolar until later in life; prior to old age they may have presented once or recurrently as cases of major depression. Those cases where the first manifestations of elevated mood do not occur until old age seem more commonly associated with brain disease or head injury (Almeida & Fenner, 2002; Shulman & Post, 1980; Young & Falk, 1989). Diagnosis and treatment of bipolar cases are discussed in Chapter 6; "undeclared" bipolar cases will not receive separate consideration in the present chapter.

Reifler (1994, p. 55) stated that "when geriatric psychiatrists talk about depression in elderly persons, they are usually referring to major depression." *DSM-IV* lists major depressive disorder, dysthymic disorder, and depressive disorder not otherwise specified (n.o.s.) as the *Depressive Disorders* (*i.e., unipolar depression*) and provides criteria for their diagnosis. If five or more from a *DSM-IV* set of symptom criteria are fulfilled (Criterion A: see Box 6.1), the diagnosis is major depression, whereas diagnoses of dysthymic disorder and depressive disorder n.o.s. can be made with fewer of these criteria fulfilled. Differentiation of unipolar depression that fulfils criteria for major depression from "normal" sadness is usually clear, whereas differentiation of so-called minor and subthreshold depressions from "normality" may prove difficult. *DSM-IV* does not categorize adjustment disorder with depressed mood as a depressive disorder (stating specifically that it is not a depressive disorder n.o.s.).

Other chapters give detailed consideration to late-life presentations of dysthymic disorder, depressive disorders n.o.s., mood disorder due to general medical conditions, and substance-induced mood disorder. The present chapter discusses the diagnosis and treatment of cases of *major depression* in late life—including those with biological changes but with no definite evidence that depression was a direct physiological consequence of such changes. The chapter includes discussion of major depression presenting in old age following loss or stress, as well as depressions extending for more than 2 months after bereavement and fulfilling criteria for major depression. It gives attention to clinical depression diagnosed as adjustment disorder, fulfilling several (but not five or more) criteria for major depression.

Box 6.1: Criterion A, Major Depressive Episode

As in younger adults, a <u>diagnosis of major depression</u> is made in late life only if relevant symptoms represent a change from previous functioning and have been present for at least two weeks. The symptoms must cause significant distress or impairment of functioning, and not be better accounted for by bereavement or direct physiological effects of a substance or general medical condition. For most of the time, the person must have had

   (i) *depressed mood and/or*
   (ii) *loss of interest or pleasure*
       together with enough of the following to add to at least 5 of the symptoms altogether:
  (iii) *significant weight/appetite change,*
   (iv) *insomnia or hypersomnia,*
    (v) *observable psychomotor agitation or retardation,*
   (vi) *fatigue or loss of energy,*
  (vii) *feeling worthless or excessively/inappropriately guilty,*
 (viii) *inability to think, decide things, or concentrate,*
   (ix) *recurrent thoughts of death or suicide*

SHORTCOMINGS OF EXISTING CLASSIFICATIONS OF DEPRESSION

The main reasons for promoting a diagnostic classification of mood disorders are to (1) facilitate communication and discussion between clinicians, so that they have the same understanding when using particular terms; (2) examine factors associated with particular disorders in order to better understand their causes; and (3) observe their course and the factors that may affect the natural history of the disorder, thus developing an awareness of what interventions and treatments are optimal, taking coincident circumstances into account.

The two most widely used classification systems for mental disorders (*The International Classification of Diseases* [ICD-10] and *DSM-IV*) have shortcomings and are in the process of revision. In particular, the *DSM-IV* diagnosis of depressive disorder does not provide a useful guide regarding management. Current proposals for *DSM-5* (accessed May 2012) on www.dsm5.org/ProposedRevision/Pages/DepressiveDisorders.aspx may add the category of mixed anxiety/depression to *DSM-5*'s section on conditions that require further research, and it would retain major depressive disorder (but removing the bereavement exclusion). Depressive disorder associated with a known general medical condition (formerly included in mood disorder due to a medical condition) is defined by the same criteria as major depression plus a requirement that the episode is thought to be a function of the direct physiological effects of "another medical condition." There is ongoing discussion of how to code depression in cases of Alzheimer's disease or other neurocognitive disorders. It is as yet unclear whether the new classification system will provide better guidance than the *DSM-IV* regarding the efficacy and effectiveness of specific management strategies in cases of depression.

Parker (2009) commented that *DSM-IV* and *ICD-10* diagnoses have low utility in pointing to causation of depressions or in guidance about treatment options. Fink and Taylor (2007) called the *DSM-IV* classification "arbitrary"; its diagnostic criteria are "imprecise, inadequate for treatment decisions, and do not assure homogeneous populations in clinical trials" (p. 14). Blazer (1994) considered that the *DSM* classification needed additional diagnostic categories to adequately classify the depressive disorders experienced by elderly people. Caine et al. (1994) argued that the syndromically defined diagnoses that had occupied nosology for the previous two decades, *while enhancing research rigour and reliability* [our italics], have also created an environment of "intentional suppression of variability"; confounding factors such as medical illnesses were being "defined out" of studies.

ICD-10 provides a partly dimensional model (depressive episodes being classified as mild, moderate, or severe), but with categorical elements (mild and moderate each being divided into cases with or without "somatic syndrome"; severe being divided into cases with or without mood-congruent or mood-incongruent psychotic symptoms). Parker (2009) referred to the *DSM-IV* model as a mixed one, with dimensions based on severity, persistence, and recurrence, but with provision for categorical second-order decisions by specifying the presence of melancholia, or psychotic or atypical features. He declared (p. 5) that "by including quite disparate expressions of depression (from slight to substantive) within broad overall categories, the causes, pathogenesis, natural history, and potential differential treatment responses of the constituent conditions are effectively blended and so are resistant to dissection." He commented (p. 6) that "an even greater problem—as it impacts on whether patients receive appropriate treatment—is to assume that a diagnosis of major depression is sufficient to dictate treatment choice."

Van Praag (2009) stated that the diagnosis "major depression" (which he considered a "pure categorical construct") covers a great many, if not most, depressive syndromes and has low validity. He agreed with Parker that data on personality structure and (dys)function, as well as a measure of stress burden, should be included in (depression) diagnosis. "It is relevant in determining whether or not structural forms of psychotherapy or social intervention should be included in the therapeutic programme" (p. 46).

Zisook (2009) noted that the *DSM-5* and *ICD-11* Committees were championing the incorporation of dimensional approaches when refining the diagnosis of all major psychiatric disorders, and he posited (p. 29) that "dimensional diagnoses have the advantage of more fully describing and delineating depressive disorders." He and Angst (2009) agreed with Parker (2009) that it would be desirable to classify depression by etiology but said that for the time being, this is simply not possible. "All we know", said Angst (2009, p. 38) "is that the etiology is multifactorial, including multiple genetic, epigenetic and environmental elements. Until we are wiser, it is advisable to apply descriptive dimensional measures as much as possible." He added that "the redefinition of melancholia by observable psychomotor disturbance" is important and should stimulate further research. Shorter (2007) declared that melancholic mood disorder should be established as one of two principal entities in *DSM-5*'s mood disorder section. Fink and Taylor (2007) argued that such a demarcation would lead to more effective treatment algorithms and better understanding of the pathophysiology of mood disorders.

CLASSIFYING LATE-LIFE DEPRESSION

The advantage of a diagnostic classification of late-life depression based on etiology would be that the diagnostic formulation would indicate which treatment approach to favor. Testing the validity of the classification would include assessing whether etiology-suggested treatments actually work. For example, a depression believed to be a response to a particular stress (be it physical or environmental) might be expected to be relieved by agents that neutralize the stress.

One hypothesized etiological category of particular relevance to late-life depression is *vascular depression*. There are abundant correlational data showing that white matter hyperintensities, seen on neuroimaging, are found more frequently in the brains of older people with depression than in a matched control population (Alexopoulos et al., 1997; Krishnan, Hays, George, & Blazer, 1998). There is robust evidence that these hyperintensities correspond to vascular changes in the brains of patients who have accompanying vascular risk factors, such as hypertension, diabetes, and dyslipidemia. The prevalence of white matter hyperintensities rises dramatically with increasing age (de Leeuw et al., 2001), as does the prevalence of hypertension, diabetes, and cardiovascular diseases (Australian Institute of Health and Welfare, 2004). However, although disputed (Snowdon, 2001), a majority of researchers appear to believe that the prevalence of depression is no higher in older than younger adults (Kessler et al., 2003), in which case there is a dissociation between the prevalence rates of cardiovascular risk factors and of depression. This suggests that vascular pathology does not cause the depression (Almeida, 2008).

Alexopoulos et al. (1997) regarded late onset of depression (after age 65 years) and evidence of vascular disease as the cardinal features of vascular depression, generally with associated disturbance in executive functioning, and with psychomotor retardation and reduced interest in activities. Krishnan et al. (2004) described the clinical characteristics of "subcortical ischaemic depression," the definition of which depends on magnetic resonance imaging findings. In a study of depressed elderly participants, Kim et al. (2011) found that geriatric depression with impaired executive function was related to cerebrovascular attacks, unlike depression without executive dysfunction. The former were significantly more likely to present with psychomotor retardation and feelings of worthlessness and guilt. Even with varying definitions, there would be good reason to expect an age-associated increase in vascular disease would lead to a higher incidence of "vascular depression" in late life. Most cases (not all) can be expected to be of late onset.

Numerous attempts have been made to differentiate people with early-onset depression (EOD) and late-onset depression (LOD) based on their clinical presentation. For example, Krishnan et al. (1995) examined differences between cases of EOD and LOD among patients aged over 60 years with unipolar depression. They first excluded from their sample patients with dementia, major neurological disorders, or depression secondary to medication or medical illnesses. They noted that LOD patients had had fewer depressive episodes, though

the frequency since their first episode was higher. Apathy was commoner in LOD. EOD patients had higher rates of family history of substance abuse and suicide, and they were more likely to report guilt feelings. Psychomotor retardation has been reported as equally common in the two groups (Brodaty et al., 1991; Krishnan, Hays, Tupler, George, & Blazer, 1995), though in the oldest old, psychomotor retardation and loss of energy are associated with vascular or neurodegenerative risk factors (Hegeman, Kok, van der Mast, & Giltay, 2012).

There is also some evidence that life events and negative social circumstances may play a more prominent role in LOD than EOD (Blazer & Hybels, 2005). However, the specificity of these associations is low and, at this stage, they cannot be used to guide the classification of depression. Noting their presence could help guide management strategies, though there are currently no data showing that their systematic assessment and management change the clinical outcome of patients. EOD patients take longer to achieve remission than LOD patients (Reynolds et al., 1998).

THE PHENOMENOLOGY OF EARLY-LIFE AND LATE-LIFE DEPRESSION

A meta-analysis of 11 reports comparing the features of major depression in older and in younger people showed more agitation, general somatic symptoms, and hypochondriasis among the older participants, but less guilt and less loss of sexual interest (Hegeman et al., 2012). On average, older people had significantly more severe depression, though the researchers questioned whether this could be explained by overlapping somatic symptoms and comorbid age-related physical disorders in older populations. Older adults with depression complain more frequently of pain (Clarke, Piterman, Byrne, & Austin, 2008) and are more likely to experience subtle cognitive deficits (Beats, Sahakian, & Levy, 1996). Brodaty et al. (1991) found psychosis to occur more often among elderly than younger people referred to a tertiary service.

SUBTYPING MAJOR DEPRESSION

Diagnosing that a person has major rather than minor depression implies greater severity. However, the diagnosis says nothing about causation—the relevance of life events, situations, vulnerabilities, comorbid conditions, genetics, or biological changes. There is good reason for postulating that cases of major depression variously have predominantly biological, psychological, or environmental causation, and for suggesting that subtyping could facilitate treatment approaches that accord with clinicians' formulations regarding etiology and factors that affect presentation.

DSM-IV specifiers allow for a subclassification of major depression into psychotic, melancholic, and other types. However, etiological and treatment studies of those with *DSM-IV*-defined melancholia have failed to generate support for its specificity as a category (Parker & Hadzi-Pavlovic, 1996). Parker (2009) pointed out that five of the eight criteria for a *DSM-IV* diagnosis of melancholia are essentially the same as those for major depression; the three non-shared criteria are mood nonreactivity, mood worse in the morning, and distinct quality of mood. Parker and colleagues (Parker & Hadzi-Pavlovic, 1996) have argued for observable psychomotor disturbance as a specific and discriminating feature of melancholia, whereas symptoms commonly regarded as markers of melancholia (so-called endogeneity symptoms) are also common in other depressive disorders. They showed that their CORE measure of noninteractiveness, agitation, and retardation was superior to assessment of endogeneity symptoms in distinguishing melancholia (redefined) from non-melancholic depressions. Parker (2011) highlighted that meta-analyses have suggested that psychotic depression, melancholia, and nonmelancholic unipolar depression have differing response rates to different types of antidepressant, combined or not with antipsychotic medication. Arguing for more consequential definitions, he proposed criteria for "clinical depression," to distinguish it from normal mood states. A diagnosis of the melancholic subtype would require at least five (from a list of eight) symptom criteria to be fulfilled in addition to those for "clinical depression." If, in addition, the person has delusions and/or hallucinations, the diagnosis would be psychotic depression.

DSM-IV also provides an atypical features specifier, but two studies found little evidence to support its status as a syndrome (Parker, 2009). Atypical depression is said to be less common in old age. It has been suggested that including age of onset and chronicity as *DSM* criteria would define a more homogeneous group that is distinct from melancholia and other depression (Stewart, McGrath,

Quitkin, & Klein, 2007). Like dysthymic disorder, it seems likely that those with major depression with atypical features are more likely to have superimposed personality disorders, which might suggest that treatment with psychotherapy may be particularly useful in the management of these cases. Unfortunately, confirmatory data are lacking.

DIFFERENTIAL DIAGNOSIS OF MAJOR DEPRESSION IN LATE LIFE

Currently, despite criticisms related to its utility in relation to planning treatment, the *DSM* system is widely used in classifying late-life depression. Differential diagnosis (see Box 6.2) depends partly on whether symptoms can be attributed to the effects of medication or bodily disease (e.g., loss of energy related to anemia). Marked psychomotor disturbance may point to the possibility of diagnosing major depression with melancholic features, while inappropriate guilt or feeling worthless may raise the possibility of psychotic depression.

Differentiating major depression from dysthymic disorder depends on assessment of severity, chronicity, and persistence. Depressed mood for more than half the days for at least 2 years, plus two or more from a list of symptoms that includes diminished self-esteem, and no symptom-free periods lasting over 2 months, allows a diagnosis of dysthymic disorder—unless the threshold number of features allowing a diagnosis of long-lasting major depression has been reached. Many of those so diagnosed can be regarded as having characterological, but often situation-related, depression. There may be evidence of coexisting personality disorder. Depression with the same features but of duration less than 2 years is diagnosed as minor depression or depression n.o.s., and it may be less often personality related.

Adjustment disorder with depressed mood is diagnosed when depression develops in response to (and within 3 months of onset of) a stressor, but it is called major depression if criteria for the latter are fulfilled. If the depression persists more than 6 months after the stressor and its consequences cease, it is no longer called "adjustment."

Because this chapter is focused on unipolar major depressive disorder, the factors contributing to causation and persistence of other types of late-life depression will not receive consideration here. It is evident, however, that the borders between major depression and other depressive disorders are not clear-cut. Diagnosis depends on the number of symptoms (from a list) and interpretations of "most of the day" and "most days." In severe cases (including most of those with psychomotor disturbance and/or psychotic manifestations, most of whom would have six to nine of the symptoms listed in Box 6.1) there is no boundary difficulty. Those manifesting just five of the symptoms may have histories and associated factors that are similar to those manifesting four of the symptoms. A large proportion is likely to report apparently relevant losses or ongoing stressful situations.

A *DSM-IV* diagnosis of major depressive episode following bereavement depends on whether the symptoms have persisted longer than 2 months or are characterized by marked functional impairment or other indicators of severity. A person responding to a major loss (but not of a loved one) and presenting five or more Criterion A symptoms (Box 6.1) for more than 2 weeks can be diagnosed as having major depression. The same does not apply to a person bereaved for between 2 weeks and 2 months and presenting five or more Criterion A symptoms, unless that person is morbidly preoccupied with worthlessness, suicidal ideas, or psychotic symptoms, or shows psychomotor retardation. Those responsible for *DSM-5* have agreed with arguments (e.g., by Zisook et al., 2010) that bereavement should no longer be an exemption criterion when considering a diagnosis of major depression. Decisions on management of such cases will not depend on diagnoses; they will depend on formulations concerning how and why an individual has responded to a loss, and the meaning of that loss.

FACTORS ASSOCIATED WITH LATE-LIFE UNIPOLAR DEPRESSION

Numerous factors are thought to play some role in the causation of depression in later life, including psychosocial factors, genetic vulnerability, biochemical imbalances, brain lesions, and medical morbidity. This complexity of associations suggests that depression is either a very heterogeneous condition or that different factors converge into a common physiological pathway that ultimately leads to the expression of a major depressive disorder. In this section, we will review the possible contribution of these factors to the causation of depression in later life (Fig. 6.1).

Genetic Vulnerability

Evidence from twins and family studies of younger adults shows that vulnerability to depression runs in families, but concordance even among identical twins is only about 40% (for review of genetic studies of depression, see Levinson, 2006). Such findings suggest that genetic factors interact with the environment to express the depressive phenotype.

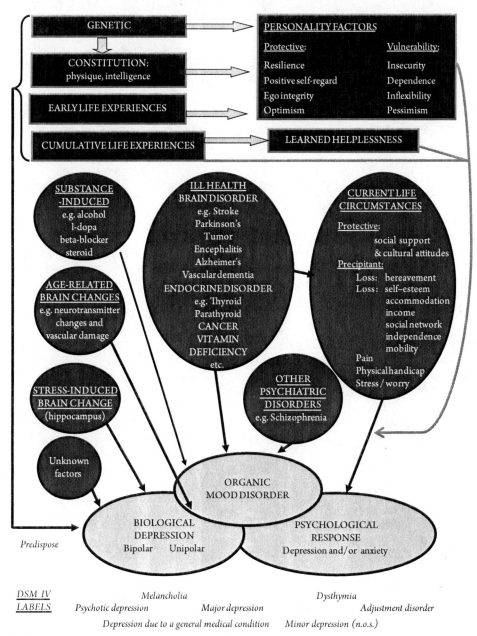

FIGURE 6.1 Factors in the development of late-life depression.

One particular genetic variation (polymorphism) that has received substantial attention over the past 10 years occurs on the serotonin transporter promoter gene (*5-HTTLPR*). Adults carrying one or two copies of the relatively low-expressing short (S, as opposed to the wild-type long L) allele are more likely to display clinically significant depressive symptoms and suicidal ideation when exposed to repetitive stress (i.e., the association between this polymorphism and depression/suicide ideation only becomes apparent when stress is present; Caspi et al., 2003). A recent meta-analysis confirmed that this polymorphism increases the risk of depression after exposure to stress (Karg, Burmeister, Shedden, & Sen, 2011), although no systematic data on this topic are currently available for older adults.

Almeida and colleagues (Almeida, Norman, et al., 2009) showed that a common polymorphism of the C-reactive protein (CRP) gene that decreases the basal serum concentration of CRP nearly doubles the risk of depression in older men. The authors speculated that carriers of this particular polymorphism were less competent at mounting allostatic responses to physiological stress, thereby triggering a chain of events that culminated with the expression of depressive symptoms and behaviors (Almeida, 2011). Like the 5-HTTLPR studies, these results suggest that the genetic vulnerability to depression may be linked to the diminished ability of carriers to cope with stress.

Recently published data suggested the existence of a possible link between variation on a neuron-specific neutral aminoacid transporter gene, hippocampal changes, and susceptibility to depression. Kohli and colleagues (2011) used an animal model and human clinical and neuroimaging data to show that variation in this particular gene decreases its expression in the hippocampus, hinders the ability of mice to cope with stress, and increases the expression of depressive symptoms in humans. These data offer a plausible link between genetic vulnerability, stress, and hippocampal changes in association with depression (see also neuroimaging findings on depression later in this chapter). However, one should also acknowledge that candidate-gene and genetic-linkage studies of depression have failed to produce consistent results to date, and that genetic data on older people with depression are very sparse.

Biochemical Changes Associated With Depression

Depression has been associated with several biochemical abnormalities over the years, although none has proven sufficiently sensitive or specific to be useful in practice. Nevertheless, it is appropriate to provide a brief review of this topic.

Broadly speaking, the biochemical changes that have been linked to depression can be grouped into two categories: (1) markers of morbidities that increase the risk of depression and (2) markers indicative of depression independent of other morbidities. The first group includes tests of thyroid dysfunction and other hormonal abnormalities, vitamin deficiencies, lipid imbalances, and inflammatory markers, among others. The second includes biochemical markers of monoamine activity, cortisol suppression, and novel approaches such as stimulated gene expression profile.

A recent investigation showed that subtle changes (up or down) in the serum concentration of thyroid-stimulating hormone and free thyroxin are not associated with greater risk of incident depression in older men (Almeida et al., 2011a). The authors concluded that their results did not support the proposed link between subclinical thyroid dysfunction and depression in later life (Helfand, 2004). There has also been some suggestion that lower serum concentrations of testosterone and estradiol increase the risk of depression (Almeida, Yeap, Hankey, Jamrozik, & Flicker, 2008), and preliminary evidence from small randomized trials of hormone replacement therapy is consistent with such a hypothesis (Soares, Almeida, Joffe, & Cohen, 2001). However, data from larger trials indicate that hormone replacement with testosterone (Idan et al., 2010) or estradiol (Heiss et al., 2008) increases morbidity and the risk of death compared with placebo.

Deficiencies of certain B vitamins, particularly folate and B12, increase the plasma concentration of total homocysteine and have been associated with depression in observational studies (Almeida, McCaul, et al., 2008). A randomized trial of supplementation with folate and vitamins B12 and B6 showed a decreased incidence of depression after stroke over a period of 10 years (Almeida et al., 2010), but such data were limited to stroke survivors and it remains unclear whether these findings can be generalized to a broader population of older adults at risk of depression. In addition, there is no compelling evidence at present that the use of B vitamins (or lowering of total plasma homocysteine) improves treatment response of older adults with depression.

Depression has also been associated with unfavorable lipid profiles, reduced high-density lipoprotein cholesterol being associated with melancholia and elevated low-density lipoprotein cholesterol with atypical depression (van Reedt Dortland et al., 2010). Observational data have also suggested that metabolic syndrome in mid and early late life may be associated with increased risk of depression (Akbaraly et al., 2011; Almeida, Calver, Jamrozik, Hankey, & Flicker, 2009), although those findings have not been replicated consistently and there is no evidence from randomized trials that lipid-lowering treatment with statins improves mood—in fact, the opposite may be true (Hyyppa, Kronholm, Virtanen, Leino, & Jula, 2003).

There is abundant animal and observational data showing that inflammatory markers (such as CRP, interleukin 6, and tumor necrosis factor alpha) tend to be raised in depression (including among older people) (Almeida, Norman, Hankey, Jamrozik, & Flicker, 2007; Dantzer, O'Connor, Freund, Johnson, & Kelley, 2008) and that cytokines may contribute to triggering symptoms such as decreased responsivity, loss of appetite, sleep disturbance, and decreased energy. However, inflammatory markers have no value in the assessment and diagnosis of depression due to their very poor specificity. Evidence from a handful of small randomized trials using anti-inflammatory drugs as adjuvants to normal antidepressant treatment have produced inconclusive results (Akhondzadeh et al., 2009; Muller et al., 2006), although no such data are yet available for older people.

Attempts to establish biochemical markers of depression have also proven unsuccessful up to now. Cerebrospinal fluid metabolites of serotonin (5-hydroxyindole acetic acid) are not consistently associated with depression, but they seem to be decreased in people with greater impulsivity (Lidberg, Tuck, Asberg, Scalia-Tomba, & Bertilsson, 1985). Similarly, the dexamethasone suppression test has unacceptably low sensitivity for the diagnosis of depression and its results change in accordance with the mental state of the individual. Absence of suppression seems to predict relapse after adequate response to treatment (Carroll, 1982).

Structural Brain Abnormalities

Subcortical and periventricular white matter hyperintensities in magnetic resonance imaging studies are the most frequent and consistent associations with depression in later life, particularly when the disorder has its onset in older age (Herrmann, Le Masurier, & Ebmeier, 2008). Neuropathological studies have demonstrated that such white matter lesions have an ischemic basis (Thomas et al., 2002), which lends support to the vascular hypothesis of depression in later life (Alexopoulos et al., 1997). However, as discussed earlier, others have argued that such changes lack specificity and are unlikely to be causally related to depression in later life (Almeida, 2008; de Leeuw et al., 2001).

Nonvascular changes to the brain have also been reported in association with depression. Findings suggest that hippocampal changes resulting from repeated stress (as happens with repeated depressive episodes) are associated with increased risk of depression and, possibly, cognitive impairment (Duman, Heninger, & Nestler, 1997; Sapolsky, 2001). Depression with later onset has been shown to be associated with decreased hippocampal volume in both cerebral hemispheres (Lloyd et al., 2004); these changes are linked to persisting cognitive deficits among older people with depression (O'Brien, Lloyd, McKeith, Gholkar, & Ferrier, 2004). Treatment with antidepressants may reverse some of these hippocampal changes (Sheline, Gado, & Kraemer, 2003), possibly because they enhance the action of brain-derived neurotrophic factor in this particular brain region (Martinowich, Manji, & Lu, 2007).

Depression in later life has also been associated with loss of frontal lobe volume or mass (Almeida, Burton, Ferrier, McKeith, & O'O'Brien, 2003; Goveas et al., 2011; Lavretsky, Ballmaier, Pham, Toga, & Kumar, 2007), and although the origin of these changes remains unclear, they are thought to contribute to some of the cognitive deficits displayed by older people with depression (Herrmann, Goodwin, & Ebmeier, 2007). Other brain changes affecting the limbic system, in particular the anterior cingulate, have also been reported in association with depression in later life (Ballmaier et al., 2004), but their relevance to the causation of symptoms is not well understood.

Taken together, these results suggest that depression in later life is associated with some brain abnormalities. The challenge must be to work out how this information can be used to improve current classification systems and the management of patients.

Medical Comorbidity

Over recent years, much has been made of the association between depression in later life and cardiovascular diseases (including coronary heart disease, cardiac failure, and strokes) (Alexopoulos et al., 1997; Musselman, Evans, & Nemeroff, 1998), although a relatively high prevalence of depression is found in association with most chronic illnesses (Krishnan et al., 2002). For example, between a quarter and a half of patients with chronic obstructive pulmonary disease display clinically significant symptoms of depression (Wilson, 2006), as do adults with cancer (Massie, 2004), neurodegenerative diseases (Reijnders, Ehrt, Weber, Aarsland, & Leentjens, 2008), and chronic pain (Bair, Robinson, Katon, & Kroenke, 2003). Depression is common among older people with dementia, with most estimates suggesting that 1 in 3 affected people will display clinically significant symptoms of depression at any one point in time (Lyketsos et al., 2002). Taken together, these findings indicate that patients with chronic medical conditions would benefit from systematic screening for depression. They also show that the association between medical morbidity and depression is not specific to a particular set of illnesses.

Prince et al. (1997, 1998) reported that higher rates of depression relate mainly to the degree of functional impairment and handicap resulting from the health problem. Handicap due to disability was found to be the most significant predictor of the development of pervasive depression, but persistence of depression was more strongly related to low levels of social support and social participation. In a community study, Beekman et al. (1997) found that chronic physical illness and functional impairment were associated with minor but not major depression, and that significant interactions between ill health and social support were found only for minor depression. They concluded that major depression has its origins in long-standing personality vulnerability.

Psychosocial Factors and Lifestyle

Depression is more prevalent in women than men (Hasin, Goodwin, Stinson, & Grant, 2005), although this gender discrepancy all but disappears in later life. Early life adversities, such as physical or sexual abuse, can also increase the risk of depression, even later in life (Almeida et al., 2011b). Limited education, psychosocial deprivation, and loss of parents during childhood contribute to enhancing the risk of depression throughout the life span; socioeconomic disadvantage increases the risk of prevalent and persistent depression

in later life (Almeida et al., 2012). It is possible that this may contribute to the adoption of hazardous lifestyle practices, such as smoking, alcohol abuse/dependence, use of substances, and physical inactivity, which in turn may facilitate the development of health hazards such as obesity, diabetes, hypertension, and social isolation (Almeida et al., 2011b). Medical comorbidities may ensue and, together with financial concerns and loss of loved ones, might tilt the balance in favor of the development of depressive symptoms (Koster et al., 2006).

We have recently suggested that some of the factors that increase the risk of depression in later life are due to chance, whereas others are a direct or indirect consequence of choices (Almeida, 2011). We have also argued that the pathways that lead to the onset of depressive symptoms are probabilistic rather than deterministic, and that observational and trial-derived data can (and should) be used to guide the introduction of consumer-tailored risk-reduction strategies. Figure 6.2 illustrates how risk factors might accumulate over time to facilitate the expression of depressive symptoms later in life.

MANAGEMENT OF LATE-LIFE DEPRESSION

Giving Attention to the Factor(s) That Led to Development of Depression

Because late-life depression commonly has a multifactorial etiology, treatment needs to be

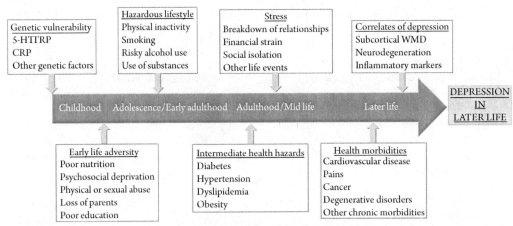

FIGURE 6.2 The figure illustrates how risk factors accumulate throughout the life span to increase the risk of depression, including later in life. Note that the placement of the vertical arrows is not meant to be accurate. WMD, white matter disease.

personalized and should take account of individual risk factors. The first step in management of unipolar depression is to try to understand why the person became and remains depressed, exploring particularly any underlying or associated medical, personality, and social factors (Figs. 6.1 and 6.2). Assessments should include gathering of full medical, psychiatric, and personal histories, together with information about current circumstances. Where indicated, medical examination should be arranged or conducted and details of recent medical examinations and investigations sought. Further tests, including neuroimaging, may be appropriate.

This chapter conforms to a biopsychosocial model of depression. If a particular factor appears likely to have been the precipitant of the mood disorder, it is appropriate to provide a relevant intervention. Thus, if a person's depression arose after beta-blocker treatment was commenced, and there were no other obvious precipitants, that medication should be ceased (if possible) and there may be no need for other treatments. If a person with depression is found to be hypothyroid, or there is good evidence of low folate levels or other medical problems, those medical problems should receive attention before embarking on antidepressant medication. The formulation can be changed later, if necessary, depending on response to interventions. If a person has undergone a recent, or even a persistent, loss or bereavement, grief therapy (counseling, ventilation and exploration of feelings, environmental change, etc.) may be the active agent—though various pharmaceutical aids may be considered at some stage. Our view is that a diagnosis of unipolar depression should not automatically lead to prescription of antidepressant medication. Antidepressive therapy is indicated, yes, but programmed according to perceived pathoplastic factors.

It is common for major depressive disorder to be undiagnosed and untreated among older adults (Gelenberg et al., APA Practice Guidelines, 2010), often being misattributed to physical illness, dementia, or the aging process. Studies in primary care have shown low rates of antidepressant treatment of older patients with probable depressive disorders (Unützer et al., 2000). Depression accompanying chronic physical illness or disability (not necessarily a physiological consequence of the medical condition) may erroneously be regarded as expected or inevitable, and therefore be overlooked.

Undertreatment may be a result of excessive caution by doctors when prescribing for elderly people, partly related to their awareness of altered pharmacodynamics in old age.

The APA guidelines include a section relating to old age, and they mention that psychosocial factors are frequent contributors to depression in this age group. They note that older patients are more likely to experience relapses and less likely to achieve a full response to treatment with antidepressants.

Efficacy and Effectiveness of Varying Approaches in Treating Late-Life Depression

Evidence for the efficacy and effectiveness of various treatments for late-life depression has been reviewed. Chiu et al. (2009) commented that the "old old" (i.e., persons aged over 75 years) have been underrepresented in randomized controlled trials of late-life depression treatment, as have physically ill and institutionalized elderly. Most such randomized controlled trials have examined use of antidepressants, whereas routine clinical management usually involves a combination of interventions. There are doubts about whether data obtained from these randomized controlled trials can be generalized, since most have involved stringent exclusion criteria, so that those selected for the trials have not been truly representative of cases of late-life depression, or even of late-life major depression. Complex questions regarding which combination of interventions best suit particular subtypes of depression remain largely unaddressed. Few studies have examined the effectiveness of antidepressants combined with psychotherapy or other nonpharmacological interventions. Schneider and Olin (1995) commented that symptom reduction was generally the only outcome assessed in clinical trials, even though (as stated by Alexopoulos, 2005) antidepressive treatment has a number of additional aims.

Table 6.1 summarizes the evidence for efficacy and effectiveness in relation to antidepressants, psychotherapy, combined treatments, electroconvulsive therapy, transcranial stimulation, and collaborative care in treating older patients. Malhi et al. (2009) have provided clinical practice recommendations, algorithms, and levels of evidence regarding treatment of depression in adults. In contrast, evidence to support recommendations specifically for treatment of late-life depression is sparse.

Table 6.1 Evidence-Based Summary of the Efficacy and Effectiveness of Various Antidepressant Treatments in Later Life

INDEX INTERVENTION	CONTROL INTERVENTION	*EVIDENCE THAT INDEX INTERVENTION IS COMPARATIVELY ASSOCIATED WITH	
		GREATER REMISSION OF SYMPTOMS	LESS RELAPSE AND/OR RECURRENCE
Antidepressants	Placebo	Level I	Level I
Non-tricyclic antidepressants	Placebo	Level I	Level I
Tricyclic antidepressants	Placebo	Level I	Level I
Tricyclic antidepressants	SSRIs	Level II	Not established
SSRIs	Tricyclic antidepressants	Level IVa	Not established
Antidepressant + psychotherapy	Antidepressant	Level IVb	Level IVb
Cognitive-behavioral therapy	Waiting list/usual care	Level I	Level IVb
Interpersonal therapy	Waiting list/usual care	Level II	Level II
Problem-solving therapy	Waiting list/usual care	Level II	Not established
Physical activity	Usual care	Level II	Level II
Omega-3	Placebo	Level IVa	Not established
Folate, B12	Placebo	Level IVa	Not established
Bibliotherapy	Usual care	Not established	Not established

*Evidence of effect:
Level I, supported by one or more meta-analyses of at least three well-conducted randomized trials.
Level II, supported by at least one well-conducted randomized trial.
Level III, supported by nonrandomized controlled trials.
Level IVa, supported by noncontrolled trials (case series with pre- and postintervention assessments).
Level IVb, supported by expert opinion without systematic critical appraisal.

Efficacy and Effectiveness of Antidepressant Treatment of Late-Life Depression

Most subjects of antidepressant drug trials are not elderly, and most have nonmelancholic depressions. Improvement rates of 30% to 60% are seen (Quitkin, 1999). The question of whether response rates are the same when *older* depressed people are given antidepressants needs consideration.

Analysis has suggested that response in antidepressant drug trials is made up of spontaneous improvement (24%), placebo effect (51%), and a "true" drug effect of about 25% (Kirsch & Sapirstein, 1998). However, improvements due to

a so-called placebo effect occur in less than 20% of cases of psychotic or melancholic depression. Malhi et al. (2005) cited evidence to suggest that only one quarter of patients with nonmelancholic and psychotic depression respond to antidepressant treatment, whereas such treatment has a stronger effect (with one half responding) in cases of melancholic depression. Parker (2002) found that nonmelancholic patients responded equally well (36% each) to tricyclics and selective serotonin reuptake inhibitors (SSRIs). Melancholia was reported to respond distinctly better to tricyclics and broader action drugs than to the SSRIs (Parker, 2002; Rudolph, 2002), but the difference was notably greater among older subjects: Of those aged over

60 years, 38% responded to tricyclics but only 9% to SSRIs (Parker, 2002). A report relating to SSRI treatment of midlife depression stated that melancholic features were associated with significantly poorer remission rates (8.4% compared to 24.1% in cases of nonmelancholic depression) (McGrath et al., 2008). Tricyclics have been reported as more effective than SSRIs in treating psychotic depression (Wijkstra, Lijmer, Balk, Geddes, & Nolen, 2006). The SSRIs are said to be of equivalent effectiveness to the psychotherapies in treating nonmelancholic depression, although it is unclear how well those who agree to engage in psychological treatment represent the population of people with depression.

Analysis restricted to older patients has been more limited. The focus has tended to be on whether and which antidepressants reduce depression in old age, rather than exploring whether psychosocial and other factors affect whether they work. A Cochrane review (Mottram, Wilson, & Strobl, 2006), relating to 32 randomized controlled trials conducted in samples of people aged at least 55 years (a majority being physically well outpatients with nonpsychotic major depression), found no difference in efficacy between different classes of antidepressants, though SSRIs were better tolerated and had lower withdrawal rates. Antidepressants were shown to be more effective than placebo, and age alone seemed not to affect response to treatment. In one randomized controlled trial of patients aged 75 years or more, citalopram showed no benefit over placebo except in those who were severely depressed (Roose et al., 2004). Reynolds et al. (1999a) showed that depression complicating bereavement can also respond to antidepressants.

Nelson et al. (2008) conducted a meta-analysis relating to 10 trials of second-generation antidepressants (five different SSRIs, plus venlafaxine, duloxetine and bupropion) in community-dwelling patients aged 60 years or more who had nonpsychotic, unipolar major depression not associated with specific medical disorders. Mean pooled response rates were 44.4% (antidepressants) and 34.7% (placebo). Those in 10- to 12-week trials had a better response rate than those in 6- to 8-week trials. The authors concluded that identification of the characteristics of responders and nonresponders would be crucial to improving treatment outcomes.

EOD patients have been found to take 5 or 6 weeks longer to achieve remission than LOD patients (Reynolds et al., 1998). The most significant predictor of long-term treatment response is early symptom resolution (Andreescu & Reynolds, 2011). Higher self-esteem was associated with faster response rates (Gildengers et al., 2005), and speed of response to paroxetine was strongly influenced by the serotonin transporter genotype (Pollock et al., 2000). Poorer response is predicted by higher levels of acute or chronic stressors, poorer social support, greater medical burden, cognitive impairment, and depression severity and chronicity (Andreescu & Reynolds, 2011; Reynolds et al., 2010). Most studies have documented a poorer response to antidepressants if subcortical vascular lesions are seen in cases of depression (Andreescu & Reynolds, 2011). There have been mixed findings about the effects of comorbid anxiety on the effectiveness of antidepressants in late-life depression (Chiu et al., 2009). Andreescu et al. (2007) found that patients with greater pretreatment anxiety took longer to respond to treatment, and in the first 2 years after recovery they had higher rates of recurrence (58% versus 29%). In a study of 1-year outcome following treatment of late-life depression using a standardized algorithm, 45% achieved remission. Nonremitted patients were more likely at baseline to use anxiolytic medication and to have lower perceived social support (Bosworth, Hays, George, & Steffens, 2002).

Driscoll et al. (2005) showed that older patients with recurrent late-onset major depression respond well to treatment but take longer to do so than patients with late-onset single episode depression. They are more likely to have cognitive and functional impairments than those with late-onset single episode depression or early-onset recurrent depression.

Little has been reported about the efficacy of antidepressants in cases where the history points to a diagnosis of late-onset depression fulfilling criteria for major depression with melancholia (commonly with psychomotor retardation).

Augmenting medications (lithium, antipsychotic medication, and thyroid hormones being the most commonly used) have been reported to improve the response of older patients to antidepressants. For example, there have been reports relating to methylphenidate with citalopram (Lavretsky, Park, Siddarth, Kumar, & Reynolds, 2006); bupropion, nortryptiline, or lithium with paroxetine (Dew et al., 2007); and aripiprazole with duloxetine or venlafaxine after a period on escitalopram (Sheffrin, Driscoll, & Lenze, 2009). Nimodipine has been found effective in augmenting fluoxetine in treating and preventing relapse of vascular depression

(Taragano, Bagnatti, & Allegri, 2005). Combining two different antidepressants has been reported as effective in 50% of treatment-resistant cases, though few data are available concerning older patients (Dodd, Horgan, Malhi, & Berk, 2005). There is a lack of structured guidance on how best to approach the management of older people with depression who fail to respond to treatment (Cooper et al., 2011).

Examining outcome, Driscoll et al. (2007) noted that 40% to 50% of older people with nonpsychotic major depressive disorder respond to a first trial of an antidepressant. Of those who do not respond, half then respond if treated by swapping to a different antidepressant or if the dose of the original antidepressant is augmented. The remainder tend to follow a chronic, treatment-resistant course. Those with recurrent depression more frequently need augmentation pharmacotherapy to achieve remission.

Researchers have found that if there is little or no improvement in the first 4 weeks on an antidepressant, recovery or remission is unlikely (Sackheim, Roose, & Burt, 2005, referring to subjects with a mean age of 67 years). Nonresponse should prompt a change in strategy.

Mock et al. (2010) noted that the factors influencing response to treatment include severity of the illness, medical burden, comorbid anxiety, cognitive impairment, and very old age. They stated that the number of trials of the different antidepressants is too small and heterogeneous to be able to make specific recommendations about using them to treat late-life depression. However, they noted that venlafaxine is reported to have efficacy comparable to that of nortriptyline, sertraline, and citalopram, though sertraline and citalopram were better tolerated. Despite the merit of these various attempts, the reality is that there are limited data on how best to proceed if an older adult fails to respond to an appropriate course of antidepressant treatment. Practice, in these cases, has been largely guided by personal preferences and trial and error. Cooper et al. (2011) commented that treatment-refractory depression in old age is understudied; the only treatment for which there was evidence from more than one methodologically sound trial was lithium augmentation.

Various studies of the efficacy of continuing treatment with antidepressants in preventing relapse of late-life depression have been conducted. A meta-analysis of eight studies showed that 117 of 467 (25%) subjects prescribed antidepressants, compared with 240 of 458 (52.4%) of those taking placebo, had recurrences (Kok, Heeren, & Nolen, 2011). The number needed to treat, for an antidepressant to prevent one additional relapse or recurrence, was 3.6 (tricyclics 2.9, SSRIs 4.2, though this difference did not reach significance). The researchers drew attention to differences in methodology between the studies, imposing limitations on the conclusions that can be drawn. An expert guideline recommended continuing treatment for at least 1 year after a single episode (Alexopoulos et al., 2001).

Efficacy and Effectiveness of Psychotherapy in Treating Late-Life Depression

Exposure to various risk factor situations was found to have been significantly more common among older persons with major depression than those with minor depression or no depression (Almeida et al., 2011b). This highlights possibilities for nonpharmacological intervention, both in prevention and in treatment of late-life depression. The odds ratios for poor social support and financial stress in cases of major depression when compared to no depression were reported as, respectively, 13.6 and 5.0, while for physical and sexual abuse the odds ratios were, respectively, 3.2 and 2.5. The probability of depression increased as the number of recorded different risk factor exposures increased. Whether the odds ratios differed between subjects with melancholic and those with nonmelancholic depression was not reported. The factors themselves were not necessarily caused by depression, nor were they necessarily the reason why depression developed, but the association suggested that their presence could make it more likely that depression would develop in certain circumstances, and therefore that attention to those risk factors could contribute to improved functional status and self-esteem.

Several studies of adult subjects have shown the advantage of cognitive-behavioral therapy over other psychological therapies and placebo, and equivalence to antidepressant medication, in treatment of unipolar depression (Thase et al., 2000). Turning to treatment of late-life depression, reviews of cognitive-behavioral therapy, psychotherapy, and psychosocial interventions have consistently concluded that they are effective, though studies commonly lacked credible control conditions and frequently included nonclinical populations (Chiu et al., 2009). Most psychotherapy studies have been of cognitively intact and medically stable patients (Baldwin & Wild, 2004). The APA Guidelines

(Gelenberg et al., 2010) state that evidence for the effectiveness of "stand-alone" psychotherapy in treating late-life depression is weak.

Interpersonal therapy can be effective in relapse prevention (Reynolds et al., 1999b). There is also evidence that problem-solving treatment can be effective (Cuijpers, van Straten, & Warmerdam, 2007; Unutzer et al., 2002). Psychotherapy was found to have an advantage over antidepressants only among subjects with non-major depression (Chiu et al., 2009). A meta-analysis of results from 37 studies, focused exclusively on major depression in late life, suggested that pharmacotherapy and psychotherapy were similarly effective in decreasing observer-rated depression (Pinquart, Duberstein, & Lyness, 2006). A Cochrane review (Wilson, Mottram, & Vassilas, 2008) included seven small trials, involving only 153 participants, when examining psychotherapeutic treatments for depression (major and minor) in older people. Five compared forms of cognitive-behavioral therapy versus controls and found cognitive-behavioral therapy more effective. Two trials comparing cognitive-behavioral therapy against psychodynamic therapy found no significant difference in effectiveness. The researchers found no randomized controlled trials relating to other psychotherapeutic approaches and techniques.

Other psychosocial interventions warrant mention. Marital and family therapy, as well as other interventions to reduce psychological stresses, can have striking effects. So, too, can environmental and social manipulations—for example, assisting in finding more appropriate accommodation. Skill training with an emphasis on emotional problem management may lead to decreased depressive symptoms and increased self-efficacy (Coon, Thompson, Steffen, Sorocco & Gallagher-Thompson, 2003). Family psychoeducation has proved effective in prevention of relapse of major depression (Shimazu et al., 2011). The importance of interventions customized for older adults suffering from various functional limitations has been emphasized (Forsman, Jane-Llopis, Scheirenbeck, & Wahlbeck, 2009), among them group discussions, social contact, and interventions to reduce loneliness. The efficacy of physical exercise in treating and preventing depression has been reported as good. Music therapy (for example, in loss situations) has its advocates, but the evidence of efficacy is limited. The same would apply to some complementary therapies.

A holistic approach is appropriate when treating depression in residential care settings (Snowdon,

2010) and in general hospitals. A majority of nursing home residents have dementia and physical illnesses, but what proportion of their depressions should be regarded as the physiological effects of dementia and/or stroke or other medical condition would be debatable. Commonly they do not respond well to antidepressants, but interventions aimed at boosting mastery and self-esteem may well be beneficial (Blanchard, Serfaty, Duckett, & Flatley, 2009; Jang, Haley, Small, & Mortimer, 2002). As in all cases of late-life depression, optimal treatment of hospital and residential care patients is dependent on understanding and interpreting the effects of factors that have caused depression to develop or persist, rather than allowing diagnoses to be the main arbiters of treatment.

Noting that less than 50% of adults with major depressive episodes achieve remission when taking first-line antidepressant treatment, Reynolds et al. (2010) examined whether interpersonal psychotherapy added to depression care management (education and support), used adjunctively in treatment of partial responders to escitalopram, would be more effective in achieving remission than escitalopram plus depression care management. The difference (58% versus 45% response) was not statistically significant.

Reynolds et al. (1999b) found evidence that prevention of relapse in cases of major depression was more effective if maintenance nortriptyline was combined with interpersonal therapy than if either of these treatments was used alone. However, maintenance paroxetine alone was not significantly more (or less) effective in preventing relapse than paroxetine plus monthly interpersonal therapy in patients aged 70 years or more. Monthly maintenance psychotherapy did not prevent recurrence of depression (Reynolds et al., 2006).

Efficacy and Effectiveness of Collaborative Care in Treating Late-Life Depression

Studies of collaborative treatment involving nurse health specialists (e.g., the IMPACT study; Katz & Coyne, 2000) have resulted in improved symptomatic and functional outcomes for primary care patients with major depression. Depression care managers have been reported as more effective than usual care in achieving remission, but it is said that such arrangements are usually not implemented (in the United States anyway) because of inadequate insurance coverage (Alexopoulos, 2005).

Another example of collaborative care is provided by PROSPECT (Prevention of Suicide in Primary Care Elderly—Collaborative Trial) (Bruce & Pearson, 1999; Mulsant et al., 2001). Health specialists work in close collaboration with primary care physicians, and an algorithm is used to guide them in selection and use of antidepressant medications. Pharmacotherapy is recommended over psychotherapy because it is said to be "often more practical in primary care settings" (Mulsant et al., 2001, p. 590). Dose and duration of treatment are seen as the major determinants of the success or failure of antidepressant trials, and the side effect profile of a drug often determines whether an appropriate dose will be taken for an appropriate duration. Discontinuation of tricyclics was reported as higher than that of SSRIs in trials, so, in the absence of strong evidence suggesting superiority of one SSRI over the others, citalopram was selected as the agent of choice, related to its reported tolerability and a paucity of drug–drug interactions. After 6 weeks of treatment, a partial response (30%–50% reduction in HDRS score) leads to a dosage increase; if the response has been less good, the drug is substituted by another, while if the response is better than 50% the same dose is maintained. If there is only partial response after 12 weeks, augmentation with bupropion, nortriptyline, or lithium is recommended, but switching antidepressant is recommended for nonresponse; bupropion, venlafaxine, nortriptyline, and mirtazapine are suggested. "Formal psychotherapy is reserved for patients who do not tolerate or do not respond to pharmacotherapy" (Mulsant et al., 2001, p. 590).

It is noteworthy, in an outcome study of 215 elderly patients with major depression, that the cumulative probability of remission (HDRS score <10) after 4 months was only 33% when PROSPECT guidelines were followed, and 16% in the usual care group. At 12 months the figures were, respectively, 54% and 45% (Alexopoulos et al., 2005). Depression with comorbid anxiety disorder, hopelessness, and/or limitations in physical and emotional functioning showed lower remission rates in both PROSPECT and usual care groups. PROSPECT proved more effective than usual care in patients with low anxiety but added little benefit for patients with severe anxiety. The researchers recommended referral to mental health professionals in those with high anxiety or with physical and emotional function limitations (Alexopoulos et al., 2005).

Physical Treatments of Late-Life Depression

Use of electroconvulsive therapy (ECT), repetitive transcranial magnetic stimulation (TMS), vagus nerve stimulation (VNS), and deep brain stimulation (DBS) are discussed in detail elsewhere in this book, and by Alexopoulos and Kelly (2009). When administered in an optimal manner, ECT is a safe, well-tolerated, and effective treatment in older patients (Flint & Gagnon, 2002). ECT is usually given in psychiatric units or hospitals, either for inpatients with severe depression or on a maintenance (continuing treatment) basis for people who present on an overnight or day-only basis. It is effective in most cases of psychotic or melancholic depression, but it is less used and less effective in the range of nonmelancholic depressions. Psychotic depression does not usually respond to an antidepressant alone, responds better to an antidepressant combined with an antipsychotic medication, and responds best of all to ECT. However, relapse or recurrence within 2 years occurred in 53% despite their being on nortriptyline (Flint & Rifat, 1998). One case-controlled study found that the cumulative probability of relapse or recurrence within 2 years of an acute course of ECT was 7% for maintenance ECT and 52% for continuation pharmacotherapy (Gagné, Furman, Carpenter, & Price, 2000). Research on the efficacy and safety of maintenance ECT in preventing recurrences of late-life depression is sparse (van Schaik et al., 2012), and whether it is used more often or with less effect in cases of LOD has not been reported. Although LOD patients may recover well with ECT, experience suggests that they (in contrast to EOD patients) are less likely to completely remit and are more likely to relapse—due, it is believed, to underlying vascular or other brain changes. Ultrabrief ECT may well prove preferable in treatment of older people with cognitive impairment, but research data are too limited, at present, to allow firm recommendations.

Daily prefrontal TMS has been found as effective as medication but not as effective as ECT in treatment-resistant patients with unipolar illness. Its place in the treatment algorithm is evolving (George & Post, 2011). Jorge et al. (2008) showed that repetitive TMS can be beneficial for vascular depression.

The evidence for VNS and DBS as treatments for late-life depression is (at present) inconclusive.

PREVENTION OF LATE-LIFE DEPRESSION

There is currently no hard evidence from randomized trials that the primary prevention of depression in later life is possible. However, there is good evidence that secondary preventive strategies may contribute to reduce the prevalence of depression in older age. Promising approaches include the continuation of treatment with antidepressants, some forms of psychotherapy and physical activity (see Table 6.1).

Another approach that has been used with some success involves "indicated prevention," a treatment strategy that targets older people at increased risk for a major depressive episode (e.g., minor or subthreshold depression) using stepped care. A stepped-care program was implemented by mental health nurses with primary care patients aged 75 years or more who displayed subthreshold symptoms, using 3 months of watchful waiting, 3 months of bibliotherapy, 3 months of problem-solving therapy, and then referral if symptoms persisted. The incidence of major depression was reduced by 50% in 1 year, compared with 12% in a control group receiving care as usual (van't Veer-Yazelaar et al., 2009).

Hindi et al. (2011) emphasize the need for pathophysiological models that will help identify how to prevent depression. They ask what are the causal mechanisms that need to be interrupted. They focus on a need to personalize depression prevention strategies and suggest that biopredictors of depression (for example, proinflammatory cytokines) may enable depression prevention to be aimed at individuals at highest risk. They have listed what is needed in order to prevent depression but also listed the methodologic challenges faced when researching the effects of such interventions. They recommend use of a structured but flexible menu of approaches—to be carried out by general medical clinicians.

LINKING DIAGNOSIS AND TREATMENT

If, as stated earlier, diagnosing cases of depression is meant to help identify what factors caused the condition to develop and/or persist, and then to use interventions that deal with those factors (get rid of them or help adjustment to them), the aim of *DSM-5* should be to improve on *DSM-IV*.

In Table 6.2 we have tried to summarize the range of types of depression for which there appear to be agreed-upon or plausibly appropriate treatments. We accept that the quality of evidence varies and no doubt will need updating in due course. Ultimately, all cases are unique and all people with depression should benefit from personalized formulations about what caused their depressions, and what factors would seem relevant to address. We believe that major depressive episode (whether single episode or recurrent) is too broad a category to be used when guiding clinicians on how best to treat unipolar depression. Including cases with a mainly biological causation (such as vascular depression, psychotic depression, and melancholic depression) in the same category as psychologically driven loss-related depression does not provide optimal opportunities for demonstrating links between diagnosis and recommended treatment.

CONCLUSION

This chapter has focussed on major depression but emphasized a need, both in treatment and in prevention, for a model that will foster strategies of treatment that relate to formulations concerning causation—in other words, for management that is more personalized than is commonly the case at present. Commenting on outcomes of research trials, Pinquart et al. (2006) noted that 50% of those treated for late-life depression but only 27% of control subjects were considerably improved or no longer depressed. Some researchers provide more optimistic views; a stepped-care protocol eventually produced improvement or recovery in over 80% of older patients (Flint & Rifat, 1996). Nelson et al's (2008) meta-analysis relating to nonpsychotic major depressions in old age showed 44.4% improving on antidepressants and 34.7% on placebo. The oldest old seem to do less well than younger people. Antidepressants appear to help in relieving late-life unipolar depression, but not much more than placebo. Why do we not do better?

Our own view parallels that of Hindi et al. (2011). It is inappropriate to talk about treatment of major depression. There are different subtypes of major depression, with majority agreement concerning what treatment works best for psychotic depression. *Vascular depression* is a diagnostic term based on formulations concerning a possible underlying etiology for depression in older age, but its

Table 6.2 Strategies for Treatment of Late-Life Depression

TYPE OF DEPRESSION	RECOMMENDED TREATMENT STRATEGY
Largely biological/organic:	
Psychotic depression	Treat with antidepressant + antipsychotic or ECT
Melancholic depression	Treat with antidepressant; can add augmenting agent or go to ECT
Vascular depression	Treat with antidepressant; may use nimodipine and/or augment; or ECT
Depression related to brain disease (e.g., Parkinson's, stroke, Alzheimer's, frontotemporal disease)	Treat the brain disease, use supportive psychotherapy, attend to caregiver needs, optimize environment, use antidepressant
Depression attributable to physiological effects of bodily disease (e.g., hypothyroid, Ca pancreas)	Treat underlying physical illness, use supportive psychotherapy and antidepressant if depression persists
Substance-related depression (alcohol, medication, other drugs)	Cease depressogenic drugs
Largely psychological/psychosocial:	
Major depressive disorder related to loss (1) health, (2) loved one, (3) stress-reducing pet, person, item, situation, (4) self-esteem	*Treat initially with psychotherapeutic approach: CBT, IPT, ventilation of feelings, and/or behavioral interventions. Add antidepressant (initially SSRI, but then dual-action drug). Consider PROSPECT or similar. Environmental support, remove stress, exercise program, etc.*
Chronic depressive disorder (1) Personality clearly a factor, (2) No obvious personality issues but ongoing situational issues	*Psychotherapeutic, environmental, or behavioral approach. If depression persists, use antidepressant.*
Unspecified depressive disorder	Treatment will depend on formulation regarding factors leading to depression. *CBT, cognitive-behavioral therapy; ECT, electroconvulsive therapy; IPT, interpersonal therapy.*

features overlap those used as criteria in defining the different subtypes of major depression, and concerns about the low specificity of the association between cardiovascular disease and depression have not been resolved. There has been disagreement between experts regarding the benefits of separating melancholia from nonmelancholic major depression, and on whether the criteria for melancholia should be revised. We draw attention also to the fact that there is no clear boundary between major and minor depression, with some cases of major and of minor depression seeming to have a psychological basis, whereas other cases of major depression more clearly are related to physiological shifts.

Most cases of unipolar depression in late life can be formulated as being of multifactorial causation, though commonly with one factor more obviously precipitant at the onset of depressive symptoms. We encourage the personalized approach, with identification of personality and experiential factors that may have shaped the development of an identified depressive disorder. We recognize the importance of medical and physical factors that may be viewed as causative or contributory, and particularly of many forms of loss (including loss of self-esteem), which also may be causative or contributory. And we recognize that depressive disorders may have an "endogenous" origin, though commonly affected by external factors. The challenge to clinicians, researchers, and classifiers is to develop a model that will facilitate appropriate (and personalized) treatment of all types of depression.

Disclosures

Professor Snowdon has conducted research which was fully or partly funded by Janssen-Cilag and Astra-Zeneca. For some years he was a member of the Janssen-Cilag Australia Dementia Drug Advisory Board. He has been a sponsored speaker and/or investigator for Organon, SmithKline Beecham, Pharmacia, Wyeth and Pfizer. He has received financial support to attend educational meetings from Novartis, Roche, Lundbeck and Janssen-Cilag.

REFERENCES

Akbaraly, T. N., Ancelin, M. L., Jaussent, I., Ritchie, C., Barberger-Gateau, P., Dufouil, C., . . . Ritchie, K. (2011). Metabolic syndrome and onset of depressive symptoms in the elderly: Findings from the three-city study. *Diabetes Care, 34,* 904–909.

Akhondzadeh, S., Jafari, S., Raisi, F., Nasehi, A. A., Ghoreishi, A., Salehi, B., . . . Kamalipour, A. (2009). Clinical trial of adjunctive celecoxib treatment in patients with major depression: A double blind and placebo controlled trial. *Depression and Anxiety, 26,* 607–611.

Alexopoulos, G. S. (2005). Depression in the elderly. *Lancet, 365,* 1961–1970.

Alexopoulos, G. S., Katz, I. R., Bruce, M. L., Heo, M., Ten Have, T., Raue, P., . . . Reynolds, C. F., III. (2005). Remission in depressed geriatric primary care patients: A report from the PROSPECT study. *American Journal of Psychiatry, 162,* 718–724.

Alexopoulos, G. S., Katz, I. R., Reynolds, C. F. III, Carpenter, D., Docherty, J. P., & Ross, R. W. (2001). Pharmacotherapy of depressive disorders in older patients. *Postgraduate Medicine,* 1–86.

Alexopoulos, G. S., & Kelly, R. E. (2009). Research advances in geriatric depression. *World Psychiatry, 8,* 140–149.

Alexopoulos, G. S., Meyers, B. S., Young, R. C., Campbell, S., Silbersweig, D., & Charlson, M. (1997). 'Vascular depression' hypothesis. *Archives of General Psychiatry, 54,* 915–922.

Almeida, O. P. (2008). Vascular depression: Myth or reality? *International Psychogeriatrics, 20,* 645–652.

Almeida, O. P. (2011). Evolution, depression and the interplay between chance and choices. *International Psychogeriatrics, 23,* 1021–1025.

Almeida, O. P., Alfonso, H., Flicker, L., Hankey, G. J., Chubb, S. A., & Yeap, B. B. (2011a). Thyroid hormones and depression: The Health in Men Study. *American Journal of Geriatric Psychiatry, 19,* 763–770.

Almeida, O. P., Alfonso, H., Pirkis, J., Kerse, N., Sim, M., Flicker, L., . . . Pfaff, J. (2011b). A practical approach to assess depression risk and to guide risk reduction strategies in later life. *International Psychogeriatrics, 23,* 280–291.

Almeida, O. P., Burton, E. J., Ferrier, N., McKeith, I. G., & O'Brien, J. T. (2003). Depression with late onset is associated with right frontal lobe atrophy. *Psychological Medicine, 33,* 675–681.

Almeida, O. P., Calver, J., Jamrozik, K., Hankey, G. J., & Flicker, L. (2009). Obesity and metabolic syndrome increase the risk of incident depression in older men: The Health in Men Study. *American Journal of Geriatric Psychiatry, 17,* 889–898.

Almeida, O. P., & Fenner, S. (2002). Bipolar disorder: Similarities and differences between patients with illness onset before and after 65 years of age. *International Psychogeriatics, 14,* 311–322.

Almeida, O. P., Marsh, K., Alfonso, H., Flicker, L., Davis, T. M., & Hankey, G. J. (2010). B-vitamins reduce the long-term risk of depression after stroke: The VITATOPS-DEP trial. *Annals of Neurology, 68,* 503–510.

Almeida, O. P., McCaul, K., Hankey, G. J., Norman, P., Jamrozik, K., & Flicker, L. (2008). Homocysteine and depression in later life. *Archives of General Psychiatry, 65,* 1286–1294.

Almeida, O. P., Norman, P. E., Allcock, R., van Bockxmeer, F., Hankey, G. J., Jamrozik, K., & Flicker, L. (2009). Polymorphisms of the CRP gene inhibit inflammatory response and increase susceptibility to depression: The Health in Men Study. *International Journal of Epidemiology, 38,* 1049–1059.

Almeida, O. P., Norman, P., Hankey, G. J., Jamrozik, K., & Flicker, L. (2007). The association between C-reactive protein concentration and depression in later life is due to poor physical health: Results from the Health in Men Study (HIMS). *Psychological Medicine, 37,* 1775–1786.

Almeida, O. P., Pirkis, J., Kerse, N., Sim, M., Flicker, L., Snowdon, J., . . . Pfaff, J. J. (2012). Socioeconomic disadvantage increases risk of prevalent and persistent depression in later life. *Journal of Affective Disorders, 138,* 322–331.

Almeida, O. P., Yeap, B. B., Hankey, G. J., Jamrozik, K., & Flicker, L. (2008). Low free testosterone concentration as a potentially treatable cause of depressive symptoms in older men. *Archives of General Psychiatry, 65,* 283–289.

American Psychiatric Association. (1994). *Diagnostic and statistical manual of mental disorders* (4th ed.). Washington, DC: Author.

Andreescu, C., Lenze, E. J., Dew, M. A., Begley, A. E., Mulsant, B. H., Dombrovski, A. Y., ... Reynolds, C. F. (2007). Effect of comorbid anxiety on treatment response and relapse risk in late-life depression: A controlled study. *British Journal of Psychiatry, 190,* 344–349.

Andreescu, C., & Reynolds, C. F. III (2011). Late-life depression: Evidence-based treatment and promising new directions for research and clinical practice. *Psychiatric Clinics of North America, 34,* 335–355.

Angst, J. (2009). Severity and subtypes of depression. In H. Herrman, M. Maj, & N. Sartorius (Eds.), *Depressive disorders* (3rd ed., pp. 37–39). Chichester, England: Wiley Blackwell.

Australian Institute of Health and Welfare. (2004). *Heart, stroke and vascular diseases: Australian facts 2004.* Canberra, Australia: Author.

Bair, M. J., Robinson, R. L., Katon, W., & Kroenke, K. (2003). Depression and pain comorbidity: A literature review. *Archives of Internal Medicine, 163,* 2433–2445.

Baldwin, R., & Wild, R. (2004). Management of depression in later life. *Advances in Psychiatric Treatment, 10,* 131–139.

Ballmaier, M., Toga, A. W., Blanton, R. E., Sowell, E. R., Lavretsky, H., Peterson, J., Pham, D., & Kumar, A. (2004). Anterior cingulate, gyrus rectus, and orbitofrontal abnormalities in elderly depressed patients: An MRI-based parcellation of the prefrontal cortex. *American Journal of Psychiatry, 161,* 99–108.

Beats, B. C., Sahakian, B. J., & Levy, R. (1996). Cognitive performance in tests sensitive to frontal lobe dysfunction in the elderly depressed. *Psychological Medicine, 26,* 591–603.

Beekman, A. T. F., Penninx, B. W. J. H., Deeg, D. J. H., Ormel, J., Braam, A. W., & van Tilburg, W. (1997). Depression and physical health in later life: Results from the Longitudinal Aging Study Amsterdam (LASA). *Journal of Affective Disorders, 46,* 219–231.

Blanchard, M., Serfaty, M., Duckett, S., & Flatley, M. (2009). Adapting services for a changing society: a reintegrative model for Old Age Psychiatry (based on a model proposed by Knight and Emanuel, 2007). *International Journal of Geriatric Psychiatry, 24,* 202–206.

Blazer, D. G., II. (1994). Epidemiology of late-life depression. In L. S. Schneider, C. F. Reynolds, III, B. D. Lebowitz, & A. F. Friedhoff (Eds.), *Diagnosis and treatment of depression in late life* (pp. 9–19). Washington, DC: American Psychiatric Press.

Blazer, D. G., II, & Hybels, C. F. (2005). Origins of depression in later life. *Psychological Medicine, 35,* 1241–1252.

Bosworth, H. B., Hays, J. C., George, L. K., & Steffens, D. C. (2002). Psychosocial and clinical predictors of unipolar depression outcome in older adults. *International Journal of Geriatric Psychiatry, 17,* 238–246.

Brodaty, H., Peters, K., Boyce, P., Hickie, I., Parker, G., Mitchell, P., & Wilhelm, K. (1991). Age and depression. *Journal of Affective Disorders, 23,* 137–149.

Bruce, M. L., & Pearson, J. L. (1999). Designing an intervention to prevent suicide: PROSPECT (Prevention of Suicide in Primary Care Elderly Collaborative Trial). *Dialogues in Clinical Neurosciences, 1,* 100–112.

Caine, E. D., Lyness, J. M., King, D. A., & Connors, L. (1994). Clinical and etiological heterogeneity of mood disorders in elderly patients. In L. S. Schneider, C. F. Reynolds, III, B. D. Lebowitz, & A. J. Friedhoff (Eds.), *Diagnosis and treatment of depression in late life* (pp. 23–53). Washington, DC: American Psychiatric Press.

Carroll, B. J. (1982). The dexamethasone suppression test for melancholia. *British Journal of Psychiatry, 140,* 292–304.

Caspi, A., Sugden, K., Moffitt, T. E., Taylor, A., Craig, I. W., Harrington, H., ... Poulton, R. (2003). Influence of life stress on depression: Moderation by a polymorphism in the 5-HTT gene. *Science, 301,* 386–389.

Chiu, E., Ames, D., Draper, B., & Snowdon, J. (2009). Depressive disorders in the elderly: A review. In H. Herrman, M. Maj, & N. Sartorius (Eds.), *Depressive disorders* (3rd ed., pp. 197–257). Chichester, England: Wiley-Blackwell.

Clarke, D. M., Piterman, L., Byrne, C. J., & Austin, D. W. (2008). Somatic symptoms, hypochondriasis and psychological distress: A study of somatisation in Australian general practice. *Medical Journal of Australia, 189,* 560–564.

Coon, D. W., Thompson, L., Steffen, A., Sorocco, K., & Gallagher-Thompson, D. (2003). Anger and depression management: Psychoeducational skill training interventions for women caregivers of a relative with dementia. *Gerontologist, 43,* 678–689.

Cooper, C., Katona, C., Lyketsos, K., Blazer, D., Brodaty, H., Rabins, P., ... Livingston, G. (2011). A systematic review of treatments for refractory depression in older people. *American Journal of Psychiatry*, 168, 681–688.

Cuijpers, P., van Straten, A., & Warmerdam, L. (2007). Problem-solving therapies for depression: A meta-analysis. *European Psychiatry*, 22, 9–15.

Dantzer, R., O'Connor, J. C., Freund, G. G., Johnson, R. W., & Kelley, K. W. (2008). From inflammation to sickness and depression: When the immune system subjugates the brain. *National Review of Neurosciences*, 9, 46–56.

De Leeuw, F. E., de Groot, J. C., Achten, E., Oudkerk, M., Ramos, L. M., Heijboer, R., ... Breteler, M. M. (2001). Prevalence of cerebral white matter lesions in elderly people: A population based magnetic resonance imaging study. The Rotterdam Scan Study. *Journal of Neurology Neurosurgery and Psychiatry*, 70, 9–14.

Dew, M. A., Whyte, E. M., Lenze, E. J., Houck, P. R., Mulsant, B. H., Pollock, B. G., ... Reynolds, C. F., III. (2007). Recovery from major depression in older adults receiving augmentation of antidepressant pharmacotherapy. *American Journal of Psychiatry*, 164, 892–899.

Dodd, S., Horgan, D., Malhi, G. S., & Berk, M. (2005). To combine or not to combine? A literature review of antidepressant combination therapy. *Journal of Affective Disorders*, 89, 1–11.

Driscoll, H. C., Basinski, J., Mulsant, B. H., Butters, M. A., Dew, M. A., Houck, P. R., ... Reynolds, C. F., III. (2005). Late-onset major depression: Clinical and treatment-response variability. *International Journal of Geriatric Psychiatry*, 20, 661–667.

Driscoll, H. C., Karp, J. F., Dew, M. A., & Reynolds, C. F., III. (2007). Getting better, getting well: Understanding and managing partial and non-response to pharmacological treatment of non-psychotic major depression in old age. *Drugs and Aging*, 24, 801–814.

Duman, R. S., Heninger, G. R., & Nestler, E. J. (1997). A molecular and cellular theory of depression. *Archives of General Psychiatry*, 54, 597–606.

Fink, M., & Taylor, M. A. (2007). Resurrecting melancholia. *Acta Psychiatrica Scandinavica*, 115 (Suppl 433), 14–20.

Flint, A. J., & Gagnon, N. (2002). Effective use of electroconvulsive therapy in late-life depression. *Canadian Journal of Psychiatry*, 47, 734–741.

Flint, A. J., & Rifat, S. L. (1996). The effect of sequential antidepressant treatment on geriatric depression. *Journal of Affective Disorders*, 36, 95–105.

Flint, A. J., & Rifat, S. L. (1998). Two-year outcome of psychotic depression in late life. *American Journal of Psychiatry*, 155, 178–183.

Forsman, A., Jane-Llopis, E., Schierenbeck, I., & Wahlbeck, K. (2009). Psychosocial interventions for prevention of depression in older people. *Cochrane Database of Systematic Reviews*, Issue 2. No. CD007804.

Gagné, G. G., Furman, M. J., Carpenter, L. L., & Price, L. H. (2000). Efficacy of continuation ECT and antidepressant drugs compared to long-term antidepressants alone in depressed patients. *American Journal of Psychiatry*, 157, 1960–1965.

Gelenberg, A. J, Freeman, M. P., Markowitz, J. C., Rosenbaum, J. R., Thase, M. E., Trivedi, M. H., & Van Rhoads, R. S. (2010). *Practice guideline for the treatment of patients with major depressive disorder* (3rd ed.). Washington, DC: American Psychiatric Association.

George, M. S., & Post, R. M. (2011). Daily left prefrontal repetitive transcranial magnetic stimulation for acute treatment of medication-resistant depression. *American Journal of Psychiatry*, 168, 356–362.

Gildengers, A. G., Houck, P. R., Mulsant, B. H., Dew, M. A., Aizenstein, H. J., Jones, B. L., ... Reynolds, C. F., III. (2005). Trajectories of treatment response in late-life depression. *Journal of Clinical Psychopharmacology*, 25, S8–S13.

Goveas, J. S., Espeland, M. A., Hogan, P., Dotson, V., Tarima, S., Coker, L. H., ... Resnick, S. (2011). Depressive symptoms, brain volumes and subclinical cerebrovascular disease in postmenopausal women: The Women's Health Initiative MRI Study. *Journal of Affective Disorders*, 132, 275–284.

Hasin, D. S., Goodwin, R. D., Stinson, F. S., & Grant, B. F. (2005). Epidemiology of major depressive disorder: Results from the National Epidemiologic Survey on Alcoholism and Related Conditions. *Archives of General Psychiatry*, 62, 1097–1106.

Heiss, G., Wallace, R., Anderson, G. L., Aragaki, A., Beresford, S. A., Brzyski, R., ... WHI Investigators.. (2008). Health risks and benefits 3 years after stopping randomized treatment with estrogen and progestin. *Journal of the American Medical Association*, 299, 1036–1045.

Hegeman, J. M., Kok, R. M., van der Mast, R. C., & Giltay, E. J. (2012). Phenomenology of depression in older compared with younger adults: Meta-analysis. *British Journal of Psychiatry*, 200, 275–281.

Helfand, M. (2004). Screening for subclinical thyroid dysfunction in nonpregnant adults: A summary of the evidence for the U.S. Preventive Services Task Force. *Annals of Internal Medicine*, 140, 128–141.

Herrmann, L. L., Goodwin, G. M., & Ebmeier, K. P. (2007). The cognitive neuropsychology of depression in the elderly. *Psychological Medicine*, 37, 1693–1702.

Herrmann, L. L., Le Masurier, M., & Ebmeier, K. P. (2008). White matter hyperintensities in late life depression: A systematic review. *Journal of Neurology Neurosurgery and Psychiatry, 79,* 619–624.

Hindi, F., Dew, M. A., Albert, S. M., Lotrich, F. E., & Reynolds, C. F., III. (2011). Preventing depression in later life: State of the art and science circa 2011. *Psychiatric Clinics of North America, 34,* 67–78.

Hyyppa, M. T., Kronholm, E., Virtanen, A., Leino, A., & Jula, A. (2003). Does simvastatin affect mood and steroid hormone levels in hypercholesterolemic men? A randomized double-blind trial. *Psychoneuroendocrinology, 28,* 181–194.

Idan, A., Griffiths, K. A., Harwood, D. T., Seibel, M. J., Turner, L., Conway, A. J., & Handelsman, D. J. (2010). Long-term effects of dihydrotestosterone treatment on prostate growth in healthy, middle-aged men without prostate disease: A randomized, placebo-controlled trial. *Annals of Internal Medicine, 153,* 621–632.

Jang, Y., Haley, W. E., Small, B. J., & Mortimer, J. A. (2002). The role of mastery and social resources in the association between disability and depression in later life. *Gerontologist, 42,* 807–813.

Jorge, R. E., Moser, D. J., Acion, L., & Robinson, R. G. (2008). Treatment of vascular depression using repetitive transcranial magnetic stimulation. *Archives of General Psychiatry, 65,* 268–276.

Karg, K., Burmeister, M., Shedden, K., & Sen, S. (2011). The serotonin transporter promoter variant (5-HTTLPR), stress, and depression meta-analysis revisited: Evidence of genetic moderation. *Archives of General Psychiatry, 68,* 444–454.

Katz, I. R., & Coyne, J. C. (2000). The public health model for mental health care for the elderly. *Journal of the American Medical Association, 283,* 1–6.

Kessler, R. C., Berglund, P., Demler, O., Jin, R., Koretz, D., Merikangas, K. R., ... National Comorbidity Survey Replication. (2003). The epidemiology of major depressive disorder: Results from the National Comorbidity Survey Replication (NCS-R). *Journal of the American Medical Association, 289,* 3095–3105.

Kim, B-S., Lee, D. H., Lee, D. W., Bae, J. N., Chang, S. M., Kim, S., & Cho, M. J. (2011). The role of vascular risk factors in the development of DED syndrome among an elderly community sample. *American Journal of Geriatric Psychiatry, 19,* 104–114.

Kirsch, I., & Sapirstein, G. (1998). Listening to Prozac but hearing placebo: A meta-analysis of antidepressant medication. *Preventative Treatment, 1,* 1–17.

Kohli, M. A., Lucae, S., Saemann, P. G., Schmidt, M. V., Demirkan, A., Hek, K., ... Binder, E. B. (2011). The neuronal transporter gene SLC6A15 confers risk to major depression. *Neuron, 70,* 252–265.

Kok, R. M., Heeren, T. J., & Nolen, W. A. (2011) Continuing treatment of depression in the elderly: A systematic review and meta-analysis of double-blinded randomized controlled trials with antidepressants. *American Journal of Geriatric Psychiatry, 19,* 249–255.

Koster, A., Bosma, H., Kempen, G. I., Penninx, B. W., Beekman, A. T., Deeg, D. J., & van Eijk, J. T. (2006). Socioeconomic differences in incident depression in older adults: The role of psychosocial factors, physical health status, and behavioral factors. *Journal of Psychosomatic Research, 61,* 619–627.

Krishnan, K. R., Delong, M., Kraemer, H., Carney, R., Spiegel, D., Gordon, C., ... Wainscott, C. (2002). Comorbidity of depression with other medical diseases in the elderly. *Biological Psychiatry, 52,* 559–588.

Krishnan, K. R., Hays, J. C., George, L. K., & Blazer, D. G. (1998). Six-month outcomes for MRI-related vascular depression. *Depression and Anxiety, 8,* 142–146.

Krishnan, K. R. R., Hays, J. C., Tupler, L. A., George, L. K., & Blazer, D. G. (1995). Clinical and phenomenological comparisons of late-onset and early-onset depression. *American Journal of Psychiatry, 152,* 785–788.

Krishnan, K. R., Taylor, W. D., McQuoid, D. R., MacFall, J. R., Payne, M. E., Provenzale, J. M., & Steffens, D. C. (2004). Clinical characteristics of magnetic resonance imaging-defined subcortical ischemic depression. *Biological Psychiatry, 55,* 390–397.

Lavretsky, H., Ballmaier, M., Pham, D., Toga, A., & Kumar, A. (2007). Neuroanatomical characteristics of geriatric apathy and depression: A magnetic resonance imaging study. *American Journal of Geriatric Psychiatry, 15,* 386–394.

Lavretsky, H., Park, S., Siddarth, P., Kumar, A., & Reynolds, C. F., III. (2006). Methylphenidate-enhanced antidepressant response to citalopram in the elderly: A double-blind, placebo-controlled pilot trial. *American Journal of Geriatric Psychiatry, 14,* 181–185.

Levinson, D. F. (2006). The genetics of depression: A review. *Biological Psychiatry, 60,* 84–92.

Lidberg, L., Tuck, J. R., Asberg, M., Scalia-Tomba, G. P., & Bertilsson, L. (1985). Homicide, suicide and

CSF 5-HIAA. *Acta Psychiatrica Scandinavica, 71*, 230–236.

Lloyd, A. J., Ferrier, I. N., Barber, R., Gholkar, A., Young, A. H., & O'Brien, J. T. (2004). Hippocampal volume change in depression: Late- and early-onset illness compared. *British Journal of Psychiatry, 184*, 488–495.

Lyketsos, C. G., Lopez, O., Jones, B., Fitzpatrick, A. L., Breitner, J., & DeKosky, S. (2002). Prevalence of neuropsychiatric symptoms in dementia and mild cognitive impairment: Results from the cardiovascular health study. *Journal of the American Medical Association, 288*, 1475–1483.

Malhi, G. S., Adams, D., Porter, R., Wignall, A., Lampe, L., O'Connor, N., et al. (2009). Clinical practice recommendations for depression. *Acta Psychiatrica Scandinavica, 119*, 8–26.

Malhi, G. S., Parker, G. B., & Greenwood, J. (2005). Structural and functional models of depression: From sub-types to substrates. *Acta Psychiatrica Scandinavica, 111*, 94–105.

Martinowich, K., Manji, H., & Lu, B. (2007). New insights into BDNF function in depression and anxiety. *Nature Neurosciences, 10*, 1089–1093.

Massie, M. J. (2004). Prevalence of depression in patients with cancer. *Journal of the Nationall Cancer Institute Monographs*, 57–71.

McGrath, P. J., Khan, A. Y., Trivedi, M. H., Stewart, J. W., Morris, D. W., Wisniewski, S. R., . . . Rush, A. J. (2008). Response to a selective serotonin reuptake inhibitor (citalopram) in major depressive disorder with melancholic features: A STAR*D report. *Journal of Clinical Psychiatry, 69*, 1847–1855.

Mock, P., Norman, T. R., & Olver, J. S. (2010). Contemporary therapies for depression in older people. *Journal of Pharmacy Practice and Research, 40*, 58–64.

Mottram, P. G., Wilson, K., & Strobl, J. J. (2006). Antidepressants for depressed elderly. *Cochrane Database of Systematic Reviews*, Issue 1., CD003491.

Muller, N., Schwarz, M. J., Dehning, S., Douhe, A., Cerovecki, A., Goldstein-Müller, B., . . . Riedel, M. (2006). The cyclooxygenase-2 inhibitor celecoxib has therapeutic effects in major depression: Results of a double-blind, randomized, placebo controlled, add-on pilot study to re. *Molecular Psychiatry, 11*, 680–684.

Mulsant, B. H., Alexopoulos, G. S., Reynolds, C. F., III, Katz, I. R., Abrams, R., Oslin, D., . . . PROSPECT Study Group. (2001). Pharmacological treatment of depression in older primary care patients: The PROSPECT algorithm. *International Journal of Geriatric Psychiatry, 16*, 585–592.

Musselman, D. L., Evans, D. L., & Nemeroff, C. B. (1998). The relationship of depression to cardiovascular disease: Epidemiology, biology, and treatment. *Archives of General Psychiatry, 55*, 580–592.

Nelson, J. C., Delucchi, K., & Schneider, L. S. (2008). Efficacy of second generation antidepressants in late-life depression: A meta-analysis of the evidence. *American Journal of Geriatric Psychiatry, 16*, 558–567.

O'Brien, J. T., Lloyd, A., McKeith, I., Gholkar, A., & Ferrier, N. (2004). A longitudinal study of hippocampal volume, cortisol levels, and cognition in older depressed subjects. *American Journal of Psychiatry, 161*, 2081–2090.

Parker, G. (2002). Differential effectiveness of newer and older antidepressants appears mediated by an age effect on the phenotypic expression of depression. *Acta Psychiatrica Scandinavica, 106*, 168–170.

Parker, G. (2009). Diagnosis of depressive disorders. In H. Herrman, M. Maj, & N. Sartorius (Eds.), *Depressive disorders* (3rd ed., pp. 1–26). Chichester, England: Wiley-Blackwell.

Parker, G. (2011). Classifying clinical depression: An operational proposal. *Acta Psychiatrica Scandinavica, 123*, 314–316.

Parker, G., & Hadzi-Pavlovic, D. (1996). *Melancholia. A disorder of movement and mood*. Cambridge, England: Cambridge University Press.

Pinquart, M., Duberstein, P. R., & Lyness, J. M. (2006). Treatments for later-life depressive conditions: A meta-analytic comparison of pharmacotherapy and psychotherapy. *American Journal of Psychiatry, 163*, 1493–1501.

Pollock, B. G., Ferrell, R. E., Mulsant, B. H., Mazumdar, S., Miller, M., Sweet, R. A., . . . Kupfer, D. J. (2000). Allelic variation in the serotonin transporter promoter affects onset of paroxetine treatment response in late-life depression. *Neuropsychopharmacology, 23*, 587–590.

Prince, M. J., Harwood, R. H., Blizard, R. A., Thomas, A., & Mann, A. H. (1997). Impairment, disability and handicap as risk factors for depression in old age. The Gospel Oak Project V. *Psychological Medicine, 27*, 311–321.

Prince, M. J., Harwood, R. H., Thomas, A., & Mann, A. H. (1998). A prospective population-based cohort study of the effects of disablement and social milieu on the onset and maintenance of late-life depression. The Gospel Oak Project VII. *Psychological Medicine, 28*, 337–350.

Quitkin, F. M. (1999). Placebos, drug effects, and study design: A clinician's guide. *American Journal of Psychiatry, 156*, 829–836.

Reifler, B. V. (1994). Depression: Diagnosis and comorbidity. In L. S. Schneider, C. F. Reynolds, III, B. D. Lebowitz, & A. J. Friedhoff (Eds.), *Diagnosis and treatment of depression in late life* (pp. 55–59). Washington, D.C.: American Psychiatric Press.

Reijnders, J. S., Ehrt, U., Weber, W. E., Aarsland, D., & Leentjens, A. F. (2008). A systematic review of prevalence studies of depression in Parkinson's disease. *Movement Disorders, 23,* 183–189; quiz 313.

Reynolds, C. F., III, Dew, M. A., Frank, E., Begley, A. E., Miller, M. D., Cornes, C., … Kupfer, D. J. (1998). Effects of age at onset of first lifetime episode of recurrent major depression on treatment response and illness course in elderly patients. *American Journal of Psychiatry, 155,* 795–799.

Reynolds, C. F., III, Dew, M. A., Martire, L. M., Miller, M. D., Cyranowski, J. M., Lenze, E., … Frank, E. (2010). Treating depression to remission in older adults: A controlled evaluation of combined escitalopram with interpersonal psychotherapy versus escitalopram with depression care management. *International Journal of Geriatric Psychiatry, 25,* 1134–1141.

Reynolds, C. F., III, Dew, M. A., Pollock, B. G., Mulsant, B. H., Frank, E., Miller, M. D., … Kupfer, D. J. (2006). Maintenance treatment of major depression in old age. *New England Journal of Medicine, 354,* 1130–1138.

Reynolds, C. F., III, Frank, E., Perel, J. M., Imber, S. D., Cornes, C., Miller, M. D., … Kupfer, D. J. (1999b). Nortriptyline and interpersonal Psychotherapy as maintenance therapies for recurrent major depression: A randomized controlled trial in patients older than 59 years. *Journal of the American Medical Association, 281,* 39–45.

Reynolds, C. F., III, Miller, M. D., Pasternak, R. E., Frank, E., Perel, J. M., Cornes, C., … Kupfer, D. J. (1999a). Treatment of bereavement-related major depressive episodes in later life: A controlled study of acute and continuation treatment with nortriptyline and interpersonal psychotherapy. *American Journal of Psychiatry, 156,* 202–208.

Roose, S. P., Sackeim, H. A., Krishnan, K. R., Pollock, B. G., Alexopoulos, G., Lavretsky, H., … Old-Old Depression Study Group.. (2004). Antidepressant pharmacotherapy in the treatment of depression in the very old. A randomized, placebo-controlled trial. *American Journal of Psychiatry, 161,* 2050–2059.

Rudolph, R. L. (2002). Achieving remission from depression with venlafaxine and venlafaxine extended release: A literature review of comparative studies with selective serotonin reuptake inhibitors. *Acta Psychiatrica Scandinavica, 106,* 24–30.

Sackeim, H. A., Roose, S. P., & Burt, T. (2005). Optimal length of antidepressant trials in late-life depression. *Journal of Clinical Psychopharmacology, 25*(Supplement 1), S34–S37.

Sapolsky, R. (2001). Depression, antidepressants, and the shrinking hippocampus. *Proceedings of the National Academy of Sciences USA, 98,* 12320–12323.

Schneider, L. S., & Olin, J. T. (1995). Efficacy of acute treatment for geriatric depression. *International Psychogeriatrics, 7,* 7–25.

Sheffrin, M., Driscoll, H. C., & Lenze, E. J. (2009). Pilot study of augmentation with aripiprazole for incomplete response in late-life depression: Getting to remission. *Journal of Clinical Psychiatry, 70,* 208–213.

Sheline, Y. I., Gado, M. H., & Kraemer, H. C. (2003). Untreated depression and hippocampal volume loss. *American Journal of Psychiatry, 160,* 1516–1518.

Shimazu, K., Shimodera, S., Mino, Y., Nishida, A., Kamimura, N., Sawada, K., … Inoue, S. (2011). Family psychoeducation for major depression: Randomised controlled trial. *British Journal of Psychiatry, 198,* 385–390.

Shorter, E. (2007). The doctrine of the two depressions in historical perspective. *Acta Psychiatric Scandinavica, 115*(Suppl 433), 5–13.

Shulman, K., & Post, F.(1980). Bipolar affective disorder in old age. *British Journal of Psychiatry, 136,* 26–32.

Snowdon, J. (2001). Is depression more prevalent in old age? *Australian and New Zealand Journal of Psychiatry, 35,* 782–787.

Snowdon, J. (2010). Depression in nursing homes. *International Psychogeriatrics, 7,* 1143–1148.

Soares, C. N., Almeida, O. P., Joffe, H., & Cohen, L. S. (2001). Efficacy of estradiol for the treatment of depressive disorders in perimenopausal women: A double-blind, randomized, placebo-controlled trial. *Archives of General Psychiatry, 58,* 529–534.

Stewart, J. W., McGrath, P. J., Quitkin, F. M., & Klein, D. F. (2007). Atypical depression: Current status and relevance to melancholia. *Acta Psychiatrica Scandinavica, 115*(Suppl 433), 58–71.

Taragano, F. E., Bagnatti, P., & Allegri, R. F. (2005). A double-blind, randomized clinical trial to assess the augmentation with nimodipine of antidepressant therapy in the treatment of 'vascualr depression'. *International Psychogeriatrics, 17,* 487–498.

Thase, M. E., Friedman, E. S., Berman, S. R., Fasiczka, A. L., Lis, J. A., Howland, R. H., & Simons, A.

D. (2000). Is cognitive behaviour therapy just a 'nonspecific' intervention for depression? A retrospective comparison of consecutive cohorts treated with cognitive behaviour therapy or supportive counselling and pill placebo. *Journal of Affective Disorders, 57,* 63–71.

Thomas, A. J., O'Brien, J. T., Davis, S., Ballard, C., Barber, R., Kalaria, R. N., & Perry, R. H. (2002). Ischemic basis for deep white matter hyperintensities in major depression: A neuropathological study. *Archives of General Psychiatry, 59,* 785–792.

Unützer, J., Simon, G., Belin, T. R., Datt, M., Katon, W., & Patrick, D. (2000). Care for depression in HMO patients aged 65 and older. *Journal of the American Geriatrics Society, 48,* 871–878.

Unützer, J., Katon, W., Callahan, C. M., Williams, J. W., Jr., Hunkeler, E., Harpole, L.et al. IMPACT Investigators. (2002). Collaborative care management of late-life depression in the primary care setting. *Journal of the American Medical Association, 288,* 2836–2845.

Van Praag, H. M. (2009). The need to functionalise psychiatric diagnosis. In H. Herrman, M. Maj, & N. Sartorius (Eds.), *Depressive disorders* (3rd ed., pp. 44–46). Chichester, England: Wiley-Blackwell.

Van Reedt Dortland, A. K., Giltay, E. J., van Veen, T., van Pelt, J., Zitman, F. G., & Penninx, B. W. (2010). Associations between serum lipids and major depressive disorder: Results from the Netherlands Study of Depression and Anxiety (NESDA). *Journal of Clinical Psychiatry, 71,* 729–736.

Van Schaik, A. M., Comijs, H. C., Sonnenberg, C. M., Beekman, A. T., Sienaert, P., & Stek, M. L.

(2012). Efficacy and safety of continuation and maintenance electroconvulsive therapy in depressed elderly patients: a systematic review. *American Journal of Geriatric Psychiatry, 20,* 5–17.

Van't Veer-Tazelaar, P. J., van Marwijk, H. W., van Oppen, P., van Hout, H. P., van der Horst, H. E., Cuijpers, P., . . . Beekman, A. T. (2009). Stepped-care prevention of anxiety and depression in late life: A randomized controlled trial. *Archives of General Psychiatry, 66,* 297–304.

Wijkstra, J., Lijmer, J., Balk, F. J., Geddes, J. R., & Nolen, W. A. (2006). Pharmacological treatment for unipolar psychotic depression: Systematic review and meta-analysis. *British Journal of Psychiatry, 188,* 410–415.

Wilson, I. (2006). Depression in the patient with COPD. *International Journal of Chronic Obstructive Pulmonary Disease, 1,* 61–64.

Wilson, K., Mottram, P. G., & Vassilas, C. (2008). Psychotherapeutic treatments for older depressed people. *Cochrane Database of Systematic Reviews,* Issue 1., CD004853.

Young, R. C., & Falk, J. R. (1989). Age, manic psychopathology and treatment response. *International Journal of Geriatric Psychiatry, 4,* 73–78.

Zisook, S. (2009). Four questions and an alternative. In H. Herrman, M. Maj, & N. Sartorius (Eds.), In *Depressive disorders* (3rd ed., pp. 27–30). Chichester, England: Wiley-Blackwell.

Zisook, S., Reynolds, C. F., III, Pies, R., Simon, N., Lebowitz, B., Madowitz, J., . . . Shear, M. K. (2010). Bereavement, complicated grief, and DSM, Part 1: Depression. *Journal of Clinical Psychiatry, 71,* 955–956.

7

BIPOLAR DISORDER

Robert C. Young and Nahla A. Mahgoub

ELDERLY PATIENTS with mania and bipolar (BP) disorders constitute a substantial subgroup among elderly patients presenting for psychiatric treatment, and they often have severe illness that requires intensive utilization of services. These patients have diverse clinical characteristics, comorbidities, and presumed etiologies and pathophysiologies. Age-associated factors contribute to this heterogeneity. Their illness courses differ widely between individuals. Responses to interventions are difficult to predict. This discussion is organized around age and age-related factors, including age at onset of illness.

Kraepelin (1921) commented on the rate of first-episode mania, depression, and mixed states across the age span. In a sample of 903 cases, he observed that mania as first episode of illness was less frequent with increased age, although it tended to increase between age 45 and 50 years. He also observed that, in contrast to depressive first episodes, mixed first episodes declined consistently with age. Yet he noted that affective episodes could appear first in old age, for

example, 80 years. Kraepelin did not differentiate unipolar depression from BP disorder, however.

Roth and colleagues (Slater & Roth, 1977) suggested that although manic syndromes in the elderly were similar qualitatively to that in younger patients, older patients demonstrate attenuation or exaggeration of particular features. Post (1965) suggested that elderly manic patients less often have typical flight of ideas, and that they more often have persecutory delusions that are not mood congruent compared to younger patients. In the experience of Slater and Roth (1977), many cases of mania in old age are "relatively mild." They observed that euphoria in older manic patients is often not "infectious," and speech and thought lack the usual "sparkle and versatility" and are commonly "threadbare and repetitious." These clinicians suggested, however, that "hostility and resentment" are often marked.

These psychiatrists also pointed out that cognitive impairments frequently accompany manic syndromes, and that impairments are particularly apparent in aged manic patients. They described disorientation and delirium in manic patients (Kraepelin, 1921; Post, 1965; Slater & Roth, 1977). Kraepelin observed that dementia was not a necessary outcome of late-onset affective episodes, however.

Early European literature also commented on manic psychopathology in the context of brain lesions and disorders (Shulman, 1997), including behavioral changes referred to as "Witzelsucht" (Oppneheim, 1890) or "pseudopsychopathic syndrome" (Blumer & Benson, 1975) associated with lesions of the orbital surface of the frontal lobes (Welt, 1888). These observations set the stage for investigations of possible neuroanatomic specificity in brain lesions associated with mania and depression. Early clinical writing also mentions the association between vascular disease and mood disorder in late life (Kraepelin, 1921). Kay et al. (Kay, Roth, & Hopkins, 1955) and Post (1965) proposed that mood disorder with onset in late life reflects in part age-associated brain changes.

In the mid-20th century, investigation of mood disorders in late life was advanced by validation of the distinction between unipolar depression and BP disorder (Marneros & Angst, 2000). The introduction of lithium salts (Cade, 1949) and other mood stabilizers reinforced the utility of the BP category across the age spectrum. It also encouraged testing, in younger patients, distinctions within BP disorder such as atypical or type II patients, and broadening the concept of BP disorder. However, investigation in aged patients is at a comparatively early stage. We will therefore emphasize research needs, and we will suggest special opportunities that are offered by studies of bipolar disorder in late life.

DIAGNOSIS

Diagnostic categories (e.g., *Diagnostic and Statistical Manual of Mental Disorders*, fourth edition; *DSM-IV-TR*; American Psychiatric Association, 1994) used in younger patients are broadly applicable to aged BP patients. The knowledge base in geriatric BP disorders has been too preliminary to warrant modification of existing nosologies. However, in what follows we discuss the differential diagnosis and comorbidity.

Differential Diagnosis of Mania

TYPE I BIPOLAR DISORDERS

Type I BP disorders are defined by idiopathic manic states. Manic states have thus far been the main focus

of clinical description and investigation of "bipolarity" in late life. Type I BP disorders in the elderly can be recurrent from young age, or they may begin in late life. Manic states can also occur in patients with a prior history of recurrent major depression, representing a change in "polarity." Idiopathic, recurrent manic states in the absence of depressive episodes, referred to as "unipolar" mania, can occur in aged patients, although relatively infrequently (Shulman & Tohen, 1994).

TYPE II BIPOLAR DISORDERS

Type II BP disorders are characterized by hypomanic states and major depressive episodes. Benazzi (2000) reported that the proportion of type II BP patients among depressed ambulatory psychiatric patients was lower among those who were aged compared to those who were younger.

MANIC STATES AND MOOD DISORDERS ASSOCIATED WITH MEDICAL CONDITIONS OR DRUG TREATMENTS

In elderly BP patients, medical and neurological disorders can be prevalent, and they may have significance for psychiatric management. Particular conditions and treatments are implicated in the etiology of manic syndromes (see later). These syndromes are sometimes referred to as "symptomatic" (Slavney, Rich, Pearlson, & McHugh, 1977), "secondary" mania (Krauthammer & Klerman, 1978), or "complicated" mania (Black, Winokur, Bell, Nasrallah, & Hulbert, 1988).

ORGANIC MENTAL DISORDERS

Delirious patients can present with manic features. Delirium has also been described as a manifestation of manic episodes of BP disorder (Kraepelin, 1921; Slater & Roth, 1977).

Patients with dementing illness can present with either manic features or manic syndromes (Burns, Jacoby, & Levy, 1990; Dorey et al., 2008; Lyketsos, Corazzini, & Steele, 1995). Manic psychopathology and manic syndromes in patients with dementia may not be correctly identified by caregivers and clinicians, and they may be treated as agitation (Folstein, 1999). Manic patients with dementia may or may not have had affective episodes prior to the onset of the dementia. This group of patients has received little investigation, except as a focus of preliminary pharmacological study (Mega et al., 2000; Tariot, Schneider et al., 2001). Patients with frontotemporal dementia can show mood changes and excess behaviors similar to bipolar mania (Agronin & Malette, 2006).

CHRONIC PSYCHOSES

BP schizoaffective disorders can present with manic syndromes in late life. Schizoaffective disorders have presented challenges for classification, and these patients have not been well described in the elderly. In an early study by Post (1971), BP and depressive subtypes were not distinguished. BP-type schizoaffective disorders may constitute a substantial proportion of geriatric schizoaffective inpatients (Yu & Young, 2001). Paranoid schizophrenic patients can have manic features, such as grandiose delusions. The differentiation of BP schizoaffective disorders and paranoid schizophrenia from BP disorder rests on longitudinal course.

SUBSTANCE ABUSE

Active substance abuse/dependence and intoxication can contribute to manic-like signs and symptoms. Alcohol, anxiolytic, and analgesic dependence in particular must be considered in the differential diagnosis of mania in the elderly.

Psychiatric Comorbidity

Substance abuse may be less prevalent with increased age among BP patients (Cassidy, Ahearn, & Carroll, 2001; Ponce, Kunik et al., 1999; Sajatovic, Popli et al., 1996). One study (Sajatovic, Blow, & Ignacio, 2006) found comorbid anxiety, substance abuse, and dementia in 29% of geriatric veterans with BP disorder. In another study, one third of manic inpatients aged >55 years had a history of substance abuse (Himmelhoch, Neil, May, Fuchs, & Licata, 1980). Comorbid adult attention-deficit disorder has been investigated in mixed-age BP disorder (Nierenberg et al., 2005), but co-occurrence of these disorders has not been examined in elders.

In summary, the assessment and differential diagnosis of mania and BP disorders in old age must consider a broad range of possibilities. An adequate history is central to management, and longitudinal assessment can help clarify the diagnosis. The fact that manic states can reflect underling medical and neurological disorders and treatments highlights the need for thorough medical evaluation.

EPIDEMIOLOGY

Epidemiological issues related to BP disorders in late life are reviewed in Chapter 3. In what follows, a few points are highlighted.

Age

In this review, the definition of aged, elderly, or geriatric is 60 years of age or older, since this is one commonly used convention. In some studies, older adults have been defined by a younger index age, and this will be indicated.

Prevalence

The lifetime and 1-year prevalence rates for mania in the elderly community detected in the Epidemiologic Catchment Area study were only 0.1% (Weissman, Bruce et al., 1990). On the other hand, the prevalence of mania at age >60 years in patients presenting for treatment to psychiatric services ranges from 5% to 19% (Dunn & Rabins, 1996; Yassa, Nair et al., 1988b). The sex distribution favors women. Comparisons in racial and ethnic groups are lacking.

Incidence

Wertham (1929) observed a decline in first psychiatric admissions of manic patients over the age of 50. Clayton (1986) concluded that the risk of new-onset mania declines, or at least does not increase, with aging. This is consistent with findings of a retrospective study of psychiatric inpatients by Loranger and Levine (1978), although these investigators excluded an unspecified number of elderly patients with medical illnesses. In contrast to this experience, the geropsychiatry literature indicates that age at onset of mania tends to be late, often in the fifth or sixth decade (Broadhead & Jacoby, 1990; Charron, Fortin, & Paguette, 2001; Glasser & Rabins, 1984; Shulman & Post, 1980; Stone, 1989). Similarly, Spicer et al. (Spicer, Hare, & Slater, 1973) found that first admissions of male manic patients increased above 60 years of age, and Eagles and Whaley (1985) observed a gradual increase with age in first hospital admissions of manic patients— especially males, an increase that was sustained past the age of 70. Angst suggested a bimodal distribution for age at onset of BP disorder based on findings in a sample of 95 mixed-age patients (Angst,

1978). Chu et al. (2010) did not, however, find demographic differences between BP elders in early versus late age at onset of illness.

Episodes of depression often predate the onset of mania in late life, and this interval can be more than a decade (Broadhead & Jacoby, 1990; Glasser & Rabins, 1984; Shulman & Post, 1980; Snowdon, 1991; Stone, 1989; Yassa, Nair et al., 1988a). There has also been speculation that the availability of antidepressant pharmacotherapies may be provoking increased rates of BP disorder in late life. On the other hand, one report suggests that a pattern of unipolar mania in late life may be linked to early age at onset of illness (Shulman & Tohen, 1994).

Ascertainment of age at onset can be challenging in late-life mood disorder. The definition of late onset differs between studies (Young & Klerman, 1992); age at onset of first mania or of first episode can be considered. Distributions of values within a sample, either using median or apparent biphasic distribution of age at onset, have been considered in some studies; other investigators have used particular ages such as 50 years.

In summary, there is fairly strong evidence for decreased community prevalence with age in BP disorder. It remains an important proportion of aged psychiatric inpatients. Among older patients presenting with BP disorder, a subgroup has onset of illness late in life.

PATHOPHYSIOLOGY AND ETIOLOGY

Overview

AGE

Age-associated factors may modify the pathophysiology of early-onset illness. They may modify the features and course of patients with BP disorders having onset in early age. The nature of such changes is not well delineated in geriatric populations. The potential mechanisms for such changes could include both physical/physiological changes within the range of "normal aging" that interact with the pathophysiology of early-onset illnesses, and disorders or illnesses. Other potential mechanisms include learning and adaptation, and changes in social context, environment, and resources. The best way to examine age effects on illness would be to compare elderly patients with early-onset BP disorder with younger BP patients, but the limited

available data have generally involved index age alone.

AGE AT ONSET

Patients who develop BP disorder in late life can be conceptualized as manifesting emergences of age-associated pathogenic factors for the disorder and/or loss of protective factors. The potential mechanisms could overlap with those listed under the section on "Age" earlier. Whether these patients differ from elders with early-onset BP disorder on a clinical, pathophysiological, or etiological level has received limited investigation. To examine age-at-onset effects requires comparison of aged patients with either early- or late-onset illness.

Late-onset illness may be differentiated from early-onset illness in regard to age-acquired factors that confer additional vulnerability and by factors that may be protective in early life. Age-associated brain changes, for example, have been proposed to mediate change from unipolar depression to BP disorder (Shulman, 1997).

Vascular Risk Factors

Elderly manic patients may have greater clinical evidence of cerebrovascular disease compared to normal elders. Berrios and Bakshi (1991) recorded high Hachinski scores in elderly patients with manic symptoms compared to elders with depressive symptoms. Broadhead and Jacoby (1990) and Snowdon (1991) indicated that some of the geriatric patients that they studied had onset of mania soon after a central neurological event.

AGE AT ONSET

Stroke risk factors may be particularly high in patients with late onset of BP disorder (Cassidy & Carroll, 2002; Wylie et al., 1999). Steffens and Krishnan (1998) proposed a vascular subtype of mania, similar to the vascular depression concept (Alexopoulos et al., 1997). This concept may have implications for studies of prevention and long-term management (Subramaniam, Dennis, & Byrne, 2007).

Brain Lesions and Mania

Studies of patients with focal brain pathology have implicated specific neural circuits with manic psychopathology. Right hemisphere lesions have been linked to mania. Sackeim and colleagues (1982) noted that pathological laughing was associated with destructive lesions of right brain, and that right hemispherectomy often produces euphoric mood. Furthermore, Starkstein and colleagues (Starkstein, Boston, & Robinson, 1988; Starkstein et al., 1990) reported preponderance of right-sided or bilateral hemispheric localization of heterogeneous brain lesions, including tumors, strokes, and head injuries in patients with mania. Some left-sided lesions, including basal ganglia lesions, have also been associated with mania, however (Liu, Wang, Fuh, Yang, & Liu, 1996; Turecki, Mari, & Del Porto, 1993).

A number of reports have linked mania and "disinhibition syndrome" with pathology of the medial orbitofrontal cortex (OFC)-subcortical circuits, including thalamus and caudate (Cummings, 1993; Starkstein, Federoff, Berthier, & Robinson, 1991). The behavioral abnormalities encompassed by disinhibition overlap with the psychopathology of mania, for example, "secondary" mania (Cummings, 1993; Shulman, 1997; Starkstein & Robinson, 1997). Involvement of OFC dysfunction in mania is supported by functional imaging studies in mixed-age manic patients (Blumberg, Charney, & Krystal, 2002). Frontotemporal dementia can present with disinhibition (Miller et al., 1991). Primate studies also link OFC lesions to disruption of social behavior (Kling & Steklis, 1976).

Basotemporal cortical lesions are also linked to mania (Starkstein et al., 1991; Starkstein & Robinson, 1997). A study of patients with head injury found predominant basotemporal injury in the 9% who developed mania (Jorge et al., 1993).

Other Abnormalities on Structural Neuroimaging

Brain morphologic abnormalities on neuroimaging may be prominent in elderly manic and BP patients treated at psychiatric services. Investigators have described both excess signal hyperintensities (SHs) on magnetic resonance imaging and loss of tissue volume. Studies of these patients have found prominent deep frontal white matter and periventricular SH (deAsis, Young et al., 1998; McDonald, Krishnan, Doraiswamy, & Blazer, 1991; McDonald et al., 1999) and subcortical gray matter SH (McDonald et al., 1999). SH in aged BP patients may reflect different processes than those seen in unipolar depressed elders. Excess "silent strokes" have

also been described in aged BP patients (Fujikawa, Yamawaki, & Touhouda, 1995).

Several studies have found decreased tissue volume on neuroimaging compared to controls in aged manic patients. These findings include excess cortical sulcal widening on computed tomography (Young, Nambudiri, Jain, de Asis, & Alexopoulos, 1999) and magnetic resonance imaging (Rabins, Aylward, Holroyd, & Pearlson, 2000). One computed tomography study found larger lateral ventricle-brain ratio in aged manic patients compared to controls (Young et al., 1999), although other studies did not (Beyer et al., 2004; Broadhead & Jacoby, 1990).

Differences in regional tissue volume compared to controls have been reported in BP older adults/elders. These findings include greater left sylvian fissure and left and right temporal sulcal widening (Rabins et al., 2000), smaller bilateral volume in the inferior frontal gray matter (Beyer et al., 2009), lower parietal cortex volume, and smaller right caudate volume (Beyer et al., 2004), and larger left hippocampus.

AGE

More severe SH scores were noted compared to controls in a mixed-age BP sample that included aged patients (McDonald et al., 1999), although there was a trend for less confluent SH in the older patients. In this study, subcortical gray nuclei SH scores were also greater than in controls, which has not been reported in studies of young BP patients. In a meta-analysis of studies of BP disorder, unipolar depression, and schizophrenia in adulthood, Beyer et al. (Beyer, Young, Kuchibhatla, & Krishnan, 2009) found greater SH in BP subjects in deep white matter and subcortical regions compared to controls. They found that SH were also increased compared to controls in unipolar depression and in schizophrenia. Caudate volume was inversely associated with age in a study of mixed-age BP patients (Brambilla et al., 2001).

AGE AT ONSET

Some abnormalities on structural neuroimaging may be particularly prominent in those BP elders with late age at onset; these may include small strokes (Fujikawa et al., 1995; McDonald et al., 1991; Young et al., 1999). Studies of SH in older patients with late-onset illness revealed greater subcortical SH than in aged controls (McDonald et al.,

1991) and greater SH in right deep frontal white matter with later age at onset of mania (deAsis et al., 2006); however, a study of a mixed-age sample did not support an association with age at onset (McDonald et al., 1999). Greater cortical sulcal widening was associated with later age at onset of illness in one study (Young et al., 1999), but not in another (Broadhead & Jacoby, 1990). Greater prevalence of white matter SHs in late-onset elderly BP patients relative to early-onset and elderly healthy volunteers were reported in deep frontal and parietal regions and in putamen (Tamashiro et al., 2008). In BP subjects, later age at onset of illness was associated with smaller brain volume, and smaller right and total caudate volume compared to earlier age at onset in patients (Beyer et al., 2004).

OTHER CLINICAL CORRELATES

One study found no significant correlations between white matter hyperintensity ratings and number of episodes in BP elders (Tamashiro et al., 2008).

Functional Neuroimaging

One study found an association between resting cerebral metabolism in the limbic, paralimbic, and prefrontal areas, and sustained attention performance during euthymia in older adults with BP; inferior frontal gyrus hypometabolism and paralimbic hypermetabolism were related to sustained attention deficits and inhibitory control during euthymia (Brooks, Bearden, Hoblyn, Woodard, & Ketter, 2010).

Other Neurological Disorders and Treatments.

Kay et al. (1955) and Post (1965) proposed that mood disorder with onset in late life reflects in part degenerative brain changes. Shulman and Post (1980) reported that the onset of manic states in the geriatric age range was associated with clinical evidence of coarse brain diseases. Stone (1989) found evidence of "organic cerebral impairment" among 24% of 92 elderly manic inpatients studied retrospectively and suggested that they had later onset of illness. Tohen, Shulman, and Satlin (1994) observed neurological comorbidity in 74% of late-onset cases.

Geriatric manic patients also have a higher prevalence of heterogeneous neurological disorders compared to age- and sex-matched unipolar depressed patients (Shulman, Tohen, Satlin, Mallya, & Kalunian, 1992) . In addition to cerebrovascular disease, degenerative brain disorders linked to BP disorders include multiple sclerosis (Joffe, Lippert, Gray, Sawa, & Horvath, 1987) and Huntington's disease (Folstein, 1989).

There has been only preliminary study of the association between Alzheimer's disease and mania or manic phenomenology. Burns et al. (1990) recorded manic features in 3.5% of Alzheimer's disease patients. Lyketsos et al. (1995) found that 2.2% of Alzheimer's patients had a manic syndrome, and that two thirds of these had had prior manic episodes prior to onset of dementia.

Gait disorder can be a particular concern in frail BP elders. In mixed-age samples gait disorder is more frequent in BP than in patients with unipolar depression (Hausdorff, Chung-Kang, Goldberger, & Stoll, 2004).

MEDICAL COMORBIDITY

Krauthammer and Klerman (1978) demonstrated that a range of medical disorders can be associated with late-onset mania. Black et al. (1988) observed that older age was a characteristic of patients with mania complicated by a broad range of medical disorders; these include endocrinopathies, nutrient deficiencies, and infections (Brooks & Hoblyn, 2005; Strakowski, McElroy, Keck, & West, 1994; Verdoux & Bourgeois, 1995). Treatments used to treat medical disorders, such as corticosteroids, also have been implicated in manic states. Roose et al. (Roose, Nurnberger, Dunner, Blood, & Fieve, 1979) cautioned that psychiatrists may be the only physicians involved with elderly BP patients despite their prevalent medical comorbidities.

Aged BP elders have a higher rate of cardiovascular, endocrine, and pulmonary disorders compared to younger patients (Lala & Sajatovic, 2012). BP elders had higher rate of endocrine, metabolic, and pulmonary disorders compared to elderly unipolar depressed patients (Gildengers et al., 2008).

Chu et al. (2010) did not find differences in medical burden based on age at onset in BP elders. Medical comorbidity presents an important focus for management in BP elders. The development and application of strategies for such interventions are discussed elsewhere (Kilbourne et al., 2008).

Familial Factors

BP disorder is strongly associated with hereditary factors. Late-onset probands have a lower rate affective disorder among their relatives than do probands with early-onset illness, both in mixed-age patient samples (Hays, 1976; Mendlewics, Fieve, Rainer, & Fleiss, 1972; Rice et al., 1987; Taylor & Abrams, 1981) and in elderly BP patients (Glasser & Rabins, 1984; Schouws et al., 2009; Shulman & Post, 1980; Snowdon, 1991; Stone, 1989). Genetic factors may contribute to late age at onset (McMahon, DePaulo et al., 1996). Genetic factors in late-life mood disorders are discussed in Chapter 37.

Life Events and Daily Routine

There is limited information concerning life events in geriatric manic or BP patients (Walter-Ryan, 1983). Yassa et al. (Yassa, Nair et al., 1988a) observed stressful events in 70% of elderly manic patients studied. In a mixed-age sample, negative life events preceding manic episode was associated with older index age (Ambelas, 1987). On the other hand, decreased conflicts and/or more regular daily routine with increased age may be protective in some individuals (Depp & Jeste, 2004).

In summary, late-age-at-onset manic syndromes and BP disorders represent models for studying age-associated constitutional and psychosocial factors in relationship to pathogenesis. Thus, familial and genetic contributions may be different and may include different balances between protective aspects and vulnerabilities. Brain changes may play an important role, particularly those arising from cerebrovascular or degenerative changes at a microscopic or clinical level. Manic and BP disorders arising out of brain lesions have implicated particular neuronal circuits in these disorders, including integrity of cortico-striato-limbic circuits, and these may have relevance to the pathophysiology of idiopathic disorders. Dementing disorders and subcortical neurological diseases present additional opportunities. Thus, models of late-life illness may be relevant to mechanisms of early-life illness.

EPISODES: AFFECTIVE FEATURES

Mania

In this syndrome the predominant affective signs and symptoms represent acceleration and/or excesses of behavior, mental activity, or emotion. These characteristics can result in harm to the patient and to others. For example, Petrie, Lawson, and Hollender (1982) observed that 9%–16% of aggressive or violent geriatric inpatients are manic.

Rating scales for manic psychopathology (Bech, Rafaelsen, Kramp, & Bolwig, 1978; Blackburn, Loudon, & Ashworth, 1977; Young, Biggs, Ziegler, & Meyer, 1978) have been applied in elderly patients, and others are available. These can be used to monitor change. Instruments for assessment of manic symptoms and other psychopathology in demented patients are also available, for example, the Dementia Signs and Symptoms Scale (Loreck, Bylsma, & Folstein, 1994).

AGE

Few studies have used rating scales to compare manic psychopathology in elderly patients to that in younger patients. Findings in existing studies have been modest. In symptomatic inpatients of mixed-age studied prospectively (Young & Falk, 1989) age was negatively associated with scores on the "activity-energy" item of the Young Mania Rating Scale (Young et al., 1978). There was a low negative correlation between age and scores on the "language-thought disorder" item and a trend for decreased "sexual interest" scores with age. Limited effects of age were again noted in subsequent analyses in mixed-age and elderly samples of BP manic patients (Young et al., 2007; Young, Marino et al., 2011). In aged manic patients, Broadhead and Jacoby (1990) found that total scores on the Modified Mania Scale (Blackburn et al., 1977) at admission to hospital were lower than those of a younger patient comparison group. Older patients had lower scores on the "religiosity" item of the scale; however, other items did not differentiate older and young patients. In an elderly subgroup of manic patients in the EMBLEM study (Oostervink, Boomsma, Nolen, & EMBLEM Advisory Board, 2009) baseline Clinical Global Impression scores were lower than in young patients.

AGE AT ONSET

In elderly manic patients, Broadhead and Jacoby (1990) found higher average item ratings for "happiness" and "cheerfulness" on the Modified Mania Scale in late- compared to early-onset cases. One study of ambulatory BP patients aged 45–85 years found less overall symptom severity in late-onset compared to early-onset patients (Depp et al., 2004). A retrospective report (Glasser & Rabins, 1984) and the prospective European Mania in Bipolar Longitudinal Evaluation of Medication study (EMBLEM) (Oostervink et al., 2009) did not detect differences in global severity between aged patients with late-onset and early-onset illness, however.

Mixed States

A mixture of depressive features occur in young adult manic patients, that is, mixed states (e.g., *DSM-IV*) or dysphoric mania (Swann, 1995). Post (1965) suggested that older manic patients exhibit concomitant depressive features more often than do younger patients, based on clinical impressions. In geriatric bipolar I manic patients, one analysis found that manic symptom ratings were similar in those with and without depressive symptoms (Sajatovic et al., 2011).

AGE

In the study by Broadhead and Jacoby (1990), there were equivalent mixed features in the elderly and the young manic patients.

AGE AT ONSET

Those investigators also found no difference in depressive features during the manic episode between late-onset and early-onset elderly manic patients.

Bipolar Depression

BP depressed states have received minimal study in elderly patients. They were part of the sample studied by Wylie et al. (1999).

AGE

BP patients older than 50 years at first psychiatric hospitalization presented less with manic psychotic episodes and more with depressive psychotic episodes compared to younger patients (Kessing, 2006).

In the study of Broadhead and Jacoby (1990) a greater proportion of elderly than younger manic patients suffered a depressive episode after resolution of mania but before hospital discharge. Greater frequency of cycling into depression with increased age was also reported in the EMBLEM study (Oostervink et al., 2009). Rapid cycling has apparently not been studied in aged patients.

Psychotic Features

Delusions and hallucinations can occur in manic and BP depressed elders. For example, 58% of the symptomatic geriatric BP patients studied by Wylie et al. (1999) were psychotic. The distinction between mood congruent and incongruent psychotic features has not been used in studies of these patients. Benazzi (1999) observed that among aged depressed patients, those who were psychotic more often had BP disorder.

AGE

A prospective assessment of mixed-age manic inpatients did not find an association between age and the presence of hallucinations and/or delusions (Young, Schreiber, & Nysewander, 1983) nor did another comparison of geriatric and younger manic patients (Broadhead & Jacoby, 1990). Benazzi (1999) did not detect an age effect on the BP preponderance among psychotic depressed patients.

AGE AT ONSET

Wylie et al. (1999) found an association between late age at onset and psychosis in a sample of aged BP patients with manic and depressed states. Tohen et al. (1994) reported delusions in 45% of their late-onset manic sample. Broadhead and Jacoby (1990) did not detect a difference in rate of delusions between early- and late-onset manic elders. There have been conflicting reports concerning age at onset and psychosis in the mixed-age BP literature (Angst et al., 1973; Rosen, Rosenthal, Van Dusen, Dunner, & Fieve, 1984).

EPISODES: COGNITIVE IMPAIRMENTS

Clinical investigation in manic elders has supported the presence of cognitive impairment (Shulman & Post, 1980; Stone, 1989). Stone (1989) reported that evidence of "cerebral organic impairment" was present in 24% of elderly manic patients and that more than 60% of these patients had memory impairment associated with the episode.

Assessment with standardized instruments during symptomatic states may be feasible if limitations of cooperation are addressed and short duration of testing is used. Testing cognitive function both during episodes of illness and on follow-up, when patients are in affective remission, permits retrospective assessment regarding state-dependent versus persistent dysfunction. Medication effects may be relevant to both symptomatic and remitted patients, however.

Consistent with cognitive test results in mixed-age BP *manic* patients, where deficits in attention and memory have been documented (Bearden, Hoffman, & Cannon, 2001; Clayton, Pitts et al., 1965; Kerry, McDermott, & Orme, 1983; Strauss, Bohannon, Stephens, & Pauker, 1984), Broadhead and Jacoby (1990) found that a greater proportion of elderly manic patients performed in the demented range on the Kendrick neuropsychological battery compared to young patients; however, they observed a large discrepancy between verbal and performance IQ in both groups. Impaired *global measures* of cognitive function have been also described in geriatric manic patients in more recent reports (Gildengers et al., 2010; Young, Murphy, Heo, Schulberg, & Alexopoulos, 2006). Cognitive dysfunction in mania can resolve with treatment and with resolution of mood symptoms (Kraepelin, 1921; Post, 1965; Slater & Roth, 1977). Similarly in elders, performance may improve with treatment of BP episodes (Wylie et al., 1999).

Cognitive impairments have also been documented in BP *depressed* elders. Burt et al. (Burt, Prudic, Peyser, Clark, & Sackeim, 2000) found greater *memory* impairment in BP depressed elders compared to aged controls, and this impairment was also greater than that in younger BP depressed patients.

Cognitive dysfunction has also been reported in studies of *remitted* mixed-age BP patients, as supported in a recent meta-analysis (Robinson et al., 2006). Findings in elderly BP patients are consistent with this (see section on "Nonaffective Outcomes").

Interest has focused on whether particular cognitive functions are impaired in aged BP patients. Overall, reported impairments have included a range of cognitive domains in various studies: attention, executive functions (set shifting, response inhibition), memory, calculation, abstraction, and psychomotor/processing speed (Bearden et al., 2001; Delaloye, Moy et al., 2009; Depp et al., 2007; Gildengers et al., 2004; Gunning-Dixon, Murphy, Alexopoulos, Majcher-Tascio, & Young, 2008; Schouws et al., 2009; Silva et al., 2009; Young et al., 2006). Impaired performance on executive tasks in manic elders can be more severe than in unipolar depressed elders (Gunning-Dixon et al., 2008). A more recent study of aged patients with BP disorder or unipolar depression concluded that cognitive function was worse in BP patients (Gildengers, Butters et al., 2012).

AGE

One study (Burt et al., 2000) documented worse memory impairment in BP depressed elders compared to young BP depressed patients.

AGE AT ONSET

In the study by Stone (1989) cerebral organic impairment was associated with late age at onset. In another report cognitive impairments were greater in elderly patients with late-onset compared to early-onset BP illness (Schouws et al., 2009). Broadhead and Jacoby (1990) did not detect an effect of age at onset.

OTHER CORRELATES

In manic BP elders, global cognitive impairment was inversely related to manic symptom severity in one report (Gildengers et al., 2010). Performance on memory tasks has been found to be negatively related to level of vascular burden in BP elders (Gildengers et al., 2010; Schouws, Stek, Comijs, & Beekman, 2010). In a functional neuroimaging study, verbal memory impairment was correlated with prefrontal hypometabolism and paralimbic hypermetabolism (Brooks et al., 2009). Cognitive performance measures have been reported to be unrelated to duration of illness (Depp et al., 2007; Gildengers et al., 2010), brain tissue volume, or white matter changes (Delaloye, de Bilbao et al., 2009; Delaloye, Moy et al., 2009; Delaloye et al., 2011).

Cognitive impairments are clinically important because they are associated with behavioral disability and quality-of-life measures, as indicated later. Also this perspective underscores the need to minimize exacerbation of cognitive dysfunction by identifying treatments that are best tolerated. In addition, a more speculative issue is the possibility of enhancement of cognition with psychotropic treatments such as mood stabilizers that may have neuro-protective/neurotrophic effects. The role, if any, for other approaches, such as cognitive rehabilitation, in impaired BP patients has not been studied.

Disability and Quality of Life

Functional impairment is described in young BP patients (Arnold et al., 2000) during illness episodes. Behavioral disability and impaired quality-of-life measures is an important dimension in BP elders (Bartels, Meuser, & Miles, 1997). Disability is linked to cognitive impairments in BP elders (Bartels et al., 1997; Depp, Davis, Mittal, Patterson, & Jeste, 2006; Gildengers et al., 2007). Treatment nonadherence has been linked to reported forgetfulness in mixed-age BP patients (Depp, Lebowitz, Patterson, Lacro, & Jeste, 2007; Sajatovic et al., 2011).

In summary, there is a broad range of mood abnormalities and other impairments associated with BP episodes in the elderly. Cognitive performance in bipolar elders may be influenced by many, potentially interrelated, factors (Fig. 7.1). Findings regarding group differences of interest are scant, particularly for depressed states. Modest attenuations of manic symptom severity with increased age may reflect modification of related pathophysiology by age-associated neurobiological and psychosocial

factors; comparison of recurrent early-onset BP disorders in late life with early-onset disorders in young adults, with controls, provides a model for studying such processes.

AFFECTIVE COURSE

Chronicity

There is some evidence that manic or depressive symptoms in BP elders are more persistent. During standardized open treatment of a small sample of BP elders, most did not experience sustained recovery (Gildengers et al., 2005).

AGE

There is little information available as to whether the rates of recovery from mania are different in elderly and younger patients. Several investigators (Lundquist, 1945; MacDonald, 1918; Wertham, 1929) have reported a positive association between age and duration of the acute manic episode in populations of mixed ages. Wertham's (1929) 2,000 patients ranged in age up to the eighth decade. In MacDonald's (1918) sample, 12 of 451 patients were 60 years of age or older, and in Lundquist's (1945) sample, 11 of 103 manic patients were older than 50 years. Chronic mania has been associated

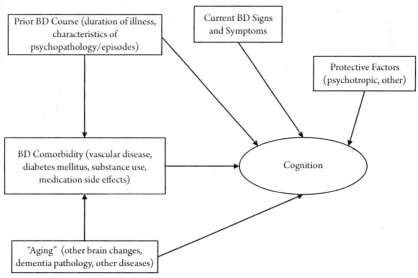

FIGURE 7.1 Factors influencing cognition in late-life bipolar disorder. Not all potential interactions are depicted. BD, bipolar disorder. (Adapted from Gildengers et al., 2010.)

with increased age (Henderson & Gillespie, 1956; Wertham, 1929). Wertham (1929) observed that seven patients with manic episodes lasting at least 5 years ranged in age from 31 to 60 years. Henderson and Gillespie (1956) reported that patients with chronic mania were frequently aged more than 40 years. Among Lundquist's (1945) patients, fewer of those aged more than 40 years recovered (84%) compared to younger patients (95%).

Roth (1955) suggested a relatively poor outcome for elderly patients with mania. He reported that among 28 geriatric inpatients, 65% of those still living at 2-year follow-up had remained in the hospital; this was a poorer outcome than that of geriatric depressed patients.

Van der Velde (1970) observed worse acute outcomes with increased age in patients receiving naturalistic lithium treatment. In a mixed-age sample of manic patients examined prospectively, older age was associated with longer duration of acute psychiatric hospitalization (Young & Falk, 1989). In that sample, consistent with clinical observation by Post (1965), older age was also associated with higher residual ratings on the Impaired Insight item of the Mania Rating Scale over 2 weeks of naturalistic lithium treatment. Berrios and Bakshi (1991) observed worse acute outcomes in geriatric mania than in unipolar geriatric depression. However, Himmelhoch et al. (1980) did not find an effect of age on recovery from mania in 81 patients studied retrospectively, although all were aged 55 years or more. In the prospective study by Broadhead and Jacoby (1990), there was no difference in duration of the index manic episode between elderly and younger patients. Stone (1989) reported episodes lasting 2–13 years in five of 92 geriatric manic patients, but only 8% of patients remained in hospital at 6 months. Glasser and Rabins (1984) found that 79% of manic elderly inpatients were discharged to home after acute treatment, which further supports an improved short-term prognosis since the era of Roth's investigations.

AGE AT ONSET

In mixed-age patients, some reports have suggested an association between greater age at onset and greater duration of episode and/or chronicity. MacDonald's (1918) patients and Lundquist's were selected on the basis of first psychiatric hospitalization. In Wertham's study (1929), four of seven chronic manic patients were aged 38–60 years at the onset of illness.

On the other hand, Perlis et al. (2009) reported that in mixed-age adults, those with early-onset BP disorder appear to be at greater risk for recurrence, chronicity of mood symptoms, and functional impairment.

In the geriatric literature, neither the report of Broadhead and Jacoby (1990) nor that of Stone (1989) indicated differences in duration of episode between late-onset and early-onset geriatric manic patients. Dhingra and Rabins (1991) and Shulman et al. (1992) did not comment on this issue.

RELAPSE/RECURRENCE

AGE

In mixed-age BP patients, MacDonald (1918) reported an association between greater age and shorter intervals between episodes. Studies in geriatric manic patients have observed further episodes in a high proportion, albeit a better prognosis than that observed by Roth. The study designs have varied in measures and duration of assessment. Shulman and Post (1980) observed further episodes in 76% of the patients in their sample. Stone (1989) reported a 52% readmission rate on a 1-month to 10-year follow-up. Dhingra and Rabins (1991) recorded relapse requiring hospitalization in 32% of patients followed up over 5–7 years. Risk of recurrence reportedly increases with the number of episodes in BP disorders, as does risk of depressive residual symptoms (Kessing, Hansen, Andersen, & Angst, 2004).

AGE AT ONSET

In mixed-age BP patients, investigators (Angst et al., 1973; Swift, 1907) have reported an association between shorter interepisode intervals and later age at onset. Among geriatric patients, Stone (1989) found increased frequency of readmission in those with histories of previous affective episodes compared to those without such a history. On the other hand, Shulman et al. (1992) found that an age at onset greater than 55 years predicted decreased time to psychiatric rehospitalization at 3- to 10-year follow-forward. Other studies have found not difference in relapse and rehospitalization in elders with early versus later age at onset of illness (Dhingra & Rabins, 1991; Lehmann & Rabins, 2006).

Suicide

Suicidal ideation or attempt, or completed suicide, are not well characterized in geriatric BP disorders. Shulman et al. (1992) did not detect suicide as a cause of mortality in his follow-up study. Given associations with age and with mood disorder in mixed-age adults, investigation in elderly BP patients is warranted.

Psychiatric Services Use and Caregiver Burden

The public health importance of BP disorders in the elderly stems not only from their clinical characteristics and the burden on patients themselves but also their impact on caregivers, families, and care systems. Among geriatric psychiatric patients discharged from hospital, BP diagnosis was a predictor of early readmission (Woo et al., 2006). Elderly BP patients use services at a high rate (Sajatovic, Vernon, & Semple, 1997). Bartels et al. (1997) reported that they use psychiatric services at an almost four-fold greater rate than do aged unipolar depressed patients.

Older BP adults with recurrent illness episodes appear to be more ill and utilize more health services than older adults with new-onset illness (Sajatovic, Blow, Ignacio, & Kales, 2004, 2005). Depp et al. (2005) cautioned that elders with BP disorder and functional decline may be at risk of being overlooked by community services. Comorbid dementia is associated with higher general medical costs in BP elders (Al Jurdi et al., 2012; Sajatovic et al., 2006). .

MODIFICATION OF COURSE BY OTHER AGE-ASSOCIATED FACTORS

Psychiatric Comorbidity

Substance abuse was associated with poorer acute therapeutic outcome in older patients with mania (Himmelhoch et al., 1980).

Medical/Neurological Comorbidity

In the study of Shulman et al. (1992) neurological disorders were associated with greater rates of subsequent psychiatric hospitalization. In the study of Berrios and Bakshi (1991) high Hatchinski scores were predictive of worse acute outcome in mania.

Patients aged >55 years with dementia accompanied by mania had poorer acute antimanic treatment response (Himmelhoch et al., 1980). Other medical disorders may contribute to poor acute outcomes in mania (Black et al., 1988). The symptomatic treatment of secondary mania in older adults is similar to the treatment of primary mania, except that treatment of the causal factors should be addressed (Brooks & Hoblyn, 2005).

Lack of Social Support

Mixed-age BP patients receive less social support than either medically ill patients or normal controls (Romans & McPherson, 1992; Speer, 1992); this lack of support has been linked to greater depressive symptoms on follow-up (Johnson, Meyer, Winett, & Small, 2000) and poorer function (O'Connell, Mayo, Flatow, Cuthbertson, & O'Brien, 1991). Geriatric BP disorder patients report less social support compared to same age controls (Beyer et al., 2003). Among geriatric BP patients (Bartels et al., 1997), lack of a spouse was associated with residence in a nursing facility rather than residing in the community.

Disability

In young BP patients disability can worsen symptom course. This has not been studied in elderly patients (Gitlin, Swendsen, Heller, & Hammen, 1995).

In summary, the course of illness in late-life mania and BP disorders is heterogeneous and may be more malignant than that of unipolar depression. Predictors of poor outcomes may include neurological disorders.

NONAFFECTIVE OUTCOMES

Nonsuicide Mortality

Mortality rates are relatively high in aged patients with BP disorder. Roth (1955) observed a mortality rate over 2 years of 11%; this was lower than that for elderly demented patients but was higher than that for elderly unipolar depressed patients. There were two deaths among nine patients followed for 2 years by Yassa et al. (Yassa, Nair et al., 1988b). Stone (1989) observed a mortality rate over 2 years of 16% for geriatric mania. In the study by Dhingra and Rabins (1991), mortality at

5- to 7-year follow-up was 34%; these authors commented that the survival rate was significantly lower than the expected rate calculated from Census data. Similarly, Shulman et al. (1992) found that the mortality rate of geriatric manic patients, 50% on an average of 6 years, exceeded that of geriatric depressed patients (20%). The mechanisms for this increased nonsuicide mortality are not clear but include effects of cerebrovascular disease (Tohen et al., 1994). Mortality was not increased by neurologic disorder in the sample of Shulman et al. (1992).

Affective episodes themselves may be lethal, and manic episodes have in the past been linked to mortality through "exhaustion." Decreased sleep, impaired nutritional status through overactivity and distraction, and decreased compliance with medical regimens all pose a threat to health. These issues carry added weight in the frail elderly patient. Although deaths from "manic exhaustion" were reported to occur most often among young patients (Derby, 1933), the age distribution of the total samples was not clear. The incidence of manic exhaustion has apparently been reduced dramatically in the psychopharmacologic era (Wendkos, 1979).

AGE

Mortality among elderly patients has apparently not been compared to that among younger BP patients in the same study. There is evidence for greater mortality among BP patients of mixed ages—at least among those with medical illness (Jamison & Goodwin, 1998)—than among the general population.

AGE AT ONSET

Late-onset mania has a high mortality rate (Tohen et al., 1994). Male patients had higher mortality than females in that sample. Neither the study by Dhingra and Rabins (1991) nor that of Shulman et al. (1992) detected differences in mortality between late-onset and early-onset illness patients.

Cognitive Impairment and Emergent Dementia

A proportion of elderly manic patients have cognitive impairment and/or dementia on follow-up. Cognitive dysfunction and accelerated cognitive decline may lead to increased reliance on family and community supports, and placement.

In one study (Savard, Rey, & Post, 1980) neuropsychological task performance of remitted BP patients aged >40 years was poorer than that of same-age controls. In ambulatory BP patients aged 45–85 years, performance on neuropsychological tests was considerably impaired, with a pattern somewhat distinct from patients with schizophrenia (Depp et al., 2007). Several groups have documented cognitive impairments in BP elders who are *remitted* (Delaloye et al., 2009; Delaloye, Moy et al., 2009; Gildengers et al., 2004; Schouws et al., 2010), including *abnormalities of memory*, *executive function* (response inhibition, set shifting), and *psychomotor/processing speed*, compared with healthy individuals. One study reported differences in cognitive performance profile in middle-aged and elderly BP elders compared to same-aged individuals with mild cognitive impairment (Silva et al., 2009).

Stone (1989) reported that 3% of 92 geriatric patients with mania went on to develop moderate to severe dementia over an average of 3 years of follow-up. Dhingra and Rabins (1991) found that at 5- to 7-year follow-up, 32% of elderly manic patients had Mini-mental State Examination (MMSE) (Folstein, Folstein, & McHugh, 1975) scores in the cognitively impaired range (less than 24), and 20% had been placed in nursing homes; they commented that this was greater than the incidence of all forms of dementia expected in this age group in the community; the rate was not greater than that of geriatric depressed patients, however. Gildengers et al. (2009) found that older adults with BP disorder have more cognitive dysfunction and more rapid cognitive decline than controls. In another study of BP disorder, the risk of diagnosis of dementia at readmission was increased by greater number of prior episodes leading to admission (Kessing & Andersen, 2004).

AGE

Emergent dementia occurs relatively infrequently in BP patients of mixed ages, but it has received limited study as an outcome (Coffman, Bornstein, Olson, Schwarzkopf, & Nasrallah, 1990), and then in combined unipolar/BP samples. In the study by Astrup, Fossum, and Holmboe (1959), less than 5% of patients with affective disorders were clinically demented on 7- to 19-year follow-up.

AGE AT ONSET

It is not known whether late-onset manic patients are at particularly high risk for development of cognitive dysfunction/dementia. Dhingra and Rabins (1991) could not detect differences in MMSE scores between late-onset mania and geriatric early-onset mania at 5- to 7-year follow-up. Charron et al. (2001) did not observe dementia on 2-year follow-up in their six late-onset cases.

Function/Behavioral Disability

While a substantial proportion of young BP patients have impaired function (behavioral disability) in remission (Coryell et al., 1993), the course of disability has not been studied in geriatric BP patients. Nursing home/chronic institutional placement is reported in 20%–30% in recent follow-up studies of elderly manic patients (Dhingra & Rabins, 1991; Shulman et al., 1992). In young BP patients, disability may be worsened by symptomatic states (Gitlin et al., 1995).

Real-world function in geriatric BP disorder is likely to be impaired. Behavioral disability needs to be assessed as an outcome in treatment studies; particular interventions might have different effects on symptoms and function. In a cross-sectional study of geriatric BP patients (Bartels et al., 1997), global cognitive performance (MMSE) accounted for a substantial proportion of interindividual differences in functional measures (activities of daily living and community living skills); psychopathology ratings accounted for little. Gildengers et al. (2007) found that in BP elders, cognitive impairments were associated with greater disability, a relationship also described by Depp et al.(2006). In older adults with BP depression, comorbid anxiety is associated with greater functional impairment and lower quality of life (Sajatovic et al., 2006).

In summary, nonaffective outcomes in mania and BP disorders in old age impose additional patient and caregiver burden. Predictors of these outcomes, and the impact of interventions, clearly warrant investigation.

MODIFIERS OF TREATMENT OUTCOMES

Existing literature related to treatment of aged BP patients deals predominantly with pharmacotherapy and includes experience with newer agents in relatively small samples (Kohen, Lester, & Lam, 2010; Robillard & Conn, 2002; Sajatovic et al., 2008, 2011) or secondary analyses of aged subgroups in larger controlled trials (Sajatovic, Calabrese, & Mullen, 2008). Recent reports have described experience with geriatric subgroups within large-scale prospective open treatment studies (STEP-BD; EMBLEM). In STEP-BD participants (Al Jurdi et al., 2008) more than one medication was often prescribed; however, while valproate was more often prescribed than lithium, 42% of recovered BP elders achieved recovery with lithium alone, compared with only 21% of the younger patients treated with lithium. There has been little information about the role of electroconvulsive therapy in BP elders (Chapter 23). There has been limited investigation of nonsomatic components of management, for example, education and psychotherapy, and for patient and family and caregivers, or rehabilitative interventions for aged BP patients, despite evidence of benefits in young BP patients. The following section outlines the still limited evidence regarding potential modifiers outcomes of pharmacological interventions in aged BP patients. Related issues, including pharmacokinetic distortions with advanced age, concentration-effect relationships, and tolerability, are discussed in Chapter 38.

Slowed or Attenuated Antimanic Response

AGE

There is limited information regarding influence of age on acute outcomes in BP disorders. Van der Velde (1970) noted poorer acute therapeutic benefit of lithium in older manic patients compared to a sample of younger (aged <60 years) patients. In fact, only 3 of 12 elderly manic patients responded to lithium, while 51 out of 63 younger patients responded. A prospective study of naturalistic lithium treatment in mixed-age manic patients suggested that benefit was attenuated by increased age (Young & Falk, 1989). In the EMBLEM study of open treatment of mania, there was no age effect on outcomes, although aged patients were more often treated with monotherapy (Oostervink et al., 2009). There are no analyses that address age effects on divalproex efficacy in mania. Okuma et al. (1990) did not separately analyze response to carbamazepine, or lithium, in aged patients. Cycling immediately into a depressive episode may occur more often after inpatient management of mania in elders than in younger patients (Broadhead & Jacoby, 1990).

AGE AT ONSET

There has been little attention paid to the relationship, if any, of age at onset to treatment outcome in geriatric BP patients (Young & Klerman, 1992). There was no effect of age at onset on outcome at endpoint in one naturalistic study of BP elderly (Wylie et al., 1999) or in a preliminary retrospective report (Lehman S. W. & Rabins, 2001). In BP patients two chronological points related to age at onset are pertinent in examination of illness, that is, first affective episode and first manic episode. The reliability of retrospective course assessment in geriatric patients is a limiting factor in research, but multiple sources of information clearly must be utilized. Ostervink et al. (2009) observed that, among BP manic elders, cases with late age at onset had better therapeutic outcome than did those with early age at onset.

OTHER FACTORS

Cognitive impairments may be associated with limitation of acute therapeutic outcomes in older BP patients. Impairments of performance on executive tasks may be associated with attenuated acute response to pharmacotherapy in a preliminary study of elderly manic patients (Young, Murphy et al., 2001). Comorbid dementia may also be associated with worse antimanic outcomes of lithium treatment (Himmelhoch et al., 1980). In one report, DVP benefited BP patients with dementia (Niedermier & Nasrallah, 1998). However, in a placebo-controlled trial in demented patients with manic symptoms, DVP reduced agitation but not mania ratings (Tariot, Schneider et al., 2001). Carbamazepine has been reported to reduce agitation in dementia, but these patients were not manic (Leibovici & Tariot, 1988). Brain mechanisms linking cognitive impairments to differences in response to particular antimanic agents await elucidation. Also, the potential impact of cognitive impairments on medication adherence suggests that targeting specific interventions for enhancing adherence (Depp, Lebowitz et al., 2007) may be one rewarding strategy in studies aimed at improving outcomes of pharmacotherapies in BP elders.

Acute treatment can improve cognitive performance in geriatric BP patients (Wylie et al., 1999; Young, Mattis et al., 1991). Alleviation of affective psychopathology can be associated with improvement of cognitive performance, a phenomenon referred to as "reversible dementia." In addition, mood stabilizers may have neuroprotective effects (Manji, Moore, & Chen, 1999; Moore, Bebchuk et al., 2000

a) and in fact may promote regeneration of cortical gray matter (Moore, Bebchuk et al., 2000

b). Systemic effects of behavioral improvement may also be relevant to cognitive improvement. However, cognitive impairments may also persist in euthymic mixed-age BP patients (Krabbendam et al., 2000; van Gorp, Altshuler, Theberge, Wilkins, & Dixon, 1998).

Elderly manic patients with neurological compromise may have worse therapeutic outcomes compared to those without compromise. Berrios and Bakshi (1991) reported an association between higher Hachinski scores, indicating cerebrovascular disease, and worse acute management outcome. Himmelhoch and colleagues (1980) observed that extrapyramidal impairment predicted poorer acute antimanic effect of lithium treatment. On the other hand, in one case series mixed-age patients with brain disease responded well with DVP (Stoll et al., 1994).

Other comorbid conditions may have negative influences on treatment outcomes in mania. Substance abuse was associated with poor antimanic response to lithium in elderly manic patients in one report (Himmelhoch et al., 1980). Comorbid medical conditions (Black et al., 1988) also can predict poor lithium response; in that mixed-age sample, patients with medical comorbidity had a mean age of 51 years, higher than that of patients without such comorbidity.

The potential relationship of symptom profile to treatment outcomes in geriatric mania has received little study. Mixed features and psychosis are clinically meaningful examples for consideration. In a retrospective study, Chen et al. (1999) observed that lithium had better therapeutic effect than DVP in patients with classic mania compared to those with mixed mania; drug levels were not provided in this comparison. Rapid cycling patients are another subgroup of elderly patients who await study from this perspective.

Response to Pharmacotherapy in Bipolar Depression

There has been minimal investigation of treatment of BP depression in late life (Chapter 21). The effect of age on outcome was not examined in a study of mixed-age patients, for example (Nemeroff et al., 2001). A recent report found that cognitive and metabolic features were associated with limited acute response to lamotrigine in BP depressed elders (Gildengers, Tatsuoka et al., 2012).

The nature of the "switch" to mania or change to a rapid cycling course during antidepressant treatment has been of long-standing clinical concern but a focus of controversy in younger patients; antidepressant-associated mania has been reported in aged patients and may be a particular issue in patients who have first episodes of mania late in life (vanScheyen & vanKammen, 1979; Young, Jain, Kiossess, & Meyers, 2003). On the other hand, one study of illness course in BP elders found lower rates of manic/mixed episodes in those treated with antidepressants compare to those who were not (Schaffer, Zuker, & Levitt, 2006).

Relapse Recurrence in Maintenance Treatment

Since aged BP patients are at risk for repeated episodes requiring treatment, continuation and maintenance pharmacotherapy and other long-term management are central to their care. There is even less literature regarding their long-term treatment than there is for acute management. Efficacy findings are summarized in Chapter 21.

AGE

Abou-Saleh and Coppen (1983) observed no age effect on affective morbidity in mixed-aged unipolar and bipolar patients; however, there were few bipolar elders in the sample. In a naturalistic study of patients aged 25 to 90 years, the affective outcome of BP patients receiving lithium treatment was independent of age (O'Connell et al., 1991). On the other hand, Van der Velde (1970) found that, over 3 years of observation, 52% of the younger and 8% of the older patients remained free of affective episodes during lithium treatment. Murray, Hopwood, Balfour, Ogston, and Hewick (1983) observed only trends for greater manic psychopathology, although no more frequent hospitalizations, among older compared to younger patients treated with lithium. Interpretation of another report (Hewick, Newburg, Hopwood, Naylor, & Moody, 1977) is confounded by differing plasma concentrations with age.

AGE AT ONSET

This factor was not evaluated as a predictor in existing reports. However, Stone (1989) found that a history of prior episodes predicted a greater rate of recurrence in geriatric mania on naturalistic follow-up.

OTHER FACTORS

Cognitive impairments may have adverse implications for long-term treatment outcomes in elderly BP patients. Bartels et al. (1997) observed that cognitive deficits were associated with poor community living skills and deficits in activities of daily living (ADLs), and with nursing home placement. In a naturalistic, prospective study, however, elderly manic patients with or without global cognitive impairment had equal risk of relapse with hospitalization (Dhingra & Rabins 1991). Shulman et al. (1992) found that patients with neurological comorbidity had a higher risk of psychiatric rehospitalization and institutionalization. Findings from controlled treatment trials are needed.

DIFFERENCES IN ADHERENCE TO PHARMACOTHERAPY CAN HAVE ADVERSE EFFECTS ON OUTCOMES

Older individuals with BP disorder are more adherent with antipsychotic medications compared to younger individuals, but a substantial proportion (39%) of older patients has difficulties with adherence (Sajatovic et al., 2007). Lehmann and Rabins (2006) identified nonadherence with psychiatric medication as a factor contributing to relapse and hospitalization in elderly patients with BP disorder. Early-onset patients were more likely to have been nonadherent with prescribed psychiatric medication.

In summary, information regarding classical mood stabilizer treatment is based on case reports, and case series regarding open treatment. These suggest modification of outcomes by dementia. Recent reports suggest a role for lamotrigine and atypical antipsychotics; these are based on small open studies or subgroups of patients with older age participating in studies of patients with broad age range. Large-scale studies focused on elderly treated with medication or convulsive therapy are under way. Recent preliminary findings provide correlates of treatment outcome in geriatric BP depression and in subgroups of patients followed prospectively during open treatment. These suggest that prescribing patterns differ by age, and they provide opportunities to explore modifiers of outcomes.

Challenges for Research in Geriatric Bipolar Disorder

It has been suggested that a number of factors have limited research in geriatric BD. First, perceptions and attitudes: The low prevalence detected in the community has led to the perception that it is unimportant; risks of studying such patients, attached to suicide and risks related to comorbidities, have lead to avoidance of such investigation; and treatments such as lithium may be perceived as "too good" and not motivating development of novel agents (although clinicians are concerned about side-effect profile and how to dose) (Lebowitz, 2007). In addition, the challenges of clinical complexity may outweigh the sense that heterogeneity provides opportunities for hypothesis generation. Second, need for multicenter studies: Generating sample sizes adequate to test hypotheses involves coordinating structure to reduce intersite variation in assessment and other procedures (although using more than one site can potentially add to the generalizability of findings). Third, assessment challenges: Methods must be selected and applied in a way that can accommodate the severity of symptom states in these patients.

Opportunities for Translational Research in Geriatric Bipolar Disorder

The perspectives on late-life BP disorder discussed herein suggests not only that there is a critical need for an age-specific evidence base that can help guide management but also that these patients present important opportunities for research that can contribute to an understanding of the nature of BP disorder across the age spectrum. One advantage within the domain of late-life mood disorder is that BP disorder may be somewhat more homogeneous than unipolar major depression. At the same time, there are suggestions that signals of abnormality on some neurobiological measures may be larger in BP disorder than in depression.

There are a number of strategies that can be envisioned. One would be to study potential neurobiological markers, including abnormalities in neural circuits (Insel et al., 2010), and vulnerability and disease expression, for example, types of BP disorders in patients with differing ages at onset of illness and differing course. Another strategy would be to examine neurobiological markers in aged patients with BP disorder and other disorders who exhibit common signs and symptoms or behavioral abnormalities. Late-life BP disorder also offers opportunities for studying markers that may be related to mechanisms of BP treatments and may have associations with treatment outcomes, that is, resistance and relapse. Additional investigation in BP elders could include designs in which combined influences of psychosocial challenges and neurobiological abnormalities can be tested.

CONCLUSIONS

Manic symptoms in late life have a broad differential diagnosis. Affective psychopathology in mania in old age is qualitatively similar to younger patients, although quantitative changes have been suggested. Cognitive impairments are prominent, and these may have both state- and trait-related components. Antecedent course includes early recurrent cases, change in polarity, and late-onset illness. Comorbidities are prevalent. Vascular pathology and other brain changes may be linked to pathogenesis in late-onset patients. The course of illness in elderly manic and BP patients appears to be characterized by excess mortality and by vulnerability to further episodes. Age-associated modifiers of treatment outcomes have been suggested, but these associations await validation in controlled treatment trials. Investigation of late-life BP illness, in addition, can provide models relevant to pathophysiology and pathogenesis of early-life BP illness.

Disclosures
Dr. Young is supported by National Institutes of Mental Health grant K02 MH067028.
Dr. Mahgoub has no disclosures.

REFERENCES

Abou-Saleh, M. T., & Coppen, A. (1983). Prognosis of depression in old age: The case for lithium therapy. *British Journal of Psychiatry 143*: 527–528.

Agronin, M. E., & Malette, G. J. (2006). *Principles and practice of geriatric psychiatry*. Baltimore, MD: Lippincott Williams & Wilkins.

Al Jurdi, R., Marangell, L., Petersen, N. J., Martinez, M., Gyulai, L., & Sajatovic, M. (2008). Prescription patterns of psychotropic medications in elderly compared with younger participants who achieved a "recovered" status in the systematic treatment enhancement program for bipolar disorder. *American Journal of Geriatric Psychiatry, 16*(11), 922–933.

Al Jurdi, R. K., Schulberg, H. C., Greenberg, R. L., Kunik, M. E., Gildengers, A., Sajatovic, M.,...GERI-BD Study Group. (2012). Characteristics associated with inpatient versus outpatient status in older adults with bipolar disorder. *Journal of Geriatric Psychiatry and Neurology, 25*(1), 62–68.

Alexopoulos, G., Meyers, B. S., Young, R. C., Kakuma, T., Silbersweig, D., & Charlson, M. (1997). Clinically defined vascular depression. *American Journal of Psychiatry, 154*, 562–565.

Ambelas, A. (1987). Life events and mania: A special relationship? *British Journal of Psychiatry, 150*, 235–240.

American Psychiatric Association. (1994). *Diagnostic and statistical manual of mental disorders* (4th ed., text rev.). Washington, DC: Author.

Angst, J. (1978). The course of affective disorders. II. Typology of bipolar manic-depressive illness. *Arch Psychiatr Nervenkr , 226*, 65–73.

Angst, J., Baastrup, P., Grof, P., Hippius, H., Pöldinger, W., & Weis, P. (1973). The course of monopolar and bipolar depression and bipolar psychosis. *Psychiat Neurol Neurochir 76*: 489–500.

Arnold, L. M., Witzeman, K. A., Swank, M. L., McElroy, S. L., & Keck, P. E., Jr. (2000). Health-related quality of life using the SF-36 in patients with bipolar disorder compared with patients with chronic back pain and the general population. *Journal of Affective Disorders, 57*(1–3), 235–239.

Astrup, C., Fossum, A., & Holmboe, R. (1959). A follow-up study of 270 patients with acute affective psychoses. *Acta Psychiatrica Scandinavica Supplement, 135*, 1–65.

Bartels, S. J., Meuser, K. T., & Miles, K. M . (1997). A comparative study of elderly patients with schizophrenia and bipolar disorder in nursing homes and the community. *Schizophrenia Research, 27*(2–3), 181–190.

Bearden, C. E., Hoffman, K. M., & Cannon, T. D. (2001). The neuropsychology and neuroanatomy of bipolar affective disorder: A critical review. *Bipolar Disorder, 3*, 106–150.

Bech, P., Rafaelsen, O. J., Kramp, P., & Bolwig, T. G. (1978). The Mania Rating Scale: Scale construction and interobserver agreement. *Neuropsychopharmacology, 17*, 430–431.

Benazzi, F. (1999). Psychotic late–life depression: A 376-case study. *International Psychogeriatrics, 11*(3), 325–332.

Benazzi, F. (2000). Late-life chronic depression: A 339-case study in private practice. *International Journal of Geriatric Psychiatry, 15*, 1–6.

Berrios, G. E., & Bakshi, N. (1991). Manic and depressive symptoms in the elderly: Their relationships to treatment outcome, cognition and motor symptoms. *Psychophathology, 24*, 31–38.

Beyer, J., Kuchibhatla, M., Looney, C., Engstrom, E., Cassidy, F., & Krishnan, K. R. (2003). Social support in elderly patients with bipolar disorder. *Bipolar Disorders, 5*(1), 22–27.

Beyer, J., Kuchibhatla, M., Payne, M. E., Macfall, J., Cassidy, F., & Krishnan, K. R. (2009). Gray and white matter brain volumes in older adults with bipolar disorder. *International Journal of Geriatric Psychiatry, 24*(12), 1445–1452.

Beyer, J., Kuchibhatla, M., Payne, M., Moo-Young, M., Cassidy, F., MacFall, J., & Krishnan, K. R. (2004). Caudate volume measurement in older adults with bipolar disorder. *International Journal of Geriatric Psychiatry, 19*(2), 109–114.

Beyer, J., Young, R. C., Kuchibhatla, M., & Krishnan, K. R. (2009). Hyperintense MRI lesions in bipolar disorder: A meta-analysis and review. *International Review of Psychiatry, 21*(4), 394–409.

Black, D. W., Winokur, G., Bell, S., Nasrallah, A., & Hulbert, J. (1988). Complicated mania. *Archives of General Psychiatry, 45*(3), 232–236.

Blackburn, J., Loudon, J., & Ashworth, C. M. (1977). A new scale for measuring mania. *Psychological Medicine, 7*, 453–458.

Blumberg, H. P., Charney, D. S., & Krystal, J. H. (2002). Frontotemporal neural systems in bipolar disorder. *Seminars in Clinical Neuropsychiatry, 7*, 243–254.

Blumer, D., & Benson, D. F. (1975). Personality changes with frontal and temporal lobe lesions. In *Psychiatric Aspects of Neurologic Disease* (pp. xx–xx). New York: Grune and Stratton.

Brambilla, P., Harensi, K., Nicoletti, M. A., Mallinger, A. G., Frank, E., Kupfer, D. J.,...Soares, J. C. (2001). Anatomical MRI study of basal ganglia in bipolar disorder patients. *Psychiatry Research, 106*, 65–80.

Broadhead, J., & Jacoby, R. (1990). Mania in old age: A first prospective study. *International Journal of Geriatric Psychiatry, 5*, 215–222.

Brooks, J., Bearden, C., Hoblyn, J. C., Woodard, S. A., & Ketter, T. A. (2010). Prefrontal and paralimbic metabolic dysregulation related to sustained attention in euthymic older adults with bipolar disorder. *Bipolar Disorders, 12*(8), 866–874.

Brooks, J., & Hoblyn, J. (2005). Secondary mania in older adults. *American Journal of Psychiatry, 162*(11), 2033–2038.

Brooks, J., Rosen, A., Hoblyn, J. C., Woodard, S. A., Krasnykh, O., & Ketter, T. A. (2009). Resting prefrontal hypometabolism and paralimbic hypermetabolism related to verbal recall deficits in euthymic older adults with bipolar disorder. *American Journal of Geriatric Psychiatry, 17*(12), 1022–1029.

Burns, A., Jacoby, R., & Levy, R. (1990). Psychiatric phenomena in Alzheimer's Disease. III: Disorders of mood. *British Journal of Psychiatry, 157*, 81–86.

Burt, T., Prudic, J., Peyser, S., Clark, J., & Sackeim, H. A.. (2000). Learning and memory in bipolar and unipolar major depression:Effects of aging. *Neuropsychiatry, Neuropsychology and Behavioral Neurology, 13*, 246–253.

Cade, J. F. J. (1949). Lithium salts in the treatment of psychotic excitement. *Medical Journal of Australia, 36*, 349–352.

Cassidy, F., Ahearn, E. P., & Carroll, B. J. (2001). Substance abuse in bipolar disorder. *Bipolar Disorders, 3*, 181–188.

Cassidy, F., & Carroll, B. J. (2002). Vascular risk factors in late-onset mania. *Psychological Medicine, 32*(2), 359–362.

Charron, M., Fortin, L., & Paguette, I. (2001). De novo mania among elderly people. *Acta Psychiatrica Scandinavica, 84*, 503–507.

Chen, S. T., Altshuler, L. L., Melnyk, K. A., Erhart, S. M., Miller, E., & Mintz, J. (1999). Efficacy of lithium vs valproate in the treatment of mania in the elderly: A retrospective study. *Journal of Clinical Psychiatry, 60*, 181–185.

Chu, D., Gildengers, A., Houck, P. R., Anderson, S. J., Mulsant, B. H., Reynolds, C. F., III, & Kupfer, D. J. (2010). Does age at onset have clinical significance in older adults with bipolar disorder? *International Journal of Geriatric Psychiatry, 25*(12), 1266–1271.

Clayton, P. J. (1986). The epidemiology of bipolar affective disorder. *Comprehensive Psychiatry, 22*, 31–43.

Clayton, P. J. (1986). Manic symptoms in the elderly. In E. Busse (Ed.), *Aspects of aging* (pp. 3–13). Philadelphia, PA: Smith Kline & French.

Clayton, P. J., & Pitts, F. N., Jr. (1965). Affective disorder IV: Mania. *Comprehensive Psychiatry, 6*, 313–322.

Coffman, J. A., Bornstein, R. A., Olson, S. C., Schwarzkopf, S. B., & Nasrallah, H. A. (1990). Cognitive impairment and cerebral structure by MRI in bipolar disorder. *Biological Psychiatry, 27*, 1188–1196.

Coryell, W., Scheffner, W., Keller, M., Endicott, J., Maser, J., & Klerman, G. L. (1993). The enduring psychosocial consequences of mania and depression. *American Journal of Psychiatry, 150*(5), 720–727.

Cummings, J. L. (1993). Fronto-subcortical circuits and human behavior. *Archives of Neurology, 50*, 873–880.

deAsis, J., Greenwald, B., Alexopoulos, G. S., Kiosses, D. N., Ashtari, M., Heo, M., & Young, R. C. (2006). Frontal signal hyperintensities in mania in old age. *American Journal of Geriatric Psychiatry, 14*(7), 598–604.

deAsis , J., Young, R. C., (1998). Signal hyperintensities in geriatric mania. *Abstract, Annual Meeting, American Association of Geriatric Psychiatry.*

Delaloye, C., de Bilbao, F., Moy, G., Baudois, S., Weber, K., Campos, L., … Gold, G. (2009). Neuroanatomical and neuropsychological features of euthymic patients with bipolar disorder. *American Journal of Geriatric Psychiatry, 17*(12), 1012–1021.

Delaloye, C., Moy, G., Baudois, S., de Bilbao, F., Remund, C. D., Hofer, F., … Giannakopoulos, P. (2009). Cognitive features in euthymic bipolar patients in old age. *Bipolar Disorders, 11*(7), 735–743.

Delaloye, C., Moy, G., de Bilbao, F., Weber, K., Baudois, S., Haller, S., … Giannakopoulos, P. (2011). Longitudinal analysis of cognitive performances and structural brain changes in late-life bipolar disorder. *International Journal of Geriatric Psychiatry, 26*(12), 1309–1318.

Depp, C. A., Davis, C. E., Mittal, D., Patterson, T. L., & Jeste, D. V. (2006). Health-related quality of life and functioning of middle-aged and elderly adults with bipolar disorder. *Journal of Clinical Psychiatry, 67*(2), 215–221.

Depp, C. A., & Jeste, D. V. (2004). Bipolar disorder in older adults: A critical review. *Bipolar Disorders, 6*(5), 343–367.

Depp, C. A., Jin, H., Mohamed, S., Kaskow, J., Moore, D. J., & Jeste, D. V. (2004). Bipolar disorder in middle-aged and elderly adults: Is age of onset important? *Journal of Nervous and Mental Disease, 192*(11), 796–799.

Depp, C. A., Lebowitz, B. D., Patterson, T. L., Lacro, J. P., & Jeste, D. V. (2007). Medication adherence skills training for middle-aged and elderly adults with bipolar disorder: development and pilot study. *Bipolar Disorders, 6,* 636–645.

Depp, C. A., Lindamer, L. A., Folsom, D. P., Gilmer, T., Hough, R. L., Garcia, P., & Jeste, D. V. (2005). Differences in clinical features and mental health service use in bipolar disorder across the lifespan. *American Journal of Geriatric Psychiatry, 13*(4), 290–298.

Depp, C. A., Moore, D. J., Sitzer, D., Palmer, B. W., Eyler, L. T., Roesch, S., . . . Jeste, D. V. (2007). Neurocognitive impairment in middle-aged and older adults with bipolar disorder: Comparison to schizophrenia and normal comparison subjects. *Journal of Affective Disorders, 101*(1–3), 201–209.

Derby, I. M. (1933). Manic depressive exhaustion deaths. *Psychiatric Quarterly,* 436–449.

Dhingra, U., & Rabins, P. V. (1991). Mania in the elderly: a five-to-seven year follow-up. *Journal of the American Geriatrics Society, 39,* 581–583.

Dorey, J-M., Beauchet, O., Thomas Antérion, C., Rouch, I., Krolak-Salmon, P., Gaucher, J., . . . Akiskal, H. S. (2008). Behavioral and psychological symptoms of dementia and bipolar spectrum disorders: Review of the evidence of a relationship and treatment implications. *CNS Spectrums, 13*(9), 796–803.

Dunn, K. L., & Rabins, P. V. (1996). Mania in old age. In K. I. Shulman, M. Tohen, & S. P. Kutcher (Eds.), *Mood disorders across the life span* (pp. 399–406). New York: Wiley.

Eagles, J. M., & Whalley, L. J. (1985). Ageing and affective disorders: The age at first onset of affective disorders in Scotland 1966–1978. *British Journal of Psychiatry, 147,* 180–187.

Folstein , M. (1999). Mania agitation and Alzheimer's disease. *Abstract AAGP Annual Meeting.*

Folstein, M. F., Folstein, S. E., & McHugh, P. R. (1975). Mini-mental state: A practical method for grading the cognitive state of patients for the clinician. *Journal of Psychiatry Research, 12,* 189–198.

Folstein, S. E. (1989). *Huntington's disease. A disorder of families.* Baltimore, MD: Johns Hopkins University Press.

Fujikawa, T., Yamawaki, S., & Touhouda, Y. (1995). Silent cerebral infarctions in patients with late-onset mania. *Stroke, 26,* 946–949.

Gildengers, A., Mulsant, B., Al Jurdi, R. K., Beyer, J. L., Greenberg, R. L., Gyulai, L., . . . GERI-BD Study Group. (2010). The relationship of bipolar disorder lifetime duration and vascular burden to cognition in older adults. *Bipolar Disorders, 12*(8), 851–858.

Gildengers, A., Tatsuoka, C., Bialko, C., Cassidy, K. A., Al Jurdi, R. K., Gyulai, L., . . . Sajatovic, M. (2012).

Correlates of treatment response in depressed older adults with bipolar disorder. *Journal of Geriatric Psychiatry and Neurology, 25*(1), 37–42.

Gildengers, A., Whyte, E., Drayer, R. A., Soreca, I., Fagiolini, A,, Kilbourne, A. M., . . . Mulsant, B. H. (2008). Medical burden in late-life bipolar and major depressive disorders. *American Journal of Geriatric Psychiatry, 16*(3), 194–200.

Gildengers, A. G., Butters, M. A., Chisholm, D., Anderson, S. J., Begley, A., Holm, M., . . . Mulsant, B. H. (2012). Cognition in older adults with bipolar disorder versus major depressive disorder. *Bipolar Disorders, 14*(2), 198–205.

Gildengers, A. G., Butters, M. A., Chisholm, D., Rogers, J. C., Holm, M. B., Bhalla, R. K., . . . Mulsant, B. H. (2007). Cognitive functioning and instrumental activities of daily living in late-life bipolar disorder. *American Journal of Geriatric Psychiatry, 15*(2), 174–179.

Gildengers, A. G., Butters, M. A., Seligman, K., McShea, M., Miller, M. D., Mulsant, B. H., . . . Reynolds, C. F., III. (2004). Cognitive functioning in late-life bipolar disorder. *American Journal of Psychiatry, 161*(4), 736–738.

Gildengers, A. G., Mulsant, B. H., Begley, A., Mazumdar, S., Hyams, A. V., Reynolds, C. F., III, . . . Butters, M. A. (2009). The longitudinal course of cognition in older adults with bipolar disorder. *Bipolar Disorders, 11*(7), 744–752.

Gildengers, A. G., Mulsant, B. H., Begley, A. E., McShea, M., Stack, J. A., Miller, M. D., . . . Reynolds, C. F., III. (2005). A pilot study of standardized treatment in geriatric bipolar disorder. *American Journal of Geriatric Psychiatry, 13*(4), 319–323.

Gitlin, M. J., Swendsen, J., Heller, T. L., & Hammen, C. (1995). Relapse and impairment in bipolar disorder. *American Journal of Psychiatry, 152*(11), 1635–1640.

Glasser, M., & Rabins, P. (1984). Mania in the elderly. *Age and Ageing, 13,* 210–213.

Gunning-Dixon, F., Murphy, C., Alexopoulos, G. S., Majcher-Tascio, M., & Young, R. C. (2008). Executive dysfunction in elderly bipolar manic patients. *American Journal of Geriatric Psychiatry, 16*(6), 506–512.

Hausdorff, J. M., Chung-Kang, P., Goldberger, A. L., & Stoll, A. L. (2004). Gait unsteadiness and fall risk in two affective disorders: A preliminary study. *BMC Psychiatry, 4,* 39.

Hays, P. (1976). Etiological factors in manic depressive psychosis. *Archives of General Psychiatry, 33,* 1187–1188.

Henderson, D., & Gillespie, R. D. (1956). *A textbook of psychiatry for students and practitioners.* London: Oxford University Press.

Hewick, D. S., Newburg, P., Hopwood, S., Naylor, G., & Moody, J. (1977). Age as a factor affecting lithium therapy. *British Journal of Clinical Pharmacology, 4*, 201–205.

Himmelhoch, J. M., Neil, J. F., May, S. J., Fuchs, C. Z., & Licata, S. M. (1980). Age, dementia, dyskinesias, and lithium response. *American Journal of Psychiatry, 137*(8), 941–945.

Insel, T., Cuthbert, B., Garvey, M., Heinssen, R., Pine, D. S., Quinn, K., ... Wang, P. (2010). Research domain criteria (RDoC): Toward a new classification framework for research on mental disorders. *American Journal of Psychiatry, 167*(7), 748–751.

Jamison, K. R., & Goodwin, F. K. (1998). Medical treatment of acute bipolar depression. *Manic Depressive Illness*, 643–651.

Joffe, R. T., Lippert, G. P., Gray, T. A., Sawa, G., & Horvath, Z. (1987). Mood disorder and multiple sclerosis. *Archives of Neurology, 44*, 376–378.

Johnson, S. L., Meyer, B., Winett, C., & Small, J. (2000). Social support and self-esteem predict changes in bipolar depression but not mania. *Journal of Affective Disorders, 58*(1), 79–86.

Jorge, R. E., Robinson, R. G., Starkstein, S. E., Arndt, S. V., Forrester, A. W., & Geisler, F. H. (1993). Secondary mania following traumatic brain injury. *American Journal of Psychiatry, 150*, 916–921.

Kay, D. W. K., Roth, M., & Hopkins, B. (1955). Affective disorders arising in the senium, I: Their association with organic cerebral degeneration. *Journal of Mental Science, 101*, 302–316.

Kerry, R. J., McDermott, C. M., & Orme, J. E. (1983). Affective disorders and cognitive performance. *Journal of Affective Disorders, 5*, 345–352.

Kessing, L. L. V., Hansen, M. M. G., Andersen, P. K., & Angst, J (2004). The predictive effect of episodes on the risk of recurrence in depressive and bipolar disorders—a life-long perspective. *Acta Psychiatrica Scandinavica, 109*(5), 339–344.

Kessing, L. V., & Andersen, P. K. (2004). Does the risk of developing dementia increase with the number of episodes in patients with depressive disorder and in patients with bipolar disorder? *Journal of Neurology, Neurosurgery and Psychiatry, 75*(12), 1662–1666.

Kessing, L. V. (2006). Diagnostic subtypes of bipolar disorder in older versus younger adults. *Bipolar Disorders, 8*(1), 56–64.

Kilbourne, A. M., Post, E. P., Nossek, A., Sonel, E., Drill, L. J., Cooley, S., & Bauer, M. S. (2008). Service delivery in older patients with bipolar disorder: A review and development of a medical care model. *Bipolar Disorders, 10*(6), 672–683.

Kling, A., & Steklis, H. D. (1976). A neural substrate for affiliative behavior in nonhuman primates. *Brain Behavior and Evolution, 13*, 216–238.

Kohen, I., Lester, P. E., & Lam, S. (2010). Antipsychotic treatement for the elderly: Efficacy and safety of Aripiprazole. *Neuropsychiatric Disease and Treatment, 6*, 47–58.

Krabbendam, L., Honig, A., Wiersma, J., Vuurman, E. F., Hofman, P. A., Derix, M. M., ... Jolles, J. (2000). Cognitive dysfunctions and white matter lesions in patients with bipolar disorder in remission. *Acta Psychiatrica Scandinavica, 101*, 274–280.

Kraepelin, E. (1921). *Manic-depressive insanity and paranoia* (G. M. Robertson, Trans.). Edinburgh, Scotland: Livingstone.

Krauthammer, C., & Klerman, G. (1978). Secondary mania. *Archives of General Psychiatry, 35*(11), 1333–1339.

Lala, S. V., & Sajatovic, M. (2012). Medical and psychiatric comorbidities among elderly individuals with bipolar disorder: **A** literature review. *J Geriatr Psychiatry Neurol, 25*(1), 20–25.

Lebowitz, B. (2007). *Bipolar disorder in late life*. Paper presented at the Annual Meeting fo the American Association for Geriatric Psychiatry,.

Lehman, S W., & Rabins, P. V. (2001). Factors influencing treatment outcomes in geriatric mania. *Biological Psychiatry, 49*(8), 12.

Lehman, S. W., & Rabins, P. V. (2006). Factors related to hospitalization in elderly manic patients with early and late-onset bipolar disorder. *International Journal of Geriatric Psychiatry, 21*(11), 1060–1064.

Leibovici, A., & Tariot, P. N. (1988). Carbamazepine treatment of agitation associated with dementia. *Journal of Geriatric Psychiatry and Neurology, 1*, 110–112.

Liu, C. Y., Wang, S. J., Fuh, J. L., Yang, Y. Y., & Liu, H. C. (1996). Bipolar disorder following a stroke involving the left hemisphere. *Australian and New Zealand Journal of Psychiatry, 30*, 688–691.

Loranger, A. W., & Levine, P. M. (1978). Age at onset of bipolar affective illness. *Archives of General Psychiatry, 35*, 345–345.

Loreck, D. J., Bylsma, F. W., & Folstein, M. F. (1994). A new scale for comprehensive assessment of psychopathology in Alzheimer's disease. *American Journal of Geriatr Psychiatry, 2*(1), 60–74.

Lundquist, G. (1945). Prognosis and course in manic depressive psychoses: A follow-up study of 319 first admissions. *Acta Psychiatrica Scandinavica Supplement, 1*, 1–96.

Lyketsos, C. G., Corazzini, K., & Steele, C. (1995). Mania in Alzheimer's disease. *Journal of Neuropsychiatry and Clinical Neuroscience, 7*, 350–352.

MacDonald, J. B. (1918). Prognosis in manic-depressive insanity. *Journal of Nervous and Mental Disorders, 47*, 20–30.

Manji, H. K., Moore, G. J., & Chen, G. (1999). Lithium at 50: Have the neuroprotective effects of this unique cation been overlooked? *Biological Psychiatry, 46*(7), 929–940.

Marneros, A., & Angst, J. (2000). Bipolar disorders: roots and evolution. In A. Marneros & J. Angst (Eds.), *Bipolar disorders* (pp. 1–35). Dordrecht, The Netherlands :.

McDonald, W. M., Krishnan, K. R., Doraiswamy, P. M., & Blazer, D. G. (1991). Occurrence of subcortical hyperintensities in elderly subjects with mania. *Psychiatric Research, 40*, 211–220.

McDonald, W. M., Tupler, L. A., Marsteller, F. A., Figiel, G. S., DiSouza, S., Nemeroff, C. B., & Krishnan, K. R. (1999). Hyperintense lesions on magnetic resonance images in bipolar disorder. *Biological Psychiatry, 45*(8), 965–971.

McMahon, F. J., DePaulo, J. R., (1996). Genetics and age at onset. In K. I. Shulman, M. Tohen, & S. P. Kutcher (Eds.), *Mood disorders across the life span* (pp. 35–48). New York: Wiley-Liss.

Mega, M. S., Dinov, I. D., Feaster, S. R., Anderson, S. M., Saviolakis, G. A., & Garcia, G. E. (2000). Orbital and dorsolateral perfusion defect associated with behavioral response to cholinesterase inhibitor therapy in Alzheimer disease. *Neuroscience, 12*, 209–218.

Mendlewics, J., Fieve, R. R., Rainer, J. D., & Fleiss, J. L. (1972). Manic depressive illness: a comparative study of patients with and without a family history. *British Journal of Psychiatry, 120*, 523–530.

Miller, B. L., Cummings, J. L., Villanueva-Meyer, J., Boone, K., Mehringer, C. M., Lesser, I. M., & Mena, I. (1991). Fontal lobe degeneration: Clinical, neuropsychological, and SPECT characteristics. *Neurology, 41*, 1374–1382.

Moore, G. J., Bebchuk, J. M., Hasanat, K., Chen, G., Seraji-Bozorgzad, N., Wilds, I. B.,...Manji, H. K. (2000a). In vivo evidence in support of bcl-2's neurotrophic effects? *Biological Psychiatry, 48*(1), 1–8.

Moore, G. J., Bebchuk, J. M., Wilds, I. B., Chen, G., & Manji, H. K. (2000b). Lithium-induced increase in human brain grey matter. *Lancet, 356*(9237), 1241–1242.

Murray, E., Hopwood, S., Balfour, D. J., Ogston, S., & Hewick, D. S. (1983). The influence of age on lithium efficacy and side-effects in out-patients. *Psychological Medicine, 13*, 53–60.

Nemeroff, C. B., Evans, D. L., Gyulai, L., Sachs, G. S., Bowden, C. L., Gergel, I. P.,...Pitts, C. D. (2001). Double-blind, placebo-controlled comparison of imipramine and paroxetine in the treatment of bipolar depression. *American Journal of Psychiatry, 158*(6), 906–912.

Niedermier, J. A., & Nasrallah, H. A. (1998). Clinical correlates of response to valproate in geriatric inpatients. *Annals of Clinical Psychiatry, 10*(4), 165–168.

Nierenberg, A., Miyahara, S., Spencer, T., Wisniewski, S. R., Otto, M. W., Simon, N.,... STEP-BD Investigators. (2005). Clinical and diagnostic implications of lifetime attention-deficit/ hyperactivity disorder comorbidity in adults with bipolar disorder: Data from the first 1000 STEP-BD participants. *Biological Psychiatry, 57*(11), 1467–1473.

O'Connell, R. A., Mayo, J. A., Flatow, L., Cuthbertson, B., & O'Brien, B. E. (1991). Outcome of bipolar disorder on long-term treatment with li. *British Journal of Psychiatry, 159*, 123–129.

Okuma, T., Yamashita, I., Takahashi, R., Itoh, H., Otsuki, S., Watanabe, S.,... Inanaga, K. (1990). Comparison of the antimanic efficacy of carbamazepine and lithium carbonate by double-blind controlled study. *Pharmacopsychiatry, 23*(3), 143–150.

Oostervink, F., Boomsma, M., Nolen, W. A., & EMBLEM Advisory Board. (2009). Bipolar disorder in the elderly; different effects of age and of age of onset. *Journal of Affective Disorders, 116*(3), 176–183.

Oppneheim, J. (1890). Zur pathologie der grosshirngeschwulste. *Arch Psychiatr Nervenkr, 21*, 560–587.

Perlis, R., Dennehy, E., Miklowitz, D. J., Delbello, M. P., Ostacher, M., Calabrese, J. R.,... Sachs, G. (2009). Retrospective age at onset of bipolar disorder and outcome during two-year follow-up: Results from the STEP-BD study. *Bipolar Disorders, 11*(4), 391–400.

Petrie, W., Lawson, E. C., & Hollender, M. H. (1982). Violence in geriatric patients. *Journal of the American Medical Association, 248*, 443–444.

Ponce, H., Kunik, M ., (1999). Divalproex sodium treatment in elderly male bipolar patients. *Journal of Geriatric Drug Therapy 12*, 55–63.

Post, F. (1965). *The clinical psychiatry of late life.* Oxford, England: Pergamon Press.

Post, F. (1971). Schizo-affective symptomatology in late life. *British Journal of Psychiatry, 118*, 437–445.

Rabins, P. V., Aylward, E., Holroyd, S., & Pearlson, G. (2000). MRI findings differentiate between late-onset schizophrenia and mood disorder. *International Journal of Geriatric Psychiatry, 15*, 954–960.

Rice, J. P., Reich, T., Andreasen, N. C., Endicott, J., Van Eerdewegh, M., Fishman, R., ... Klerman, G. L. (1987). The familial transmission of bipolar illness. *Archives of General Psychiatry, 44*, 441–447.

Robillard, M., & Conn, D. K. (2002). Lamotrigine use in geriatric patients with bipolar depression. *Canadian Journal of Psychiatry, 47*(8), 767–770.

Robinson, L. J., Thompson, J. M., Gallagher, P., Goswami, U., Young, A. H., Ferrier, I. N., & Moore, P. B. (2006). A meta-analysis of cognitive deficits in euthymic patients with bipolar disorder. *Journal of Affective Disorders, 93*(1–3), 105–115.

Romans, S. E., & McPherson, H. M. (1992). The social networks of bipolar affective disorder patients. *Journal of Affective Disorders, 25*(4), 221–228.

Roose, S. P., Nurnberger, J., Dunner, D. L., Blood, D. K., & Fieve, R. R. (1979). Cardiac sinus node dysfunction during lithium treatment. *American Journal of Psychiatry, 136*, 804–806.

Rosen, L. N., Rosenthal, N. E., Van Dusen, P. H., Dunner, D. L., & Fieve, R. R. (1984). Age at onset and number of psychotic symptoms in bipolar I and schizoaffective disorder. *American Journal of Psychiatry, 140*, 1523–1524.

Roth, M. (1955). The natural history of mental disorder in old age. *Journal of Mental Science, 101*, 281–301.

Sackeim, H. A., Greenberg, M. S., Weiman, A. L., Gur, R. C., Hungerbuhler, J. P., & Geschwind, N. (1982). Hemispheric assymmetry in the expression of positive and negative emotions. *Archives of Neurology, 39*, 210–218.

Sajatovic, M., Blow, F. C., & Ignacio, R. V. (2006). Psychiatric comorbidity in older adults with bipolar disorder. *International Journal of Geriatric Psychiatry, 21*(6), 582–587.

Sajatovic, M., Blow, F. C., Ignacio, R. V., & Kales, H. C. (2004). Age-related modifiers of clinical presentation and health service use among veterans with bipolar disorder. *Psychiatric Services, 55*(9), 1014–1021.

Sajatovic, M., Blow, F. C., Ignacio, R. V., & Kales, H. C. (2005). New-onset bipolar disorder in later life. *American Journal of Geriatric Psychiatry, 13*, 282–289.

Sajatovic, M., Blow, F. C., Kales, H. C., Valenstein, M., Ganoczy, D., & Ignacio, R. V. (2007). Age comparison of treatment adherence with antipsychotic medications among individuals with bipolar disorder. *International Journal of Geriatric Psychiatry, 22*(10), 992–998.

Sajatovic, M., Calabrese, J. R., & Mullen, J. (2008). Quetiapine for the treatment of bipolar mania in older adults. *Bipolar Disorders, 10*(6), 662–671.

Sajatovic, M., Coconcea, N., Ignacio, R. V., Blow, F. C., Hays, R. W., Cassidy, K. A., & Meyer, W. J. (2008). Aripiprazole therapy in 20 older adults with bipolar disorder: A 12-week, open-label trial. *Journal of Clinical Psychiatry, 69*(1), 41–46.

Sajatovic, M., Gildengers, A., Al Jurdi, R. K., Gyulai, L., Cassidy, K. A., Greenberg, R. L., ... Young, R. C. (2011). Multisite, open-label, prospective trial of lamotrigine for geriatric bipolar depression: A preliminary report. *Bipolar Disorders, 13*(3), 294–302.

Sajatovic, M., Jurdi, R. A., Gildengers, A., Greenberg, R. L., Tenhave, T., Bruce, M. L., ... Young, R. C. (2011). Depression symptom ratings in geriatric patients with bipolar mania. *International Journal of Geriatric Psychiatry, 26*, 1201–1208.

Sajatovic, M., Levin, J., Fuentes-Casiano, E., Cassidy, K. A., Tatsuoka, C., & Jenkins, J. H. (2011). Illness experience and reasons for nonadherence among individuals with bipolar disorder who are poorly adherent with medication. *Comprehensive Psychiatry, 3*, 280–287.

Sajatovic, M., Popli, A., (1996). Health resource utilization over a ten-year period by geriatric veterans with schizophrenia and bipolar disorder. *Journal of Geriatric Psychiatry and Neurology, 15*, 128–133.

Sajatovic, M., Vernon, L., & Semple, W. (1997). Clinical characteristics and health resource use of men and women veterans with serious mental illness. *Psychiatric Services, 48*(11), 1461–1463.

Savard, R. J., Rey, C., & Post, R. M. (1980). Halstead-Reitan Category Test in bipolar and unipolar affective disorders: Relationship to age and phase of illness. *Journal of Nervous and Mental Disorders, 168*, 297–304.

Schaffer, A., Zuker, P., & Levitt, A. (2006). Randomized, double-blind pilot trial comparing lamotrigine versus citalopram for the treatment of bipolar depression. *Journal of Affective Disorders, 96*(1–2), 95–99.

Schouws, S. N. T. M., Comijs, H., Stek, M. L., Dekker, J., Oostervink, F., Naarding, P., ... Beekman, A. T. (2009). Cognitive impairment in early and late bipolar disorder. *American Journal of Geriatric Psychiatry, 17*(6), 508–515.

Schouws, S. N. T. M., Stek, M., Comijs, H. C., & Beekman, A. T. (2010). Risk factors for cognitive impairment in elderly bipolar patients. *Journal of Affective Disorders, 125*(1–3), 330–335.

Shulman, K., & Post, F. (1980). Bipolar affective disorders in old age. *British Journal of Psychiatry, 136*, 26–32.

Shulman, K. I. (1997). Disinhibition syndromes, secondary mania and bipolar disorder in old age. *Journal of Affective Disorders, 46*, 175–182.

Shulman, K. I., & Tohen, M. (1994). Unipolar mania reconsidered: Evidence from an elderly cohort. *British Journal of Psychiatry, 164*, 547–549.

Shulman, K. I., Tohen, M., Satlin, A., Mallya, G., & Kalunian, D. (1992). Mania compared with unipolar depression in old age. *American Journal of Psychiatry, 149*(3), 341–345.

Silva, D., Santana, I., do Couto, F. S., Maroco, J., Guerreiro, M., & de Mendonça, A. (2009). Cognitive deficits in middle-aged and older adults with bipolar disorder and cognitive complaints: Comparison with mild cognitive impairment. *International Journal of Geriatric Psychiatry, 24*(6), 624–631.

Slater, E., & Roth, M. (1977). *Mayer-Gross, Slater, and Roth's clinical psychiatry*. London: Bailliere, Tindall and Cassell.

Slavney, P. R., Rich, G. B., Pearlson, G. D., & McHugh, P. R. (1977). Phencyclidine abuse and symptomatic mania. *Biological Psychiatry, 12*, 697–700.

Snowdon, J. (1991). A retrospective case-note study of bipolar disorder in old age. *British Journal of Psychiatry, 158*, 485–490.

Speer, D. C. (1992). Differences in social resources and treatment history among diagnostic groups of older adults. *Hospital and Community Psychiatry, 43*(3), 270–274.

Spicer, C. C., Hare, E. H., & Slater, E. (1973). Neurotic and psychotic forms of depressive illness:Evidence from age incidence in a national sample. *British Journal of Psychiatry, 123*, 535–541.

Starkstein, S. E., Boston, J. D., & Robinson, R. G. (1988). Mechanisms of mania after brain injury: twelve case reports and review of the literature. *Journal of Nervous and Mental Disorders, 176*, 87–100.

Starkstein, S. E., Federoff, P., Berthier, M. L., & Robinson, R. G. (1991). Manic depressive and pure manic states after brain lesions. *Biological Psychiatry, 29*, 773–782.

Starkstein, S. E., Mayberg, H. S., Berthier, M. L., Fedoroff, P., Price, T. R., Dannals, R. F.,…Robinson, R. G. (1990). Mania after brain injury: Neuroradiological and metabolic findings. *Annals of Neurology, 27*, 652–659.

Starkstein, S. E., & Robinson, R. G. (1997). Mechanism of disinhibition after brain lesions. *Journal of Nervous and Mental Disorders, 185*, 108–114.

Steffens, D. C., & Krishnan, K. R. (1998). Structural neuroimaging and mood disorders: Recent findings, implications for classification, and future directions. *Social Biological Psychiatry, 43*, 705–712.

Stoll, A. L., Banov, M., Kolbrener, M., Mayer, P. V., Tohen, M., Strakowski, S. M.,…Cohen, B. M. (1994). Neurologic factors predict a favorable valproate response in bipolar and schizoaffective disorders. *Journal of Clinical Psychopharmacology, 14*, 311–313.

Stone, K. (1989). Mania in the elderly. *British Journal of Psychiatry, 155*, 220–224.

Strakowski, S. M., McElroy, S. L., Keck, P. W., Jr., & West, S. A. (1994). The co-occurrence of mania with medical and other psychiatric disorders. *International Journal of Psychiatry in Medicine, 24*, 305–328.

Strauss, M. E., Bohannon, W. E., Stephens, J. H., & Pauker, N. E. (1984). Perceptual span in schizophrenia and affective disorders. *Journal of Nervous and Mental Disorders, 172*, 431–435.

Subramaniam, H., Dennis, M., & Byrne, E. J. (2007). The role of vascular risk factors in late onset bipolar disorder. *International Journal of Geriatric Psychiatry, 22*(8), 733–737.

Swann, A. C. (1995). Mixed or dysphoric manic states: Psychopathology and treatment. *Journal of Clinical Psychiatry, 56*(S3), 6–10.

Swift, H. M. (1907). The prognosis of recurrent insanity of the manic depressive type. *American Journal of Insanity, 64*, 311–326.

Tamashiro, J., Zung, S., Zanetti, M. V., de Castro, C. C., Vallada, H., Busatto, G. F., & de Toledo Ferraz Alves, T. C. (2008). Increased rates of white matter hyperintensities in late-onset bipolar disorder. *Bipolar Disorders, 10*(7), 765–775.

Tariot, P. N., Schneider, L. S., (2001). Safety and tolerability of divalproex sodium in the treatment of signs and symptoms of mania in elderly patients with dementia: Results of a double-blind, placebo-controlled trial. *Current Therapy Research, 62*(1), 51–67.

Taylor, M. A., & Abrams, R. (1981). Prediction of treatment response in mania. *Archives of General Psychiatry, 38*, 800–803.

Tohen, M., Shulman, K. I., & Satlin, A (1994). First-episode mania in late life. *American Journal of Psychiatry, 151*, 130–132.

Turecki, G., Mari, J. D. J., & Del Porto, J. A. (1993). Bipolar disorder following left basal ganglia stroke. *British Journal of Psychiatry, 163*, 690.

van der Velde, C. D. (1970). Effectiveness of lithium carbonate in the treatment of manic-depressive illness. *American Journal of Psychiatry, 123*, 345–351.

van Gorp, W. G., Altshuler, L., Theberge, D. C., Wilkins, J., & Dixon, W. (1998). Cognitive impairment in euthymic bipolar patients with and without prior alcohol dependence. *Archive of General Psychiatry, 55*, 41–46.

vanScheyen, J. D., & vanKammen, D. P. (1979). Clomipramine-induced mania in unipolar depression. *Archives of General Psychiatry, 36*, 560–565.

Verdoux, H., & Bourgeois, M. (1995). Manies secondaires a des pathologies organiques cerebrales. *Annals of Medical Psychology, 153*, 161–168.

Walter-Ryan, W. G. (1983). Mania with onset in the ninth decade. *Journal of Clinical Psychiatry, 44*(11), 430–431.

Weissman, M. M., Bruce, M. L ., (1990). Affective disorders. In L. N. Robins & D. A. Regier (Eds.), *Psychiatric disorders in America: The Epidemiologic Catchment Area Study* (pp. 53–80). New York: Free Press.

Welt, L. (1888). Uber characterveranderungen der menschen infolge von lasionen des stirnhirn. *Arch f Klin Med , 42*, 339–390.

Wendkos, M. H. (1979). Exhaustive mania. In *Sudden death in psychiatric illness*. New York: SP Medical & Scientific Books.

Wertham, F. I. (1929). A group of benign chronic psychoses:prolonged manic excitements with a statisticalstudy of age,duration and frequency in 2,000 manic attacks. *American Journal of Psychiatry, 86*, 17–78.

Woo, B. K., Golshan, S., Allen, E. C., Daly, J. W., Jeste, D. V., & Sewell, D. D. (2006). Factors associated with frequent admissions to an acute geriatric psychiatric inpatient unit. *Journal of Geriatric Psychiatry and Neurology, 19*(4), 226–230.

Wylie, M. E., Mulsant, B. H., Pollock, B. G., Sweet, R. A., Zubenko, G. S., Begley, A. E.,...Kupfer, D. J. (1999). Age at onset in geriatric bipolar disorder. *American Journal of Geriatric Psychiatry, 7*(1), 77–83.

Yassa, R., Nair, N. P. V., & Iskandar, H. (1988b). Late onset bipolar disorder. *Psychiatric Clinics of North America, 11*, 117–131.

Yassa, R., Nair, V., Nastase, C., Camille, Y., & Belzile, L. (1988a). Prevalence of bipolar disorder in a psychogeriatric population. *Journal of Affective Disorders, 14*, 197–201.

Young, R. C., Biggs, J. T., Ziegler, V. E., & Meyer, D. A. (1978). A rating scale for mania: Reliability, validity, and sensitivity. *British Journal of Psychiatry, 133*, 429–435.

Young, R. C., & Falk, J. R. (1989). Age, manic psychopathology and treatment response. *International Journal of Geriatric Psychiatry, 4*, 73–78.

Young, R. C., Jain, H., Kiossess, D. N., & Meyers, B. S. (2003). Antidepressant-associated mania in late life. *International Journal of Geriatric Psychiatry, 18*(5), 421–424.

Young, R. C., Kiosses, D., Heo, M., Schulberg, H. C., Murphy, C., Klimstra, S.,...Alexopoulos, G. S. (2007). Age and ratings of manic psychopathology. *Bipolar Disorders, 9*(3), 301–304.

Young, R. C., & Klerman, G. L. (1992). Mania in late life: focus on age at onset. *American Journal of Psychiatry, 149*(7), 867–876.

Young, R. C., Marino, P ., (2011). *YMRS Scores: demographic and clinical correlates in bipolar manic elders.* Paper presented at the Annual Meeting of the International Society Bipolar Disorders,.

Young, R. C., Mattis, S., (1991). *Manic states in late life: A prospective study.* Paper presented at the Annual Meeting of the Society of Biological Psychiatry, New Orleans, LA.

Young, R. C., Murphy, C. F., (2001). *Executive function and treatment outcome in geriatric mania.* Abstract presented for the New Research Program at the Annual Meeting of the American Psychiatric Association .

Young, R. C., Murphy, C. F., Heo, M., Schulberg, H. C., & Alexopoulos, G. S. (2006). Cognitive impairment in bipolar disorder in old age: Literature review and findings in manic patients. *Journal of Affective Disorders, 92*(1), 125–131.

Young, R. C., Nambudiri, D. E., Jain, H., de Asis, J. M., & Alexopoulos, G. S. (1999). Brain computed tomography in geriatric manic disorder. *Biological Psychiatry, 45*, 1063–1065.

Young, R. C., Schreiber, M. T., & Nysewander, R. W. (1983). Psychotic mania. *Biological Psychiatry, 18*, 1167–1173.

Yu, X. L., & Young, R. C. (2001). Geriatric schizoaffective disorders. *Biological Psychiatry, 49*(8S), 12s.

8

NON-MAJOR DEPRESSION

Ipsit V. Vahia, Ganesh Kulkarni, Thomas W. Meeks, and Dilip V. Jeste

OVER THE past decade, there has been growing recognition of non-major (or subthreshold or sub-syndromal) depression as a clinical entity of significant relevance, as more is learned about its impact on health-related quality of life and successful aging. However, this clinical syndrome remains an understudied area and, as a result, is infrequently given the clinical attention that it merits. One reason for this may be the lack of agreement on definitions and nomenclature of non-major depressive syndromes, making it difficult to generalize research findings. As such, non-major depression encompasses multiple clinical entities, including minor depression (MinD), subsyndromal depression (SSD), subthreshold depression (SubD), and brief recurrent depression. In this chapter, we use the term *non-major depression* to represent minor depression, subsyndromal depression, and subthreshold depression. We do not include dysthymic disorder in our conceptualization, since it has well-defined criteria established by the *Diagnostic and Statistical Manual of Mental Disorders* (DSM) and has been studied as

a distinct diagnosis, usually not as a component of non-major depression.

THE ISSUE OF NOMENCLATURE

With the introduction of the *DSM-III*, psychiatry increased the reliability of diagnoses. However, the definition of a "threshold" that constituted major psychopathology has remained a contentious issue. When possible, thresholds have been based on empirical data, but otherwise, nonempirical "expert opinion" is invariably involved in separating the "ill" from the "well." Non-major depression (NMD) has sometimes been divided into distinct categories (e.g., MinD) but at other times studied as a single entity. Based on the diagnostic criteria used in existing studies, overlap among these constructs is common. In 1992, Wells et al. (1989) reported that depressive symptoms not meeting criteria for major depressive disorder (MDD) were associated with more social disability than many medical illnesses. Soon thereafter, Judd et al. (1994), using data from the Epidemiological Catchment Area (ECA) study, reported a 1-month prevalence of SSD in the general adult population of 11.8%. *DSM-IV* later listed criteria for MinD in the section on Depression Not Otherwise Specified. These were similar to those for MDD except requiring only two to four symptoms and no prior history of MDD; however, it has been subsequently demonstrated that *DSM*-defined MinD misses several people who suffer morbidity from other variants of SSD. For instance, Judd et al. noted that among the SSD subjects in the ECA study, less than a third met criteria for MinD because neither depressed mood nor anhedonia (MDD Criterion A symptoms) was present (Judd, Rapaport, Paulus, & Brown, 1994). They found virtually no differences between SSD subjects with versus without Criterion A symptoms. Angst and colleagues (1990) proposed another variant of NMD—recurrent brief depression—in which the only reason for failing to meet MDD criteria was that symptoms did not persist uninterrupted for 2 consecutive weeks.

Despite variable definitions and criteria, NMD consistently exacts major consequences on affected individuals (e.g., increased disability, poorer quality of life) and on society (e.g., increased health care costs) (Broadhead, Blazer, George, & Tse, 1990; Hybels, Pieper, & Blazer, 2009; Koenig, 1998a; Spitzer et al., 1995; Xavier et al., 2002). The concept of NMD has resonated strongly in geriatric psychiatry (Jeste et al., 1999; Jeste, Blazer, & First, 2005), along with a speculation that MDD prevalence among older adults was inaccurate in the ECA study because of diagnostic ascertainment procedures (Judd & Akiskal, 2002). In a reanalysis of the ECA data, Judd and Kunovac (1998) noted that among adults ≥65 years old, SubD (MinD + SSD) prevalence was 31.1%, versus 6.3% for MDD—a five-fold difference. In a subsequent review summarizing prevalence of variously defined NMD, Meeks and colleagues (2011) estimated the prevalence to be approximately three times that of MDD. Meeks and colleagues also made the distinction between the two most frequently used terms among the NMDs—subsyndromal depression (SSD) and subthreshold depression (SubD). SSD and SubD have had variable definitions ranging from clinically significant depressive symptoms that do not meet clinical or manual-defined criteria for MDD to cutoff scores on a validated scale (e.g., Hamilton Depression Rating Scale [HAM-D] or Center for Epidemiological Studies Depression Scale [CES-D]) intermediate

between syndromal depression and normal mood. It is important to note that the studies described herein use differing criteria for NMD; while general conclusions drawn from a study using a particular definition may apply across definitions, cognizance of the criteria and definition used in a study must always be considered when making clinical conclusions drawn from studies. Throughout this chapter, we have used the terms *MDD*, *MinD*, *SubD*, and *SSD* as reported in parent studies, and we use *NMD* as a general term to represent this class of disorders.

EPIDEMIOLOGY

Community-Based Studies

In their review of NMD, Meeks and colleagues (2011) differentiate epidemiological descriptions of SSD depending on the clinical setting where depressive symptoms were studied—principal settings being community-dwelling settings, primary care (PC) clinics, and long-term care (LTC) institutions. They note that 12 of the 17 CD studies reviewed reported point prevalence, with SSD point prevalence ranging from 4.0% to 22.9% (median point prevalence, 9.8%). All CD studies reported MDD or "syndromal depression" prevalence as well, and the ratio of SSD:MDD prevalence ranged from 1.1 to 6.9 (median 2.5). Studies assessing more than one variant of SSD (e.g., MinD *and* SSD) yielded higher than the median prevalence rates of SSD and ratios of SSD:MDD. Although many studies did not report these data, the female:male prevalence ratios of SSD ranged from 1.0 to 2.4:1 (median 1.6:1), in comparison to the 2:1 ratio noted in most studies of MDD.

Four community-based investigations assessed 1-month prevalence: (a) SubD (SSD + MinD) prevalence of 31.1% (Judd & Kunovac, 1998); (b) 16.5% SSD prevalence (Geiselmann, Linden, & Helmchen, 2001); (c) 12.9% MinD prevalence (Beekman et al., 1995); and (d) 8.8% SSD prevalence (Chen, Chong, & Tsang, 2007). The first three studies reported similar rates of various NMD syndromes, whereas the fourth study was noted to have employed more stringent criteria, and as a result, likely reported lower rates.

Meeks and colleagues noted that prevalence of late-life NMD appeared to be lower in the community as compared to PC and inpatient hospitals, and highest in institutional settings, similar to the epidemiological pattern of MDD. However, it remains difficult to comment on whether this represents a progressive increase across populations, due to the heterogeneity of criteria. The work of Lyness and colleagues, conducted chiefly in primary care settings, represents the majority of all research in this area and remains a benchmark for NMD research (Lyness, Chapman, McGriff, Drayer, & Duberstein, 2009; Lyness, King, Cox, Yoediono, & Caine, 1999; Lyness et al., 2007). Overall, employing varying definitions, Lyness and colleagues have reported a prevalence range from 15.1% to 35.9% in primary care samples. The definitions used have included *DSM*-defined MinD, Hamilton Depression Rating Scale scores (>10), criteria defined by Judd and colleagues, and alternative criteria proposed by Lyness et al. The highest prevalence reported by Lyness and colleagues was 35.9%, in a study that combined MinD, SSD (Lyness et al criteria), and also dysthymia. The SSD:MDD ratio among the Lyness et al. primary care studies ranged from 2.3 to 7.5:1. The female:male prevalence ratio from two studies (2.1–2.3:1) was higher than that seen in the community. It is also notable that in other PC studies (Aranda, Lee, & Wilson, 2001; Williams, Kerber, Mulrow, Medina, & Aguilar, 1995) that included ≥50% Mexican Americans or exclusively Latinos, the NMD prevalence (16.0%–20.1%) and ratio of SSD:MDD (4.0–5.0:1) were comparable to the range reported in the aforementioned, predominantly Caucasian samples, despite the use of more restrictive criteria. Findings from studies that employed *International Classification of Disease* (*ICD*) criteria are somewhat more varied. One study by Berardi and colleagues (2002) employed *ICD* "current depressive episode" (CDE) criteria (similar but not identical to *DSM*-defined MDD) and found CDE almost twice as common as SSD. A separate study, also conducted in Europe (in the Netherlands; Licht-Strunk et al., 2005), observed a notably lower point prevalence of SubD (10.2%) than that observed in American PC clinics. Meeks and colleagues note that these differences between European and American PC studies may be attributable to differences in populations as well as criteria and definitions.

Meeks and colleagues report four epidemiological studies of NMD among older medical inpatients. Three reported higher point prevalence of SSD than MDD; while three of these studies used *DSM* criteria for MinD (Koenig et al., 1991, 1997; McCusker et al., 2005), a fourth study (Schneider, Kruse, Nehen, Senf, & Heuft, 2000) examined SSD prevalence (determined by an *ICD* checklist) using inclusive versus exclusive approaches to depression

diagnosis. The prevalence reported using an inclusive approach ranged from 27.9% to 32.1%, while the exclusive approach employed by Schneider and colleagues reported a prevalence of 17.6%. Among inpatients, ratios of SSD:MDD ranged from 1.3 to 2.2:1, and the estimated female:male prevalence ratio was 1.9:1.

The review by Meeks and colleagues reports multiple studies that examined SSD point prevalence in LTC settings. The prevalence of MinD ranged from 4.0% to 30.5%, with studies using more rigorous criteria yielding similar rates of 16.8% and 14.1% (Jongenelis et al., 2004; Morrow-Howell et al., 2008; Østbye et al., 2005; Parmelee, Katz, & Lawton, 1992; Teresi, Abrams, Holmes, Ramirez, & Eimicke, 2001). There were two investigations (Meeks, Vahia, Lavretsky, Kulkarni, & Jeste, 2010) which reported that approximately 33%–61% of LTC residents experienced SSD at any given point in time. This high rate may be attributed, in part, to a high prevalence of cognitive impairment in this population. Notably, only one study has assessed prevalence of NMD in hospice settings. This study estimated prevalence to be 9.2% (in comparison to 16.9% for MDD; Chochinov, Wilson, Enns, & Lander, 1994). Three studies among older home health care recipients reported comparable point prevalence of NMD (7.0%, 8.2%, and 10.8%; Meeks et al. 2010).

ILLNESS COURSE

Risk of Developing Major Depression

A major focus of NMD research has been to identify whether this condition serves as a prodrome to major depression. Two large studies in general adult populations found 1-year and 2-year rates of conversion to MDD to be 10% and 25%, respectively (Broadhead et al., 1990; Wells, Burnam, Rogers, Hays, & Camp, 1992). A comprehensive review by Cuijpers et al. evaluated multiple studies and estimated relative risk to range from 1.15 to 9.73 (median, 4.43; Cuijpers, Beekman, Smit, & Deeg, 2006). Two community-based studies assessed MDD risk in late-life NMD. One study reported that at 6-year follow-up, 20% of older adults with SSD developed a *DSM-IV* mood disorder—5.8% developed MDD, 12.3% developed dysthymia, and 1.9% developed comorbid MDD and dysthymia (Cuijpers et al., 2006). A separate study reported the 3-year relative risk of developing MDD among

Table 8.1. Rates of conversion of Non-major depression to Major Depression

AUTHOR/YEAR	STUDY POPULATION	FOLLOW-UP PERIOD	FORM OF NON-MAJOR DEPRESSION STUDIED	CONVERSION RATE/RISK (DENOMINATOR)
Broadhead et al., 1990	US community-dwelling adults	1 year	SubD →MDD	10% (1 year)
Wells et al., 1992	US Adults	2 year	SubD →MDD	25% (2 years)
Cuijpers et al., 2006	Netherlands community-dwelling adults	3–6 years	SubD →MDD SubD →DYS	5.8% (end of study) 12.8% (end of study)
Schoevers et al., 2006	Netherlands community-dwelling adults	3 years	SSD →MDD	30% absolute risk
Lyness et al., 2006	US primary care	1 year	MinD/SSD →MDD	Odds ratio of 5.5
Lyness et al., 2002	US primary care	1.5 years	SubD →MDD	10% (1 year)
Vuorilehto, Melartin, & Isometsä, 2009	US primary care	1.5 years	MinD/SSD →MDD	25% (18 months)

DYS, dsythymia; MDD, major depressive disorder; MinD, minor depression; SSD, subsyndromal depression; SubD, subthreshold depression

older adults with SSD versus nondepressed peers to be 2.43 (3-year absolute risk 29.3%; Schoevers et al., 2006), overall suggesting the 1-year conversion rate of SubD to MDD among older adults is approximately 10%.

Among PC populations, Lyness et al. (2006) reported that 8.8% of older adults with MinD or SSD had MDD after 1 year, consistent with a 16.2% 2-year absolute risk of MDD in another PC study of late-life NMD (Cui, Lyness, Tang, Tu, & Conwell, 2008). These results were consistent with 10%/year conversion rate from SSD to MDD in a separate PC study (Lyness et al., 2002). Vuorilehto and colleagues (2009) reported that at 18 months, 25% of those diagnosed with MinD had developed MD. A different PC study addressed the issue of whether outcomes differed according to past history of MDD. This study observed that after 3 months, more than twice the number of patients with SSD and a past history of MDD developed a *DSM*-diagnosed depressive disorder, in comparison to those without a history of MDD (24% vs. 10%) (Meeks et al., 2010).

There are few data on longitudinal risk of developing MDD following NMD in other populations. However, two studies conducted on specific clinical populations bear mentioning, since they may be indicative of higher risk of conversion to MDD among persons with vascular disease. One study noted that among post-acute myocardial infarction patients, 14% of persons with MinD had MDD versus only 6% among persons with no depression at baseline (Schleifer et al., 1989). Another study of persons with coronary heart disease found that of the 17% of persons with MinD at baseline, 42% developed MDD at 1-year follow-up. Table 8.1 summarizes reported rates of conversion of MinD to MDD. One study assessing SSD occurrence after remission of MDD in late life found that longer prevalence of SSD predicted significantly higher risk of MDD relapse (Kiosses et al., 2012).

Stability of Longitudinal Diagnosis

In addition to studies of conversion to MDD, much of the longitudinal literature dealing with NMD has focused on diagnostic stability. In the Longitudinal Aging Study Amsterdam (LASA; Beekman et al., 2002), it was noted that among community-dwelling older adults with MDD, dysthymia, or SSD those with "double depression" (MDD/DYS) fared the worst, with only 5% achieving remission. While SSD had the best prognosis among the diagnoses assessed (26% remission rate), 61% of older adults with SSD had a chronic or chronic-intermittent course. Among primary care patients with SSD, stability of diagnosis at 1 year was similar to the LASA results (62%–70%) (Cui et al., 2008; Lyness et al., 2009). Cohen and colleagues (2009) reported strikingly similar numbers (65% diagnostic stability) among a very different population of mostly urban, community-dwelling African Americans of Caribbean heritage, Studies of the longitudinal course of SSD in PC have yielded a somewhat more favorable prognosis than in the community, although the number of studies is limited in both settings.

Studies on the longitudinal course of NMD in medical inpatients have shown inconsistent results. In one study, older medical inpatients with NMD showed a fluctuant 1-year course—4% maintained a stable diagnosis of MinD, 28% maintained stable recovery, and 68% vacillated between diagnoses (Cole et al., 2006). However, another investigation that measured severity of symptoms, rather than change in diagnoses, showed a stable 1-year symptom course (McCusker et al., 2007). Another study of inpatients with congestive heart failure reported faster recovery time for MinD (3 weeks) versus MDD (20 weeks) (Koenig, 1998a). A separate study of post-myocardial infarction older patients noted that those with MinD have higher rates of being non-depressed at follow-up compared to those with MDD and also suggested a fluctuating illness course.

Evidence from other older populations supports the notion that MinD has a more favorable prognosis than MDD but that its course varies and is certainly less favorable than for those without depression. Among LTC residents, the rate of being depression-free 1 year after baseline assessment was 88% for those with no depression, but less than 4% for those with NMD or MDD at baseline. The longitudinal course of SSD has also been examined among persons with recent bereavement. Evaluations conducted 2–25 months after the loss showed that prognosis varied from best to worst in the following order: ND→SSD→MinD→MDD (Zisook, Paulus, Shuchter, & Judd, 1997). Despite having a better prognosis than MDD patients, spousally bereaved older adults with SSD still spent more than 40% of their time in a persistent state of SSD over 2 years. In a study of persons with dementia, 23.6% of patients had MinD at baseline, and they spent on average 25% of the next 9 months with symptomatic depression (Ballard, Patel, Solis, Lowe, & Wilcock, 1996).

HEALTH OUTCOMES

Studies have demonstrated associations between NMD and multiple negative medical and psychosocial conditions similar to MDD. Most investigations have been cross-sectional, limiting cause-and-effect interpretations. Meeks and colleagues have noted the possibility of certain conditions being both consequences as well as risk factors for NMD. Similar to Meeks and colleagues' report, we first outline the following.

Cross-Sectional Associations

Even in cross-sectional studies, certain variables are clearly risk factors rather than consequences (e.g., gender). Many epidemiological studies indicated female gender as a risk factor for late-life NMD (Kvaal, McDougall, Brayne, Matthews, & Dewey, 2008). Other variables reported as risk factors include past depression history (Beekman et al., 1995; McCusker et al., 2005) and family history of depression/psychiatric illness (Beekman et al., 1995).

Certain medical illnesses associated with MDD have been identified as possible risk factors for SSD, for example, visual impairment (Horowitz, Reinhardt, & Kennedy, 2005), end-stage renal disease requiring hemodialysis (Drayer et al., 2006), Parkinson's disease (Starkstein et al., 2008), cardiac disease/coronary heart disease (Penninx et al., 2001), and stroke (Saxena, Ng, Yong, Fong, & Koh, 2008). Cognitive disorders also increase risk of SSD; four studies of cognitively impaired older adults (two with Alzheimer's disease, two with mild cognitive impairment) reported similar point prevalence of MinD—17.2%, 26%, 26.5%, and 27% (versus median community prevalence of 9.8%; Meeks et al., 2010).

Variables cross-sectionally associated with late-life SSD that may be antecedents, consequences, or both include the following: (a) being unmarried, (b) low socioeconomic status, (c) lower education, (d) executive function and verbal recall impairment, (e) increased medical burden, (f) disability, (g) decreased social support/loneliness/conflicted relationships, and (h) negative life events and loss (Meeks et al., 2010).

Prospective Studies: Risk Factors

Prospective findings point to medical burden, functional disability, negative life events, past depression history, and decreased social support as risk factors for persistence or worsening of NMD among older medical inpatients (Cui et al., 2008; Koenig, 1998a; Koenig, Vandermeer, Chambers, Burr-Crutchfield, & Johnson, 2006b). These findings have been replicated in PC populations (Lyness et al., 2009).

Prospective Studies: Consequences

Several prospective studies have demonstrated significant adverse public health outcomes in late-life SSD. The majority of these have identified increased health care utilization as a consequence of NMD (Beekman, Deeg, Braam, Smit, & van Tilburg, 1997; Creed, Cooper-Patrick, & Ford, 2002; Koenig, 1998a).

At the individual level, prospective investigations of late-life SSD have identified the following adverse consequences in comparison with nondepressed older adults: (a) increased cognitive impairment among cognitively intact medical inpatients (Han, McCusker, Cole, Abrahamowicz, & Capek, 2008); (b) elevated risk of dementia or cognitive disorder NOS (Boyle, Porsteinsson, Cui, King, & Lyness, 2010); (c) poorer physical health (Beekman et al., 1997); (d) future functional disability (Allen, Agha, Duthie, & Layde, 2004), including more impairment in activities of daily living (Hybels et al., 2009; Barry, Allore, Bruce., & Gill, 2009); and (e) decline on physical performance tests (e.g., balance and walking speed; Penninx et al., 1998).

There are inconsistent data regarding the impact of NMD on mortality. SSD increases suicidal ideation (Angst, Merikangas, Scheidegger, & Wicki, 1990; Chopra et al., 2005; Montross et al., 2008), and one retrospective study found that among completed suicides the odds ratio for completed suicide among persons age ≥75 was significantly elevated for those with MinD (Waern, Rubenowitz, & Wilhelmson, 2003). This finding is echoed by a study conducted in Sweden, which noted a higher odds ratio for suicide attempts among older persons with MinD (Wiktorsson, Runeson, Skoog, Ostling, & Waern, 2010). NMD has also been linked to increased nonsuicide mortality among several late-life disorders (Katon et al., 2008), including coronary heart disease (Whang et al., 2009), congestive heart failure (Rafanelli, Roncuzzi, & Milaneschi, 2006), and diabetes mellitus (Lin et al., 2009). One hypothesis is that at least part of the reason for increased mortality in chronic medical illness maybe be due to poorer self-care.

COMORBIDITY

Non-major depressions, especially SSD, have been reported as comorbid conditions in a broad range of medical and psychiatric illnesses. Almost uniformly, the presence of SSD is associated with poorer health outcomes in persons with medical and psychiatric illnesses.

Medical Comorbidity

Several studies have found association between SSD and adverse cardiovascular events, most notably with congestive heart failure and myocardial infarction. Prevalence of SSD in patients with myocardial infarction and congestive heart failure are similar and vary from 10% to 40%, with higher rates found in those with more severe congestive heart failure (Freedland et al., 2003). Koenig (1998b) has demonstrated higher rates of congestive heart failure in inpatients with MinD compared to those with no depression. Follow-up studies have noted that changes in depression and physical illness track closely with each other in a longitudinal study of inpatients with congestive heart failure (Koenig et al., 2006b) and that severity of depression is proportional to increased medical comorbidity and decreased physical functioning (Koenig, Vandermeer, Chambers, Burr-Crutchfield, & Johnson, 2006a). Depressive symptoms in congestive heart failure may respond to nonpharmacological treatments; a trial comparing cognitive-behavioral therapy and supportive stress management (Freedland et al., 2009) found both these modalities to be efficacious compared to usual care, with cognitive-behavioral therapy demonstrating greater and more sustained improvement in depressive outcomes.

Presence of minor depressive symptoms in myocardial infarction patients poses increased risk of future cardiac events (Rafanelli et al., 2006) and is associated with higher mortality (Romanelli, Fauerbach, Bush, & Ziegelstein, 2002), possibly due to poorer adherence to post- myocardial infarction treatments. As with congestive heart failure, greater severity of depressive symptoms is associated with poorer functional recovery in myocardial infarction (Schleifer et al., 1989). In outpatients with chronic obstructive pulmonary disease, SSD is associated with lower physical functioning, lower quality of life, and increased mortality (Yohannes, Baldwin, & Connolly, 2003).

In diabetes mellitus, global studies suggest that the presence of MinD is associated with lower mental health-related quality of life and lower self-perceived health (McCollum, Ellis, Regensteiner, Zhang, & Sullivan, 2007), but not physical health-related quality of life or functioning. A separate study of minor depressive symptoms in diabetes mellitus (Viinamaki, Niskanen, & Uusitupa, 1995) suggests that presence/severity of depressive symptoms may be related to specific symptoms. This study noted that albuminuria and neuropathy were both independently associated with minor depressive symptoms.

In addition to functioning, SSD may impact response to rehabilitative treatment. Presence of SSD/MinD has been shown to decrease likelihood of functional independence in older adults undergoing physical rehabilitation (Allen et al., 2004) and greater functional disability and poorer self-rated health in older persons in rehabilitation for age-related vision loss (Horowitz et al., 2005).

Neuropsychiatric Illness

In persons with cerebrovascular accidents, prevalence of depressive symptoms has been estimated as high as 50% (Eastwood, Rifat, Nobbs, & Ruderman, 1989), likely a consequence of neuroanatomical changes resulting from vascular insult (Paradiso & Robinson, 1999). Effects of SSD on post-cerebrovascular accident functioning exist on a continuum with MDD, with greater severity associated with slower recovery (Parikh et al., 1990), impairment in activities of daily living (Parikh et al., 1990; Saxena, Ng, Koh, Yong, & Fong, 2007), and higher risk of cerebrovascular accident recurrence (Saxena et al., 2007).

In studies of Parkinson's disease, minor or subsyndromal depressive symptoms are more common than major depression (Tandberg, Larsen, Aarsland, & Cummings, 1996) and likewise appear to exist on a continuum with MDD (Costa, Peppe, Carlesimo, Pasqualetti, & Caltagirone, 2006). Depressive symptoms in Parkinson's disease have been associated in a proportional manner with functional deficits (Starkstein et al., 2008) and parkinsonian symptoms.

Multiple studies involving various clinical populations have noted an association between depressive symptoms and impaired cognitive function. In both cerebrovascular accidents and Parkinson's disease, SubD is associated with increased severity of cognitive deficits (Costa et al., 2006; Parikh et al., 1990; Saxena et al., 2007; Starkstein et al., 2008; Uekermann et al., 2003). In persons with dementia, the prevalence of SSD is estimated to range from 22% to 27% (median, 26%) (Devanand et al., 1997; Gabryelewicz et al., 2004; Geiselmann et al., 2001; Klembara, 2001; Lyketsos et al., 1997; Starkstein, Jorge, Mizrahi, & Robinson, 2005). Comorbid SSD has been commonly observed in mild cognitive impairment, vascular dementia, and Alzheimer's disease. Prevalence rates of SSD in mild cognitive impairment, vascular dementia, and Alzheimer's disease dementia appear similar. Mood disorders likely exist on a continuum of severity in Alzheimer's disease, and greater severity is associated with increased functional impairment, behavioral disturbances such as agitation and wandering, and greater cognitive deficits (Meeks et al., 2010). However, two longitudinal studies have noted that depressive symptoms in Alzheimer's disease are less likely to persist and may resolve spontaneously (Devanand et al., 1997; Li, Meyer, & Thornby, 2001), while in mild cognitive impairment and vascular dementia depressive symptoms were more persistent and may be resistant to treatment (Li et al., 2001). In a trial among Alzheimer's disease patients, Devanand and colleagues (2003) found moderate response to sertraline in persons with minor depressive symptoms in Alzheimer's disease, although there was little improvement in cognitive symptoms.

In community studies, presence of SSD is associated with higher prevalence of anxiety symptoms (Geiselmann et al., 2001; Heun, Papassotiropoulos, & Ptok, 2000), illicit drug use (Geiselmann et al., 2001), and somatic illnesses (Geiselmann et al., 2001). A secondary analysis of data from the Epidemiological Catchment Area study by Crum and colleagues (1994) found that presence of depressive symptoms in primary care patients was associated with increased 1-year incidence rates of MDD, anxiety disorder, schizophrenia, and alcohol/illicit drug use.

Studies of comorbid SSD in older adults with schizophrenia have noted that depressive symptoms are associated with higher overall positive and negative symptoms (i.e., more severe psychopathology; Diwan et al., 2007; Zisook et al., 2007), higher frequency of anxiety symptoms (Hu, Pepper, & Goldman, 1991), poorer physical health (Kneale, Sorahan, & Stewart, 1991), decreased physical and mental functioning (Acquavella, 1991), and lower quality of life (Kneale et al., 1991). Suicidality is also more common in schizophrenia patients with SSD (Cohen, Abdallah, & Diwan, 2010; Zisook et al., 2007). A study by Zisook and colleagues (2007) noted that 24% of older schizophrenia patients with SSD had current suicidal ideation and almost 50% reported a past suicide attempt, suggesting that older schizophrenia patients with depressive symptoms merit great clinical vigilance for suicidal thoughts.

ASSOCIATION WITH SUCCESSFUL AGING

Recently there has been an increased research and clinical focus in geriatric psychiatry on successful (or healthy) aging. It has been suggested that, among older persons, trajectories of successful physical aging, cognitive aging, emotional aging, and psychosocial aging may differ (Jeste, Wolkowitz, & Palmer, 2011). Successful aging is therefore increasingly being conceptualized as a multiple dimensional entity, which comprises both objectively measurable domains such as cognition and absence of clinically significant depression, as well as subjective factors such as ratings of older persons' attitudes toward their own aging and self-rated successful aging.

In one study conducted in a sample of postmenopausal women, Vahia and colleagues (2010) observed that SSD was associated with poorer outcomes on nearly every successful aging-related measure used in their study, including worse self-rated successful aging, worse physical and emotional functioning, lower optimism, more negative attitudes toward aging, lower personal mastery and self-efficacy, and greater anxiety and hostility. They also noted that subjects with NMD had higher self-reported rates of previous diagnosis, treatment, and hospitalization for mental health problems. Importantly, they found that NMD lies on a continuum where those with NMD had worse outcomes than those with no depressive symptoms, but better outcomes than those with MDD. Their finding is supported by another study by Grabovich and colleagues (2010), who noted that at 1-year follow-up, presence of SSD was associated with a broad range of adverse outcomes. While this study did not specifically target successful aging-related outcomes, they found higher rates of suicidality, anxiety, cognitive impairment, and functional decline in SSD versus nondepressed older adults. These studies point to a potential role for clinical investigation into NMD as a target for interventions to promote successful aging by leading to a cascading improvement in a broad range of outcomes.

NEUROBIOLOGY

Research on the neurobiology underlying depressive disorders in general has exploded in the past two decades. The concomitant research on neurobiology of late-life depression has lagged behind slightly, while neurobiological research on NMD in late life can be still regarded as in its infancy. A full summary of the neurobiology of late-life depression is beyond the scope of this chapter. However, the biological systems implicated in late-life NMD are not very different from those summarized in reviews of biological findings of major depression in general (Maletic, Robinson, & Oakes, 2007) and share similarities with the findings of the neurobiology of NMD among general adult populations. For example, in terms of genetics, polymorphisms in the serotonin transporter promoter region (l vs. s alleles) have been associated with depressive symptoms among adults without *DSM* depressive disorders in a pattern similar to that seen in MDD (symptom severity: $(s)/(s) > (l)/(s) > (l)/(l)$) (Gonda, Juhasz, Laszik, Rihmer, & Bagdy, 2005). Likewise, via family history methods, there were no significant differences in risk of affective disorders for first-degree relatives of persons with MDD versus MinD (Remick, Sadovnick, Lam, Zis, & Yee, 1996).

TREATMENT

There remains a lack of consensus regarding effective treatments for NMD. There have been studies of pharmacological interventions, psychotherapy, and other psychosocial and physical activity–based interventions. However, there have been no known randomized studies that compared various treatment modalities against each other.

Pharmacological Interventions

Results of pharmacological trials for treatment of NMD have been inconclusive. Studies in this area have also been limited by poor evidence, with a paucity of randomized controlled trials. In two studies that included older patients with NMD as well as MDD, Devanand and colleagues (2005) observed only limited improvement in NMD with both fluoxetine and sertraline. These studies included persons with dysthymia. While the studies were placebo controlled, other than modest improvement over placebo in raw scores of HAM-D and some improvement in cognition, the investigators did not note changes in any other measures of outcome, including quality of life. An open-label trial of citalopram by Kasckow and colleagues (2002) and an open trial comparing sertraline and citalopram by Rocca and colleagues (2005) both noted significantly improved HAM-D scores in older persons with MinD, which were sustained up to 1 year. A multisite randomized controlled trial by Williams and colleagues (2000) comparing placebo and clinical treatment to paroxetine also noted a modest improvement in functioning in older adults with MinD. However, this study had a large variability in site effects, impairing its generalizability. In contrast, an open trial of amitriptyline by Paykel and colleagues (1988) found that use of this medication led to significant symptomatic improvement in MDD but not in MinD. Summarizing available evidence in a review of 10 clinical trials for NMD, Oxman and Sengupta (2002) observed that pharmacological treatment appears to lead, at best, to a minimal improvement in minor depressive symptoms.

Notably, however, Zisook and colleagues have found in a two-site, randomized controlled study that citalopram leads to significant improvement in depressive symptoms, as well as suicidality, in comparison to placebo in older persons with schizophrenia who suffer from subsyndromal depression (Kasckow et al., 2010).

Psychotherapy

The evidence regarding efficacy of psychotherapeutic interventions for NMD appears to be more substantial than that for pharmacotherapy. At least two trials have documented the efficacy for cognitive-behavioral therapy for NMD among older adults (California Health and Safety Code, 2003; Miranda & Munoz, 1994). Efficacy of problem-solving therapy and also of telephone-delivered psychotherapy has also been demonstrated for NMD in older adults (Lynch, Tamburrino, & Nagel, 1997; Mossey, Knott, Higgins, & Talerico, 1996).

Physical Activity

Two randomized trials that included a population of older persons have pointed to a beneficial effect of physical activity interventions—either aerobic exercise or strength training—for alleviating NMD (Brenes et al., 2007; Singh, Clements, & Fiatarone, 1997). An interesting open, noncontrolled pilot study by Rosenberg and colleagues (2010) employed "exergames" as an intervention for older adults with NMD, in which participants played Wii "virtual" sports games for 30 minutes a day, three times a week. At the end of 12 weeks, the investigators noted statistically significant improvement in depressive symptoms, which was sustained at 24 weeks.

PREVENTION

As described previously in this chapter, non-major depression is comorbid with a wide range of medical and neuropsychiatric conditions. Interventions aimed at reducing the incidence of NMD in these populations, and conversion of NMD to major depression across clinical and community-dwelling samples, can significantly reduce comorbidity related to depression. While there is limited evidence specifically on preventing development of NMD, both pharmacological and psychosocial interventions have found to be effective in reducing conversion of minor to major depression, in community-dwelling persons as well as specific clinical samples such as stroke survivors or persons with macular degeneration. Clinical trials have demonstrated the effectiveness of escitalopram as a preventative agent in conversion of non-major to major depression (Robinson et al., 2008). In a meta-analysis Cuijpers and colleagues (2007) note that problem-solving therapy, cognitive-behavioral therapy, and interpersonal therapy may all be effective preventative interventions. All these treatments have been found effective in clinical trials (Rovner & Casten, 2008; Rovner, Casten, Hegel, Leiby, & Tasman, 2007; Sriwattanakomen et al., 2010). There remains a lack of consensus, however, on the cost-effectiveness of interventions to prevent NMD (Romeo et al., 2011). The broader issue of prevention of depression in late life is beyond the scope of this chapter, and it is discussed in greater depth in Chapter 25.

SUMMARY

Clinically significant non-major depression encompasses a range of clinical entities, including minor depression, subsyndromal and subthreshold depression, and recurrent brief depression. While lack of consistency in nomenclature and definitions has impaired research in this area, prevalence among older adults is estimated to be three to five times greater than that of major depression and is further increased in certain specific populations (e.g., long-term care residents, persons with cardiovascular disease). Late-life NMD appears to increase the likelihood of developing major depressive disorder and to be associated with a wide range of medical and neuropsychiatric comorbidity, including coronary heart disease, dementia, and diabetes mellitus. NMD also negatively impacts prospects for successful aging. While there is a general lack of solid empirical evidence to guide treatment, clinical vigilance for MDD is recommended, and psychotherapy and physical exercise may be prioritized over pharmacotherapy for management of late-life NMD.

Disclosures

To my knowledge, all of my possible conflicts of interest and those of my coauthors, financial or otherwise, including direct or indirect financial or personal relationships, interests, and affiliations, whether or not directly related to the subject of the chapter, are listed in the following:

Ipsit V. Vahia, MD, has no conflicts of interest to disclose. He receives partial support from the John A. Hartford Foundation.

Ganesh Kulkarni, MBBS, has no conflicts of interest or sources of support to disclose.

Thomas W. Meeks, MD, has no conflicts of interest or sources of support to disclose.

Dilip V. Jeste, MD, has no conflicts to disclose. He is funded by NIMH and the University of California, San Diego. Grant Support: National Institute of Mental Health (NIMH), NIMH (P30 MH080002).

REFERENCES

Acquavella, J. F. (1991). Re: "Are non-whites at greater risk for occupational cancer?" *American Journal of Industrial Medicine, 20,* 811, 813–814.

Allen, B. P., Agha, Z., Duthie, E. H., Jr., & Layde, P. M. (2004). Minor depression and rehabilitation outcome for older adults in subacute care. *Journal of Behavioral Health Services and Research, 31,* 189–198.

Angst, J., Merikangas, K., Scheidegger, P., & Wicki, W. (1990). Recurrent brief depression: A new subtype of affective disorder. *Journal of Affective Disorders, 19,* 87–98.

Aranda, M. P., Lee, P. J., & Wilson, S. (2001). Correlates of depression in older Latinos. *Home Health Care Services Quarterly, 20,* 1–20.

Ballard, C. G., Patel, A., Solis, M., Lowe, K., & Wilcock, G. (1996). A one-year follow-up study of depression in dementia sufferers. *British Journal of Psychiatry, 168,* 287–291.

Barry, L. C., Allore, H. G., Bruce, M. L., & Gill, T. M. (2009). Longitudinal association between depressive symptoms and disability burden among older persons. *Journals of Gerontology Series A: Biological Sciences and Medical Sciences, 64,* 1325–1332.

Beekman, A. T., Deeg, D. J., Braam, A. W., Smit, J. H., & van Tilburg, W. (1997). Consequences of major and minor depression in later life: A study of disability, well-being and service utilization. *Psychological Medicine, 27,* 1397–1409.

Beekman, A. T., Deeg, D. J., van Tilburg, T., Smit, J. H., Hooijer, C., & van Tilburg, W. (1995). Major and minor depression in later life: A study of prevalence and risk factors. *Journal of Affective Disorders, 36,* 65–75.

Beekman, A. T., Geerlings, S. W., Deeg, D. J., Smit, J. H., Schoevers, R. S., de Beurs, E., . . . van Tilburg, W. (2002). The natural history of late-life depression: A 6-year prospective study in the community. *Archives of General Psychiatry, 59,* 605–611.

Berardi, D., Menchetti, M., De Ronchi, D., Rucci, P., Leggieri, G., & Ferrari, G. (2002). Late-life depression in primary care: A nationwide Italian epidemiological survey. *Journal of the American Geriatrics Society, 50,* 77–83.

Boyle, L. L., Porsteinsson, A. P., Cui, X., King, D. A., & Lyness, J. M. (2010). Depression predicts cognitive disorders in older primary care patients. *Journal of Clinical Psychiatry, 71,* 74–79.

Brenes, G. A., Williamson, J. D., Messier, S. P., Rejeski, W. J., Pahor, M., Ip, E., & Penninx, B. W. (2007) Treatment of minor depression in older adults: A pilot study comparing sertraline and exercise. *Aging and Mental Health, 11,* 61–68.

Broadhead, W. E., Blazer, D. G., George, L. K., & Tse, C. K. (1990). Depression, disability days, and days lost from work in a prospective epidemiologic survey. *Journal of the American Medical Association, 264,* 2524–2528.

California Health and Safety Code: Section 24178. 2003.

Chen, C. S., Chong, M. Y., & Tsang, H. Y. (2007). Clinically significant non-major depression in a community-dwelling elderly population: Epidemiological findings. *International Journal of Geriatric Psychiatry, 22,* 557–562.

Chochinov, H. M., Wilson, K. G., Enns, M., & Lander, S. (1994). Prevalence of depression in the terminally ill: Effects of diagnostic criteria and symptom threshold judgments. *American Journal of Psychiatry, 151,* 537–540.

Chopra, M. P., Zubritsky, C., Knott, K., Ten Have, T., Hadley, T., Coyne, J. C., & Oslin, D. W. (2005). Importance of subsyndromal symptoms of depression in elderly patients. *American Journal of Geriatric Psychiatry, 13,* 597–606.

Cohen, C. I., Abdallah, C. G., & Diwan, S. (2010). Suicide attempts and associated factors in older adults with schizophrenia. *Schizophrenia Research, 119,* 253–257.

Cohen, C. I., Goh, K. H., & Yaffee, R. A. (2009). Depression outcome among a biracial sample of depressed urban elders. *American Journal of Geriatric Psychiatry, 17,* 943–952.

Cole, M. G., McCusker, J., Ciampi, A., Windholz, S., Latimer, E., & Belzile, E. (2006). The prognosis of major and minor depression in older medical inpatients. *American Journal of Geriatric Psychiatry, 14,* 966–975.

Costa, A., Peppe, A., Carlesimo, G. A., Pasqualetti, P., & Caltagirone, C. (2006). Major and minor depression in Parkinson's disease: A neuropsychological investigation. *European Journal of Neurology, 13,* 972–980.

Creed, F., Morgan, R., Fiddler, M., Marshall, S., Guthrie, E., & House, A. (2002). Depression and anxiety impair health-related quality of life and are associated with increased costs in general medical inpatients. *Psychosomatics, 43,* 302–309.

Crum, R. M., Cooper-Patrick, L., & Ford, D. E. (1994). Depressive symptoms among general medical patients: Prevalence and one-year outcome. *Psychosomatic Medicine, 56,* 109–117.

Cui, X., Lyness, J. M., Tang, W., Tu, X., & Conwell, Y. (2008). Outcomes and predictors of late-life depression trajectories in older primary care patients. *American Journal of Geriatric Psychiatry* 16:406–415, 2008.

Cuijpers, P., Beekman, A., Smit, F., & Deeg, D. (2006). Predicting the onset of major depressive disorder and dysthymia in older adults with subthreshold depression: A community based study. *International Journal of Geriatric Psychiatry, 21,* 811–818.

Cuijpers, P., Smit, F., & van Straten, A. (2007). Psychological treatments of subthreshold depression: A meta-analytic review. *Acta Psychiatrica Scandinavica, 115,* 434–441.

Devanand, D. P., Jacobs, D. M., Tang, M. X., Del Castillo-Castaneda, C., Sano, M., Marder, K., ... Stern, Y. (1997). The course of psychopathologic features in mild to moderate Alzheimer disease. *Archives of General Psychiatry, 54,* 257–263.

Devanand, D. P., Nobler, M. S., Cheng, J., Turret, N., Pelton, G. H., Roose, S. P., & Sackeim, H. A. (2005). Randomized, double-blind, placebo-controlled trial of fluoxetine treatment for elderly patients with dysthymic disorder. *American Journal of Geriatric Psychiatry, 13,* 59–68.

Devanand, D. P., Pelton, G. H., Marston, K., Camacho, Y., Roose, S. P., Stern, Y., & Sackeim, H. A. (2003). Sertraline treatment of elderly patients with depression and cognitive impairment. *International Journal of Geriatric Psychiatry, 18,* 123–130.

Diwan, S., Cohen, C. I., Bankole, A. O., Vahai, I., Kehn, M., & Ramirez, P. M. (2007). Depression in older adults with schizophrenia spectrum disorders: Prevalence and associated factors. *American Journal of Geriatric Psychiatry, 15,* 991–998.

Drayer, R. A., Piraino, B., Reynolds, C. F., III, Houck, P. R., Mazumdar, S., Bernardini, J., ... Rollman, B. L. (2006). Characteristics of depression in hemodialysis patients: Symptoms, quality of life and mortality risk. *General Hospital Psychiatry, 28,* 306–312.

Eastwood, M. R., Rifat, S. L., Nobbs, H., & Ruderman, J. (1989). Mood disorder following cerebrovascular accident. *British Journal of Psychiatry, 154,* 195–200.

Freedland, K. E., Rich, M. W., Skala, J. A., Carney, R. M., Dávila-Román, V. G., & Jaffe, A. S. (2003). Prevalence of depression in hospitalized patients with congestive heart failure. *Psychosomatic Medicine, 65,* 119–128.

Freedland, K. E., Skala, J. A., Carney, R. M., Rubin, E. H., Lustman, P. J., Dávila-Román, V. G., ... Hogue, C. W., Jr. (2009). Treatment of depression after coronary artery bypass surgery: A randomized controlled trial. *Archives of General Psychiatry, 66,* 387–396.

Gabryelewicz, T., Styczynska, M., Pfeffer, A., Wasiak, B., Barczak, A., Luczywek, E., ... Barcikowska, M. (2004). Prevalence of major and minor depression in elderly persons with mild cognitive impairment—MADRS factor analysis. *International Journal of Geriatric Psychiatry, 19,* 1168–1172.

Geiselmann, B., Linden, M., & Helmchen, H. (2001). Psychiatrists' diagnoses of subthreshold depression in old age: Frequency and correlates. *Psychological Medicine, 31,* 51–63.

Gonda, X., Juhasz, G., Laszik, A., Rihmer, Z., & Bagdy, G. (2005). Subthreshold depression is linked to the functional polymorphism of the 5HT transporter gene. *Journal of Affective Disorders, 87*, 291–297.

Grabovish, A., Lu, N., Tang, W., Tu, X., & Lyness, J. M. (2010). Outcomes of subsyndromal depression in older primary care patients. *American Journal of Geriatric Psychiatry, 18*, 227–235.

Han, L., McCusker, J., Cole, M., Abrahamowicz, M., & Capek, R. (2008). 12-month cognitive outcomes of major and minor depression in older medical patients. *American Journal of Geriatric Psychiatry, 16*, 742–751.

Heun, R., Papassotiropoulos, A., & Ptok, U. (2000). Subthreshold depressive and anxiety disorders in the elderly. *European Psychiatry, 15*, 173–182.

Horowitz, A., Reinhardt, J. P., & Kennedy, G. J. (2005). Major and subthreshold depression among older adults seeking vision rehabilitation services. *American Journal of Geriatric Psychiatry, 13*, 180–187.

Hu, H., Pepper, L., & Goldman, R. (1991). Effect of repeated occupational exposure to lead, cessation of exposure, and chelation on levels of lead in bone. *American Journal of Industrial Medicine, 20*, 723–735.

Hybels, C. F., Pieper, C. F., & Blazer, D. G. (2009). The complex relationship between depressive symptoms and functional limitations in community-dwelling older adults: The impact of subthreshold depression. *Psychological Medicine, 9*, 1–12.

Jeste, D. V., Blazer, D. G., & First, M. (2005). Aging-related diagnostic variations: Need for diagnostic criteria appropriate for elderly psychiatric patients. *Biological Psychiatry, 58*, 265–271.

Jeste, D. V., Wolkowitz, O. M., & Palmer, B. W. (2011). Divergent trajectories of physical, cognitive and psychosocial aging in schizophrenia. *Schizophrenia Bulletin, 37*, 451–455.

Jeste, D. V., Alexopoulos, G. S., Bartels, S. J., Cummings, J. L., Gallo, J. J., Gottlieb, G. L.,...Lebowitz, B. D. (1999). Consensus statement on the upcoming crisis in geriatric mental health: Research agenda for the next two decades. *Archives of General Psychiatry, 56*, 848–853.

Jongenelis, K., Pot, A. M., Eisses, A. M., Beekman, A. T., Kluiter, H., & Ribbe, M. W. (2004). Prevalence and risk indicators of depression in elderly nursing home patients: The AGED study. *Journal of Affective Disorders, 83*, 135–142.

Judd, L. L., & Akiskal, H. S. (2002). The clinical and public health relevance of current research on subthreshold depressive symptoms to elderly patients. *American Journal of Geriatric Psychiatry, 10*, 233–238.

Judd, L. L., & Kunovac, J. L. (1998). Bipolar and unipolar depressive disorders in geriatric patients: Mental disorders in the elderly: New therapeutic approaches. *International Academy of Biomedical and Drug Research (Basel, Karger), 13*, 1–10.

Judd, L. L., Rapaport, M. H., Paulus, M. P., & Brown, J. L. (1994). Subsyndromal symptomatic depression: A new mood disorder? *Journal of Clinical Psychiatry, 55*(Suppl), 18–28.

Kasckow, J., Fellows, I., Golshan, S., Solorzano, E., Meeks, T., & Zisook, S. (2010). Treatment of subsyndromal depressive symptoms in middle-age and older patients with schizophrenia: Effect of age on response. *American Journal of Geriatric Psychiatry, 18*, 853–857.

Kasckow, J. W., Welge, J., Carroll, B. T., Thalassinos, A., & Mohamed, S. (2002). Citalopram treatment of minor depression in elderly men: An open pilot study. *American Journal of Geriatric Psychiatry, 10*, 344–347.

Katon, W., Fan, M. Y., Unützer, J., Taylor, J., Pincus, H., & Schoenbaum, M. (2008). Depression and diabetes: A potentially lethal combination. *Journal of General Internal Medicine, 23*, 1571–1575.

Kiosses, D. N., & Alexopoulos, G. S. (2012). The prognostic significance of subsyndromal symptoms emerging after remission of late-lifedepression. *Psychological Medicine*, May 21:1–10. (ePub ahead of print).

Klembara, J (2001). Postparietal and prehatching ontogeny of the supraoccipital in Alligator mississippiensis (Archosauria, Crocodylia). *Journal of Morphology, 249*, 147–153.

Kneale, G. W., Sorahan, T., & Stewart, A. M. (1991). Evidence of biased recording of radiation doses of Hanford workers. *American Journal of Industrial Medicine, 20*, 799–803.

Koenig, H. G. (1997). Differences in psychosocial and health correlates of major and minor depression in medically ill older adults. *Journal of the American Geriatrics Society, 45*, 1487–1495.

Koenig, H. G. (1998a). Depression in hospitalized older patients with congestive heart failure. *General Hospital Psychiatry, 20*, 29–43.

Koenig, H. G. (1998b). Depression in hospitalized older patients with congestive heart failure. *General Hospital Psychiatry, 20*, 29–43.

Koenig, H. G., Meador, K. G., Shelp, F., Goli, V., Cohen, H. J., & Blazer, D. G. (1991). Major depressive disorder in hospitalized medically ill patients: An examination of young and elderly male veterans. *Journal of the American Geriatrics Society, 39*, 881–890.

Koenig, H. G., Vandermeer, J., Chambers, A., Burr-Crutchfield, L., & Johnson, J. L. (2006a).

Comparison of major and minor depression in older medical inpatients with chronic heart and pulmonary disease. *Psychosomatics, 47,* 296–303.

Koenig, H. G., Vandermeer, J., Chambers, A., Burr-Crutchfield, L., & Johnson, J. L. (2006b). Minor depression and physical outcome trajectories in heart failure and pulmonary disease. *Journal of Nervous and Mental Disorders, 194,* 209–217.

Kvaal, K., McDougall, F. A., Brayne, C., Matthews, F. E., & Dewey, M. E. (2008). Co-occurrence of anxiety and depressive disorders in a community sample of older people: Results from the MRC CFAS (Medical Research Council Cognitive Function and Ageing Study). *International Journal of Geriatric Psychiatry, 23,* 229–237.

Li, Y. S., Meyer, J. S., & Thornby, J. (2001). Longitudinal follow-up of depressive symptoms among normal versus cognitively impaired elderly. *International Journal of Geriatric Psychiatry, 16,* 718–727.

Licht-Strunk, E., van der Kooij, K. G., van Schaik, D. J., van Marwijk, H. W., van Hout, H. P., de Haan, M., & Beekman, A. T. (2005). Prevalence of depression in older patients consulting their general practitioner in The Netherlands. *International Journal of Geriatric Psychiatry, 20,* 1013–1019.

Lin, E. H., Heckbert, S. R., Rutter, C. M., Katon, W. J., Ciechanowski, P., Ludman, E. J., ... Von Korff, M. (2009). Depression and increased mortality in diabetes: Unexpected causes of death. *Annals of Family Medicine, 7,* 414–421.

Lyketsos, C. G., Steele, C., Baker, L., Galik, E., Kopunek, S., Steinberg, M., & Warren, A. (1997). Major and minor depression in Alzheimer's disease: Prevalence and impact. *Journal of Neuropsychiatry and Clinical Neuroscience, 9,* 556–561.

Lynch, D. J., Tamburrino, M. B., & Nagel, R. (1997). Telephone counseling for patients with minor depression: Preliminary findings in a family practice setting. *Journal of Family Practice, 44,* 293–298.

Lyness, J. M., Caine, E. D., King, D. A., Conwell, Y., Duberstein, P. R., & Cox, C..(2002). Depressive disorders and symptoms in older primary care patients: One-year outcomes. *American Journal of Geriatric Psychiatry, 10,* 275–282.

Lyness, J. M., Chapman, B. P., McGriff, J., Drayer, R., & Duberstein, P. R. (2009). One-year outcomes of minor and subsyndromal depression in older primary care patients. *International Psychogeriatrics, 21,* 60–68.

Lyness, J. M., Heo, M., Datto, C. J., Ten Have, T. R., Katz, I. R., Drayer, R., ... Bruce, M. L. (2006).

Outcomes of minor and subsyndromal depression among elderly patients in primary care settings. *Annals of Internal Medicine, 144,* 496–504.

Lyness, J. M., Kim, J., Tang, W., Tu, X., Conwell, Y., King, D. A., & Caine, E. D. (2007). The clinical significance of subsyndromal depression in older primary care patients. *American Journal of Geriatric Psychiatry, 15,* 214–223.

Lyness, J. M., King, D. A., Cox, C., Yoediono, Z., & Caine, E. D. (1999). The importance of subsyndromal depression in older primary care patients: Prevalence and associated functional disability. *Journal of the American Geriatrics Society, 47,* 647–652.

Maletic, V., Robinson, M., & Oakes, T., (2007). Neurobiology of depression: An integrated view of key findings. *International Journal of Clinical Practice, 61,* 2030–2040.

McCollum, M., Ellis, S. L., Regensteiner, J. G., Zhang, W., & Sullivan, P. W. (2007). Minor depression and health status among US adults with diabetes mellitus. *American Journal of Managed Care, 13,* 65–72.

McCusker, J., Cole, M., Ciampi, A., Latimer, E., Windholz, S., Elie, M., & Belzile, E. (2007). Twelve-month course of depressive symptoms in older medical inpatients. *International Journal of Geriatric Psychiatry, 22,* 411–417.

McCusker, J., Cole, M., Dufouil, C., Dendukuri, N., Latimer, E., Windholz, S., & Elie, M. (2005). The prevalence and correlates of major and minor depression in older medical inpatients. *Journal of the American Geriatrics Society, 53,* 1344–1353.

Meeks, T. W., Vahia, I. V., Lavretsky, H., Kulkarni, G., & Jeste, D. V. (2011). A tune in "a minor" can "b major": A review of epidemiology, illness course, and public health implications of subthreshold depression in older adults. *Journal of Affective Disorders, 129,* 126–142.

Miranda, J., & Munoz, R. (1994). Intervention for minor depression in primary care patients. *Psychosomatic Medicine, 56,* 136–141.

Montross, L. P., Kasckow, J., Golshan, S., Solorzano, E., Lehman, D., & Zisook, S. (2008). Suicidal ideation and suicide attempts among middle-aged and older patients with schizophrenia spectrum disorders and concurrent subsyndromal depression. *Journal of Nervous and Mental Disorders, 196,* 884–890.

Morrow-Howell, N., Proctor, E., Choi, S., Lawrence, L., Brooks, A., Hasche, L., ... Blinne, W. (2008). Depression in public community long-term care: Implications for intervention development. *Journal of Behavioral Health Services and Research, 35,* 37–51.

Mossey, J. M., Knott, K. A., Higgins, M., & Talerico, K. (1996). Effectiveness of a psychosocial intervention, interpersonal counseling, for subdysthymic depression in medically ill elderly. *Journals of Gerontology Series A: Biological Sciences and Medical Sciences, 51,* M172-M178.

Østbye, T., Kristjansson, B., Hill, G., Newman, S. C., Brouwer, R. N., & McDowell, I. (2005). Prevalence and predictors of depression in elderly Canadians: The Canadian Study of Health and Aging. *Chronic Diseases in Canada, 26,* 93–99.

Oxman, T. E., & Sengupta, A. (2002). Treatment of minor depression. *American Journal of Geriatric Psychiatry, 10,* 256–264.

Paradiso, S., & Robinson, R. G. (1999). Minor depression after stroke: An initial validation of the DSM-IV construct. *American Journal of Geriatric Psychiatry, 7,* 244–251.

Parikh, R. M., Robinson, R. G., Lipsey, J. R., Starkstein, S. E., Federoff, J. P., & Price, T. R. (1990). The impact of poststroke depression on recovery in activities of daily living over a 2-year follow-up. *Archives of Neurology, 47,* 785–789.

Parmelee, P. A., Katz, I. R., & Lawton, M. P. (1992). Incidence of depression in long-term care settings. *Journal of Gerontology, 47,* M189-M196.

Paykel, E. S., Freeling, P., & Hollyman, J. A. (1988). Are tricyclic antidepressants useful for mild depression? A placebo controlled trial. *Pharmacopsychiatry, 21,* 15–18.

Penninx, B. W., Guralnik, J. M., Ferrucci, L., Simonsick, E. M., Deeg, D. J., & Wallace, R. B. (1998). Depressive symptoms and physical decline in community-dwelling older persons. *Journal of the American Medical Association, 279,* 1720–1726.

Penninx, B. W. J., Beekman, A. T. F., Honig, A., Deeg, D. J., Schoevers, R. A., van Eijk, J. T., & van Tilburg, W. (2001). Depression and cardiac mortality. *Archives of General Psychiatry, 58,* 221–227.

Rafanelli, C., Roncuzzi, R., & Milaneschi, Y. (2006). Minor depression as a cardiac risk factor after coronary artery bypass surgery. *Psychosomatics, 47,* 289–295.

Remick, R. A., Sadovnick, A. D., Lam, R. W., Zis, A. P., & Yee, I. M. (1996). Major depression, minor depression, and double depression: Are they distinct clinical entities? *American Journal of Medical Genetics, 67,* 347–353.

Robinson, R. G., Jorge, R. E., Moser, D. J., Acion, L., Solodkin, A., Small, S. L., ... Arndt, S. (2008). Escitalopram and problem-solving therapy for prevention of poststroke depression: A randomized controlled trial. *Journal of the American Medical Association, 299,* 2391–2400.

Rocca, P., Calvarese, P., Faggiano, F., Marchiaro, L., Mathis, F., Rivoira, E., ... Bogetto, F. (2005). Citalopram versus sertraline in late-life nonmajor clinically significant depression: A 1-year follow-up clinical trial. *Journal of Clinical Psychiatry, 66,* 360–369.

Romanelli, J., Fauerbach, J. A., Bush, D. E., & Ziegelstein, R. C. (2002). The significance of depression in older patients after myocardial infarction. *Journal of the American Geriatrics Society, 50,* 817–822.

Romeo, R., Knapp, M., Banerjee, S., Morris, J., Baldwin, R., Tarrier, N., ... Burns, A. (2011). Treatment and prevention of depression after surgery for hip fracture in older people: Cost-effectiveness analysis. *Journal of Affective Disorders, 128,* 211–219.

Rosenberg, P. B., Drye, L. T., Martin, B. K., Frangakis, C., Mintzer, J. E., Weintraub, D., ... DIADS-2 Research Group. (2010). Sertraline for the treatment of depression in Alzheimer disease. *American Journal of Geriatric Psychiatry, 18,* 136–145.

Rovner, B. W., & Casten, R. J. (2008). Preventing late-life depression in age-related macular degeneration. *American Journal of Geriatric Psychiatry, 16,* 454–459.

Rovner, B. W., Casten, R. J., Hegel, M. T., Leiby, B. E., & Tasman, W. S. (2007). Preventing depression in age-related macular degeneration. *Archives of General Psychiatry, 64,* 886–892.

Saxena, S. K., Ng, T. P., Koh, G., Yong, D., & Fong, N. P. (2007). Is improvement in impaired cognition and depressive symptoms in post-stroke patients associated with recovery in activities of daily living? *Acta Neurologica Scandinavica, 115,* 339–346.

Saxena, S. K., Ng, T. P., Yong, D., Fong, N. P., & Koh, G. (2008). Subthreshold depression and cognitive impairment but not demented in stroke patients during their rehabilitation. *Acta Neurologica Scandinavica, 117,* 133–140.

Schleifer, S. J., Macari-Hinson, M. M., Coyle, D. A., Slater, W. R., Kahn, M., Gorlin, R., & Zucker, H. D. (1989). The nature and course of depression following myocardial infarction. *Archives of Internal Medicine, 149,* 1785–1789.

Schneider, G., Kruse, A., Nehen, H. G., Senf, W., & Heuft, G. (2000). The prevalence and differential diagnosis of subclinical depressive syndromes in inpatients 60 years and older. *Psychotherapy and Psychosomatics, 69,* 251–260.

Schoevers, R. A., Smit, F., Deeg, D. J., Cuijpers, P., Dekker, J., van Tilburg, W., & Beekman, A. T. (2006). Prevention of late-life depression in primary care: Do we know where to begin? *American Journal of Psychiatry, 163,* 1611–1621.

Singh, N. A., Clements, K. M., & Fiatarone, M. A. (1997). A randomized controlled trial of progressive resistance training in depressed elders. *Journals of Gerontology Series A: Biological Sciences and Medical Sciences, 52,* M27-M35.

Spitzer, R. L., Kroenke, K., Linzer, M., Hahn, S. R., Williams, J. B., deGruy, F. V., III, ... Davies, M. (1995). Health-related quality of life in primary care patients with mental disorders. Results from the PRIME-MD 1000 Study. *Journal of the American Medical Association, 274,* 1511–1517.

Sriwattanakomen, R., McPherron, J., Chatman, J., Morse, J. Q., Martire, L. M., Karp, J. F., ... Reynolds, C. F., III. (2010). A comparison of the frequencies of risk factors for depression in older black and white participants in a study of indicated prevention. *International Psychogeriatrics, 22,* 1240–1247.

Starkstein, S. E., Jorge, R., Mizrahi, R., & Robinson, R. G. (2005). The construct of minor and major depression in Alzheimer's disease. *American Journal of Psychiatry, 162,* 2086–2093.

Starkstein, S. E., Merello, M., Jorge, R., Brockman, S., Bruce, D., Petracca, G., & Robinson, R. G. (2008). A validation study of depressive syndromes in Parkinson's disease. *Movement Disorders, 23,* 538–546.

Tandberg, E., Larsen, J. P., Aarsland, D., & Cummings, J. L. (1996). The occurrence of depression in Parkinson's disease. A community-based study. *Archives of Neurology, 53,* 175–179.

Teresi, J., Abrams, R., Holmes, D., Ramirez, M., & Eimicke, J. (2001). Prevalence of depression and depression recognition in nursing homes. *Social Psychiatry and Psychiatric Epidemiology, 36,* 613–620.

Uekermann, J., Daum, I., Peters, S., Wiebel, B., Przuntek, H., & Müller, T. (2003). Depressed mood and executive dysfunction in early Parkinson's disease. *Acta Neurologica Scandinavica, 107,* 341–348.

Vahia, I. V., Meeks, T. W., Thompson, W. K., Depp, C. A., Zisook, S., Allison, M., ... Jeste, D. V. (2010). Subthreshold depression and successful aging in older women. *American Journal of Geriatric Psychiatry, 18,* 212–220.

Viinamaki, H., Niskanen, L., & Uusitupa, M. (1995). Mental well-being in people with non-insulin-dependent diabetes. *Acta Psychiatrica Scandinavica, 92,* 392–397.

Vuorilehto, M. S., Melartin, T. K., & Isometsä, E. T. (2009). Course and outcome of depressive disorders in primary care: A prospective 18-month study. *Psychological Medicine, 39,* 1697–1707.

Waern, M., Rubenowitz, E., & Wilhelmson, K. (2003). Predictors of suicide in the old elderly. *Gerontology, 49,* 328–334.

Wells, K. B., Burnam, M. A., Rogers, W., Hays, R., & Camp, P. (1992). The course of depression in adult outpatients. Results from the Medical Outcomes Study. *Archives of General Psychiatry, 49,* 788–794.

Wells, K. B., Stewart, A., Hays, R. D., Burnam, M. A., Rogers, W., Daniels, M., ... Ware, J. (1989). The functioning and well-being of depressed patients. Results from the Medical Outcomes Study. *Journal of the American Medical Association, 262,* 914–919.

Whang, W., Kubzansky, L. D., Kawachi, I., Rexrode, K. M., Kroenke, C. H., Glynn, R. J., ... Albert, C. M. (2009). Depression and risk of sudden cardiac death and coronary heart disease in women: Results from the Nurses' Health Study. *Journal of the American College of Cardiology, 53,* 950–958.

Wiktorsson, S., Runeson, B., Skoog, I., Ostling, S., & Waern, M. (2010). Attempted suicide in the elderly: Characteristics of suicide attempters 70 years and older and a general population comparison group. *American Journal of Geriatric Psychiatry, 18,* 57–67.

Williams, J. W., Jr., Barrett, J., Oxman, T., Frank, E., Katon, W., Sullivan, M., ... Sengupta, A. (2000). Treatment of dysthymia and minor depression in primary care: A randomized controlled trial in older adults. *Journal of the American Medical Association, 284,* 1519–1526.

Williams, J. W., Jr., Kerber, C. A., Mulrow, C. D., Medina, A., & Aguilar, C. (1995). Depressive disorders in primary care: Prevalence, functional disability, and identification. *Journal of General Internal Medicine, 10,* 7–12.

Xavier, F. M., Ferraza, M. P., Argimon, I., Trentini, C. M., Poyares, D., Bertollucci, P. H., ... Moriguchi, E. H. (2002). The DSM-IV 'minor depression' disorder in the oldest-old: Prevalence rate, sleep patterns, memory function and quality of life in elderly people of Italian descent in Southern Brazil. *International Journal of Geriatric Psychiatry, 17,* 107–116.

Yohannes, A. M., Baldwin, R. C., & Connolly, M. J. (2003). Prevalence of sub-threshold depression in elderly patients with chronic obstructive pulmonary disease. *International Journal of Geriatric Psychiatry, 18,* 412–416.

Zisook, S., Montross, L., Kasckow, J., Mohamed, S., Palmer, B. W., Patterson, T. L., ... Solorzano, E. (2007). Subsyndromal depressive symptoms in middle-aged and older persons with schizophrenia. *American Journal of Geriatric Psychiatry, 15,* 1005–1014.

Zisook, S., Paulus, M., Shuchter, S. R., & Judd, L. L. (1997). The many faces of depression following spousal bereavement. *Journal of Affective Disorders, 45,* 85–94.

9

ANXIOUS DEPRESSION

APPLICATION OF A UNIFIED MODEL OF EMOTIONAL DISORDERS TO OLDER ADULTS

Andrew J. Petkus, Eric J. Lenze, and Julie Loebach Wetherell

Mood and anxiety disorders are two of the most common psychiatric disorders in later life. These disorders commonly co-occur, with the majority of depressed older adults also experiencing significant symptoms of anxiety (Kvaal, McDougall, Brayne, Matthews, & Dewey, 2008). Depression with anxiety is important as it has been associated with a number of adverse outcomes, including higher rates of suicide (Bartels et al., 2002), somatic complaints (Lenze et al., 2000), and functional impairment (Brenes et al., 2008). Largely due to the current classification system of psychiatric disorders, research with depressed and anxious older adults has treated these disorders as if they were separate and distinct. Theories of the etiology, presentation, and pharmacological treatment of depression and anxiety, however, suggest that these disorders may be more similar than different. These models posit that depression and anxiety may be different manifestations of a broader underlying affective disturbance that is central to both.

This chapter will review the literature examining the co-occurrence of depression and anxiety later in life. The prevalence of these problems along with the negative outcomes associated with anxious depression will be examined. Current explanations and biological evidence for comorbidity will be presented. Theories that conceptualize depression and anxiety as emotional disorders characterized by disrupted emotional experience and regulation that have been largely developed with younger adults will be applied to older adults. Lastly, newly developed etiological models and transdiagnostic psychotherapy treatment recommendations for depression and anxiety disorders will be reviewed and applied to older adults.

PREVALENCE AND NEGATIVE OUTCOMES OF DEPRESSION WITH ANXIETY

Research with younger adults suggests that anxiety symptoms as well as anxiety disorders commonly co-occur with mood disorders (Kessler, Berglund, et al., 2005; Kessler, Chiu, Demler, Merikangas, & Walters, 2005). These studies suggest that as many as 63% of adults with major depressive disorder (MDD) also meet criteria for a current anxiety disorder. In one study, 42% of individuals with MDD or dysthymia reported social phobia and 18% reported panic disorder (Brown, Campbell, Lehman, Grisham, & Mancill, 2001). The diagnostic criteria for generalized anxiety disorder (GAD) includes a hierarchy rule in which a diagnosis of GAD cannot be made if the anxiety symptoms do not occur outside of a major depressive episode. In one study, using this rule, only 5% of participants with current MDD also met criteria for GAD (Brown, Di Nardo, Lehman, & Campbell, 2001). If this rule was not applied, however, 72% of those with MDD had co-occurring GAD. When examining lifetime diagnoses, rates of comorbidity are even higher. Of those with current MDD or dysthymia, 71% of individuals in one sample had met criteria for an anxiety disorder at some point in their lives.

Similar rates of comorbidity have also been reported in older adults, although most of the epidemiological studies have been limited to Canadian or European samples. Of adults aged 55–85 years from the Longitudinal Aging Study Amsterdam, 47.5% of adults with MDD met criteria for a co-occurring anxiety disorder in the past 6 months (Beekman et al., 2000). Research with 1,873 older adults in France found that 22.4% of those with current MDD also met criteria for current GAD, whereas 34.5% met criteria for a specific phobia (Ritchie et al., 2004). Similar rates have been found in epidemiological studies of adults aged 55 and older in Canada, with 23.0% of adults with MDD also meeting criteria for social phobia, agoraphobia, or panic disorder (Cairney, Corna, Veldhuizen, Herrmann, & Streiner, 2008). Research from the National Comorbidity Survey-Replication in the United States examined current and lifetime comorbidity of anxiety with depression (King-Kallimanis, Gum, & Kohn, 2009). Using 12-month prevalence rates, they found that 51.8% of older adults with MDD also met criteria for an anxiety disorder. Similarly, approximately half (48.4%) of those with a diagnosis of MDD at some point in their lives also met criteria for a lifetime anxiety disorder. This investigation also examined differences in rates of comorbidity between those aged 65 and older and those aged 18–64. They found that rates of comorbidity were consistent across the life span, with little differences between younger and older adults.

The prevalence of anxious depression (significant anxiety symptoms co-occurring with symptoms of depression) in older adulthood is even higher. Research suggests that as many as 60.1% of older adults with depression also experience significant symptoms of anxiety (Kvaal et al., 2008). Taken together, these findings suggest that the majority of depressed older adult patients also will present with significant anxiety.

In addition to being common, anxious depression has been associated with a number of adverse outcomes in later life. Older adults with comorbid anxiety and depression exhibit more somatic symptoms and greater health care utilization (Lenze et al., 2000; Vasiliadis et al., 2012). Additionally, adults with anxious depression have higher rates of suicidal ideation (Bartels et al., 2002) as well as completed suicide (Allgulander & Lavori, 1993). These older adults also tend to be in poorer physical health (Lenze et al., 2001) and be more disabled than those without depression or anxiety (Brenes et al., 2008; Lenze, 2003). Comorbid GAD and depression was associated with worse social functioning and greater disability after experiencing a stroke (Schultz, Castillo, Kosier, & Robinson, 1997; Shimoda & Robinson, 1998). Depression with anxiety is associated with poorer treatment outcome for late-life depression (Andreescu et al., 2007; Andreescu, Lenze, et al., 2009; Dombrovski et al., 2007; Greenlee et al., 2010; Saghafi et al., 2007). In an open-label trial of escitalopram for MDD in adults aged 60 and over, higher levels of anxiety at baseline were associated with lower rates of response to treatment after 6 weeks (Saghafi et al., 2007). Following this 6-week open-label trial, individuals who partially responded to the escitalopram remained on the drug for 16 weeks and were randomized to receive depression care management or interpersonal psychotherapy (Greenlee et al., 2010). This study found that adults with more severe symptoms of anxiety following the 6-week open-label phase were less likely to respond and took longer to remit. Symptoms of worry rather than physiological symptoms may be more highly associated with longer response and earlier relapse (Andreescu, Lenze, et al., 2009).

Less research has examined the long-term outcomes of anxious depression with older adults in the realm of cognitive functioning. Research has documented that late-life depression is highly associated with deficits in cognitive functioning, particularly in the domains of executive functioning (Kindermann,

Kalayam, Brown, Burdick, & Alexopoulos, 2000), attention (Lockwood, Alexopoulos, Kakuma, & Van Gorp, 2000), and working memory (Nebes et al., 2000). Anxiety has been associated with similar declines in cognitive performance in older adulthood, particularly in the domains of executive functioning, working memory, and processing speed (Beaudreau & O'Hara, 2008). Little research, however, has examined the impact of comorbid depression and anxiety on cognitive functioning. One study followed 79 older adults with lifetime MDD alone and those with MDD and history of panic disorder or GAD over a span of 4 years (DeLuca et al., 2005). This study found that the older adults with history of co-occurring anxiety disorders exhibited greater decline in memory than those individuals who were only depressed.

In summary, epidemiological studies suggest that the majority of depressed older adults also suffer from significant symptoms of anxiety. Additionally, older adults with anxious depression tend to have greater symptom severity, higher risk of suicide, more severe somatic symptoms, and greater disability and functional impairment.

EXPLANATIONS OF CO-OCCURRENCE

There are a number of potential explanations for the co-occurrence of anxiety and depression later in life. According to the *Diagnostic and Statistical Manual of Mental Disorders* (*DSM-IV*), symptoms of MDD overlap considerably with symptoms of several anxiety disorders, particularly GAD (American Psychiatric Association, 1994). Symptoms that are characteristic of both disorders include sleep disturbance, difficulty concentrating, fatigue, and psychomotor agitation. Older adults typically have longer histories of psychiatric illness than do younger adults, and as a result, disentangling the temporal precedence of anxiety and depression may be difficult when diagnosing GAD (Wetherell, Ruberg, & Petkus, 2010). Additionally, many older adults have difficulty identifying mental health problems (Gum et al., 2009) and symptoms (Wetherell, Petkus, et al., 2009a). All of these factors contribute to the challenge of making accurate diagnoses with older adults who report symptoms of both depression and anxiety.

Another explanation for the high rates of comorbidity is that these are not separate disorders; rather,

mood and anxiety disorders are different manifestations of the same underlying emotional dysfunction. This broad category has been labeled by some as "general neurotic syndrome" (Andrews, 1990) or "negative affect syndrome" (Barlow, Allen, & Choate, 2004). Research on the nature and presentation of depression and anxiety suggests that these disorders may be more alike than different. Similar biological processes have been implicated in both depression and anxiety. Additionally, although treatment may not work as quickly for older adults with anxious depression, treatment designed to alleviate depression also tends to alleviate symptoms of anxiety and vice versa.

Studies investigating the physiology of mood and anxiety disorders suggest that similar biological processes occur in both disorders. First, both depression and anxiety may have similar genetic vulnerability. Studies have shown that the short form of the serotonin transporter gene (5-HTTLPR) may be implicated as a vulnerability factor for late-life depression and anxiety (Gerretsen & Pollock, 2008; E. J. Lenze et al., 2005, 2010). Additionally, dysfunction in the hypothalamic-pituitary-adrenal (HPA) axis has been implicated in both mood and anxiety disorders. Under conditions of stress, the hormone cortisol is released by the adrenal cortex of the kidneys; it flows throughout the bloodstream and is eventually terminated via a negative feedback loop (Bremner, 2006). Older adults with anxiety and mood disorders typically have hyperactive HPA activation and higher cortisol levels under stress (E. J. Lenze et al., 2011; Penninx et al., 2007).

In addition to similar genetic and endocrine pathways, mood and anxiety disorders may share similar neurobiology (Ressler & Mayberg, 2007). Both depression and anxiety are associated with disruptions to limbic and cortical brain circuits that are responsible for emotional regulation and stress responsiveness. Disruptions to the serotonin and noradrenergic systems have also been associated with emotional disorders (Ressler & Nemeroff, 2000). Specifically, in anxiety and depression the noradrenergic (excitatory) system appears overactivated, whereas the serotonin system has decreased activation. These pathways interact with each other, such that under stress, norepinephrine (NE) neurons from the locus coeruleus (LC) activate the amygdala. Normally, 5-HT neurons from the raphe nuclei (RN) project to the amygdala to balance and modulate amygdala activation. The amygdala has important connections to the prefrontal cortex; in particular, it has inhibitory connections to the dorsal prefrontal cortex and excitatory connections to the orbital prefrontal cortex, which are associated with inhibition of fear and tolerance of adverse events. Under normal mood, amygdala activation is modulated by both excitatory NE and inhibitory 5-HT, resulting in normal activation in the dorsal and orbital prefrontal cortices.

Similar to the amygdala, NE neurons from the LC also activate the hippocampus under stress. The hippocampus plays an important role in learning, and this structure is hypothesized to be activated under stress in order to increase learning of aversive stimuli. With normal mood, inhibitory 5-HT neurons from the RN play a role in decreasing this learning of aversive material. Under normal mood states, the NE and 5-HT systems interact to balance each other.

Research has suggested that the NE and 5-HT functional pathways may be disrupted in individuals with depression and/or anxiety disorders. Ressler and Nemeroff (2000) suggest that depression and anxiety are associated with hyper-response to stress, whereas the 5-HT system is hypo-responsive to stress. As a result, under stress, the limbic system experiences increased activation and decreased inhibition. Increased NE release, in combination with decreased 5-HT inhibition to the amygdala, results in overall increased amygdala activation. This increased activation of the amygdala activates the hypothalamus, resulting in increased corticotrophin-releasing factor and eventually corticosteroid release. Additionally, increased amygdala activation results in increased inhibition of the dorsal and orbital prefrontal cortex. The inhibition of the prefrontal cortex results in decreased attention, concentration, problem solving, and inhibition of aversive emotions characteristic of both anxiety and depressive disorders. Additionally, the inhibition of prefrontal cortex results in increased inhibition of RN and 5-HT release. Increased NE from the LC also activates the hippocampus, which results in increased rate of memory formation. Therefore, individuals are more likely to learn that the stimulus in the environment should be feared. As a result, individuals with depression or anxiety may be more likely to avoid these stressful stimuli. Additionally, the deregulation of the NA and 5-HT systems is thought to disrupt sleep, approach behaviors, concentration, and energy (causing fatigue), which are common symptoms of depressive and anxiety disorders.

The neurobiology of anxiety and depression also provides evidence that individuals with depression or anxiety may have altered brain structures, particularly in the limbic and prefrontal cortex. The anterior cingulate is an important area associated with the modulation of emotional behavior and fear learning (Drevets, Savitz, & Trimble, 2008). Research has suggested that reduced gray matter in the anterior cingulate may be present in individuals with major depression (Drevets, Price, & Furey, 2008), posttraumatic stress disorder (Corbo, Clement, Armony, Pruessner, & Brunet, 2005), panic disorder (Massana et al., 2003), and obsessive-compulsive disorder (Radua, van den Heuvel, Surguladze, & Mataix-Cols, 2010). Structural changes in the amygdala also appear to be common between anxiety and depressive disorders as studies have found either disrupted amygdala volume in depression (Drevets, Price, et al., 2008), posttraumatic stress disorder (Wignall et al., 2004), panic disorder (Massana et al., 2003), GAD (Schienle, Ebner, & Schafer, 2011), and obsessive-compulsive disorder (Radua, Via, Catani, & Mataix-Cols, 2011).

Research with depressed older adults has found similar patterns of activity in the amygdala and prefrontal cortex as have been found with younger adults (Aizenstein et al., 2005; Alexopoulos et al., 2007; Murphy et al., 2007). Less research has been conducted to investigate the neurobiology of late-life anxiety. One study found that adults with comorbid anxiety and depression had different patterns of activation in the anterior and posterior cingulate when compared with older adults with depression alone (Andreescu, Butters, et al., 2009). Although studies with younger adults suggest that the physiology of depression and anxiety are similar, given age-related physiological changes in the brain, more research is needed to examine the physiology of anxiety and anxious depression in older adults.

Chronically elevated cortisol levels via the overactivation of the HPA axis may be one mechanism causing changes in brain structures. Elevated cortisol levels have been shown to damage the hippocampus (Lupien et al., 1998), which in turn may explain deficits in learning and memory. The prefrontal cortex may also be vulnerable to damage from cortisol as documented by recent research. Data from the Vietnam Twin Study of Aging found that elevated cortisol was associated with damage to the frontal cortex and not the hippocampus (Kremen et al., 2010). Elevated cortisol was associated with worse visuospatial ability, abstract reasoning, processing speed, and executive functioning. Furthermore, those with higher cortisol levels had significantly thinner prefrontal cortices (Kremen et al., 2010).

Interventions research, both psychopharmacological and psychosocial, provides evidence that depression and anxiety are alike. Typically when depression is treated, anxiety symptoms also improve. Selective serotonin reuptake inhibitor (SSRI) medication is an effective pharmacological treatment for late-life MDD (Alexopoulos et al., 2001, 2005; Unutzer, et al., 2002) and GAD (Lenze et al., 2009; Wetherell, Stoddard, et al., 2010). Research examining the effects of psychosocial treatments for depression such as cognitive-behavioral therapy (CBT) commonly reports that treatment also decreases anxiety symptoms in addition to the targeted depressive symptoms. In younger adults, CBT for anxiety also alleviates symptoms of depression. Although CBT for late-life anxiety may be less effective in older adults (Wetherell, Ruberg, et al., 2010; Wolitzky-Taylor, Castriotta, Lenze, Stanley, & Craske, 2010), studies show that depressive symptoms tend to decrease along with anxiety symptoms (Stanley et al., 2003, 2009; Wetherell et al., 2011; Wetherell, Ayers, et al., 2009; Wetherell, Gatz, & Craske, 2003). It is unclear whether psychosocial treatment for late-life depression also improves symptoms of anxiety later in life. Unfortunately, most studies investigating psychosocial treatments, such as problem-solving therapy, for late-life mood disorders do not assess or report the effect of treatment on symptoms of anxiety (Alexopoulos, Raue, & Arean, 2003; Arean, Hegel, Vannoy, Fan, & Unutzer, 2008; Arean et al., 1993, 2010). Two studies that did assess for anxiety found that problem-solving therapy for late-life depression in older home care patients with cardiovascular disease (Gellis & Bruce, 2010), and CBT for depressed primary care patients (Serfaty et al., 2009), did not improve symptoms of anxiety, consistent with other evidence that anxiety symptoms are resistant to treatment.

One explanation for the finding that psychotherapy for depression tends to alleviate symptoms of anxiety and vice versa is that skills learned in the context of one problem may generalize to solving other problems. An alternative explanation is that successful treatment targets two general factors, negative affect and maladaptive emotional regulation, which are common to both depression and anxiety (Aldao & Nolen-Hoeksema, 2010; Brown & Barlow, 2009).

DEPRESSION AND ANXIETY AS MALADAPTIVE EMOTIONAL EXPERIENCE AND EMOTION DYSREGULATION

Depression and anxiety are emotional disorders characterized by increased experience of negative emotions, and in some cases decreased experience of positive emotions. The tripartite model of depression and anxiety was an early approach to such a conceptualization (Clark & Watson, 1991). This model posits that three broad factors are characteristic of mood and anxiety disorders: negative affect (NA), positive affect (PA), and autonomic arousal (AA). In this conceptualization, NA is a higher order factor common to both depression and anxiety. Depression is characterized by high NA, low PA, and normal AA, whereas anxiety is characterized by high NA, normal PA, and high AA.

Recent modifications to this model (Mineka, Watson, & Clark, 1998) suggest that high AA may not discriminate anxiety and depression as originally posited. AA may be more indicative of panic disorder while not being associated with other DSM-IV diagnoses. Research has largely supported this model. Using structural equation modeling, Brown, Chorpita, and Barlow (1998) tested the tripartite model with younger treatment-seeking outpatients with mood and anxiety disorders. These authors found that NA was strongly associated with depression, GAD, panic/agoraphobia, obsessive-compulsive disorder, and social phobia. Additionally, lower levels of PA were associated with depression and social phobia. AA was highly associated with NA and with panic disorder, whereas it was not associated with depression or other anxiety disorders.

The tripartite model of anxiety and depression appears to be valid across the life span. Cook et al. (2004) found a good fit for this model with older adult psychiatric outpatients. This study also found that high NA was associated with depression and anxiety, whereas low PA was uniquely associated with depression. Additionally, although including an AA factor in the model improved model fit, consistent with research in younger adults (Brown et al., 1998), it was mainly associated with panic disorder. In another investigation, Teachman,

Siedlecki, and Magee (2007) compared the tripartite model across younger, middle-aged, and older community-dwelling adults and found a good fit for all three age groups. Importantly, no differences in overall model fit or individual pathways between constructs were found between groups, suggesting that this model is stable across the life span. In summary, the structure of depression and anxiety can be characterized by one overarching factor, mainly high NA. Low PA is implicated in depression but not in anxiety. This model has validity across adulthood into older adulthood.

In addition to experiencing alterations in negative and positive emotions, individuals with emotional disorders may have problems regulating these emotions (Hofmann, Sawyer, Fang, & Asnaani, 2012). Emotional regulation is the conscious and unconscious processes by which individuals attempt to control their affective experience (Aldao, Nolen-Hoeksema, & Schweizer, 2010). Research has implicated poor emotional regulation in MDD (Nolen-Hoeksema, 2000) and anxiety disorders (Mennin, Holaway, Fresco, Moore, & Heimberg, 2007). Individuals suffering from emotional disorders may be less likely to use adaptive regulation strategies such as positive appraisal, while utilizing more maladaptive strategies such as thought suppression and avoidance (for review, see Aldao et al., 2010).

Positive reappraisal is a form of adaptive emotion regulation that entails viewing stressful situations as positive or neutral. Reappraising situations as positive has been associated with lower rates of psychopathology, including depression and anxiety (Aldao et al., 2010). Conversely, both depressive and anxiety disorders are associated with negative appraisals of situations. Depressed and/or anxious individuals with emotional disorders commonly interpret events as negative and uncontrollable (Allen, McHugh, & Barlow, 2008; Britton, Lissek, Grillon, Norcross, & Pine, 2011). In addition to viewing situations as out of their control, two fundamental misappraisals are common to both depression and anxiety: (1) overestimating the probability of negative events happening, and (2) catastrophizing the negative consequences of the negative event if it were to occur. Thus, anxious and depressed individuals, when faced with a stressful situation, will be more likely to believe that the worst outcome will occur and that this outcome will be disastrous.

Older adults have often been shown to exhibit what has been called a "positivity bias," in which positive appraisal is more common than earlier in life (Charles & Carstensen, 2010). Older adults are more likely to interpret stimuli as positive and to remember positive rather than negative events. This positivity bias may explain why rates of both depression and anxiety decrease in older adulthood. Despite this general bias toward positive information in normal aging, negative appraisals are still associated with late-life depression and anxiety. Depressed and anxious older adults are more likely to view stressful situations as out of their control, overestimate the probability that negative things will happen, and see negative events as their fault. Additionally, biases toward negative stimuli may be associated with increased anxiety (Lee & Knight, 2009) and poorer response to SSRI treatment in older GAD patients (Steiner, Petkus, Nguyen, & Wetherell, in press).

Maladaptive emotion regulation strategies in response to stress, such as thought suppression, have been implicated in both depression and anxiety (Aldao & Nolen-Hoeksema, 2010). Thought suppression has been repeatedly shown to be a maladaptive coping strategy that paradoxically results in increases in the frequency and duration of unwanted thoughts. Briefly, when trying to suppress unwanted thoughts, two processes occur: (1) a search for distracters to focus on to divert attention away from the target, and (2) a process which monitors the suppressed thought/emotion to see whether the first process was successful. This typically results in what is call a "rebound effect" in which the target thought or emotion is commonly experienced with greater severity and frequency (Wegner & Zanakos, 1994). This in turn may result in increased distress and more utilization of suppression, creating a vicious cycle of distress for the individual (Lynch, Cheavens, Morse, & Rosenthal, 2004).

The association between thought suppression and adverse outcomes persists into older adulthood. Thought suppression has been associated with decreased meaning in life in community-dwelling older adults (Krause, 2007), suicidal ideation in depressed older adults with personality disorders (Cukrowicz, Ekblad, Cheavens, Rosenthal, & Lynch, 2008), and poorer outcomes following depression treatment (Rosenthal, Cheavens, Compton, Thorp, & Lynch, 2005). In a cross-sectional investigation with homebound older adults, increased use of thought suppression was associated with depressive and anxiety symptoms and disorders (Petkus, Gum, & Wetherell, 2012). Another investigation found that in older survivors of trauma, avoidance of trauma-related thoughts and situations was associated with greater depressive and anxiety symptoms (Dulin & Passmore, 2010).

Using avoidance to down-regulate emotions is another maladaptive emotional regulation strategy central to depression and anxiety. Avoidance can be manifested in a number of ways: cognitive, behavioral, and the use of "safety signals." Cognitive avoidance is diverting one's attention in order to dampen unpleasant thoughts or emotions. Behavioral avoidance involves escaping or evading situations that elicit a strong emotional response.

Cognitive avoidance is more challenging to observe and measure than behavioral avoidance or the use of safety signals. One form of cognitive avoidance is rumination, a process in which the individual persistently, repetitively, and passively focuses on the consequences and occurrence of emotions and symptoms (Stroebe et al., 2007). The focus of attention during rumination is typically past events, such as the causes of current negative emotions. Rumination is most characteristic of depression (Allen et al., 2008). It is considered a form of cognitive avoidance because it allows the individual to disengage from the current environment (Moulds, Kandris, Starr, & Wong, 2007). Attempts at adaptive problem solving can increase distress, at least temporarily; rumination is an alternative behavior that can appear constructive (e.g., "If only I could understand why I am feeling so depressed, I would feel better") while allowing the individual to avoid confronting the stressful situation and resulting negative emotions. Additionally, sharing ruminative thoughts may increase sympathy and support from others, thus positively reinforcing the behavior.

Worry is a cognitive avoidance strategy most characteristic of anxiety, especially GAD (Borkovec, Alcaine, & Behar, 2004; Borkovec, Hazlett-Stevens, & Diaz, 1999). Whereas rumination is a process in which attention is focused on the past, worry is a process in which attention is fixed on threatening things that may happen in the future. Theories of worry have posited that worry may be a form of cognitive avoidance in a number of ways. First, the avoidance model of worry suggests that worry is a verbal process which decreases autonomic arousal and the extinction of the anxious response (Borkovec et al., 2004). Thus, focusing on the future prevents the individual from experiencing negative emotions in the present as well as allows the individual to feel more prepared for negative consequences if they were to occur. Additionally, when an undesirable event occurs, worry enables the individual to avoid unwanted emotions in the present by focusing on negative events that may happen in the future (Borkovec et al., 1999). Research does not fully support this theory, however, in that worry tends to lead to sustained emotional response. These mixed findings have led to the development of different models of characterizing worry as avoidance, such as the avoidance of negative emotion contrast model (Newman & Llera, 2011). This theory posits that worry allows for prolonged activation of negative emotional states in order to avoid the unpleasantness of shifting from a positive emotional state to a negative emotional state. More research needs to be done to validate this theory; however, taken together, these theories of worry suggest that the function of worry most likely is related to cognitive avoidance of distressing emotions.

An extensive literature documents that rumination and worry are highly correlated forms of negative repetitive thinking, although some studies find them differentiable by factor analysis or by their effects on other variables (de Jong-Meyer, Beck, & Riede, 2009; Ehring & Watkins, 2008; Heimberg, Fresco, Frankel, Mennin, & Turk, 2002; Kim, Yook, Suh, & Lee, 2010; Muris, Roelofs, Rassin, Franken, & Mayer, 2005; Roberts & Calmes, 2007; Segerstrom, Stanton, Alden, & Shortridge, 2003; Segerstrom, Tsao, Alden, & Craske, 2000; Watkins, Moulds, & Mackintosh, 2005). Other anxiety disorders are also characterized by forms of cognitive avoidance (Allen et al., 2008). For example, individuals with social phobia may engage in cognitive avoidance by "tuning out" or disengaging during conversations with others as a way to regulate unpleasant emotions arising during social interactions.

Like cognitive avoidance, behavioral avoidance is also common in depression and anxiety. Distressed individuals avoid situations associated with increases in negative emotions. Depression is characterized by anhedonia and withdrawal from social and other activities. Under stress or following changes in life circumstances, activities and social situations that were once pleasurable may instead elicit negative emotions, resulting in avoidance. This may be particularly true for older adults. Depressed older adults are more likely to present with what has been called "depression without sadness," chiefly characterized by anhedonia rather than depressed mood (Gallo & Rabins, 1999). According to a behavioral avoidance model of depression, due to age-related changes (i.e., decline in physical and cognitive abilities, death of loved ones, changing roles), formerly enjoyed activities may begin to evoke negative emotion. For example, gardening may once have been an important source of pleasure. However, due to age-related functional changes or disability, this activity may begin to evoke negative emotions when former performance expectations are not met. Thus, the older person may begin to avoid gardening to avoid distress, putting himself or herself at risk for developing depression.

Anxiety is also associated with behavioral avoidance. For example, individuals with GAD typically engage in avoidance behaviors such as procrastination. One investigation found that older adults with GAD who engaged in avoidant coping had more anxiety over the year following treatment with cognitive-behavioral therapy (Ayers, Petkus, Liu, Patterson, & Wetherell, 2010). GAD patients may also engage in behavior that serves the purpose of avoiding negative emotions, such as excessive planning or frequent checking. Checking behaviors include calling loved ones to inquire about their well-being and frequent contacts with health care providers to obtain reassurance about symptoms or side effects from medications. These behaviors alleviate anxiety and unpleasant emotions associated with uncertainty about the future.

The last type of avoidance involves use of "safety signals." Safety signals serve the purpose of alleviating or protecting individuals from unpleasant emotions. Anxious individuals of all ages often carry benzodiazepine medications with them at all times in case they feel an onset of anxiety. This safety signal may be particularly dangerous for older adults, as benzodiazapines have been associated with significantly increased risk of falling in older people (Titler, Shever, Kanak, Picone, & Qin, 2011). Noninvasive oxygen monitors and frequent checking with home blood pressure monitors are common safety signals for older adults with anxiety accompanying physical health conditions. Likewise, older adults with significant fear of falling may use hand-holding as a safety signal, even when it is done in such a way as to provide no physical security against a fall.

UNIFIED MODELS OF DEPRESSION AND ANXIETY DISORDERS

The "triple vulnerabilities model" provides a framework for describing the etiology of depression and anxiety disorders (Brown & Barlow, 2009). This model posits that three factors increase the risk of developing depression and anxiety: biological vulnerability, a generalized psychological vulnerability, and specific psychological vulnerability. Under stress, these factors interact with each other, and individuals with sufficient vulnerability factors present will manifest either depression and/or anxiety. We describe each of these vulnerabilities as well as new components and considerations to adapt this model to older adults.

The generalized biological vulnerability is hypothesized to be genetically driven. Behavioral genetic studies suggest that shared genetic factors exist for depression and anxiety disorders (Domschke & Reif, 2012; Kendler et al., 2011). Additionally, specific genes such as the 5-HTTLPR allele are associated with both depression and anxiety (Gerretsen & Pollock, 2008; Sen, Burmeister, & Ghosh, 2004). Personality factors that are thought to be influenced by genetics are also considered part of this biological vulnerability. For example, neuroticism is a personality trait strongly associated with increased experience of negative affect and emotion. This personality trait is common to both anxiety and depression. Low levels of openness to experience (i.e., low extraversion), another personality trait, are thought to be related to the low positive affect that is characteristic of depression. Studies suggest that these personality factors remain important vulnerability factors for the development of negative affect, depression, and anxiety later in life (de Beurs et al., 2001, 2005). To adapt this model to older adults, we propose to add cognitive decline as an additional biological vulnerability factor. Studies have repeatedly shown that individuals with cognitive impairment are at higher risk for both mood and anxiety disorders (Fiske, Wetherell, & Gatz, 2009; Wolitzky-Taylor et al., 2010).

General psychological vulnerability is driven by the fundamental belief that one has little control over stress or negative events. Maladaptive coping mechanisms such as avoidance are also part of this risk factor. According to the model, the general psychological vulnerability typically develops early in life. This vulnerability typically develops through the experience of early life stress, during which the individual learns that stressful life experiences are uncontrollable. Additionally, psychologically vulnerable people may learn to avoid stressful situations by modeling the behavior of other people around them.

Under the triple vulnerabilities model, these two general vulnerabilities describe the etiology of MDD and GAD. When under stress, individuals will present with GAD if they have the biological vulnerability of neuroticism as well as sufficient psychological vulnerability. Individuals with a biological vulnerability of neuroticism as well as low openness to experience, along with general psychological vulnerability, will present primarily as depressed, with or without anxiety. Although these two vulnerability factors describe the development of GAD and MDD, a third specific vulnerability factor is needed to explain the etiology of other anxiety disorders.

Specific psychological vulnerability develops from learning to fear certain experiences, typically early in life. Development of social phobia is associated with learning that social situations are threatening, typically via strict parents, bullying, or other traumatic social experiences. Individuals who learn that somatic and physiological symptoms are dangerous may develop panic disorder. Similarly, learning that intrusive thoughts are dangerous may be associated with obsessive-compulsive disorder. Learning experiences in which specific animals or situations are associated with danger may lead to the development of specific phobias. Lastly, traumatic events such as combat or assault are associated with posttraumatic stress disorder. Figure 9.1 displays this model and how the three vulnerability factors theoretically interact in the development of the various disorders.

PHARMACOLOGICAL TREATMENT OF LATE-LIFE ANXIOUS DEPRESSION

Few studies have specifically tested medications for efficacy in late-life anxious depression. They have generally found that antidepressant medications, including selective serotonin reuptake inhibitors (SSRIs), are less efficacious than they are in nonanxious depression. This has been found in research examining acute treatment response (Greenlee et al., 2010; Saghafi et al., 2007; Steffens & McQuoid, 2005), response to treatment augmentation (Dew et al., 2007), relapse prevention (Andreescu et al., 2007), and even in prevention of cognitive decline following remission from depression (DeLuca et al., 2005). Thus, the literature as a whole suggests that anxious depression is a more medication-resistant illness (Whyte et al., 2004), although some

research disputes this finding (Nelson, Delucchi, & Schneider, 2009).

It is counterintuitive that medications which are efficacious at treating both depressive and anxiety disorders would somehow be less effective in anxious depression. One theory suggests that comorbid anxiety symptoms are more persistent, reducing remission probability and increasing relapse risk (Dombrovski et al., 2007). Another suggests that anxious depression may have a differential pathophysiology at a neural systems level than nonanxious depression in older adults (Andreescu, Butters, et al., 2009; Andreescu et al., 2011). These various theories are largely untested, and it is unlikely that the true nature of this treatment resistance will be understood in the near future.

Typical first-line treatment for anxious depression is with an SSRI, with escitalopram, citalopram, and sertraline being the preferred agents because of their lack of drug interactions. Of the other SSRIs, paroxetine has several drug interactions and also is anticholinergic, potentially adversely affecting memory; fluoxetine has an exceedingly long half-life and several drug interactions; and fluvoxamine has some drug interactions and is infrequently used. Aside from these observations, the specific medication chosen does not appear to matter; there is no known difference in efficacy of these SSRIs.

In terms of tolerability, sertraline is associated with more gastrointestinal side effects, and citalopram with more sedative side effects at higher doses, but these differences are often not clinically relevant. Most side effects from SSRIs are temporary and benign. Some concern has been raised about potential long-term risks of these medications, particularly with respect to increasing rates of bone loss (Haney, Warden, & Bliziotes, 2010) and bleeding (Andrade, Sandarsh, Chethan, & Nagesh, 2010); however, the clinical significance of these risks is unknown and (in the case of bone loss) may more reflect confound by the underlying depressive or anxious illness.

It would also be considered appropriate practice to initiate a serotonin-norepinephrine reuptake inhibitor such as venlafaxine XR, desvenlafaxine, duloxetine, or milnacepran; these have similar side effects as SSRIs plus higher rates of sweating, dry mouth, and other "sympathetic" or noradrenergic side effects, but they are possibly more efficacious than SSRIs for depression, although proving this has been elusive. Finally, the atypical antidepressants

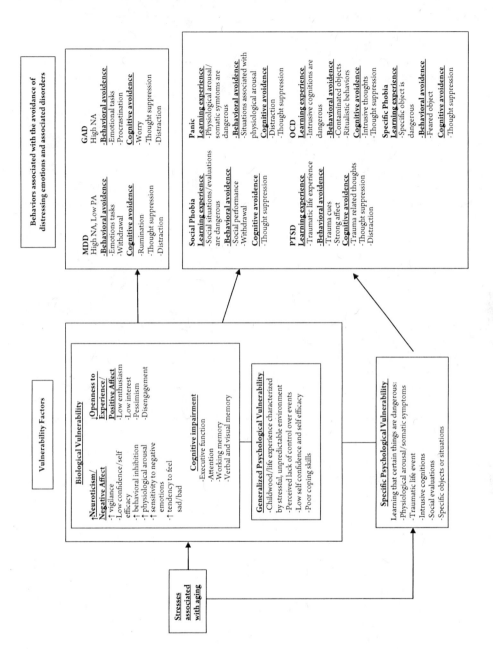

FIGURE 9.1 Triple vulnerabilities transdiagnostic model of depression and anxiety disorders.

vilazodone or mirtazapine are appropriate first-line (or augmentation) antidepressants, with mirtazapine having the side effects of increased appetite and sedation but usually lacking in intolerability problems sometimes seen with SSRIs (Schatzberg, Kremer, Rodrigues, & Murphy, 2002).

Although it is typical to start these medications in older adults at low doses, approximately 50% of the normal dosage, it is often necessary to push the dose to the highest tolerated one in anxious depression. Guidelines also suggest that after 12 weeks of first-line treatment, if the patient has not responded it is recommended to switch to a different class of antidepressants or to augment with a second agent in the case of partial or incomplete response. Augmentation agents can include the atypical antipsychotic drugs quetiapine and aripiprazole, although their use is often hampered by increased appetite and weight gain, tricyclic antidepressants, bupropion, and in some cases lithium or thyroid supplementation.

More important than the specific medication chosen is the management strategy accompanying it (Lenze, 2007). First, older adults with anxiety tend to exhibit poor tolerance to medication side effects, possibly resulting from increased physiological vigilance and catastrophic beliefs that side effects are indicative of serious harm. Because of the low tolerance of side effects, it is recommended that the clinician provide education about side effects and ensure patients are aware that side effects may occur but are likely to be benign and self-limited. In addition, it is important to educate patients on how the medications typically do not provide immediate relief; rather, results are typically seen after taking the medications for a number of weeks, with dose adjustments and augmentation likely.

Lastly, clinicians will often find that their patients are also taking a benzodiazepine. This may be problematic for a number of reasons in older adults, as benzodiazepine use has been linked with increased risk of falls and with cognitive impairment (particularly memory and attentional impairment). High rates of benzodiazepine use in anxious and depressed older adults suggest that clinicians will need to speak with the patient about the risks versus benefits of this medication. Generally, issues such as an unsteady gait, recent falls, or obvious memory impairment or sedation would move such an issue to front and center of treatment. Benzodiazepines have significant and even dangerous withdrawal reactions, so their sudden discontinuation is discouraged except in cases where the dose is low or where the medications are only used as needed and not daily.

PSYCHOTHERAPY BASED ON UNIFIED MODELS

Taken together, this research suggests that depression and anxiety disorders may be more alike than different, with similar biological processes, maladaptive experience of affect, poor emotion regulation, and general psychological vulnerability. Given these commonalities, transdiagnostic therapies designed to target the factors that are central to both depression and anxiety may be an efficient approach to psychotherapeutic treatment of anxious depression. We will describe three models of transdiagnostic treatment, problem-solving therapy, acceptance and commitment therapy (ACT; Hayes, Strosahl, & Wilson, 1999), and a variant of CBT, which is entitled the unified approach to emotional disorders (Allen, McHugh, & Barlow, 2008).

Problem-solving therapy has become the "gold standard" psychosocial treatment for late-life depression (Alexopoulos et al., 2003; P. Arean et al., 2008; P. A. Arean et al., 1993, 2010). Problem-solving therapy teaches skills and attempts to engage the depressed older adult in more adaptive problem solving, thus decreasing avoidance (D'Zurilla & Nezu, 2007). See Figure 9.2 for a diagram of the seven steps of problems solving that are taught in problem-solving therapy. Although problem-solving therapy has never been applied to individuals with anxiety disorders without depression, Arean and colleagues found that the presence of GAD did not influence the effectiveness of problem-solving therapy in a sample of depressed, cognitively impaired older adults (Arean et al., 2010).

ACT is a relatively new psychosocial approach to the treatment of emotional disorders. Broadly, the goals of this treatment are to increase acceptance of emotions, decrease avoidance of emotions, and increase behaviors that are consistent with one's values. Figure 9.3 is a diagram of the ACT hexaflex, which provides an overview of the main components of the ACT model. In a pilot study, Wetherell et al. (2011) found preliminary evidence that ACT is effective for worry and depression in older adults with GAD. Petkus and Wetherell (2011) discuss the potential usefulness of ACT as a transdiagnostic treatment for depressed and/or anxious older adults. Gerontological research and theory, particularly important theories of

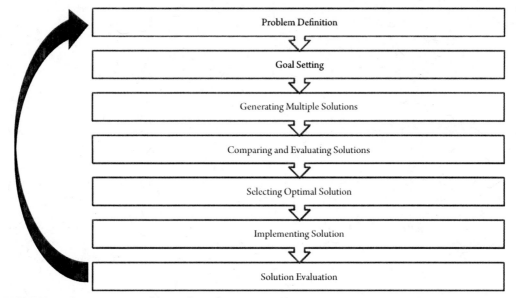

FIGURE 9.2 Seven steps in problem-solving therapy.

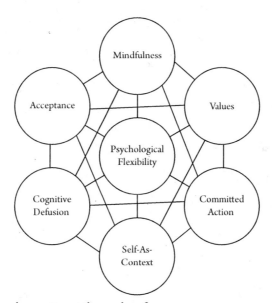

FIGURE 9.3 Acceptance and commitment therapy hexaflex.

successful aging such as the Selective Optimization and Compensation model (Baltes, 1997), suggest that an ACT approach to treatment may be useful with older adults. Additionally, the goal of ACT is not to decrease depression or anxiety, but rather to increase engagement in behaviors that are consistent with the individual's core values. Given that research suggests that older adults tend to have poor recognition or understanding of mental health symptoms (Fisher & Goldney, 2003; Wetherell, Petkus, et al., 2009), older adults may be more likely to engage in and understand an intervention that stresses their core values rather than alleviation of anxiety or depression. More research is needed to test transdiagnostic ACT interventions with older adults.

The unified approach to emotional disorders (Allen et al., 2008; Wilamoska et al., 2010) is another potentially promising transdiagnostic cognitive-behavioral approach to the treatment of depression and anxiety that targets features central to both depression and anxiety. This treatment, as outlined in Wilamoska et al. (2010), contains five modules aimed at modifying maladaptive methods of coping with emotional distress. The first module involves increasing awareness of emotions. This is typically done through education, mindfulness exercises, and role-playing exercises designed to elicit negative emotions. The second module aims to modify negative appraisals. This is done through cognitive restructuring techniques. The third module involves decreasing emotional avoidance. The goals of this module are to identify avoidance behaviors and teach more adaptive alternatives. The fourth module contains activities geared toward increasing awareness of physical and somatic symptoms as they relate to depression and anxiety. The final module entails cognitive and/or behavioral exposure to emotionally arousing situations. This may be done via behavioral activation for depressed or withdrawn individuals or exposure to feared situations for anxious individuals. Although data are still being gathered to support this new treatment approach, preliminary research suggests that it holds promise for treating mood and anxiety disorders (Wilamowska et al., 2010). It has not yet been implemented with older adults. See Figure 9.4 for a basic overview of the unified approach to emotional disorders.

For older patients with anxious depression who are interested in psychotherapy, a transdiagnostic approach may be particularly efficient for several reasons. First, as discussed, the majority of older adults with depression also have concurrent anxiety symptoms. A transdiagnostic approach will therefore potentially be better able to address the complex needs of distressed older adults. Second, a transdiagnostic approach may be easier to implement because it may make assessment and treatment planning more efficient. Currently, psychotherapists need to determine whether the older adult client's problem is primarily depression or anxiety. This process may be difficult, particularly with older patients. After determining the patient's primary problem, the therapist then has to choose the most appropriate treatment. With respect to behavioral therapy, this means that the psychotherapist must be familiar with a wide range of specific techniques to treat depression, panic disorder, posttraumatic stress disorder, social phobia, GAD, obsessive-compulsive disorder, and so on. Under a transdiagnostic model, determining whether the patient's main problem is anxiety or depression is not as important. Instead, the focus is on conducting a functional analysis of the person's thoughts and behavior to identify broad problem areas. Therapists would need to know a few general strategies for addressing these core problems, rather than many, often highly specialized, disorder-specific techniques.

Moreover, depressed and/or anxious older adults typically present to primary care rather than to specialty mental health providers. Additionally, many subpopulations of older adults who are at high risk for emotional disorders, such as nursing home residents (Smalbrugge, Pot, Jongenelis, Beekman, & Eefsting, 2005; Thakur & Blazer, 2008) and older adults receiving home care services (Bruce et al.,

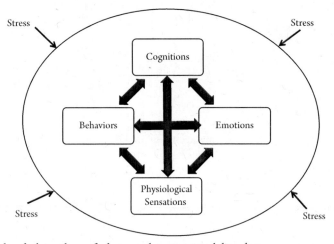

FIGURE 9.4 Model underlying the unified approach to emotional disorders.

2002), face many barriers to receiving care. As a result, efforts are under way to implement psychotherapeutic treatments for depression and anxiety in primary care, home health care, and aging services. Transdiagnostic approaches are a potential way to increase the accessibility of psychosocial treatment for depressed and anxious older adults because professionals in these settings who may not be trained psychotherapists can learn a smaller set of basic principles for cognitive and behavioral change rather than the ever-expanding menu of treatment manuals for specific disorders.

CONCLUSIONS

Mood and anxiety disorders commonly co-occur in older adulthood, with the most common presentation consisting of co-occurring symptoms of anxiety and depression. The neurobiology of depression and anxiety are very similar, and both involve disruptions to the HPA axis, noradrenergic, and serotonin systems, as well as possible disruptions to the limbic system and frontal cortex. Treatments, both pharmacological and psychosocial, also suggest that these disorders may be more similar than different.

SSRI medications, particularly escitalopram, citalopram, and sertraline, are the first-line agents of choice for anxious depression. Because this condition may respond more poorly to pharmacotherapy than depression without comorbid anxiety, doses may need to be pushed to the highest tolerable level. Augmentation with atypical antidepressants, atypical antipsychotics, tricyclic antidepressants, bupropion, and in some cases lithium or thyroid supplementation, or with psychotherapy, may be indicated in the case of partial response. Appropriate medication management is probably more important than the specific agent(s), and clinicians will often need to address benzodiazepine use.

With respect to psychotherapy, given the similarities between depression and anxiety, it may increase treatment efficacy, eventual implementation, and accessibility to develop and test transdiagnostic treatments that target the factors that are shared by these disorders. Transdiagnostic approaches may be particularly beneficial with older adults. Older adults typically are not as good as younger adults in identifying their own symptoms (Gum et al., 2009) or classifying accurately what is depression and what is anxiety (Wetherell, Petkus, et al., 2009). This may add to the already

challenging task of accurate diagnosis facing therapists working with older adults. A transdiagnostic approach would make the assessment process potentially more efficient, as well increase therapists' ability to address all of the complex concerns of older adults.

Disclosures

Mr. Petkus has no conflicts to disclose. He is funded by NIA only. Grant Support: National Institute on Aging (NIA) F31AG042218.

Dr. Lenze receives grant support from Lundbeck, Roche, and Johnson & Johnson.

Dr. Wetherell received research funding from Forest Laboratories, which ended in 2011. She currently receives grant support from the National Institutes of Health and the Veteran's Health Administration Office of Research and Development.

REFERENCES

Aizenstein, H. J., Butters, M. A., Figurski, J. L., Stenger, V. A., Reynolds, C. F., III, & Carter, C. S. (2005). Prefrontal and striatal activation during sequence learning in geriatric depression. *Biological Psychiatry, 58,* 290–296.

Aldao, A., & Nolen-Hoeksema, S. (2010). Specificity of cognitive emotion regulation strategies: A transdiagnostic examination. *Behavior Research and Therapy, 48,* 974–983.

Aldao, A., Nolen-Hoeksema, S., & Schweizer, S. (2010). Emotion-regulation strategies across psychopathology: A meta-analytic review. *Clinical Psychology Review, 30,* 217–237.

Alexopoulos, G. S., Katz, I. R., Bruce, M. L., Heo, M., Ten Have, T., Raue, P., ... PROSPECT Group. (2005). Remission in depressed geriatric primary care patients: a report from the PROSPECT study. *American Journal of Psychiatry, 162,* 718–724.

Alexopoulos, G. S., Katz, I. R., Reynolds, C. F., III, Carpenter, D., Docherty, J. P., & Ross, R. W. (2001). Pharmacotherapy of depression in older patients: A summary of the expert consensus guidelines. *Journal of Psychiatric Practice, 7,* 361–376.

Alexopoulos, G. S., Murphy, C. F., Gunning-Dixon, F. M., Kalayam, B., Katz, R., Kanellopoulos, D., ... Foxe, J. J. (2007). Event-related potentials in an emotional go/no-go task and remission of geriatric depression. *Neuroreport, 18,* 217–221.

Alexopoulos, G. S., Raue, P., & Arean, P. (2003). Problem-solving therapy versus supportive therapy in geriatric major depression with executive dysfunction. *American Journal of Geriatric Psychiatry, 11*, 46–52.

Allen, L. B., McHugh, K., & Barlow, D. H. (2008). Emotional disorders: A unified protocol. In D. H. Barlow (Ed.), *Clinical handbook of psychological disorders* (Vol. 4, pp. 216–249). New York: Guilford Press.

Allgulander, C., & Lavori, P. W. (1993). Causes of death among 936 elderly patients with "pure" anxiety neurosis in Stockholm County, Sweden, and in patients with depressive neurosis or both diagnoses. *Comparative Psychiatry, 34*, 299–302.

American Psychiatric Association. (1994). *Diagnostic and statistical manual of mental disorders: DSM-IV* (4th ed.). Washington, DC: Author.

Andrade, C., Sandarsh, S., Chethan, K. B., & Nagesh, K. S. (2010). Serotonin reuptake inhibitor antidepressants and abnormal bleeding: A review for clinicians and a reconsideration of mechanisms. *Journal of Clinical Psychiatry, 71*, 1565–1575.

Andreescu, C., Butters, M., Lenze, E. J., Venkatraman, V. K., Nable, M., Reynolds, C. F., III, & Aizenstein, H. J. (2009). fMRI activation in late-life anxious depression: A potential biomarker. *International Journal of Geriatric Psychiatry, 24*, 820–828.

Andreescu, C., Lenze, E. J., Dew, M. A., Begley, A. E., Mulsant, B. H., Dombrovski, A. Y., ... Reynolds, C. F. (2007). Effect of comorbid anxiety on treatment response and relapse risk in late-life depression: Controlled study. *British Journal of Psychiatry, 190*, 344–349.

Andreescu, C., Lenze, E. J., Mulsant, B. H., Wetherell, J. L., Begley, A. E., Mazumdar, S., & Reynolds, C. F., III. (2009). High worry severity is associated with poorer acute and maintenance efficacy of antidepressants in late-life depression. *Depression and Anxiety, 26*, 266–272.

Andreescu, C., Wu, M., Butters, M. A., Figurski, J., Reynolds, C. F., III, & Aizenstein, H. J. (2011). The default mode network in late-life anxious depression. *American Journal of Geriatric Psychiatry, 19*, 980–983.

Andrews, G. (1990). Classification of neurotic disorders. *Journal of the Royal Society of Medicine, 83*, 606–607.

Arean, P., Hegel, M., Vannoy, S., Fan, M. Y., & Unuzter, J. (2008). Effectiveness of problem-solving therapy for older, primary care patients with depression: Results from the IMPACT project. *Gerontologist, 48*, 311–323.

Arean, P. A., Perri, M. G., Nezu, A. M., Schein, R. L., Christopher, F., & Joseph, T. X. (1993). Comparative effectiveness of social problem-solving therapy and reminiscence therapy as treatments for depression in older adults.

Journal of Consulting and Clinical Psychology, 61, 1003–1010.

Arean, P. A., Raue, P., Mackin, R. S., Kanellopoulos, D., McCulloch, C., & Alexopoulos, G. S. (2010). Problem-solving therapy and supportive therapy in older adults with major depression and executive dysfunction. *American Journal of Psychiatry, 167*, 1391–1398.

Ayers, C., Petkus, A. J., Liu, L., Patterson, T. L., & Wetherell, J. L. (2010). Negative life events and avoidant coping are associated with poorer long-term outcome in older adults treated for generalized anxiety disorder. *Journal of Experimental Psychopathology, 1*, 312–316.

Baltes, P. (1997). On the incomplete architecture of human ontogeny: Selection, optimization, and compensation as foundation of developmental theory. *American Psychologist, 52*, 366–380.

Barlow, D. H., Allen, L. B., & Choate, M. L. (2004). Toward a unified treatment for emotional disorders. *Behavior Therapy, 35*, 205–230.

Bartels, S. J., Coakley, E., Oxman, T. E., Constantino, G., Oslin, D., Chen, H., ... Sanchez, H. (2002). Suicidal and death ideation in older primary care patients with depression, anxiety, and at-risk alcohol use. *American Journal of Geriatric Psychiatry, 10*, 417–427.

Beaudreau, S. A., & O'Hara, R. (2008). Late-life anxiety and cognitive impairment: A review. *American Journal of Geriatric Psychiatry, 16*, 790–803.

Beekman, A. T., de Beurs, E., van Balkom, A. J., Deeg, D. J., van Dyck, R., & van Tilburg, W. (2000). Anxiety and depression in later life: Co-occurrence and communality of risk factors. *American Journal of Psychiatry, 157*, 89–95.

Borkovec, T. D., Alcaine, O., & Behar, E. (2004). Avoidance theory of worry and generalized anxiety disorder. In R. G. Heimberg, C. L. Turk, & D. S. Mennin (Eds.), *Generalized anxiety disorder: Advances in research and practice* (pp. 77–109). New York: Guilford Press.

Borkovec, T. D., Hazlett-Stevens, H., & Diaz, M. L. (1999). The role of positive beliefs about worry in generalized anxiety disorder and its treatment. *Clinical Psychology and Psychotherapy, 1999*, 126–138.

Bremner, J. D. (2006). Traumatic stress: effects on the brain. *Dialogues of Clinical Neurosciences, 8*, 445–461.

Brenes, G. A., Penninx, B. W., Judd, P. H., Rockwell, E., Sewell, D. D., & Wetherell, J. L. (2008). Anxiety, depression and disability across the lifespan. *Aging and Mental Health, 12*, 158–163.

Britton, J. C., Lissek, S., Grillon, C., Norcross, M. A., & Pine, D. S. (2011). Development of anxiety: The role of threat appraisal and fear learning. *Depression and Anxiety, 28*, 5–17.

Brown, T. A., & Barlow, D. H. (2009). A proposal for a dimensional classification system based on the shared features of the DSM-IV anxiety and mood disorders: Implications for assessment and treatment. *Psychological Assessment, 21*, 256–271.

Brown, T. A., Chorpita, B. F., & Barlow, D. H. (1998). Structural relationships among dimensions of the DSM-IV anxiety and mood disorders and dimensions of negative affect, positive affect, and autonomic arousal. *Journal of Abnormal Psychology, 107*, 179–192.

Brown, T. A., Di Nardo, P. A., Lehman, C. L., & Campbell, L. A. (2001). Reliability of DSM-IV anxiety and mood disorders: Implications for the classification of emotional disorders. *Journal of Abnormal Psychology, 110*, 49–58.

Bruce, M. L., McAvay, G. J., Raue, P. J., Brown, E. L., Meyers, B. S., Keohane, D. J., ... Weber, C. (2002). Major depression in elderly home health care patients. *American Journal of Psychiatry, 159*, 1367–1374.

Cairney, J., Corna, L. M., Veldhuizen, S., Herrmann, N., & Streiner, D. L. (2008). Comorbid depression and anxiety in later life: Patterns of association, subjective well-being, and impairment. *American Journal of Geriatric Psychiatry, 16*, 201–208.

Charles, S. T., & Carstensen, L. L. (2010). Social and emotional aging. *Annual Review of Psychology, 61*, 383–409.

Clark, L. A., & Watson, D. (1991). Tripartite model of anxiety and depression: Psychometric evidence and taxonomic implications. *Journal of Abnormal Psychology, 100*, 316–336.

Cook, J. M., Orvaschel, H., Simco, E., Hersen, M., & Joiner, T. (2004). A test of the tripartite model of depression and anxiety in older adult psychiatric outpatients. *Psychology and Aging, 19*, 444–451.

Corbo, V., Clement, M. H., Armony, J. L., Pruessner, J. C., & Brunet, A. (2005). Size versus shape differences: Contrasting voxel-based and volumetric analyses of the anterior cingulate cortex in individuals with acute posttraumatic stress disorder. *Biological Psychiatry, 58*, 119–124.

Cukrowicz, K. C., Ekblad, A. G., Cheavens, J. S., Rosenthal, M. Z., & Lynch, T. R. (2008). Coping and thought suppression as predictors of suicidal ideation in depressed older adults with personality disorders. *Aging and Mental Health, 12*, 149–157.

D'Zurilla, T., & Nezu, A. (2007). *Problem-solving therapy: A positive approach to clinical intervention* (3rd ed.). New York: Springer.

de Beurs, E., Beekman, A., Geerlings, S., Deeg, D., Van Dyck, R., & Van Tilburg, W. (2001). On becoming depressed or anxious in late life: Similar vulnerability factors but different effects of stressful life events. *British Journal of Psychiatry, 179*, 426–431.

de Beurs, E., Comijs, H., Twisk, J. W., Sonnenberg, C., Beekman, A. T., & Deeg, D. (2005). Stability and change of emotional functioning in late life: Modelling of vulnerability profiles. *Journal of Affective Disorders, 84*, 53–62.

de Jong-Meyer, R., Beck, B., & Riede, K. (2009). Relationships between rumination, worry, intolerance of uncertainty and metacognitive beliefs. *Personality and Individual Differences, 46*, 547–551.

DeLuca, A. K., Lenze, E. J., Mulsant, B. H., Butters, M. A., Karp, J. F., Dew, M. A., ... Reynolds, C. F., III. (2005). Comorbid anxiety disorder in late life depression: Association with memory decline over four years. *International Journal of Geriatric Psychiatry, 20*, 848–854.

Dew, M. A., Whyte, E. M., Lenze, E. J., Houck, P. R., Mulsant, B. H., Pollock, B. G., ... Reynolds, C. F., III. (2007). Recovery from major depression in older adults receiving augmentation of antidepressant pharmacotherapy. *American Journal of Psychiatry, 164*, 892–899.

Domschke, K., & Reif, A. (2012). Behavioral genetics of affective and anxiety disorders. *Current Topics in Behavioral Neurosciences, 12*, 463–502.

Dombrovski, A. Y., Mulsant, B. H., Houck, P. R., Mazumdar, S., Lenze, E. J., Andreescu, C., ... Reynolds, C. F., III. (2007). Residual symptoms and recurrence during maintenance treatment of late-life depression. *Journal of Affective Disorders, 103*, 77–82.

Drevets, W. C., Price, J. L., & Furey, M. L. (2008). Brain structural and functional abnormalities in mood disorders: Implications for neurocircuitry models of depression. *Brain Structure and Function, 213*, 93–118.

Drevets, W. C., Savitz, J., & Trimble, M. (2008). The subgenual anterior cingulate cortex in mood disorders. *CNS Spectrums, 13*, 663–681.

Dulin, P. L., & Passmore, T. (2010). Avoidance of potentially traumatic stimuli mediates the relationship between accumulated lifetime trauma and late-life depression and anxiety. *Journal of Traumatic Stress, 23*, 296–299.

Ehring, T., & Watkins, E. R. (2008). Repetitive negative thinking as a transdiagnostic process. *International Journal of Cognitive Therapy, 1*, 192–205.

Fisher, L. J., & Goldney, R. D. (2003). Differences in community mental health literacy in older and younger Australians. *International Journal of Geriatric Psychiatry, 18*, 33–40.

Fiske, A., Wetherell, J. L., & Gatz, M. (2009). Depression in older adults. *Annual Review in Clinical Psychology, 5*, 363–389.

Gallo, J. J., & Rabins, P. V. (1999). Depression without sadness: Alternative presentations of depression in late life. *American Family Physician, 60*, 820–826.

Gellis, Z. D., & Bruce, M. L. (2010). Problem solving therapy for subthreshold depression in home healthcare patients with cardiovascular disease. *American Journal of Geriatric Psychiatry, 18*, 464–474.

Gerretsen, P., & Pollock, B. G. (2008). Pharmacogenetics and the serotonin transporter in late-life depression. *Expert Opinion in Drugs, Metabolism and Toxicology, 4*, 1465–1478.

Greenlee, A., Karp, J. F., Dew, M. A., Houck, P., Andreescu, C., & Reynolds, C. F., III. (2010). Anxiety impairs depression remission in partial responders during extended treatment in late-life. *Depression and Anxiety, 27*, 451–456.

Gum, A. M., Petkus, A., McDougal, S. J., Present, M., King-Kallimanis, B., & Schonfeld, L. (2009). Behavioral health needs and problem recognition by older adults receiving home-based aging services. *International Journal of Geriatric Psychiatry, 24*, 400–408.

Haney, E. M., Warden, S. J., & Bliziotes, M. M. (2010). Effects of selective serotonin reuptake inhibitors on bone health in adults: Time for recommendations about screening, prevention and management? *Bone, 46*, 13–17.

Hayes, S. C., Strosahl, K., & Wilson, K. (1999). *Acceptance and commitment therapy: An experiential approach to behavior change.* New York: Guilford Press.

Heimberg, R. G., Fresco, D. M., Frankel, A. N., Mennin, D. S., & Turk, C. L. (2002). Distinct and overlapping features of rumination and worry: The relationship of cognitive production to negative affective states. *Cognitive Therapy and Research, 26*, 179–188.

Hofmann, S. G., Sawyer, A. T., Fang, A., & Asnaani, A. (2012). Emotion dysregulation model of mood and anxiety disorders. *Depression and Anxiety, 29*, 409–416.

Kendler, K. S., Aggen, S. H., Knudsen, G. P., Roysamb, E., Neale, M. C., & Reichborn-Kjennerud, T. (2011). The structure of genetic and environmental risk factors for syndromal and subsyndromal common DSM-IV axis I and all axis II disorders. *American Journal of Psychiatry, 168*, 29–39.

Kessler, R. C., Berglund, P., Demler, O., Jin, R., Merikangas, K. R., & Walters, E. E. (2005). Lifetime prevalence and age-of-onset distributions of DSM-IV disorders in the National Comorbidity Survey Replication. *Archives of General Psychiatry, 62*, 593–602.

Kessler, R. C., Chiu, W. T., Demler, O., Merikangas, K. R., & Walters, E. E. (2005). Prevalence, severity, and comorbidity of 12-month DSM-IV disorders in the National Comorbidity Survey Replication. *Archives of General Psychiatry, 62*, 617–627.

Kim, K. H., Yook, K., Suh, S. Y., & Lee, K. S. (2010). Intolerance of uncertainty, worry, and rumination in major depressive disorder and generalized anxiety disorder. *Journal of Anxiety Disorders, 24*, 623–628.

Kindermann, S. S., Kalayam, B., Brown, G. G., Burdick, K. E., & Alexopoulos, G. S. (2000). Executive functions and P300 latency in elderly depressed patients and control subjects. *American Journal of Geriatric Psychiatry, 8*, 57–65.

King-Kallimanis, B., Gum, A. M., & Kohn, R. (2009). Comorbidity of depressive and anxiety disorders for older Americans in the national comorbidity survey-replication. *American Journal of Geriatric Psychiatry, 17*, 782–792.

Krause, N. (2007). Thought suppression and meaning in life: A longitudinal investigation. *International Journal of Aging and Human Development, 64*, 67–82.

Kremen, W. S., O'Brien, R. C., Panizzon, M. S., Prom-Wormley, E., Eaves, L. J., Eisen, S. A., ... Franz, C. E. (2010). Salivary cortisol and prefrontal cortical thickness in middle-aged men: A twin study. *Neuroimage, 53*, 1093–1102.

Kvaal, K., McDougall, F. A., Brayne, C., Matthews, F. E., & Dewey, M. E. (2008). Co-occurrence of anxiety and depressive disorders in a community sample of older people: Results from the MRC CFAS (Medical Research Council Cognitive Function and Ageing Study). *International Journal of Geriatric Psychiatry, 23*, 229–237.

Lee, L. O., & Knight, B. G. (2009). Attentional bias for threat in older adults: Moderation of the positivity bias by trait anxiety and stimulus modality. *Psychology and Aging, 24*, 741–747.

Lenze, E. (2007). Anxious depression in the elderly. *The Psychiatric Times, 24*, 3–6.

Lenze, E. J. (2003). Comorbidity of depression and anxiety in the elderly. *Current Psychiatry Reports, 5*, 62–67.

Lenze, E. J., Goate, A. M., Nowotny, P., Dixon, D., Shi, P., Bies, R. R., ... Pollock, B. G. (2010). Relation of serotonin transporter genetic variation to efficacy of escitalopram for generalized anxiety disorder in older adults. *Journal of Clinical Psychopharmacology, 30*, 672–677.

Lenze, E. J., Mantella, R. C., Shi, P., Goate, A. M., Nowotny, P., Butters, M. A., ... Rollman,

B. L. (2011). Elevated cortisol in older adults with generalized anxiety disorder is reduced by treatment: A placebo-controlled evaluation of escitalopram. *American Journal of Geriatric Psychiatry, 19*, 482–490.

Lenze, E. J., Mulsant, B. H., Shear, M. K., Schulberg, H. C., Dew, M. A., Begley, A. E., ... Reynolds, C. F., III. (2000). Comorbid anxiety disorders in depressed elderly patients. *American Journal of Psychiatry, 157*, 722–728.

Lenze, E. J., Munin, M. C., Ferrell, R. E., Pollock, B. G., Skidmore, E., Lotrich, F., ... Reynolds, C. F., III. (2005). Association of the serotonin transporter gene-linked polymorphic region (5-HTTLPR) genotype with depression in elderly persons after hip fracture. *American Journal of Geriatric Psychiatry, 13*, 428–432.

Lenze, E. J., Rogers, J. C., Martire, L. M., Mulsant, B. H., Rollman, B. L., Dew, M. A., ... Reynolds, C. F., III. (2001). The association of late-life depression and anxiety with physical disability: A review of the literature and prospectus for future research. *American Journal of Geriatric Psychiatry, 9*, 113–135.

Lenze, E. J., Rollman, B. L., Shear, M. K., Dew, M. A., Pollock, B. G., Ciliberti, C., ... Reynolds, C. F., III. (2009). Escitalopram for older adults with generalized anxiety disorder: A randomized controlled trial. *Journal of the American Medical Association, 301*, 295–303.

Lockwood, K. A., Alexopoulos, G. S., Kakuma, T., & Van Gorp, W. G. (2000). Subtypes of cognitive impairment in depressed older adults. *American Journal of Geriatric Psychiatry, 8*, 201–208.

Lupien, S. J., de Leon, M., de Santi, S., Convit, A., Tarshish, C., Nair, N. P., ... Meaney, M. J. (1998). Cortisol levels during human aging predict hippocampal atrophy and memory deficits. *Nature Neuroscience, 1*, 69–73.

Lynch, T. R., Cheavens, J. S., Morse, J. Q., & Rosenthal, M. Z. (2004). A model predicting suicidal ideation and hopelessness in depressed older adults: The impact of emotion inhibition and affect intensity. *Aging and Mental Health, 8*, 486–497.

Massana, G., Serra-Grabulosa, J. M., Salgado-Pineda, P., Gasto, C., Junque, C., Massana, J., & Mercader, J. M. (2003a). Parahippocampal gray matter density in panic disorder: A voxel-based morphometric study. *American Journal of Psychiatry, 160*, 566–568.

Massana, G., Serra-Grabulosa, J. M., Salgado-Pineda, P., Gasto, C., Junque, C., Massana, J., ... Salamero, M. (2003b). Amygdalar atrophy in panic disorder

patients detected by volumetric magnetic resonance imaging. *Neuroimage, 19*, 80–90.

Mennin, D. S., Holaway, R. M., Fresco, D. M., Moore, M. T., & Heimberg, R. G. (2007). Delineating components of emotion and its dysregulation in anxiety and mood psychopathology. *Behavior Therapy, 38*, 284–302.

Mineka, S., Watson, D., & Clark, L. A. (1998). Comorbidity of anxiety and unipolar mood disorders. *Annuual Reviews in Psychology, 49*, 377–412.

Moulds, M. L., Kandris, E., Starr, S., & Wong, A. C. (2007). The relationship between rumination, avoidance and depression in a non-clinical sample. *Behavior Research and Therapy, 45*, 251–261.

Muris, P., Roelofs, J., Rassin, E., Franken, I., & Mayer, B. (2005). Mediating effects of rumination and worry on the links between neuroticism, anxiety and depression. *Personality and Individual Differences, 39*, 1105–1111.

Murphy, C. F., Gunning-Dixon, F. M., Hoptman, M. J., Lim, K. O., Ardekani, B., Shields, J. K., ... Alexopoulos, G. S. (2007). White-matter integrity predicts stroop performance in patients with geriatric depression. *Biological Psychiatry, 61*, 1007–1010.

Nebes, R. D., Butters, M. A., Mulsant, B. H., Pollock, B. G., Zmuda, M. D., Houck, P. R., & Reynolds, C. F., III. (2000). Decreased working memory and processing speed mediate cognitive impairment in geriatric depression. *Psychological Medicine, 30*, 679–691.

Nelson, J. C., Delucchi, K., & Schneider, L. S. (2009). Anxiety does not predict response to antidepressant treatment in late life depression: Results of a meta-analysis. *International Journal of Geriatric Psychiatry, 24*, 539–544.

Newman, M. G., & Llera, S. J. (2011). A novel theory of experiential avoidance in generalized anxiety disorder: A review and synthesis of research supporting a contrast avoidance model of worry. *Clinical Psychology Reviews, 31*, 371–382.

Nolen-Hoeksema, S. (2000). The role of rumination in depressive disorders and mixed anxiety/depressive symptoms. *Journal of Abnormal Psychology, 109*, 504–511.

Penninx, B. W., Beekman, A. T., Bandinelli, S., Corsi, A. M., Bremmer, M., Hoogendijk, W. J., ... Ferrucci, L. (2007). Late-life depressive symptoms are associated with both hyperactivity and hypoactivity of the hypothalamo-pituitary-adrenal axis. *American Journal of Geriatric Psychiatry, 15*, 522–529.

Petkus, A. J., Gum, A., & Wetherell, J. L. (2012). Thought suppression is associated with psychological distress in homebound older adults. *Depression and Anxiety, 29*, 219–225.

Petkus, A. J., & Wetherell, J. L. (2011). Acceptance and commitment therapy with older adults: Rationale and considerations. *Cognitive and Behavioral Practice*, Early view online. DOI: 10.1016/j.cbpra.2011.07.004

Radua, J., van den Heuvel, O. A., Surguladze, S., & Mataix-Cols, D. (2010). Meta-analytical comparison of voxel-based morphometry studies in obsessive-compulsive disorder vs other anxiety disorders. *Archives of General Psychiatry, 67*, 701–711.

Radua, J., Via, E., Catani, M., & Mataix-Cols, D. (2011). Voxel-based meta-analysis of regional white-matter volume differences in autism spectrum disorder versus healthy controls. *Psychological Medicine, 41*, 1539–1550.

Ressler, K. J., & Mayberg, H. S. (2007). Targeting abnormal neural circuits in mood and anxiety disorders: From the laboratory to the clinic. *Nature and Neuroscience, 10*, 1116–1124.

Ressler, K. J., & Nemeroff, C. B. (2000). Role of serotonergic and noradrenergic systems in the pathophysiology of depression and anxiety disorders. *Depression and Anxiety, 12*(Suppl 1), 2–19.

Ritchie, K., Artero, S., Beluche, I., Ancelin, M. L., Mann, A., Dupuy, A. M., ... Boulenger, J. P. (2004). Prevalence of DSM-IV psychiatric disorder in the French elderly population. *British Journal of Psychiatry, 184*, 147–152.

Roberts, J. E., & Calmes, C. A. (2007). Repetitive thought and emotional distress: Rumination and worry as prospective predictors of depressive and anxious symptomatology. *Cognitive Therapy and Research, 31*, 343–356.

Rosenthal, M. Z., Cheavens, J. S., Compton, J. S., Thorp, S. R., & Lynch, T. R. (2005). Thought suppression and treatment outcome in late-life depression. *Aging and Mental Health, 9*, 35–39.

Saghafi, R., Brown, C., Butters, M. A., Cyranowski, J., Dew, M. A., Frank, E., ... Reynolds, C. F., III. (2007). Predicting 6-week treatment response to escitalopram pharmacotherapy in late-life major depressive disorder. *International Journal of Geriatric Psychiatry, 22*, 1141–1146.

Schatzberg, A. F., Kremer, C., Rodrigues, H. E., & Murphy, G. M., Jr. (2002). Double-blind, randomized comparison of mirtazapine and paroxetine in elderly depressed patients. *American Journal of Geriatric Psychiatry, 10*, 541–550.

Schienle, A., Ebner, F., & Schafer, A. (2011). Localized gray matter volume abnormalities in generalized anxiety disorder. *European Archives Psychiatry Clinical Neurosciences, 261*, 303–307.

Schultz, S. K., Castillo, C. S., Kosier, J. T., & Robinson, R. G. (1997). Generalized anxiety and depression. Assessment over 2 years after stroke. *American Journal of Geriatric Psychiatry, 5*, 229–237.

Segerstrom, S. C., Stanton, A. L., Alden, L. E., & Shortridge, B. E. (2003). A multidimensional structure for repetitive thought: What's on your mind, and how, and how much? *Journal of Personality and Social Psychology, 85*, 909–921.

Segerstrom, S. C., Tsao, J. C. I., Alden, L. E., & Craske, M. G. (2000). Worry and rumination: Repetitive thought as a concomitant and predictor of negative mood. *Cognitive Therapy and Research, 24*, 671–688.

Sen, S., Burmeister, M., & Ghosh, D. (2004). Meta-analysis of the association between a serotonin transporter promoter polymorphism (5-HTTLPR) and anxiety-related personality traits. *American Journal of Medical Genetics B Neuropsychiatry and Genetics, 127B*, 85–89.

Serfaty, M. A., Haworth, D., Blanchard, M., Buszewicz, M., Murad, S., & King, M. (2009). Clinical effectiveness of individual cognitive behavioral therapy for depressed older people in primary care: A randomized controlled trial. *Archives of General Psychiatry, 66*, 1332–1340.

Shimoda, K., & Robinson, R. G. (1998). Effects of anxiety disorder on impairment and recovery from stroke. *Journal of Neuropsychiatry and Clinical Neuroscience, 10*, 34–40.

Smalbrugge, M., Pot, A. M., Jongenelis, K., Beekman, A. T., & Eefsting, J. A. (2005). Prevalence and correlates of anxiety among nursing home patients. *Journal of Affective Disorders, 88*, 145–153.

Stanley, M. A., Beck, J. G., Novy, D. M., Averill, P. M., Swann, A. C., Diefenbach, G. J., & Hopko, D. R. (2003). Cognitive-behavioral treatment of late-life generalized anxiety disorder. *Journal of Consulting and Clinical Psychology, 71*, 309–319.

Stanley, M. A., Wilson, N. L., Novy, D. M., Rhoades, H. M., Wagener, P. D., Greisinger, A. J., ... Kunik, M. E. (2009). Cognitive behavior therapy for generalized anxiety disorder among older adults in primary care: A randomized clinical trial. *Journal of the American Medical Association, 301*, 1460–1467.

Steffens, D. C., & McQuoid, D. R. (2005). Impact of symptoms of generalized anxiety disorder on the course of late-life depression. *American Journal of Geriatric Psychiatry, 13*, 40–47.

Steiner, A., Petkus, A. J., Nguyen, H., & Wetherell, J. L. (in press). Attention bias and SSRI treatment in older adults with Generalized Anxiety Disorder. *Journal of Anxiety Disorders*.

Stroebe, M., Boelen, P. A., van den Hout, M., Stroebe, W., Salemink, E., & van den Bout, J. (2007). Ruminative coping as avoidance: A reinterpretation of its function in adjustment to bereavement. *European Archives of Psychiatry and Clinical Neuroscience, 257*, 462–472.

Teachman, B. A., Siedlecki, K. L., & Magee, J. C. (2007). Aging and symptoms of anxiety and depression: Structural invariance of the tripartite model. *Psychology and Aging, 22*, 160–170.

Thakur, M., & Blazer, D. G. (2008). Depression in long-term care. *Journal of the American Medical Directors Association, 9*, 82–87.

Titler, M. G., Shever, L. L., Kanak, M. F., Picone, D. M., & Qin, R. (2011). Factors associated with falls during hospitalization in an older adult population. *Research Theory Nursing Practice, 25*, 127–148.

Unutzer, J., Katon, W., Callahan, C. M., Williams, J. W., Jr., Hunkeler, E., Harpole, L., ... IMPACT Investigators. (2002). Collaborative care management of late-life depression in the primary care setting: A randomized controlled trial. *Journal of the American Medical Association, 288*, 2836–2845.

Vasiliadis, H. M., Dionne, P. A., Preville, M., Gentil, L., Berbiche, D., & Latimer, E. (2012). The excess healthcare costs associated with depression and anxiety in elderly living in the community. *American Journal of Geriatric Psychiatry*. ePub ahead of print.

Watkins, E., Moulds, M., & Mackintosh, B. (2005). Comparisons between rumination and worry in a non-clinical population. *Behaviour Research and Therapy, 43*, 1577–1585.

Wegner, D., & Zanakos, S. (1994). Chronic thought suppression. *Journal of Personality, 62*, 615–640.

Wetherell, J. L., Afari, N., Ayers, C. R., Stoddard, J. A., Ruberg, J., Sorrell, J. T., ... Patterson, T. L. (2011). Acceptance and commitment therapy for generalized anxiety disorder in older adults: A preliminary report. *Behavior Therapy, 42*, 127–134.

Wetherell, J. L., Ayers, C. R., Sorrell, J. T., Thorp, S. R., Nuevo, R., Belding, W., ... Patterson, T. L. (2009). Modular psychotherapy for anxiety in older primary care patients. *American Journal of Geriatric Psychiatry, 17*, 483–492.

Wetherell, J. L., Gatz, M., & Craske, M. G. (2003). Treatment of generalized anxiety disorder in older adults. *Journal of Consulting and Clinical Psychology, 71*, 31–40.

Wetherell, J. L., Petkus, A. J., McChesney, K., Stein, M. B., Judd, P. H., Rockwell, E., ... Patterson, T. L. (2009). Older adults are less accurate than younger adults at identifying symptoms of anxiety and depression. *Journal of Nervous and Mental Disordes, 197*, 623–626.

Wetherell, J. L., Ruberg, J. L., & Petkus, A. J. (2011). Generalized anxiety disorder. In K. H. Sorocco & S. Lauderdale (Eds.), *Cognitive behavior therapy with older adults: Innovations across care settings* (pp. 157–188). New York: Springer.

Wetherell, J. L., Stoddard, J. A., White, K. S., Kornblith, S., Nguyen, H., Andreescu, C., ... Lenze, E. J. (2010). Augmenting antidepressant medication with modular CBT for geriatric generalized anxiety disorder: A pilot study. *International Journal of Geriatric Psychiatry, 26*(8), 869–875.

Whyte, E. M., Dew, M. A., Gildengers, A., Lenze, E. J., Bharucha, A., Mulsant, B. H., & Reynolds, C. F. (2004). Time course of response to antidepressants in late-life major depression: Therapeutic implications. *Drugs Aging, 21*, 531–554.

Wignall, E. L., Dickson, J. M., Vaughan, P., Farrow, T. F., Wilkinson, I. D., Hunter, M. D., & Woodruff, P. W. (2004). Smaller hippocampal volume in patients with recent-onset posttraumatic stress disorder. *Biological Psychiatry, 56*, 832–836.

Wilamoska, Z., Thompson-Hollands, J., Fairholme, C., Ellard, K., Farchione, T., & Barlow, D. H. (2010). Conceptual background, development, and preliminary data from the unified protocol for transdiagnostic treatment of emotional disorders. *Depression and Anxiety, 27*, 882–890.

Wolitzky-Taylor, K. B., Castriotta, N., Lenze, E. J., Stanley, M. A., & Craske, M. G. (2010). Anxiety disorders in older adults: A comprehensive review. *Depression and Anxiety, 27*, 190–211.

10

THE SOCIAL DETERMINANTS OF DEPRESSION IN OLDER ADULTHOOD

Stephen E. Gilman, Hannah Carliner, and Alex Cohen

IN 1855, in a report commissioned by the Massachusetts legislature, Jarvis published one of the earliest findings on the social determinants of mental illness (Jarvis, 1971). He tabulated the numbers of individuals residing in state mental hospitals according to their status—either independent or pauper—and determined that "the pauper class furnishes, in ratio of its numbers [in the population], sixty-four times as many cases of insanity as the independent classes" (Jarvis, 1971, pp. 52–53). He concluded that "insanity is, then, part and parcel of poverty" (Jarvis, 1971, p. 53).

Since Jarvis's time, after important advances in sampling, assessment methods, and statistics, landmark studies in psychiatric epidemiology have come to the same general conclusion—that risk for the most common psychiatric disorders, including depression, is significantly higher among individuals exposed to adverse social environments (e.g., Murphy et al., 1991).

We review in this chapter the evidence on the types of adverse social environments that are most strongly related to depression in older adulthood.

The chapter is organized in two parts: (1) evidence for the social determinants of the development of depression in older adulthood; and (2) evidence for the social determinants of the receipt of depression treatment and depression treatment outcomes. In the first part, we present the evidence from a life course perspective, which means that we also address the extent to which the social determinants of late-life depression result from the cumulative lifetime exposure to environmental adversity. In the second part, we focus on intervention studies that provide evidence that is relevant to reducing social inequalities in late-life depression.

EVIDENCE FOR THE SOCIAL DETERMINANTS OF DEPRESSION IN OLDER ADULTHOOD

Theoretical Models of the Social Determinants of Depression

The social and environmental risk factors for depression in older adulthood, reviewed previously (Areán

& Reynolds, 2005; Bruce, 2002; Cole & Dendukuri, 2003; Djernes, 2006; Fiske, Wetherell, & Gatz, 2009; Vink, Aartsen, & Schoevers, 2008), span multiple, overlapping domains. A challenge consolidating the evidence reviewed previously and studies published since these reviews is the absence of any widely accepted "taxonomy" to provide an organizing framework of the social environment. As a result, there have been divergent conceptualizations and operationalizations of social and environmental risk factors across studies. Where constellations of risk factors are located along the causal pathways to late-life depression remains unclear.

Existing theoretical models tend to focus more narrowly on specific types of environmental effects. For example, stress-diathesis theory posits that social and environmental stressors activate an individual's preexisting vulnerability (or diathesis) and subsequently increase an individual's risk for depression. Research on gene–environment interactions has been motivated by stress-diathesis theory and has attempted to determine whether environmental stressors activate individuals' genetic vulnerability to depression. One of the most frequently investigated genetic variants is a length polymorphism in the serotonin transporter gene (5-HTTLPR), the short version of which has been associated with increased risk of depression in the context of environmental adversity. Substantial controversy has arisen over the replication or nonreplication of findings in this area (Monroe & Reid, 2008), and one of the major problems has been the lack of any coherent organizing framework over how the "environment" has been defined and assessed across studies.

Broad frameworks in social epidemiology provide some guidance in identifying social and environmental risk factors for late-life depression. For example, Kaplan (1999) articulated a model of the social determinants of health, which depicts individual health outcomes as a function of increasingly broader levels of organization, ranging from pathophysiologic pathways to neighborhoods and communities, and social and economic policies. Of particular relevance to late-life depression, Berkman et al. proposed a model explaining how social integration impacts health: via social-structural conditions, social networks, psychosocial mechanisms, and individual (psychological and physiologic) pathways (Berkman, Glass, Brissette, & Seeman, 2000). Finally, life course epidemiology demonstrates how social and environmental exposures at each stage of the life course impact health and well-being at subsequent stages (Gilman & McCormick, 2010).

We highlight here two features that these frameworks share in common. First, the social determinants of health are inherently multilevel; this means that policies and interventions to reduce the public health burden of depression via targeting psychosocial risk factors will, to be successful, need to expand their focus beyond the individual. Examples of this include interventions that attempt to change health care delivery systems, such as primary care practices; that address contextual-level risk factors; and that attempt to remove barriers to care that are common among disadvantaged groups (Bruce et al., 2004; Miranda et al., 2003).

Second, the patterning of the social determinants of health varies systematically according to the societal distribution of resources. In part, this reflects the continuity throughout the life course of stressors associated with ascribed statuses such as gender and race/ethnicity. For example, analyses of data from the first National Comorbidity Survey demonstrated not only that higher rates of depression among females persisted throughout the life span, but that these differences were due largely to gender differences in the first onset of depression (which often occurred during adolescence or young adulthood) (Kessler, McGonagle, Swartz, Blazer, & Nelson, 1993). This also reflects the differential exposure to (and possibly also, susceptibility to) both acute and chronic stressors associated with socioeconomic disadvantage. Thus, Miech and Shanahan (2009) reported that socioeconomic differences in depression widened with age, and that this widening gap was due to higher levels of physical health problems associated with lower socioeconomic status in older adulthood. Similarly, Cairney and Krause (2005) reported that differences in late-life depression associated with factors such as gender and socioeconomic status were explained by social stressors to which women and individuals of lower socioeconomic status are disproportionately exposed.

We present a prototypical model that illustrates these concepts in Figure 10.1. It depicts the emergence of the social determinants of depression early in the life course, and the continuities of risk and resilience processes into older adulthood, influencing both the onset of depression, depression treatment, and the likelihood of recurrent depressive episodes. The specific components of the model are based on the evidence reviewed next.

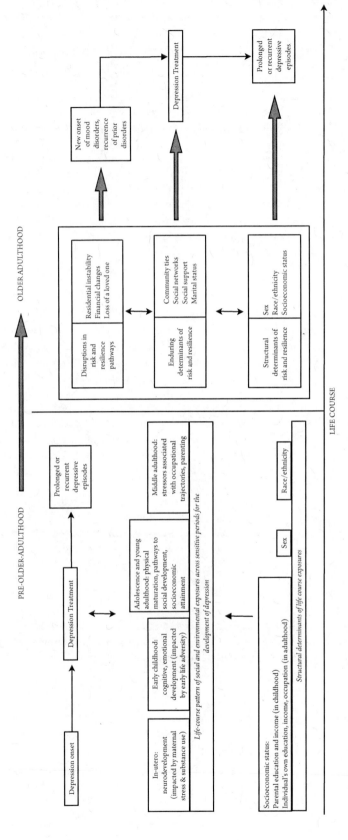

FIGURE 10.1 Conceptual model of the social and environmental determinants of depression in older adulthood. The figure depicts a conceptual model of the social and environmental determinants of depression in older adulthood. The left-hand panel, *Pre-Older-Adulthood*, illustrates that risk factors for depression in older adulthood often arise during developmentally sensitive periods earlier in the life course, and that depression in older adulthood is often preceded by a prior history of depression (Kim-Cohen et al., 2003). Moreover, the social determinants of depression vary across developmental stages, a trend that persists into older adulthood. The social determinants influence depression onset and its subsequent course, in part through associations with the likelihood of receiving and the effectiveness of depression treatment. Thus, among older adults there are significant continuities linking current disease risk with prior disease history and risk factors. Consistent with our focus in this chapter, the right-hand panel, *Older Adulthood*, illustrates the multilevel nature of the social determinants of depression. Structural factors such as socioeconomic status provide a context that shapes patterns of enduring, or stable, risk and protective factors; disruptions in these enduring risk or protective factors have been shown to be of particular importance in late-life depression. Arrows linking the multiple levels are bidirectional, indicating dynamic effects over time between levels that may have long-lasting influences. Factors at each level may in turn directly impact the development and course of depression (depicted in the figure by the three arrows leading to depression onset and recurrence, depression treatment, and the risk of subsequent episodes).

Socioeconomic and Demographic Factors and the Social Determinants of Depression in Older Adulthood

GENDER

Elevated levels of depression (both depressive symptoms and diagnoses of major depressive disorder) among females remain one of the more robust findings in psychiatric epidemiology (Kessler et al., 2003). Most of the studies in Djernes's and Vink et al.'s reviews reported higher rates of depression among females than males. However, the epidemiology of gender differences in depression in later stages of the life course remains unsettled, as several studies in these reviews indicate a narrowing of gender differences in depression with increasing age, particularly among the oldest old. It is generally established that gender differences in depression emerge for the first time during adolescence, a critical period for physical maturation as well as social and psychological development. Incidence studies among older adults are rare. Norton et al. (2006), using data from the Cache County study, reported 3-year incidence rates of first-onset depression that were 1.5 times higher among women than men, suggesting that incidence rates remain elevated among females throughout the life span. This may reflect both differential stress exposure and vulnerability, including to factors such as spousal bereavement which are common in later life (Williams, Baker, Allman, & Roseman, 2006).

In addition to elevated incidence rates, there is some evidence that recurrence rates of depressive episodes are also higher among women. Kessler et al. (2003), in the National Comorbidity Survey Replication, reported that among lifetime cases of depression, women were at a higher risk than men of depression during the past year (odds ratio = 1.4; 95% confidence interval = 1.1–1.8), an indirect meter of depression chronicity. However, longitudinal studies on gender differences in the course of depression among the elderly generally have not found large differences.

An important methodological consideration in investigating gender differences in late-life depression is the effect of depression on mortality. When Norton et al. (2006) supplemented their Cache County analyses with proxy interviews from relatives of participants who had died, gender differences in incidence rates were no longer statistically significant. This finding is consistent with reports from the Stirling County study and the Three-City study demonstrating that depression-related mortality is gender dependent, with higher risks among men than women (Murphy et al., 2010; Ryan et al., 2008).

It remains important to determine whether there are true gender differences in the onset and recurrence of depression in older adulthood, because such differences would motivate studies to identify gender-specific risk factors. However, this work will require overcoming several methodological challenges, including sex differences in the measurement and reporting of depressive symptoms (particularly in cross-sectional studies), the potential underrecognition of depression among men, and selection factors, including differential mortality (Wilhelm & Parker, 1994).

RACE/ETHNICITY

Epidemiologic studies of depression in the United States remain confronted with an apparent paradox regarding race/ethnicity (Keyes, Barnes, & Bates, 2011). Rates of lifetime major depressive disorder have been found to be lower among minority racial/ethnic minorities, in contrast to what would be expected based on racial/ethnic differences in physical health conditions (Breslau et al., 2006). While there is evidence of racial/ethnic differences in the psychometric properties of instruments used to assess depression in epidemiologic studies, these differences do not seem to account for the lower rates of depressive disorders among minorities (Yang, Tommet, & Jones, 2009). Psychological theories regarding racial/ethnic differences in coping have been put forward to explain this supposed paradox, but empirical tests of these theories have had mixed success (Keyes et al., 2011). Others have drawn on homophily-type theories—that is, the presumed differences in social support or social cohesion among racial/ethnic groups (Musick, Koenig, Hays, & Cohen, 1998). Guided by this theory, Mair et al. (2010) investigated racial/ethnic differences in mean levels of depressive symptoms according to the racial/ethnic composition of neighborhoods. They reported that African Americans living in neighborhoods with higher proportions of other African Americans had higher levels of depressive symptoms; in contrast, Hispanics enjoyed mental health benefits from living in neighborhoods with higher proportions of other Hispanics. More work is needed to follow up on the possibility that race/

ethnicity-specific risk or protective factors exist to account for true differences in disorder rates between groups, or whether the differences in rates observed are simply artifacts of instrumentation, reporting differences, or sampling.

SOCIOECONOMIC STATUS

An individual's socioeconomic status is defined as his or her location within the societal hierarchy of resources and prestige. Most often in medical research, socioeconomic status is measured by a respondent's income, education, occupation, or some composite of these. It is important to pay special attention to the assessment of socioeconomic status among older adults (Grundy & Holt, 2001). Current income and occupation are likely to be less accurate indicators of socioeconomic status among retired individuals, though indicators of current economic deprivation are generally associated with worse health, including major depression, both in the United States and cross-nationally (Back & Lee, 2011; Carvalhais et al., 2008). This includes poverty status, financial strain, and poor housing conditions (Kahn & Pearlin, 2006; Mojtabai & Olfson, 2004). Indicators of lifetime occupation and accumulated wealth might be more relevant in studies of older adults, given evidence that many years of exposure to financial hardship may take a pronounced toll on mental health (Kahn & Pearlin, 2006; Szanton, Thorpe, & Whitfield, 2010). In addition, it is important to differentiate individuals' cumulative lifetime exposure to financial hardship from changes in socioeconomic status that occurs in older adulthood. Contextual measures of socioeconomic status, such as neighborhood-level poverty, have also been linked with depression among older adults (Cohen et al., 2006, 2010; Cohen, Gilman, Houck, Szanto, & Reynolds, 2009). These findings may indicate that neighborhood-level poverty is a useful proxy for an individual's socioeconomic status (Wight, Cummings, Karlamangla, & Aneshensel, 2009); they may also indicate that attributes of neighborhoods exert independent influences on mental health (Paczkowski & Galea, 2010). Finally, educational attainment is one of the most commonly used indicators of socioeconomic status (Lee, 2011). It is stable over the life course, and in older adults, has the advantage of not being subject to "reverse causation" or other health selection processes by which poor health reduces an individual's socioeconomic status. However, in older adults, education differences in health may be confounded by cohort effects and are not reflective of cumulative and/or varying levels of socioeconomic effects on health over time. In their meta-analysis, Cole and Dendukuri (2003) found inconsistent results across studies for educational differences in depression.

Social Integration and Depression in Older Adulthood: A Unifying Framework

As mentioned earlier, the lack of a validated taxonomy of the social environment in epidemiologic research has led to divergent conceptualizations and operationalizations of social and environmental risk factors across studies. One of the most important consequences of this for research on the social determinants of late-life depression concerns the range, from macro to micro, in which various aspects of social connectedness are measured and examined. Various terms are used across studies for overlapping constructs—for example, small social networks, social isolation, bereavement, widowhood, and marital status. In addition, changes in social connectedness are often included in studies of "stressful life events" as one of many stressors in prediction models for depression, often without investigating the individual meaning and context of the events, and their role in the etiology of depression. We have known since Brown and Harris's seminal work in the United Kingdom that the context in which specific types of events occur plays a major role in moderating their depressogenic effects (Brown & Harris, 1978). This work has been replicated and extended by Kendler and his colleagues, who have demonstrated the importance of the psychological impact and meaning of events in the development of depression (Kendler, Hettema, Butera, Gardner, & Prescott, 2003).

Development of a unifying framework, or taxonomy, of the domains of social connectedness and depression would aid not only in generating greater consistencies in methods across studies but also in the discovery of etiologic processes and identification of intervention points. For example, it is probably not sufficient to know that the loss of a loved one is a risk factor for depression in order to develop optimally effective intervention strategies. Though the effects of bereavement on depression have been demonstrated empirically for decades, what remains less clear is how to investigate the myriad consequences of experiencing the loss of a loved one— ranging from the psychological consequences of the loss on an individual's sense of self, to the impact of the loss and attendant bereavement process on an individual's social network, to the relief experienced after the death of a spouse one had been a caregiver to throughout a chronic illness, to the financial strain or change in housing conditions following this loss. In other words, discrete events such as the loss of a loved one (which in the context of long-lasting medical conditions may not be discrete events at all) may have disruptive effects at the levels of physiologic systems through social well-being. The model presented in Figure 10.1, and Berkman et al.'s (2000) model of social networks and health, are the types of model that could be developed and tested in the area of late-life depression. These models encompass the multilevel nature of social integration, from community-level social ties to individual relationships, as well as both the qualitative and quantitative aspects of social integration (i.e., the strength of social ties as well as their number). A key feature of these models is that they posit specific, and empirically testable, causal mechanisms attached to each domain. We focus next on aspects of social integration that have particular relevance for depression in older adulthood.

SOCIAL NETWORKS AND SOCIAL SUPPORT

Social networks are structures of ties linking individuals, and they serve as conduits for the transmission of both risk and protection. For example, Rosenquist et al.'s analysis of data on depressive symptoms in the social networks of participants in the Framingham Heart Study revealed that depressive symptoms tended to spread throughout an individual's network (Rosenquist, Fowler, & Christakis, 2011). In contrast, strong social networks (and based on Rosenquist et al., social networks characterized by low levels of depressive symptoms) have consistently been found to be protective against depressive disorders and symptoms among the elderly (Wilby, 2011). One of the important functions of social networks is that they provide a source of social support, which is of particular importance in late-life depression (Berkman & Glass, 2000). Opportunities for social support may be patterned by socioeconomic and cultural factors; for example, Sicotte et al. reported that social supports received from living with extended family members among

the elderly in Cuba were associated with lower levels of depression and reduced impact on depression of financial strain (Sicotte, Alvarado, León, & Zunzunegui, 2008). Longitudinal studies demonstrate that impaired social support is associated with increased depressive symptoms (Henderson et al. 1997). The causal effect of social support on depression is often difficult to identify, however, because of dynamic effects over time between changes in social support and changes in depressive symptoms (Lynch & George, 2002). Social support interventions overcome this methodological challenge, and there is promising evidence that providing depressed individuals with social support will lead to at least a modest reduction in depressive symptoms (Mead, Lester, Chew-Graham, Gask, & Bower, 2010).

DISRUPTIONS IN SOCIAL CONNECTIONS

Attachments are central to psychological well-being and to the development of depression beginning in childhood. Throughout the life span the loss of a loved one, which disrupts attachments, remains a significant predictor of depression (Kendler et al., 2003). In older adulthood, spousal loss is the most common form and is one of the strongest risk factors for subsequent depression (Alexopoulos 2005; Cole & Dendukuri, 2003). Depressive symptoms are very common immediately after a loss, though a much smaller proportion of individuals develop clinically significant depressive symptoms, and depression following bereavement frequently remits within a year of the loss. In addition, those with a prior history of major depression have a heightened risk for a subsequent depressive episode in the context of a loss (Zisook, Paulus, Shuchter, & Judd, 1997). Though the loss of a loved one is often considered in research on late-life depression as one of many stressful life events that are hypothesized to cause depression, the mental health consequences of bereavement and the disruptions in social support can have widespread effects across multiple dimensions of one's social connections (Stroebe, Folkman, Hansson, & Schut, 2006).

BEREAVEMENT, SOCIAL DETERMINANTS, AND DEPRESSION NOSOLOGY

The consequences of bereavement on depression illustrate an ongoing controversy in depression nosology that is fundamental to research on the social determinants of depression. That is because, in the case of bereavement, aspects of the social environment are incorporated directly into the diagnostic criteria for major depressive disorder, thereby building a potential circularity into studies of loss and depression. The introduction to the *Diagnostic and Statistical Manual of Mental Disorders*, fourth edition (*DSM-IV*) states that a psychiatric diagnosis should not be given to individuals experiencing "an expectable and culturally sanctioned response to a particular event, for example, the death of a loved one" (American Psychiatric Association, 2000, p. xxxi). This is incorporated into the diagnostic criteria for depression by excluding from a diagnosis episodes occurring in the context of bereavement unless they are severe or prolonged.

As discussed at length by Horwitz and Wakefield (2007), there is an asymmetry in the diagnostic criteria, wherein depressions associated with the loss of a loved one are excluded from a diagnosis, but not depressions associated with other stressors. Their book has sparked a series of studies investigating the similarity of depressive episodes associated with the loss of a loved one and episodes associated with other stressors; these studies revealed far more similarities than differences between the different types of episodes (Karam et al., 2009; Wakefield, Schmitz, First, & Horwitz, 2007; Zisook & Kendler, 2007). Wakefield and colleagues' solution to the asymmetry is to extend the bereavement exclusion to cover other stressors (Wakefield et al., 2007). This has some conceptual appeal, because it entails diagnosing only those episodes that reflect disproportionate reactions to stressors. For example, they might argue that depression following the loss of a job should only qualify for a psychiatric diagnosis if symptoms are more severe than what is commonly observed following a job loss. Clearly there are practical difficulties with such a proposal, not the least of which is the lack of evidence to justify multiple diagnostic criteria sets corresponding to the range of social conditions associated with depression.

The validity of the bereavement exclusion also rests on the validity of its exception. It is generally accepted that some bereavement reactions can evolve into psychiatric disorders (what prior versions of the *DSM* termed "complicated bereavement"). It is therefore important to differentiate bereavement-related depressions that are nonpathological from those that have evolved into psychopathology. Unfortunately, there is little evidence to

support the validity of the *DSM-IV*'s criteria for making this distinction. For example, Karam et al. (2009) found that the *DSM-IV*'s conditional criteria (e.g., marked functional impairment, suicidal ideation, duration >2 months) used to demarcate diagnosable bereavement-related depression were not valid markers of depression severity. Similarly, Gilman et al. (2011) investigated bereavement-related depression in a large national sample; they reported that individuals whose bereavement-related depression did not qualify for a depression diagnosis were no different in terms of a wide range of diagnostic validators than individuals with bereavement-related depression who did qualify for a diagnosis. It is important to point out here that a distinct form of bereavement-induced disorder, termed *prolonged grief disorder*, is also being proposed for consideration as a psychiatric diagnosis (Prigerson et al., 2009).

While the field of psychiatry aims to advance toward an etiologically based system of classifying disorders, evidence does not yet support such an approach for depression. Therefore, we conclude based on the aforementioned evidence that diagnoses of depression should not be made contingent on the social context in which a depressive episode occurs. In other words, excluding clinically significant depressive episodes from receiving a psychiatric diagnosis because of their connection to bereavement detracts from the utility of a theory-neutral diagnostic system (Wakefield, 1998), hinders rather than facilitates research that aims to determine the causal connections between social factors and depressive illness, and could reduce the likelihood of receiving psychiatric treatment (Zisook, Shuchter, Pedrelli, Sable, & Deaciuc, 2001).

SOCIAL DETERMINANTS OF DEPRESSION ACROSS THE LIFE COURSE

Many of the social determinants of late-life depression involve aspects of the social environment that are often features of older adulthood (e.g., the financial conditions surrounding retirement, spousal loss). However, the social determinants associated with depression later in life do not always emerge de novo in old age but may have persisted for decades, including since childhood. Catastrophic events experienced during childhood, such as exposure to violence during World War II, have been linked with elevated risks of depression in late life (Kraaij & de Wilde, 2001). More common risk factors such as low socioeconomic status during childhood and adolescence, as well as childhood abuse, have also been associated with depression in late life (Kraaij & de Wilde, 2001). Linkages between social factors early in the life course and depression in older adulthood might be contingent on intervening events (Luo & Waite, 2005; Wainwright & Surtees, 2002). Finally, childhood adversity has been shown to sensitize individuals to depression in the context of adult adversity in some but not all studies (Comijs et al., 2007).

SOCIAL DETERMINANTS OF DEPRESSION TREATMENT IN OLDER ADULTS

Substantial evidence exists to suggest that the social determinants of depression onset and recurrence observed in epidemiologic studies also exist in clinical samples and, moreover, have significant influences on the receipt and effectiveness of depression treatments. With respect to the receipt of treatment, evidence comes from studies of social inequalities in treatment seeking, and in the provision of treatments among those who have sought care. As for treatment effectiveness, evidence comes largely from antidepressant treatment studies (using either medication, psychotherapy, or both) in which social variables were associated with treatment outcomes.

Social Determinants of Receiving and Using Antidepressant Treatment

In the older adult population generally, the diagnosis and treatment of depression over the past three decades has increased almost two-fold (Crystal, Sambamoorthi, Walkup, & Akincigil, 2003). However, this trend is not reflected to the same degree in population subgroups. Despite higher levels of depressive symptomatology, older adult minorities (African Americans, Asian Americans, and Hispanics) were significantly less likely to have accessed mental health services in the 2005 California Health Interview Survey (Sorkin, Pham, & Ngo-Metzger, 2009). Treatment rates for depression based on health care claims data indicate disparities according to sex, educational attainment, income, and race/ethnicity (Akincigil et al., 2011). Melfi et al. analyzed Medicaid claims data between 1989 and 1994 and reported that African Americans with a diagnosis of a depressive disorder had half the

odds of receiving antidepressant medication than Whites; furthermore, among those receiving antidepressant therapy, African Americans had a 20% lower odds of receiving a selective serotonin reuptake inhibitor than a tricyclic antidepressant (Melfi, Croghan, Hanna, & Robinson, 2000). In 1998 Medicaid claims data, older African Americans with a primary diagnosis of depression had almost half the odds of being treated with antidepressants than their White counterparts (Strothers et al., 2005). Even in Medicare claims data, covering a wider population, minority racial/ethnic groups (African Americans, Hispanics, and Asian Americans) had lower rates of antidepressant use and received substantially less follow-up care after being hospitalized for a mental illness (Virnig et al., 2004).

One factor that may contribute to social inequalities in the diagnosis and treatment of depression is access to insurance that supplements Medicare, which has been shown to vary by socioeconomic status (Crystal et al., 2003). A recent study has found that the Medicare Part D drug benefits have improved access to antidepressants, but this research did not examine social inequalities (Donohue et al., 2011).

In general, relatively fewer ethnic minorities access mental health services for treatment of depressive disorders (Areán et al., 2005). Furthermore, older individuals of racial/ethnic minorities tend to seek care in primary care settings in which levels of treatment are liable to be less intensive (Pingitore, Snowden, Sansone, & Klinkman, 2001). The Improving Mood-Promoting Access to Collaborative Treatment (IMPACT) study, a multisite clinical trial of the treatment of late-life depression attendees of primary care practices provides evidence that these inequalities, at least in part, can be addressed (Unutzer et al., 2002). Randomization to the collaborative care arm of the trial improved rates of antidepressant use and psychotherapy among Hispanics and African Americans, compared to randomization to usual care (Areán & Reynolds, 2005).

Social Determinants of Depression Treatment Outcomes

There is increasing evidence supporting highly effective treatment of late-life depression (Andreescu & Reynolds, 2011). However, given the social inequalities in risks for the development of late-life depression (e.g., educational levels, income, employment status, and stressful social environments), it is important to determine whether these same factors negatively impact the effectiveness of interventions (Cohen et al., 2006).

The Sequenced Treatment Alternatives to Relieve Depression (STAR*D) study, a large clinical trial that was conducted in primary care practices and psychiatric outpatient clinics, has produced evidence on social inequalities in response to specific treatment protocols. Higher income and having a college degree were both associated with higher rates of depression remission (Trivedi et al., 2006), while African Americans and Hispanics had poorer responses to treatments (Lesser et al., 2007). In addition, being African American or having less than a college education was associated with worsened depression during the course of the trial (Friedman et al., 2009).

In a trial on maintenance treatments for late-life depression, Dew et al. (1997) determined that poor social support was predictive of relatively poorer response to a combination of antidepressant medication and. Cohen et al. (2006) later examined social inequalities in treatment outcomes in this and a subsequent trial and found that, even when controlling for a range of sociodemographic and clinical characteristics, subjects living in middle and high income neighborhoods, as compared to subjects living in low-income neighborhoods, were more likely to respond to treatment and less likely to experience suicidal ideation during the course of treatment. Because subsequent analyses of these same data suggested that levels of comorbid anxiety at baseline were predictive of treatment outcomes (Andreescu et al., 2007), Cohen et al. (2009) reanalyzed the data to examine whether social inequalities were due, at least in part, to anxiety symptoms among residents of low-income neighborhoods. However, this did not prove to be the case and living in a low-income neighborhood remained an independent predictor of response to treatment and the likelihood of experiencing suicidal ideation. Surprisingly, education status was not predictive of response to treatment or experience of suicidal ideation in any of the analyses conducted by Cohen and colleagues.

As noted earlier, the IMPACT intervention improved the use of antidepressants and psychotherapy among African Americans and Hispanics. This increased use of treatment options resulted in improved outcomes for African Americans and Hispanics: Compared to minority status participants who received usual care, those in the collaborative care arm of the trial displayed lower depression severity, higher rates of treatment response, and higher rates of remission (Areán & Reynolds, 2005). Analyses that examined possible inequalities in outcomes according to income status among IMPACT participants had similar results, suggesting all income groups enjoyed similar benefits from the intervention (Areán, Gum, Tang, & Unützer, 2007).

In sum, there is substantial evidence from observational studies on the existence of social inequalities in both access to and effectiveness of treatments for late-life depression. Promising, emerging evidence from intervention studies such as IMPACT suggests that these inequalities can be mitigated by collaborative care strategies in primary care settings and by interventions that specifically target disadvantaged populations (Areán & Reynolds, 2005; Bao et al., 2011).

CONCLUSIONS

We began this chapter by citing Jarvis's work on disparities in mental illness to provide a historical context to the social determinants of late-life depression. This research has shown an intricate connection between mental illness and the social environment. Methodological advances in sampling, assessment of psychopathology, and statistical modeling have since enabled researchers to uncover the extent of these connections. An individual's position in the social hierarchy, from birth through old age, correlates with the risk of depression onset and persistence, access to treatment, and treatment outcomes. The current challenge for the field is to understand the etiologic role of social and environmental exposures in the risk of late-life depression. This will require further refining theoretical models of social determinants that articulate testable hypotheses concerning the meaning and consequences of social environments to older adults, and the ways in which environmental exposures disrupt or protect mental health and functioning. This work will contribute to advancing the nosology of mood disorders by moving toward an etiologically based classification rather than a purely descriptive or phenomenologically based classification. Finally, this work will identify points of intervention at all stages of the disease process—from preventing depression onset to reducing its chronicity. Such interventions may target social and environmental risk factors directly or may adapt existing psychopharmacologic and psychotherapeutic treatments to population subgroups at risk for poor treatment response.

Disclosures

Dr. Gilman has no conflicts of interest to disclose. He has received funding from the National Institute of Mental Health.

Ms. Carliner has no conflicts to disclose.

Dr. Cohen has no conflicts to disclose. He is funded only by NIMH and Wellcome Trust. Grant Support: NIH (1R21MH093304) and Wellcome Trust (090287).

ACKNOWLEDGMENTS

This work was supported in part by grants MH83335 and MH087544 from the National Institutes of Health.

REFERENCES

Akincigil, A., Olfson, M., Walkup, J. T., Siegel, M. J., Kalay, E., Amin, S., ... Crystal, S. (2011). Diagnosis and treatment of depression in older community-dwelling adults: 1992–2005. *Journal of the American Geriatrics Society, 59*(6), 1042–1051.

Alexopoulos, G. S. (2005). Depression in the elderly. *Lancet, 365*(9475), 1961–1970.

American Psychiatric Association. (2000). *Diagnostic and statistical manual of mental disorders* (4th ed., text rev.). Washington, DC.

Andreescu, C., Lenze, E. J., Dew, M. A., Begley, A. E., Mulsant, B. H., Dombrovski, A. Y., ... Reynolds, C. F. (2007). Effect of comorbid anxiety on treatment response and relapse risk in late-life depression: Controlled study. *British Journal of Psychiatry, 190*, 344–349.

Andreescu, C., & Reynolds, C. F., III. (2011). Late-life depression: Evidence-based treatment and promising new directions for research and clinical practice. *Psychiatric Clinics of North America, 34*(2), 335–355.

Areán, P. A., Ayalon, L., Hunkeler, E., Lin, E. H., Tang, L., Harpole, L., ... IMPACT Investigators. (2005). Improving depression care for older, minority patients in primary care. *Medical Care, 43*(4), 381–390.

Areán, P. A., Gum, A. M., Tang, L., & Unützer, J. (2007). Service use and outcomes among elderly persons with low incomes being treated for depression. *Psychiatric Services, 58*(8), 1057–1064.

Areán, P. A., & Reynolds, C. F., III. (2005). The impact of psychosocial factors on late-life depression. *Biological Psychiatry, 58*(4), 277–282.

Back, J. H., & Lee, Y. (2011). Gender differences in the association between socioeconomic status (SES) and depressive symptoms in older adults. *Archives of Gerontology and Geriatrics, 52*(3), e140–144.

Bao, Y., Alexopoulos, G. S., Casalino, L. P., Ten Have, T. R., Donohue, J. M., Post, E. P., ... Bruce, M. L. (2011). Collaborative depression care management and disparities in depression treatment and outcomes. *Archives of General Psychiatry, 68*(6), 627–636.

Berkman, L. F., & Glass, T. (2000). Social integration, social networks, social support, and health. In L. F. Berkman & I. Kawachi (Eds.), *Social epidemiology* (pp. 137–173). New York: Oxford University Press.

Berkman, L. F., Glass, T., Brissette, I., & Seeman, T. E. (2000). From social integration to health: Durkheim in the new millennium. *Social Science and Medicine, 51*(6), 843–857.

Breslau, J., Aguilar-Gaxiola, S., Kendler, K. S., Su, M., Williams, D., & Kessler, R. C. (2006). Specifying race-ethnic differences in risk for psychiatric disorder in a USA national sample. *Psychological Medicine, 36*(1), 57–68.

Brown, G. W., & Harris, T. O. (1978). *Social origins of depression: A study of psychiatric disorder in women.* London: Tavistock.

Bruce, M. L. (2002). Psychosocial risk factors for depressive disorders in late life. *Biological Psychiatry, 52*(3), 175–184.

Bruce, M. L., Ten Have, T. R., Reynolds, C. F., III, Katz, I. I., Schulberg, H. C., Mulsant, B. H., ... Alexopoulos, G. S. (2004). Reducing suicidal ideation and depressive symptoms in depressed older primary care patients: A randomized controlled trial. *Journal of the American Medical Association, 291*(9), 1081–1091.

Cairney, J., & Krause, N. (2005). The social distribution of psychological distress and depression in older adults. *Journal of Aging and Health, 17*(6), 807–835.

Carvalhais, S. M., Lima-Costa, M. F., Peixoto, S. V., Firmo, J. O., Castro-Costa, E., & Uchoa, E. (2008). The influence of socio-economic conditions on the prevalence of depressive symptoms and its covariates in an elderly population with slight income differences: The Bambui Health and Aging Study (BHAS). *International Journal of Social Psychiatry, 54*(5), 447–456.

Cohen, A., Chapman, B. P., Gilman, S. E., Delmerico, A. M., Wieczorek, W., Duberstein, P. R., & Lyness, J. M. (2010). Social inequalities in the occurrence of suicidal ideation among older primary care patients. *American Journal of Geriatric Psychiatry, 18*(12), 1146–1154.

Cohen, A., Gilman, S. E., Houck, P. R., Szanto, K., & Reynolds, C. F., III. (2009). Socioeconomic status and anxiety as predictors of antidepressant treatment response and suicidal ideation in older adults. *Social Psychiatry and Psychiatric Epidemiology, 44*(4), 272–277.

Cohen, A., Houck, P. R., Szanto, K., Dew, M. A., Gilman, S. E., & Reynolds, C. F., III. (2006). Social inequalities in response to antidepressant treatment in older adults. *Archives of General Psychiatry, 63*(1), 50–56.

Cole, M. G., & Dendukuri, N. (2003). Risk factors for depression among elderly community subjects: A systematic review and meta-analysis. *American Journal of Psychiatry, 160*(6), 1147–1156.

Comijs, H. C., Beekman, A. T., Smit, F., Bremmer, M., van Tilburg, T., & Deeg, D. J. (2007). Childhood adversity, recent life events and depression in late life. *Journal of Affective Disorders, 103*(1–3), 243–246.

Crystal, S., Sambamoorthi, U., Walkup, J. T., & Akincigil, A. (2003). Diagnosis and treatment of depression in the elderly medicare population: Predictors, disparities, and trends. *Journal of the American Geriatrics Society, 51*(12), 1718–1728.

Dew, M. A., Reynolds, C. F., III., Houck, P. R., Hall, M., Buysse, D. J., Frank, E., & Kupfer, D. J. (1997). Temporal profiles of the course of depression during treatment. Predictors of pathways toward recovery in the elderly. *Archives of General Psychiatry, 54*(11), 1016–1024.

Djernes, J. K. (2006). Prevalence and predictors of depression in populations of elderly: A review. *Acta Psychiatrica Scandinavica, 113*(5), 372–387.

Donohue, J. M., Zhang, Y., Aiju, M., Perera, S., Lave, J. R., Hanlon, J. T., & Reynolds, C. F., III. (2011). Impact of Medicare Part D on antidepressant treatment, medication choice, and adherence among older adults with depression. *American Journal of Geriatric Psychiatry,19*(12), 989–997.

Fiske, A., Wetherell, J. L., & Gatz, M. (2009). Depression in older adults. *Annual Review of Clinical Psychology, 5*, 363–389.

Friedman, E. S., Wisniewski, S. R., Gilmer, W., Nierenberg, A. A., Rush, A. J., Fava, M., … Trivedi, M. H. (2009). Sociodemographic, clinical, and treatment characteristics associated with worsened depression during treatment with citalopram: Results of the NIMH STAR(*)D trial. *Depression and Anxiety, 26*(7), 612–621.

Gilman, S. E., Breslau, J., Trinh, N. H., Fava, M., Murphy, J. M., & Smoller, J. W. (2011). Bereavement and the diagnosis of major depressive episode in the National Epidemiologic Survey on Alcohol and Related Conditions. *Journal of Clinical Psychiatry, 73*(2), 208–215.

Gilman, S. E., & McCormick, M. C. (2010). Insights from life course epidemiology. *Academy of Pediatrics, 10*(3), 159–160.

Grundy, E., & Holt, G. (2001). The socioeconomic status of older adults: How should we measure it in studies of health inequalities? *Journal of Epidemiology and Community Health, 55*(12), 895–904.

Henderson, A. S., Korten, A. E., Jacomb, P. A., Mackinnon, A. J., Jorm, A. F., Christensen, H., & Rodgers, B. (1997). The course of depression in the elderly: A longitudinal community-based study in Australia. *Psychological Medicine, 27*(1), 119–129.

Horwitz, A. V., & Wakefield, J. C. (2007). *The loss of sadness: How psychiatry transformed normal sorrow into depressive disorder.* New York: Oxford University Press.

Jarvis, E. (1971). *Insanity and idiocy in Massachusetts: Report of the Commission on Lunacy, 1855.* Cambridge, MA: Harvard University Press.

Kahn, J. R., & Pearlin, L. I. (2006). Financial strain over the life course and health among older adults. *Journal of Health and Social Behavior, 47*(1), 17–31.

Kaplan, G. A. (1999). What is the role of the social environment in understanding inequalities in health? *Annals of the New York Academy of Sciences, 896*, 116–119.

Karam, E. G., Tabet, C. C., Alam, D., Shamseddeen, W., Chatila, Y., Mneimneh, Z., … Hamalian, M. (2009). Bereavement related and non-bereavement related depressions: A comparative field study. *Journal of Affective Disorders, 112*(1–3), 102–110.

Kendler, K. S., Hettema, J. M., Butera, F., Gardner, C. O., & Prescott, C. A. (2003). Life event dimensions of loss, humiliation, entrapment, and danger in the prediction of onsets of major depression and generalized anxiety. *Archives of General Psychiatry, 60*(8), 789–796.

Kessler, R. C., Berglund, P., Demler, O., Jin, R., Koretz, D., Merikangas, K. R., … National Comorbidity Survey Replication. (2003). The epidemiology of major depressive disorder: Results from the National Comorbidity Survey Replication (NCS-R). *Journal of the American Medical Association, 289*(23), 3095–3105.

Kessler, R. C., McGonagle, K. A., Swartz, M., Blazer, D. G., & Nelson, C. B. (1993). Sex and depression in the National Comorbidity Survey. I: Lifetime prevalence, chronicity and recurrence. *Journal of Affective Disorders, 29*(2–3), 85–96.

Keyes, K. M., Barnes, D. M., & Bates, L. M. (2011). Stress, coping, and depression: Testing a new hypothesis in a prospectively studied general population sample of U.S.-born Whites and Blacks. *Social Science and Medicine, 72*(5), 650–659.

Kim-Cohen, J., Caspi, A., Moffitt, T. E., Harrington, H., Milne, B. J., & Poulton, R. (2003). Prior juvenile diagnoses in adults with mental disorder: Developmental follow-back of a prospective-longitudinal cohort. *Archives of General Psychiatry, 60*(7), 709–717.

Kraaij, V., & de Wilde, E. J. (2001). Negative life events and depressive symptoms in the elderly: A life span perspective. *Aging and Mental Health, 5*(1), 84–91.

Lee, J. (2011). Pathways from education to depression. *Journal of Cross-Cultural Gerontology, 26*(2), 121–135.

Lesser, I. M., Castro, D. B., Gaynes, B. N., Gonzalez, J., Rush, A. J., Alpert, J. E., ... Wisniewski, S. R. (2007). Ethnicity/race and outcome in the treatment of depression: Results from STAR*D. *Medical Care, 45*(11), 1043–1051.

Luo, Y., & Waite, L. J. (2005). The impact of childhood and adult SES on physical, mental, and cognitive well-being in later life. *Journals of Gerontology Series B, Psychological Sciences and Social Sciences, 60*(2), S93-S101.

Lynch, S. M., & George, L. K. (2002). Interlocking trajectories of loss-related events and depressive symptoms among elders. *Journals of Gerontology Series B, Psychological Sciences and Social Sciences, 57*(2), S117-125.

Mair, C., Diez Roux, A. V., Osypuk, T. L., Rapp, S. R., Seeman, T., & Watson, K. E. (2010). Is neighborhood racial/ethnic composition associated with depressive symptoms? The multi-ethnic study of atherosclerosis. *Social Sciences and Medicine, 71*(3), 541–550.

Mead, N., Lester, H., Chew-Graham, C., Gask, L., & Bower, P. (2010). Effects of befriending on depressive symptoms and distress: Systematic review and meta-analysis. *British Journal of Psychiatry, 196*(2), 96–101.

Melfi, C. A., Croghan, T. W., Hanna, M. P., & Robinson, R. L. (2000). Racial variation in antidepressant treatment in a Medicaid population. *Journal of Clinical Psychiatry, 61*(1), 16–21.

Miech, R. A., & Shanahan, M. J. (2000). Socioeconomic status and depression over the life course. *Journal of Health and Social Behavior, 41*, 162–176.

Miranda, J., Chung, J. Y., Green, B. L., Krupnick, J., Siddique, J., Revicki, D. A., & Belin, T. (2003). Treating depression in predominantly low-income young minority women: A randomized controlled trial. *Journal of the American Medical Association, 290*(1), 57–65.

Mojtabai, R., & Olfson, M. (2004). Major depression in community-dwelling middle-aged and older adults: Prevalence and 2- and 4-year follow-up symptoms. *Psychological Medicine, 34*(4), 623–634.

Monroe, S. M., & Reid, M. W. (2008). Gene-environment interactions in depression research: Genetic polymorphisms and life-stress polyprocedures. *Psychological Sciences, 19*(10), 947–956.

Murphy, J. M., Gilman, S. E., Lesage, A., Horton, N. J., Rasic, D., Trinh, N. H., ... Smoller, J. W. (2010). Time trends in mortality associated with depression: Findings from the stirling county study. *Canadian Journal of Psychiatry/Revue Canadienne de Psychiatrie, 55*(12), 776–783.

Murphy, J. M., Olivier, D. C., Monson, R. R., Sobol, A. M., Federman, E. B., & Leighton, A. H. (1991). Depression and anxiety in relation to social status. A prospective epidemiologic study. *Archives of General Psychiatry, 48*(3), 223–229.

Musick, M. A., Koenig, H. G., Hays, J. C., & Cohen, H. J. (1998). Religious activity and depression among community-dwelling elderly persons with cancer: The moderating effect of race. *Journals of Gerontology Series B, Psychological Sciences and Social Sciences, 53*(4), S218-227.

Norton, M. C., Skoog, I., Toone, L., Corcoran, C., Tschanz, J. T., Lisota, R. D., ... Cache County Investigators. (2006). Three-year incidence of first-onset depressive syndrome in a population sample of older adults: The Cache County study. *American Journal of Geriatric Psychiatry, 14*(3), 237–245.

Paczkowski, M. M., & Galea, S. (2010). Sociodemographic characteristics of the neighborhood and depressive symptoms. *Current Opinion in Psychiatry, 23*(4), 337–341.

Pingitore, D., Snowden, L., Sansone, R. A., & Klinkman, M. (2001). Persons with depressive symptoms and the treatments they receive: A comparison of primary care physicians and psychiatrists. *International Journal of Psychiatry in Medicine, 31*(1), 41–60.

Prigerson, H. G., Horowitz, M. J., Jacobs, S. C., Parkes, C. M., Aslan, M., Goodkin, K., ... Maciejewski, P. K. (2009). Prolonged grief disorder: Psychometric validation of criteria proposed for DSM-V and ICD-11. *PLoS Med 6*(8), e1000121.

Rosenquist, J. N., Fowler, J. H., & Christakis, N. A. (2011). Social network determinants of depression. *Molecular Psychiatry, 16*(3), 273–281.

Ryan, J., Carriere, I., Ritchie, K., Stewart, R., Toulemonde, G., Dartigues, J. F., ... Ancelin, M. L. (2008). Late-life depression and mortality:

Influence of gender and antidepressant use. *British Journal of Psychiatry, 192*(1), 12–18.

Sicotte, M., Alvarado, B. E., León, E. M., & Zunzunegui, M. V. (2008). Social networks and depressive symptoms among elderly women and men in Havana, Cuba. *Aging and Mental Health, 12*(2), 193–201.

Sorkin, D. H., Pham, E., & Ngo-Metzger, Q. (2009). Racial and ethnic differences in the mental health needs and access to care of older adults in California. *Journal of the American Geriatrics Society, 57*(12), 2311–2317.

Stroebe, M. S., Folkman, S., Hansson, R. O., & Schut, H. (2006). The prediction of bereavement outcome: Development of an integrative risk factor framework. *Social Science and Medicine, 63*(9), 2440–2451.

Strothers, H. S., III., Rust, G., Minor, P., Fresh, E., Druss, B., & Satcher, D. (2005). Disparities in antidepressant treatment in Medicaid elderly diagnosed with depression. *Journal of the American Geriatrics Society, 53*(3), 456–461.

Szanton, S. L., Thorpe, R. J., & Whitfield, K. (2010). Life-course financial strain and health in African-Americans. *Social Science and Medicine, 71*(2), 259–265.

Trivedi, M. H., Rush, A. J., Wisniewski, S. R., Nierenberg, A. A., Warden, D., Ritz, L., … STAR*D Study Team. (2006). Evaluation of outcomes with citalopram for depression using measurement-based care in STAR*D: Implications for clinical practice. *American Journal of Psychiatry, 163*(1), 28–40.

Unutzer, J., Katon, W., Callahan, C. M., Williams, J. W., Jr., Hunkeler, E., Harpole, L., … IMPACT Investigators. (2002). Collaborative care management of late-life depression in the primary care setting: A randomized controlled trial. *Journal of the American Medical Association, 288*(22), 2836–2845.

Vink, D., Aartsen, M. J., & Schoevers, R. A. (2008). Risk factors for anxiety and depression in the elderly: A review. *Journal of Affective Disorders, 106*(1–2), 29–44.

Virnig, B., Huang, Z., Lurie, N., Musgrave, D., McBean, A. M., & Dowd, B. (2004). Does Medicare managed care provide equal treatment for mental illness across races? *Archives of General Psychiatry, 61*(2), 201–205.

Wainwright, N. W. J., & Surtees, P. G. (2002). Childhood adversity, gender and depression over the life-course. *Journal of Affective Disorders, 72*, 33–44.

Wakefield, J. C. (1998). The DSM's theory-neutral nosology is scientifically progressive: Response to Follette and Houts (1996). *Journal of Consulting and Clinical Psychology, 66*(5), 846–852.

Wakefield, J. C., Schmitz, M. F., First, M. B., & Horwitz, A. V. (2007). Extending the bereavement exclusion for major depression to other losses: Evidence from the National Comorbidity Survey. *Archives of General Psychiatry, 64*(4), 433–440.

Wight, R. G., Cummings, J. R., Karlamangla, A. S., & Aneshensel, C. S. (2009). Urban neighborhood context and change in depressive symptoms in late life. *Journals of Gerontology Series B, Psychological Sciences and Social Sciences, 64*(2), 247–251.

Wilby, F. (2011). Depression and social networks in community dwelling elders: A descriptive study. *Journal of Gerontological Social Work, 54*(3), 246–259.

Wilhelm, K., & Parker, G. (1994). Sex differences in lifetime depression rates: Fact or artefact? *Psychological Medicine, 24*(1), 97–111.

Williams, B. R., Baker, P. S., Allman, R. M., & Roseman, J. M. (2006). The feminization of bereavement among community-dwelling older adults. *Journal of Women and Aging, 18*(3), 3–18.

Yang, F. M., Tommet, D., & Jones, R. N. (2009). Disparities in self-reported geriatric depressive symptoms due to sociodemographic differences: An extension of the bi-factor item response theory model for use in differential item functioning. *Journal of Psychiatric Research, 43*(12), 1025–1035.

Zisook, S., & Kendler, K. S. (2007). Is bereavement-related depression different than non-bereavement-related depression? *Psychological Medicine, 37*(6), 779–794.

Zisook, S., Paulus, M., Shuchter, S. R., & Judd, L. L. (1997). The many faces of depression following spousal bereavement. *Journal of Affective Disorders, 45*(1–2), 85–95.

Zisook, S., Shuchter, S. R., Pedrelli, P., Sable, J., & Deaciuc, S. C. (2001). Bupropion sustained release for bereavement: Results of an open trial. *Journal of Clinical Psychiatry, 62*(4), 227–230.

11

DEPRESSION IN DEMENTIA

Christopher M. Marano, Paul B. Rosenberg, and Constantine G. Lyketsos

CLINICIANS HAVE long struggled with the problem of how to help patients with dementia and their families in the absence of a definitive and curative treatment. To optimize current treatment, one must recognize the importance of neuropsychiatric symptoms of dementia, including depression, agitation, hallucinations, delusions, insomnia, and behavioral symptoms. Among these, depression is one of the most troubling and prominent. Depression in dementia is clearly worth diagnosing and treating given its substantial adverse effects on patient and caregiver quality of life. A crucial question is whether the symptoms of depression in dementia differ from those of a typical major depressive episode.

As the most common cause of dementia and the subject of the vast majority of dementia research, this chapter will focus on depression in Alzheimer's dementia (AD) as a prototype for the evaluation and management of depression in dementia. We will briefly review the epidemiology and noncognitive manifestations of AD and then discuss current evidence regarding the presentation, etiology, diagnosis, and treatment of depression in AD.

BRIEF OVERVIEW OF ALZHEIMER'S DEMENTIA
Epidemiology

Alzheimer's disease is a neurodegenerative disorder associated with aging that is a major cause of disability and burden to society and caregivers. As the most common cause of dementia (estimated to account for 60%–80% of all dementia cases), most epidemiologic studies focus on AD. Vascular dementia is considered to be the second most common cause of dementia, though it is important to note that Alzheimer's and brain vascular pathology often coexist, and it can be difficult to distinguish between the two conditions (Langa, Foster, & Larson 2004). Approximately 5 million people in the United States have AD with an expected increase to about 15 million by 2050 (Hebert, Scherr, Bienias, Bennett, & Evans, 2003).

AD patients become fully dependent for their activities of daily living (ADLs) as the disease progresses and many require institutional care. Aggregate costs of health care payments for AD and other dementias is estimated at $183 billion/year in the United States alone with an additional estimated $202 billion of unpaid care provided by families and other caregivers (Alzheimer's Association, Thies, & Bleiler, 2011). Moreover, the emotional costs to caregivers are incalculable with the increasing burden of caregiving leading to frail physical and mental health for the caregiver (Rabins, Lyketsos, & Steele, 2006).

Alzheimer's disease is largely a disease of old age. Prevalence estimates increase from about 1% at ages 60–64 to 43%–68% at ages >95 (Franceschi, Colombo, Rossi, & Canal, 1997; Kukull & Bowen, 2002). Lower prevalence estimates in the very old were found in a population sample from Cache County, Utah, with a prevalence of 28% above age 90 (Breitner et al., 1999). Evidence also exists that incidence declines after age 90 (Miech et al., 2002).

Clinical Course

AD presents slowly and insidiously, and families often interpret cognitive changes as changes in personality, mood, or attitude. In the clinic, the chief complaint is equally likely to be mood disorder or cognitive change. Typical neuropsychological findings in early AD include deficits in verbal episodic memory and executive function (Binetti et al., 1996; Collie & Maruff, 2000) with accumulating deficits in verbal fluency, comprehension, gnosis, and praxis developing as the disease progresses (Petersen et al., 1999). Neurologic symptoms, including parkinsonism and frontal release signs (i.e., grasp, palmomental, snout, and glabellar reflexes), often occur in AD, particularly in the later stages. Average survival time from diagnosis for patients over 65 is 4 to 8 years, though some may live up to 20 years (Alzheimer's Association et al., 2011).

RELATIONSHIP BETWEEN PREMORBID DEPRESSION AND DEMENTIA

The relationship between depression prior to the onset of dementia and the subsequent development of dementia is an area of active investigation (Steffens et al., 2006). A detailed discussion is beyond the scope of this chapter, though extensively covered in several recent reviews (Butters et al., 2008, Byers & Yaffe, 2011; Ownby, Crocco, Acevedo, John, & Loewenstein, 2006). Briefly, cognitive impairment is a common feature of late-life depression and often persists after mood symptom remission (Alexopoulos, Young, Mattis, & Kakuma, 1993; Alexopoulos, Young, & Meyers, 1993; Bhalla et al., 2006). Furthermore, substantial evidence suggests late-life depression is both a risk factor for and a prodrome of dementia. A recent meta-analysis estimated that depression doubles the risk of subsequent AD (Ownby et al., 2006).

There are two predominant (though not exclusive) constructs regarding the relationship between late-life depression and dementia. The first construct centers on Alzheimer's disease. As a prodrome, late-life depression represents an initial, noncognitive manifestation of AD pathology. Evidence for late-life depression as AD prodrome is the high conversion rate to dementia in individuals with late-life depression and co-occurring cognitive impairment (Alexopoulos, Meyers, et al., 1993; Alexopoulos, Young, & Meyers, 1993). Evidence for depression as a risk factor for AD includes the following: (1) dementia risk increases as the time between diagnosis of first depression and diagnosis of AD increases (Ownby et al., 2006); and (2) increased Alzheimer's pathology (amyloid plaques and neurofibrillary tangles) in AD patients with a lifetime depression history (Rapp et al., 2006). The second construct is the vascular depression hypothesis, first postulated by both Alexopoulos and Krishnan (Alexopoulos et al., 1997; Krishnan, Hays, & Blazer, 1997) and substantiated by considerable supporting evidence (as reviewed in Culang-Reinlieb et al., 2010). The hypothesis states that brain vascular disease can predispose, precipitate, or perpetuate depression in a subset of late-life depression patients. This brain vascular disease damages critical corticostriatal circuits, resulting in depression with cognitive impairment, particularly executive dysfunction, and poor antidepressant response.

NEUROPSYCHIATRIC SYMPTOMS OF DEMENTIA

While AD is often described as a purely cognitive disorder, patients frequently, almost universally, suffer from a multitude of neuropsychiatric symptoms. There are several population-based epidemiologic studies examining NPS in AD. For example, in the Cache County study of memory and aging, 56% of participants with dementia exhibited at least one neuropsychiatric disturbance on the neuropsychiatric inventory in the past month (Lyketsos et al., 2000). Symptoms included (in order of prevalence) apathy, delusions, agitation/aggression, and depression. The Cardiovascular Health Study reported similar results (Lyketsos et al., 2002) with depression being the most prevalent neuropsychiatric symptom (32.3%). Comparable population-based studies in the United Kingdom found similar symptom frequencies (Burns, Jacoby, & Levy, 1990). The cumulative prevalence of depression over 5 years was 77% (Steinberg et al., 2008). The *incidence* of depression over an 18-month follow-up period in the Cache County study was comparably high (18%). Neuropsychiatric symptoms in AD are not benign variants within a broader illness but can lead to significant functional disability and caregiver stress above and beyond that caused by cognitive decline (Schulz & Martire, 2004). Patients with AD are struggling to make best use of their remaining cognitive skills, but the development of depression, delusions, and anxiety limits their ability to utilize these skills in daily life. Similarly, there is no question that these neuropsychiatric symptoms detract from quality of life for both patients and caregivers.

The differentiation of neuropsychiatric symptoms in AD is important to the targeting of therapies and critical in the discussion of depression in dementia. Several groups have used factor analytic methods to subtype neuropsychiatric symptoms. Most investigators agree that at least two groups of disturbance are distinguishable, one with predominately affective symptoms and one with predominately psychotic symptoms (delusions and hallucinations) (Lyketsos, Breitner, & Rabins, 2001). Affective symptoms are most common and troubling to caregivers, especially in earlier dementia (Schulz & Martire, 2004). Affective symptoms are often referred to using the term "depression" but often have a different mix of symptoms than what is seen in depressed older patients without dementia. Specifically, those with dementia are more anxious, agitated, delusional, or inattentive. They also exhibit less guilt, less self-deprecation, and are rarely suicidal (Zubenko et al., 2003).

EPIDEMIOLOGY OF DEPRESSION IN DEMENTIA

Many studies have estimated the rates of depression in dementia with widely varying reported prevalence

based on depression criteria utilized and the population studied. Table 11.1 lists representative studies. Risk factors for developing depression in AD include a prior history of depressive episodes (Garre-Olmo et al., 2003; Migliorelli et al., 1995), family history of depression (Lyketsos, Tune, Pearlson, & Steele, 1996; Pearlson et al., 1990), younger onset of dementia (Rosness, Barca, & Engedal, 2010; Savva et al., 2009), and possibly low educational level (Hargrave, Reed, & Mungas, 2000). Depressive symptoms are relatively persistent with several studies showing about half of depressed patients with dementia remaining depressed 1 year later (Garre-Olmo et al., 2003, Starkstein, Mizrahi, & Garau, 2005).

ASSESSMENT OF DEPRESSION IN DEMENTIA

Symptom Clusters and Diagnostic Dilemmas

These varying rates reflect the diagnostic dilemma of diagnosing dementia in AD. Several studies have compared symptom clusters in depressed patients with and without dementia. Janzing et al. found that dementia patients had more "motivation" symptoms and fewer "mood" symptoms than a group without dementia, despite comparable severity of depressive symptoms. The motivation factor included fatigue, slowness of thinking and movement, lack of interest in activities, and decreased affective response to pleasurable activities. The mood factor included worry, depressed mood, tearfulness, hopelessness, and suicidal thoughts. Their cohort included patients with subsyndromal depression and is representative of patients typically seen in practice (Janzing, Hooijer, van't Hof, & Zitman, 2002). Li, Meyer, and Thornby (2001) similarly noted that motivational symptoms predominate among depressive symptoms of AD. Zubenko et al. (2003) found depressed AD patients to be more likely than depressed nondemented patients to have delusions, hallucinations, and complaints of concentration difficulties and less likely to report guilt or suicidal ideation. Tractenberg et al. (2003) and Bassiony et al. (2002) concur that delusions and depression cluster together in AD. In these studies insomnia and weight loss were equally common in AD and nondemented patients. In contrast, Purandare et al. (2001) reported that neurovegetative signs did discriminate depressed AD patients from nondepressed patients. Rubin et al. (2001)

Table 11.1 Representative Studies of the Prevalence of Depression in Dementia

REFERENCE	ESTIMATED PREVALENCE OF DEPRESSIVE SYMPTOMS IN DEMENTIA (%)	COMMENTS
Garre-Olmo et al., 2003	50	NPI depressive symptoms 55% persistence at 12-month follow-up Clinical sample
Migliorelli et al., 1995	51	28% dysthymia 23% major depression Clinical sample
Weiner, Edland, & Luszczynska, 1994	1.3–1.5	Strict criteria (*DSM-III-R* major depressive episode) Clinical sample
Starkstein, Jorge, Mizrahi, & Robinson, 2005	52	Strict criteria (*DSM-IV* major and minor depression) 26% major depression 26% minor depression Clinical sample (tertiary care dementia clinic
Lyketsos et al., 2000 Cache County Study	24 (20% for AD)	NPI depressive symptoms Population sample
Lyketsos et al., 2002 Cardiovascular Health Study	32	NPI depressive symptoms Population sample
Burns, Jacoby, & Levy, 1990	24	Trained observer, 43% rated as depressed by relatives 63% had at least one depressive symptom Case registry sample

NPI, Neuropsychiatric Inventory.

noted that indecision and fatigue are particularly helpful in discriminating depressed from nondepressed AD patients.

Noting the different symptoms of depression, Lyketsos and colleagues used latent class analysis to propose the "affective syndrome of Alzheimer's disease" (Lyketsos, Breitner, & Rabins, 2001), which includes one or more symptoms of a core affective disturbance (defined as depression, irritability, anxiety, or euphoria) combined with one or more less prominent associated symptoms (defined as aggression, psychomotor agitation, delusions, hallucinations, sleep disturbance, or appetite disturbance). A later National Institute of Mental Health (NIMH) consensus conference of experts in the field proposed provisional diagnostic criteria for depression of Alzheimer's disease (Olin, Katz, Meyers, Schneider, & Lebowitz, 2002; Olin, Schneider, et al., 2002). Derived from the *DSM-IV* criteria for a major depressive episode, the criteria propose several changes in an effort to avoid overlap with cognitive deficits and/ or chronic medical illness: (1) requires only three (not five) symptoms of a major depressive episode; (2) does not require the presence of symptoms most of the day, nearly every day; (3) adds criteria for irritability and social isolation or withdrawal; and (4) revises the loss of interest criteria to reflect decreased positive affect or pleasure from social contact and usual activities. Table 11.2 lists the Provisional Diagnostic Criteria for Depression of Alzheimer's Disease.

Subsequent studies have compared the provisional diagnostic criteria to other diagnostic criteria,

Table 11.2 Summary of the National Institute of Mental Health Provisional Diagnostic Criteria for Depression of Alzheimer's Disease

CRITERION

1. Clinically significant depressed mood (e.g., depressed, sad, hopeless, discouraged, tearful)
2. Decreased positive affect or pleasure in response to social contacts and usual activities
3. Social isolation or withdrawal
4. Disruption in appetite
5. Disruption in sleep
6. Psychomotor changes (e.g., agitation or retardation)
7. Irritability
8. Fatigue or loss of energy

including *DSM-IV* criteria for major depression. An observational study of patients referred to a memory clinic found 13.4% of patients met *DSM-IV* criteria for a major depression, and 27.4% met the provisional diagnostic criteria (Vilalta-Franch et al., 2006). A later study of research subjects from Alzheimer's Disease Research Centers reported that 44% met provisional diagnostic criteria, 14% met *DSM-IV* major depression criteria, and 36% met *DSM-IV* criteria for major or minor depression. The provisional criteria correctly identified all participants meeting *DSM-IV* criteria for major depression and correlated well with major or minor depression (Teng et al., 2008). A more recent latent class analysis of patients referred to a memory clinic reported three symptom clusters considered to represent *DSM-IV* major depression, *DSM-IV* minor depression (a more heterogeneous group), and no depression (Starkstein, Dragovic, Jorge, Brockman, & Robinson, 2011). Based on these studies, there appear to be at least two types of clinically significant depressive symptoms in AD—a core group meeting more stringent *DSM-IV* criteria for a major depressive episode and a second less well-defined group who has been variably identified using different diagnostic criteria. Regardless of diagnostic criteria, patients in either group could have clinically significant depressive symptoms that necessitate treatment and can be diagnosed with a careful clinical assessment as described in the following section.

Caregiver Input and Caregiver Bias in Depression Assessment

Caregiver input is essential for adequate assessment of depressive symptoms in dementia. Deficits in short-term recall may rob a patient of the sense of time passing, of accurate recall of daily functioning, and of the severity of symptoms. In addition, AD patients have deficits in abstract thinking and executive functioning, which diminish their capacity to integrate emotions and behavioral reactions over time. Thus, they often have difficulty articulating a depressed mood, even though they may have profound sadness or anhedonia. AD patients often answer questions about their mood with cliché "empty" responses, possibly due to decreased verbal fluency (Cerhan et al., 2002, Storey, Slavin, & Kinsella, 2002). However, caregiver report may be biased by caregiver symptoms (Rosenberg, Mielke, & Lyketsos, 2005). For example, caregivers may tend to see the situation as "all bad" due to stress, just as patients may see the situation as "all good" due to not recalling problems. Thus, caregivers may overreport and AD patients may underreport symptoms. Burke et al. (1998) administered a modified Geriatric Depression Scale (GDS) to both patients and caregivers and found that caregivers rated depressive symptoms higher on all items. Teri and Truax (1994) found a moderate correlation between caregiver depression and patient depression. Moreover, depressed caregivers nearly always rated the patient as depressed, whereas nondepressed caregivers gave a more balanced assessment. Rubin et al. (2001) reported different symptom constellations arising out of factor analysis of caregiver and patients reports. These correlations between caregiver and patient mood are consistent enough to suggest a causal relationship. However, since there is no "gold standard" rating scale for depression of AD, they do not clarify whether patients underreport or caregivers overreport mood symptoms in AD. Thus, the clinician is advised to utilize *both* caregiver and patient input in assessing mood symptoms in AD, but not to take an average of the two. The clinician may need to factor in caregiver stress as a bias in reporting and utilize clinical judgment in how to incorporate caregiver input, patient report, and observation into a coherent whole. This complex process involves considerably more time and judgment than routine office management of major depressive episodes in adults.

Apathy Versus Depression

Apathy refers to deficits in motivation without appearing sad or depressed. Patient apathy is a common presenting complaint by caregivers who feel frustrated and upset that the patient "just doesn't want to do anything." In institutional settings there is a converse problem, where apathy, which can lead to serious deconditioning, may remain undiagnosed because patients are passive and easier to manage. The distinction between apathy and depression is often difficult. In practice, apathy is often treated as a symptom of mood disorder rather than a separate syndrome. In the initial Cache County study it was the most frequent neuropsychiatric symptom of dementia and was often present in the absence of other depressive symptoms (Steinberg et al., 2003). In a large clinical sample of AD patients, 37% were significantly apathetic with many (24%) not suffering from coexisting major depression (Starkstein, Petracca, Chemerinski, & Kremer, 2001). Apathy is also associated with poorer cognitive functioning as well as worse ADL impairment (Landes, Sperry, Strauss, & Geldmacher, 2001) and may be a symptom of preclinical AD (Berger, Fratiglioni, Forsell, Winblad, & Backman, 1999). Since apathy is better associated with measures of executive dysfunction than with mood measures (Stout, Wyman, Johnson, Peavy, & Salmon, 2003), it was not included as a criterion in the provisional diagnostic criteria for depression of Alzheimer's disease.

CLINICAL EVALUATION OF DEPRESSION IN DEMENTIA

In the clinical setting, patients with depression in dementia may present with a variety of complaints, including depression, anxiety, "nerves," memory problems, lack of motivation, and loss of interest. As discussed in the previous section, complaints come more often from the family than from the patient. Therefore, caregiver input is needed both for proper diagnosis and for treatment planning, and no evaluation should be considered complete without caregiver input. This input may take various forms such as individual interviews with the patient and caregiver separately, telephone interview with the caregiver, or formal or informal treatment planning meetings with institutional staff (such as in an assisted living or nursing home environment). It is particularly valuable to interview the patient and caregiver separately whenever possible, which allows both to candidly express their feelings and concerns without worrying about causing greater conflict or friction, particularly in a family dyad. The very behaviors that a caregiver spouse might feel uncomfortable discussing in an interview with the couple—such as disrobing, aggression, incontinence, or inappropriate sexual behavior—are likely to be the behaviors causing maximal stress. The clinician should also be alert to the cultural and educational backgrounds of patients and caregivers, particularly in phrasing questions and interpreting responses. Some patients and families may use terms such as "depression" and "anxiety" with a meaning similar to the clinician's, but frequently the clinician needs to explore what the patient and family are trying to express. These communication issues may be due to cultural differences or to the patient's cognitive deficits. The clinician should be alert to either possibility.

Many medical and neurologic conditions as well as medication toxicities can confound diagnosis by mimicking depressive symptoms (Table 11.3). Common neurologic confounds include flat affect, bradykinesia, and bradyphrenia of Parkinson's disease; pathologic tearfulness due to pseudobulbar palsy in multiple sclerosis; and "amotivation" from apraxia or executive dysfunction in many dementias. Psychomotor retardation is common to many medical conditions, including congestive heart failure, chronic obstructive pulmonary disease, malignancy, and drug toxicity. Diminished concentration or sustained attention to task is common to many neurologic illnesses and delirium and is often misdiagnosed as depression.

The diagnostic workup for suspected depression in dementia should be individualized to the patient's presentation but also based on routine evaluation for dementia itself (Table 11.4). A thorough physical and neurologic examination is a must for clues to medical confounds. A review of medications is equally essential. Clinicians should be particularly alert for the cognitive toxicity of anticholinergic medications (Mulsant et al., 2003; Sunderland et al., 1987) and sedation from benzodiazepines or opioid analgesics. If the mood change is relatively acute, the clinician must rule out common causes of delirium in demented patients, including urinary tract infection, pneumonia, metabolic disturbances, and recent medication changes.

When in doubt about the diagnosis or severity of depression, reliable and valid rating scales can help clarify the clinical picture. Numerous rating scales have been used in research and clinical care

Table 11.3 Medical Conditions and Medications That Can Mimic Depression in Dementia

MEDICAL CONDITION	MEDICATION
Parkinson's disease	Corticosteroids
Multiple sclerosis	Benzodiazepines
Hypothyroidism	Chemotherapeutic agents
Neurosyphilis	Lithium toxicity
Cancer	Digoxin toxicity
Congestive heart failure	Phenytoin toxicity
Chronic obstructive pulmonary disease	Opioid analgesics
Delirium	Carbamazepine
	Tricyclic antidepressants
	Anticholinergic medications (benztropine, antihistamines, chlorpromazine, thioridazine)

Table 11.4 Diagnostic Workup for Suspected Depression in Dementia

DIAGNOSTIC TEST	RATIONALE
Complete blood count (CBC)	Rule out anemia (as cause of fatigue)
Metabolic panel	Rule out hyperglycemia, hypernatremia, uremia
Liver function tests	Rule out hepatic encephalopathy (also check ammonia if high suspicion)
Thyroid panel	Rule out hypothyroidism
Vitamin B12 level	Rule out B12 deficiency (usually from decreased absorption due to achlorhydria in elderly)
Urine toxicology screen	Rule out occult ingestion, sedative abuse
Serum drug levels (i.e., lithium phenytoin, carbamazepine, digoxin)	Rule out inattention and reduced state of alertness due to toxicity
Rapid plasma reagin (RPR)	Rule out neurosyphilis
Magnetic resonance imaging (MRI) or computerized tomography (CT)	Rule out stroke, subdural hematoma, brain tumor, occult closed-head injury
Lumbar puncture	Only if infection is suspected (tuberculosis, HIV, herpetic encephalitis)
Electroencephalogram	Only if seizure or delirium is suspected

of depression in dementia. Table 11.5 summarizes the features and psychometric properties of the major rating scales. We recommend the Cornell Scale for Depression in Dementia (CSDD) as the most appropriate scale for general clinical use given its ease of administration and greatest sensitivity to change compared to other rating scales (Mayer et al., 2006). Administering the CSDD involves interviewing both patient and caregiver; the clinician then integrates observation and reports into item scores. In more advanced dementia the patient's report becomes increasingly unreliable due to difficulties in comprehending the questions and responding with expressive language, and also due

Table 11.5 Assessment Instruments for Depression in Dementia

INSTRUMENT	ASSESSMENT	RATER	NO. OF ITEMS	RANGE	PSYCHOMETRIC PROPERTIES IN AD	COMMENTS
Hamilton Depression Rating Scale (HAM-D) (Hamilton, 1960)	Depression severity	Patient, interviewer	17 (most commonly used) or 21	0–52	Reliability approximately 0.9 (Gottlieb, Gur, & Gur, 1988). Sensitivity 90% but specificity varied 9%–63% for diagnosis of depression in AD (Vida, Des Rosiers, Carrier, & Gauthier, 1994; Lichtenberg, Marcopulos, Steiner, & Tabscott, 1992).	Most widely used scale in nonelderly but does not incorporate caregiver input. Optimal cutoff for depression in AD is >9.
Cornell scale for depression in dementia (CSDD) (Alexopoulos, Abrams, Young, & Shamoian, 1988)	Depression severity	Patient, caregiver, interviewer	19	0–38	Reliability 0.63–0.84 (Kurlowicz, Evans, Strumpf, & Maislin, 2002). Correlation with HAM-D 0.86. Sensitivity 90% and specificity 75% for diagnosis of depression in AD (Vida et al., 1994).	Most widely used scale

Scale	Measure	Administered by	Number of items	Range	Reliability/validity	Comments
Geriatric depression scale (GDS) (Yesavage et al., 1982)	Depression severity	Patient	15 (short version) 30 (long version)	0–15 (short version) 0–30 (long version)	Reliability >0.9. Correlation with HAM-D >0.8 (Lichtenberg et al., 1992).	Easy to administer but heavily dependent on patient comprehension of items
Montgomery-Asberg Depression Rating Scale (MADRS) (Montgomery & Asberg, 1979)	Depression severity	Patient, interviewer	10	0–60	Reliability 0.86. Correlation with HAM-D 0.82.	Designed to be sensitive to mood change. Minimal data for validity in depression in AD
Zung Depression Rating Scale (Zung, 1965)	Depression severity	Patient (self-administered)	20	0–80	Reliability 0.8–0.9. Significant correlation with HAM-D but only for early stages of dementia (Gottlieb et al., 1988).	Self-administered scale of questionable validity in dementia due to patients' tendency to underreport symptoms

AD, Alzheimer's dementia.

to difficulties with abstractions posed in questions about emotional state; thus, the clinician relies more on observations and caregiver report.

CAUSES OF DEPRESSION IN DEMENTIA

Depression usually appears to have multiple risk factors rather than a single unitary cause. Depression in dementia is no exception as there are significant psychosocial and biologic factors that increase risk for depression. Knowledge of these risk factors may present opportunities for early intervention and education.

Psychosocial Factors

"Who wouldn't be depressed if they had AD?" It is often assumed that the diagnosis itself should lead to depression, particularly if the patient is aware of the diagnosis. But since even the highest prevalence estimates for depression of AD are around 50%, an equal number of AD patients lack mood disorder. The relationship between awareness of deficits and depression is complex. For example, it is often assumed that awareness of deficits is a major risk for depression, and that lack of awareness in advanced disease is protective against depression. AD patients tend to have insight into their cognitive deficits early in the course of disease (McDaniel, Edland, & Heyman, 1995), yet several studies report no association between insight into AD and depression (Verhey, Ponds, Rozendaal, & Jolles, 1995). Additionally, several recent prospective studies report little change in depressive symptoms before and after the diagnosis of AD (Wilson, Arnold, Beck, Bienias, & Bennett, 2008; Wilson et al., 2010). Conversely, two studies report an association between insight and depression as well as hopelessness (Harwood, Sultzer, & Wheatley, 2000; Harwood & Sultzer, 2002). Therefore, awareness of deficits can contribute to depression in some, but not all, of dementia patients with depression.

Individuals with dementia, especially younger individuals, experience major social stresses early in the illness, particularly involving loss of occupational function and diminished ability to socialize. Families may make strenuous efforts to minimize the impact of these changes and to keep them out of the patient's awareness so as not to confront the patient with his or her functional deficits. For example, many patients with dementia will sign checks that their spouses have made out to maintain the illusion of still being in charge of the finances. There are instances where patients maintain the illusion of working even with significant cognitive deficits, for example, going to the office daily to "work" at his or her old desk even if the patient no longer can perform any functional work. Another stressor is the AD patient's knowledge, however cloudy, that he or she has increased dependency needs. Even patients with advanced stages of AD will frequently resist care because of denial and anger regarding their functional dependency.

Beyond these general stressors of dependency and functional decline, specific cognitive deficits may be detrimental to patients' self-image and self-esteem. One common and poignant example is diminished verbal fluency as evidenced by word-finding deficits (Cerhan et al., 2002; Storey, Slavin, & Kinsella, 2002). When patients cannot speak fluently, they often feel frustrated and embarrassed in social situations and may avoid social contacts to avoid these conflicts. In more advanced stages of dementia, AD patients frequently suffer from agnosia (Storey, Slavin, & Kinsella, 2002). Patients may wander hazardously due to lack of cognizance of the distinction between different rooms in a facility or between indoors and outdoors, and they may require placement in a locked dementia unit. Even patients with fairly advanced disease are often aware of the locked nature of the facility and become demoralized as a result. Disorientation to time, date, and situation can lead to profound mood changes. It is not uncommon for AD patients to be tearful, sad, and beseeching because they cannot fathom where they live, or why they live there, or what the purpose of living there is, particularly if they are in a dementia unit or skilled nursing setting. The clinician should be sensitive to the interaction between the patient's awareness of functional limitations and vulnerability to depression.

Biologic Factors

NEUROCHEMISTRY

Several pathologic studies suggest that neuronal degeneration in monoaminergic (serotoninergic and norepinephrinergic) brainstem nuclei is associated with depression in AD. Zubenko and Moossy (1988) studied 37 brains from patients with pathologic diagnoses of AD and found that depressive symptoms in these patients were associated with decreased numbers of pigmented cell bodies in the locus coeruleus (LC) and substantia nigra (SN), which supply the majority of the monoaminergic innervation to the brain. Indeed, these changes in cell number were associated with a marked decrease in norepinephrine in the neocortex and hippocampus as well (Zubenko, Moossy, & Kopp, 1990). There are two comparable studies supporting these findings in LC though not SN (Forstl et al., 1992; Zweig et al., 1988). These findings were considered supportive of the hypothesis that depression was due to decreased monoaminergic activity. However, a subsequent report failed to replicate these findings and highlighted the methodologic problems of earlier studies (Hoogendijk et al., 1999). These results may be due to cell loss in LC and SN being associated with cognitive decline in AD rather than specifically with depression. A more recent postmortem study found that loss of serotonin 1A receptors in the hippocampus of AD patients specifically correlated with depressive symptoms. Given the mixed findings as well as the failure of monoaminergic antidepressants in recent clinical trials (as discussed later), the monoaminergic theory of depression in AD is uncertain.

GENETICS

Cognitive and mood symptoms of AD appear to have different genetic vulnerabilities and differ from the genetic vulnerabilities to depression in younger life. The e4 allele of the apolipoprotein E gene has been well established as a risk factor for the development of AD and for earlier age of onset of AD (Khachaturian et al., 2004; Tanzi & Bertram, 2001). As such, the role of the e4 allele in the neuropsychiatric symptoms of AD has also been extensively studied, as recently reviewed by Panza et al. (2011). In summary, studies examining the effect of the e4 allele on depression in AD have been mixed with several studies showing a relationship between the e4 allele and depression but most studies failing to find a relationship. However, many negative studies are hindered by small sample size and limited evaluation of depressive symptoms (Panza et al., 2011). Interestingly, although the e2 allele appears to protect against development of both AD and lifetime unipolar depressive disorder, it has been associated with vulnerability to depression in AD (Holmes et al., 1998).

Brain-derived neurotrophic factor (BDNF) is implicated in the pathogenesis of depression. The BDNF Vall66Met allele is associated with late-life depression (Taylor et al., 2007). This relationship appears to extend to depression in AD (Borroni, Archetti, et al., 2009) in addition to the relationship between the BDNF 11757C allele and depression in AD (Borroni, Grassi, et al., 2009; Zhang et al., 2011).

NEUROIMAGING

The vascular depression hypothesis of late-life depression postulates that brain vascular disease damages critical cortico-striatal circuits, resulting in depression with cognitive impairment. This damage can be visualized on imaging via white matter lesions. In dementia, some, but not all, studies support the role of white matter disease in the development of depression. O'Brien et al. (2000) noted a correlation between frontal lobe white matter hypodensities on brain computerized tomography (CT) scan and depression in AD. Similarly, Mueller et al. (2010) reported an association between frontal white matter lesions and depressed mood in AD and vascular dementia. Starkstein et al. (2009) reported increased parietal white matter lesions in AD patients with depression compared to nondepressed AD patients. The study also noted an association between frontal white matter lesions and apathy (Starkstein et al., 2009). Lind et al. (2006) found no relationship between white matter lesions and depression in a series of patients with a variety of dementias (Lind et al., 2006).

Functional neuroimaging studies are more limited with less robust findings. Hirono et al. (1998) reported that frontal lobe hypometabolism was associated with depressive symptoms in 53 patients with AD. In addition, anterior cingulate hypometabolism was also associated with depressive symptoms, similar to Migneco et al.'s (2001) report associating apathy with depression in AD. Sultzer et al. (1995) found a correlation between parietal hypometabolism and anxiety/depression in 21 patients with AD.

TREATMENT OF DEPRESSION IN DEMENTIA

Medications

Table 11.6 summarizes the results of controlled trials of antidepressant medications for depression in

Table 11.6 Controlled Studies of Antidepressant Medications for Depression in Dementia

REFERENCE	DESIGN	N (TOTAL)	DEPRESSION DIAGNOSIS	TREATMENTS	EFFECT OF TREATMENT ON MOOD OUTCOMES	EFFECT OF TREATMENT ON NON-MOOD OUTCOMES	SAFETY FINDINGS
(Reifler et al., 1989)	8-week, parallel, masked RCT	61	DSM-III major depression HAM-D >14	Imipramine (Mean = 82–83 mg/day), Placebo	0	– Cognitive function declined with drug	Drowsiness and dizziness equally reported for both groups
(Nyth & Gottfries, 1990)	4-week, parallel, masked RCT	98	None Baseline PDD MADRS = 8.0	Citalopram (30 mg/day max), Placebo	0	+ Irritability improved with drug	Mild, expected side effects more common on citalopram
(Nyth et al., 1992)	6-week, parallel, masked RCT	149 (but only 29 with depression and AD)	HAM-D > 13 74% met criteria for DSM-III major depression (total sample)	Citalopram (30 mg/day max), Placebo	+	+ Cognitive function improved with drug	Side effects reported >10% for entire sample: tiredness, sedation, tension
(Petracca, Teson, Chemerinski, Leiguarda, & Starkstein, 1996)	12-week, crossover, RCT	21	DSM-III-R major depression or dysthymia HAM-D >10	Clomipramine (100 mg/day max), Placebo	+	– Cognitive function declined with drug	Dry mouth, dizziness, sleep problems, tremor more frequent in clomipramine

Citation	Design	N	Diagnostic criteria	Medication	Efficacy	Secondary outcomes	Side effects/tolerability
(Roth, Mountjoy, & Amrein, 1996)	6-week, parallel, masked RCT	726	DSM-III major depressive episode HAM-D >13	Moclobemide (400 mg/day max), Placebo	+	+ Cognitive function improved with drug	No significant differences in side effects, ECG, vital signs
(Taragano, Lyketsos, Mangone, Allegri, & Comesana-Diaz, 1997)	45-day, parallel, masked RCT	37	DSM-III major depressive episode	Fluoxetine (25 mg/day max), Amitriptyline (10 mg/day max)	+ (No difference between drugs)	+ Cognitive function improved in both groups	42% completion for amitriptyline; 78% for fluoxetine
(Katona, Hunter, & Bray, 1998)	8-week, parallel, masked RCT	198	RDC major or minor depression MADRS >19	Paroxetine (40 mg/day max), Imipramine (100 mg/day max)	+ (No difference between drugs)	Not Assessed	Paroxetine better tolerated, but marginally so
(Magai, Kennedy, Cohen, & Gomberg, 2000)	8-week, parallel, masked RCT	31	DSM-IV major or minor depression CSDD >2 Gestalt scale >0	Sertraline (100 mg/day max), Placebo	0	+ "Knit-brow face" improved with drug (trend)	Not reported
(Petracca, Chemerinski, & Starkstein, 2001)	6-week, parallel, masked RCT	41	DSM-IV major or minor depression HAMD >13	Fluoxetine (40 mg/day max), Placebo	0	0	Mild tremor more common on fluoxetine
(Lyketsos et al., 2003)	12-week, parallel, masked RCT	44	DSM-IV major depressive episode	Sertraline (150 mg/day max), Placebo	+	+ Placebo group declined more than drug group in ADLs (trend)	No difference between sertraline and placebo
(de Vasconcelos Cunha et al., 2007)	6-week, parallel, masked RCT	31	DSM-IV major depressive episode	Venlafaxine (131.25 mg/day max dose), Placebo	0	Not assessed	No difference between venlafaxine and placebo

(Continued)

Table 11.6 (Continued)

REFERENCE	DESIGN	N (TOTAL)	DEPRESSION DIAGNOSIS	TREATMENTS	EFFECT OF TREATMENT ON MOOD OUTCOMES	EFFECT OF TREATMENT ON NON-MOOD OUTCOMES	SAFETY FINDINGS
(Rosenberg et al., 2010; Weintraub et al., 2010)	12-week, multicenter, masked, parallel RCT with a 24-week extension phase	131	NIMH consensus criteria for Depression of AD	Sertraline (125 mg/day max), Placebo	0	Improvement in neuropsychiatric symptoms and quality of life in both groups. No change in cognition or ADLs in both groups	GI side effects, dizziness, tremor more common on sertraline. Pulmonary serious adverse events in 12.1% of sertraline patients
(Banerjee et al., 2011)	13-week, multicenter, masked, parallel RCT	335	CSDD > 7	Sertraline (150 mg/day max), Mirtazapine (45 mg/day max) Placebo	0	+ Fewer neuropsychiatric symptoms and higher carer-rated quality of life scores for mirtazapine group at 13 weeks (did not persist at 39 weeks)	GI side effects more common on sertraline. Sedation more common on mirtazapine

AD, Alzheimer's dementia; ADL, activities of daily living; CSDD, Cornell Scale for Depression in Dementia; GI, gastrointestinal; HAM-D, Hamilton Rating Scale for Depression; MADRS, Montgomery-Asberg Depression Rating Scale; RCT, randomized controlled trial dementia. The efficacy of antidepressants in these studies is varied. Most of the "negative" studies reported substantial improvements in the patients in the placebo arms. Importantly, two recent large multicenter randomized controlled trials failed to demonstrate efficacy of antidepressants in the treatment of depression in dementia. The Depression in Alzheimer's Disease-2 (DIADS-2) study compared sertraline dosed to 125 mg daily to placebo in patients meeting NIMH consensus criteria for depression of Alzheimer's disease. Both groups also received a standardized psychosocial treatment. At 12 weeks (Rosenberg et al., 2010) and in a 24-week extension (Weintraub et al., 2010), sertraline failed to separate from placebo. Of note, a secondary analysis failed to show any difference in efficacy in participants meeting *DSM-IV* criteria for major or minor depression (Drye et al., 2011). The Health Technology Assessment Study of the Use of Antidepressants for Depression in Dementia (HTA-SADD) study compared sertraline (maximum dose 150 mg daily) to mirtazapine (maximum dose 45 mg daily) to placebo in patients with AD and depression (CSDD score of 8 or more). Again, neither sertraline nor mirtazapine separated from placebo (Banerjee et al., 2011).

Though antidepressant medications are generally well tolerated in patients with dementia (see recent reviews by Henry, Williamson, & Tampi, 2011; Nelson & Devanand, 2011), these two recent negative trials occur with the background of several new safety concerns regarding antidepressants in the elderly. The Food and Drug Administration recently issued a Drug Safety Communication for citalopram with a new maximum recommended dose of 20 mg daily in individuals greater than 60 years of age due to the potential for dose-dependent QT interval prolongation and Torsade de Pointes (US Food and Drug Administration). A large UK population-based study found no evidence for reduced risk of adverse events studied with newer antidepressants (including selective serotonin reuptake inhibitors [SSRIs]) compared to tricyclic antidepressants (TCAs). Furthermore, SSRIs had an increased hazard ratio for falls and hyponatremia compared to TCAs (Coupland et al., 2011).

Nonpharmacologic Therapies

Table 11.7 summarizes findings from controlled trials of behavioral treatments for dementia. Of note, few studies have specifically targeted depression in

dementia. Teri and colleagues found that two behavioral treatment programs, one based on problem-solving strategies and the other using the Pleasant Events Schedule (Logsdon & Teri, 1997), both led to greater mood improvement in patients and controls as opposed to a waiting-list control group (Teri, Logsdon, Uomoto, & McCurry, 1997). Similar results were seen with a similar intervention combining an individualized exercise program for the AD patient with problem-solving strategies for the caregiver; mood improvement was reported both in a general AD population and in a depressed subgroup. A trial of depressed nursing home residents with moderate to severe dementia reported improved mood and observed affect in all three behavioral interventions tested (comprehensive exercise program vs. supervised walking vs. social conversation) with a trend favoring exercise (Williams & Tappen, 2008).

These intriguing findings suggest that in treating depression in dementia, there may be value to therapeutic activities such as reminiscence therapy, focusing on pleasant events such as with the Pleasant Events Schedule (Logsdon & Teri, 1997), music, and so on. A good alternative may be an individualized exercise program designed to suit the patient's degree of mobility. These may be best implemented in the context of adult day health care or a senior citizens center. It is sensible to target the activities to a patient's cognitive strengths and work around cognitive deficits (i.e., patients with language deficits may respond better to nonverbal programs involving music and exercise).

Proposed Treatment Strategy

1. *Consider watchful waiting for milder depressive symptoms.* The authors of the HTA-SADD trial recommend 13 weeks watchful waiting based on the 43% reduction in CSDD score in the placebo group at 13 weeks in the study (Brodaty, 2011).

2. *Implement a psychosocial treatment program.* Optimal care of depression in AD starts with good dementia care (Lyketsos et al., 2006). The mixed results from controlled trials of medications are in part related to substantial improvements in the patients on placebo. This finding probably reflects the responsiveness of depression in AD, at least in its milder forms, to nonpharmacologic interventions. In addition, medication therapies alone are often not always acceptable to patients. For example, in a medication-alone study of fluoxetine, no patients completed the trial (Stevens, Katona, Manela, Watkin,

Table 11.7 Controlled Studies of Psychosocial Treatments Assessing Depression in Dementia

REFERENCE	DESIGN	N (TOTAL)	DEPRESSION DIAGNOSIS	TREATMENTS	EFFECT OF TREATMENT ON MOOD OUTCOMES	EFFECT OF TREATMENT ON NON-MOOD OUTCOMES
Teri et al., 1997	Parallel, RCT Community-dwelling patients with AD	72	*DSM-III-R* major depressive disorder or minor depressive disorder	(1) Patient intervention: "Pleasant events" (2) Caregiver intervention: "Problem solving" (3) Wait-list control (4) Typical care	+ Behavioral treatments both better than wait-list or typical care	+ Caregiver depression symptoms improved with both behavioral treatments
Teri et al., 2003	Parallel, RCT Community-dwelling patients with AD	153 total AD Unknown no. in depressed subgroup	Depression not inclusion criteria Subgroup with CSDD >5	Behavioral intervention with caregivers + exercise program vs. usual care	+	N/A
Graff et al., 2007	Parallel, RCT Community-dwelling patients with mild to moderate dementia	135	Depression not inclusion criteria Geriatric Depression Scale >14 excluded	Ten OT sessions: Patients taught "compensatory" and "environmental" strategies; caregivers taught "effective supervision, problems solving, and, coping strategies" vs. usual care	+ Decreased CSDD scores at 6 and 12 weeks	Improved quality of life and health status in patients and caregivers. Decreased depression scores in caregivers.

Study	Design	N	Inclusion criteria	Intervention	Result	Outcome	
Williams & Tappen, 2008	Parallel, RCT Nursing home residents with moderate to severe AD	45	CSDD >6	16 weeks of comprehensive exercise program vs. supervised walking vs. social conversation	+	Improved mood and observed affect in all three groups with trend favoring exercise	N/A
Conradsson, Littbrand, Lindelof, Gustafson, & Rosendahl, 2010	Parallel, cluster RCT Patients aged 65–100 in residential care facilities, MMSE >10	191 (100 with dementia)	Depression not inclusion criteria (though 61% diagnosed with depression and 49% on antidepressants)	3 months of high-intensity weight bearing exercise program vs. recreational activity	0	No improvement overall and in depressed subgroup. Improved morale in dementia subgroup.	N/A

AD, Alzheimer's dementia; CSDD, Cornell Scale for Depression in Dementia; OT, occupational therapy; RCT, randomized-controlled trial.

& Livingston, 1999). Thus, the clinician should consider a wide range of psychosocial interventions and individualize the treatment plan according to the patient's and caregiver's needs and strengths. However, traditional psychotherapy is clearly not directly applicable to cognitively impaired patients, since most models of psychotherapy depend on the patient's ability to recall insights from session to session. A popular strategy is to combine behavioral interventions for the patient and education, with problem-solving strategies for the caregiver (Stevens et al., 1999). We present a sample caregiver-targeted intervention below under "Caregiver Intervention."

3. *For more severe symptoms or if psychosocial treatments fail, start medications.* Given the lack of evidence for any particular medication, utilize standard "commonsense" principles in the use of pharmacotherapy in the elderly when choosing a medication. More detailed recommendations appear below under "Choosing a Medication."

4. *Consider electroconvulsive therapy (ECT) for the treatment-refractory patient.* In a case series of 31 patients with depression and dementia, ECT improved mood to a clinically significant extent with minimal reports of worsening cognition or prolonged postictal delirium (Rao & Lyketsos, 2000). A later case series concluded ECT is effective and well tolerated in geriatric depressed inpatients with mild cognitive impairment and dementia (Hausner, Damian, Sartorius, & Frolich, 2011).

Choosing a Medication

1. *Pay careful attention to comorbid medical conditions, medications (including over-the-counter medications and supplements), and physical examination (including vital signs).* For example, avoid the use of TCAs in patients with significant cardiac disease. Orthostatic hypotension may be exacerbated by a medication with alpha-adrenergic antagonism such as mirtazapine. If a concurrent medication is extensively metabolized by certain isoenzymes of cytochrome P450 system, avoid antidepressants which are strong 2D6 inhibitors of that isoenzyme, as the combination could result in dangerous elevations of the concurrent medication. As an example, if considering an SSRI, a drug with limited 2D6 inhibition (such as sertraline, citalopram, or escitalopram) may be preferable to one with extensive 2D6 inhibition (such as fluoxetine or paroxetine). As another example, patients taking diuretics are more likely to experience hyponatremia with serotonergic antidepressants (including SSRIs, serotonin norepinephrine reuptake inhibitors [SNRIs], and TCAs).

2. *As much as possible utilize the medication side-effect profile to therapeutic advantage based on target symptoms.* For example, if insomnia and poor appetite are target symptoms, mirtazapine may be a good choice given its side effects of sedation and weight gain. Buproprion may be a good choice for a patient with low energy but not for a patient with significant anxiety or insomnia as these are known side effects of bupropion.

3. *Avoid anticholinergic medications.* Anticholinergic medications are more likely to further impair cognition and potentially induce delirium in patients with dementia. For instance, the tricyclic antidepressant amitriptyline is strongly anticholinergic (in addition to multiple potential P450 drug–drug interactions). Therefore, if considering a TCA, an agent such as nortriptyline (which is less anticholinergic and has lower propensity for drug–drug interaction) is a better choice. Even SSRIs show differential anticholinergic effects as paroxetine has mild anticholinergic properties.

4. *Obtain informed consent from the patient and caregiver.* Especially in light of recent negative trial results for antidepressants in dementia and increasing awareness of the potential adverse effects of psychotropic medications in patients with dementia, it is crucial to review risks, benefits, indications, and alternatives to medication treatment. Educate patients and caregivers regarding what to expect from the medication, including potential side effects and expected time to response.

5. *"Start low and go slow" but get to the right dose.* Though medication trials of depression in dementia demonstrate that higher doses can be tolerated (and are often needed for response), maximize tolerability and adherence by starting with a low dose and titrating the dose slowly. For example, the starting dose of sertraline in younger adults is often 50 mg daily, whereas 25 mg daily may be a more appropriate starting dose when treating an older individual with dementia.

6. *Continually reassess the need for treatment.* Given the lack of evidence-based medication treatments and the fact the dementia is a "moving target" (as continuing neurodegeneration may affect both symptoms and medication tolerability), it is important to continually assess the need for continued medication treatment and taper/discontinue as indicated.

7. *Antipsychotic medications are not indicated for every report of delusions and hallucinations, particularly*

if they seem less prominent than the core mood syndrome. For example, a randomized clinical trial of citalopram versus perphenazine demonstrated comparable efficacy in treating agitation and psychosis in demented nursing home patients (Pollock et al., 2002). This recommendation has particular salience in light of the multiple studies showing a small but consistent increased risk of death when using antipsychotics to treat the behavioral disturbances of dementia (Kales et al., 2012) and the subsequent FDA black box warning for the increased risk of mortality for the use of antipsychotics on dementia. Though antipsychotics are not completely contraindicated in dementia care, their use should be limited to symptoms that are particularly distressing or dangerous and should always be accompanied by adequate informed consent (Rabins & Lyketsos, 2005).

8. *Psychostimulants may be helpful for the apathetic, amotivated patient.* In addition to their established role in the treatment of depression in the medically ill, emerging evidence suggests that psychostimulants may benefit apathy in AD (Herrmann et al., 2008; Padala et al., 2010) though their niche has not been well defined due to lack of controlled data (Dolder, Davis, & McKinsey, 2010). We recommend short-acting methylphenidate given at breakfast and lunch, rather than long-acting preparations, because of safety of short-acting drugs and ability to titrate finely to response. The advantage of psychostimulants is that if a patient is going to respond, the response will be rapid (within days).

Caregiver Intervention

Important components of a caregiver program include teaching caregivers the skills of caregiving, including practical approaches to handle problem behaviors. Table 11.8 presents a sample caregiver-targeted intervention used in the DIADS-2 trial and the checklist utilized appears in the Appendix. Note that this intervention covers problem behaviors and social issues, and it addresses the emotional needs of the caregiver. Other aspects of this interventions include the following: (1) validating the caregiver's accomplishments and altruism; (2) encouraging realistic expectations;

Table 11.8 Sample Caregiver Intervention for Depression in Dementia

FIRST VISIT (UP TO 30 MIN)

1. Explain the purpose of the intervention:
   To improve the day-to-day quality of life of Mr./Ms. X (person with dementia)
   To improve the caregiver's ability to care for them, and
   To help sustain the caregiver in her/his difficult task.
2. Overview of the intervention: A brief counseling session lasting up to 30 min today, and then at all follow-up visits up to 20 min. At each session, the clinician will review and update the care plan using the patient and caregiver checklists, provide educational materials, discuss specific issues in depth, work on caregiving skills, and make any necessary referrals (e.g., physical therapy, support groups, home health, and so on)
3. Provide information in writing as to how to reach the care team on a 24/7 basis to deal with crises (see example "Availability Form" provided).
4. Provide and discuss caregiver educational materials: (a) 36-hr day and (b) JHU Family Guidelines.
5. Review systematically the "JHU Supportive Care Checklists" first for patient and then for caregiver. Record the elements of the plan on the checklist.
6. Provide illness teaching about depression in AD, its recognition, causes, and treatment. Hand out the article from the Johns Hopkins Memory Bulletin on *Depression in AD* .
7. Special topic of the day: Choose a care problem (or issue) to focus on during this visit. Begin by asking: "What is the biggest care problem you are having right now?" Might also focus the discussion around one of the JHU Family Guidelines, parts of the Supportive Care checklists, or from the recent history that the caregiver provided. Discuss this topic in depth with the caregiver with an eye to teaching caregiving skills and problem-solving strategies. Tailor to the caregiver's level of sophistication.

(Continued)

Table 11.8 Continued

8. Document duration of the intervention, the topics covered, and place the completed checklists in the source document.

FOLLOW-UP VISIT (UP TO ABOUT 20–30 MIN)

1. Remind of the purpose and overview of the ongoing intervention.
2. Remind of team's 24/7 availability and how to access it.
3. Prompt for and answer questions about any of the written materials provided in the past (e.g., 36-hr day, JHU Guidelines, Memory Bulletin article on depression in AD) or any other issues the caregiver has questions about.
4. Review and update the "JHU Supportive Care Checklists" first for patient and then for caregiver. Update as necessary the elements of the plan on the checklist.
5. Update, as needed, illness teaching about depression in AD, its recognition, causes, and treatment.
6. Special topic of the day: Choose a care problem (or issue) to focus on during this visit. Begin by asking: "What is the biggest care problem you are having right now?" Might also focus the discussion around one of the JHU Family Guidelines, parts of the Supportive Care checklists, or from the recent history that the caregiver provided. Discuss this topic in depth with the caregiver with an eye to teaching caregiving skills and problem-solving strategies. Tailor to the caregiver's level of sophistication.
7. Document duration of the intervention, the topics covered, and place the completed checklists in the source document.

and (3) addressing safety issues such as wandering, driving, leaving the stove on, and so on. It is clear that patients with AD become significant driving risks as dementia advances (Dubinsky, Stein, & Lyons, 2000) and timely referrals to a formal occupational therapy/driving evaluation may help guide the decision about whether a patient can still safely drive within a limited geographic distance. The intervention also involves (4) giving caregivers' permission to ventilate their feelings of grief, disappointment, and anger in the context of a safe, therapeutic interaction; and (5) planning placement to a higher level of care such as an assisted living or skilled nursing home. Most caregivers feel very conflicted about placement and express fears that they are abandoning their loved ones and will no longer be involved in their care. In fact, caregivers continue to feel involved and stressed after placement in a nursing home (Schulz et al., 2004), and the transition process continues throughout life. In many cases, placement is the best solution to relieve the stress of a seemingly impossible care situation, and the role of the clinician is to give the caregiver permission and professional validation to "let go."

CONCLUSION

Depression is a major neuropsychiatric complication of dementia and a source of distress to patients and caregivers alike. Depression in AD has a unique constellation of symptoms that differs from depression in other populations, with more motivational and less overt mood complaints. Caregiver input is essential in the assessment process, but caregiver depression and burden must be taken into account as possible biases in reporting. The neurobiologic bases of depression in AD are not necessarily identical to those that lead to the cognitive symptoms. Antidepressant medications show mixed results in treating depression in dementia. Psychosocial interventions are crucial components of a treatment plan.

Disclosures

Dr. Marano has received research grant support from the NIMH.

Dr. Rosenberg has received grant support from Lilly, Merck, Janssen, Pfizer, Elan, American Federation for Aging Research, and the National Institute of Aging. He is a consultant and advisor for Janssen and Pfizer.

Dr. Lyketsos has received grant support from NIMH, NIA, Associated Jewish Federation of Baltimore, Weinberg Foundation, Forest, Glaxo-Smith Kline, Eisai, Pfizer, Astra-Zeneca, Lilly, Ortho-McNeil, Bristol-Myers, Novartis, National Football League, and Elan. He is a consultant and advisor for Astra-Zeneca, Glaxo-Smith Kline, Eisai, Novartis, Forest, Supernus, Adlyfe, Takeda, Wyeth, Lundbeck, Merz, Lilly, Pfizer, Genentech, Elan, NFL Players Association, and the NFL Benefits Office. He has received honorarium or travel support from Pfizer, Forest, Glaxo-Smith Kline, and Health Monitor.

APPENDIX: SAMPLE CAREGIVER INTERVENTION

Supportive Care Checklist: Caregiver

PATIENT——————— DATE —/ —/ —CAREGIVER

RELATIONSHIP

Who are caregivers?

____Primary(-ies):

____Back-up plan:

TOPIC	Y/N	DATE COMPLETED	INTERVENTION	COMMENT
Education			___Verbal (specify) ___The 36-Hour Day[140] ___Dementia Care Family Guidelines ___Resource list and telephone numbers ___Inventory of important documents	
Resource referral			___Alzheimer's Association ___Eldercare Attorney ___Office on Aging/Social Services ___Geriatric Case Management	
Caregiver mental health assessment			___Network/activity encouragement ___Support group ___Counseling referral ___Psychiatric referral	
Caregiver physical health assessment			___Primary care	
Caregiver skills counseling			___Activities ___Meds/side effects ___Supervision ___Night time ___Behaviors ___ADLs ___Skills lab referral	
Respite counseling			___Other caregivers ___Family/friends ___Professional aides ___Weekly time off ___Monthly time off ___Annual vacation	

Supportive Care Checklist: Patient

PATIENT——————— DATE —/ —/ —CAREGIVER RELATIONSHIP

TOPIC	DATE Y/N	COMPLETED	INTERVENTION	COMMENT
Diagnostic awareness ___Patient aware ___Patient not aware				
Advanced directives ___Healthcare agent: ___Other POA ___Will				
Illness education targeted at the patient			Topics covered: 1. 2. 3.	
Daily life schedule review			___Sample calendar	Schedule in place
Safety review Driving Wandering risk Level of care issues Home safety issues Fall risk Medication administration			___Advised to stop ___Driving eval. ___Level of care eval. ___Home safety eval. ___PT referral ___Devise (specify) ___Supervision ___Administration	
General medical care			Primary care: Last seen:	
Referrals			___OT ___PT ___Speech ___Home health ___Dental ___Vision ___Hearing	

*It is recognized that not all caregivers need detailed counseling at every visit and that many refuse to be counseled at specific time points. Such refusals should be honored. All caregivers should be offered the educational materials and information about the study team's 24-h availability. As well, occasional visits will be short, lasting much less than the suggested time frame. This too is appropriate. It is left to clinical judgment to determine the exact length of each counseling session. If a caregiver requires more support or counseling than can be provided during these sessions, they should be referred to the appropriate resources in the area, as usual care would dictate.

Source: From *Depression in Alzheimer's Disease Study-2* [DIADS-2] Handbook, version 1.0, 2004.

REFERENCES

Alexopoulos, G. S., Abrams, R. C., Young, R. C., & Shamoian, C. A. (1988). Cornell Scale for Depression in Dementia, *Biological Psychiatry*, *23*(3), 271–284.

Alexopoulos, G. S., Meyers, B. S., Young, R. C., Campbell, S., Silbersweig, D., & Charlson, M. (1997). 'Vascular depression' hypothesis, *Archives of General Psychiatry*, *54*(10), 915–922.

Alexopoulos, G. S., Meyers, B. S., Young, R. C., Mattis, S., & Kakuma, T. (1993). The course of geriatric depression with reversible dementia: A controlled study, *American Journal of Psychiatry*, *150*(11), 1693–1699.

Alexopoulos, G. S., Young, R. C., & Meyers, B. S. (1993). Geriatric depression: Age of onset and dementia, *Biological Psychiatry*, *34*(3), 141–145.

Alzheimer's Association, Thies, W., & Bleiler, L. (2011). 2011 Alzheimer's disease facts and figures, *Alzheimer's and Dementia*, *7*(2), 208–244.

Banerjee, S., Hellier, J., Dewey, M., Romeo, R., Ballard, C., Baldwin, R., ...Burns, A. (2011). Sertraline or mirtazapine for depression in dementia (HTA-SADD): A randomised, multicentre, double-blind, placebo-controlled trial. *Lancet*, *378*(9789), 403–411.

Bassiony, M. M., Warren, A., Rosenblatt, A., Baker, A., Steinberg, M., Steele, C. D., ...Lyketsos, C. G. (2002). The relationship between delusions and depression in Alzheimer's disease. *International Journal of Geriatric Psychiatry*, *17*(6), 549–556.

Berger, A. K., Fratiglioni, L., Forsell, Y., Winblad, B., & Backman, L. (1999). The occurrence of depressive symptoms in the preclinical phase of AD: A population-based study. *Neurology*, *53*(9), 1998–2002.

Bhalla, R. K., Butters, M. A., Mulsant, B. H., Begley, A. E., Zmuda, M. D., Schoderbek, B., ...Becker, J. T. (2006). Persistence of neuropsychologic deficits in the remitted state of late-life depression. *American Journal of Geriatric Psychiatry*, *14*(5), 419–427.

Binetti, G., Magni, E., Padovani, A., Cappa, S. F., Bianchetti, A., & Trabucchi, M. (1996) Executive dysfunction in early Alzheimer's disease. *Journal of Neurology, Neurosurgery, and Psychiatry*, *60*(1), 91–93.

Borroni, B., Archetti, S., Costanzi, C., Grassi, M., Ferrari, M., Radeghieri, A., ...ITINAD Working Group. (2009). Role of BDNF Val66Met functional polymorphism in Alzheimer's disease-related depression. *Neurobiology of Aging*, *30*(9), 1406–1412.

Borroni, B., Grassi, M., Archetti, S., Costanzi, C., Bianchi, M., Caimi, L., ...Padovani, A. (2009). BDNF genetic variations increase the risk of Alzheimer's disease-related depression. *Journal of Alzheimer's Disease*, *18*(4), 867–875.

Breitner, J. C., Wyse, B. W., Anthony, J. C., Welsh-Bohmer, K. A., Steffens, D. C., Norton, M. C., ...Khachaturian, A. (1999). APOE-epsilon4 count predicts age when prevalence of AD increases, then declines: The Cache County Study. *Neurology*, *53*(2), 321–331.

Brodaty, H. (2011). Antidepressant treatment in Alzheimer's disease. *Lancet*, *378*(9789), 375–376.

Burke, W. J., Roccaforte, W. H., Wengel, S. P., McArthur-Miller, D., Folks, D. G., & Potter, J. F. (1998). Disagreement in the reporting of depressive symptoms between patients with dementia of the Alzheimer type and their collateral sources. *American Journal of Geriatric Psychiatry*, *6*(4), 308–319.

Burns, A., Jacoby, R., & Levy, R. (1990). Psychiatric phenomena in Alzheimer's disease. III: Disorders of mood. *British Journal of Psychiatry*, *157*, 81–86, 92–94.

Butters, M. A., Young, J. B., Lopez, O., Aizenstein, H. J., Mulsant, B. H., Reynolds, C. F., III, ...Becker, J. T. (2008). Pathways linking late-life depression to persistent cognitive impairment and dementia. *Dialogues in Clinical Neuroscience*, *10*(3), 345–357.

Byers, A. L., & Yaffe, K. (2011). Depression and risk of developing dementia. *Nature Reviews Neurology*, *7*(6), 323–331.

Cerhan, J. H., Ivnik, R. J., Smith, G. E., Tangalos, E. C., Petersen, R. C., & Boeve, B. F. (2002). Diagnostic utility of letter fluency, category fluency, and fluency difference scores in Alzheimer's disease. *Clinical Neuropsychologist*, *16*(1), 35–42.

Collie, A., & Maruff, P. (2000). The neuropsychology of preclinical Alzheimer's disease and mild cognitive impairment. *Neuroscience and Biobehavioral Reviews*, *24*(3), 365–374.

Conradsson, M., Littbrand, H., Lindelof, N., Gustafson, Y., & Rosendahl, E. (2010). Effects of a high-intensity functional exercise programme on depressive symptoms and psychological well-being among older people living in residential care facilities: A cluster-randomized controlled trial. *Aging and Mental Health*, *14*(5), 565–576.

Coupland, C., Dhiman, P., Morriss, R., Arthur, A., Barton, G., & Hippisley-Cox, J. (2011). Antidepressant use and risk of adverse outcomes in older people: Population based cohort study. *British Medical Journal*, *343*, d4551.

Culang-Reinlieb, M. E., Johnert, L. C., Brickman, A. M., Steffens, D. C., Garcon, E., & Sneed, J. R. (2010). MRI-defined vascular depression: A review of the construct. *International Journal of Geriatric Psychiatry*, ePub ahead of print.

de Vasconcelos Cunha, U. G., Lopes Rocha, F., Avila de Melo, R., Alves Valle, E., de Souza Neto, J. J., Mendes Brega, R.,...Sakurai, E. (2007). A placebo-controlled double-blind randomized study of venlafaxine in the treatment of depression in dementia. *Dementia and Geriatric Cognitive Disorders*, 24(1), 36–41.

Dolder, C. R., Davis, L. N., & McKinsey, J. (2010). Use of psychostimulants in patients with dementia. *Annals of Pharmacotherapy*, 44(10), 1624–1632.

Drye, L. T., Martin, B. K., Frangakis, C. E., Meinert, C. L., Mintzer, J. E., Munro, C. A.,...DIADS-2 Research Group. (2011). Do treatment effects vary among differing baseline depression criteria in depression in Alzheimer's disease study +/- 2 (DIADS-2)? *International Journal of Geriatric Psychiatry*, 26(6), 573–583.

Dubinsky, R. M., Stein, A. C., & Lyons, K. (2000). Practice parameter: Risk of driving and Alzheimer's disease (an evidence-based review): Report of the quality standards subcommittee of the American Academy of Neurology. *Neurology*, 54(12), 2205–2211.

Forstl, H., Burns, A., Luthert, P., Cairns, N., Lantos, P., & Levy, R. (1992). Clinical and neuropathological correlates of depression in Alzheimer's disease. *Psychological Medicine*, 22(4), 877–884.

Franceschi, M., Colombo, B., Rossi, P., & Canal, N. (1997). Headache in a population-based elderly cohort. An ancillary study to the Italian Longitudinal Study of Aging (ILSA). *Headache*, 37(2), 79–82.

Garre-Olmo, J., Lopez-Pousa, S., Vilalta-Franch, J., Turon-Estrada, A., Hernandez-Ferrandiz, M., Lozano-Gallego, M.,...Cruz-Reina, M. M. (2003). Evolution of depressive symptoms in Alzheimer disease: One-year follow-up. *Alzheimer Disease and Associated Disorders*, 17(2), 77–85.

Gottlieb, G. L., Gur, R. E., & Gur, R. C. (1988). Reliability of psychiatric scales in patients with dementia of the Alzheimer type. *American Journal of Psychiatry*, 145(7), 857–860.

Graff, M. J., Vernooij-Dassen, M. J., Thijssen, M., Dekker, J., Hoefnagels, W. H., & Olderikkert, M. G. (2007). Effects of community occupational therapy on quality of life, mood, and health status in dementia patients and their caregivers: A randomized controlled trial. *Journals of Gerontology Series A, Biological Sciences and Medical Sciences*, 62(9), 1002–1009.

Hamilton, M. (1960). A rating scale for depression. *Journal of Neurology, Neurosurgery, and Psychiatry*, 23, 56–62.

Hargrave, R., Reed, B., & Mungas, D. (2000). Depressive syndromes and functional disability in dementia. *Journal of Geriatric Psychiatry and Neurology*, 13(2), 72–77.

Harwood, D. G., & Sultzer, D. L. (2002). Life is not worth living: Hopelessness in Alzheimer's disease. *Journal of Geriatric Psychiatry and Neurology*, 15(1), 38–43.

Harwood, D. G., Sultzer, D. L., & Wheatley, M. V. (2000). Impaired insight in Alzheimer disease: Association with cognitive deficits, psychiatric symptoms, and behavioral disturbances. *Neuropsychiatry, Neuropsychology, and Behavioral Neurology*, 13(2), 83–88.

Hausner, L., Damian, M., Sartorius, A., & Frolich, L. (2011). Efficacy and cognitive side effects of electroconvulsive therapy (ECT) in depressed elderly inpatients with coexisting mild cognitive impairment or dementia. *Journal of Clinical Psychiatry*, 72(1), 91–97.

Hebert, L. E., Scherr, P. A., Bienias, J. L., Bennett, D. A., & Evans, D. A. (2003). Alzheimer disease in the US population: Prevalence estimates using the 2000 census. *Archives of Neurology*, 60(8), 1119–1122.

Henry, G., Williamson, D., & Tampi, R. R. (2011). Efficacy and tolerability of antidepressants in the treatment of behavioral and psychological symptoms of dementia, a literature review of evidence. *American Journal of Alzheimer's Disease and Other Dementias*, 26(3), 169–183.

Herrmann, N., Rothenburg, L. S., Black, S. E., Ryan, M., Liu, B. A., Busto, U. E., & Lanctot, K. L. (2008). Methylphenidate for the treatment of apathy in Alzheimer disease: Prediction of response using dextroamphetamine challenge. *Journal of Clinical Psychopharmacology*, 28(3), 296–301.

Hirono, N., Mori, E., Ishii, K., Ikejiri, Y., Imamura, T., Shimomura, T.,...Sasaki, M. (1998). Frontal lobe hypometabolism and depression in Alzheimer's disease. *Neurology*, 50(2), 380–383.

Holmes, C., Russ, C., Kirov, G., Aitchison, K. J., Powell, J. F., Collier, D. A., & Lovestone, S. (1998). Apolipoprotein E: Depressive illness, depressive symptoms, and Alzheimer's disease. *Biological Psychiatry*, 43(3), 159–164.

Hoogendijk, W. J., Sommer, I. E., Pool, C. W., Kamphorst, W., Hofman, M. A., Eikelenboom, P., & Swaab, D. F. (1999). Lack of association between depression and loss of neurons in the locus coeruleus in Alzheimer disease. *Archives of General Psychiatry*, 56(1), 45–51.

Janzing, J. G., Hooijer, C., van't Hof, M. A., & Zitman, F. G. (2002). Depression in subjects with and without dementia: A comparison using GMS-AGECAT. *International Journal of Geriatric Psychiatry, 17*(1), 1–5.

Kales, H. C., Kim, H. M., Zivin, K., Valenstein, M., Seyfried, L. S., Chiang, C., … Blow, F. C. (2012). Risk of mortality among individual antipsychotics in patients with dementia. *American Journal of Psychiatry, 169*(1), 71–79.

Katona, C. L., Hunter, B. N., & Bray, J. (1998). A double-blind comparison of the efficacy and safely of paroxetine and imipramine in the treatment of depression with dementia. *International Journal of Geriatric Psychiatry, 13*(2), 100–108.

Khachaturian, A. S., Corcoran, C. D., Mayer, L. S., Zandi, P. P., Breitner, J. C., & Cache County Study Investigators. (2004). Apolipoprotein E epsilon4 count affects age at onset of Alzheimer disease, but not lifetime susceptibility: The Cache County Study. *Archives of General Psychiatry, 61*(5), 518–524.

Krishnan, K. R., Hays, J. C., & Blazer, D. G. (1997). MRI-defined vascular depression. *American Journal of Psychiatry, 154*(4), 497–501.

Kukull, W. A., & Bowen, J. D. (2002). Dementia epidemiology. *Medical Clinics of North America, 86*(3), 573–590.

Kurlowicz, L. H., Evans, L. K., Strumpf, N. E., & Maislin, G. (2002). A psychometric evaluation of the Cornell Scale for Depression in Dementia in a frail, nursing home population. *American Journal of Geriatric Psychiatry, 10*(5), 600–608.

Landes, A. M., Sperry, S. D., Strauss, M. E., & Geldmacher, D. S. (2001). Apathy in Alzheimer's disease. *Journal of the American Geriatrics Society, 49*(12), 1700–1707.

Langa, K. M., Foster, N. L., & Larson, E. B. (2004). Mixed dementia: Emerging concepts and therapeutic implications. *Journal of the American Medical Association, 292*(23), 2901–2908.

Li, Y. S., Meyer, J. S., & Thornby, J. (2001). Longitudinal follow-up of depressive symptoms among normal versus cognitively impaired elderly. *International Journal of Geriatric Psychiatry, 16*(7), 718–727.

Lichtenberg, P. A., Marcopulos, B. A., Steiner, D. A., & Tabscott, J. A. (1992). Comparison of the Hamilton Depression Rating Scale and the Geriatric Depression Scale: Detection of depression in dementia patients. *Psychological reports, 70*(2), 515–521.

Lind, K., Jonsson, M., Karlsson, I., Sjogren, M., Wallin, A., & Edman, A. (2006). Depressive symptoms and white matter changes in patients with dementia. *International Journal of Geriatric Psychiatry, 21*(2), 119–125.

Logsdon, R. G., & Teri, L. (1997). The Pleasant Events Schedule-AD: Psychometric properties and relationship to depression and cognition in Alzheimer's disease patients. *Gerontologist, 37*(1), 40–45.

Lyketsos, C. G., Breitner, J. C., & Rabins, P. V. (2001). An evidence-based proposal for the classification of neuropsychiatric disturbance in Alzheimer's disease. *International Journal of Geriatric Psychiatry, 16*(11), 1037–1042.

Lyketsos, C. G., Colenda, C. C., Beck, C., Blank, K., Doraiswamy, M. P., Kalunian, D. A., … Task Force of American Association for Geriatric Psychiatry. (2006). Position statement of the American Association for Geriatric Psychiatry regarding principles of care for patients with dementia resulting from Alzheimer disease. *American Journal of Geriatric Psychiatry, 14*(7), 561–572.

Lyketsos, C. G., DelCampo, L., Steinberg, M., Miles, Q., Steele, C. D., Munro, C., … Rabins, P. V. (2003). Treating depression in Alzheimer disease: Efficacy and safety of sertraline therapy, and the benefits of depression reduction: The DIADS. *Archives of General Psychiatry, 60*(7), 737–746.

Lyketsos, C. G., Lopez, O., Jones, B., Fitzpatrick, A. L., Breitner, J., & DeKosky, S. (2002). Prevalence of neuropsychiatric symptoms in dementia and mild cognitive impairment: Results from the cardiovascular health study. *Journal of the American Medical Association, 288*(12), 1475–1483.

Lyketsos, C. G., Sheppard, J. M., Steinberg, M., Tschanz, J. A., Norton, M. C., Steffens, D. C., & Breitner, J. C. (2001). Neuropsychiatric disturbance in Alzheimer's disease clusters into three groups: The Cache County study. *International Journal of Geriatric Psychiatry, 16*(11), 1043–1053.

Lyketsos, C. G., Steinberg, M., Tschanz, J. T., Norton, M. C., Steffens, D. C., & Breitner, J. C. (2000). Mental and behavioral disturbances in dementia: Findings from the Cache County Study on Memory in Aging. *American Journal of Psychiatry, 157*(5), 708–714.

Lyketsos, C. G., Tune, L. E., Pearlson, G., & Steele, C. (1996). Major depression in Alzheimer's disease. An interaction between gender and family history. *Psychosomatics, 37*(4), 380–384.

Magai, C., Kennedy, G., Cohen, C. I., & Gomberg, D. (2000). A controlled clinical trial of sertraline in the treatment of depression in nursing home patients with late-stage Alzheimer's disease. *American Journal of Geriatric Psychiatry, 8*(1), 66–74.

Mayer, L. S., Bay, R. C., Politis, A., Steinberg, M., Steele, C., Baker, A. S., ... Lyketsos, C. G. (2006). Comparison of three rating scales as outcome measures for treatment trials of depression in Alzheimer disease: Findings from DIADS. *International Journal of Geriatric Psychiatry, 21*(10), 930–936.

McDaniel, K. D., Edland, S. D., & Heyman, A. (1995). Relationship between level of insight and severity of dementia in Alzheimer disease. CERAD Clinical Investigators. Consortium to Establish a Registry for Alzheimer's Disease. *Alzheimer Disease and Associated Disorders, 9*(2), 101–104.

Miech, R. A., Breitner, J. C., Zandi, P. P., Khachaturian, A. S., Anthony, J. C., & Mayer, L. (2002). Incidence of AD may decline in the early 90s for men, later for women: The Cache County study. *Neurology, 58*(2), 209–218.

Migliorelli, R., Teson, A., Sabe, L., Petracchi, M., Leiguarda, R., & Starkstein, S. E. (1995). Prevalence and correlates of dysthymia and major depression among patients with Alzheimer's disease. *American Journal of Psychiatry, 152*(1), 37–44.

Migneco, O., Benoit, M., Koulibaly, P. M., Dygai, I., Bertogliati, C., Desvignes, P., ... Darcourt, J. (2001). Perfusion brain SPECT and statistical parametric mapping analysis indicate that apathy is a cingulate syndrome: A study in Alzheimer's disease and nondemented patients. *NeuroImage, 13*(5), 896–902.

Montgomery, S. A., & Asberg, M. (1979). A new depression scale designed to be sensitive to change. *British Journal of Psychiatry, 134*, 382–389.

Mueller, S. G., Mack, W. J., Mungas, D., Kramer, J. H., Cardenas-Nicolson, V., Lavretsky, H., ... Weiner, M. W. (2010). Influences of lobar gray matter and white matter lesion load on cognition and mood. *Psychiatry Research, 181*(2), 90–96.

Mulsant, B. H., Pollock, B. G., Kirshner, M., Shen, C., Dodge, H., & Ganguli, M. (2003). Serum anticholinergic activity in a community-based sample of older adults: Relationship with cognitive performance. *Archives of General Psychiatry, 60*(2), 198–203.

Nelson, J. C., & Devanand, D. P. (2011). A systematic review and meta-analysis of placebo-controlled antidepressant studies in people with depression and dementia. *Journal of the American Geriatrics Society, 59*(4), 577–585.

Nyth, A. L., & Gottfries, C. G. (1990). The clinical efficacy of citalopram in treatment of emotional disturbances in dementia disorders. A Nordic multicentre study. *British Journal of Psychiatry, 157*, 894–901.

Nyth, A. L., Gottfries, C. G., Lyby, K., Smedegaard-Andersen, L., Gylding-Sabroe, J., Kristensen, M., ... Syversen, S. (1992). A controlled multicenter clinical study of citalopram and placebo in elderly depressed patients with and without concomitant dementia. *Acta Psychiatrica Scandinavica, 86*(2), 138–145.

O'Brien, J., Perry, R., Barber, R., Gholkar, A., & Thomas, A. (2000). The association between white matter lesions on magnetic resonance imaging and noncognitive symptoms. *Annals of the New York Academy of Sciences, 903*, 482–489.

Olin, J. T., Katz, I. R., Meyers, B. S., Schneider, L. S., & Lebowitz, B. D. (2002). Provisional diagnostic criteria for depression of Alzheimer disease: Rationale and background. *American Journal of Geriatric Psychiatry, 10*(2), 129–141.

Olin, J. T., Schneider, L. S., Katz, I. R., Meyers, B. S., Alexopoulos, G. S., Breitner, J. C., ... Lebowitz, B. D. (2002). Provisional diagnostic criteria for depression of Alzheimer disease. *American Journal of Geriatric Psychiatry, 10*(2), 125–128.

Ownby, R. L., Crocco, E., Acevedo, A., John, V., & Loewenstein, D. (2006). Depression and risk for Alzheimer disease: Systematic review, meta-analysis, and metaregression analysis. *Archives of General Psychiatry, 63*(5), 530–538.

Padala, P. R., Burke, W. J., Shostrom, V. K., Bhatia, S. C., Wengel, S. P., Potter, J. F., & Petty, F. (2010). Methylphenidate for apathy and functional status in dementia of the Alzheimer type. *American Journal of Geriatric Psychiatry, 18*(4), 371–374.

Panza, F., Seripa, D., D'Onofrio, G., Frisardi, V., Solfrizzi, V., Mecocci, P., & Pilotto, A. (2011). Neuropsychiatric symptoms, endophenotypes, and syndromes in late-onset Alzheimer's disease: Focus on APOE gene. *International Journal of Alzheimer's Disease, 2011*, 721457.

Pearlson, G. D., Ross, C. A., Lohr, W. D., Rovner, B. W., Chase, G. A., & Folstein, M. F. (1990). Association between family history of affective disorder and the depressive syndrome of Alzheimer's disease. *American Journal of Psychiatry, 147*(4), 452–456.

Petersen, R. C., Smith, G. E., Waring, S. C., Ivnik, R. J., Tangalos, E. G., & Kokmen, E. (1999). Mild cognitive impairment: Clinical characterization and outcome. *Archives of Neurology, 56*(3), 303–308.

Petracca, G., Teson, A., Chemerinski, E., Leiguarda, R., & Starkstein, S. E. (1996). A double-blind placebo-controlled study of clomipramine in depressed patients with Alzheimer's disease. *Journal of Neuropsychiatry and Clinical Neurosciences, 8*(3), 270–275.

Petracca, G. M., Chemerinski, E., & Starkstein, S. E. (2001). A double-blind, placebo-controlled study of fluoxetine in depressed patients with Alzheimer's disease. *International Psychogeriatrics*, 13(2), 233–240.

Pollock, B. G., Mulsant, B. H., Rosen, J., Sweet, R. A., Mazumdar, S., Bharucha, A., ... Chew, M. L. (2002). Comparison of citalopram, perphenazine, and placebo for the acute treatment of psychosis and behavioral disturbances in hospitalized, demented patients. *American Journal of Psychiatry*, 159(3), 460–465.

Purandare, N., Burns, A., Craig, S., Faragher, B., & Scott, K. (2001). Depressive symptoms in patients with Alzheimer's disease. *International Journal of Geriatric Psychiatry*, 16(10), 960–964.

Rabins, P. V., & Lyketsos, C. G. (2005). Antipsychotic drugs in dementia: What should be made of the risks? *Journal of the American Medical Association*, 294(15), 1963–1965.

Rabins, P. V., Lyketsos, C. G., & Steele, C. D. (2006). *Practical dementia care* (2nd ed.). New York: Oxford University Press.

Rao, V., & Lyketsos, C. G. (2000). The benefits and risks of ECT for patients with primary dementia who also suffer from depression. *International Journal of Geriatric Psychiatry*, 15(8), 729–735.

Rapp, M. A., Schnaider-Beeri, M., Grossman, H. T., Sano, M., Perl, D. P., Purohit, D. P., ... Haroutunian, V. (2006). Increased hippocampal plaques and tangles in patients with Alzheimer disease with a lifetime history of major depression. *Archives of General Psychiatry*, 63(2), 161–167.

Reifler, B. V., Teri, L., Raskind, M., Veith, R., Barnes, R., White, E., & McLean, P. (1989). Double-blind trial of imipramine in Alzheimer's disease patients with and without depression. *American Journal of Psychiatry*, 146(1), 45–49.

Rosenberg, P. B., Drye, L. T., Martin, B. K., Frangakis, C., Mintzer, J. E., Weintraub, D., ... DIADS-2 Research Group. (2010). Sertraline for the treatment of depression in Alzheimer disease. *American Journal of Geriatric Psychiatry*, 18(2), 136–145.

Rosenberg, P. B., Mielke, M. M., & Lyketsos, C. G. (2005). Caregiver assessment of patients' depression in Alzheimer disease: Longitudinal analysis in a drug treatment study. *American Journal of Geriatric Psychiatry*, 13(9), 822–826.

Rosness, T. A., Barca, M. L., & Engedal, K. (2010). Occurrence of depression and its correlates in early onset dementia patients. *International Journal of Geriatric Psychiatry*, 25(7), 704–711.

Roth, M., Mountjoy, C. Q., & Amrein, R. (1996). Moclobemide in elderly patients with cognitive decline and depression: An international double-blind, placebo-controlled trial. *British Journal of Psychiatry*, 168(2), 149–157.

Rubin, E. H., Veiel, L. L., Kinscherf, D. A., Morris, J. C., & Storandt, M. (2001). Clinically significant depressive symptoms and very mild to mild dementia of the Alzheimer type. *International Journal of Geriatric Psychiatry*, 16(7), 694–701.

Savva, G. M., Zaccai, J., Matthews, F. E., Davidson, J. E., McKeith, I., Brayne, C., & Medical Research Council Cognitive Function and Ageing Study. (2009). Prevalence, correlates and course of behavioural and psychological symptoms of dementia in the population. *British Journal of Psychiatry*, 194(3), 212–219.

Schulz, R., Belle, S. H., Czaja, S. J., McGinnis, K. A., Stevens, A., & Zhang, S. (2004). Long-term care placement of dementia patients and caregiver health and well-being. *Journal of the American Medical Association*, 292(8), 961–967.

Schulz, R., & Martire, L. M. (2004). Family caregiving of persons with dementia: Prevalence, health effects, and support strategies. *American Journal of Geriatric Psychiatry*, 12(3), 240–249.

Starkstein, S. E., Dragovic, M., Jorge, R., Brockman, S., & Robinson, R. G. (2011). Diagnostic criteria for depression in Alzheimer disease: A study of symptom patterns using latent class analysis. *American Journal of Geriatric Psychiatry*, 19(6), 551–558.

Starkstein, S. E., Jorge, R., Mizrahi, R., & Robinson, R. G. (2005). The construct of minor and major depression in Alzheimer's disease. *American Journal of Psychiatry*, 162(11), 2086–2093.

Starkstein, S. E., Mizrahi, R., Capizzano, A. A., Acion, L., Brockman, S., & Power, B. D. (2009). Neuroimaging correlates of apathy and depression in Alzheimer's disease. *Journal of Neuropsychiatry and Clinical Neurosciences*, 21(3), 259–265.

Starkstein, S. E., Mizrahi, R., & Garau, L. (2005). Specificity of symptoms of depression in Alzheimer disease: A longitudinal analysis. *American Journal of Geriatric Psychiatry*, 13(9), 802–807.

Starkstein, S. E., Petracca, G., Chemerinski, E., & Kremer, J. (2001). Syndromic validity of apathy in Alzheimer's disease. *American Journal of Psychiatry*, 158(6), 872–877.

Steffens, D. C., Otey, E., Alexopoulos, G. S., Butters, M. A., Cuthbert, B., Ganguli, M., ... Yesavage, J. (2006). Perspectives on depression, mild cognitive impairment, and cognitive decline. *Archives of General Psychiatry*, 63(2), 130–138.

Steinberg, M., Shao, H., Zandi, P., Lyketsos, C. G., Welsh-Bohmer, K. A., Norton, M. C., ... Cache

County Investigators. (2008). Point and 5-year period prevalence of neuropsychiatric symptoms in dementia: The Cache County Study. *International Journal of Geriatric Psychiatry*, 23(2), 170–177.

Steinberg, M., Sheppard, J. M., Tschanz, J. T., Norton, M. C., Steffens, D. C., Breitner, J. C., & Lyketsos, C. G. (2003). The incidence of mental and behavioral disturbances in dementia: The cache county study. *Journal of Neuropsychiatry and Clinical Neurosciences*, 15(3), 340–345.

Stevens, T., Katona, C., Manela, M., Watkin, V., & Livingston, G. (1999). Drug treatment of older people with affective disorders in the community: Lessons from an attempted clinical trial. *International Journal of Geriatric Psychiatry*, 14(6), 467–472.

Storey, E., Slavin, M. J., & Kinsella, G. J. (2002). Patterns of cognitive impairment in Alzheimer's disease: Assessment and differential diagnosis. *Frontiers in Bioscience*, 7, e155–184.

Stout, J. C., Wyman, M. F., Johnson, S. A., Peavy, G. M., & Salmon, D. P. (2003). Frontal behavioral syndromes and functional status in probable Alzheimer disease. *American Journal of Geriatric Psychiatry*, 11(6), 683–686.

Sultzer, D. L., Mahler, M. E., Mandelkern, M. A., Cummings, J. L., Van Gorp, W. G., Hinkin, C. H., & Berisford, M. A. (1995). The relationship between psychiatric symptoms and regional cortical metabolism in Alzheimer's disease. *Journal of Neuropsychiatry and Clinical Neurosciences*, 7(4), 476–484.

Sunderland, T., Tariot, P. N., Cohen, R. M., Weingartner, H., Mueller, E. A., III, & Murphy, D. L. (1987). Anticholinergic sensitivity in patients with dementia of the Alzheimer type and age-matched controls. A dose-response study. *Archives of General Psychiatry*, 44(5), 418–426.

Tanzi, R. E., & Bertram, L. (2001). New frontiers in Alzheimer's disease genetics. *Neuron*, 32(2), 181–184.

Taragano, F. E., Lyketsos, C. G., Mangone, C. A., Allegri, R. F., & Comesana-Diaz, E. (1997). A double-blind, randomized, fixed-dose trial of fluoxetine vs. amitriptyline in the treatment of major depression complicating Alzheimer's disease. *Psychosomatics*, 38(3), 246–252.

Taylor, W. D., Zuchner, S., McQuoid, D. R., Steffens, D. C., Speer, M. C., & Krishnan, K. R. (2007). Allelic differences in the brain-derived neurotrophic factor Val66Met polymorphism in late-life depression. *American Journal of Geriatric Psychiatry*, 15(10), 850–857.

Teng, E., Ringman, J. M., Ross, L. K., Mulnard, R. A., Dick, M. B., Bartzokis, G., . . . Alzheimer's Disease Research Centers of California-Depression in Alzheimer's Disease Investigators. (2008). Diagnosing depression in Alzheimer disease with the national institute of mental health provisional criteria. *American Journal of Geriatric Psychiatry*, 16(6), 469–477.

Teri, L., Gibbons, L. E., McCurry, S. M., Logsdon, R. G., Buchner, D. M., Barlow, W. E., . . . Larson, E. B. (2003). Exercise plus behavioral management in patients with Alzheimer disease: A randomized controlled trial. *Journal of the American Medical Association*, 290(15), 2015–2022.

Teri, L., Logsdon, R. G., Uomoto, J., & McCurry, S. M. (1997). Behavioral treatment of depression in dementia patients: A controlled clinical trial. *Journals of Gerontology Series B, Psychological Sciences and Social Sciences*, 52(4), P159–166.

Teri, L., & Truax, P. (1994). Assessment of depression in dementia patients: Association of caregiver mood with depression ratings. *Gerontologist*, 34(2), 231–234.

Tractenberg, R. E., Weiner, M. F., Patterson, M. B., Teri, L., & Thal, L. J. (2003). Comorbidity of psychopathological domains in community-dwelling persons with Alzheimer's disease. *Journal of Geriatric Psychiatry and Neurology*, 16(2), 94–99.

US Food and Drug Administration. *FDA Drug Safety Communication: Abnormal heart rhythms associated with high doses of Celexa (citalopram hydrobromide)*. Date of release 3/28/2012. http://www.fda.gov/Drugs/DrugSafety/ucm297391.htm Accessed 10/22/2012.

Verhey, F. R., Ponds, R. W., Rozendaal, N., & Jolles, J. (1995). Depression, insight, and personality changes in Alzheimer's disease and vascular dementia. *Journal of Geriatric Psychiatry and Neurology*, 8(1), 23–27.

Vida, S., Des Rosiers, P., Carrier, L., & Gauthier, S. (1994). Depression in Alzheimer's disease: Receiver operating characteristic analysis of the Cornell Scale for Depression in Dementia and the Hamilton Depression Scale. *Journal of Geriatric Psychiatry and Neurology*, 7(3), 159–162.

Vilalta-Franch, J., Garre-Olmo, J., Lopez-Pousa, S., Turon-Estrada, A., Lozano-Gallego, M., Hernandez-Ferrandiz, M., . . . Feijoo-Lorza, R. (2006). Comparison of different clinical diagnostic criteria for depression in Alzheimer disease. *American Journal of Geriatric Psychiatry*, 14(7), 589–597.

Weiner, M. F., Edland, S. D., & Luszczynska, H. (1994). Prevalence and incidence of major depression in Alzheimer's disease. *American Journal of Psychiatry, 151*(7), 1006–1009.

Weintraub, D., Rosenberg, P. B., Drye, L. T., Martin, B. K., Frangakis, C., Mintzer, J. E., ... DIADS-2 Research Group. (2010). Sertraline for the treatment of depression in Alzheimer disease: Week-24 outcomes. *American Journal of Geriatric Psychiatry, 18*(4), 332–340.

Williams, C. L., & Tappen, R. M. (2008). Exercise training for depressed older adults with Alzheimer's disease. *Aging and Mental Health, 12*(1), 72–80.

Wilson, R. S., Arnold, S. E., Beck, T. L., Bienias, J. L., & Bennett, D. A. (2008). Change in depressive symptoms during the prodromal phase of Alzheimer disease. *Archives of General Psychiatry, 65*(4), 439–445.

Wilson, R. S., Hoganson, G. M., Rajan, K. B., Barnes, L. L., Mendes de Leon, C. F., & Evans, D. A. (2010). Temporal course of depressive symptoms during the development of Alzheimer disease. *Neurology, 75*(1), 21–26.

Yesavage, J. A., Brink, T. L., Rose, T. L., Lum, O., Huang, V., Adey, M., & Leirer, V. O. (1982). Development and validation of a geriatric depression screening scale: A preliminary report. *Journal of Psychiatric Research, 17*(1), 37–49.

Zhang, L., Fang, Y., Zeng, Z., Lian, Y., Wei, J., Zhu, H., ... Xu, Y. (2011). BDNF gene polymorphisms are associated with Alzheimer's disease-related depression and antidepressant response. *Journal of Alzheimer's Disease, 26*(3), 523–530.

Zubenko, G. S., & Moossy, J. (1988). Major depression in primary dementia. Clinical and neuropathologic correlates. *Archives of Neurology, 45*(11), 1182–1186.

Zubenko, G. S., Moossy, J., & Kopp, U. (1990). Neurochemical correlates of major depression in primary dementia. *Archives of Neurology, 47*(2), 209–214.

Zubenko, G. S., Zubenko, W. N., McPherson, S., Spoor, E., Marin, D. B., Farlow, M. R., ... Sunderland, T. (2003). A collaborative study of the emergence and clinical features of the major depressive syndrome of Alzheimer's disease. *American Journal of Psychiatry, 160*(5), 857–866.

Zung, W. W. (1965). A self-rating depression scale. *Archives of General Psychiatry, 12,* 63–70.

Zweig, R. M., Ross, C. A., Hedreen, J. C., Steele, C., Cardillo, J. E., Whitehouse, P. J., ... Price, D. L. (1988). The neuropathology of aminergic nuclei in Alzheimer's disease. *Annals of Neurology, 24*(2), 233–242.

12

THE CHALLENGE OF SUICIDE PREVENTION IN LATER LIFE

Yeates Conwell and Alisa O'Riley

"TO MY friends. My work is done. Why wait?" Having written these words on a notepad by his bed, George Eastman ended his own life with a gunshot wound to the chest in his Rochester, New York, mansion on March 14, 1932. Founder of the Eastman Kodak Company, he was a leading industrialist and philanthropist of his day, a self-made man accustomed to being in charge. It seemed almost natural then that he should end his life the way he had lived it, in an autonomous and decisive manner. Having completed his work, it was time to go.

The image of George Eastman's self-determined death is almost a comforting one; we badly want our elders to be autonomous and in charge because the alternative evokes fears of aging, debility, and pain. Of course, older adults generally find great pleasure and meaning in their advanced years, even in the face of the many challenges that aging brings (Carstensen et al., 2011). Yet Mr. Eastman's suicide note belies the reality of his final days—racked with pain and increasing disability due to a degenerative spinal condition, cut off from the work and

friends that had given life meaning, and increasingly despondent (Bayer, 1996). His was a scenario typical in every respect, except his wealth and privilege, of suicide in older adults.

In many countries throughout the world, radical demographic shifts are under way. As life expectancy increases and fertility rates decline, the proportion of populations that is over 65 years of age is rapidly increasing. In the United States, for example, over 71 million people, or 20% of the population, will be older adults by the year 2030, fueled by aging of the large post–World War II baby boomer cohort (CDC & The Merck Company Foundation, 2007). As the proportion of older adults in the population rises, so too will the number of suicides among this cohort.

Our objectives with this chapter are three-fold. First, we will review the scale of the problem of suicidal behavior in older adults. Second, we will review current knowledge about risk and protective factors for late-life suicide using a multiaxial framework analogous to that used by psychiatry's *Diagnostic and Statistical Manual of Mental Disorders (DSM;*

APA, 2000) to organize these data. Finally, we will consider the approaches to late-life suicide prevention that both show great promise and represent a necessary mix of high-risk and population-oriented approaches.

EPIDEMIOLOGY OF SUICIDE IN OLDER ADULTS

Suicide rates tend to rise inexorably with age across the life course in countries throughout the world (WHO, 2000). As depicted in Figure 12.1 using statistics compiled by the World Health Organization, that pattern is true for both men and women, although there is wide variation from region to region. The pattern in the United States (Fig. 12.2) is distinctive in several ways (CDC, 2012). First, rates tend to be higher across the life cycle for Whites than non-Whites. Second, rates of suicide for women tend to peak in midlife and level off or drop thereafter. Among White men, rates rise to an initial peak in middle adulthood, drop slightly, then increase dramatically into old, old adulthood while a later-life peak for non-White men is blunted. The dramatic rise in rates with age in the United States, therefore, is largely accounted for by older White men.

Figure 12.3 depicts recent temporal changes in suicide rates as a function of age (men and women, all races combined) in the United States between 1981 and 2007 (CDC, 2012). Speculatively, the marked drop in rates among older adults during that time frame can be ascribed to improved access to health care and other social resources, and to large increases in prescription of antidepressant medications during that time. Of concern is the recent increase in rates among those aged 35–64 years, including many of those in the baby boom generation, which as a cohort has carried with it relatively high suicide rates at each stage of life course development. There is reason for concern, therefore, that as this group enters older adulthood, when suicide rates tend to peak among men, suicide rates in older adulthood will once again begin to rise.

FACTORS ASSOCIATED WITH RISK FOR SUICIDE IN LATER LIFE

Suicide is a complex, multidetermined phenomenon at any age. Observations from a series of retrospective, case-controlled, psychological autopsy (PA) studies in recent years have yielded strong evidence, complemented by findings on determinants of risk in longitudinal cohort studies, with which to guide the design and implementation of preventive interventions. Managing that complexity, however, is key. No single factor has sufficient predictive power to be of clinical utility. Rather, while any one factor may serve to raise a clinician's awareness of potential

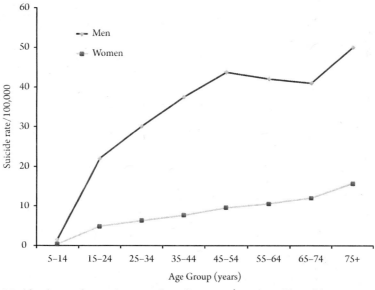

FIGURE 12.1 Worldwide suicide rates by age and gender, 2000. (From World Health Organization [WHO]. http://www.who.int/mental_health/prevention/suicide/suicide_rates_chart/en/index.html)

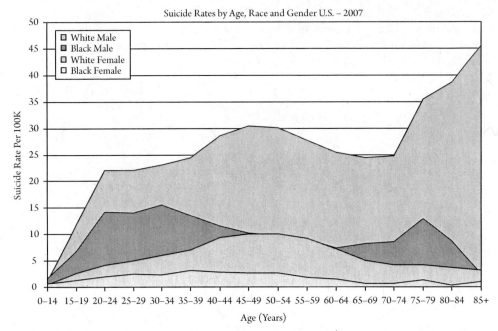

FIGURE 12.2 Suicide rates by age, race, and gender, United States, 2007. (From Centers for Disease Control [CDC]. WISQARS TM [Web-based Injury Statistics Query and Reporting System]. http://www.cdc.gov/ncipc/wisqars/default.htm)

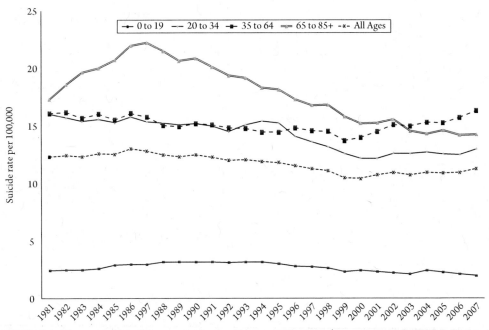

FIGURE 12.3 Changes in United States suicide rates, by age, 1981–2007. (From Centers for Disease Control [CDC]. WISQARS TM [Web-based Injury Statistics Query and Reporting System]. http://www.cdc.gov/ncipc/wisqars/default.htm)

risk, it is the confluence of multiple factors and the context in which they occur that will ultimately best inform clinical as well as public health preventive interventions. To organize that complexity, we utilize a multiaxial format, adapted from psychiatry's *DSM* (APA, 2000), as depicted in Figure 12.4.

Axis I: Psychopathology

The PA method employs interviews of people who knew an older adult who died by suicide to reconstruct the psychiatric status of the decedent in the days, months, and years leading up to the death (Hawton et al., 1998). Although limited by its retrospective nature and the powerful impact that bereavement by suicide may have on a proxy informant, the PA method has been shown to be valid and reliable (Kelly & Mann, 1996). Numerous PA studies, including several that compared individuals who died by suicide with matched comparison groups of older people who were either living in the community or had died of natural causes, have been conducted (see for, e.g., Barraclough, 1971; Beautrais, 2002; Carney, Rich, Burke, & Fowler, 1994; Chiu et al., 2004; Conwell et al., 2000, 2009; Harwood, Hawton, Hope, & Jacoby, 2001; Henriksson et al., 1995; Waern, Runeson, et al., 2002). All show that diagnosable psychopathology was present in 85% or more of older adults who took their own lives, with odds ratios ranging from 44 to over 113 for any Axis I diagnosis. Affective disorders, especially major depression, are the most common psychiatric illnesses among older adults who died by suicide, present in 54%–87% of cases. Odds ratios for suicide associated with any mood disorder range in controlled studies from 4 to over 180. Primary psychotic disorders, including schizophrenia, schizoaffective illness, and delusion disorder, tend to be present in lower proportions among older adult suicides (0 to 9% of cases); anxiety disorders are present in 1%–24% of cases; and alcohol and drug use disorders are present in 3%–45% of suicides. In case-control studies, while the evidence is unequivocal for increased relative risk associated with psychiatric illness in general and mood disorders in particular, results are mixed with regard to other disorders, reflecting the limitations of small sample size and the limitations of needing to rely on proxy respondents (Beautrais, 2002; Chiu et al., 2004; Conwell et al., 2009; Harwood et al., 2001; Waern, Runeson, et al., 2002).

Given the psychological distress, affective instability, problem-solving impairments, and profound social stress associated with dementia diagnoses, one would expect suicide risk to be high in people with Alzheimer's disease and related disorders. Indeed, epidemiological studies indicate that dementia is associated with suicide, particularly in the period soon after diagnosis (Erlangsen, Zarit, & Conwell, 2008; Haw, Harwood, & Hawton, 2009). However,

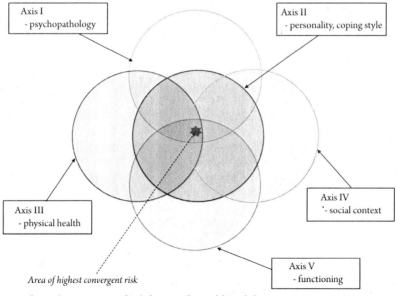

FIGURE 12.4 Multiaxial assessment of risk for suicide in older adults.

it is rarely observed in PA studies of older people. In four studies comparing the prevalence of dementia or delirium in suicides and controls (Chiu et al., 2004; Conwell et al., 2009; Harwood et al., 2001; Waern, Runeson, et al., 2002), only one reported a significant difference (Harwood et al., 2001); Harwood and colleagues found dementia to be a protective factor (lower prevalence in suicides than controls). This counterintuitive finding may be explained by their use of older adults who died in hospital, where delirium is so common, as a comparison group. Other limitations of the PA method, which relies on informant reports and retrospective recall, are likely barriers to detection of cognitive changes necessary for dementia diagnosis, especially early in the course of illness. At more advanced stages of the dementing process, functional disabilities and the requirement for closer supervision may preclude suicidal acts.

Although of little clinical utility at this stage, evidence continues to accumulate for associations between suicidal behavior and a range of neurobiological and neuropsychological processes in younger adult, mixed age, and some older adult samples (Ernst, Mechawar, & Turecki, 2009). Indices of central neurotransmitter and neuroendocrine systems have distinguished suicidal subjects from controls in many studies. Mann and colleagues articulated the stress-diathesis model of suicide in which neurobiological characteristics make some individuals susceptible to impulsivity, aggression, and ultimately suicide in the face of psychiatric illness (Mann, Waternaux, Haas, & Malone, 1999). In all likelihood, these abnormalities are the result of both genetic vulnerabilities and exposure to environmental factors. Linking this model to the distinctive age- and gender-associated epidemiology of completed suicide is difficult, however, because relatively few studies have examined neurobiological parameters in later life and because the baseline prevalence of medical illness and medications that may affect the necessary assays makes such studies very difficult.

Accumulating evidence does implicate specific neurocognitive processes in suicide among older adults, however. Frontal executive dysfunction may be especially important for a number of reasons. First, it has been closely tied to late-life depression (Alexopoulos, Kiosses, Klimstra, Kalayam, & Bruce, 2002), and several investigators have reported abnormalities in neuropsychological measures of frontal executive function among older adult suicide attempters compared with matched controls (King et al., 2000). Most recently, for example,

Dombrovski and colleagues found impaired reward/punishment learning in older adult suicide attempters, but not ideators (Dombrovski et al., 2010). They posit that this cognitive processing deficit may indicate that older adults who attempt suicide overemphasize present reward/punishment contingencies to the exclusion of past experiences. These findings complement postmortem studies of late-life suicide that implicate ventral prefrontal cortical regions as neurosubstrates of processes involved in suicidal behavior. Hwang and colleagues used voxel-based morphometric techniques to examine differences in cortical and subcortical structures, comparing older adults with late-onset major depression and a history of suicidal behavior, late-life depression without a history of suicidal behavior, and community controls (Hwang et al., 2010). A history of suicidal behavior was associated with decreased brain volume across several regions, most notably the dorsal medial prefrontal cortex. More research is needed that links studies of brain structure and functioning, refined measures of discrete cognitive processes, and carefully characterized samples of older adults with and without suicidal behavior. It is important also to keep in mind that studies of suicidal ideation and attempts in late life may not fully apply to completed suicide. Much work remains to be done.

Axis II: Personality and Coping Style

Although personality disorders, particularly in Cluster B, have been linked to completed suicide in mixed-age samples, little evidence is available regarding a role for Axis II disorders in late-life suicide. However, several studies have examined enduring traits associated with suicidal thoughts and behaviors in older adults, characteristics that may signal predisposition in the face of other accumulated stress factors. Descriptive studies have linked suicide in older adults with characteristics of hypochondriasis, shy reclusiveness, hostility, and a rigid independent style (Batchelor & Napier, 1953; Clark, 1993). Harwood and colleagues found in their case-controlled psychological autopsy study that older adults who took their own lives had significantly more anxious and obsessive traits than controlled subjects (Harwood et al., 2001), and our group has identified increased neuroticism and low scores on the Openness to Experience (OTE) factor of the NEO-Personality Inventory (Costa & McCrae, 1992) as distinguishing persons over 50 years of age who took their own lives from matched, living controls (Duberstein, 1995). Low OTE is characteristic of individuals with a constricted range of interests and muted affective and hedonic responses, a rigid style that may make adaptation to challenges of aging more difficult for some.

Other frameworks for investigation may address related factors. For instance, Marty and colleagues have studied coping strategies associated with resilience against the development of suicidal ideation (Marty, Segal, & Coolidge, 2010). They found that both "problem-focused" and "emotion-focused" coping protect against suicidal ideation, while "dysfunctional coping" elevated the risk in older adults. Gibbs and colleagues in a similar vein examined problem-solving skills in three groups of older adults—depressed suicide attempters, depressed nonattempters, and controls (Gibbs et al., 2009). Depressed attempters reported negative problem-solving orientations and greater tendencies to engage in impulsive or careless problem-solving strategies than the other two groups. Whether conceived as an enduring personality trait, coping or problem-solving style, or the manifestation of underlying neurocognitive processing, the characteristic style with which an older adult manages the inevitable challenges of aging may either exacerbate risk or serve as a buffer to mitigate it.

Axis III: Physical Health and Illness

Physical health problems are present in the great majority of older people who take their own lives (Henriksson et al., 1995; Waern, Rubenowitz, et al., 2002). However, because the base rate of physical disorders is so high in older people in general, its predictive value for suicide is poor. That said, understanding the association between late-life suicide and physical illness is critical because ill health may serve as an important stressor contributing to the accumulative risk for a vulnerable individual, it may influence where individuals at risk might best be detected, and it may guide the design and implementation of preventive interventions specific to older adults.

Data concerning the association between physical illness and suicide come from a variety of sources. First, linkage of disease registries with death registries has been a useful strategy revealing, for example, that cancers increase relative risk for suicide by a factor of approximately two (Harris & Barraclough, 1994). Other conditions have also been associated with increased suicide risk in some studies, including HIV/AIDS, epilepsy (particularly of the temporal lobe), renal and peptic ulcer disease, heart and lung disease, spinal cord injury, and systemic lupus erythematosus (Juurlink, Herrmann, Szalai, Kopp, & Redelmeier, 2004; Quan, Arboleda-Florez, Fick, Stuart, & Love, 2002). Controlled PA studies have also yielded results linking suicide to specific illnesses, including malignancy (Conwell et al., 2009; Waern, Rubenowitz, et al., 2002), serious vision problems (Waern, Rubenowitz, & Wilhelmson, 2003), and neurological diseases (Conwell et al., 2009; Waern, Rubenowitz, et al., 2002).

Although the relative risk for suicide associated with any one condition may be small, Juurlink and colleagues have shown their cumulative impact (Juurlink et al., 2004). They linked province-wide prescription records in Ontario, Canada, with provincial coroners' reports to show that relative risk of suicide increased in proportion to the number of illnesses being treated. For older adults who had seven or more illnesses, for example, the relative risk of suicide was approximately nine times higher than those who had no such diagnosis.

The relationship between physical illness and suicide can be explained by a variety of mechanisms. Physical illness may result in affective disorder, either acting as a psychological stressor or direct biological precipitant (e.g., depression due to hypothyroidism), which in turn leads to development of the suicidal state. In addition, illness may be associated with pain, which also has been associated with increased suicide risk in a number of studies. The impact of pain may in fact be particularly salient among older men. Juurlink and colleagues, for example, reported in their linkage study that the association between treatment for severe pain and suicide was somewhat stronger for men than women (Juurlink et al., 2004). Other investigators have reported similar associations (Li & Conwell, 2010). Physical illness may have profound impact on an older person's social network (see Axis IV) and functioning (Axis V), cutting them off from loved ones and, like George Eastman, their sources of meaning in life. In addition, physical illness and its treatments may have extreme financial consequences. The potential etiological pathways are many and complex, and they warrant further study.

Axis IV: Social Context

There is clear evidence from PA studies for a role of social-contextual factors in the pathogenesis of, and protection against, suicidal behavior in older people.

Stressful life events tend to be more numerous and severe in the time preceding suicide, the events being those characteristic of normal aging and development—threats to independence associated with ill health and functional impairment, losses through bereavement and age-associated role change, rupture of relationships with family members and other sources of support, and financial problems.

The themes of social isolation and family discord as a risk factor for late-life suicide, and social connectedness as a buffer, emerge most strongly. Serious relationship problems distinguished older adults with near fatal suicide attempts from controls in New Zealand (Beautrais, 2002), and, in Sweden, family discord was significantly more common in the lives of older adult suicides than a matched, living comparison sample (Rubenowitz, Waern, Wilhelmson, & Allebeck, 2001). Our group has also reported that family discord distinguished suicides from controls over the age of 50 years after adjusting for sociodemographic characteristics and mental disorders (Duberstein, Conwell, Conner, Eberly, & Caine, 2004; Duberstein, Conwell, Conner, Eberly, Evinger, et al., 2004), and evidence suggests that individuals who report a strong family connection are less likely to report suicide ideation (Purcell et al., 2011). Other retrospective studies have reported that older adult suicides were significantly less likely to have a confidante than controls (Miller, 1977), they were also more likely to live alone than their peers in the community (Barraclough, 1971), and they were less likely to participate in community activities (Duberstein, Conwell, Conner, Eberly, Evinger, et al., 2004), be active in organizations, or have a hobby (Rubenowitz et al., 2001). Turvey and colleagues examined these same issues in analyses of data from a prospective cohort study, demonstrating that having a greater number of friends and relatives in whom to confide was associated with significantly reduced suicide risk in older adults (Turvey et al., 2002).

Axis V: Functioning and Disability

Disability generally refers to the difficulties that result from functional limitations in the conduct of activities of daily life. Because physical illness is so common in older people, assessment of functional capacity and any resulting disablement is a necessary component of any comprehensive assessment. Evidence now shows that functional limitations and disablement make substantial independent contributions to suicide risk in older people and therefore represent potential targets for preventive interventions.

For example, Tsoh and colleagues found that older adults who had attempted or completed suicide had greater functional impairment than nonsuicidal older adult controls (Tsoh et al., 2005). In their case-controlled study of suicide in later life, Waern and colleagues reported a significant association between suicide and need for help with activities of daily living in those over age 75 years (Waern et al., 2003). The relationship was evident, however, in univariate but not multivariate analyses. In a similar study our group also found that deficits in instrumental activities of daily living significantly differentiated suicides from controls, even after controlling for presence of psychiatric disorders (Conwell et al., 2009). Hospitalization for medical or surgical reasons as well as use of visiting nurse or home health aide services increased risk as well.

The relationship between functional impairment and suicide in late life may be partially explained by the effect such impairment can have on some older adults' perceptions of their relationships with others. For example, some evidence based on work examining the interpersonal theory of suicide suggests people at great risk for suicidal desire experience high levels of perceived burdensomeness, or a belief that others in their lives would be "better off" if they were dead (Cukrowicz et al., 2011; Joiner, 2005; Van Orden et al., 2010). If an individual who is particularly susceptible to perceived burdensomeness develops a functional impairment that necessitates help from others, that individual may experience a direct threat to his or her sense of autonomy and personal control (Van Orden et al., 2010). Individuals who perceive themselves as a burden on those around them, according to the interpersonal theory of suicide, begin to see their deaths as worth more than their lives and are at higher risk for death by suicide. Indeed, some evidence suggests that feelings of perceived burdensomeness and loss of autonomy are associated with suicide risk in late life (Conwell et al., 2009; Cukrowicz et al., 2011; Jahn et al., 2011).

PREVENTION OF LATE-LIFE SUICIDE

As noted at the outset, the rapid increase in numbers of older adults, coupled with the increased risk for suicide associated with older age, makes the design and implementation of effective preventive intervention strategies an urgent public health priority. By determining factors associated with increased suicide risk among older adults, research has laid a firm foundation upon which to base prevention programming (Erlangsen et al., 2011). In this final section, we discuss approaches that have shown some promise in reducing suicide risk in later life, framing that discussion in terms of special characteristics of suicide at this point in the life course that pose challenges and represent potential barriers to prevention that must be overcome.

Barriers to Late-Life Suicide Prevention

The lethality of suicidal behavior is far higher in older adulthood than at younger ages, an observation that has critical implications for prevention. Whereas the estimated ratio of completed to attempted suicides in the general population is approximately 30:1, and as high as 200:1 in subpopulations of younger adults, there are as few as two or four attempted suicides for each completed suicide in older people (Crosby, Cheltenham, & Sacks, 1999; Fremouw, dePerczel, & Ellis, 1990). When an older adult attempts suicide, he is far more likely to die from his injuries than a younger person because of several distinct factors. The older suicidal person is ordinarily frail with multiple medical conditions that make any self-inflicted injury more likely to be lethal. The suicidal older adult is also more likely to live alone and be socially isolated, and therefore less likely to be recognized as in distress or rescued after initiating a self-destructive act. Finally, suicidal older people use firearms at a substantially higher rate than younger people, who act to harm themselves and implement their suicidal behavior in more planful and determined ways (Conwell et al., 1998).

Another characteristic of older suicidal people that must be taken into account in designing preventive interventions is the relatively greater difficulty caregivers and providers have in detecting the distress of an older adult at risk for suicide and engaging the older person in treatment. Older adults are less likely to express symptoms of depression or suicidal ideation than younger and middle-aged adults (Lyness, Cox, Curry, Conwell, & King, 1995). Perhaps more than at other ages, mental illness is a source of stigma for older people. Mental health concerns and suicide are rarely spoken of, and even those few older adults who may recognize their distress as a psychological rather than physical or social disorder are reluctant to see a mental health professional. Ageist attitudes are prevalent, including among older people and their caregivers. Myths, for example, that it is "normal" to feel depressed or to wish for an early death, are commonly accepted. As a consequence, the distressed older person and her caregivers and providers may misinterpret signals of increased suicide risk as expected or inevitable consequences of aging. Barriers to effective management of suicide risk exist at the practice and service system levels as well. Primary care providers may have insufficient time to sort through the multiple, complex medical conditions with which their older patients present in order to reveal their more covert psychological pain and suicidal thoughts.

Therefore, not only are the "signals" of suicide risk muted in older people, but the "noise" interfering with their reception is high. As a result, the likelihood of an older adult being recognized as in trouble before entering a suicidal crisis is reduced; and once in a suicidal crisis, the likelihood of survival is greatly diminished. Although daunting, these challenges provide important clues with which to guide development of preventive interventions at this stage of the life course.

Implications for Preventive Interventions

Terminology developed by the Institute of Medicine usefully characterizes approaches to suicide prevention at three distinct levels (IOM, Mrazek, & Haggerty, 1994).

INDICATED APPROACHES

First is "indicated" prevention, which targets individuals with detectable symptoms of mental illness or suicidal ideation. A typical objective of indicated preventive interventions is to diagnose and treat psychiatric illness in order to prevent the expression of suicidal behavior. The use of antidepressant medications or evidence-based psychotherapies are prime examples (see, e.g., Bhar & Brown, 2012; Gibbons et al., 2007; Heisel et al., 2009; Stone et al., 2009).

The characteristics of late-life suicide noted earlier have two important implications for use of indicated preventive interventions in this population. First, because suicidal behavior is so often lethal in older people, clinicians who detect suicidal ideation or developing suicidal crisis in their older patients should be aggressive in intervening to assure timely assessment, treatment, and the patient's safety. Limiting access to lethal means, mobilizing family supports, conducting a detailed risk assessment, and assuring safety while diagnosis and treatment are under way are all indicated.

Second, because older people rarely utilize mental health specialty services, indicated preventive interventions should also be mounted in other settings where older adults in or nearing suicidal crises are more likely to surface. Primary care clinics have been most intensively studied. Bruce, Alexopoulos, and colleagues, for example, reported results of the Prevention of Suicide in Primary Care Elderly: Collaborative Trial (PROSPECT) designed to test a primary care-based collaborative depression care management intervention (Alexopoulos et al., 2009; Bruce et al., 2004). Older adults with major depression, minor depression, or dysthymia were recruited from primary care practices and randomly assigned to receive either care as usual or the PROSPECT intervention. The latter included algorithm-driven treatment with antidepressants, patient/family and provider education, interpersonal therapy as a treatment option, and coordination of care by a depression care specialist. Rates of suicidal ideation declined significantly faster in intervention patients than controls, with greater reduction sustained over 24 months. Intervention patients also had significantly better outcomes over 2 years of follow-up with regard to major depressive symptoms. Unützer and colleagues tested a similar approach to collaborative, stepped care management for late-life depression in primary care practices using an intervention titled Improving Mood-Promoting Access to Collaborative Treatment (IMPACT), and observed similar benefits with regard to depression and suicidal ideation (Unutzer et al., 2002, 2006). In both of these important studies the incidence of suicide attempts was too small to judge the interventions' impact on that outcome. Nevertheless, the consistent associations observed among depression, suicidal ideation, and death by suicide provide powerful reinforcement for further study and implementation of preventive approaches targeting depression in late-life primary care.

In addition to primary care settings, other community sites that serve large numbers of older adults should also be considered sites in which indicated prevention may be beneficial. These include home health care and community-based social service agencies where rates of depression and suicidal ideation have also been found to be high (Bruce et al., 2002; Raue, Meyers, Rowe, Heo, & Bruce, 2007; Richardson, He, Podgorski, Tu, & Conwell, in press). Unfortunately, no examples of indicated preventive intervention in such settings have as yet been examined using clinical trials methods.

Perhaps the most important implication of the characteristic lethality of late-life suicide, however, is that indicated preventive interventions alone are likely to be insufficient to substantially reduce suicide mortality among older people. Instead, we must look to approaches that interrupt the development of suicidal states. These approaches according to the IOM rubric include selective and universal preventive interventions.

SELECTIVE APPROACHES

The second "level" of prevention according to the IOM framework is called "selective." Selective interventions target asymptomatic or presymptomatic individuals or groups with a greater than average risk of developing high-risk suicidal states due to presence of more distal risk factors.

The demonstrated close association between social disconnectedness, impaired social supports and family relationships, physical illness, pain, and functional impairment suggests that selective interventions targeting these risk factors should reduce late-life suicide as well. Within this framework many existing medical and social services could be considered selective suicide prevention strategies. For example, comprehensive geriatric assessment clinics that provide thorough diagnostic and treatment services to older adults may have the additional benefit of reducing health burden, optimizing functioning, and more effectively managing pain. Social services that provide outreach to isolated older people in the community and care management services that address other social needs, support active engagement with others, and support older adults in maintaining functional independence in their homes may also lower suicide risk.

We are not aware of any randomized controlled trials testing selective preventive interventions' effectiveness in reducing suicide per se. However, DeLeo and colleagues' Tele-Help/Tele-Check service addressed this question using a quasi-experimental design (De Leo, Dello Buono, & Dwyer, 2002). The service, based in Padua, Italy, provided telephone-based outreach, evaluation, and support by social work staff to more than 18,000 frail older adults at risk for institutional care. Over 11 years of service delivery, there were significantly fewer suicides among clients in the program than were expected in a comparable elder population of that region.

UNIVERSAL APPROACHES

Finally, "universal" preventive interventions target an entire population regardless of any individual's risk status. Their objective is to implement broadly directed initiatives to prevent suicide-related morbidity through reducing risk and enhancing protective factors at a population level. Examples might include education programs for the general public, clergy, or health care providers concerning normal aging and the potential benefits of depression diagnosis and treatment; or policies governing access to firearms and assuring access to affordable health care and community-based supportive services. Several "natural experiments" provide ecological evidence for the effect of such interventions. For example, when the United Kingdom implemented legislation requiring that paracetamol and salicylates be sold as blister packs in limited quantities, morbidity and mortality from overdose with those medications decreased significantly (Hawton et al., 2001). And, in the United States, passage of the Brandy Handgun Violence Prevention Act in 1994 resulted in a significant reduction in handgun suicides by people over the age of 55 years in those states that newly implemented background checks and waiting periods for gun purchases as compared to those states in which no new changes in procedures were required (Ludwig & Cook, 2000).

COMPREHENSIVE APPROACHES

Given that there are multiple pathways to suicide and that universal, selective, and indicated preventive interventions interrupt that process at different levels, it is likely that the most effective program for reducing suicide mortality in later life would be one that integrates elements from all three. A series of interventions tested by Oyama and colleagues in rural Japanese communities with high rates of late-life suicide may provide the best example of a multilevel, comprehensive intervention in older adults to date (Oyama, Fujita, Goto, Shibuya, & Sakashita, 2006; Oyama, Goto, Fujita, Shibuya, & Sakashita, 2006; Oyama, Koida, Sakashita, & Kudo,

2004; Oyama, Ono, et al., 2006; Oyama et al., 2005, 2010). Details differed somewhat between studies. Each, however, was implemented over 5- to 10-year periods and included systematic community-wide screening, referral to primary care or mental health care as indicated, and, to varying degrees, public education and social engagement programs for older adults. Late-life suicide rates in these communities following the intervention period were compared both with rates preceding the intervention and with rates of suicide in neighboring reference regions of similar size and character. Overall risk was significantly reduced in men and women when follow-up was conducted by a psychiatrist, but only in women when follow-up was conducted by general practitioners. While the studies' success lends reason for optimism regarding our ability to reduce suicide mortality in older adults, this pattern of relative resistance by men to preventive interventions at any level remains a major, unsolved challenge.

CONCLUSIONS

The size of the older adult population is growing dramatically and will continue to do so in coming decades. With this "aging tsunami" will inevitably come an increase in the number of older people who take their own lives. In recent years, research has yielded important new knowledge about factors that place older adults at risk for suicide, and it therefore provides guidance for the development of strategies to reduce late-life suicide morbidity and mortality. As reviewed here, approaches that optimize detection and management of psychiatric illness, and mood disorders in particular, are necessary but not sufficient. Selective preventive interventions that target vulnerable individuals and groups prior to development of acute clinical states must be emphasized as well. Rather than mounting prevention in mental health care settings, the preferred approach will target older adults in primary care, other ambulatory medical and surgical settings, and community-based long-term care. Integration of mental health providers into those settings to facilitate detection and management of older adults at risk with psychiatric, medical, and social comorbidities will be an important objective for services research and development.

Nonetheless, many challenges remain. The predictive value of variables in any one domain is too low to be of reliable use in assessing risk; instead, we must learn more about how combinations of risk and protective factors across domains interact to determine an individual's risk status. Referring again to Figure 12.3, for example, we can best understand George Eastman's suicide as resulting from the convergence of risk. He did not kill himself because he was in ill health or depressed, but rather because he was a man with closely held values of autonomy (Axis II) who, in the face of physical illness and mounting pain (Axis III) became increasingly disabled (Axis V), isolated from others, and cut off from activities that gave meaning to life (Axis IV). In that context, he became hopeless, depressed, and demoralized (Axis I). Underlying neurobiological changes associated with illness in aging may also have played a role. This complex interwoven set of factors then made death his chosen option.

Despite advances in our understanding of factors that place older people at risk for suicide, insufficient attention has thus far been paid to protective factors, variables that interact with risk factors to mitigate their impact. Religious participation and spirituality are examples. Virtually no research has yet explored, however, whether social connectedness serves as a buffer in the face of potentially toxic stressors, and, if so, which components, in what dose, and administered at what point in the pathway to suicide.

Finally, the greatest remaining challenge to late-life suicide prevention may be the need for political and social will, attitudes held by individuals, families, providers, and society about the relative value of years of life lost at the end of the life course. It is in this realm that universal preventive interventions will have a critical role to play in addressing the impending public health crisis of late-life suicide.

Disclosures

Dr. Conwell has no conflicts to disclose. His support comes from the University of Rochester and grants from NIH and CDC only. Grant support: CDC U01CE001942, NIMH R24071604, NIMH U24MH094284, and NIH/FIC D43 TW009101.

Dr. O'Riley has no conflicts to disclose. Her support comes from the University of Rochester and a grant from NIMH only. Grant support: NIMH T32MH20061.

REFERENCES

Alexopoulos, G. S., Kiosses, D. N., Klimstra, S., Kalayam, B., & Bruce, M. L. (2002). Clinical presentation of the "depression-executive dysfunction syndrome" of late life. *American Journal of Geriatric Psychiatry, 10*(1), 98–106.

Alexopoulos, G. S., Reynolds, C. F., III, Bruce, M. L., Katz, I. R., Raue, P. J., Mulsant, B. H., ... Ten Have, T. (2009). Reducing suicidal ideation and depression in older primary care patients: 24-month outcomes of the PROSPECT study. *American Journal of Psychiatry, 166*(8), 882–890.

American Psychiatric Association (APA). (2000). *Diagnostic and statistical manual of mental disorders* (4th ed., text rev.). Washington, DC: Author.

Barraclough, B. M. (1971). Suicide in the elderly: Recent developments in psychogeriatrics. *British Journal of Psychiatry, Spec. Suppl. 6*, 87–97.

Batchelor, I. R. C., & Napier, M. B. (1953). Attempted suicide in old age. *British Medical Journal, 2*, 1186–1190.

Bayer, E. (1996). *George Eastman: A biography*. Baltimore, MD: Johns Hopkins University Press.

Beautrais, A. L. (2002). A case control study of suicide and attempted suicide in older adults. *Suicide an Life Threatening Behavior, 32*(1), 1–9.

Bhar, S. S., & Brown, G. K. (2012). Treatment of depression and suicide in older adults. *Cognitive and Behavioral Practice, 19*, 116–125.

Bruce, M. L., McAvay, G. J., Raue, P. J., Brown, E. L., Meyers, B. S., Keohane, D. J., ... Weber, C. (2002). Major depression in elderly home health care patients. *American Journal of Psychiatry, 159*(8), 1367–1374.

Bruce, M. L., Ten Have, T., Reynolds, C. F., III, Katz, I. R., Schulberg, H. C., Mulsant, B. H., ... Alexopoulos, G. S. (2004). Reducing suicidal ideation and depressive symptoms in depressed older primary care patients: A randomized controlled trial. *Journal of the American Medical Association, 291*(9), 1081–1091.

Carney, S. S., Rich, C. L., Burke, P. A., & Fowler, R. C. (1994). Suicide over 60: The San Diego study. *Journal of the American Geriatrics Society, 42*(2), 174–180.

Carstensen, L. L., Turan, B., Scheibe, S., Ram, N., Ersner-Hershfield, H., Samanez-Larkin, G. R., ... Nesselroade, J. R. (2011). Emotional experience improves with age: Evidence based on over 10 years of experience sampling. *Psychology and Aging, 26*(1), 21–33.

Centers for Disease Control and Prevention (CDC). (2011). *WISQARS TM (Web-based Injury Statistics Query and Reporting System)*. Retrieved June 2, 2011, from http://www.cdc.gov/injury/wisqars/index.html

Centers for Disease Control and Prevention & The Merck Company Foundation. (2007). *The state of aging and health in America*. Witehouse Station, NJ: CDC & The Merck Company Foundation.

Chiu, H. F., Yip, P. S., Chi, I., Chan, S., Tsoh, J., Kwan, C. W.,…Caine, E. (2004). Elderly suicide in Hong Kong—a case-controlled psychological autopsy study. *Acta Psychiatrica Scandinavica, 109*(4), 299–305.

Clark, D. C. (1993). Narcissistic crises of aging and suicidal despair. *Suicide and Life-Threatening Behavior, 23*(1), 21–26.

Conwell, Y., Duberstein, P. R., Cox, C., Herrmann, J., Forbes, N., & Caine, E. D. (1998). Age differences in behaviors leading to completed suicide. *American Journal of Geriatric Psychiatry, 6*(2), 122–126.

Conwell, Y., Duberstein, P. R., Hirsch, J. K., Conner, K. R., Eberly, S., & Caine, E. D. (2009). Health status and suicide in the second half of life. *International Journal of Geriatric Psychiatry, 25*(4), 371–379.

Conwell, Y., Lyness, J. M., Duberstein, P., Cox, C., Seidlitz, L., DiGiorgio, A., & Caine, E. D. (2000). Completed suicide among older patients in primary care practices: A controlled study. *Journal of the American Geriatrics Society, 48*(1), 23–29.

Costa, P. T., & McCrae, R. R. (1992). *Revised NEO Personality Inventory and NEO Five Factor Inventory: Professional manual*. Odessa, FL: PAR.

Crosby, A. E., Cheltenham, M. P., & Sacks, J. J. (1999). Incidence of suicidal ideation and behavior in the United States, 1994. *Suicide and Life-Threatening Behavior, 29*(2), 131–140.

Cukrowicz, K. C., Cheavens, J. S., Van Orden, K. A., Ragain, R. M., & Cook, R. L. (2011). Perceived burdensomeness and suicide ideation in older adults. *Psychology and Aging, 26*(2), 331–338.

De Leo, D., Dello Buono, M., & Dwyer, J. (2002). Suicide among the elderly: The long-term impact of a telephone support and assessment intervention in northern Italy. *British Journal of Psychiatry, 181*, 226–229.

Dombrovski, A. Y., Clark, L., Siegle, G. J., Butters, M. A., Ichikawa, N., Sahakian, B. J., & Szanto, K. (2010). Reward/punishment reversal learning in older suicide attempters. *American Journal of Psychiatry, 167*(6), 699–707.

Duberstein, P. R. (1995). Openness to experience and completed suicide across the second half of life. *International Psychogeriatrics, 7*(2), 183–198.

Duberstein, P. R., Conwell, Y., Conner, K. R., Eberly, S., & Caine, E. D. (2004). Suicide at 50 years of age and older: Perceived physical illness, family discord and financial strain. *Psycholological Medicine, 34*(1), 137–146.

Duberstein, P. R., Conwell, Y., Conner, K. R., Eberly, S., Evinger, J. S., & Caine, E. D. (2004). Poor social integration and suicide: Fact or artifact? A case-control study. *Psychological Medicine, 34*(7), 1331–1337.

Erlangsen, A., Nordentoft, M., Conwell, Y., Waern, M., De Leo, D., Lindner, R…Lapierre, S. (2011). Key considerations for preventing suicide in older adults: Consensus opinions of an expert panel. *Crisis, 32*(2), 106–109.

Erlangsen, A., Zarit, S. H., & Conwell, Y. (2008). Hospital-diagnosed dementia and suicide: A longitudinal study using prospective, nationwide register data. *American Journal of Geriatric Psychiatry, 16*(3), 220–228.

Ernst, C., Mechawar, N., & Turecki, G. (2009). Suicide neurobiology. *Progress in Neurobiology, 89*(4), 315–333.

Fremouw, W. J., dePerczel, M., & Ellis, T. E. (1990). *Suicide risk: Assessment and response guidelines*. New York: Pergamon Press.

Gibbons, R. D., Brown, C. H., Hur, K., Marcus, S. M., Bhaumik, D. K., & Mann, J. J. (2007). Relationship between antidepressants and suicide attempts: An analysis of the Veterans Health Administration data sets. *American Journal of Psychiatry, 164*(7), 1044–1049.

Gibbs, L. M., Dombrovski, A. Y., Morse, J., Siegle, G. J., Houck, P. R., & Szanto, K. (2009). When the solution is part of the problem: Problem solving in elderly suicide attempters. *International Journal of Geriatric Psychiatry, 24*(12), 1396–1404.

Harris, E. C., & Barraclough, B. M. (1994). Suicide as an outcome for medical disorders. *Medicine (Baltimore), 73*(6), 281–296.

Harwood, D., Hawton, K., Hope, T., & Jacoby, R. (2001). Psychiatric disorder and personality factors associated with suicide in older people: A descriptive and case-control study. *International Journal of Geriatric Psychiatry, 16*(2), 155–165.

Haw, C., Harwood, D., & Hawton, K. (2009). Dementia and suicidal behavior: A review of the literature. *International Psychogeriatrics, 21*(3), 440–453.

Hawton, K., Appleby, L., Platt, S., Foster, T., Cooper, J., Malmberg, A., & Simkin, S. (1998). The psychological autopsy approach to studying suicide: A review of methodological issues. *Journal of Affective Disorders, 50*(2–3), 269–276.

Hawton, K., Townsend, E., Deeks, J., Appleby, L., Gunnell, D., Bennewith, O., & Cooper, J. (2001). Effects of legislation restricting pack sizes of paracetamol and salicylate on self poisoning in the United Kingdom: Before and after study. *British Medical Journal, 322*(7296), 1203–1207.

Heisel, M. J., Duberstein, P. R., Talbot, N. L., King, D. A., & Tu, X. M. (2009). Adapting interpersonal psychotherapy for older adults at risk for suicide: Preliminary findings. *Professional Psychology: Research and Practice, 40*(2), 156–164.

Henriksson, M. M., Marttunen, M. J., Isometsa, E. T., Heikkinen, M. E., Aro, H. M., Kuoppasalmi, K. I., & Lonnqvist, J. K. (1995). Mental disorders in elderly suicide. *International Psychogeriatrics, 7*(2), 275–286.

Hwang, J. P., Lee, T. W., Tsai, S. J., Chen, T. J., Yang, C. H., Lirng, J. F., & Tsai, C. F. (2010). Cortical and subcortical abnormalities in late-onset depression with history of suicide attempts investigated with MRI and voxel-based morphometry. *Journal of Geriatric Psychiatry and Neurology, 23*(3), 171–184.

Institute of Medicine (IOM), Mrazek, P. J., & Haggerty, R. J. (1994). *Reducing risks for mental disorders: Frontiers for preventive intervention research.* Washington, DC: National Academy Press.

Jahn, D. R., Cukrowicz, K. C., Linton, K., & Prabhu, F. (2011). The mediating effect of perceived burdensomeness on the relation between depressive symptons and suicide ideation in a community sample of older adults. *Aging and Mental Health, 15*(2), 214–220.

Joiner, T. E. J. (2005). *Why people die by suicide.* Cambridge, MA: Harvard University Press.

Juurlink, D. N., Herrmann, N., Szalai, J. P., Kopp, A., & Redelmeier, D. A. (2004). Medical illness and the risk of suicide in the elderly. *Archives of Internal Medicine, 164*(11), 1179–1184.

Kelly, T. M., & Mann, J. J. (1996). Validity of DSM-III-R diagnosis by psychological autopsy: A comparison with clinician ante-mortem diagnosis. *Acta Psychiatrica Scandinavica, 94*(5), 337–343.

King, D. A., Conwell, Y., Cox, C., Henderson, R. E., Denning, D. G., & Caine, E. D. (2000). A neuropsychological comparison of depressed suicide attempters and nonattempters. *Journal of Neuropsychiatry and Clinical Neurosciences, 12*(1), 64–70.

Li, L. W., & Conwell, Y. (2010). Pain and self-injury ideation in elderly men and women receiving home care. *Journal of the American Geriatric Society, 58*(11), 2160–2165.

Ludwig, J., & Cook, P. J. (2000). Homicide and suicide rates associated with implementation of the Brady Handgun Violence Prevention Act. *Journal of the American Medical Association, 284*(5), 585–591.

Lyness, J. M., Cox, C., Curry, J., Conwell, Y., & King, D. A. (1995). Older age and the underreporting of depressive symptoms. *Journal of the American Geriatrics Society, 43*(3), 216–221.

Mann, J. J., Waternaux, C., Haas, G. L., & Malone, K. M. (1999). Toward a clinical model of suicidal behavior in psychiatric patients. *American Journal of Psychiatry, 156*(2), 181–189.

Marty, M. A., Segal, D. L., & Coolidge, F. L. (2010). Relationships among dispositional coping strategies, suicidal ideation, and protective factors against suicide in older adults. *Aging and Mental Health, 14*(8), 1015–1023.

Miller, M. (1977). A psychological autopsy of a geriatric suicide. *Journal of Geriatric Psychiatry, 10*(2), 229–242.

Oyama, H., Fujita, M., Goto, M., Shibuya, H., & Sakashita, T. (2006). Outcomes of community-based screening for depression and suicide prevention among Japanese elders. *Gerontologist, 46*(6), 821–826.

Oyama, H., Goto, M., Fujita, M., Shibuya, H., & Sakashita, T. (2006). Preventing elderly suicide through primary care by community-based screening for depression in rural Japan. *Crisis, 27*(2), 58–65.

Oyama, H., Koida, J., Sakashita, T., & Kudo, K. (2004). Community-based prevention for suicide in elderly by depression screening and follow-up. *Community Mental Health Journal, 40*(3), 249–263.

Oyama, H., Ono, Y., Watanabe, N., Tanaka, E., Kudoh, S., Sakashita, T., … Yoshimura, K. (2006). Local community intervention through depression screening and group activity for elderly suicide prevention. *Psychiatry and Clinical Neurosciences, 60*(1), 110–114.

Oyama, H., Sakashita, T., Hojo, K., Ono, Y., Watanabe, N., Takizawa, T., … Tanaka, E. (2010). A community-based survey and screening for depression in the elderly: The short-term effect on suicide risk in Japan. *Crisis, 31*(2), 100–108.

Oyama, H., Watanabe, N., Ono, Y., Sakashita, T., Takenoshita, Y., Taguchi, M., … Kumagai, K. (2005). Community-based suicide prevention through group activity for the elderly successfully reduced the high suicide rate for females. *Psychiatry and Clinical Neurosciences, 59*(3), 337–344.

Purcell, B., Marnin, H. Speice, J., Franus, N., Conwell, Y., & Duberstein, P. R. (2011). Family connectedness moderates the association between living alone and suicide ideation in a clinical sample of adults 50 years and older. *American Journal of Geriatric Psychiatry.* ePub ahead of print, doi: 10.1097/JGP.0b013e31822ccd79

Quan, H., Arboleda-Florez, J., Fick, G. H., Stuart, H. L., & Love, E. J. (2002). Association between physical illness and suicide among the elderly. *Social Psychiatry and Psychiatric Epidemiology*, 37(4), 190–197.

Raue, P. J., Meyers, B. S., Rowe, J. L., Heo, M., & Bruce, M. L. (2007). Suicidal ideation among elderly homecare patients. *International Journal of Geriatric Psychiatry*, 22(1), 32–37.

Richardson, T. M., He, H., Podgorski, C., Tu, X., & Conwell, Y. (2010). Screening for depression in aging services clients. *American Journal of Geriatric Psychiatry*, 18(12), 1116–1123.

Rubenowitz, E., Waern, M., Wilhelmson, K., & Allebeck, P. (2001). Life events and psychosocial factors in elderly suicides—a case-control study. *Psychological Medicine*, 31(7), 1193–1202.

Stone, M., Laughren, T., Jones, M. L., Levenson, M., Holland, P. C., Hughes, A., ... Rochester, G. (2009). Risk of suicidality in clinical trials of antidepressants in adults: Analysis of proprietary data submitted to US Food and Drug Administration. *British Medical Journal*, 339, 1–10.

Tsoh, J., Chiu, H. F., Duberstein, P. R., Chan, S. S., Chi, I., Yip, P. S., & Conwell, Y. (2005). Attempted suicide in elderly Chinese persons: A multi-group, controlled study 2. *American Journal of Geriatric Psychiatry*, 13(7), 562–571.

Turvey, C. L., Conwell, Y., Jones, M. P., Phillips, C., Simonsick, E., Pearson, J. L., & Wallace, R. (2002). Risk factors for late-life suicide: A prospective, community-based study. *American Journal of Geriatric Psychiatry*, 10(4), 398–406.

Unutzer, J., Katon, W., Callahan, C. M., Williams, J. W., Jr., Hunkeler, E., Harpole, L., ... IMPACT Investigators. (2002). Collaborative care management of late-life depression in the primary care setting: A randomized controlled trial. *Journal of the American Medical Association*, 288(22), 2836–2845.

Unutzer, J., Tang, L., Oishi, S., Katon, W., Williams, J. W., Jr., Hunkeler, E., ... IMPACT Investigators. (2006). Reducing suicidal ideation in depressed older primary care patients. *Journal of the American Geriatrics Society*, 54(10), 1550–1556.

Van Orden, K., Witte, T. K., Cukrowicz, K. C., Braithwaite, S. R., Selby, E. A., & Joiner, T. E. J. (2010). The interpersonal theory of suicide. *Psychological Review*, 117, 575–600.

Waern, M., Rubenowitz, E., Runeson, B., Skoog, I., Wilhelmson, K., & Allebeck, P. (2002). Burden of illness and suicide in elderly people: Case-control study. *British Medical Journal*, 324(7350), 1355.

Waern, M., Rubenowitz, E., & Wilhelmson, K. (2003). Predictors of suicide in the old elderly. *Gerontology*, 49(5), 328–334.

Waern, M., Runeson, B. S., Allebeck, P., Beskow, J., Rubenowitz, E., Skoog, I., & Wilhelmsson, K. (2002). Mental disorder in elderly suicides: A case-control study. *American Journal of Psychiatry*, 159(3), 450–455.

World Health Organization (WHO). (2000). *Distribution of suicides rates (per 100 000) by gender and age, 2000.* Retrieved May 16, 2011, from http://www.who.int/mental_health/prevention/suicide/suicide_rates_chart/en/index.html

13

BEREAVEMENT AND COMPLICATED GRIEF IN OLDER ADULTS

M. Katherine Shear, Angela Ghesquiere, and Michael Katzke

OLDER PEOPLE know that loss is a part of life, but bereavement can still surprise them with its intensity and unfamiliarity. In the widely quoted words of author C.S. Lewis,

> No one ever told me that grief felt so like fear. I am not afraid, but the sensation is like being afraid. The same fluttering in the stomach, the same restlessness, the yawning. I keep on swallowing. At other times it feels like being mildly drunk, or concussed. There is a sort of invisible blanket between the world and me. I find it hard to take in what anyone says. Or perhaps, hard to want to take it in. It is so uninteresting. Yet I want others to be about me. I dread the moments when the house is empty. If only they would talk to one another and not to me. (C.S. Lewis, *A Grief Observed*, p. 15)

Lewis was 61 when he wrote these famous lines. Like many older people he had been bereaved before, having lost both of his parents and several close friends.

Yet neither his previous experience with grief nor his knowledge of her terminal illness prepared him for the loss of the wife he adored. Moreover, his famous strong religious faith provided little guidance during the painful and disorienting experience of acute grief.

Losing a loved one is widely understood as one of life's most painful and disruptive experiences. As Lewis poignantly describes, such a loss often creates an uncomfortable sense of distance from others and a sense of confusion about oneself—a feeling of being no longer whole. Bereavement can leave a person feeling adrift, cut loose from an anchor. About 75% of the 2.5 million people who die every year in the United States occur among people 65 years of age or older. Their close friends and relatives are most affected by bereavement; many of these are also older adults. Typically people have a convoy of close relationships throughout their lives that can be identified using a visual diagram of concentric circles as "close," "closer," and "closest." Usually there are 1–5 people in the closest group (Antonucci et al., 2004). When a person dies, it is this convoy of closest friends and relatives who suffer most and who most need support from friends and relatives.

Loss of a loved one is an experience that is shared by all humanity. Scores of bereaved people, young and old, share the experience of grief as an acute and devastating assault to mind and body. Yet acute grief can leave us feeling more alone, confused, and unsettled than any other experience. The purpose of this chapter is to outline a framework for understanding bereavement and grief in general and in older people specifically, to describe the healing process, and to point to some possible pitfalls in its course, especially those that might be more common among older adults.

BEREAVEMENT

Bereavement is defined here as the loss of someone close, not as the reaction to that loss. Bereavement is an especially common experience in later life. Recent statistics indicate there are about 37 million people age 65 and over in the United States and about 30% of them are widowed (Federal Interagency Forum on Aging Related Statistics, 2008). Though statistics on rates of loss of parents, friends, and other family members are not compiled as systematically, older adults often experience multiple losses (Williams et al., 2006). Estimates suggest that more than 40% of adults over 60 experience sibling loss and 10% experience the death of an adult child (Williams, Baker, & Allman, 2005). In another study, friends or nonspousal relatives accounted for 97% of the losses reported by the older adults they surveyed (Williams, Baker, & Allman, 2007). This survey documented that loss of nonspousal relatives was associated with mental and physical health problems and is clearly of importance for older adults. However, this chapter focuses primarily on loss of a person's closest relationships. For most people the number of very close relationships is small and their impact monumental. Most people respond to such a loss with a period of acute grief that is painful and disruptive.

Bereavement experiences vary across gender. Considering spousal loss in the United States, 42% of women 65 years of age and older are widowed, including 25% of 65–74 year olds, 52% of those aged 75–84, and 76% of those 85 and older. In contrast, only 13% of men over 65 are widowed, 8% of the 65–74 year old men are widowed, 17% of those aged 75–84, and 34% of those 85 and older (Federal Interagency Forum on Aging Related Statistics, 2008). Williams et al. conducted a 30-month observation of 839 subjects aged 65 and over who were in the University of Alabama at Birmingham Study of Aging. They demonstrated that women disproportionately bear the burden of bereavement events (Williams, Baker, Allman, & Roseman, 2006). The authors concluded that bereavement research should focus on the burden of loss on women and further consider how bereavement may impact the health and well-being of older women. In addition, they recommended that clinicians develop interventions to meet the psychosocial needs of this at-risk group. Yet, even though spousal bereavement is more prevalent among women, it may be a more difficult problem for men.

Studies of death rates following bereavement generally show more vulnerability for men than women (e.g., Shor et al., 2012) including higher suicide rates (Ajdacic-Gross et al., 2008). There are other gender differences as well. Smith et al. (1991) found that widowed men over 60, compared to women over 60, were 10 times more likely to remarry. Schneider et al. (1996) also found higher rates of remarriage among widowed men. Desire for social support may partially explain this trend; Carr (2004a) conducted a reanalysis of data from the Changing Lives of Older Couples (CLOC) study, which was conducted in the 1980s, and found that older men with strong social support resembled women in being less likely to remarry. Moreover, men and women with more conflicted relationships with the deceased had greater interest in remarrying. Notwithstanding gender-based and culture-based similarities, bereavement is a unique experience for every individual. Symptoms vary in quality, intensity, and progression over time, based on a range of factors. For example, loss of a very close, identity-defining relationship is more painful and enduring than loss of a more distant friend or relative. Loss of a very loving and deeply satisfying relationship is more difficult than loss of a conflicted relationship. For example, spouses in the CLOC study who were more dependent on their deceased spouse were more likely to experience positive outcomes than their fellow mourners who were more independent. Dependent women reported an increase in self-esteem after the death of their partners, while dependent men reported more personal growth (Carr, 2004b). Overall, a subgroup of bereaved spouses in the CLOC study experienced a chronic form of problematic grief. The bereaved people find that when a close loved one is lost, a form of acute grief that does not progress results. In these cases, grief symptoms can be prolonged and impairing.

GRIEF

We define grief as the psychobiological response to bereavement. Grief progresses over time, roughly following a trajectory from acute to integrated symptoms. Acute grief is usually characterized by prominent feelings of yearning and sorrow, a feeling of distance or disinterest in the everyday world, and thoughts strongly centered on the person who died. A range of other negative emotions can also occur, and there can be feelings of uncertainty about how to go on without the deceased. Positive emotions are also usually present during acute grief, especially in connection with cherished memories of the person who died.

The intensity of grief symptoms varies widely depending on factors such as the closeness of the relationship and the circumstances and consequences of the death. Each person's grief follows a unique course, guided by factors related to the bereaved person, her relationship to the deceased, the circumstances of the death, and the context in which the bereaved person mourns. It is a tribute to human resilience that most people weather the storm of loss without any severe detriment to their mental or physical states, often absorbing this most unwanted reality in a way that deepens their humanity and opens their hearts to the suffering of others.

Grief is permanent after a loved one dies, though the degree to which sadness and yearning continue is, in part, culturally determined. As discussed earlier, there is wide variability in expectations for sadness. Cultures and religions differ in how they see the relationship between life and death. However, in general, death is naturally anxiety provoking. Several studies in younger adults suggest that those who have experienced a loss experience greater death anxiety than those who have not. However, a recent study in older Israeli adults (Azaiza et al., 2011) did not find that bereaved parents had more death anxiety than those who had not lost a child. In any case, bereaved people need to find a way to think about death that reduces anxiety. Religious beliefs are a common way to do so.

Given the intensity of the natural response to losing a loved one, mourning usually takes some time in order to facilitate the transformation of grief to a place where the loss is integrated into our minds and lives. Rituals can be very helpful in facilitating this process, but even without them, people face a psychological problem that must be solved. Sometimes, though, grief is complicated by ruminations over the circumstances or consequences of the death, excessive avoidance and/or proximity seeking, or persistent disruptive difficulty with emotion regulation. The presence of these complications can interfere with the natural healing process and prolong acute grief.

MOURNING

Mourning is the natural healing process, defined here as the set of psychological processes set in motion by bereavement that leads to coming to terms with the loss. Mourning practices are very influenced by cultural and religious background, and these, in turn, impact grief symptoms. In general, though, adjusting to the loss of a close companion requires fully acknowledging the finality and consequences of the loss, revising the internalized mental representations of the person who died, and redefining life goals and plans without the loved one present. People we love give meaning and purpose to our lives and are often the source of our most important happiness. When someone we love dies, we must find a way to restore a sense of meaning and purpose and the possibility of joy and satisfaction in ongoing life. Mourning rituals and beliefs about the relationship between life and death can help us do this.

Grief symptoms may manifest somewhat differently across cultural groups. Rituals vary across cultures, and with them expectations for the process of mourning. In some cultures sadness and yearning is expected to last only a few days, while in others these feelings are prolonged, lasting many years. Clements et al. (2003) describe rituals common among different cultural groups, providing examples of this variability. These authors describe a general picture of grief practices in Latino, African American, Navajo, Jewish, and Hindu groups. The authors take care to point out that there is considerable heterogeneity within as well as between these groups. They urge clinicians to explore beliefs and practices of each grieving family in order to treat them respectfully and to optimize support. Most cultural groups draw upon close family and friends to provide support after a death, though the manner in which they provide this support varies. To introduce cultural practices, we briefly summarize Clements and colleagues' descriptions.

In traditional Latino culture, there can be a strict status hierarchy based on age and gender. It may be considered healthy and appropriate for women to express grief by crying openly, whereas machismo dictates that men must be strong and stoic. Many Latino families practice Catholicism and believe in continuity of life and death. Prayer, church services, and burial are very important. Physical touch is used to comfort mourners.

African Americans are a particularly heterogeneous group and Clements et al. (2003) focuses on a group of non-Catholic Christians who also retain some traditional African beliefs about death. According to these beliefs, death is a commemoration and a time of transition from one existence to another. Birth, life, and death are considered to be circular and continuous. This group often utilizes group activities at churches to assist in mourning. The concept of reunion with family and friends in heaven may be comforting. Also notable is the significant kin-based social networks enjoyed by many older African Americans (Ajrouch, Antonucci, & Janevic, 2001). Perhaps for this reason, a recent study found nonspousal loss was more prevalent in African Americans than Caucasians (Williams, Baker, & Allman, 2005). Widows who suffer higher rates of nonspousal losses also report more mental and physical health problems (Williams, Baker, & Allman, 2007). Losing a close relationship is clearly a significant stressor.

Clements and colleagues (2003) also review bereavement practices in other diverse cultures. The authors note that in traditional Navajo culture, there is a strict traditional ritual around death. Ceremonies take up to 4 days and must be honored in order to ensure the deceased completes his or her journey to the next world. At the end of these rituals, members of the family wash themselves to symbolize cleansing themselves from the burial, and from that time, discussion about the deceased is considered to be harmful to the spirit of the deceased and can be harmful to the remaining family as well. This very abbreviated mourning ritual can seem strange to western Europeans.

However, orthodox Judaism provides another example of strictly ritualized mourning. Jewish law prescribes rituals for preparing the body and mourning rituals. According to this tradition, the funeral and burial should both occur as soon after the death as possible, preferably by sundown the day of the death. The body is washed and cared for by members of the religious community and placed in a simple pine box without embalming. The Jewish belief is that the soul returns to God and the body should be returned to the earth. The family does not view the body but spends the period prior to the funeral in a period of deep grief and prayer during which an article of clothing or a ribbon is torn and mirrors are turned backward. Cut flowers are not sent but rather donations to charity in the name of the deceased. After the funeral the family begins a 7-day period of sitting shivah, followed by another period of mourning for 30 days during which they may return to work but do not visit the grave. A headstone is placed at the grave after 1 year.

People who practice forms of Hinduism believe in reincarnation. Death is accompanied by ritual bath and dress and is quickly created in order to free the soul to transition to the next world. Rituals and ceremonies are observed for the next 10 days in order to help the departed soul on its journey. At the end of this time the immediate family washes in a ritual bath and other ceremonies and on day 12 they gather with friends and family to honor their deceased loved one.

BEREAVEMENT, GRIEF, AND MOURNING AMONG OLDER ADULTS

Most studies of bereavement have not discriminated between those with and without complicated grief, making results difficult to interpret. There is strong evidence that negative health and mental health consequences of bereavement are significantly more prevalent in those with complicated grief when compared to other bereaved individuals. In studies which looked at bereaved individuals as a whole, a large body of literature has found that losing a spouse is related to increased mortality (e.g., Bowling, 1987). A meta-analysis (Moon et al., 2011) of longitudinal studies that followed participants from the time of bereavement identified 15 studies with a total of 2,263,888 participants. The authors found that the association between widowhood and mortality was statistically significant, but that the association was much stronger within the first 6 months after bereavement than after 6 months. Strikingly, increased mortality was associated with widowhood regardless of the widowed person' age, income, education, race/ethnicity, place of birth, health behavior, social class, occupation, and number of children. Risks also did not differ between studies conducted in the United States, Europe, or Japan. However, there were differences in mortality by gender, with men having much greater risk of mortality after widowhood than women. There may, however, be some cultural variability in the association between mortality and bereavement.

Manor and Eisenbach (2003) linked records in the Israeli census and found higher mortality among the bereaved in their sample, with an increased mortality rate of 50% among women and 40% among men. Interestingly, for men, the effect of bereavement decreased with age, so that younger bereaved men had a higher relative risk of mortality. And in a sample of several hundred widowed Japanese adults, widowhood did not have an impact on mortality. In fact, the data suggested that women who had been widowed 3 years or more actually had a decreased mortality rate (Nagata, Takatsuka, & Shimizu, 2003). Greater understanding of the mechanisms behind this difference is needed.

Studies have also found that loss of a loved one can have a major impact on physical health and functioning. Lee and Carr (2007) followed older adults prior to spousal loss and 6, 18, and 28 months after spousal loss. They found group differences in long-term physical functioning based on several factors. First, decreased physical functioning only occurred among bereaved men, not bereaved women. Second, on average, those whose spouses had severe, chronic health problems before they died had more severe impairment in daily activities both 18 and 48 months after the loss, even when age was considered. Those widowed people who were not with their spouses at the time of death also were at risk for greater physical limitations. The researchers posit that the decrease in physical functioning could be related to stress surrounding the death; sudden death is generally thought to be the most stressful type of loss, as is, on the other extreme, witnessing one's partner in severe distress.

Widowhood also appears to affect use of health care services and medications. Using data from two nationwide registry of 6,421 adults age 60 and over in Denmark, Oksuzyan et al. (2011) collected data on average number of visits to general practitioners per year within 1 year before and up to 4 years after spousal death, and frequency and cause of all medication prescribed for 1 year before and 5 years after spousal death. The authors posited that less health care use may be a possible partial explanation for the increased mortality and more adverse health outcomes among widowers compared to widows. The authors found that average dosage for all medications increased from 1 year before to 1 year after widowhood for the entire sample. Average number of general practitioner visits also increased after the loss but remained constant after 3–4 years. The authors had also hypothesized that widowers would use health care less than widows. However, they found no significant differences in medication use and number of general practitioner visits after the loss across genders. Therefore, health care use did not appear to account for differences in health outcomes and mortality. It should be noted, however, this increased service use was identified in a nation with universal health care coverage; in nations where health care coverage requires additional payment, it is possible health care utilization patterns may differ after widowhood. Similarly, Charlton et al. (2001) studied the general practitioner medical records of 100 British adults whose spouses had died for the year before and after the death. Between these two periods, the average number of doctors' visits increased significantly and were primarily for physical illness.

Mild cognitive impairment has been associated with bereavement in older adults. Xavier et al. examined cognitive functioning and found decreased memory functioning among those who were bereaved compared to those who were not. Ward, Mathias, and Hitchings (2007) examined whether there was association between spousal bereavement and performance on a range of cognitive tasks. Bereaved and nonbereaved adults aged 65 to 80, matched on age, gender, education, intellectual functioning, and general cognitive ability, were given a battery of tests that assessed verbal fluency, memory, attention, and visual-spatial ability. These researchers measured depression, stress, and anxiety. Though the bereaved group performed more poorly on tests of attention, information-processing speed, and verbal fluency, hierarchical regressions showed that depression, anxiety, and stress accounted for the group difference in four of the five cognitive tests. The bereaved group still performed more poorly on an attention-switching task, though this may have been explained by complicated grief, if this condition had been measured.

OTHER ASPECTS OF LOSS

It is also important to recognize that older adults often take on extended periods of caregiving before their loved one dies. The nature of the caregiving experience (i.e., difficult or strenuous experience as compared to a generally positive experience) has received limited research attention, and most studies on caregiving focus on caregiver depression. Boerner, Schulz, and Horowitz (2004) found that positive aspects of caregiving of a family member suffering from dementia affected bereavement adaptation by older adults in terms of both depression and complicated grief. Somewhat surprisingly, a more positive experience with caregiving was associated with higher levels of complicated grief. The authors speculate that the loss of a meaningful and important role might explain this association.

Burton Haley, and Small (2006) focused upon depression in a study examining the effects of the circumstances of death. These investigators compared depression during 18 months among people bereaved by unexpected death to those whose loved one's death was expected. When death was expected, the bereaved person's caregiving role was categorized as no caregiving, low-stress caregiving, or high-stress caregiving. Those who experienced an unexpected death were the only group who showed worsening depression over the study period. Highly stressed caregivers had an increased risk of social isolation and no increase in social well-being over the 18-month study assessment period.

Older adults' loss of a child may be associated with special grief reactions. Smith et al. (2011) used qualitative methods to examine the experience of grieving among 31 adults age 60 and older who had lost an adult child. Participants who were recruited through posters, word of mouth, and advertisements participated in 10 focus groups that met once for approximately 90 minutes. Four major themes emerged: losses, limited influence/decision-making power, regrets, and decreased quality of life.

Death of an adult child entailed a range of losses, including loss of a special relationship with their child, seeing their child achieve or contribute to society, a purpose in life, and loss of their present/future caregiver. These bereaved parents were troubled by limited influence and decision-making power concerning their adult child's behavior before the death, as well as a lack of opportunity to be present at the time of death, and less involvement than they hoped for in funeral arrangements. These parents experienced regrets such as sadness that they never got to say good-bye or tell their child they loved them, thoughts of times they did not do enough for their child, or feeling they did not allow terminally ill children the opportunity to express to their friends about their impending death. They reported a reduction in quality of life related to feeling they had a a broken heart and loss of joy. They also experienced survivor guilt and had reduced involvement in or increased worry or responsibilities concerning their grandchildren's lives. Participating parents expressed common grief reactions, including sadness, anger, guilt, regret, being overwhelmed, and loneliness, as well as experiences specifically related to loss of a child, including a sense of unfulfilled dreams, emotional loneliness, and decreased social and financial support. Participants also reported that having someone listen to them via the focus group format was helpful. The authors suggest older adults who experience the death of an adult child can benefit from attentive listening, storytelling, and the use of metaphors.

STRENGTHS AND RESOURCES IN BEREAVED OLDER ADULTS

Researchers have identified factors that enhance the ability to adjust adaptively to the loss of a loved one. Religious and spiritual beliefs are often a source of comfort. Hebert, Dang, and Schulz (2007) examined the relationship between religious beliefs and practices and mental health in a sample of 225 caregivers of persons with moderate to severe dementia as part of the Resources for Enhancing Alzheimer's Caregiver Health (REACH) study, a study of simple support interventions for Alzheimer's disease caregivers across the United States. After controlling for caregiver age, caregiver physical health, and level of caregiver social integration, the frequency of negative interactions with others, and caregiver depression at study entry, higher frequency of attendance at religious services was significantly associated with lower depression symptoms and less intense grief.

Though religious attendance is generally thought to serve as a form of social support, the association remained in this sample even when social support variables were controlled for. The authors argue that religious attendance may be a marker for a unique set of processes, including providing an opportunity to interact with those with similar values and increased support in adapting religious principles to their lives.

Engagement in leisure activities may also enhance the ability to adapt to bereavement. Janke, Nimrod, and Kleiber (2008) examined change in leisure time involvement in 154 widowed adults aged 50 and older (mean age = 69) using data from the American Changing Lives (ACL) dataset collected across the United States. Average time since widowhood at follow-up was about 2 years. Both number of leisure activities engaged in and frequency of involvement in each activity were examined and widows were classified as either "reducers" or "nonreducers" of leisure activities based on behavioral patterns after bereavement. "Reducers" were those who decreased both their total number of leisure activities and their overall frequency of participation after widowhood. Most widowed participants (61.7%) were characterized as "reducers." Mean depressive scores were significantly higher among the reducers when compared to the nonreducers ($p < .01$). However, the direction of this effect is not clear. Path analyses indicated that those who reported less of a sense of recovery from the loss of their spouse, more depressive symptoms, and more functional limitations were more likely to reduce their leisure activities.

Patterson (1996) examined leisure activities among a sample of 60 recently bereaved widowed older adults (mean age = 64), using a combination of quantitative and qualitative methods. These investigators found that the most frequent leisure activities among widows and widowers were home-based activities, involving socializing with family and friends. Similar to Janke and colleagues' findings, greater participation in leisure activities was negatively correlated with stress scores on a standardized questionnaire. However, there was no significant association between participation in leisure activities and adaptation after the death.

Bisconti et al. assessed emotional well-being in widows beginning in the first month after a spouse's death, specifically examining the relationship between social support and emotional well-being (Bisconti, Bergeman, & Boker, 2006). They argue that adaptation to loss is not a linear process, but rather a dynamic experience that is often in flux. Measurement of social support included frequency and amount of support received as well as functional parts of support received, such as perceived control over the elicitation of support and support seeking for instrumental and emotional needs. The researchers found that emotional support-seeking behaviors in the widows led to a greater sense of well-being. Ong, Bergeman, and Bisconti (2005) used the same sample of widows over time to examine the relationship between adjustment after bereavement and perceived control more closely. They discovered that the correlation between stress and anxiety was significantly reduced and there was slightly less

depression on days when greater perceived control was present.

There is now considerable evidence that positive emotions are healthy. Positive emotions are associated with greater physical health, including cardiovascular and immune function, as well as mental health and well-being. Positive emotions also assist in problem solving, opening the mind to creativity and new solutions. Again using the same older widowed sample, Ong and colleagues (2006) found that daily positive emotions in recently bereaved widows served to moderate stress reactivity and mediate stress recovery.

Utz et al. (2011) examined the effect of personal resources, forewarning of the death, and aspects of the relationship with the deceased spouse on widows' perceived self-competency at managing tasks of daily life. These investigators analyzed baseline interviews from 328 widowed participants in the Living After Loss project, a bereavement intervention study for recently widowed adults aged 50 and above (average age = 69.5) living in the San Francisco and Salt Lake City areas. Results indicated that perceived self-competency was generally high in the sample, with at least 40% of the sample reporting "a lot" of ability across 24 specific daily activities. Higher competency was associated with significantly lower levels of grief, depression, and loneliness in correlation analyses, across all four competency domains. Results suggest that restoring life activities (along with coping with the sadness associated with the loss) may be an important part of coping with grief, though the directionality (whether low competency increases mental health distress or whether mental health distress decreases competency) cannot be discerned in these cross-sectional analyses.

Lund, Caserta, Utz, and DeVries (2010a) conducted another set of analyses of the same sample in the Living After Loss study, examining differences between the 328 participants who enrolled in the study across the two study recruitment areas. They compared the participants' sociodemographic characteristics, bereavement outcomes, and social support to determine whether participants in these diverse areas reported similar grief experiences. Though there were some differences between the samples in racial, ethnic, and religious diversity, length of marriage, level of education, and size and quality of social networks, measures of depression, grief, loneliness, coping self-efficacy, self-esteem, mastery, and stress-related growth were similar across both groups. Across both samples, greater social support was significantly associated with lower depression, grief, loneliness, and increased growth and coping self-efficacy ($p < .05$). The strongest association was found between high support satisfaction from friends and experiencing lower degrees of loneliness ($r = -.53$). When sources of support were considered, having more positive assessments of support from friends (rather than family) was significantly associated with lower levels of depression and loneliness.

Using a sample of 292 widowed participants who had completed baseline interviews in the Living After Loss study at the time of the analyses, Lund, Utz, Caserta, and DeVries (2008) examined both the perceived importance and actual experience of having positive emotions in participants' daily lives and considered how these variables might impact bereavement adjustment. Experiences of humor, happiness, and laughter were measured by a five-item scale developed by the authors, while degree of importance that the bereaved persons placed on these positive emotions in their daily lives was assessed by two statements. The authors found that most of the bereaved spouses rated humor and happiness as being very important in their daily lives. Moreover, on the five-item scale of experiences of humor, happiness, and laughter, more than 75% of respondents said that they strongly agreed or agreed with each statement. Experiencing humor, laughter, and happiness was strongly negatively correlated with both grief ($r = -.37$) and depression outcomes ($r = -.49$) associated with favorable bereavement adjustments (lower grief and depression). Regression analyses indicated that daily experiences of humor, laughter, and happiness were more strongly associated with more favorable grief and depression outcomes than whether the bereaved person valued those emotions.

Brown, Brown, House, and Smith (2008) examined the role of self-reported helping behavior among the elderly bereaved. Using data from the same sample as Ong et al., these researchers found that among bereaved men and women who had experienced high grief, helping behavior toward others was associated with greater rate of decline in depressive symptoms over a period of 6 to 19 months after their spouse died. The relationship between helping behavior and declines in depression symptoms was independent of physical health, demographics, perceived social support, received emotional support, and social integration. The research therefore seems to indicate that social support, helping behavior,

perceived control, personality traits, and the experience of positive emotions can all influence emotional states after a death.

Carr et al. (2000) focused on pre-loss variables. They examined the impact of marital quality on psychological adjustment after widowhood, focusing on three aspects of the relationship: closeness, conflict, and dependence. They found that the relationship between widowed people and their spouses had an impact on emotional functioning after the spouse's death. Specifically, those who were highly dependent on their spouses had greater anxiety after the death compared to married controls. High levels of yearning were also expressed in those whose marriages that had high levels of warmth, high levels of dependence, and low levels of conflict. There were no significant differences between men and women.

THE SYNDROME OF COMPLICATED GRIEF

Loss of a loved one is always a wrenching and difficult experience. A sudden, unexpected death can cause intense pain with physical, mental, and behavioral manifestations. Following his famous interviews of survivors of the Chestnut Grove fire, Lindemann (1944) depicted the clinical state of acute grief as including somatic distress, preoccupation with images of the deceased, feelings of guilt, a loss of warmth for others, and a tendency for restless, searching behavior. When bereavement is anticipated, the reaction is sometimes less dramatic, though any death can evoke profound acute grief symptoms. Mercifully though, as is the case with other stressors, most people mourn successfully and find a way to move forward in a life that again has meaning and purpose and the possibility for joy and satisfaction.

Since Lindemann's landmark paper, much has been written about coping with loss, the goals of mourning, and the process that needs to occur for acute grief symptoms to subside. Most famous and insightful is John Bowlby's treatise on loss (Bowlby, 1980). Bowlby used an attachment theory perspective and suggested the goals of successful mourning are to acknowledge the finality and consequences of the loss, revise the attachment working model, and redefine life plans and goals. These three objectives provide a useful scaffold for thinking about the mourning process.

The suffering imposed by chronic grief has been observed by numerous authors, including Freud (1917), Lindemann (1979), Bowlby (1980), Parkes (1986), Raphael (1975, 1983), Horowitz and colleagues (1997), and Jacobs and colleagues (1986). Within this literature there is general agreement about the type of symptoms that would comprise a disorder of grief. Yet defining precise boundaries of problematic grief has been daunting. For decades, clinicians and researchers interested in helping the bereaved have expressed frustration over the lack of standardized diagnostic criteria. Recently this problem has been addressed.

Several groups, including ours (Shear et al., 2011), have proposed diagnostic criteria. While these are similar, there are some important differences. Horowitz et al. (1997) were the first to suggest criteria. This group has been studying grief for a number of years, and results of their empirical studies indicated that a putative complicated grief disorder includes intrusive thoughts, strong pangs of severe emotions, strong yearnings, feeling alone and empty, avoidance of people and places that act as reminders of the loss, and loss of interest in personal activities. Prigerson et al. (1995) found a similar criteria set for the syndrome variously named complicated grief, traumatic grief, or prolonged grief disorder. Importantly, this group also developed a rating scale, the Inventory of Complicated Grief (Prigerson et al., 1995), derived in part from symptom clusters in older adults. Our own criteria are similar but include symptoms related to rumination about the circumstances or consequences of the loss, not included in the other criteria sets. Additionally, we focus on two putative groups of symptoms, those attributable to complications (rumination, behavioral changes, and emotion dysregulation) as well as prolonged acute grief symptoms. Notably, though, the group of symptoms identified by the Inventory of Complicated Grief meets several of the criteria outlined by Robins and Guze (1970) that are needed to confirm validity of a new diagnostic entity as well as a more recent criteria set proposed by Stein and colleagues (2010).

Complicated grief comprises a replicable, identifiable clinical description. Symptoms include grief complications that prolong acute grief. The resulting syndrome typically includes inability to accept the death, with persistent intense yearning and longing and sadness; intrusive images of the deceased, often accompanied by feelings of guilt, anger, or anxiety; preoccupation with thoughts or images of the deceased, including a tendency to enter states of reverie; being upset by reminders of the deceased, with avoidance of situations that trigger these reminders; difficulty trusting and/or caring about others, sometimes accompanied by feelings of unfairness, bitterness, envy of others, and feeling very lonely and estranged from others.

It is possible to clearly delimitate complicated grief from other disorders. There is strong evidence that complicated grief is distinguishable from depression and posttraumatic stress disorder (PTSD). When comparing complicated grief and major depressive disorder (MDD), the two disorders have different risk factors, clinical correlates, temporal course, and response to antidepressant medication and to interpersonal psychotherapy. In a community sample of widows and widowers, 46% of subjects who have syndromal-level complicated grief did not meet criteria for a diagnosis of MDD. In our ongoing study, only 60% meet SCID criteria for current MDD. Complicated grief also differs from PTSD. First, complicated grief occurs following loss of an important relationship, rather than exposure to a life-threatening event. PTSD does not include yearning or searching for the deceased, and the primary emotional reaction is fear, not the sadness and anguish of grief. Many people with complicated grief do not meet criteria for PTSD. In our current study, only about 30% meet SCID criteria for PTSD. Additionally, complicated grief can be distinguished from adjustment disorder by reviewing Criterion D for adjustment disorder, which explicitly states that the symptoms cannot be a consequence of bereavement. Follow-up studies provide further support for the validity of the syndrome.

Complicated grief symptoms predict onset of cancer, heart trouble, high blood pressure, substance abuse, and suicidal ideation in the aftermath of the loss. Suicidality, a growing public health problem among the elderly, is twice as common in bereaved spouses over the age of 50, with complicated grief, as opposed to those without complicated grief. Laboratory findings are more limited, but a very interesting report describing the relationship between grief and corticosteroid secretion in parents of leukemic children describes complicated grief clearly in parents with elevated urinary cortisol. Individuals with complicated grief have electroencephalographic sleep patterns that differ from individuals with major depression. There is some indication of impaired immune function. Another study suggests there is activation in the nucleus accumbens in women with, compared to without, complicated grief upon exposure to cues of their deceased sister or mother (O'Connor et al., 2008).

EPIDEMIOLOGY, RISK, AND PROTECTIVE FACTORS

There are few population-based studies of complicated grief. Studies of spousal bereavement indicate an overall rate of complicated grief of about 10% among those who are bereaved. Studies of suicide, homicide, and disaster-related bereavement come from smaller samples and generally report higher rates, ranging from 20% to 40%. In Western countries, death of a child is particularly difficult and rates of complicated grief in parents bereaved of a child may be as high as 60%. A small study conducted in China and the United States suggested that complicated grief rates following loss of a child may be lower in China (Bonanno et al., 2005). Most studies of complicated grief indicate that there is a female preponderance. In clinical studies this is as high as 80%–90%. One study suggests that complicated grief may be more prevalent in African Americans compared to European Americans (Laurie & Neimeyer, 2008).

Prevalence rates of bereavement-related depression or bereavement-related PTSD are also not available from large-scale epidemiologic studies. It appears that bereavement triggers depression in about 20%–30% of cases. Rates of PTSD vary, depending on the nature of the death, with higher prevalence of PTSD following violent, compared to natural, causes.

Definitive information about risk factors for complicated grief requires a prospective epidemiologic study. When the person who died was exceptionally close; when the death was sudden, unexpected, or violent; or when there were troubling concerns about the timing or manner in which the death occurred, these can become a focus for counterfactual thinking and derail the mourning process. Additionally, people who experienced adversity in childhood, and those whose relationships with primary caregivers were not secure, are likely to be at risk for complicated grief, especially if they lose someone with whom they did have a satisfying attachment/caregiving relationship. People with complicated grief frequently have a strong caregiving orientation and many find it difficult to ask for or receive help from others. Additionally, if there is a history of mood or anxiety disorders, and especially if such a disorder is actively present at, or shortly after the death, this can also predispose

to complicated grief. Concurrent physical health problems or environmental stressors, such as financial problems, or relationship problems, can also be a distracting focus of attention that predisposes to complicated grief. Female gender, low education, and low socioeconomic status may be risk factors. It is likely that situational factors interact with personal and relationship vulnerabilities to lead to complicated grief. If there are important financial or social consequences of the death, these can also become a focus of worry and concern that interferes with the mourning process.

Major depression, PTSD, and other anxiety disorders, insomnia, or substance abuse can all occur in the wake of an important loss. Serious illness or death of a loved one is a profound stressor and, as such, can trigger the onset or worsening of almost any psychiatric or physical health problem. When any of these occurs during bereavement, they need to be diagnosed and treated. In part, these are debilitating disorders themselves, and in part, if they are untreated, they can impede the natural mourning process and lead to complicated grief.

Importantly, these same risk factors pertain to complicated grief and, again, it is likely that complicated grief at least partially accounted for these impairment findings. Indeed, a few studies have shown unique physical health concerns among those with complicated grief. Prigerson et al. found that the risk of hypertension is 10 times greater among widowed subjects who met criteria for complicated grief compared to those who do not (Prigerson et al., 1997.). Complicated grief has also been associated with increased risk for smoking (Neria et al., 2007) and sleep impairment (Prigerson et al., 1995).

In one of the few studies to examine health service use in those with complicated grief, Prigerson and colleagues found that those with complicated grief were 17 times less likely to have visited a physician in the months since the death than those without complicated grief (Prigerson et al., 2001), suggesting that this condition, rather than bereavement in general, may account for these findings.

It is possible that the general trend of increased mortality is accounted for by those who have complicated grief, but this question has not yet been examined. There is some evidence, however, that complicated grief increases risk for suicidality, which may partially account for the association between bereavement and mortality. In one study, 57% of participants with high complicated grief scores expressed suicidal ideation, and having both complicated grief and depressive symptoms made the bereaved more vulnerable to suicidal ideation (Szanto, Prigerson, Houck, Ehrenpreis, & Reynolds, 1997).

TREATMENT OF COMPLICATED GRIEF

Considering the importance of the problem, the existing literature on grief interventions is remarkably small. Reported interventions include two main strategies. The first is preventative and based on observations that greater social support predicts better adjustment to spousal loss. Supportive psychotherapy, self-help groups, and widow-to-widow programs show moderate success. However, a meta-analysis (Jordan & Neimeyer, 2003) showed a strikingly low effect size (0.15) for grief interventions that have been tested. A recent treatment study by Lund et al. (2010b) also failed to show strong evidence of efficacy. Other reports describe treatments targeting pathological grief. These authors consistently recommend a focus on the loss, as does complicated grief. Two studies of guided mourning compared a brief exposure intervention with an anti-exposure treatment, where patients were encouraged to avoid thinking about the deceased and avoid doing anything upsetting. These showed a significant treatment effect on only a few measures, none of which was a measure of complicated grief. The third study compared psychodynamic psychotherapy with a self-help support group and found no difference. A study of bereavement-related depression showed lack of efficacy for interpersonal psychotherapy (Reynolds et al., 1999). We developed the first treatment targeting complicated grief and confirmed its efficacy (Shear et al., 2005). Several groups have now published small studies that show promise for ameliorating symptoms of complicated grief (Acierno et al., 2012; Boelen et al., 2007; Maccullum & Bryant, 2011; Wagner et al., 2006). There is clearly a need to find efficacious treatments for this debilitating condition.

Psychotherapy for the elderly is almost certainly underutilized, as many therapists consider the elderly not amenable to therapeutic intervention. Furthermore, many older patients are reluctant to seek psychological treatments. Garner (2003) suggests that this view was perhaps influenced by Freud, who wrote that the "elasticity of the mental processes, on which the treatment depends, is as a rule lacking—old people are no longer educable" (p. 264). Ageism has been pervasive in the thinking of mental health professionals. Garner further observes that Western culture "deprives older adults of an acknowledged emotional life and subjects them to negative stereotypes, even in the minds of those employed to provide services" (p. 537). She suggests that, in fact, older individuals have a good capacity to recall emotion-related information, even when there is a decrease in working memory, and that the elderly are often motivated to accelerate psychological change.

Given this capacity for psychological mindedness, and given the frequent occurrence of concomitant medical problems and their accompanying medications, an older patient may be particularly well suited for a psychotherapy intervention. Such interventions, when tested, are generally efficacious. As Gum and Arean point out, research has demonstrated that psychotherapy is an appropriate modality for older people with psychiatric disorders, and one that elderly people often prefer. Nevertheless, some modifications need to be made when treating the elderly.

Changes in appearance with aging; physical disabilities, when present; and mild cognitive impairment all need to be acknowledged and considered as a part of the therapeutic context. Goals and potential may be different in the elderly. Often older people have less potential and more constraints. Elderly people may be socially isolated and may find it more difficult than their younger counterparts to develop new relationships. Older people do better when social relations build upon familiar people, if possible.

Understanding aspects of aging is important in doing psychotherapy with the elderly, though this does not require major modification of most existing therapies. The therapy we developed for complicated grief always takes personal life context into consideration. A series of studies with interpersonal therapy for the elderly shows this is a well-developed treatment. Complicated grief therapy uses an interpersonal therapy base and has also been used successfully in the elderly. However, given the reticence of many clinicians to utilize psychotherapy to treat older patients, the dearth of psychotherapy studies focused on the older age group, and the possibility that there are different factors related to response in older age groups, it is important to study complicated grief therapy targeted specifically for geriatric patients. Such a study is currently nearing completion. Data are not yet available, but anecdotally, many older people have responded to this treatment.

Complicated grief is an important and greatly underrecognized public health problem across the life span, but this problem is especially pertinent for the elderly, among whom loss is very common. Ten to twenty percent of bereaved seniors develop complicated grief. Clinical reports of pathological grief reactions attest to the fact that clinicians see patients whose primary problem is abnormal grief. However, as noted by a recent author (Robak, 1999), "empirical studies of psychotherapy [of bereavement] are fewer than could be reasonably expected…This is a troubling state of affairs…[that] indicates that practitioners are practicing without being informed" (p. 702). This includes studies focused on older adults, the group most likely to experience bereavement. Several authors acknowledge a pressing need for proper scientific testing of interventions. Our recent study included a mixed age range and approximately equal representation of people who lost parents, spouse, child, or other friend or relatives; and people who have lost loved ones to suicide, homicide, accident, cancer, and other acute and prolonged medical illness. Complicated grief therapy was effective and flexible enough to accommodate this diversity, and preliminary data indicated that older people can benefit from this treatment.

Twenty-nine individuals 60 years of age or older (mean age 68; range 60–85) were included in our first complicated grief therapy study or in the pilot phase that preceded that study (Shear et al., 2001; Shear et al., 2005). Twenty-two of these were treated with complicated grief therapy and seven with interpersonal therapy. Compared with 163 younger adults, the older group was less likely to be employed full time (14% vs. 33%; $p = .04$) and more likely to live alone (63% vs. 34%, $p = .01$). Complicated grief scores were lower in the older patients (42.6 ± 9.2 vs. 47.6 ± 9.7; $p = .01$) though this difference is not clinically significant. The older group was somewhat less likely to have a concurrent *DSM-IV* anxiety disorder (55% vs. 78%; $p = .01$), though more than half of the older participants did suffer from these disorders. No other demographic or clinical measures showed a significant difference.

Twenty-two older individuals (mean age, 67 years) were treated with complicated grief therapy, as well as 63 younger adults (mean age, 44 years). This includes participants in our pilot study (elderly $n = 10$; young $n = 13$), individuals who participated as therapist training cases (elderly $n = 2$; young $n = 11$), and participants randomized to receive complicated grief therapy in the randomized controlled trial (elderly $n = 10$; young $n = 39$). Among those assessed, eligible older individuals were more likely than younger adults to enter treatment (18/23; 78%) vs. 34/61; 56%) and less likely to drop out (2/22 vs. 27/61). Mean decrease in complicated grief in older participants was 16.4 and for the completers ($n = 19$) and 14.9 for the intent to treat group ($n = 22$). This compared to a decrease of 23.6 for younger adult completers ($n = 36$) and 16.7 for the intent to treat group ($n = 63$).

Seven older participants and 39 younger adults were treated with interpersonal therapy. Mean decrease in complicated grief in the older group was 8.8 for the completers ($n = 6$) and 7.3 for the intent to treat group ($n = 7$). This decrease is very similar to the change in complicated grief score in older adults who participated in our prior study of bereavement-related depression (mean decrease, 8.75) and compares to a mean decrease of 13.6 for younger adult completers ($n = 28$) and 13.8 for the intent to treat group ($n = 39$).

These results suggest complicated grief therapy is a promising treatment for older as well as younger adults. However, data for older seniors and those with physical, mental, and social infirmity are still lacking. Given the high prevalence of bereavement in aging individuals and the marked impairment and increased suicide risk associated with complicated grief, it is important to have good therapeutic tools to help people suffering from this syndrome.

CONCLUSIONS

Bereavement is a universal co-traveler with aging. Older people regularly face loss of their closest friends and relatives and, not infrequently, even their adult children. Though larger population studies need to be conducted, complicated grief appears to be present in a sizable minority of older adults who have suffered loss. Complicated grief may account for many of the physical and mental health consequences observed in bereaved older adult samples. However, more research that focuses specifically on those with complicated grief, and compares their physical and mental health to those without complicated grief, is needed. In particular, the association between complicated grief and mortality and cognitive impairment requires more exploration. The possible role of religious participation and helping behavior in reducing the risk of developing complicated grief also needs attention. Greater understanding of risk factors for complicated grief in older adults, especially in large, population-based samples, is important as well.

It appears that people with complicated grief benefit from specific treatment; however, only a few treatments have been developed and tested for this condition. Ours is one of the few studies with a large sample and tested in a randomized controlled trial that showed clear evidence of improving complicated grief symptoms. Preliminary results in older adults are promising. We are currently adapting and disseminating this treatment in a number of populations and have nearly completed a study testing its efficacy specifically in older adults. In the meantime, professionals working with such bereaved older adults might consider using this treatment, along with the inclusion of culturally relevant practices to aid in the mourning process. With greater understanding of complicated grief and its treatment, the emotional and physical burdens experienced by many bereaved older adults can be significantly reduced.

Disclosures

Dr. Ghesquiere and Mr. Katzke have no conflicts or funding to disclose.

ACKNOWLEDGMENTS

Dr. Shear is affiliated with the Columbia University School of Social Work and the Columbia University College of Physicians and Surgeons. Dr. Ghesquiere is affiliated with Weill Cornell Medical College, while Mr. Katzke is in a private legal practice.

This work was supported by a grant from the National Institute of Mental Health MH70741.

REFERENCES

Acierno, R., Rheingold, A., Amstadter, A., Kurent, J., Amella, E., Resnick, H. et al. (2012). Behavioral activation and therapeutic exposure for bereavement in older adults. *American Journal of Hospice and Palliative Care, 29*(1), 13–25. doi: 10.1177/1049909111411471

Ajdacic-Gross, V., Ring, M., Gadola, E., Lauber, C., Bopp, M., Gutzwiller, F., & Rossler, W. (2008). Suicide after bereavement: An overlooked problem. *Psychological Medicine, 38*(5), 673–676. doi: 10.1017/S0033291708002754

Ajrouch, K. J., Antonucci, T. C., & Janevic, M. R. (2001). Social networks among blacks and whites: The interaction between race and age. *Journals of Gerontology. Series B, Psychological Sciences and Social Sciences, 56*(2), S112–118.

Antonucci, T. C., Akiyama, H., & Takahashi, K. (2004). Attachment and close relationships across the life span. *Attachment and Human Development, 6*(4), 353–370.

Azaiza, F., Rona, P., Shohama, M. & Tinsky-Roimia, T. (2011). Death and dying anxiety among bereaved and nonbereaved elderly parents, *Death Studies, 35*, 610–624. doi: 10.1080/07481187.2011.553325

Bisconti, T. L., Bergeman, C. S., & Boker, S. M. (2006). Social support as a predictor of variability: an examination of the adjustment trajectories of recent widows. *Psychology and Aging, 21*(3), 590–599.

Boelen, P. A., de Keijser, J., van den Hout, M. A., & van den Bout, J. (2007). Treatment of complicated grief: A comparison between cognitive-behavioral therapy and supportive counseling. *Journal of Consulting and Clinical Psychology, 75*(2), 277–284. doi: 10.1037/0022–006X.75.2.277

Boerner, K., Schulz, R., & Horowitz, A. (2004). Positive aspects of caregiving and adaptation to bereavement. *Psychology and Aging, 19*(4), 668–675.

Bonanno, G. A., Papa, A., Lalande, K., Zhang, N., & Noll, J. G. (2005). Grief processing and deliberate grief avoidance: a prospective comparison of bereaved spouses and parents in the United States and the People's Republic of China. *Journal of Consulting and Clinical Psychology, 73*(1), 86–98. doi: 10.1037/0022-006X.73.1.86

Bowlby, J. (1980). *Attachment and loss, volume III: Loss.* New York: Basic Books.

Bowling, A. (1987). Mortality after bereavement: A review of the literature on survival periods and factors affecting survival. *Social Science and Medicine, 24*(2), 117–124.

Brown, S. L., Brown, R. M., House, J. S., & Smith, D. M. (2008). Coping with spousal loss: Potential buffering effects of self-reported helping behavior. *Personality and Social Psychology Bulletin, 34*(6), 849–861. doi: 10.1177/0146167208314972

Burton, A. M., Haley, W. E., & Small, B. J. (2006). Bereavement after caregiving or unexpected death: Effects on elderly spouses. *Aging & Mental Health, 10*(3), 319–326.

Carr, D. (2004a). The desire to date and remarry among older widows and widowers. *Journal of Marriage and Family, 66*, 1051–1068.

Carr, D. (2004b). Gender, preloss marital dependence, and older adults' adjustment to widowhood. *Journal of Marriage and Family, 66*, 220–235.

Carr, D., House, J. S., Kessler, R. C., Nesse, R. M., Sonnega, J., & Wortman, C. (2000). Marital quality and psychological adjustment to widowhood among older adults: A longitudinal analysis. *Journals of Gerontology. Series B, Psychological Sciences and Social Sciences, 55*(4), S197–207.

Charlton, R., Sheahan, K., Smith, G., & Campbell, I. (2001). Spousal bereavement – Implications for health. *Family Practice, 18*(6), 614–618.

Clements, P. T., Vigil, G. J., Manno, M. S., Henry, G. C., Wilks, J., Das, S. et al. (2003). Cultural perspectives of death, grief, and bereavement. . *Journal of Psychosocial Nursing and Mental Health Services, 41*(7), 18–26.

Federal Interagency Forum on Aging Related Statistics (2008). *Older Americans 2008: Key indicators of well-being.* Retrieved October 12, 2011 from http://www.aoa.gov/Agingstatsdotnet/Main_Site/Data/2008_Documents/Population.aspx.

Freud, S. (1917). Mourning and melancholia. *Internationale Zeitschrift fur arzliche Psychoanalyse, 4,* 288–301.

Garner, J. (2003). Psychotherapies and older adults. *Australian & New Zealand Journal of Psychiatry, 37*(5), 537–548. doi: 1198 [pii]

Hebert, R. S., Dang, Q., & Schulz, R. (2007). Religious beliefs and practices are associated with better mental health in family caregivers of patients with dementia: Findings from the REACH study. *American Journal of Geriatric Psychiatry, 15*(4), 292–300. doi: 10.1097/01.JGP.0000247160.11769.ab

Horowitz, M.J. et al. (1997). Diagnostic criteria for complicated grief disorder. *American Journal of Psychiatry, 154,* 904–910.

Jacobs, S. C., Kasl, S. V., Ostfeld, A. M., Berkman, L., Kosten, T. R., & Charpentier, P. (1986). The measurement of grief: Bereaved versus non-bereaved. *Hospice Journal, 2*(4), 21–36.

Janke, M. C., Nimrod, G., & Kleiber, D. A. (2008). Reduction in leisure activity and well-being during the transition to widowhood. *Journal of Women and Aging, 20*(1–2), 83–98. doi: 10.1300/J074v20n01_07

Jordan, J. R., & Neimeyer, R. A. (2003). Does grief counseling work? *Death Studies, 27*(9), 765–786.

Laurie, A., & Neimeyer, R. A. (2008). African Americans in bereavement: Grief as a function of ethnicity. *Omega (Westport), 57*(2), 173–193.

Lee, M., & Carr, D. (2007). Does the context of spousal loss affect the physical functioning of older widowed persons? A longitudinal analysis. *Research on Aging, 29*(5), 457–487.

Lewis C.S. (1961). *A grief observed.* New York: Harper and Row.

Lindemann, E. (1944). Symptomatology and management of acute grief. *American Journal of Psychiatry, 101,* 141–148.

Lindemann, E. (1979). *Beyond grief: Studies in crisis intervention.* New York: Jason Aronson, Inc.

Lund, D., Caserta, M., Utz, R., & Devries, B. (2010a). A tale of two counties: Bereavement in socio-demographically diverse Places. *Illness, Crisis, and Loss, 18*(4), 301–321.

Lund, D., Caserta, M., Utz, R., & De Vries, B. (2010b). Experiences and early coping of bereaved spouses/partners in an intervention based on the dual process model (DPM). *Omega (Westport), 61*(4), 291–313.

Lund, D. A., Utz, R., Caserta, M. S., & De Vries, B. (2008). Humor, laughter, and happiness in the daily lives of recently bereaved spouses. *Omega (Westport), 58*(2), 87–105.

Maccallum, F. & Bryant, R.A. (2011). Autobiographical memory following cognitive behaviour therapy for complicated grief. *Journal of Behavior Therapy and Experimental Psychiatry, 42*(1), 26–31.

Manor, O., & Eisenbach, Z. (2003). Mortality after spousal loss: Are there socio-demographic differences? *Social Science and Medicine, 56*(2), 405–413.

Moon, J. R., Kondo, N., Glymour, M. M., & Subramanian, S. V. (2011). Widowhood and mortality: A meta-analysis. *PLoS One, 6*(8), e23465. doi: 10.1371/journal.pone.0023465

Nagata, C., Takatsuka, N., & Shimizu, H. (2003). The impact of changes in marital status on the mortality of elderly Japanese. *Annals of Epidemiology, 13*(4), 218–222.

Neria, Y., Gross, R., Litz, B., Maguen, S., Insel, B., Seirmarco, G. et al. (2007). Prevalence and psychological correlates of complicated grief among bereaved adults 2.5–3.5 years after September 11th attacks. *Journal of Traumatic Stress, 20*(3), 251–262.

O'Connor, M. F., Wellisch, D. K., Stanton, A. L., Eisenberger, N. I., Irwin, M. R., & Lieberman, M. D. (2008). Craving love? Enduring grief activates brain's reward center. *Neuroimage, 42*(2), 969–972. doi: 10.1016/j.neuroimage.2008.04.256

Oksuzyan, A., Jacobsen, R., Glaser, K., Tomassini, C., Vaupel, J. W., & Christensen, K. (2011). Sex differences in medication and primary healthcare use before and after spousal bereavement at older ages in Denmark: Nationwide register study of over 6000 bereavements. *Journal of Aging Research.* doi: 10.4061/2011/678289

Ong, A. D., Bergeman, C. S., & Bisconti, T. L. (2005). Unique effects of daily perceived control on anxiety symptomology during conjugal bereavement. *Personality and Individual Differences, 38*, 1057–1067.

Ong, A. D., Bergeman, C. S., Bisconti, T. L., & Wallace, K. A. (2006). Psychological resilience, positive emotions, and successful adaptation to stress in later life. *Journal of Personality and Social Psychology, 91*(4), 730–749. doi: 10.1037/0022-3514.91.4.730

Parkes, C. M. (1986). *Bereavement: Studies of grief in adult life* (2nd ed.). Madison, CT: International Universities Press, Inc.

Patterson, I. (1996). Participation in leisure activities by older adults after a stressful life event: The loss of a spouse. *International Journal of Aging and Human Development, 42*(2), 123–142.

Prigerson, H. G., Maciejewski, P. K., Reynolds, C. F., 3rd, Bierhals, A. J., Newsom, J. T., Fasiczka, A. et al. (1995). Inventory of Complicated Grief: A scale to measure maladaptive symptoms of loss. *Psychiatry Research, 59*(1–2), 65–79.

Prigerson, H. G., Bierhals, A. J., Kasl, S. V., Reynolds, C. F., 3rd, Shear, M. K., Day, N. et al. (1997). Traumatic grief as a risk factor for mental and physical morbidity. *American Journal of Psychiatry, 154*(5), 616–623.

Prigerson, H. G., Frank, E., Kasl, S. V., Reynolds, C. F., 3rd, Anderson, B., Zubenko, G. S. et al. (1995). Complicated grief and bereavement-related depression as distinct disorders: Preliminary empirical validation in elderly bereaved spouses. *American Journal of Psychiatry, 152*(1), 22–30.

Prigerson, H., Silverman, G. K., Jacobs, S., Maciejewski, P., Kasi, S., & Rosenheck, R. (2001). Traumatic grief, disability and the underutilization of health services: A preliminary examination *Primary Psychiatry, 8*, 712–718.

Raphael, B. (1975). The management of pathological grief. *Australian and New Zealand Journal of Psychiatry, 9* (3), 173–180.

Raphael, B. (1983). *The anatomy of bereavement.* New York, NY: Basic Books. pp. 33–73

Reynolds, C. F., 3rd, Miller, M. D., Pasternak, R. E., Frank, E., Perel, J. M., Cornes, C. (1999). Treatment of bereavement-related major depressive episodes in later life: A controlled study of acute and continuation treatment with nortriptyline and interpersonal psychotherapy. *American Journal of Psychiatry, 156*(2), 202–208.

Robins, E., & Guze, S. B. (1970). Establishment of diagnostic validity in psychiatric illness: Its application to schizophrenia. *American Journal of Psychiatry, 126*(7), 983–987.

Schneider, D. S., Sledge, P. A., Shuchter, S. R., & Zisook, S. (1996). Dating and remarriage over the first two years of widowhood. *Annals of Clinical Psychiatry, 8*(2), 51–57.

Shear, M. K., Frank, E., Foa, E., Cherry, C., Reynolds, C. F., 3rd, Vanderbilt, J., & Masters, S. (2001). Traumatic grief treatment: A pilot study. *American Journal of Psychiatry, 158*(9), 1506–1508.

Shear, M. K., Frank, E., Houck, P. R., & Reynolds, C. F., 3rd. (2005). Treatment of complicated grief: a randomized controlled trial. *Journal of the American Medical Association, 293*(21), 2601–2608.

Shear, M. K., Simon, N., Wall, M., Zisook, S., Neimeyer, R., Duan, N., et al. (2011). Complicated grief and related bereavement issues for DSM-5. *Depression and Anxiety, 28*(2), 103–117. doi: 10.1002/da.20780

Shor, E., Roelfs, D.J., Curreli, M., Clemow, L., Burg, M.M., Schwartz, J.E. (2012). Widowhood and mortality: A meta-analysis and meta-regression. *Demography, 49*, 575–606.

Smith, K. R., Zick, C. D., & Duncan, G. J. (1991). Remarriage patterns among recent widows and widowers. *Demography, 28*(3), 361–374.

Smith, M. E., Nunley, B. L., Kerr, P. L., & Galligan, H. (2011). Elders' experiences of the death of an adult child. *Issues in Mental Health Nursing, 32*(9), 568–574. doi: 10.3109/01612840.2011.576802

Stein, D. J., Phillips, K. A., Bolton, D., Fulford, K. W., Sadler, J. Z., & Kendler, K. S. (2010). What is a mental/psychiatric disorder? From DSM-IV to DSM-V. *Psychological Medicine, 40* (11), 1759–1765. doi: 10.1017/S0033291709992261

Szanto, K., Prigerson, H., Houck, P., Ehrenpreis, L., & Reynolds, C. F., 3rd. (1997). Suicidal ideation in elderly bereaved: The role of complicated grief. *Suicide and Life Threatening Behaviors, 27*(2), 194–207.

Utz, R. L., Lund, D. A., Caserta, M. S., & Devries, B. (2011). Perceived self-competency among the recently bereaved. *Journal of Social Work in End of Life and Palliative Care, 7*(2–3), 173–194. doi: 10.1080/15524256.2011.593154

Wagner, B., Knaevelsrud, C., & Maercker, A. (2006). Internet-based cognitive-behavioral therapy for complicated grief: A randomized controlled trial. *Death Studies, 30*(5), 429–453.

Ward, L., Mathias, J. L., & Hitchings, S. E. (2007). Relationships between bereavement and cognitive functioning in older adults. *Gerontology, 53*(6), 362–372. doi: 10.1159/000104787

Williams, B. R., Baker, P. S., Allman, R. M., & Roseman, J. M. (2007). Bereavement among African American and White older adults. *Journal of Aging and Health, 19*(2), 313–333. doi: 10.1177/0898264307299301

Williams, B., Baker, P. S., & Allman, R. (2005). Nonspousal family loss among community-dwelling older adults. *Omega, 51,* 125–142.

Williams, B. R., Baker, P. S., Allman, R. M., & Roseman, J. M. (2006). The feminization of bereavement among community-dwelling older adults. *Journal of Women and Aging, 18*(3), 3–18. doi: 10.1300/J074v18n03_02

14

CURRENT ISSUES IN INFORMAL CAREGIVING RESEARCH

PREVALENCE, HEALTH EFFECTS, AND INTERVENTION STRATEGIES

Richard Schulz

FAMILY MEMBERS are an essential resource to older individuals with chronic illness and disability. Without the care and support provided by friends or relatives, it would be difficult and often impossible for persons with disability to avoid institutional placement. Informal caregivers are also a major resource to society, saving the formal health care system hundreds of billions of dollars annually, although often at considerable cost to the caregiver's well-being. The prevalence and importance of informal caregiving has spawned a large research enterprise that continues to grow and expand with hundreds of studies being published annually.

The goal of this chapter is to provide an up-to-date overview of the current status of informal caregiving with a focus on key unresolved issues in this literature. We begin with a discussion of prevalence of caregiving in the United States and show how rates can vary by several orders of magnitude depending on definitions used and populations sampled. Relying on national surveys of caregivers, we next characterize who they are, whom they care

for, and the types of tasks carried out by caregivers. This is followed by detailed discussion of both the detrimental and potentially beneficial health effects of caregiving, their causes, and methodological challenges associated with this research. We conclude with a brief discussion of the caregiver intervention literature with a focus on emerging innovative treatment strategies.

PREVALENCE OF CAREGIVING

There are no exact estimates of the number of informal caregivers in the United States. Prevalence estimates vary widely depending on definitions used and populations sampled. At one extreme are estimates that 28.5% of the US adult population, or 65.7 million Americans, provided unpaid care to an adult relative in 2009, with the majority (83%) of this care being delivered to people age 50 years or older (NAC & AARP, 2009). This number approximates the estimated 59 million adults with a disability in the United States, based on the

Behavioral Risk Factor Surveillance System survey (CDC, 2006). At the other extreme, data from the National Long-Term Care survey suggest that as few as 3.5 million informal caregivers provided instrumental activities of daily living (IADL) or activities of daily living (ADL) assistance to people age 65 and over. Intermediate estimates of 28.8 million caregivers ("persons aged 15 or over providing personal assistance for everyday needs of someone age 15 and older") are reported by the Survey on Income and Program Participation (NFCA & FCA, 2006). A recent national survey of individuals age 45 and older yielded a caregiving rate of 12% or 14.9 million adults (Roth, Perkins, Wadley, Temple, & Haley, 2009).

These differences are in part attributable to when the data were collected, the age range of the population sampled, and care recipient populations targeted, but most important to the definition of caregiving. Thus, the high-end estimates are generated when broad and inclusive definitions of caregiving are used (e.g., "Unpaid care may include help with personal needs or household chores. It might be managing a person's finances, arranging for outside services, or visiting regularly to see how they are doing") (NAC & AARP, 2009), and low-end estimates are generated when definitions require the provision of specific ADL or IADL assistance (e.g., Wolff & Kasper, 2006). A related issue is that definitions of caregiving do not clearly distinguish caregiving for chronic disability from caregiving for acute care episodes that might follow a hospitalization event. However, most definitions used emphasize chronic disability; intermittent episodes of caregiving are not well represented in the existing data.

Although there are some encouraging signs that age-related disability is declining in the United States, this will be offset by the rapid growth of the senior population to an estimated 70 million in 2035. It is projected that the number of older adults with functional deficits will grow from 22 million in 2005 to 38 million by 2030, assuming no changes in disability rates from current levels (Field & Jette, 2007). The challenges posed by this demographic shift will be exacerbated by the decreasing ability of existing formal care systems to care for older adults because of a shortage of nurses and other health care workers, and increasing costs of hospitalization and long-term care (Talley & Crews, 2007). Changes in family size and composition and the increased labor force participation of women will make informal caregivers less available. Thus, the convergence of three factors in the decades ahead—increased need for care, decreased availability of formal care, and decreased number of adult children to provide care—has the makings of a perfect storm that will challenge policy makers for the decades ahead.

CHARACTERISTICS OF INFORMAL CAREGIVERS AND THEIR CARE RECIPIENTS

Nearly everyone serves as an unpaid caregiver at some point during the life span, and some individuals enact this role over extended periods of time lasting months and often years. Providing care to an individual with chronic illness and disability is generally viewed as a major life stressor, and its effects on the health and well-being of the caregiver have been intensively studied over the last three decades. Because informal caregivers are often called upon to provide highly demanding and complex care over long periods of time, the question inevitably arises: Who ends up in this role and how able are they to address care recipients' needs?

Relatively few population-based studies have been carried out to characterize the population of caregivers. One of the most comprehensive national caregiving studies to date (NAC & AARP, 2009) estimates that among adults age 18 and over, 28.5% or 65.7 million individuals provide unpaid care in any given year to an adult family member or friend who is also age 18 and over. The typical caregiver in the United States is a 48-year-old female, has some college education, works, and spends more than 20 hours per week providing unpaid care to her mother. Sixty-six percent of caregivers are women, and most work either full or part-time (59%). Education level of caregivers is slightly higher than the US adult population, with more than 90% having completed high school, and 43% being college graduates (compared to 85% and 27%, respectively) (Stoops, 2004).

Although caregivers are predominantly middle-aged or older, there is growing recognition that even children can be cast in the caregiver role. As many as 1.4 million children in the United States between the ages of 8 and 18 provide care for an older adult. These caregiving children are more likely to come from households with lower incomes, are less likely to live in a two-parent home, and are more likely to experience depression and anxiety when compared to their noncaregiving counterparts (Levine et al., 2005).

Care recipients are typically female (66%) and older (80% are age 50 or older), and their main presenting problems or illnesses are "old age" (12%), followed by Alzheimer's disease or other dementia (10%), cancer (7%), mental/emotional illness (7%), heart disease (5%), and stroke (5%). Among younger care recipients (age 18–49) the primary health problem requiring assistance is mental illness or depression (23%). Caregivers provide assistance with a wide range of IADLs, including helping with transportation (83%), housework (75%), grocery shopping (75%), and preparing meals (65%). Fifty-six percent of all caregivers also provide ADL assistance, primarily in helping the care recipient to get in and out of bed (40%), dress (32%), and bathe (26%). The average length of time caregivers report providing care is 4.6 years (NAC & AARP, 2009).

ROLES AND RESPONSIBILITIES OF CAREGIVERS

The delivery of effective health-related care in the home requires caregivers to play multiple roles. To varying degrees, caregivers must communicate and negotiate with family members about care decisions, provide companionship and emotional support, interact with physicians and other health care providers about patient status and care needs, drive care recipients to appointments, do housework, shop, complete paperwork and manage finances, hire nurses and aides, help with personal care and hygiene, lift and maneuver the care recipient, and assist with complex medical and nursing tasks (e.g., infusion therapies, tube feedings, medication monitoring) necessitated by the care recipient's health condition. In addition, caregivers are also

called upon to coordinate services from health and human service agencies, to make difficult decisions about service needs, and to figure out how to access needed services. Inasmuch as caregiving tasks are physically, cognitively, and emotionally demanding, we can anticipate that older, low-income, and chronically ill or disabled individuals who are cast in the caregiving role will be particularly vulnerable to adverse outcomes.

Figure 14.1 illustrates a typical caregiving trajectory involving an older individual with disability living in the community. Caregiving often begins when that individual is no longer able to perform IADL tasks such as cooking, cleaning, or managing finances because of a chronic health condition. Thus, the early stages of a caregiving career involve tasks such as monitoring symptoms and medications, helping with household tasks and finances, providing emotional support, and communicating with health professionals. As the health condition of the care recipient worsens and disabilities increase, the caregiver typically provides assistance with ADL tasks such as dressing, bathing, ambulating, and toileting. Caregivers may also be required to closely monitor the care recipient's activity in order to assure his or her safety. It is important to note that the tasks performed by caregivers are cumulative.

Thus, in the later stages of a caregiving career, caregivers typically help with ADL tasks in addition to those tasks they performed earlier. For some caregivers the need for care exceeds their ability to provide it, resulting in the placement of the care recipient into a long-term care facility, but even under these circumstances, caregiving does not end. Many caregivers continue to provide high levels of ADL assistance (e.g., feeding, grooming)

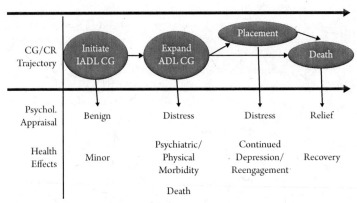

FIGURE 14.1 Caregiver (CG)/care recipient (CR) trajectory and health. ADL, activities of daily living; IADL, instrumental activities of daily living.

to their institutionalized relative and must in addition acquire new skills associated with navigating long-term care systems. Given the demands and duration of long-term caregiving, it should come as no surprise that caregivers experience relief when the care recipient dies (Schulz et al., 2003).

One of the biggest challenges facing informal caregivers is the coordination of services to support care recipients in the home or as they transition from one care setting to another. Caregivers may need to negotiate roles among family members who disagree on care options, identify relevant available services, assess eligibility requirements, and communicate and negotiate with health professionals and insurance companies. Even seasoned health professionals with detailed knowledge of and experience with health care systems find care coordination for care recipients a formidable challenge.

Coordinating care is particularly problematic for caregivers providing support to older individuals. The spectrum of formal support options available to care recipients and caregivers is broad, complex, and disorganized, with different access points and eligibility criteria. Access to information about options for care such as respite services, adult day care, support groups, Meals on Wheels, transportation services, and financial help is one of the major unmet needs of informal caregivers (NAC & AARP, 2004). This is particularly problematic among Hispanic, African American, and Asian American caregivers, who are much more likely to say they need help obtaining, processing, and understanding health information than White caregivers (NAC & AARP, 2004).

Health literacy, or the ability to obtain, process, and understand basic health information and service needs in order to make appropriate health decisions, is associated with poverty, limited education, minority status, immigration, and older age. Results from a recent national survey in the United States suggest that 36% of the adult population has limited health literacy skills (Kutner, Greenberg, Jin, & Paulsen, 2006), which have been consistently associated with lower health outcomes (i.e., poorer disease management) and increased rates of hospitalization and mortality (Hironaka & Paasche-Orlow, 2008; Kripalani et al., 2006).

One example of the magnitude of care coordination challenges was recently demonstrated in a study to evaluate the ability of relatively well-educated adults with computer experience to use the Medicare.gov website to make decisions about eligibility for services and prescription drug plans (Czaja, Sharit, & Nair, 2008). Participants were asked to determine eligibility for home health care services, select a home health agency to meet specified needs, make decisions about enrollment in Medicare Part D, and select a drug plan and determine associated costs based on a specified medication regime. Most participants were unable to specify all eligibility criteria for home health services (68.8%), choose the correct home health agency (80.4%), or execute computation procedures needed for making a plan enrollment decision (83.9%).

To help address the need for coordinated and comprehensive care, one-stop service programs such as PACE (Program for All-Inclusive Care for the Elderly) have been developed to provide integrated and seamless total care, including both social and medical services. These programs, however, have eligibility criteria that make them inaccessible to the majority of individuals with chronic disability and their caregivers (e.g., PACE participants must be age 55 or older and meet criteria for nursing facility level of care). Thus, the need in this area remains great.

In sum, the complexity of identifying and accessing health and social service options that might be useful to caregivers is daunting even to experienced health professionals cast in an informal caregiving role. The average lay person has little chance of optimizing formal support services to minimize the burdens of caregiving.

DETRIMENTAL HEALTH EFFECTS OF CAREGIVING

Clinical observation and early empirical research on family caregiving strongly suggested that assuming a caregiving role is stressful and burdensome to family members. Researchers and clinicians were quick to note that caregiving had all the features of a chronic stress experience; providing care generates physical and psychological strain over extended periods of time, is accompanied by high levels of unpredictability and uncontrollability, has the capacity to generate secondary stress in multiple life domains, and frequently requires high levels of vigilance on the part of the caregiver. Indeed, caregiving fits the recipe for chronic stress so well it came to be viewed as an ideal platform for studying the health effects of chronic stress exposure (Vitaliano, Zhang, & Scanlan, 2003).

It should come as no surprise that the dominant conceptual model for caregiving assumes that the onset and progression of chronic illness and physical disability is stressful for both care recipient and caregiver and, as such, can be studied within the framework of traditional stress-coping models. Within this framework, objective stressors include measures of care recipients' physical disability, cognitive impairment, and problem behaviors, as well as the type and intensity of care provided. These objective stressors in turn generate psychological stress, impair health behaviors, and perturb physiological systems within the body that cause illness and death (Vitaliano et al., 2003).

Table 14.1 Physical Health Measures

TYPE OF MEASURE	SPECIFIC INDICATORS	COMMENT
Global health measures		
	Self-reported health (current health, health compared to others, changes in health status)	Overall, effects are small; self-report measures are most common and show largest effects; one prospective study reports increased mortality for strained caregivers when compared to noncaregivers; higher age, lower socioeconomic status, and lower levels of informal support related to poorer health; greater negative effects found for dementia vs. nondementia caregiver and spouses vs. nonspouses
	Chronic conditions (chronic illness checklists)	
	Physical symptoms (Cornell Medical Index) (Brodman, Erdmann, Lorge, Wolff, & Broadbent, 1949)	
	Medications (number and types)	
	Health service utilization (clinic visits, days in hospital, physician visits)	
	Mortality	
Physiological measures		
	Antibodies and functional immune measures (immunoglobulin, Epstein Barr virus, T-cell proliferation, responses to mitogens, response to cytokine stimulation, lymphocyte counts)	Effect sizes for all indicators are generally small; stronger relationships found for stress hormones and antibodies than other indicators; evidence linking caregiving to metabolic and cardiovascular measures is weak. Men exhibit greater negative effects on most physiological indicators
	Stress hormones and neurotransmitters (ACTH, epinephrine, norepinephrine, cortisol, prolactin)	
	Cardiovascular measures (blood pressure, heart rate)	
	Metabolic measures (body mass, weight, cholesterol, insulin, glucose, transferin)	
	Speed of wound healing	
Health habits		
	Sleep, diet, exercise	
	Self-care, medical compliance	

Magnitude of Physical and Mental Health Effects

Several recent reviews document the link between caregiving and health (Gouin, Hantsoo, & Kiecolt-Glaser, 2008; Pinquart & Sörensen, 2003a; Vitaliano et al., 2003). For example, Vitaliano et al. (2003) reviewed 23 studies to compare the physical health of dementia caregivers with demographically similar noncaregivers, and across 11 health categories caregivers exhibited a slightly greater risk of health problems than did noncaregivers. We briefly summarize in Tables 14.1 and 14.2 the wide range of outcome variables represented in the literature. All of these variables have been linked to stressors such as the duration and type of care provided and functional and cognitive disabilities of the care recipient, as well as secondary stressors such as finances and family conflict. As a result of these stressors, providing care has been linked to psychological distress, health habits, physiological responses, psychiatric and physical illness, and mortality (Christakis & Allison, 2006; Haley, Roth, Howard, & Safford, 2010; Pinquart & Sörensen, 2003a, 2003b; Pinquart & Sörensen, 2007; Schulz & Beach, 1999; Schulz, O'Brien, Bookwala, & Fleissner, 1995; Schulz, Visintainer, & Williamson, 1990; Vitaliano et al., 2003).

Measures of psychological well-being such as depression, stress, and burden have been most frequently studied in the caregiving literature and generally yield consistent and relatively large health effects (Marks, Lambert, & Choi, 2002; Pinquart

& Sörensen, 2003a; Schulz et al., 1995, 1997; Teri, Logsdon, Uomoto, & McCurry, 1997). The effects of caregiving on depression are most pronounced for dementia caregivers where nearly half of caregivers report clinically meaningful depressive symptomatology (i.e., score 16 or higher on the Center for Epidemiologic Studies Depression Scale, CES-D), and approximately 25% of caregivers meet criteria for depressive disorder (Schulz et al., 1995). Similarly, a recent review shows that clinically significant anxiety is found in about 25% of caregivers for people with dementia (Cooper, Balamurali, Selwood, & Livingston, 2007). These effects are moderated by age, socioeconomic status (SES), and the availability of informal support. Specifically, older caregivers, low SES caregivers, and caregivers with limited support networks report lower levels of health than caregivers who are younger and have more economic and interpersonal resources (Vitaliano et al., 2003).

Detrimental physical health effects of caregiving are generally smaller than psychological health effects, regardless of whether they are measured by global self-report instruments or physiological measures such as stress hormones (Vitaliano et al., 2003). Although relatively few studies have focused on the association between caregiving and self-care behaviors, there is evidence to suggest that individuals engaged in heavy-duty caregiving manifest impaired self-care (Lee, Colditz, Berkman, & Kawachi, 2003; Schulz et al., 1997). Several recent large population studies further support

Table 14.2 Psychological Health Measures

TYPE OF MEASURE		COMMENT
Depression	Clinical diagnosis, symptom checklists, antidepressant medication use	Most frequently studied caregiver outcomes with largest effects; greater
Anxiety	Clinical diagnosis, symptom checklists, anxiolytic medication use	negative effects found for dementia vs. nondementia caregivers; higher age, lower
Stress	Burden	socioeconomic status, and
Subjective well-being	Global self-ratings; global quality of life ratings	lower levels of informal support related to poorer
Positive aspects of caregiving	Self-ratings of benefit finding	mental health
Self-efficacy	Self-ratings	

the relationship between caregiving and physical health. Fredman and colleagues (2008) found among healthy community-dwelling elderly adults, caregivers had modestly elevated rates of mortality and incident mobility limitations when compared to noncaregivers. In another study they found that older women who were long-term caregivers (4 years or more) and/or who cared for a person with dementia, considered to be a highly stressful type of caregiving, declined more in walking speed, a risk factor for mortality, than short-term or noncaregivers (Fredman, Doros, Cauley, Hillier, & Hochberg, 2010). Similar findings were recently reported in a study by Haley and colleagues (2010), who showed that caregiving strain among spousal caregivers was significantly associated with higher estimated stroke risk.

The high prevalence of depressive symptoms, clinical depression, and reduced quality of life among caregivers make caregiving an important public health issue in the United States, particularly given the fact that depression is the second leading cause of disability worldwide. Moreover, even if the detrimental effects of caregiving on physical health are relatively small, the large number of people affected means that the overall impact is significant. Recognition of these facts, coupled with the knowledge that caregivers represent a major national health resource, has resulted in national policy aimed at supporting caregivers.

Causes of Physical and Mental Health Effects

The data clearly show that providing care for a close relative with illness and disability causes distress in caregivers and may compromise their health and well-being. The negative effects of caregiving are typically attributed to a variety of illness-related factors, including patient functional disability, cognitive impairment and confusion, problem behaviors, and the care demands engendered by the illness. For example, depression, stress, and low subjective well-being are consistently associated with patient behavior problems, cognitive impairment, functional disabilities, duration and amount of care provided, and being older, a spouse, and female.

Recent research carried out by our group has emphasized the role that patient distress or suffering may play in generating caregiver distress and impaired health. In close relationships, suffering

can be contagious. Numerous studies have shown strong associations between husbands' and wives' emotional distress, even after controlling for the effects of sociodemographic factors, functional and health statuses of both members of the dyad, and shared life events (Bookwala & Schulz, 1996; Gaugler et al., 2005; Tower & Kasl, 1995, 1996). People are physiologically reactive to witnessing close others' pain (Block, 1981; Singer et al., 2004), and there is evidence that partners' suffering, conceptualized as physical symptoms, psychological distress, and existential or spiritual distress, directly influences caregivers' depression and prevalence of cardiovascular disease (Schulz et al., 2008; Schulz, Beach, et al., 2009).

Methodological Issues in Assessing Health Effects

Although the literature on caregiving is vast, much of it is based on cross-sectional analyses of relatively small (i.e., N < 100) nonprobability opportunity samples. Confounding effects are often not controlled through study design or statistical analysis. Thus, caution is advised before concluding unequivocally that caregiving leads to adverse health effects. Even large, longitudinal, or case control studies are subject to a number of biases. Differences in illness rates between caregivers and noncaregivers are not necessarily the result of caregiving experience and may instead reflect differences that likely existed prior to taking on the caregiving role. For example, individuals of low SES are more likely to take on the caregiving role than persons of high SES, and low SES is also a risk factor for poor health status. Higher rates of illness in spousal caregivers also may be the result of assortative mating (people tend to choose others who are similar to them) and because of shared health habits (e.g., diet, exercise) and life circumstances (e.g., access to medical care, job stress). As a result, older spouses tend to develop illness and disability conjointly; when one individual develops health problems requiring a caregiver, chances are his or her partner also has health problems, although they may be less severe.

Prospective studies (Schulz & Beach, 1999; Shaw et al., 1997) that link caregiver health declines to increasing care demands provide more compelling evidence of the health effects of caregiving. Since family caregiving cannot be experimentally manipulated, the best alternative study design is one in which individuals are followed longitudinally and their health is assessed as they move into and out of a caregiving role. A handful of studies have assessed caregiver outcomes such as depression and physical health status before and after taking on the caregiving role (Burton, Zdaniuk, Schulz, Jackson & Hirsch, 2003; Hirst, 2005; Lawton, Moss, Hoffman, & Perkinson, 2000; Seltzer & Li, 2000). Burton et al. (2003) and more recently Hirst (2005) provide compelling evidence that moving into a demanding caregiving role, defined as providing assistance with basic activities of daily living for 20 hours or more of care per week, results in increased depression and psychological distress, impaired self-care, and lower self-reported health. The fact that transitioning to lesser amounts of care provision has little impact on the health of the caregiver suggests that a threshold of care demands has to be reached before negative health effects are observed. Note, too, hours of care provided is associated with several other factors, including the level of illness and disability, and the amount of suffering experienced by the care recipients, as well as restrictions in freedom of the caregiver, all of which may contribute to the negative health effects among caregivers. Findings on the effects of transitioning out of the caregiving role because of patient improvement, institutionalization, or death help to complete the picture on the association between caregiving and health. Improved care recipient functioning is associated with reductions in caregiver distress (Nieboer et al., 1998), and the death of the care recipient has been found to reduce caregiver depression, enabling the caregiver to return to normal levels of functioning within a year of the care recipient's death (Schulz et al., 2003). In the short term, the effects of the transition to nursing homes are less positive as caregivers continue to exhibit high levels of psychiatric morbidity after placement (Schulz et al., 2004). While institutionalizing typically reduces the amount of hands-on care provided by the caregiver, it does not necessarily reduce the perceived suffering of the care recipient, and possibly introduces new stressors such as feelings of guilt about institutionalizing their loved one.

A related shortcoming of the existing literature is that while researchers have been able to link caregiving stressors to caregiver responses, they have rarely shown the sequential progression of illness effects. For example, while many studies show that caregiving causes psychological distress, virtually none have shown within persons over time that stress results in physiological dysregulation such as increased cortisol secretion or changes in immune function. Similarly, researchers interested in the effects of caregiving on health behaviors or physiological responses have not yet demonstrated within persons that these effects are directly linked to the emergence of illnesses. To be sure, demonstrating sequential causal relationships among variables thought to be critical in the path from caregiver stress to illness is challenging, but such efforts should receive high priority. Large-sample longitudinal studies that include a rich array of biological, psychosocial, and behavioral measures would be required to achieve this goal.

BENEFICIAL HEALTH EFFECTS OF CAREGIVING

Caregiving is not always a negative experience. In studies of caregiving that use large population-based samples, a significant proportion of caregivers report neither strain nor negative health effects (Schulz et al., 1997). This is particularly true for caregivers in the early stages of a caregiving career (Burton et al., 2003; Hirst, 2005). Even when caregiving demands become more intense and are associated with high levels of distress and depression, caregivers acknowledge positive aspects of the caregiving experience. They report that it makes them feel good about themselves, makes them feel useful and needed, gives meaning to their lives, enables them to learn new skills, and strengthens relationships with others. Because studies on the positive aspects of caregiving are typically given short shrift in the review literature on caregiving, we focus in detail here on recent studies suggesting that caregiving can have beneficial effects on the health of the caregiver. We begin with studies suggesting that caregiving may decrease the risk of mortality.

Caregiving and Decreased Risk of Mortality

There is an emerging literature showing that caregiving is associated with a lower risk of mortality (Brown, Nesse, Vinokur, & Smith, 2003; Brown et al., 2009; O'Reilly, Connolly, Rosato, & Patterson, 2008). These effects remain even when controlling for caregivers' baseline health status, decreasing the possibility of a "healthy caregiver" effect—"that those in a caring role may be self-selected because of their current 'healthiness' and thus present with lower mortality risks" (O'Reilly et al., 2008, p. 1284). Instead, the positive effects of caregiving found in these studies are generally attributed to the benefits of helping (Brown et al., 2003).

These beneficial effects of caregiving are contradictory to those from other studies that show increased risk of mortality among caregivers (Christakis & Allison, 2006; Schulz & Beach, 1999). What might account for this inconsistency? One reason may be that researchers have found negative effects more consistently with strained caregivers (Schulz & Beach, 1999), whereas positive effects have been found with relatively less burdened caregivers. For example, O'Reilly and colleagues (2008) found that caregivers from the 2001 Northern Ireland Census had lower risk of mortality than noncaregivers, but risk increased with the time spent caregiving. Beneficial mortality effects were larger among those who spent 1–19 hours a week providing care compared to those providing care more than 20 hours a week. Those providing 1–19 hours of care were also most affluent, suggesting that they had more resources to deal with the burden of providing care. In contrast to the O'Reilly and colleagues study (2008), Brown and colleagues (2009) found that high numbers of caregiving hours (more than 14 hours per week) were associated with decreased mortality risk, whereas low numbers of caregiving hours (1–14 hours per week) were not associated with mortality, even after controlling for spousal impairments, age, employment status, and caregiver health at baseline.

Another important difference between studies demonstrating positive versus negative health effects concerns the conceptualization and measurement of caregiving. Studies showing positive effects tend to define caregiving more broadly, whereas studies showing negative effects focus on the provision of care to a particular close relationship partner. For example, the O'Reilly study (2008) assessed caregiving with the Census question: "Do you look after, or give any help or support to family members, friends, neighbors or others because of: long term physical or mental ill-health or disability; problems related to old age?" This question makes it unclear who exactly is receiving support or what is the nature of the relationship between caregiver and recipient. Brown and colleagues (2003) measured instrumental support given to others (friends, relatives, and neighbors), excluding relationship partners. It is possible that those who are able to give support to others are least involved in caring for a close relationship partner. Being responsible for the care of a close relationship partner is presumably a very different experience than providing support to others in one's social network.

O'Reilly and colleagues (2008) did try to assess whether caregiving relationships were between spouses by examining marital status, but one cannot be certain that those who were married were necessarily taking care of their spouse. Also, Brown and colleagues (2003) examined emotional support given to spouses; however, they measured emotional support with a scale that typically assesses relationship quality, the Dyadic Adjustment Scale (Spanier, 1976), and two items asking participants whether they made their spouse feel loved and cared for and whether they were willing to listen if their spouse needed to talk. This conceptualization of caregiving with its emphasis on relationship quality and emotional as opposed to instrumental support is different from what is used in most other studies examining the association between caregiving and mortality. Finally, Brown and colleagues' (2009) study that shows decreased mortality among spousal caregivers assessed caregiving based on the spouse's report of help received rather than the caregiver's report of help provided. It is unclear whether the same results would have emerged if the caregiver's perspective was measured instead.

Positive Physical and Psychological Health Outcomes

Although the majority of studies show that caregiving is associated with poor health and impaired psychological functioning (Dunlop et al., 2005; Ory, Yee, Tennstedt, & Schulz, 2000; Schulz et al., 1997), there are also some studies showing positive health correlates (Beach, Schulz, Yee, & Jackson, 2000; Brown, Consedine, & Magai, 2005; Jenkins, Kabeto, & Langa, 2009; Taylor, Ford, & Dunbar, 1995). Like the mortality studies, most of these studies control for sociodemographic factors and baseline health status, decreasing the probability of a "healthy caregiver" effect.

As with the mortality studies, inconsistencies with previous studies showing negative psychological and physical health effects may stem from differences in caregiver strain. For example, Beach and colleagues (2000) found that helping in the context of caregiving is associated with better health outcomes (decreased anxiety and depression); however, caregivers who experience more strain and who have highly impaired partners suffer from poorer health outcomes (Beach et al., 2000).

Sociodemographic characteristics may also serve as a proxy for caregiver strain. Jenkins and colleagues (2009) found that once age, education, and net worth were controlled, the negative association between caregiving and health (ADL/IADL functioning and self-rated health) disappeared. Those who were older, less educated, and had a lower net worth were more likely to suffer the negative consequences of being a caregiver. Conversely, younger caregivers with low levels of strain may experience better health outcomes than noncaregivers. For example, Taylor and colleagues (1995) found a tendency for caregivers to report better health and functioning than noncaregivers over a 3-year period; however, the median number of caregiving hours per week was 7, caregivers were on average 55 years old, and many of the caregivers discontinued providing care over the 3-year period of their study. In sum, the combination of feeling strained in the caregiving role and other vulnerabilities such as advanced age and low SES consistently yield negative health effects. At this time, a definitive single, well-designed study that shows that SES, age, caregiving hours, and strain produce different (positive vs. negative) health effects is lacking. Such a study would show positive health effects for relatively high SES, younger, less strained caregivers who spend relatively few hours providing care, and negative health effects for relatively low SES, older, more strained caregivers who spend a large number of hours providing care.

Why Might Caregiving Be Beneficial to Health?

The positive health effects of caregiving have mainly been attributed to the benefits of helping (Brown et al., 2003). This is based on empirical evidence that helping is associated with reduced stress (Cialdini, Darby, & Vincent, 1973; Midlarsky, 1991) and improved health (Schwartz & Sendor, 2000), and that older adults who volunteer have a reduced risk of morbidity and mortality (Brown et al., 2005; Krause, Herzog, & Baker, 1992; Musik, Herzog, & House, 1999; Oman, Thoresen, & McMahon, 1999). Brown and colleagues (2009) hypothesize that helping can serve as a stress buffer, citing prior findings that increased instrumental support given to other people accelerated recovery from depressive symptoms (Brown, House, Brown, & Smith, 2008).

Suggested mechanisms for the stress buffering effect include increased positive emotion (Cialdini & Kenrick, 1976), which can speed cardiovascular recovery from the effects of negative emotion (Fredrickson, Mancuso, Branigan, & Tugade, 2000), and hormones, such as oxytocin, which decreases activity in the hypothalamic-pituitary-adrenal axis and contribute to cellular repair and storage of nutrients (Heaphy & Dutton, 2008).

Brown and colleagues (2003) also provide an evolutionary explanation for the association between helping and longevity. They refer to kin selection theory (Hamilton, 1964a, 1964b) and reciprocal-altruism theory (Trivers, 1971) that suggest that human reproductive success was contingent upon the ability to give resources to relationship partners, which triggers a desire for self-preservation on the part of the giver and enables prolonged investment in kin (De Catanzaro, 1986) and reciprocal altruists.

Other researchers have emphasized the role of caregiving in enhancing relationships and providing personal strength and meaning to caregivers. For example, Motenko (1989) noted that "caregiving is an expression of bonds which tie people to their loved ones" (p. 166), and it is an important way of expressing intimacy, love, and basic emotions to another person. Motenko (1989) suggested that this expression is necessary to maintain continuity in values, self-respect, and identity, and this may be especially true for women who often define their identity based on caring and nurturing others (Baker-Miller, 1976; Chodorow, 1978; Gilligan, 1982). Consistent with this, O'Reilly and colleagues (2008) found that decreased mortality associated with caregiving was enhanced for women.

Caring for a loved one can also provide meaning to the lives of caregivers. Farran and colleagues (1991) emphasized that the caregiving experience can provide opportunities for creative expression, as seen when caregivers develop innovative approaches to solving day-to-day challenges. Also, caregivers often feel a sense of fulfillment knowing that they are taking care of someone they love. Finding personal strength and fulfilling a duty to a loved one may promote caregivers' health, psychological well-being, and life satisfaction. Similarly, researchers have found that a sense of usefulness in old age is associated with better self-rated health and decreased mortality (Okamoto & Tanaka, 2004).

To capture the positive aspects of caregiving, researchers have developed scales such as the Caregiving Satisfaction Scale (Lawton, Kleban, Moss, Rovine, & Glickman, 1989), which includes items such as "You really enjoy being with (care recipient)?" and "Helping has made you feel closer to (care recipient)?" and the Positive Aspects of Caregiving measure (Tarlow et al., 2004) which includes two factors: Self-Affirmation (e.g., "Providing help to (care recipient) has made me feel useful") and Outlook on Life (e.g., "Providing help to (care recipient) has enabled me to develop a more positive attitude toward life"). Using these scales as well as more specific questions, studies have shown that many caregivers experience satisfaction (Lawton et al., 1989), pleasure and rewards (Donelan et al., 2002; Wolff, Dy, Frick, & Kasper, 2007), enjoyment (Cohen, Gold, Shulman, & Zucchero, 1994), and uplifts and daily events that evoke joy (Pruchno, Michaels, & Potashnik, 1990) when caring for their family members (see Kramer, 1997, and Tarlow et al., 2004 for reviews).

Measures assessing positive aspects of caregiving have been linked with enhanced well-being and health for caregivers (Cohen, Colantonio, & Vernich, 2002; Motenko, 1989; Pinquart & Sörenson, 2003a; see Kramer, 1997 for a review). For example, in a national sample of caregivers derived from the Canadian Study of Health and Aging, positive feelings about caring, such as companionship and a sense of fulfillment, were associated with fewer depressive symptoms, a reduced sense of burden, and better self-rated health (Cohen et al., 2002). In a meta-analysis, Pinquart and Sörensen (2003b) found that perceived uplifts of caregiving, such as feeling useful or experiencing increased closeness to the care recipient, were associated with lower levels of caregiver burden and depression. They also found that perceived uplifts were largely independent of objective caregiving stressors. Motenko (1989) found that among women caring at home for a husband with dementia, gratification was associated with greater well-being, and wives who perceived continuity in marital closeness since their partners' illness had greater gratification than those who perceived change. Thus, there is reason to believe that caregiving is not only a source of stress but also has the potential to provide benefits to caregivers and enhance relationships. This may be especially true for caregivers who are in the early stages of caregiving careers, are less strained, and provide care to family members who are less impaired.

Reconciling Positive and Negative Caregiving Effects

Family caregiving is a dynamic process that at any point can be characterized by multiple factors. Although its onset may be insidious, it has a time dimension typically measured in months or years, and an endpoint marked by the death of the care recipient, sometimes preceded by placement in a long-term care facility. It also has an intensity dimension, measured in hours of care provided, or the amount and type of care provided. Duration and intensity tend to covary; inasmuch as the illness and disability in late life typically increase over time, the intensity of care provided increases as well, as the caregiver moves through the middle and late stages of a caregiving episode. Finally, because caregiving is an intensely interpersonal experience, it has a strong emotional component. The attitudes, behaviors, and emotions of both caregiver and care recipient undoubtedly play a key role in defining the caregiving experience.

Our own recent work draws attention to the effects of suffering of the care recipient and the role this plays in shaping the caregiver's response to caregiving, and it, too, tends to increase with time and intensity of care provided (Monin & Schulz, 2009; Schulz, Beach, et al., 2009; Schulz et al., 2007, 2008). We differentiate three types of suffering—physical, psychological, and existential/spiritual—and in several studies show that each independently contributes to caregiver psychological and physical morbidity. Expressions of suffering provide important signals of the need for help, which activate responses in humans through mechanisms such as cognitive empathy, mimicry, and conditioned learning. From an evolutionary perspective, it is critical that mammals have well-developed distress signaling and response systems. Young children need to be able to communicate when they are suffering, and their parents need to respond to signs of suffering for the survival and optimal development of their offspring. Signaling systems such as the expression of pain are clearly innate, although they are likely to become more elaborated and nuanced through experience and learning. Some components of the response system such as mimicry may also be innate but are likely developed through experience and learning. By middle and late adulthood both systems are highly entrenched and serve as part of the motivational system that underlies caregiving. What makes caregiving in late life uniquely challenging is that the ability to effectively respond to suffering may be compromised, particularly in the late stages of a caregiving career when there is little that anyone can do to alleviate the suffering of the care recipient.

In general, we would expect the negative effects of caregiving to be greatest when all three factors—duration of caregiving, intensity of caregiving, and the magnitude of care recipient suffering—are at their peak. This combination is most likely to lead to chronic stress experiences characterized by high demand but low control, and a mismatch between effort and reward (Dimsdale, 2008). Caregivers faced with prolonged and daunting care demands with little reward in terms of reducing care recipient suffering should be at highest risk for negative outcomes. Our views here diverge somewhat from the perspective of S. L. Brown and W. M. Brown and colleagues (2003, 2005, respectively) who argue that the act of helping is fulfilling in its own right; from our perspective, helping that fails to reduce care recipient suffering is perceived as futile and has little benefit to the caregiver. Conversely, the benefits of helping should be maximized when they effectively relieve the suffering of another individual. A more detailed description of these ideas can be found in our recent theoretical discussion of suffering in the context of caregiving (Monin & Schulz, 2009).

The predominantly negative effects observed in the caregiving literature are likely due to the fact that most caregiving studies selectively focus on caregivers in the middle to late stages of a caregiving episode when both care demands and care recipient suffering are high, with little control over care recipient outcomes and little reward for the time and effort expended. Conversely, studies that show positive effects of caregiving likely reflect caregiving experiences that afford high levels of control over care recipient outcomes such as suffering and favorable effort-reward ratios. Identifying how and when caregivers transition from a positive to a negative caregiving experience are important unresolved questions that should receive high priority in future research. Finding an answer to these questions will require fine-grained longitudinal studies of caregiving in which caregiver behavior and emotion regulation strategies as well as care recipient response are studied.

INTERVENTIONS FOR CAREGIVERS

Despite the recent research suggesting that caregiving can be beneficial under some circumstances, there is strong consensus among researchers and clinicians that for most individuals caregiving is a major chronic stressor that exacts a high price on the health and well-being of the caregiver. This conclusion has spawned dozens of caregiver intervention studies and numerous reviews and meta-analysis of this literature (e.g., Cooper et al., 2007; Schulz, Martire, & Klinger, 2005; Sörensen, Duberstein, Gill, & Pinquart, 2006).

Caregiving poses multiple, diverse challenges. As a result, a broad array of intervention strategies has been evaluated, either in combination or as individual treatments. For example, psychotherapeutic approaches include individual or group-based psychodynamic behavioral and cognitive-behavioral therapies. These strategies are designed to enable the caregiver to focus on unproductive thoughts and behaviors and help them develop new alternative behavioral responses to the challenges they face. Psychoeducation is a common feature of most interventions and is aimed at providing information about the care recipient's disease and its course, stress management, and methods for managing patient behaviors. Information can be delivered either in person or via computer or other communication technologies. Enhanced support interventions are frequently used to enable sharing of feelings, concerns, and patient management strategies among caregivers, and they can be delivered in person or via communication technologies. Case management or care coordination strategies include practical advice and information on how to access services and support organizations, while respite interventions are designed to give the caregiver a break by offering substitute care through group day care, home respite, or institutional respite.

Several recent meta-analyses show that these interventions are effective overall, but the effect sizes are small to medium. Thus, psychoeducational interventions are generally effective in increasing caregiver knowledge and somewhat less effective in reducing burden, depression, and increasing subjective well-being. Psychotherapeutic approaches, particularly cognitive-behavioral therapy, are effective treatments for burden, depression, and anxiety, and several studies have achieved clinically significant improvements in treating depression, anxiety, and enhancing quality of life. Overall, treatments tend to be more effective to the extent that they engage the caregiver in active participation through role playing, homework assignments, and demonstration of newly acquired skills.

Because most caregivers must simultaneously face multiple challenges, recent intervention strategies have emphasized multicomponent treatment strategies that combine psychoeducational approaches with problem solving, skills training, enhancing support, and managing emotional problems (Belle et al., 2006; Nichols, Martindale-Adams, Burns, Graney, & Zuber, 2011; Schulz, Czaja, et al., 2009). These strategies have been further refined to emphasize tailoring of the intervention to the need profile of the caregiver. Caregivers are administered a risk assessment to determine their levels of need in multiple areas and the intervention is then tailored to the unique risk profile of that individual (Czaja et al., 2009). These strategies have resulted in moderate to large effects in enhancing caregiver quality of life (Belle et al., 2006; Nichols et al., 2011).

Another recent refinement of the caregiver intervention literature has been the introduction of dyadic treatment strategies in which the caregiver and care recipient are treated simultaneously (Martire, Lustig, Schulz, Miller, & Helgeson, 2004; Martire, Schulz, Helgeson, Small, & Saghafi, 2010; Schulz, Czaja, et al., 2009). This approach assumes there are important synergies to be attained by simultaneously treating the caregiver and care recipient. For individuals with disability embedded in supportive personal relationships, it is important to consider the reciprocal impact that providers and recipients of care have on each other (Bookwala & Schulz, 1996). Interventions targeting both patient and family caregiver may have added benefit as compared to interventions aimed at only one of these individuals. For example, while both single and dyadic interventions may improve the emotional well-being and health behaviors of either individual, dyadic intervention has greater potential due to its effects on factors such as effective support seeking and support provision within the dyad (Martire & Schulz, 2007). The dyadic approach sensitizes us as well to the fact that it is important to focus on the dyad as the unit of analysis and the possibility that a positive outcome for the care recipient may not necessarily be positive for the caregiver. This approach is illustrated in a recent study of caregivers of older spinal cord injured patients in which we compared outcomes between treatment as usual, caregiver-only treatment, and dyadic treatment in which both caregivers and patients received complementary interventions. We found that dyads enrolled in the dyadic treatment condition were significantly less depressed and had fewer health problems when compared to participants in the caregiver-only treatment condition (Schulz, Czaja, et al., 2009).

CONCLUSION

Informal caregiving is a central feature of our health care landscape and will become even more prominent in the decades ahead. The demand and need for care will increase dramatically over the next three decades as a result of the aging of the population, infant and childhood survival, health behaviors that increase disabling health conditions such as obesity, and returning war veterans suffering from polytrauma. This will happen in a context where the availability of informal support is declining, the costs of formal care and support are already too high and unsustainable, and there is a growing shortfall of health care professionals with relevant expertise. Resolving this supply-demand dilemma will require efficiencies in both the informal and formal health care systems that greatly exceed current practice. Important research and policy issues need to be addressed before we move forward on this agenda. By no means exhaustive, we present five recommendations that should receive high priority.

1. Adopt a standard definition of what it means to be an informal caregiver and use it consistently in surveys of the US population in order to accurately assess the prevalence of caregiving, the public health burden associated with caregiving, and a full range of issues such as those discussed earlier. We need to have accurate and consistent data on who is providing care, what types of care are provided, for how long, at what costs to the caregiver, and the probable downstream costs to society. Having such data is an important requisite to developing policy on support programs for caregivers. The value of this recommendation is evident in Australia, Japan, and the United Kingdom, for example, all of which have adopted standard definitions of caregiving that are linked to eligibility for caregiver and care recipient services. Variations of the standard definition may be necessary for different populations of caregivers and care recipients, and levels of care should also be consistently defined.

2. A recurrent theme of this chapter is that we need better coordination between formal and informal health care systems to assure a close match between home care demands and the informal caregiver's ability to provide that care. This will require a clear understanding of the task demands of home

care and assessment of caregiver capabilities, including their motivation to provide care, their physical, sensory, motor, and cognitive ability to perform caregiving tasks, their levels of distress and depression, and the quantity and quality of other support available to them. Assessments of the caregiver should be a routine feature during care recipient and health care provider encounters, and these data should inform decisions about whether a caregiver is capable of taking on the caregiver role, the types of training needed, and the intensity of monitoring and external support required to assure adequate care that does not unduly compromise the caregiver's own functioning. A related need concerns the development of decision rules for terminating caregiving responsibilities when caregivers are no longer able to carry out their assignments. Implementing these strategies will require that we expand the training of health care and social service providers to give them the skills and tools to carry out these types of assessments (FCA, 2006a, 2006b). Detailed recommendations on who should do assessments, what should be assessed, and when and where are available from the National Consensus Development Conference on Caregiver Assessment (FCA, 2006a, 2006b). Although intended for caregivers of older care recipients, these recommendations serve as a good starting point for developing assessment procedures and tools for all caregiving populations.

3. From a scientific perspective there remain important unanswered questions about caregiving that have far-reaching policy implications. For example, we need a deeper understanding of what causes distress in the caregiving experience and how best to help the caregiver. Although numerous studies point to the importance of various functional disabilities and associated care demands as causes of caregiver burden, we may be underestimating the role that factors such as care recipient suffering play in the life of a caregiver. Making these distinctions is important because it may lead to different policy responses (e.g., providing respite to ease the burdens of care provision as well as treatments to decrease the suffering of the care recipient or to help the caregiver come to terms with the suffering of his or her loved one).

4. Technology has the potential of calming the waters of the emerging storm by increasing the efficiency and effectiveness of formal and informal care providers, enhancing the functioning and autonomy of individuals with disability, preventing premature decline, and generally enhancing the quality of life of elders. Implementing technology-based solutions will require that we develop user-friendly and highly reliable systems that are able to both identify needs and respond to them. We have made considerable progress in recent years in developing and deploying sensing and monitoring technology useful in identifying individuals experiencing or at risk for adverse outcomes. Computer, sensing, and communication technologies have also been effectively used for caregiver training and performance monitoring. Research on enabling technologies that extend the functional capability of humans is still in the early stages of development and should receive high priority.

5. Because caregiving is so prevalent in our society and integral to the health and well-being of the population, all adults need to be educated about the likelihood of becoming a caregiver and a care recipient, the roles and responsibilities of caregiving, and rudimentary caregiving skills. A recent survey of 1,018 adults aged 18 and over commissioned by Johnson and Johnson Consumer Products Co. (Schulz, Czaja, Belle, and Lewin, unpublished data) found that adults have realistic expectations about becoming caregivers in the future but are less able to see themselves as care recipients. Nearly two-thirds of American adults expect to be caregivers in the future, but nearly half believe that they will not need any care in the future. Indeed, more than one third of adults have *never* thought about needing care in the future, and few have made any preparations for future care such as talking with family or friends about care needs in the future (34%), setting aside funds to cover additional expenses (41%), signing living wills or health care power of attorney (40%), or purchasing disability or long-term care insurance. When asked how prepared they are to provide care to others, the majority (56%) were unprepared to carry out basic caregiving tasks such as bathing, dressing, and toileting; 35% said they were only somewhat or not at all (28%) prepared to handle health insurance matters; 56% said they were unprepared to assist with medications; and most worried about handling financial matters for a loved one. These data suggest that caregiving and care receiving should be a normative component of adult education. The goal of such efforts should be to inform adults about the likelihood of caregiving and care receiving, ways in which one can plan for these eventualities, and rudimentary skills needed to enact and/or cope in these roles.

Disclosures

Dr. Schulz has no conflicts of interest to disclose.

REFERENCES

Baker Miller, J. (1976). *Toward a new psychology of women*. Boston, MA: Beacon Press.

Beach, S. R., Schulz, R., Yee, J. L., & Jackson, S. (2000). Negative and positive health effects of caring for a disabled spouse: Longitudinal findings from the Caregiver Health Effects Study. *Psychology and Aging, 15,* 259–271.

Belle, S. H., Burgio, L., Burns, R., Coon, D., Czaja, S. J., Gallagher-Thompson, D.,… Zhang, S. (2006). Enhancing the quality of life of dementia caregivers from different ethnic or racial groups. *Annals of Internal Medicine, 145*(10), 727–738.

Block, A. R. (1981). Investigation of the response of the spouse to chronic pain behavior. *Psychosomatic Medicine, 43,* 415–422.

Bookwala, J., & Schulz, R. (1996). Spousal similarity in subjective well-being. The cardiovascular health study. *Psychology and Aging, 11,* 582–591.

Brown, S. L., House, J. S., Brown, R. M., & Smith, D. M. (2008). Coping with spousal loss: The buffering effects of helping behavior. *Personality and Social Psychology Bulletin, 34,* 849–861.

Brown, S. L., Nesse, R. M., Vinokur, A., & Smith, D. M. (2003). Providing social support may be more beneficial than receiving it: Results from a prospective study of mortality. *Psychological Science, 14,* 320–327.

Brown, S. L., Smith, D. M., Schulz, R., Kabeto, M. U., Ubel, P. A., Poulin, M.,… Langa, K. M. (2009). Caregiving behavior is associated with decreased mortality risk. *Psychological Science, 20*(4), 488–494.

Brown, W. M., Consedine, N. S., & Magai, C. (2005). Altruism relates to health in an ethnically diverse sample of older adults. *Journal of Gerontology: Social Sciences, 60B*(3), 143–152.

Burton, L. C., Zdaniuk, B., Schulz, R., Jackson, S., & Hirsch, C. (2003). Transitions in spousal caregiving. *Gerontologist, 43,* 230–241.

Centers for Disease Control and Prevention (CDC). (2006). *Disability and health state chartbook, 2006: Profiles of health for adults with disabilities*. Atlanta, GA: Centers for Disease Control and Prevention.

Chodorow, N. (1978). *The reproduction of mothering*. Berkeley and Los Angeles: University of California Press.

Christakis, N., & Allison, P. D. (2006). Mortality after the hospitalization of a spouse. *New England Journal of Medicine, 354*(7), 719–730.

Cialdini, R. B., & Kenrick, D. T. (1976). Altruism as hedonism: A social development perspective on the relationship of negative mood state and helping. *Journal of Personality and Social Psychology, 34,* 907–914.

Cialdini, R. B., Darby, B. K., & Vincent, J. E. (1973). Transgression and altruism: A case for hedonism. *Journal of Experimental Social Psychology, 9,* 502–516.

Cohen, C. A., Colantonio, A., & Vernich, L. (2002). Positive aspects of caregiving: Rounding out the caregiving experience. *International Journal of Geriatric Psychiatry, 17*(2), 184–188.

Cohen, C. A., Gold, D. P., Shulman, K. I., & Zucchero, C. A. (1994). Positive aspects in caregiving: An overlooked variable in research. *Canadian Journal on Aging, 13,* 378–391.

Cooper, C., Balamurali, T. B. S., Selwood, A., & Livingston, G. (2007). A systematic review of intervention studies about anxiety in caregivers of people with dementia. *International Journal of Geriatric Psychiatry, 22,* 181–188.

Czaja, S. J., Gitlin, L. N., Schulz, R., Zhang, S., Burgio, D., Stevens, A. B.,… Gallagher-Thompson, D. (2009). Development of the Risk Appraisal Measure (RAM): A brief screen to identify risk areas and guide interventions for dementia caregivers. *Journal of the American Geriatrics Society, 57,* 1064–1072.

Czaja, S. J., Sharit, J., & Nair, S. N. (2008). Usability of the Medicare health web site. *Journal of the American Medical Association, 300*(7), 790–792.

De Cantanzaro, D. (1986). A mathematical model of evolutionary pressures regulating self-preservation and self-destruction. *Suicide and Life-Threatening Behavior, 16,* 166–181.

Dimsdale, J. E. (2008). Psychological stress and cardiovascular disease. *Journal of the American College of Cardiology, 51*(13), 1237–1246.

Donelan, K., Hill, C. A., Hoffman, C., Scoles, K., Hollander Feldman, P., Levine, C., & Gould, D. (2002). Challenged to care: Informal caregivers in a changing health system. *Health Affairs, 21*(4), 222–231.

Dunlop, D. D., Semanik, P., Song, J., Manheim, L. M., Shih, V., & Chang, R. W. (2005). Risk factors for functional decline in older adults with arthritis. *Arthritis and Rheumatism, 52*(4), 1274–1282.

Family Caregiver Alliance (FCA). (2006a). *Caregiver assessment: Principals, guidelines, and strategies for change*. Report from a National Consensus Development Conference (Vol. I). San Francisco, CA: Author.

Family Caregiver Alliance (FCA). (2006b). *Caregiver assessment: Voices and views from the field*. Report from a National Consensus Development Conference (Vol. II). San Francisco, CA: Author.

Farran, C. J., Keane-Hagerty, E., Salloway, S., Kupferer, S., & Wilken, C. S. (1991). Finding meaning: An alternative paradigm for Alzheimer's disease family caregivers. *Gerontologist, 31*(4), 483–489.

Field, M., & Jette, A. M., (Eds.). (2007). *The future of disability in America.* Washington, DC: National Academies Press.

Fredman, L., Cauley, J. A., Satterfield, S., Simonsick, E., Spencer, S. M., Ayonayon, H. N., & Harris, T. B. (2008). Caregiving, mortality, and mobility decline. *Archives of Internal Medicine, 168*(19), 2154–2162.

Fredman, L., Doros, G., Cauley, J. A., Hillier, T. A., & Hochberg, M. C. (2010). Caregiving, metabolic syndrome indicators, and 1-year decline in walking speed: Results of caregiver-SOF. *Journals of Gerontology Series A, Biological Sciences Medical Sciences, 65A*(5), 565–572.

Fredrickson, B. L., Mancuso, R. A., Branigan, C., & Tugade, M. M. (2000). The undoing effect of positive emotions. *Motivation and Emotion, 24,* 237–258.

Gaugler, J. E., Hanna, N., Linder, J., Given, C. W., Tolbert, V., Kataria, R., & Regine, W. F. (2005). Cancer caregiving and subjective stress: A multi-site, multi-dimensional analysis. *Psycho-oncology, 14*(9), 771–785.

Gilligan, C. (1982). *In a different voice.* Cambridge, MA: Harvard University Press.

Gouin, J. P., Hantsoo, L., & Kiecolt-Glaser, J. K. (2008). Immune dysregulation and chronic stress among older adults: A review. *Neuroimmunomodulation, 15*(4–6), 251–259.

Haley, W. E., Roth, D. L., Howard, G., & Safford, M. M. (2010). Caregiving strain and estimated risk for stroke and coronary heart disease among spouse caregivers. *Stroke, 41*(2), 331–336.

Hamilton, W. D. (1964a). The genetic evolution of social behavior: I. *Journal of Theoretical Biology, 7,* 1–16.

Hamilton, W. D. (1964b). The genetic evolution of social behavior: II. *Journal of Theoretical Biology, 7,* 17–52.

Heaphy, E. D., & Dutton, J. E. (2008). Positive social interactions and the human body at work. Linking organizations and physiology. *Academy of Management Review, 33,* 137–162.

Hironaka, L. K., & Paasche-Orlow, M. K. (2008). The implications of health literacy on patient-provider communication. *Archives of Disease in Childhood, 93*(5), 428–432.

Hirst, M. (2005). Career distress: A prospective, population-based study. *Social Science and Medicine, 61,* 697–708.

Jenkins, K. R., Kabeto, M. U., & Langa, K. M. (2009). Does caring for your spouse harm one's health? Evidence from a United States nationally-representative sample of older adults. *Ageing and Society, 29,* 277–293.

Kramer, B. J. (1997). Gain in the caregiving experience: Where are we? What next? *Gerontologist, 37*(2), 218–32.

Krause, N., Herzog, A. R., & Baker, E. (1992). Providing support to others and well-being in later life. *Journal of Gerontology: Social Sciences, 47*(5), 300–311.

Kripalani, S., Henderson, L. E., Chiu, E. Y., Robertson, R., Kolm, P., & Jacobson, T. A. (2006). Predictors of medication self-management skill in a low-literacy population. *Journal of General Internal Medicine, 21*(8), 852–856.

Kutner, M., Greenberg, E., Jin, Y., & Paulsen, C. (2006). The health literacy of America's adults: Results from the 2003 National Assessment of Adult Literacy. Washington, DC: US Department of Education, National Center for Education Statistics.

Lawton, M. P., Kleban, M. H., Moss, M., Rovine, M., & Glickman, A. (1989). Measuring caregiving appraisal. *Journal of Gerontology: Social Sciences, 44,* 61–71.

Lawton, M. P., Moss, M., Hoffman, C., & Perkinson, M. (2000). Two transitions in daughters' caregiving careers. *Gerontologist, 40,* 437–448.

Lee, S., Colditz, G., Berkman, L., & Kawachi, I. (2003). Caregiving and risk of coronary heart disease in U.S. women: A prospective study. *American Journal of Preventive Medicine, 24*(2), 113–119.

Levine, C., Gibson Hunt, G., Halper, D., Hart, A. Y., Lautz, J., & Gould, D. A. (2005). Young adult caregivers: A first look at an unstudied population. *American Journal of Public Health, 95*(11), 2071–2075.

Marks, N. E., Lambert, J. D., & Choi, H. (2002). Transitions to caregiving, gender and psychological: A prospective U.S. national study. *Journal of Marriage and Family, 64,* 657–667.

Martire, L. M. & Schulz, R. (2007). Involving family in psychosocial interventions for chronic illness. *Current Directions in Psychological Science, 16*(2), 90–94.

Martire, L. M., Lustig, A. P., Schulz, R., Miller, G. E., & Helgeson, V. S. (2004). Is it beneficial to involve a family member? A meta-analytic review of psychosocial interventions for chronic illness. *Health Psychology, 23*(6), 599–611.

Martire, L. M., Schulz, R., Helgeson, V. S., Small, B. J., & Saghafi, E. (2010). Review and meta-analysis of couple-oriented interventions for chronic illness. *Annals of Behavioral Medicine, 40*, 325–342.

Midlarsky, E. (1991). Helping as coping. In M. S. Clark (Ed.), *Prosocial behavior* (pp. 238–264). Thousand Oaks, CA: Sage.

Monin, J. K., & Schulz, R. (2009). Interpersonal effects of suffering in older adult caregiving relationships. *Psychology and Aging, 24*(3), 681–695.

Motenko, A. K. (1989). The frustrations, gratifications, and well-being of dementia caregivers. *Gerontologist, 29*, 166–172.

Musik, M., Herzog, A. R., & House, J. S. (1999). Volunteering and mortality among older adults: Findings from a national sample. *Journal of Gerontology: Social Sciences, 54B*, S137-S180.

National Alliance for Caregiving (NAC) & American Association of Retired Persons (AARP). (2004). *Caregiving in the U.S.* Washington, DC: National Alliance for Caregiving.

National Alliance for Caregiving (NAC) & American Association of Retired Persons (AARP). (2009). *Caregiving in the U.S.* Washington, DC: National Alliance for Caregiving.

National Family Caregivers Association (NFCA) & Family Caregiver Alliance (FCA). (2006). *Prevalence, hours and economic value of family caregiving, updated state-by-state analysis of 2004 national estimates.* Kensington, MD: NFCA and San Francisco, CA: FCA.

Nichols, L. O., Martindale-Adams, J., Burns, R., Graney, M. J., & Zuber, J. (2011). Translation of a dementia caregiver support program in a health care system—REACH VA. *Archives of Internal Medicine, 171*(4), 353–359.

Nieboer, A. P., Schulz, R., Matthews, K. A., Scheier, M. F., Ormel, J., & Lindenberg, S. M. (1998). Spousal caregivers' activity restriction and depression: A model for changes over time. *Social Science and Medicine, 47*(9), 1361–1371.

O'Reilly, D., Connolly, S., Rosato, M., & Patterson, C. (2008). Is caring associated with an increased risk of mortality? A longitudinal study. *Social Science and Medicine, 67*, 1282–1290.

Okamoto, K., & Tanaka, Y. (2004). Subjective usefulness and 6-year mortality risks among elderly persons in Japan. *Journal of Gerontology: Social Sciences, 59B*(5), 246–249.

Oman, D., Thoresen, C., & McMahon, K. (1999). Volunteerism and mortality among the community dwelling elderly. *Journal of Health Psychology, 4*, 301–316.

Ory, M. G., Yee, J. L., Tennstedt, S. L., & Schulz, R. (2000). The extent and impact of dementia care: Unique challenges experienced by family caregivers. In R. Schulz (Ed.), *Handbook of dementia caregiving: Evidence-based interventions for family caregivers* (pp. 1–32). New York: Springer.

Pinquart, M., & Sörensen, S. (2007). Correlates of physical health of informal caregivers: A meta-analysis. *Journals of Gerontology Series B, Psychological Science Social Science, 62*(2), P126–137.

Pinquart, M., & Sörensen, S. (2003a). Associations of stressors and uplifts of caregiving with caregiver burden and depressive mood: A meta-analysis. *Journals of Gerontology Series B, Psychological Science Social Science, 58*, P112–128.

Pinquart, M., & Sörensen, S. (2003b). Differences between caregivers and noncaregivers in psychological health and physical health: a meta-analysis. *Psychology and Aging, 18*(2), 250–267.

Pruchno, R. A., Michaels, J. E., & Potashnik, S. L. (1990). Predictors of institutionalization among Alzheimer's disease victims with caregiving spouses. *Journal of Gerontology: Social Sciences, 45*, 259–266.

Roth, D., Perkins, M., Wadley, V., Temple, E., & Haley, W. (2009). Family caregiving and emotional strain: Associations with quality of life in a large national sample of middle-aged and older adults. *Quality of Life Research, 18*(6), 679–688.

Schulz, R., & Beach, S. R. (1999). Caregiving as a risk factor for mortality: The Caregiver Health Effects Study. *Journal of the American Medical Association, 282*(23), 2215–2219.

Schulz, R., Beach S. R., Hebert, R., Martire, L. M., Monin, J. K, Tompkins, C. A., & Albert, S. M. (2009). Spousal suffering and partner's depression and cardiovascular disease: The Cardiovascular Health Study. *American Journal of Geriatric Psychiatry, 17*(3), 246–254.

Schulz, R., Belle, S. H., Czaja, S. J., McGinnis, K. A., Stevens, A., & Zhang, S. (2004). Long-term care placement of dementia patients and caregiver health and well-being. *Journal of the American Medical Association, 292*, 961–967.

Schulz, R., Czaja, S. J., Lustig, A., Zdaniuk, B., Martire, L. M., & Perdomo, D. (2009). Improving the quality of life of caregivers of persons with spinal cord injury: A randomized controlled trial. *Rehabilitation Psychology, 54*(1), 1–15.

Schulz, R., Hebert, R. S., Dew, M. A., Brown, S. L., Scheier, M. F., Beach, S. R., … Nichols, L. (2007). Patient suffering and caregiver compassion: New opportunities for research, practice, and policy. *Gerontologist, 47*(1), 4–13.

Schulz, R., Martire, L. M., & Klinger, J. (2005). Evidence-based caregiver interventions in geriatric psychiatry. *Psychiatry Clinics of North America*, 28(4), 1007–1038.

Schulz, R., McGinnis, K. A., Zhang, S., Martire, L. M., Hebert, R. S., Beach, S. R.,... Belle, S. H. (2008). Dementia patient suffering and caregiver depression. *Alzheimer Disease and Associated Disorders*, 22(2), 170–176.

Schulz, R., Mendelsohn, A. B., Haley, W. E., Mahoney, D., Allen, R. S., Zhang, S.,... Belle, S. H. (2003). End of life care and the effects of bereavement on family caregivers of persons with dementia. *New England Journal of Medicine*, 349(20), 1936–1942.

Schulz, R., Newsom, J., Mittelmark, M., Burton, L. Hirsch, C., & Jackson, S. (1997). Health effects of caregiving: The Caregiver Health Effects Study: An ancillary study of the Cardiovascular Health Study. *Annals of Behavioral Medicine*, 19(2), 110–116.

Schulz, R., O'Brien, A. T., Bookwala, J., & Fleissner, K. (1995). Psychiatric and physical morbidity effects of dementia caregiving: Prevalence, correlates, and causes. *Gerontologist*, 35(6), 771–791.

Schulz, R., Visintainer, P., & Williamson, G. M. (1990). Psychiatric and physical morbidity effects of caregiving. *Journal of Gerontology*, 45(5), P181–191.

Schwartz, C., & Sendor, M. (2000). Helping others helps oneself: Response shift effects in peer support. In K. Schmaling (Ed.), *Adaptation to changing health: Response shift in quality-of-life research* (pp. 43–70). Washington, DC: American Psychological Association.

Seltzer, M. M, & Li, W. (2000). The dynamics of caregiving: Transitions during a three-year prospective study. *Gerontologist*, 40(2), 165–178.

Shaw, W. S., Patterson, T. L., Semple, S. J., Ho, S., Irwin, M. R., Hauger, R. L., & Grant, I. (1997). Longitudinal analysis of multiple indicators of health decline among spousal caregivers. *Annals of Behavioral Medicine*, 19, 101–109.

Singer, T., Seymour, B., O'Doherty, J., Kaube, H., Dolan, R. J., & Frith, C. D. (2004). Empathy for pain involves the affective but not sensory components of pain. *Science*, 303, 1157–1161.

Sörensen, S., Duberstein, P., Gill, D., & Pinquart, M. (2006). Dementia care: Mental health effects, intervention strategies, and clinical implications. *Lancet Neurology*, 5(11), 961–973.

Spanier, G. B. (1976). Measuring dyadic adjustment: New scales for assessing the quality of marriage and similar dyads. *Journal of Marriage and the Family*, 38, 15–28.

Stoops, N. (2004). *Current population reports. Educational attainment in the United States: 2003.* Washington, DC: US Department of Commerce, Economics and Statistics Administration, US Census Bureau. http://www.census.gov/prod/2004pubs/p20-550.pdf

Talley, R. C., & Crews, J. E. (2007). Framing the public health of caregiving. *American Journal of Public Health*, 97(2), 224–228.

Tarlow, B. J., Wisniewski, S., Belle, S., Rubert, M., Ory, M. G., & Gallagher-Thompson, D. (2004). Positive aspects of caregiving: Contributions of the REACH project to the development of new measures for Alzheimer's caregiving. *Research on Aging*, 26(4), 429–453.

Taylor, R., Ford, G., & Dunbar, M. (1995). The effects of caring on health: A community-based longitudinal study. *Social Science and Medicine*, 40(10), 1407–1415.

Teri, L., Logsdon, R. G., Uomoto, J., & McCurry, S. M. (1997). Behavioral treatment of depression in dementia patients: A controlled clinical trial. *Journals of Gerontology Series B, Psychological Science Social Sciene*, 52(4), P159–166.

Tower, R. B., & Kasl, S. V. (1995). Depressive symptoms across older spouses and the moderating effect of marital closeness. *Psychology and Aging*, 10(4), 625–638.

Tower, R. B., & Kasl, S. V. (1996). Depressive symptoms across older spouses: Longitudinal influences. *Psychology and Aging*, 11(4), 683–697.

Trivers, R. L. (1971). The evolution of reciprocal altruism. *Quarterly Review of Biology*, 46, 35–57.

Vitaliano, P., Zhang, J., & Scanlan, J. M. (2003). Is caregiving hazardous to one's physical health? A meta-analysis. *Psychological Bulletin*, 129(6), 946–972.

Wolff, J. L., & Kasper, J. D. (2006). Caregivers of frail elders: Updating a national profile. *Gerontologist*, 46(3), 344–356.

Wolff, J. L., Dy, S. M., Frick, K. D., & Kasper, J. D. (2007). End-of-life care: Findings from a national survey of informal caregivers. *Archives of Internal Medicine*, 167, 40–46.

15

POST-STROKE DEPRESSION AND VASCULAR DEPRESSION

Sarah Volk and David C. Steffens

THE RELATIONSHIP between cerebrovascular disease and depression is complex. Both acute stroke and silent cerebrovascular disease have been associated with depression. The corresponding diagnostic entities—post-stroke depression and vascular depression—have been linked to cognitive impairment, disability, and mortality. Though the underlying mechanisms are not fully understood and may be similar, the literature to date supports two distinct constructs based on differences in clinical features, risk factors, prognosis, and treatment.

POST-STROKE DEPRESSION

Definition and Clinical Features

There is no single accepted definition for post-stroke depression (PSD). The *Diagnostic and Statistical Manual of Mental Disorders*, fourth edition, text revision (*DSM-IV-TR*) lists stroke among the general medical conditions that cause depression as a "direct physiological consequence." PSD is therefore considered "mood disorder due to stroke, with depressive features" or "with major depressive-like episode" (*DSM-IV-TR*, American Psychiatric Association, 2000). Though there is some evidence supporting a pathophysiological relationship between stroke and depression, some authors have argued for a definition that does not imply a purely biological mechanism. Whyte and Mulsant defined PSD as "depression occurring in the context of a clinically apparent stroke (as opposed to silent vascular disease)" (2002, p. 254). This definition allows for psychosocial as well as biological factors, and it relies on a temporal rather than an etiopathophysiologic relationship between stroke and depression (Newberg, Davydow, & Lee, 2006).

For research purposes, a variety of diagnostic criteria have been used to identify PSD. For major depression, most have used diagnostic criteria for a major depressive episode based on either *DSM* or research diagnostic criteria (Spitzer et al., 1975). However, many studies have also included patients with less severe depression. Some used the *DSM* criteria for dysthymia, with the time requirement shortened from 2 years to 2 weeks (Whyte & Mulsant, 2002). Others have used *DSM-IV* research criteria for minor depression (Robinson & Spalletta, 2010), which differs from *DSM* criteria for major depression only in the number of symptoms (two to four rather than five or more). Of note, the *DSM-IV* diagnosis "mood disorder due to stroke, with depressive features" does not specify any criteria aside from depressed mood (*DSM-IV-TR*).

There has also been debate about how to apply diagnostic criteria to stroke patients. Some authors have expressed concern about the reliability of assessing depressive symptoms in stroke patients because of neurologic sequelae that could mimic or mask depressive symptoms, for example, aphasia, anosognosia, cognitive deficits or complaints, somatic complaints, slowing of speech and motor activity, loss of motivation, and emotionalism (Aben, Verhey, Honig, Lodder, Lousberg, & Maes, 2001; Johnson, 1991; Spencer, Tompkins, & Schulz 1997). Although no study has found a reliable way of examining patients with fluent or global aphasia (Robinson, 2010), many studies have validated the reliability of applying standard *DSM* criteria as assessed in a structured interview (Fedoroff, Starkstein, et al., 1991; Paradiso, Ohkubo, & Robinson, 1997; Spalletta, Ripa, & Caltagirone, 2005).

Several studies have examined depression among stroke patients for clinical features that distinguish it from depression in other populations. Using the Present State Examination, Lipsey et al. compared depressive symptoms in patients with PSD and patients with endogenous or "functional" depression (no identified medical cause). In this study, only "slowness" was more frequent in PSD; lack of interest and concentration were less frequent (Lipsey, Spencer, Rabins, & Robinson, 1986). Another study found that patients with PSD had more "motivated" or reactive symptoms compared with patients with functional depression (Gainotti, Azzoni, & Marra, 1999). In comparing stroke patients to patients with other severe medical or neurologic conditions, Fedoroff, Lipsey, et al. (1991) found that depressed stroke patients had higher scores for generalized anxiety and ideas of reference compared to depressed patients with myocardial infarction or spinal cord injury. However, most authors have concluded that the symptom profiles are similar between PSD and endogenous depression (Newberg, Davydow, &

Lee, 2006; Provinciali & Coccia, 2002; Whyte & Mulsant, 2002).

Prevalence

Measurements of the prevalence of PSD vary based on the diagnostic criteria, assessment tools, study population, and evaluation time after stroke (Aben, 2001; Newberg, 2006). Based on pooled prevalence studies, Robinson and Spalletta concluded that the overall prevalence of major depression was 21.7% using *DSM-IV* diagnostic criteria for "mood disorder due to a general medical condition with major depressive-like episode." The overall prevalence of minor depression was 19.5% using *DSM-IV* research criteria for minor depression. These studies assessed depressive symptoms using a structured interview, so most excluded patients with fluent or global aphasias. Many also excluded patients with hemorrhagic or other atypical stroke, fatigue, decreased level of consciousness, or systemic illnesses (Robinson & Spaletta, 2010). The prevalence of PSD is higher among patients in acute and rehabilitation hospitals and outpatient settings compared to community settings. The prevalence of depression varies with time following the stroke, with the prevalence of major depression peaking 3–6 months post-stroke (Whyte & Mulsant, 2002). A 3-year longitudinal study of Swedish stroke survivors found that the prevalence of major depression was 25% during the acute stage, 31% at 3 months, 16% at 12 months, and 19% at 2 years (Aström, Adolfsson, & Asplund, 1993).

Risk Factors

In general, the risk factors for PSD are considered to be similar to those for endogenous depression. Studies have identified history of previous depression (Andersen, Vestergaard, Ingemann-Nielsen, & Lauritzen, 1995; Leentjens, Aben, Lodder, & Verhey, 2006; Paolucci et al., 2006), family history of depression (Leentjens et al., 2006), female gender (Andersen et al., 1995; Leentjens et al., 2006; Paolucci et al., 2006), somatic comorbidity (Leentjens et al., 2006), living alone (Andersen et al., 1995) or being divorced (Burvill et al., 1997), pre-stroke social distress (Andersen et al., 1995) or major life event (Bush, 1999), pre-stroke alcohol intake (Burvill, Johnson, Jamrozik, Anderson, & Stewart-Wynne, 1997), and disability (Burvill et al., 1997; Paolucci et al., 2006). However, Aström et al. found that risk factors for major depression change over time. Acutely, the most important predictors were left anterior brain lesion (see next section for further discussion of lesion location), dysphasia, and living alone. At 3 months, dependence in one's activities of daily living was most important. After 12 months, few social contacts outside the family became most important, and cerebral atrophy contributed after 3 years. Apart from stroke, cerebrovascular risk factors have not been consistently correlated with risk for PSD (Chatterjee, Fall, & Barer, 2010; Leentjens et al., 2006; Mast et al., 2004).

Mechanism

The primary cause of PSD has been a source of debate, particularly regarding the relative contributions of biological versus psychosocial factors (Whyte & Mulsant, 2002). Whyte and Mulsant thoroughly discussed the key elements of this debate in their 2002 review. Evidence for a biological mechanism included the occurrence of depression in patients with anosognosia (Starkstein, Berthier, Fedoroff, Price, & Robinson, 1990; Starkstein, Fedoroff, Price, Leiguarda, & Robinson 1992). The increased frequency of depression in stroke compared to other disabling medical illnesses (Folstein, Maiberger, McHugh, 1977), association of specific lesion locations with occurrence of depression, and better response to noradrenergic than serotonergic antidepressants were also cited as evidence for a biological mechanism, though it was acknowledged that these latter findings have not been consistent across studies. They noted that the temporal relationship between stroke and depression has been used to argue both for and against a biological mechanism, since a similar temporal relationship exists with psychological stressors and depression. The similar symptom profile between functional and PSD has been considered evidence against a biological mechanism (Gainotti et al., 1999; House, 1996).

Though extensively studied, the relationship between lesion location and depression risk has remained controversial. Locations that have been linked to increased risk include left anterior (Morris, Robinson, Raphael, & Hopwood, 1996; Robinson, Kubos, Starr, Rao, & Price, 1984; Starkstein, Robinson, & Price, 1987; Starkstein et al., 1991) and left basal ganglia lesions (Morris et al., 1996; Starkstein et al., 1991). Furthermore, studies have found correlation between the severity of depressive

symptoms and the distance of the lesion from the frontal pole in patients with left hemisphere stroke (Narushima, Kosier, & Robinson, 2003; Starkstein et al., 1987). However, these findings have not been consistently replicated (Agrell & Dehlin, 1994; Bozikas et al., 2005; Carson et al., 2000; Gainotti et al., 1997; Schwartz et al., 1993; Singh, Hermann, & Black, 1998). Some have observed that lesion location is more relevant in early depression (Aström et al., 1993; Narushima et al., 2003; Shimoda & Robinson, 1999).

On a neurochemical level, the two main proposed mechanisms have been the biogenic amine hypothesis and the proinflammatory cytokine hypothesis (Spalletta et al., 2006). In the biogenic amine model, Robinson and Bloom postulated that ischemic lesions may interrupt the biogenic amine-containing axons ascending from the brainstem to the cerebral cortex, leading to a decreased production of serotonin (5HT) and norepinephrine (NE) in limbic structures (Robinson & Bloom, 1977). The finding of reduced 5-hydroxyindoleacetic acid (5-HIAA) in the cerebrospinal fluid of patients with PSD supported this hypothesis (Bryer et al., 1992). In the proinflammatory cytokine model, cerebral ischemia causes proinflammatory cytokines (IL-1β, IL-6, IL-18, and TNF-α 20–22) to activate indolamine 2,3-dioxygenase, which metabolizes tryptophan to kynurenin and results in depletion of serotonin (Spalletta et al., 2006). Aside from these two mechanisms, PSD has also been associated with specific serotonin transporter polymorphisms (5-HTTLPR and STin2 VNTR) (Kohen et al., 2008).

See Figure 15.1 for a model of the mechanism of PSD.

Prognosis and Course

PSD has been associated with poorer outcomes for survival, functional status, and cognition. Several studies have found increased all-cause mortality rates among patients with PSD (Ellis, Zhao, & Egede, 2010; Jorge, Robinson, Arndt, & Starkstein, 2003; Morris, Robinson, Andrzejewski, Samuels, & Price, 1993; Ried et al., 2011; Williams, Ghose, & Swindle, 2004). Morris et al. found that patients with major or minor depression were 3.4 times more likely to die during a 10-year follow-up period, independent of age, sex, social class, type of stroke, lesion location, and level of social functioning (Morris et al., 1993).

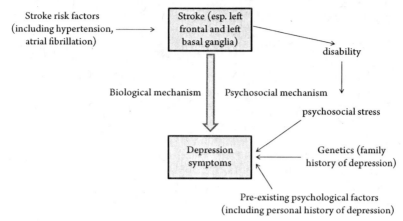

FIGURE 15.1 Model of post-stroke depression.

Studies have consistently shown that PSD is correlated with poorer functional status after stroke (Chemerinski, Robinson, & Arndt, 2001; Donnellan, Hickey, Hevey, & O'Neill, 2010; Herrmann, Black, Lawrence, Szekely, & Szalai, 1998; Morris, Raphael, & Robinson, 1992; Parikh et al., 1990). In a prospective study of the impact of depression on activities of daily living (ADLs), during the acute post-stroke hospitalization, depressed and nondepressed patients had similar impairment in ADLs, neurologic findings, lesion location and volume, demographic variables, cognitive impairment, and social functioning. However, 2 years after the stroke, the patients with in-hospital diagnosis of major or minor depression had significantly more impairment in physical activities and language functioning compared to nondepressed patients (Parikh et al., 1990). This study found that patients with major depression had significantly more impairment even after remission of depression; however, other evidence suggests that patients who achieve remission show greater improvement in ADLs (Chemerinski et al., 2001). Although most authors have concluded that depression impairs recovery of ADLs following a stroke (Hadidi, Treat-Jacobson, & Lindquist, 2009), disability is also a strong risk factor for depression (Burvill et al., 1997; Whyte & Mulsant, 2002).

PSD is also correlated with increased cognitive impairment (Downhill & Robinson, 1994; Morris et al., 1992; Robinson, Bolla-Wilson, Kaplan, Lipsey, & Price, 1986; Starkstein, Robinson, & Price, 1988), with some studies suggesting greater association between depression and cognitive impairment in left hemispheric stroke (Downhill & Robinson,

1994; Spalletta et al., 2002). Though it has been suggested that cognitive impairment worsens the course of depression (Downhill & Robinson, 1994), cognitive impairment is not generally considered a risk factor for PSD (Burvill et al., 1997; Murata, Kimura, & Robinson, 2000; Whyte & Mulsant, 2002).

Evidence suggests that the natural course of the depression is related to the time of onset. A 3-year longitudinal study found that patients who developed depressive symptoms within a few weeks of a stroke were more likely to have spontaneous remission in the first year (Aström et al., 1993). Andersen et al. observed a 50% remission rate within 1 month of placebo treatment among patients who developed depression in the first 6 weeks post-stroke. The same study found that patients with later onset of symptoms (7 weeks or more after the stroke) had a more persisting course (Andersen et al., 1994).

Treatment

Most studies have found that antidepressants are effective in treating PSD, with about 60% of patients responding to antidepressant treatment. One randomized, placebo-controlled trial found significant improvement with nortriptyline (Lipsey, Robinson, Pearlson, Rao, & Price, 1984), and a second randomized controlled trial found an intention-to-treat response rate of 63% (10 of 16) for nortriptyline, 9% (2 of 23) for fluoxetine, and 24% (4 of 17) for placebo (Robinson et al., 2000). In the second study, although neither group showed a significant difference in the Mini-Mental State Examination, the nortriptyline group had greater improvement in Functional Independence Measure scores at 9 and

12 weeks. Based on these two studies, Robinson and Spalleta (2010) consider nortriptyline the treatment of choice for PSD in the absence of any contraindications.

However, other authors have cautioned against concluding that tricyclic antidepressants are more effective than selective serotonin reuptake inhibitors (SSRIs). Whyte and Mulsant noted that the apparent superiority of nortriptyline over fluoxetine in the latter study may have been an artifact of the study design, in which some patients received placebo before crossing over to active treatment. The fluoxetine group had significantly more patients who did not respond to placebo during the initial phase, suggesting that their depression may have been more difficult to treat (Whyte & Mulsant, 2002). Other studies have found that SSRIs result in response rates that are similar to response rates with nortriptyline. These studies have included a randomized placebo-controlled trial of fluoxetine 20 mg/day (Wiart, Petit, Joseph, Mazaux, & Barat, 2000); a randomized placebo-controlled trial of citalopram 10–40 mg/day (Andersen et al., 1994); and an open-label study of sertraline 50–100 mg/day (Spalletta & Caltagirone, 2003).

Although they have not been studied in a randomized controlled trial, stimulants have been reported to be effective in two retrospective chart reviews (Johnson, Roberts, Ross, & Witten, 1992; Masand, Murray, & Pickett, 1991) and one open-label trial (Lazarus et al., 1992). Electroconvulsive therapy has also been reported to be helpful in two retrospective chart reviews (Currier, Murray, & Welch, 1992; Murray, Shea, & Conn, 1986), and in a preliminary study, repetitive transcranial magnetic stimulation (rTMS) resulted in significant reduction in depressive symptoms compared with sham treatments (Jorge et al., 2004). In a randomized controlled trial of cognitive-behavioral therapy (CBT) versus attention placebo intervention or standard care, patients with PSD who received CBT showed no significant differences in mood, independence in instrumental ADLs, or disability (Lincoln & Flannaghan, 2003).

Prevention

Prevention studies have yielded mixed results. Although individual studies have found significant benefit, a systematic review that included results from 10 trials found no clear effect of antidepressant medications on prevention of depression. The same systematic review did find a small but significant benefit for psychotherapy (Hackett, Anderson, House, & Halteh, 2008). Since that review, another study compared double-blind treatment with escitalopram or placebo with nonblinded problem-solving therapy group. Using intention-to-treat analysis and adjusting for confounders, only escitalopram was significantly better than placebo (Robinson et al., 2008). Another recent study by Ried et al. found that SSRI treatment before and after stroke was associated with reduced mortality compared with SSRI treatment only before the stroke. These authors recommended initiating or resuming SSRI treatment in patients with a history of depression or who were taking an SSRI before their stroke (Ried et al., 2011). Other evidence has suggested that antidepressant treatment is associated with decreased mortality poststroke, regardless of depression status (Jorge et al., 2003).

VASCULAR DEPRESSION

Definition and Clinical Features

In contrast to PSD, vascular depression occurs in the context of vascular disease without clinically apparent stroke. Also, while the *DSM* classifies PSD as a mood disorder due to a general medical condition, vascular depression has been considered a subtype of major depressive disorder (Hickie et al., 1995; Steffens & Krishnan, 1998).

Several different definitions for vascular depression have been proposed. In 1997, Alexopoulos proposed clinical and/or cerebrovascular disease and depression onset after age 65 as cardinal features, with secondary features of cognitive impairment, psychomotor retardation, limited depressive ideation, poor insight, disability, and absent family history of mood disorders (Alexopoulos et al., 1997a). Steffens and Krishnan proposed a similar definition but classified neuropsychological impairment as a cardinal feature, along with clinical and/or neuroimaging evidence of cerebrovascular disease. Secondary features included age of onset >50, marked loss of interest or pleasure, psychomotor retardation, lack of family history of mood disorder, and disability as supporting features (Steffens & Krishnan, 1998).

From these definitions, two overlapping constructs emerged (Sneed, 2011). The so-called depression-executive dysfunction (DED) syndrome focused on the frontostriatal dysfunction that contributes to the development of both depression and executive dysfunction, and did not specifically require evidence of cerebrovascular disease. In one effort to further characterize the syndrome, Alexopoulos et al. included patients who were at least 60 years old, met research diagnostic criteria and *DSM-IV* criteria for unipolar major depressive disorder and had an HAM-D $\geq$ 18. Executive dysfunction was defined as a Mattis Dementia Rating Scale Initiation-Perseveration score that was one standard deviation below the mean. They found that patients who met criteria for the DED syndrome had impaired verbal fluency and visual naming, paranoia, loss of interest in activities, and psychomotor retardation (Alexopoulos et al., 2002).

Krishnan et al. coined the term "subcortical ischemic depression" for the second construct (Krishnan et al., 2004), which required only magnetic resonance imaging (MRI) evidence of cerebrovascular disease. In a study of the associated clinical features, Krishnan et al. defined MRI evidence of subcortical ischemic depression as a Coffey classification score of at least 2 for deep white matter hyperintense lesions (beginning confluence of foci) or 3 for subcortical gray matter hyperintensities (diffuse). In this elderly depressed population, 54% of patients met criteria for subcortical ischemic depression based on the Coffey classification. Compared with patients without subcortical ischemic depression, these patients were more likely to be older and to report lassitude and history of hypertension. They were less likely to report family history of mental illness and loss of libido. There was no significant difference in age of depression onset, psychomotor agitation, or instrumental ADL impairment.

Though criteria for vascular depression have varied across studies, MRI hyperintensities, executive dysfunction, and late age at onset have all been considered markers of vascular depression. Sneed et al. applied latent class analysis to two large clinical samples to determine which features most accurately identify the illness, with proposed features, including deep white matter hyperintensity burden, late-onset depression, response inhibition component of executive functions, and subcortical hyperintensity burden (Sneed, Rindskopf, Steffens, Krishnan, & Roose, 2008). Of these, deep white matter lesion burden detected vascular depression

with the greatest sensitivity and specificity (1.00 and 0.95, respectively), though all were found to be useful indicators. This study not only provided support for specific diagnostic criteria but also was considered evidence for internal validity of the vascular depression subtype of major depressive disorder.

Despite clear evidence for the validity of MRI-defined vascular depression, a consistent method of measuring the lesions has not been firmly established. In both clinical samples used in the Sneed study, deep white matter hyperintensity burden was measured using the Coffey modified Fazekas Rating Scale and scored as 0 (absent), 1 (punctate foci), 2 (beginning confluence of foci), and 3 (large confluent areas). The Scheltens rating is another visual measure of the severity of MRI hyperintensities that includes measurement of size. Although automated methods may be faster and better able to quantify the lesion volume, there is concern for radiological artifacts. Consistent criteria should also be applied to classification of deep white, periventricular, and subcortical gray matter lesions (Culang-Reinleib et al., 2010), as well as to the evaluation of associated neuropsychological features.

Mechanism

Both clinical and epidemiological studies provide considerable evidence linking late-life depression and cerebrovascular disease. Early MRI studies found that patients with late-onset depression had more subcortical hyperintensities compared with patients with early onset (Hickie et al., 1995; Krishnan, Hays, & Blazer, 1997; O'Brien et al., 1996; Salloway et al., 1996). In a systematic review of 30 studies, Herrmann et al. found that the odds of white matter hyperintensities were 4.33 times greater in patients with late-onset depression compared to patients with early-onset depression (Herrmann et al., 2008). Moreover, subcortical hyperintensities have been found more commonly in elderly depressed subjects compared with elderly controls (Coffey et al., 1993; Greenwald et al., 1996; Krishnan et al., 1993). In the Cardiovascular Health Study, a study of 3,236 participants 65 years and older, depressive symptoms were associated with lesions in both the white and subcortical gray matter on MRI (Steffens, Helms, Krishnan, & Burke, 1999).

Most early studies did not differentiate between the effects of deep white matter hyperintensities and periventricular hyperintensities, but more recent evidence has suggested a stronger association between depression and deep white matter hyperintensities compared to periventricular hyperintensities (Krishnan et al., 2006; Nebes et al., 2001). However, this pattern has not been consistent across all studies (Iidaka et al., 1996). In a large population-based study, patients in the upper quintile of white matter lesion severity were 3 to 5 times more likely to have depressive symptoms compared to those in the lowest quintile (de Groot et al., 2000), with a periventricular odds ratio of 3.3 (95% CI 1.2–9.5) and subcortical odds ratio of 5.4 (95% CI 1.8–16.5).

In the brain, frontal-subcortical circuits connect the prefrontal cortex to the caudate, globus pallidus, dorsomedial thalamus, and back to the prefrontal cortex (Alexander, DeLong, & Strick, 1986). The deep white matter hyperintensities characteristic of vascular depression appear to predominantly affect these anterior circuits, particularly those originating in the dorsolateral prefrontal cortex, the anterior cingulate, and the orbitofrontal prefrontal cortex (Alexopoulos et al., 1997). In one study, elderly depressed subjects had significantly greater total frontal white matter lesion volume compared to elderly controls (Firbank, Lloyd, Ferrier, & O'Brien, 2004). In another study, hyperintensities in different brain regions were rated according to the Scheltens rating scale in elderly subjects with and without depression. Using logistic regression analysis, the authors found that left frontal hyperintensity rating was the best predictor of depressive group assignment ($p < .005$, Greenwald et al., 1998). Another MRI study found that in patients with late-life depression, there was a significant association between age and deep white matter hyperintensities in bilateral frontal and left parietal regions; in control subjects, the association was significant for bilateral parieto-temporal, but not frontal, regions (Taylor, MacFall, et al., 2003). MacFall et al. compared MRI images from 88 elderly depressed subjects with those of 47 elderly controls and found two major regions of increased lesion density in the medial orbital prefrontal white matter. Severity of depression was correlated with lesions in the medial orbital region (MacFall, Payne, Provenzale, & Krishnan, 2001).

Other studies have shown that these white matter hyperintensities are associated with decreased cortical and subcortical gray nuclei volume in other parts of the circuit. For example, in one MRI study comparing depressed and nondepressed elderly subjects, the depressed subjects had smaller orbitofrontal cortex volumes, and white matter lesion volume was significantly negatively associated with orbitofrontal cortex volume (Taylor, MacFall, et al., 2007). In another study, white matter lesion volume was negatively associated with right caudate volume in patients with late-life depression, and the association was stronger for white matter lesions in the anterior half of the brain (Hannestad et al., 2006). In imaging studies, gray matter volume reductions have been shown to affect the caudate (Beyer & Krishnan 2002; Hannestad et al., 2006; Krishnan et al., 1993), the anterior cingulate (Ballmaier et al., 2004), the gyrus rectus (Ballmaier et al., 2004), the orbitofrontal cortex (Ballmaier et al., 2004; Lai, Payne, Byrum, Steffens, & Krishnan, 2000; Taylor et al., 2003), dorsolateral prefrontal cortex (Chang et al., 2011), and the hippocampus (Steffens, Payne, et al., 2002). Some postmortem studies of cellular pathology have found decreased neuronal density in the dorsolateral prefrontal cortex (Khundakar, Morris, Oakley, McMeekin, & Thomas, 2009), orbitofrontal cortex (Rajkowska et al., 2005), and caudate nucleus (Khundakar, Morris, Oakley, & Thomas, 2011), but these results have not been consistent across all studies (Khundakar et al., 2011; Van Otterloo et al., 2009).

Diffusion tensor imaging studies can assess fractional anisotropy, a measure of white matter integrity. One of these studies measured white matter fractional anisotropy in the superior and middle frontal gyri of the bilateral dorsolateral prefrontal cortex of elderly subjects with and without depression. Microstructural changes in the white matter of the right superior frontal gyrus were associated with late-life depression (Taylor et al., 2004). In another study, Bae et al. measured fractional anisotropy of the white matter of the dorsolateral prefrontal cortex, anterior cingulate cortex, corpus callosum, and internal capsule. Compared with elderly subjects without depression, elderly depressed subjects had significantly lower fractional anisotropy values in white matter of the right anterior cingulate cortex, bilateral superior frontal gyri, and left middle frontal gyrus (Bae et al., 2006). Nobuhara et al. also used diffusion tensor imaging to compare patients with late-life depression and elderly controls. They found a significant reduction in white matter fractional anisotropy values in widespread regions of the frontal and temporal lobes. They also found that white matter fractional anisotropy values of the inferior frontal brain appeared to be inversely related to the severity of depression (Nobuhara et al., 2006). These studies suggest that depression is associated not just with specific brain regions but also with impaired connectivity between those regions.

The abnormal frontal-subcortical circuitry is thought to account for not only the mood symptoms but also the executive dysfunction characteristic of vascular depression (Alexopoulos et al., 1997; Lesser et al., 1996; Salloway et al., 1996). Among elderly subjects with and without depression, the number of perseverative errors on the Benton Visual Retention Test was negatively associated with left orbitofrontal cortex volume for only the depressed sample (Steffens, McQuoid, Welsh-Bohmer, & Krishnan, 2003). In another study, elderly depressed patients were assessed with the Stroop Color-Word test as a measure of response inhibition, and diffusion tensor imaging was used to determine white matter integrity in frontostriatal-limbic regions. Executive dysfunction as measured with Stroop Color-Word Interference was significantly associated with reduced fractional anisotropy in the prefrontal, insular, and parahippocampal regions as well as in white matter lateral to the anterior and posterior cingulate cortex (Murphy et al., 2007).

Although the causes of hyperintense lesions are heterogeneous, there is evidence that ischemic cerebrovascular disease accounts for the majority of deep white matter hyperintensities in depressed elderly subjects. In a study comparing postmortem brain tissue from 20 elderly subjects with history of depression and 20 elderly controls, Thomas et al. found that all the deep white matter hyperintensities in the depressed group resulted from ischemia, compared with less than a third in the control group (Thomas et al., 2002). In another study, Thomas et al. used intercellular adhesion molecule-1 (ICAM-1) and vascular adhesion molecule-1 (VCAM-1) to detect microvascular disease and ischemia in tissue from the dorsolateral prefrontal cortex, anterior cingulate cortex, and occipital cortex (control area) of elderly depressed and control subjects. A significant increase in ICAM-1 in the deep white matter of the dorsolateral prefrontal cortex, along with a trend toward increase in VCAM-1, was considered further evidence for a cerebrovascular basis of late-life depression, with lesions to the dorsolateral prefrontal cortex specifically implicated (Thomas et al., 2003). Elevations in other inflammatory markers, including interleukin-1beta (Diniz, Teixeira, Talib, Gattaz, & Forlenza, 2010; Thomas et al., 2005), interleukin-6 (Bremmer et al., 2008), and interleukin-1alpha (Lee et al., 2009), have suggested involvement of cytokines in the mechanism of late-life depression.

The role for psychosocial factors in the development of vascular depression is unclear (Ramasubbu, 2000). Alexopoulos et al. proposed two broad mechanisms of vascular depression. The first was that lesions disrupting critical pathways could precipitate depression, and the second was that the accumulation of lesions exceeding a threshold could confer vulnerability to depression. The latter hypothesis allows for the possibility that the executive dysfunction associated with those lesions could also be a predisposing factor, and that the depressive episode could be triggered by a psychosocial stressor (Alexopoulos et al., 1997). Although evidence is limited in this area, Oldehinkel et al. conducted a case-control study to evaluate the association of psychosocial stressors and vascular risk factors with onset of depression. They found a significantly greater effect of vascular risk in depressive episodes that were not precipitated by a stressful life event, and they concluded that vascular risk factors represent an independent pathway to depression (Oldehinkel, Ormel, Brilman, & van den Berg, 2003). In contrast, Holley et al. found that the depressogenic effect of stress was stronger in the presence of significant vascular risk (Holley, Murrell, & Mast, 2006).

See Figure 15.2 for a model of the mechanism of vascular depression.

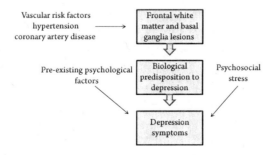

FIGURE 15.2 Model of vascular depression.

Prognosis and Treatment

Considerable evidence suggests a poor prognosis for patients with vascular depression. The presence of subcortical white and gray matter hyperintensities has been associated with nonresponse to antidepressant treatment and to ECT (Hickie et al., 1995; Simpson, Baldwin, Jackson, & Burns, 1998), though this finding has not been consistent across all studies (Krishnan et al., 1998; Salloway et al., 2002; Sneed et al., 2007). Diffusion tensor imaging studies have also found an association between antidepressant nonresponse and reduced fractional anisotropy in select frontal-subcortical and limbic regions (Alexopoulos et al., 2002, 2008). Longer term studies also suggest that white matter hyperintensities are associated with a more chronic course of depression (Hickie et al., 1997; O'Brien et al., 1998; Steffens, Krishnan, Crump, & Burke, 2002; Yanai, Fujikawa, Horiguchi, Yamawaki, & Touhouda, 1998). Not only the baseline white matter burden but also the change over time appears to affect treatment outcome. In a 2-year naturalistic study of elderly depressed subjects, Taylor et al. found that an increase in white matter hyperintensity volume over time was associated with failure to sustain remission (Taylor et al., 2003). Subcortical hyperintensities have also been associated with increased functional impairment (Krishnan et al., 1997; Steffens, Bosworth, Provenzale, & MacFall, 2002), mortality (Levy et al., 2003), and dementia (Hickie et al., 1997; O'Brien et al., 1998).

Executive dysfunction is also associated with nonresponse to antidepressant treatment (Alexopoulos et al., 2000, 2004, 2005; Dunkin et al., 2000; Kalayam & Alexopoulos 1999; McLennan & Mathias, 2010; Potter, Kittinger, Wagner, Steffens, & Krishnan, 2004; Sheline et al., 2010) and functional disability (Kiosses, Alexopoulos, & Murphy, 2000; Kiosses, Klimstra, Murphy, & Alexopoulos, 2001). In one study, executive dysfunction, but not memory impairment, disability, medical burden, social support, and history of previous episodes, was found to be significantly associated with recurrent and residual depressive symptoms (Alexopoulos et al., 2000). Specifically, impairment in response inhibition (Alexopoulos et al., 2005; Sneed et al., 2007, 2008) and initiation perseveration (Alexopoulos et al., 2005; Kalayam & Alexopoulos, 1999; Morimoto et al., 2011) tasks are associated with poor response to antidepressants. However, it is not clear that the executive dysfunction itself accounts for a more chronic course (Butters et al., 2004; Cui, Lyness, Tu, King, & Caine, 2007).

Randomized controlled trials of other therapies for vascular depression are scant, but a variety of modalities have shown benefit. Alexopoulos et al. found that in elderly patients with depression and executive dysfunction, problem-solving therapy was associated with greater remission of depression, fewer posttreatment depressive symptoms, and decreased disability (Alexopoulos, Raue, & Areán, 2003, Alexopoulos, Raue, et al., 2011). Another group found superior response and remission rates with rTMS compared to placebo in elderly patients with clinically defined vascular depression (Jorge et al., 2008, statistically significant only at higher rTMS dose). Two studies have found that augmentation with the calcium channel blocker nimodipine resulted in higher remission rates and lower recurrence rates compared to placebo augmentation (Taragano, Allegri, Vicario, Bagnatti, & Lyketsos, 2001; Taragano, Bagnatti, & Allegri, 2005).

Disclosures
Dr. Volk has no conflicts to disclose.
Dr. Steffens has no conflicts to disclose.

REFERENCES

Aben, I., Verhey, F., Honig, A., Lodder, J., Lousberg, R., & Maes, M. (2001). Research into the specificity of depression after stroke: a review on an unresolved issue. *Progress in Neuropsychopharmacology and Biological Psychiatry*, 25(4), 671–689.

Agrell, B., & Dehlin, O. (1994). Depression in stroke patients with left and right hemisphere lesions. A study in geriatric rehabilitation in-patients. *Aging (Milano)*, 6(1), 49–56.

Alexander, G. E., DeLong, M. R., & Strick, P. L. (1986). Parallel organization of functionally segregated circuits linking basal ganglia and cortex. *Annual Review of Neuroscience*, 9, 357–381.

Alexopoulos, G. S., Kiosses, D. N., Choi, S. J., Murphy, C. F., & Lim, K. O. (2002). Frontal white matter microstructure and treatment response of late-life depression: A preliminary study. *American Journal of Psychiatry*, 159(11), 1929–1932.

Alexopoulos, G. S., Kiosses, D. N., Heo, M., Murphy, C. F., Shanmugham, B., & Gunning-Dixon, F. (2005). Executive dysfunction and the course of geriatric depression. *Biological Psychiatry*, 58(3), 204–210.

Alexopoulos, G. S., Kiosses, D. N., Klimstra, S., Kalayam, B., & Bruce, M. L. (2002). Clinical presentation of the "depression-executive dysfunction syndrome" of late life. *American Journal of Geriatric Psychiatry, 10*(1), 98–106.

Alexopoulos, G. S., Kiosses, D. N., Murphy, C., Heo, M. (2004). Executive dysfunction, heart disease burden, and remission of geriatric depression. *Neuropsychopharmacology, 29*(12), 2278–2284.

Alexopoulos, G. S., Meyers, B. S., Young, R. C., Campbell, S., Silbersweig, D., & Charlson, M. (1997a). "Vascular depression" hypothesis. *Archives of General Psychiatry, 54*(10), 915–922.

Alexopoulos, G. S., Meyers, B. S., Young, R. C., Kakuma, T., Silbersweig, D., & Charlson, M. (1997b). Clinically defined vascular depression. *American Journal of Psychiatry, 154*(4), 562–565.

Alexopoulos, G. S., Meyers, B. S., Young, R. C., Kalayam, B., Kakuma, T., Gabrielle, M., ... Hull, J. (2000). Executive dysfunction and long-term outcomes of geriatric depression. *Archives of General Psychiatry, 57*(3), 285–290.

Alexopoulos, G. S., Murphy, C. F., Gunning-Dixon, F. M., Latoussakis, V., Kanellopoulos, D., Klimstra, S., ... Hoptman, M. J. (2008). Microstructural white matter abnormalities and remission of geriatric depression. *American Journal of Psychiatry, 165*(2), 238–244.

Alexopoulos, G. S., Raue, P., & Areán, P. (2003). Problem-solving therapy versus supportive therapy in geriatric major depression with executive dysfunction. *American Journal of Geriatric Psychiatry, 11*(1), 46–52.

Alexopoulos, G. S., Raue, P. J., Kiosses, D. N., Mackin, R. S., Kanellopoulos, D., McCulloch, C., & Areán, P. A. (2011). Problem-solving therapy and supportive therapy in older adults with major depression and executive dysfunction: Effect on disability. *Archives of General Psychiatry, 68*(1), 33–41.

American Psychiatric Association. (2000). *Diagnostic and statistical manual of mental disorders.* (4th ed., Text rev.). Washington, DC: Author.

Andersen, G., Vestergaard, K., Ingemann-Nielsen, M., & Lauritzen, L. (1995). Risk factors for post-stroke depression. *Acta Psychiatrica Scandinavica, 92*(3), 193–198.

Andersen, G., Vestergaard, K., & Lauritzen, L. (1994). Effective treatment of poststroke depression with the selective serotonin reuptake inhibitor citalopram. *Stroke, 25*(6), 1099–1104.

Aström, M., Adolfsson, R., & Asplund, K. (1993). Major depression in stroke patients. A 3-year longitudinal study. *Stroke, 24*(7), 976–982.

Bae, J. N., MacFall, J. R., Krishnan, K. R., Payne, M. E., Steffens, D. C., & Taylor, W. D. (2006). Dorsolateral prefrontal cortex and anterior cingulate cortex white matter alterations in late-life depression. *Biological Psychiatry, 60*(12), 1356–1363.

Ballmaier, M., Toga, A. W., Blanton, R. E., Sowell, E. R., Lavretsky, H., Peterson, J., ... Kumar, A. (2004). Anterior cingulate, gyrus rectus, and orbitofrontal abnormalities in elderly depressed patients: An MRI-based parcellation of the prefrontal cortex. *American Journal of Psychiatry, 161*(1), 99–108.

Beyer, J. L., & Krishnan, K. R. (2002). Volumetric brain imaging findings in mood disorders. *Bipolar Disorder, 4*(2), 89–104.

Bozikas, V. P., Gold, G., Kövari, E., Herrmann, F., Karavatos, A., Giannakopoulos, P., & Bouras, C. (2005). Pathological correlates of poststroke depression in elderly patients. *American Journal of Geriatric Psychiatry, 13*(2), 166–169.

Bremmer, M. A., Beekman, A. T., Deeg, D. J., Penninx, B. W., Dik, M. G., Hack, C. E., & Hoogendijk, W. J. (2008). Inflammatory markers in late-life depression: Results from a population-based study. *Journal of Affective Disorders, 106*(3), 249–255.

Bryer, J. B., Starkstein, S. E., Votypka, V., Parikh, R. M., Price, T. R., & Robinson, R. G. (1992). Reduction of CSF monoamine metabolites in poststroke depression: A preliminary report. *Journal of Neuropsychiatry and Clinical Neuroscience, 4*(4), 440–442.

Burvill, P., Johnson, G., Jamrozik, K., Anderson, C., & Stewart-Wynne, E. (1997). Risk factors for post-stroke depression. *International Journal of Geriatric Psychiatry, 12*(2), 219–226.

Bush, B. A. (1999). Major life events as risk factors for post-stroke depression. *Brain Injury, 13*(2), 131–137.

Butters, M. A., Bhalla, R. K., Mulsant, B. H., Mazumdar, S., Houck, P. R., Begley, A. E., ... Reynolds, C. F., 3rd. (2004). Executive functioning, illness course, and relapse/recurrence in continuation and maintenance treatment of late-life depression: Is there a relationship? *American Journal of Geriatric Psychiatry, 12*(4), 387–394.

Carson, A. J., MacHale, S., Allen, K., Lawrie, S. M., Dennis, M., House, A., & Sharpe, M. (2000). Depression after stroke and lesion location: a systematic review. *Lancet, 356*(9224), 122–126.

Chang, C. C., Yu, S. C., McQuoid, D. R., Messer, D. F., Taylor, W. D., Singh, K., ... Payne, M. E. (2011). Reduction of dorsolateral prefrontal cortex gray matter in late-life depression. *Psychiatry Research, 193*(1), 1–6.

Chatterjee, K., Fall, S., & Barer, D. (2010). Mood after stroke: A case control study of biochemical, neuro-imaging and socio-economic risk factors for major depression in stroke survivors. *BMC Neurology, 10,* 125.

Chemerinski, E., Robinson, R. G., Arndt, S., & Kosier, J. T. (2001). The effect of remission of poststroke depression on activities of daily living in a double-blind randomized treatment study. *Journal of Nervous and Mental Disorders, 189*(7), 421–425.

Coffey, C. E., Wilkinson, W. E., Weiner, R. D., Parashos, I. A., Djang, W. T., Webb, M. C.,... Spritzer, C. E. (1993). Quantitative cerebral anatomy in depression. A controlled magnetic resonance imaging study. *Archives of General Psychiatry, 50*(1), 7–16.

Cui, X., Lyness, J. M., Tu, X., King, D. A., & Caine, E. D. (2007). Does depression precede or follow executive dysfunction? Outcomes in older primary care patients. *American Journal of Psychiatry, 164*(8), 1221–1228.

Culang-Reinlieb, M. E., Johnert, L. C., Brickman, A. M., Steffens, D. C., Garcon, E., & Sneed, J. R. (2010, December 29). MRI-defined vascular depression: A review of the construct. *International Journal of Geriatric Psychiatry,* ePub ahead of print.

Currier, M. B., Murray, G. B., & Welch, C. C. (1992). Electroconvulsive therapy for post-stroke depressed geriatric patients. *Journal of Neuropsychiatry and Clinical Neuroscience, 4*(2), 140–144.

de Groot, J. C., de Leeuw, F. E., Oudkerk, M., Hofman, A., Jolles, J., & Breteler, M. M. (2000). Cerebral white matter lesions and depressive symptoms in elderly adults. *Archives of General Psychiatry, 57*(11), 1071–1076.

Diniz, B. S., Teixeira, A. L., Talib, L., Gattaz, W. F., & Forlenza, O. V. (2010). Interleukin-1beta serum levels is increased in antidepressant-free elderly depressed patients. *American Journal of Geriatric Psychiatry, 18*(2), 172–176.

Donnellan, C., Hickey, A., Hevey, D., & O'Neill, D. (2010). Effect of mood symptoms on recovery one year after stroke. *International Journal of Geriatric Psychiatry, 25*(12), 1288–1295.

Downhill, J. E., Jr., & Robinson, R. G. (1994). Longitudinal assessment of depression and cognitive impairment following stroke. *Journal of Nervous and Mental Disorders, 182*(8), 425–431.

Dunkin, J. J., Leuchter, A. F., Cook, I. A., Kasl-Godley, J. E., Abrams, M., & Rosenberg-Thompson, S. (2000). Executive dysfunction predicts nonresponse to fluoxetine in major depression. *Journal of Affective Disorders, 60*(1), 13–23.

Ellis, C., Zhao, Y., & Egede, L. E. (2010). Depression and increased risk of death in adults with stroke. *Journal Psychosomatic Research, 68*(6), 545–551.

Fedoroff, J. P., Lipsey, J. R., Starkstein, S. E., Forrester, A., Price, T. R., & Robinson, R. G. (1991). Phenomenological comparisons of major depression following stroke, myocardial infarction or spinal cord lesions. *Journal of Affective Disorders, 22*(1–2), 83–89.

Fedoroff, J. P., Starkstein, S. E., Parikh, R. M., Price, T. R., & Robinson, R. G. (1991). Are depressive symptoms nonspecific in patients with acute stroke? *American Journal of Psychiatry, 148*(9), 1172–1176.

Firbank, M. J., Lloyd, A. J., Ferrier, N., & O'Brien, J. T. (2004). A volumetric study of MRI signal hyperintensities in late-life depression. *American Journal of Geriatric Psychiatry, 12*(6), 606–612.

Folstein, M. F., Maiberger, R., & McHugh, P. R. (1977). Mood disorder as a specific complication of stroke. *Journal of Neurology, Neurosurgery, and Psychiatry, 40*(10):1018–1020.

Gainotti, G., Azzoni, A., Gasparini, F., Marra, C., & Razzano, C. (1997). Relation of lesion location to verbal and nonverbal mood measures in stroke patients. *Stroke, 28*(11), 2145–2149.

Gainotti, G., Azzoni, A., & Marra, C. (1999). Frequency, phenomenology and anatomical-clinical correlates of major post-stroke depression. *British Journal of Psychiatry, 175,* 163–167.

Greenwald, B. S., Kramer-Ginsberg, E., Krishnan, R. R., Ashtari, M., Aupperle, P. M., & Patel, M. (1996). MRI signal hyperintensities in geriatric depression. *American Journal of Psychiatry, 153*(9), 1212–1215.

Greenwald, B. S., Kramer-Ginsberg, E., Krishnan, K. R., Ashtari, M., Auerbach, C., & Patel, M. (1998). Neuroanatomic localization of magnetic resonance imaging signal hyperintensities in geriatric depression. *Stroke, 29*(3), 613–617.

Hackett, M. L., Anderson, C. S., House, A., & Halteh, C. (2008). Interventions for preventing depression after stroke. *Cochrane Database of Systematic Review,* (3), CD003689.

Hadidi, N., Treat-Jacobson, D. J., & Lindquist, R. (2009). Poststroke depression and functional outcome: A critical review of literature. *Heart Lung, 38*(2), 151–162.

Hannestad, J., Taylor, W. D., McQuoid, D. R., Payne, M. E., Krishnan, K. R., Steffens, D. C., & Macfall, J. R. (2006). White matter lesion volumes and caudate volumes in late-life depression. *International Journal of Geriatric Psychiatry, 21*(12), 1193–1198.

Herrmann, N., Black, S. E., Lawrence, J., Szekely, C., & Szalai, J. P. (1998). The Sunnybrook Stroke Study:

A prospective study of depressive symptoms and functional outcome. *Stroke, 29*(3), 618–624.

Herrmann, L. L., Le Masurier, M., & Ebmeier, K. P. (2008). White matter hyperintensities in late life depression: A systematic review. *Journal of Neurology, Neurosurgery, and Psychiatry, 79*(6), 619–624.

Hickie, I., Scott, E., Mitchell, P., Wilhelm, K., Austin, M. P., & Bennett, B. (1995). Subcortical hyperintensities on magnetic resonance imaging: Clinical correlates and prognostic significance in patients with severe depression. *Biological Psychiatry, 37*(3), 151–160.

Hickie, I., Scott, E., Wilhelm, K., & Brodaty, H. (1997). Subcortical hyperintensities on magnetic resonance imaging in patients with severe depression—a longitudinal evaluation. *Biological Psychiatry, 42*(5), 367–374.

Holley, C., Murrell, S. A., & Mast, B. T. (2006). Psychosocial and vascular risk factors for depression in the elderly. *American Journal of Geriatric Psychiatry, 14*(1), 84–90.

House, A. (1996). Depression associated with stroke. *Journal of Neuropsychiatry and Clinical Neuroscience, 8*(4), 453–457.

Iidaka, T., Nakajima, T., Kawamoto, K., Fukuda, H., Suzuki, Y., Maehara, T., & Shiraishi, H. (1996). Signal hyperintensities on brain magnetic resonance imaging in elderly depressed patients. *European Neurology, 36*(5), 293–299.

Johnson, G. A. (1991). Research into psychiatric disorder after stroke: the need for further studies. *Australia New Zealand Journal of Psychiatry, 25*(3), 358–370.

Johnson, M. L., Roberts, M. D., Ross, A. R., & Witten, C. M. (1992). Methylphenidate in stroke patients with depression. *American Journal of Physical Medicine and Rehabilitation, 71*(4), 239–241.

Jorge, R. E., Moser, D. J., Acion, L., & Robinson, R. G. (2008). Treatment of vascular depression using repetitive transcranial magnetic stimulation. *Archives of General Psychiatry, 65*(3), 268–276.

Jorge, R. E., Robinson, R. G., Arndt, S., & Starkstein, S. (2003). Mortality and poststroke depression: A placebo-controlled trial of antidepressants. *American Journal of Psychiatry, 160*(10), 1823–1829.

Jorge, R. E., Robinson, R. G., Tateno, A., Narushima, K., Acion, L., Moser, D., ... Chemerinski, E. (2004). Repetitive transcranial magnetic stimulation as treatment of poststroke depression: A preliminary study. *Biological Psychiatry, 55*(4), 398–405.

Kalayam, B., & Alexopoulos, G. S. (1999). Prefrontal dysfunction and treatment response in geriatric depression. *Archives of General Psychiatry, 56*(8), 713–718.

Khundakar, A., Morris, C., Oakley, A., McMeekin, W., & Thomas, A. J. (2009). Morphometric analysis of neuronal and glial cell pathology in the dorsolateral prefrontal cortex in late-life depression. *British Journal of Psychiatry, 195*(2), 163–169.

Khundakar, A., Morris, C., Oakley, A., & Thomas, A. J. (2011). Morphometric analysis of neuronal and glial cell pathology in the caudate nucleus in late-life depression. *American Journal of Geriatric Psychiatry, 19*(2), 132–141.

Kiosses, D. N., Alexopoulos, G. S., & Murphy, C. (2000). Symptoms of striatofrontal dysfunction contribute to disability in geriatric depression. *International Journal of Geriatric Psychiatry, 15*(11), 992–999.

Kiosses, D. N., Klimstra, S., Murphy, C., & Alexopoulos, G. S. (2001). Executive dysfunction and disability in elderly patients with major depression. *American Journal of Geriatric Psychiatry, 9*(3), 269–274.

Kohen, R., Cain, K. C., Mitchell, P. H., Becker, K., Buzaitis, A., Millard, S. P., ... Veith, R. (2008). Association of serotonin transporter gene polymorphisms with poststroke depression. *Archives of General Psychiatry, 65*(11), 1296–1302.

Krishnan, K. R., Hays, J. C., & Blazer, D. G. (1997). MRI-defined vascular depression. *American Journal of Psychiatry, 154*(4), 497–501.

Krishnan, K. R., Hays, J. C., George, L. K., & Blazer, D. G. (1998). Six-month outcomes for MRI-related vascular depression. *Depression and Anxiety, 8*(4), 142–146.

Krishnan, K. R., McDonald, W. M., Doraiswamy, P. M., Tupler, L. A., Husain, M., Boyko, O. B., ... Ellinwood, E. H., Jr. (1993). Neuroanatomical substrates of depression in the elderly. *European Archives of Psychiatry and Clinical Neuroscience, 243*(1), 41–46.

Krishnan, M. S., O'Brien, J. T., Firbank, M. J., Pantoni, L., Carlucci, G., Erkinjuntti, T., ... LADIS Group. (2006). Relationship between periventricular and deep white matter lesions and depressive symptoms in older people. The LADIS Study. *International Journal of Geriatric Psychiatry, 21*(10), 983–989.

Krishnan, K. R., Taylor, W. D., McQuoid, D. R., MacFall, J. R., Payne, M. E., Provenzale, J. M., & Steffens, D. C. (2004). Clinical characteristics of magnetic resonance imaging-defined subcortical ischemic depression. *Biological Psychiatry, 55*(4), 390–397.

Lai, T., Payne, M. E., Byrum, C. E., Steffens, D. C., & Krishnan, K. R. (2000). Reduction of orbital frontal cortex volume in geriatric depression. *Biological Psychiatry, 48*(10), 971–975.

Lazarus, L. W., Winemiller, D. R., Lingam, V. R., Neyman, I., Hartman, C., Abassian, M.,...Fawcett, J. (1992). Efficacy and side effects of methylphenidate for poststroke depression. *Journal of Clinical Psychiatry, 53*(12), 447–449.

Lee, K. S., Chung, J. H., Lee, K. H., Shin, M. J., Oh, B. H., Lee, S. H., & Hong, C. H. (2009). Simultaneous measurement of 23 plasma cytokines in late-life depression. *Neurological Sciences, 30*(5), 435–438.

Leentjens, A. F., Aben, I., Lodder, J., & Verhey, F. R. (2006). General and disease-specific risk factors for depression after ischemic stroke: A two-step Cox regression analysis. *International Psychogeriatrics, 18*(4), 739–748.

Lesser, I. M., Boone, K. B., Mehringer, C. M., Wohl, M. A., Miller, B. L., & Berman, N. G. (1996). Cognition and white matter hyperintensities in older depressed patients. *American Journal of Psychiatry, 153*(10), 1280–1287.

Levy, R. M., Steffens, D. C., McQuoid, D. R., Provenzale, J. M., MacFall, J. R., & Krishnan, K. R. (2003). MRI lesion severity and mortality in geriatric depression. *American Journal of Geriatric Psychiatry, 11*(6), 678–682.

Lincoln, N. B., & Flannaghan, T. (2003). Cognitive behavioral psychotherapy for depression following stroke: A randomized controlled trial. *Stroke, 34*(1), 111–115.

Lipsey, J. R., Robinson, R. G., Pearlson, G. D., Rao, K., & Price, T. R. (1984). Nortriptyline treatment of post-stroke depression: A double-blind study. *Lancet, 1*(8372), 297–300.

Lipsey, J. R., Spencer, W. C., Rabins, P. V., & Robinson, R. G. (1986). Phenomenological comparison of poststroke depression and functional depression. *American Journal of Psychiatry, 143*(4), 527–529.

MacFall, J. R., Payne, M. E., Provenzale, J. E., & Krishnan, K. R. (2001). Medial orbital frontal lesions in late-onset depression. *Biological Psychiatry, 49*(9), 803–806.

Masand, P., Murray, G. B., & Pickett, P. (1991). Psychostimulants in post-stroke depression. *Journal of Neuropsychiatry and Clinical Neuroscience, 3*(1), 23–27.

Mast, B. T., MacNeill, S. E., & Lichtenberg, P. A. (2004). Post-stroke and clinically-defined vascular depression in geriatric rehabilitation patients. *American Journal of Geriatric Psychiatry, 12*(1), 84–92.

McLennan, S. N., & Mathias, J. L. (2010). The depression-executive dysfunction (DED) syndrome and response to antidepressants: A meta-analytic review. *International Journal of Geriatric Psychiatry, 25*(10), 933–944.

Morimoto, S. S., Gunning, F. M., Murphy, C. F., Kanellopoulos, D., Kelly, R. E., & Alexopoulos, G. S. (2011). Executive function and short-term remission of geriatric depression: The role of semantic strategy. *American Journal of Geriatric Psychiatry, 19*(2), 115–122.

Morris, P. L., Raphael, B., & Robinson, R. G. (1992). Clinical depression is associated with impaired recovery from stroke. *Medical Journal of Australia, 157*(4), 239–242.

Morris, P. L., Robinson, R. G., Andrzejewski, P., Samuels, J., & Price, T. R. (1993). Association of depression with 10-year poststroke mortality. *American Journal of Psychiatry, 150*(1), 124–129.

Morris, P. L., Robinson, R. G., Raphael, B., & Hopwood, M. J. (1996). Lesion location and poststroke depression. *Journal of Neuropsychiatry and Clinical Neuroscience, 8*(4), 399–403.

Murata, Y., Kimura, M., & Robinson, R. G. (2000). Does cognitive impairment cause post-stroke depression? *American Journal of Geriatric Psychiatry, 8*(4), 310–317.

Murphy, C. F., Gunning-Dixon, F. M., Hoptman, M. J., Lim, K. O., Ardekani, B., Shields, J. K.,...Alexopoulos, G. S. (2007). White-matter integrity predicts Stroop performance in patients with geriatric depression. *Biological Psychiatry, 61*(8), 1007–1010.

Murray, G. B., Shea, V., & Conn, D. K. (1986). Electroconvulsive therapy for poststroke depression. *Journal of Clinical Psychiatry, 47*(5), 258–260.

Narushima, K., Kosier, J. T., & Robinson, R. G. (2003). A reappraisal of poststroke depression, intra- and inter-hemispheric lesion location using meta-analysis. *Journal of Neuropsychiatry and Clinical Neuroscience, 15*(4), 422–430.

Nebes, R. D., Vora, I. J., Meltzer, C. C., Fukui, M. B., Williams, R. L., Kamboh, M. I.,...Reynolds, C. F., 3rd. (2001). Relationship of deep white matter hyperintensities and apolipoprotein E genotype to depressive symptoms in older adults without clinical depression. *American Journal of Psychiatry, 158*(6), 878–884.

Newberg, A. R., Davydow, D. S., & Lee, H. B. (2006). Cerebrovascular disease basis of depression: Post-stroke depression and vascular depression. *International Review of Psychiatry, 18*(5), 433–441.

Nobuhara, K., Okugawa, G., Sugimoto, T., Minami, T., Tamagaki, C., Takase, K.,...Kinoshita, T. (2006). Frontal white matter anisotropy and symptom severity of late-life depression: A magnetic resonance diffusion tensor imaging study. *Journal of Neurology, Neurosurgery, and Psychiatry, 77*(1), 120–122.

O'Brien, J., Ames, D., Chiu, E., Schweitzer, I., Desmond, P., & Tress, B. (1998). Severe deep white matter lesions and outcome in elderly patients with major depressive disorder: Follow up study. *British Medical Journal, 317*(7164), 982–984.

O'Brien, J., Desmond, P., Ames, D., Schweitzer, I., Harrigan, S., & Tress, B. (1996). A magnetic resonance imaging study of white matter lesions in depression and Alzheimer's disease. *British Journal of Psychiatry, 168*(4), 477–485.

Oldehinkel, A. J., Ormel, J., Brilman, E. I., & van den Berg, M. D. (2003). Psychosocial and vascular risk factors of depression in later life. *Journal of Affective Disorders, 74*(3), 237–246.

Paolucci, S., Gandolfo, C., Provinciali, L., Torta, R., Toso, V., & DESTRO Study Group. (2006). The Italian multicenter observational study on post-stroke depression (DESTRO). *Journal of Neurology, 253*(5), 556–562.

Paradiso, S., Ohkubo, T., & Robinson, R. G. (1997). Vegetative and psychological symptoms associated with depressed mood over the first two years after stroke. *International Journal of Psychiatry in Medicine, 27*(2), 137–157.

Parikh, R. M., Robinson, R. G., Lipsey, J. R., Starkstein, S. E., Fedoroff, J. P., & Price, T. R. (1990). The impact of poststroke depression on recovery in activities of daily living over a 2-year follow-up. *Archives of Neurology, 47*(7), 785–789.

Potter, G. G., Kittinger, J. D., Wagner, H. R., Steffens, D. C., & Krishnan, K. R. (2004). Prefrontal neuropsychological predictors of treatment remission in late-life depression. *Neuropsychopharmacology, 29*(12), 2266–2271.

Provinciali, L., & Coccia, M. (2002). Post-stroke and vascular depression: A critical review. *Neurological Sciences, 22*(6), 417–428.

Rajkowska, G., Miguel-Hidalgo, J. J., Dubey, P., Stockmeier, C. A., & Krishnan, K. R. (2005). Prominent reduction in pyramidal neurons density in the orbitofrontal cortex of elderly depressed patients. *Biological Psychiatry, 58*(4), 297–306.

Ramasubbu, R. (2000). Relationship between depression and cerebrovascular disease: Conceptual issues. *Journal of Affective Disorders, 57*(1–3), 1–11.

Ried, L. D., Jia, H., Feng, H., Cameon, R., Wang, X., Tueth, M., & Wu, S. S. (2011). Selective serotonin reuptake inhibitor treatment and depression are associated with poststroke mortality. *Annals of Pharmacotherapy, 45*(7–8), 888–897.

Robinson, R. G. (2003). Poststroke depression: prevalence, diagnosis, treatment, and disease progression. *Biological Psychiatry, 54*(3), 376–387.

Robinson, R. G., & Bloom, F. E. (1977). Pharmacological treatment following experimental cerebral infarction: Implications for understanding psychological symptoms of human stroke. *Biological Psychiatry, 12*(5), 669–680.

Robinson, R. G., Bolla-Wilson, K., Kaplan, E., Lipsey, J. R., & Price, T. R. (1986). Depression influences intellectual impairment in stroke patients. *British Journal of Psychiatry, 148*, 541–547.

Robinson, R. G., Jorge, R. E., Moser, D. J., Acion, L., Solodkin, A., Small, S. L., ... Arndt, S. (2008). Escitalopram and problem-solving therapy for prevention of poststroke depression: A randomized controlled trial. *Journal of the American Medical Association, 299*(20), 2391–2400.

Robinson, R. G., Kubos, K. L., Starr, L. B., Rao, K., & Price, T. R. (1984). Mood disorders in stroke patients. Importance of location of lesion. *Brain, 107*(Pt. 1), 81–93.

Robinson, R. G., Schultz, S. K., Castillo, C., Kopel, T., Kosier, J. T., Newman, R. M., ... Starkstein, S. E. (2000). Nortriptyline versus fluoxetine in the treatment of depression and in short-term recovery after stroke: A placebo-controlled, double-blind study. *American Journal of Psychiatry, 157*(3), 351–359.

Robinson, R. G., & Spalletta, G. (2010). Poststroke depression: A review. *Canadian Journal of Psychiatry, 55*(6), 341–349.

Salloway, S., Boyle, P. A., Correia, S., Malloy, P. F., Cahn-Weiner, D. A., Schneider, L., ... Nakra, R. (2002). The relationship of MRI subcortical hyperintensities to treatment response in a trial of sertraline in geriatric depressed outpatients. *American Journal of Geriatric Psychiatry, 10*(1), 107–111.

Salloway, S., Malloy, P., Kohn, R., Gillard, E., Duffy, J., Rogg, J., ... Westlake, R. (1996). MRI and neuropsychological differences in early- and late-life-onset geriatric depression. *Neurology, 46*(6), 1567–1574.

Schwartz, J. A., Speed, N. M., Brunberg, J. A., Brewer, T. L., Brown, M., & Greden, J. F. (1993). Depression in stroke rehabilitation. *Biological Psychiatry, 33*(10), 694–699.

Sheline, Y. I., Pieper, C. F., Barch, D. M., Welsh-Bohmer, K., McKinstry, R. C., MacFall, J. R., ... Doraiswamy, P. M. (2010). Support for the vascular depression hypothesis in late-life depression: Results of a 2-site, prospective, antidepressant treatment trial. *Archives of General Psychiatry, 67*(3), 277–285.

Shimoda, K., & Robinson, R. G. (1999). The relationship between poststroke depression and lesion location in long-term follow-up. *Biological Psychiatry, 45*(2), 187–192.

Simpson, S., Baldwin, R. C., Jackson, A., & Burns, A. S. (1998). Is subcortical disease associated with a poor response to antidepressants? Neurological, neuropsychological and neuroradiological findings in late-life depression. *Psychological Medicine, 28*(5), 1015–1026.

Singh, A., Herrmann, N., & Black, S. E. (1998). The importance of lesion location in poststroke depression: A critical review. *Canadian Journal of Psychiatry, 43*(9), 921–927.

Sneed, J. R., & Culang-Reinlieb, M. E. (2011). The vascular depression hypothesis: An update. *American Journal of Geriatric Psychiatry, 19*(2), 99–103.

Sneed, J. R., Keilp, J. G., Brickman, A. M., Roose, S. P. (2008). The specificity of neuropsychological impairment in predicting antidepressant non-response in the very old depressed. *International Journal of Geriatric Psychiatry, 23*(3), 319–323.

Sneed, J. R., Rindskopf, D., Steffens, D. C., Krishnan, K. R., (2008). Roose, S. P. The vascular depression subtype: Evidence of internal validity. *Biological Psychiatry, 64*(6), 491–497.

Sneed, J. R., Roose, S. P., Keilp, J. G., Krishnan, K. R., Alexopoulos, G. S., & Sackeim, H. A. (2007). Response inhibition predicts poor antidepressant treatment response in very old depressed patients. *American Journal of Geriatric Psychiatry, 15*(7), 553–563.

Spalletta, G., & Caltagirone, C. (2003). Sertraline treatment of post-stroke major depression: An open study in patients with moderate to severe symptoms. *Functional Neurology, 18*(4), 227–232.

Spalletta, G., Bossù, P., Ciaramella, A., Bria, P., Caltagirone, C., & Robinson, R. G. (2006). The etiology of poststroke depression: a review of the literature and a new hypothesis involving inflammatory cytokines. *Molecular Psychiatry, 11*(11), 984–991.

Spalletta, G., Guida, G., De Angelis, D., & Caltagirone, C. (2002). Predictors of cognitive level and depression severity are different in patients with left and right hemispheric stroke within the first year of illness. *Journal of Neurology, 249*(11), 1541–1551.

Spalletta, G., Ripa, A., & Caltagirone, C. (2005). Symptom profile of DSM-IV major and minor depressive disorders in first-ever stroke patients. *American Journal of Geriatric Psychiatry, 13*(2), 108–115.

Spencer, K. A., Tompkins, C. A., & Schulz, R. (1997). Assessment of depression in patients with brain pathology: The case of stroke. *Psychology Bulletin, 122*(2), 132–152.

Spitzer, R. L., Endicott, J., & Robins, E. (1975). Research diagnostic criteria. *Psychopharmacology Bulletin, 11*(3), 22–25.

Starkstein, S. E., Berthier, M. L., Fedoroff, P., Price, T. R., & Robinson, R. G. (1990). Anosognosia and major depression in 2 patients with cerebrovascular lesions. *Neurology, 40*(9), 1380–1132.

Starkstein, S. E., Bryer, J. B., Berthier, M. L., Cohen, B., Price, T. R., & Robinson, R. G. (1991). Depression after stroke: The importance of cerebral hemisphere asymmetries. *Journal of Neuropsychiatry and Clinical Neuroscience, 3*(3), 276–285.

Starkstein, S. E., Fedoroff, J. P., Price, T. R., Leiguarda, R., & Robinson, R. G. (1992). Anosognosia in patients with cerebrovascular lesions. A study of causative factors. *Stroke, 23*(10), 1446–1453.

Starkstein, S. E., Robinson, R. G., & Price, T. R. (1987). Comparison of cortical and subcortical lesions in the production of poststroke mood disorders. *Brain, 110*(Pt 4), 1045–1059.

Starkstein, S. E., Robinson, R. G., & Price, T. R. (1988). Comparison of patients with and without poststroke major depression matched for size and location of lesion. *Archives of General Psychiatry, 45*(3), 247–252.

Steffens, D. C., Bosworth, H. B., Provenzale, J. M., & MacFall, J. R. (2002). Subcortical white matter lesions and functional impairment in geriatric depression. *Depression and Anxiety, 15*(1), 23–28.

Steffens, D. C., Helms, M. J., Krishnan, K. R., & Burke, G. L. (1999). Cerebrovascular disease and depression symptoms in the cardiovascular health study. *Stroke, 30*(10), 2159–2166.

Steffens, D. C., & Krishnan, K. R. (1998). Structural neuroimaging and mood disorders: Recent findings, implications for classification, and future directions. *Biological Psychiatry, 43*(10), 705–712.

Steffens, D. C., Krishnan, K. R., Crump, C., & Burke, G. L. (2002). Cerebrovascular disease and evolution of depressive symptoms in the cardiovascular health study. *Stroke, 33*(6), 1636–1644.

Steffens, D. C., McQuoid, D. R., Welsh-Bohmer, K. A., & Krishnan, K. R. (2003). Left orbital frontal cortex volume and performance on the benton visual retention test in older depressives and controls. *Neuropsychopharmacology, 28*(12), 2179–2183.

Steffens, D. C., Payne, M. E., Greenberg, D. L., Byrum, C. E., Welsh-Bohmer, K. A., Wagner, H. R., &

MacFall, J. R. (2002). Hippocampal volume and incident dementia in geriatric depression. *American Journal of Geriatric Psychiatry, 10*(1), 62–71.

Taragano, F. E., Allegri, R., Vicario, A., Bagnatti, P., & Lyketsos, C. G. (2001). A double blind, randomized clinical trial assessing the efficacy and safety of augmenting standard antidepressant therapy with nimodipine in the treatment of "vascular depression." *International Journal of Geriatric Psychiatry, 16*(3), 254–2560.

Taragano, F. E., Bagnatti, P., & Allegri, R. F. (2005). A double-blind, randomized clinical trial to assess the augmentation with nimodipine of antidepressant therapy in the treatment of "vascular depression." *International Psychogeriatrics, 17*(3), 487–498.

Taylor, W. D., MacFall, J. R., Payne, M. E., McQuoid, D. R., Provenzale, J. M., Steffens, D. C., & Krishnan, K. R. (2004). Late-life depression and microstructural abnormalities in dorsolateral prefrontal cortex white matter. *American Journal of Psychiatry, 161*(7), 1293–1296.

Taylor, W. D., MacFall, J. R., Steffens, D. C., Payne, M. E., Provenzale, J. M., & Krishnan, K. R. (2003). Localization of age-associated white matter hyperintensities in late-life depression. *Progress in Neuropsychopharmacology and Biological Psychiatry, 27*(3), 539–544.

Taylor, W. D., Steffens, D. C., MacFall, J. R., McQuoid, D. R., Payne, M. E., Provenzale, J. M., & Krishnan, K. R. (2003). White matter hyperintensity progression and late-life depression outcomes. *Archives of General Psychiatry, 60*(11), 1090–1096.

Taylor, W. D., Steffens, D. C., McQuoid, D. R., Payne, M. E., Lee, S. H., Lai, T. J., & Krishnan, K. R. (2003). Smaller orbital frontal cortex volumes associated with functional disability in depressed elders. *Biological Psychiatry, 53*(2), 144–149.

Taylor, W. D., MacFall J. R., Payne M. E., McQuoid D. R., Steffens D. C., Provenzale J. M., & Krishnan K. R. (2007). Orbitofrontal cortex volume in late-life depression: Influence of hyperintense lesions and genetic polymorphisms. *Psychological Medicine, 37*(12):1763–1773.

Thomas, A. J., Davis, S., Morris, C., Jackson, E., Harrison, R., & O'Brien, J. T. (2005). Increase in interleukin-1beta in late-life depression. *American Journal of Psychiatry, 162*(1), 175–177.

Thomas, A. J., O'Brien, J. T., Davis, S., Ballard, C., Barber, R., Kalaria, R. N., & Perry, R. H. (2002). Ischemic basis for deep white matter hyperintensities in major depression: A neuropathological study. *Archives of General Psychiatry, 59*(9), 785–792.

Thomas, A. J., Perry, R., Kalaria, R. N., Oakley, A., McMeekin, W., & O'Brien, J. T. (2003). Neuropathological evidence for ischemia in the white matter of the dorsolateral prefrontal cortex in late-life depression. *International Journal of Geriatric Psychiatry, 18*(1), 7–13.

Van Otterloo, E., O'Dwyer, G., Stockmeier, C. A., Steffens, D. C., Krishnan, R. R., & Rajkowska, G. (2009). Reductions in neuronal density in elderly depressed are region specific. *International Journal of Geriatric Psychiatry, 24*(8), 856–864.

Whyte, E. M., & Mulsant, B. H. (2002). Post stroke depression: Epidemiology, pathophysiology, and biological treatment. *Biological Psychiatry, 52*(3), 253–264.

Wiart, L., Petit, H., Joseph, P. A., Mazaux, J. M., & Barat, M. (2000). Fluoxetine in early poststroke depression: A double-blind placebo-controlled study. *Stroke, 31*(8), 1829–1832.

Williams, L. S., Ghose, S. S., Swindle R. W. (2004), Depression and other mental health diagnoses increase mortality after stroke. *American Journal of Psychiatry, 161*(6), 1090–1095.

Yanai, I., Fujikawa, T., Horiguchi, J., Yamawaki, S., & Touhouda, Y. (1998). The 3-year course and outcome of patients with major depression and silent cerebral infarction. *Journal of Affective Disorders, 47*(1–3), 25–30.

16

DEPRESSION AND MEDICAL ILLNESS IN LATE LIFE

RACE, RESOURCES, AND STRESS

Briana Mezuk and Joseph J. Gallo

THERE IS no health without mental health (Prince et al., 2007). The co-occurrence of depression with medical conditions is arguably the distinguishing feature of depression in late life. Medical comorbidity is more than merely the background on which depression plays out—medical conditions such as cardiovascular disease and diabetes interact with depression in ways that are key to optimal patient-centered management. For most chronic medical conditions such as diabetes, increasing attention has been given to the principle that day-to-day management should be in the hands of patients themselves, in the context of their own culture and community. Self-care activities (e.g., checking one's own finger-stick blood sugar), health behaviors (e.g., smoking, alcohol use, diet, physical activity), and patient choice (e.g., whether to undergo a procedure) all profoundly affect quality of life in chronic illness and all are strongly influenced by psychiatric states such as depression. Individual behaviors and choices also occur within a specified context, including access to and quality of health care, neighborhood resources that influence the ability to engage in health promotion activities (e.g., access to fresh fruits and vegetables, proximity to safe areas to exercise outside, availability of tobacco and alcohol products), exposure to stressors (e.g., financial strain, community and interpersonal violence, racial discrimination), and cultural values, resources, and norms (Jackson, Knight, & Rafferty, 2010).

Several community-based studies suggest that major depression is common among older adults, affecting up to 15% of older persons (Copeland et al., 1987, 1992; Gallo, Rabins, Lyketsos, Tien, & Anthony, 1997; Heeren, van Hemert, Lagaay, & Rooymans, 1992; Skoog, 1993). In an analysis from the 13-year follow-up of the participants of the Baltimore Epidemiologic Catchment Area (ECA) study, the life course distribution of the incidence of *DSM-III* major depression appeared to be bimodal, with a primary peak in the third decade and a secondary peak in the sixth decade (Eaton et al., 1997). Based on continued follow-up of the ECA cohort (Eaton, Kalaydjian, Scharfstein, Mezuk, & Ding, 2007; Eaton et al., 2008) and on population projections (Heo, Murphy, Fontaine, Bruce, & Alexopolous, 2008), the prevalence of depression appears to be rising, especially in middle age. The second peak in depressive onset occurring in later life may be due to medical morbidity, particularly cardiovascular disease and associated white-matter lesions (Hoptman et al., 2009). Similarly, the increase in the prevalence of depression over time among middle-aged adults is undoubtedly tied to increasingly common chronic medical conditions that impair quality of life but are not immediately life threatening, such as arthritis and diabetes.

Studies indicate that depressive symptoms that do not meet clinical diagnostic criteria are also relevant to health and functioning. Subsyndromal, or minor depression, has no standard operational criteria across studies; nevertheless, minor depression is particularly common among older adults and is associated with medical comorbidity (Broadhead, Blazer, George, & Tse, 1990; Judd et al., 2004; Katon & Schulberg, 1992; Meeks, Vahia, Lavretsky, Kulkarni, & Jeste, 2011; Tannock & Katona, 1995). Population-based studies have also indicated that although racial and ethnic minorities tend to report greater symptoms of general distress and higher burden of medical comorbidity (Jackson, 2002; Mezuk et al., 2010), they are *less likely* to meet diagnostic criteria for major depression relative to non-Hispanic Whites (Breslau et al., 2006; Jackson, Rafferty, & Knight, 2010); this unexpected discrepancy between distress and prevalence of major depression is not due to measurement error of depression across racial/ethnic groups (Breslau, Aguilar-Gaxiola, & Kendler, 2006; Williams et al., 2007). Also, a robust association between depression and mortality has been reported even when symptoms are relatively mild (Bush et al., 2001; Gallo et al., 1997; Lesperance, Frasure-Smith, Talajic, & Bourassa, 2002) or when psychological factors that map to depression but are not strictly a component of standard criteria are studied (e.g., hopelessness, pessimism; Kubzansky, Davidson, & Rozanski, 2005). Over the course of a 2-year follow-up interval, depression contributed as much to mortality as did myocardial infarction or diabetes, with the population attributable fraction of mortality due to depression approximately 13% (similar to the attributable risk associated with heart attack at 11%, and diabetes at 9%; Gallo, Bogner, Morales,

Post, et al., 2005). Together these findings indicate that in order to understand the relationship between depression and medical illness in later life, it is necessary to consider depressive symptoms regardless of whether diagnostic criteria are met.

In this chapter we set the stage for understanding the dynamic relationship between depression and medical conditions in later life by discussing the growing diversity of the aging population and the wide racial disparities in the burden of medical illness over the life course. We provide and discuss a conceptual framework that emphasizes the potential psychological, behavioral, social, and biological mechanisms through which depression and medical illness interact to cause disability and death. The intersection of stress, resources, depression, health behaviors, medical morbidity, and mortality across the life course provides an opportunity to synthesize our understanding of the sources of health disparities. This model has implications for development of new service delivery models that integrate the care of depression into the care of chronic medical conditions.

DIVERSITY OF THE OLDER POPULATION

The two most pronounced aspects of US demographic change over the next 50 years will be population aging and an increase in racial and ethnic diversity (Shrestha & Heisler, 2011). Currently approximately 13% of the US population is aged 65 and older, but by 2030 that proportion is projected to increase to 20% (Vincent & Velkoff, 2010). By 2042 non-Hispanic Whites will constitute a "minority majority" in the United States—that is, the majority of individuals in the United States will be from a racial/ethnic group other than non-Hispanic Whites (primarily Hispanic, Black, and Asian; Shrestha & Heisler, 2011). While among older adults non-Hispanic Whites will remain a clear majority, the face of aging is also becoming more diverse. For example, in 2000 non-Hispanic Whites comprised 82% of the population aged 55 and older, but this proportion is projected to decline to 75% by 2015; conversely, the proportion of Blacks and Hispanics aged 55 and older is projected to increase over this period by 1 and 4 percentage points, respectively (US Census Bureau, 2008). Twin changes—increasing diversity and size of the aging population—present both challenges and opportunities for clinicians, health care professionals, and public health officials. The opportunity to develop novel models of preventive and clinical strategies that reflect the needs of the changing aging population, as well as the challenge of implementing strategies that effectively meet the needs of diverse older adults, will intersect with practically every aspect of health care policy over the next 50 years.

The increasing diversity of the US aging population has highlighted the need to explicitly understand the sources of variation in health not just *between* population groups (e.g., comparing Whites and Blacks), but *within* population groups. Critical examination of how factors contribute to health within groups over the life course, and assessing whether these relationships vary across groups, can provide insight regarding how factors interact with race, gender, socioeconomic position, cultural norms, and place (Neighbors & Jackson, 1996; Whitfield & Hayward, 2003). For example, perceived stigma is a strong deterrent for seeking mental health services among all persons with depression; however, a recent study found that the relationship between perceived stigma and unwillingness to seek psychiatric care was particularly strong among older Black adults with depression (Conner et al., 2010). Other research suggests that minority elders may not attribute psychiatric symptoms to emotional health and thus may be less likely to seek mental health treatment for these symptoms (Kim et al., 2011). Older adults may also be less likely to endorse symptoms thought to be salient for depression (e.g., dysphoria or anhedonia; Gallo, Anthony, & Muthén, 1994; Gallo et al., 1997), particularly among ethnic minorities (Dahlberg, Barg, Gallo, & Wittink, 2009; Gallo, Bogner, Morales, & Ford, 2005; Gallo, Cooper-Patrick, & Lesikar, 1998). Such knowledge can inform models of clinical care and prevention that account for differences in beliefs about the sources of psychiatric symptoms; these findings also suggest that psychological *functioning* can be disaggregated from psychiatric *disorder*, which may inform the identification of factors that promote functioning among persons with depression.

THE BURDEN OF DEPRESSION AND MEDICAL COMORBIDITY

Cardiovascular disease, cancer, and diabetes are the leading causes of mortality for all adults in industrialized nations, but the burden of these conditions is disproportionately high among racial/ethnic minorities and socioeconomically disadvantaged groups. For example, the mortality rate from diabetes for non-Hispanic White women is 33% lower than that of Black women (22.5 deaths per 100,000 versus 33.3 deaths per 100,000; Xu, Kochanek, Murphy, & Tejada-Vera, 2010). These mortality estimates reflect a combination of disease incidence, disease severity (particularly at the point of first identification by a clinician), and access to treatment, all of which in the United States are patterned by socioeconomic position and race/ethnicity. Similarly, life expectancy for Black men born in 2010 is 70.2 years—non-Hispanic White men have not had a life expectancy this low since 1980 (Xu et al., 2010).

How these pronounced disparities interact with psychiatric-medical comorbidity in later life is generally understudied and not well understood. Overall medical burden as indicated by a count of conditions, or functional impairment regardless of cause, may be associated with depression (Bartels, 2004; Katon, 2003; Lyness, Niculescu, Tu, Reynolds, & Caine, 2006). In our analysis of data from the National Comorbidity Survey and the Health and Retirement Study (Fig. 16.1), among both Blacks and Whites, as the cumulative burden of health conditions increases the prevalence of major depression also tends to increase. However, the relationship between number of conditions and depression appears to be less consistent for Blacks (Fig. 16.1). Several factors may contribute to these apparent differences, such as the degree of functional impairment due to medical illness (Xie et al., 2008), disparities in access to care (Hammond et al., 2011; Saha et al., 2008; Shippee, Ferraro, & Thorpe, 2011), and availability of social support (De Leon et al., 2009) and coping resources (Neighbors & Jackson, 1996). Figure 16.1 also illustrates the utility of conceptualizing medical and psychiatric comorbidity from a life course perspective. For example, although Blacks have higher overall burden of medical comorbidity at all ages, this is particularly apparent earlier in the life course; only 35% of Blacks aged 45–54 years have no medical conditions, as compared to 55% of Whites. These findings illustrate the value of explicitly incorporating race and ethnicity into conceptual models of how depression and medical illness intersect in later life.

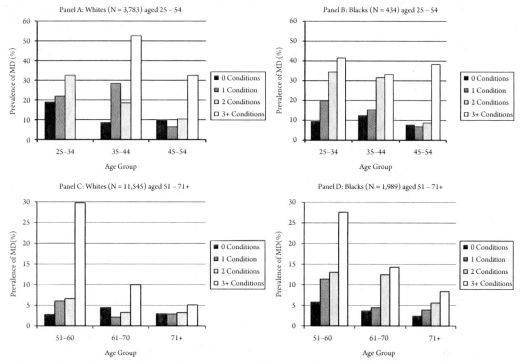

Panel A: Whites (N = 3,783) aged 25 – 54

Prevalence of MD (%) — Age Group: 25–34, 35–44, 45–54

Legend: ■ 0 Conditions ▨ 1 Condition ▤ 2 Conditions ☐ 3+ Conditions

Panel B: Blacks (N = 434) aged 25 – 54

Prevalence of MD (%) — Age Group: 25–34, 35–44, 45–54

Legend: ■ 0 Conditions ▨ 1 Condition ▤ 2 Conditions ☐ 3+ Conditions

Panel C: Whites (N = 11,545) aged 51 – 71+

Prevalence of MD(%) — Age Group: 51–60, 61–70, 71+

Legend: ■ 0 Conditions ▨ 1 Condition ▤ 2 Conditions ☐ 3+ Conditions

Panel D: Blacks (N = 1,989) aged 51 – 71+

Prevalence of MD(%) — Age Group: 51–60, 61–70, 71+

Legend: ■ 0 Conditions ▨ 1 Condition ▤ 2 Conditions ☐ 3+ Conditions

FIGURE 16.1 Lifetime prevalence of major depression by age, number of health conditions, and race.

EXCESS MORBIDITY AND MORTALITY ASSOCIATED WITH DEPRESSION

The World Health Organization estimates that by 2020 major depression will be second only to cardiovascular disease as a contributor to disability worldwide (Murray & Lopez, 1996). Ample clinical and epidemiologic evidence has accumulated that the risk for depression is higher with increasing levels of medical burden, that depression is associated with the onset of medical illness and vice versa, and that medical illness accompanied by depression is associated with more functional impairment and mortality than when depression is not present. We review the clinical and epidemiologic evidence here. In the next section we tackle the pathways that help explain *how* these consequences of depression come about.

Depression has been reported to be a risk factor for cardiovascular disease (Ford et al., 1998; Pratt et al., 1996), type 2 diabetes (Eaton, Armenian, Gallo, Pratt, & Ford, 1996; Mezuk, Eaton, Albrecht, & Golden, 2008), cancer (Gallo, Armenian, Ford, Eaton, & Khachaturian, 2000; Gross, Gallo, & Eaton, 2010), migraine headache (Swartz, Pratt,

Armenian, Lee, & Eaton, 2000), and other medical conditions (de Vries, Northington, & Bogner 2011). In the Baltimore Epidemiologic Catchment Area study, community-dwelling adults without a history of heart disease who met criteria for major depression in 1981 were four times as likely to have nonfatal cardiovascular disease 13 years later when compared to persons without depression (Pratt et al., 1996). In the Precursors Study, whose participants were recruited as medical students at Johns Hopkins University between 1948 and 1964, depression reported in early life was found to be an independent risk factor for incident coronary artery disease prospectively—even several decades after the onset of the depressive episode (Ford et al., 1998).

Several meta-analyses have summarized data showing that depression and diabetes are closely linked (Ali, Stone, Peters, Davies, & Khunti, 2006; Anderson, Freedland, Clouse, & Lustman, 2001; Mezuk et al., 2008). Persons with diabetes were about twice as likely to report depressive symptoms than were persons without diabetes (Ali et al., 2006; Anderson et al., 2001; Atlantis, Browning, Sims, & Kendig, 2010; Eaton, 2002; Rustad, Musselman, & Nemeroff, 2011). Summarizing 13 studies, Mezuk and colleagues estimated that baseline depression predicted type 2 diabetes with a hazard ratio of 1.60 (95% CI [1.37, 1.88]) and the hazard ratio for depression associated with baseline diabetes estimated from seven studies was 1.15 (95% CI [1.02, 1.30]; Mezuk et al., 2008). The evidence is less clear that impaired glucose tolerance (IGT), or undiagnosed diabetes, is associated with increased risk of depression. In the Finnish D2D Survey, a population-based study of over 2,700 Finns, only diagnosed diabetes was associated with depression while IGT was not (Mantyselka et al., 2011). Similar findings were reported from the Multi-Ethnic Study of Atherosclerosis: Treated diabetes was associated with increased risk of depression, while IGT and undiagnosed diabetes was not (Golden et al., 2008). These studies suggest that the psychological distress associated with diabetes management, complications, and comorbidity leads to increased depression, rather than this association solely reflecting a direct effect of hyperglycemia.

The association between chronic illness and depression may vary as a function of disease pathology and time since diagnosis. Polsky and colleagues reported that risk of depression was increased 2 years after diagnosis of cancer (3.5-fold), chronic lung disease (2.2-fold), and heart disease (1.3-fold); the risk of depression declined over time for cancer and chronic lung disease, but not for heart disease (Polsky et al., 2005). Similarly, Kendler et al. reported that heart disease was associated with a nearly 3-fold risk of major depression in the year of diagnosis and about a 2-fold risk subsequently, without attenuation over time (Kendler, Gardner, Fiske, & Gatz, 2009). In contrast, the association of major depression with newly incident heart disease was strongest in the year of depression onset (increasing the risk of heart disease about 2.5-fold) but was not associated with heart disease onset over longer periods of time (Kendler et al., 2009). This suggests that the experience of a life-threatening health event such as a heart attack is strongly associated with depression over time, but that the increased risk of heart disease associated with depression is focused in a short period of time around the onset of the depressive episode.

Unlike the fairly consistent literature on the relationships between depression and risk of cardiovascular and metabolic conditions, the relationship between depression and cancer risk is more conflicting. Some studies have found that depression is associated with increased risk for cancer prospectively, particularly hormonal cancers such as of the breast and prostate (Gallo et al., 2000; Gross, Gallo, & Eaton, 2010; Linkins & Comstock, 1990; Penninx et al., 1998; Persky, Kempthorne-Rawson, & Shekelle, 1987; Shekelle et al., 1981; Whitlock & Siskind, 1979), although several others have not reported an association (Aromaa et al., 1994; Friedman, 1990, 1994; Kaplan & Reynolds, 1988; Nguyen, Kitner-Triolo, Evans, & Zonderman, 2004; Whooley, Browner, & for the Study of Osteoporotic Fractures Research Group, 1998). Nevertheless, depression in persons with cancer and cancer survivors exceeds rates in the general population, depending on the stage of cancer, the patient's past history of depression, and other factors (Weinberger, Bruce, Roth, Breitbart, & Nelson, 2011).

Prospective studies have consistently shown a relationship between depression and overall mortality in older adults, with depression associated with a 2-fold increase in risk of death. Suicide alone does not account for the increased mortality among older persons with depression—the vast majority of older persons with depression die of cardiovascular disease and other medical conditions. Depression also influences quality of life in the context of medical illness; patients with co-occurring depression and medical conditions experience more functional impairment and mortality than expected from the severity of the medical condition alone. For example, depression in diabetes confers increased functional impairment (Egede, 2004), complications of diabetes (de Groot, Anderson, Freedland, Clouse, & Lustman, 2001; Williams et al., 2010), and mortality (Black, Markides, & Ray, 2003; Egede, Nietert, & Zheng, 2005; Katon et al., 2005; Rubin, Ciechanowski, Egede, Lin, & Lustman, 2004; Silber et al., 2003). The studies of Frasure-Smith drew attention to the prognostic importance of depression among persons who had sustained a myocardial infarction (Frasure-Smith, Lesperance, & Talajic, 1993, 1995). Subsequent follow-up studies have borne out the increased risk conferred by depression on the mortality of patients with cardiovascular disease (Frasure-Smith et al., 2009; Glassman, Bigger, & Gaffney, 2009; Lesperance et al., 2002). Anhedonia may confer increased risk of death among patients with acute coronary syndrome independently of depressed mood (Davidson et al., 2010). Possible pathways through which depression leads to excess morbidity and mortality are the focus of the next section.

PATHWAYS LINKING DEPRESSION AND MEDICAL ILLNESS

Older adults usually do not present to their doctor with a single medical condition, although research and practice guidelines often only focus on uncomplicated cases (Boyd et al., 2005). Rather than organizing our discussion around mediating factors pertaining to specific medical conditions, we instead frame the discussion around potential psychological, social, behavioral, and biological links between depression and general medical morbidity. As a heuristic device, we think of these four domains as pathways—with bidirectional links—between depression and medical comorbidity. This framework moves away from the particulars of individual cases that may present to a physician, and instead considers the broader factors that may be salient for promoting overall health and well-being of the older patient. While the contribution of these mediating factors may vary according to the specific medical condition (e.g., diabetes versus arthritis) and stage of disorder (early versus late cancer), by not framing our discussion as instructions for one illness after another and incorporating the implications of the earlier discussion of the increasing diversity of the aging population, we hope to make meaningful conceptual progress for research and practice.

Most studies of the relationship between depression and medical comorbidity are cross-sectional, but we need to keep in mind that these relationships are dynamic, not static. As difficult as it can be to conceptualize, we need to think of depression as both an "effect" of medical conditions (i.e., as a possible consequence) and as a "cause" (i.e., as an antecedent). The life course framework provides a unifying approach to understanding how depression may act as an antecedent in one situation and a consequence in another, even within the same person's life trajectory. For example, growing up in poverty is associated with increased exposure to unstable home environments; exposure to an unstable home environment is associated with depression risk in adolescence; behaviors such as smoking, alcohol misuse, and eating so-called comfort foods may be used to cope both with depressive symptoms and external stressors in young adulthood; exposure to stressors and access to substances such as cigarettes, alcohol, and high-fat and high-carbohydrate foods is greater in disadvantaged neighborhoods; these behaviors, along with biological alterations

associated with depression and perceived stress, such as inflammation and hypercortisolism, are associated with atherosclerosis and insulin resistance; onset of overt cardiovascular and metabolic disease is associated with risk of depression; finally, depression is associated with increased risk of complications and mortality. In this manner the specific links between depression and medical comorbidity change over the life course and may vary according to factors such as family history, environmental context, and culture. The intersection across the life course of stress, resources, mental health, health behaviors, and medical morbidity provides an opportunity to synthesize our understanding of the relationship between depression and medical conditions, and to explain the differences we observe in the prevalence of depression across racial/ethnic groups (described in the section on "An Integrated Model of Depression, Stress, Resources, and Behaviors").

We define a *stressor* as any external demand that threatens homeostasis (that is, requires an organism to respond in order to maintain or regain homeostasis; Lazarus & Folkman, 1984). We acknowledge this definition of stress is inadequate, primarily because it requires that a stressor almost always be identified post hoc rather than a priori. This is true because if a purported stressor (e.g., preparing for a medical licensure exam) does not invoke a stress response, it was not, by this definition, a stressor. The advantage of this type of definition is that it explicitly acknowledges that there is heterogeneity in what different individuals find stressful (although we would agree that practically everyone would find a licensure exam stressful to some degree, there will be marked heterogeneity in the quantity and quality of individual responses to this experience; for example, someone who was balancing studying with caregiving duties at home would likely find this exam more stressful than someone who had the resources to hire outside caregivers while he or she studied). Second, stressors evoke a feeling of psychological distress, a state of anxious, somatic, and depressive symptoms best indexed in primary care settings by scales such as the General Health Questionnaire (Goldberg & Hillier, 1979). However, the relationship between stressors and distress is not linear; one may feel distress in anticipation of a stressor (e.g., preoccupation with the threat of being laid off during a time of economic instability), and feelings of distress may linger long after a stressor has been resolved (e.g., rumination over a romantic breakup).

Stressors and psychological distress are both associated with a cascade of neuroendocrine changes that facilitate a response to the stressor (e.g., the mobilization of the sympathetic nervous system that is the *flight or fight* response [Jansen, Van Nguyen, Karpitskiy, Mettenleiter, & Loewy, 1995] and activation of the hypothalamic-pituitary-adrenal axis with resultant hypercortisolism within 20 to 30 minutes). Together, the experience of stressors, psychological distress, and the accompanying biological cascade represent the *stress process*. Finally, the concept of *coping* denotes the ways in which individuals respond to the stress process (Lazarus & Folkman, 1984). Stressors, distress, and depression are related, but distinct, constructs that are linked to medical comorbidity through *psychological, social, behavioral, and biological pathways*.

Psychological Pathways

The relationship between psychological factors and depression is important to consider in the context of medical comorbidity because attitudes and beliefs about the condition and one's ability to cope are key to effectively engaging the health care system, adhering to medical regimens, and implementing personal behavioral changes. The most familiar psychological constellation related to depression is the "cognitive triad" of hopelessness (Beck, Weissman, Lester, & Trexler, 1974), low self-esteem (Brown, Bifulco, Veil, & Andrews, 1990; Brown, Bifulco, & Andrews 1990), and the wish to die (often described as negative thoughts about oneself, the world, and the future; Beevers & Miller, 2004).

Behavior is often a logical extension of beliefs about the illness and what to do about it, no matter how "wrong" and unreasoned the beliefs seem to a health professional (Good, 1992). Patients' perceptions of their medical conditions have long been postulated to act as important mediators of illness-related behaviors such as treatment acceptability and adherence (Kleinman, 1980; Leventhal, Nerenz, & Steele, 1984). Both Leventhal and Kleinman contended that it is the components of such personal illness models that play a large role in determining patient responses and behaviors related to illness such as seeking medical help, interacting with health care providers, complying with professionally recommended treatment, and performing self-care behaviors (Kleinman, 1988; Leventhal, Leventhal, & Contrada, 1998). A cultural model for an illness such as depression consists of largely unspoken attitudes, stances, and beliefs about the source of mental illness and the way it should be treated that are shared among a group of people. For example, older adults describe a cultural model for the role of individual responsibility for the management of depression in which one must "pull yourself up by your bootstraps" to recover (Switzer, Wittink, Karsch, & Barg, 2006). Cultural models have been used to understand beliefs about diabetes (Loewe & Freeman, 2000), AIDS (Baer, Weller, Garcia de alba Garcia, & Salcedo Rocha, 2004), breast cancer (Coreil, Wilke, & Pintado, 2004), cervical cancer (Chavez, Hubbell, McMullin, Martinez, & Mishra, 1995), and depression among older adults (Switzer et al., 2006). Beliefs and attitudes about depression and its relationship to medical conditions may be important in understanding what underlies lack of adherence to treatment (Bogner, Dahlberg, de Vries, Cahill, & Barg, 2008; Bogner, Cahill, Frauenhoffer, & Barg, 2009; Cooper et al., 2003; Zivin & Kales, 2008), and the need physicians feel for trying to convince the patient of the "biomedical model" of depression (Wittink, Givens, Knott, Coyne, & Barg, 2011).

Hopelessness has been studied as a risk factor independent of depression for the onset of suicidal ideation (Kuo, Gallo, & Eaton, 2004), cardiovascular disease, and mortality (Anda et al., 1993; Everson et al., 1996; Eaton, Kaplan, Goldberg, Salonen, & Salonen, 1997). Among 534 patients who had undergone percutaneous insertion of a paclitaxel-eluting stent, hopelessness was associated with markedly increased risk of death or nonfatal myocardial infarction 3 years after the procedure (Pedersen, Denollet, Erdman, Serruys, & van Domburg, 2009). In combination with diabetes, hopelessness was particularly adverse for mortality compared to patients without risk factors (HR = 4.9, 95% CI [1.9, 12.8]; Pedersen et al., 2009). Negative life events such as disability and illness, death of a spouse and friends, financial difficulties, and the loss of professional roles can lead to hopelessness and depression (Byrne & Raphael, 1999; Rubenowitz, Waern, Wilhelmson, & Allebeck, 2001). Older people who live alone or have multiple medical conditions may be particularly vulnerable, endorsing significantly higher levels of psychological loss, low self-esteem, and negative attitudes toward aging and the future. Hopelessness is a signal of suicidal thoughts or risk for suicidal thoughts that may be more readily reported by older adults, particularly African Americans. Numerous prospective studies have linked hopelessness to completed suicide in adults and older adults (Beck, Brown, Berchick, Stewart, & Steer, 1990; Brown, Beck, Steer, & Grisham, 2000; Kuo, Gallo, & Eaton, 2004). Self-efficacy is tightly linked but distinct from hopelessness. Self-efficacy refers to the sense that one can control or adapt to environmental demands, including management of physical illness. Among women with breast cancer, women with high self-efficacy were higher on a measure of emotional well-being at 12 months follow-up (Rottmann, Dalton, Christensen, Frederiksen, & Johansen, 2010). Poor self-efficacy and feelings of helplessness in dealing with the functional impairment and self-care activities required by medical conditions may interfere with adherence to medical regimens (Bane, Hughes, & McElnay, 2006; Chao, Nau, Aikens, & Taylor, 2005).

Thoughts of death, wanting to die, or that one would be better off dead are not uncommon among older persons with medical illness but may be poorly communicated to physicians and other health care providers. Among consecutive cases of suicide, Jurrlink et al. found an association between suicide and several medical conditions (congestive heart failure, chronic lung disease, and seizures) and depression (Juurlink, Herrmann, Szalai, Kopp, & Redelmeier, 2004). Kaplan and colleagues found that persons with physical illness and functional impairment were at high suicide risk (Kaplan, McFarland, Huguet, & Newsom, 2007). Callahan and coworkers systematically screened older primary care patients and estimated the prevalence of suicidal ideation to be 0.7% to 1.2% with most suffering from a current affective disorder accompanied by functional impairment (Callahan, Hendrie, Nienaber, & Tierney, 1996). Bartels and colleagues reported prevalence estimates of 27.5% for death ideation and 10.5% for suicidal ideation in older primary care patients with depression, anxiety, and at-risk alcohol abuse (Bartels et al., 2002). Among older primary care patients, myocardial infarction, stroke, urinary incontinence, and falls were associated with a wish to die (Kim, Bogner, Brown, & Gallo, 2006). The wish to die was associated with mortality after 5 years of follow-up among older primary care patients, even among patients who did not meet standard criteria for major depression and over and above the effects of hopelessness (Raue et al., 2010). The wish to die may act on medical conditions through poor self-efficacy, self-care activities, and health behaviors (O'Connell, Chin, Cunningham, & Lawlor, 2004).

Social Pathways

Although it is not yet fully understood how social factors "get under the skin" to influence health (Krieger 2004; Miller, Chen, & Cole, 2009), epidemiologic studies have demonstrated robust associations between social support, social integration, and loneliness with medical morbidity and mortality. These factors are important for researchers and clinicians alike because they intersect with other pathways in meaningful ways (e.g., social networks have been associated with uptake of poor health behaviors, such as smoking; Christakis & Fowler, 2008), and there are effective programs to promote social connections, particularly for older adults (Fried et al., 2004; Hong & Morrow-Howell, 2010).

Social support is one mechanism for how one's social network can influence health and health behaviors. Social support is a multifactorial construct that consists of emotional support (e.g., how much one feels loved and cared for by family and friends), instrumental support (e.g., ability of one's social network to provide assistance with tangible needs such as trips to the doctor), and appraisal support (e.g., aid from friends and family in decision making, including clinical decisions; Berkman, Glass, Brissette, & Seeman, 2000). Emotional social support is positively associated with a broad range of health outcomes, including greater survivorship following cancer treatment (Pinquart & Duberstein, 2010) and lower overall mortality (Berkman, 1995; Holt-Lunstad, Smith, & Layton, 2010). However, randomized controlled trials aimed at promoting social support among patients with established heart disease have not shown a beneficial effect on mortality (Lett et al., 2007). It is also important to note that not all social support is positive (Berkman et al., 2000). Caregiving is a common form of social support in later life, as older adults care for their partners who may have developed chronic medical conditions or dementia. Caregiving is a particularly taxing form of social support, and older adults who care for a spouse or partner are at increased risk of cognitive decline, depression, and social isolation (Vitaliano, Murphy, Young, Echeverria, & Borson, 2011). Social support intersects with gender, culture, and environmental resources; for example, an elder's willingness to be a caretaker, despite the stress incurred by this social role, may reflect the cultural value of familism (Knight & Sayegh, 2010; Sayegh & Knight, 2011). This example shows that while we often consider cultural factors "resources" that protect health (Clark & Smith, 2011), they may also increase the likelihood that an older adult takes on social roles that are inherently stressful.

Social isolation—loneliness—is a subjective experience; one does not have to be alone in order to feel lonely (Miller, 2011). Older adults may be more inclined to describe depression symptoms in terms of loneliness. The literature on the relationship between loneliness and depression in older adults emphasizes social support factors (Pinquart & Sorensen, 2001) and the growing number of losses that older adults experience (Alpass & Neville, 2003; Andersson, 1998; van Baarsen, 2002), personality factors such as neuroticism and extraversion (or introversion; Long & Martin, 2000; Pinquart & Sorensen, 2001), and differences between the experience of being alone and feeling lonely (Adams, Sanders, & Auth, 2004). When depression is experienced as loneliness, it may be classified, by older adults and by their doctors, as a normal outcome of aging. As such, "depression as loneliness" may not trigger further diagnostic assessment. Older adults may view loneliness as a gateway or precursor to depression; that is, if left unaddressed, loneliness can lead to mental illness (Barg et al., 2006; Luborsky & Riley, 1997; Wittink, Dahlberg, Biruk, & Barg, 2008). Loneliness may be a more acceptable, less stigmatizing way to express depressive symptoms.

Behavioral Pathways

Major depression is strongly correlated with behavioral disorders such as nicotine and alcohol dependence (Hasin, Stinson, Ogburn, & Grant, 2007; John, Meyer, Rumpf, & Hapke, 2004). However, the robustness of the associations between less severe depressive symptoms and more normative health behaviors such as regular smoking (Benjet, Wagner, Borges, & Medina-Mora, 2004; Sachs-Ericsson et al., 2009), alcohol use (Golding, Burnam, Wells, & Benjamin, 1993), and overall (as opposed to visceral) obesity (Sachs-Ericsson et al., 2007) are less clear and vary by characteristics such as age, gender, socioeconomic status, and race/ethnicity. Part of this inconsistency may be due to how these behaviors interact with the neuroendocrine stress response, a system that has been implicated in the pathophysiology of both depression and medical conditions such as diabetes and cardiovascular disease.

In the past two decades a growing body of research has begun to elucidate the neurobiology underlying the stress response and stress-coping strategies, including the neurobiology of health behaviors that are the leading causes of preventable morbidity and mortality in the world. Many of the neurobiological systems that drive the physiologic stress response have also been implicated in depression (McEwen & Seeman, 1999; Sapolsky, 2002). Animal and human research has identified palatable foods, cigarette smoking, and alcohol consumption as behaviors initiated and used to cope with the psychological stress experience (Adam & Epel, 2007; Kalivas & Volkow, 2005; Marinelli & Piazza, 2002; Uhart & Wand, 2009; Volkow & Wise, 2005). The interactions between stress and these poor health behaviors are complex, and although the exact mechanisms are not completely understood, evidence suggests that these substances simultaneously activate the body's stress response system and elicit rewarding and reinforcing effects when consumed in response to stress (Jackson & Knight, 2006).

As described next, the hypothalamic-pituitary-adrenal (HPA) axis is a major pathway through which the body responds to stress (McEwen & Seeman, 1999; Sapolsky, 2002). Intake of nicotine (the main active ingredient in cigarettes), alcohol, and many illicit drugs (e.g., cocaine) has been shown to activate the HPA axis, creating a biological reaction similar to that seen in response to stress (Armario, 2010). While acute exposure to substances activates the HPA axis, chronic exposure to substances, as with any stressor, may dysregulate the HPA axis, with the nature of this dysregulation varying by substance. The HPA axis of habitual cigarette smokers remains responsive to nicotine, suggesting that chronic use does not alter the ability of nicotine to activate the HPA axis (Kirschbaum, Wust, & Strasburger, 1992); however, persistent nicotine use dampens the response of the HPA axis to psychosocial stressors (Rohleder & Kirschbaum, 2006). Similarly, a study assessing cortisol in low and high alcohol users found that alcohol use was positively correlated with cortisol levels among low-level users but unrelated to cortisol among high-level users (Thayer, Hall, Sollers, & Fischer, 2006), suggesting the HPA axis was desensitized to alcohol after chronic exposure.

Recent evidence suggests that consuming high-fat and/or high-sugar foods may also alter the HPA axis and the brain's reward systems (Adam & Epel, 2007; Gearhardt et al., 2011). Diets high in these palatable foods have been shown to be associated with higher levels of inflammatory markers (e.g. C-reactive protein and interleukin-6) that are associated with risk of cardiovascular disease and diabetes (Kiecolt-Glaser, 2010). Glucocorticoid release in response to chronic stress stimulates the ingestion of palatable foods and the deposition of fat in the abdomen; these abdominal fat depots are thought to stimulate the metabolic inhibitory feedback signal on corticotropin-releasing hormone (CRH), thereby reducing HPA activity (Dallman et al., 2003; Foster et al., 2009). Palatable food consumption also increases dopamine release into the nucleus accumbens, similar to illicit drugs (Gearhardt et al., 2011; Volkow & Wise, 2005). This is thought to be driven by the endogenous opioid system. Mu-opioids augment the intake of palatable foods; they also prevent GABAergic neurons from inhibiting the dopaminergic system, leading to increased dopamine release in the nucleus accumbens and related regions, heightening the rewarding or reinforcing effects of these foods (Gearhardt et al., 2011; Ulrich-Lai et al., 2010). Studies have shown that stress exposure elicits increased food intake when offered highly palatable food (e.g., lard and sugar) among rats, particularly if they have been exposed to such a diet prior to the stress (Foster et al., 2009). Human research studies indicate cortisol reactivity profiles may also explain differences in eating behaviors during times of stress. Women with higher cortisol reactivity were shown to consume more calories than a low reactivity group shortly after a stressor, while there was no difference in caloric intake between the groups in the absence of the stressor (Epel, Lapidus, & McEwen, 2001). Together these findings suggest that part of the reason that the literature is inconsistent regarding the relationship between mild depressive symptoms and health behaviors is because in the context of stressors (and in environments in which there is limited access to positive coping outlets) such behaviors may serve as a kind of coping strategy via the dampening of the biological stress response, thereby alleviating the psychological experience of distress (Steptoe, Wardle, Pollard, Canaan, & Davies, 1996). Thus, the total effect of such poor health behaviors in the context of stress may be to alleviate feelings of psychological distress while damaging physical health (Jackson, Knight, & Rafferty, 2010).

It is important to acknowledge that health behaviors may also act through psychological and social pathways. For example, eating behavior is influenced by whether one is eating alone or with others (Davis, Murphy, & Meuhaus, 1988; Nestle et al., 1998; Redd & de Castro, 1992). Smokers may experience a physiologic relief when they take a smoke break, but this break also provides a psychological break from work, and potentially an opportunity to socialize with other smokers. Even though the biological correlates of these behaviors are now coming into focus, we cannot assume behaviors link depression and medical comorbidity only through biological pathways.

A robust literature links depression to reduced adherence to medical care regimens and preventative health behaviors (Gonzalez et al., 2008), including poor adherence to aspirin regimens, smoking cessation, healthy dietary habits, antihypertensive regimens, and physical rehabilitation (Anda et al., 1990; DiMatteo, Lepper, & Croghan, 2000; Kiecolt-Glaser, 2010). Among those with diabetes, depression is associated with poor adherence to oral hypoglycemic agents (Ciechanowski, Katon, & Russo, 2000), self-care regimens (Gonzalez et al., 2008), poor glycemic control, increased risk of complications (de Groot et al., 2001), and progression of micro- and macro-vascular complications (Black, Markides, & Ray, 2003). Persons with mental illness are just as likely as others to want to quit smoking (Hall & Prochaska, 2009) but are much less successful at long-term abstinence (Prochaska, 2011). Clinical care models are needed that explicitly account for the influence depression can have on a patient's ability to adhere to regimens for medical conditions (Bogner & de Vries, 2010; Zivin & Kales, 2008).

Biological Pathways

Investigators seeking to understand the biological mechanisms linking depression and medical conditions have drawn attention to cardiovascular, immunologic, inflammatory, metabolic, and neuroendocrine mediators (Alexopoulos et al., 2002). Much of the inference linking depression with biological factors has been based on cross-sectional studies comparing levels of a purported mediator in persons with depression to persons without depression. Reliance on cross-sectional studies is understandable from a logistical point of view, but we must recognize the limitations from such evidence. Persons with depression may differ in many ways from persons without depression, which could account for observed differences in a purported mediator. Since depression as currently diagnosed and understood may represent as yet poorly characterized diverse subtypes, no single biological mechanism is likely to account for all associations of depression with medical illness. The relationship between depression and medical comorbidity is *dynamic*—the product of a trajectory of biological mechanisms but also of social, psychological, and behavioral factors. Sorting the biological pathways linking depression and medical illness into cardiovascular, immunologic, inflammatory, metabolic, and neuroendocrine channels is a simplification. In late life, we cannot afford the simplicity of considering "mind" as separate from "body." Depression is best conceptualized as a "whole-body" disorder (Wolkowitz, Epel, & Mellon, 2008; Wolkowitz, Epel, Reus, & Mellon, 2010).

In the 1930s, Hans Selye recognized the role of the HPA axis in the response and adaptation of an organism to stress. Perception of stress is transmitted to the hypothalamus and begins a cascade of events: CRH from the hypothalamus stimulates the pituitary to release corticotropin into plasma (corticotropin is also called adrenocorticotropic hormone, ACTH), and circulating corticotropin results in cortisol release from the adrenal cortex (McEwen, 1998). Hypothalamic cortisol receptors exposed to the circulation decrease CRH production to maintain homeostasis. Depression is associated with HPA axis dysregulation (Ehlert, Gaab, & Heinrichs, 2001; Maas et al., 1994). Patients with depression may have elevated cortisol levels in plasma (Burke, Davis, Otte, & Mohr, 2005), elevated CRH levels in cerebrospinal fluid, and increased CRH messenger RNA and protein in limbic brain regions (Merali et al., 2004). Chronic stress-related HPA dysregulation leads to several neuroendocrine changes, including increased CRH, decreased BDNF (brain-derived neurotropic factor), decreased DHEA (dihydroepiandrosterone), and decreased anti-inflammatory cytokines (IL-10). HPA dysregulation leads to changes in gene expression and neurotoxic effects in prefrontal cortex and hippocampus (Wolkowitz et al., 2010; Wolkowitz, Epel, & Mellon, 2008).

Elevated cortisol associated with depression has wide-ranging consequences. A review of the evidence on cortisol, depression, and medical illness found the evidence was strong for an association between major depression and cognitive impairment, hippocampal atrophy, increased waist-hip ratio, decreased bone mineral density, hypertension, and type 2 diabetes mellitus (Brown, Varghese, & McEwen, 2004). Elevated cortisol levels increase visceral fat and could increase the risk of cardiovascular disease among persons with depression

(Brown, Varghese, & McEwen, 2004). Low bone mineral density is associated with HPA axis dysregulation and is disproportionately represented among persons with depression (Williams et al., 2009). While depression may influence bone mineral density through smoking, alcohol consumption, diet, and physical activity, cytokines may play a role (Penninx et al., 2003). In diabetes, depression-associated changes such as increased glucocorticoids contribute to insulin resistance and poor glycemic control (Musselman, Betan, Larsen, & Phillips, 2003).

The idea that emotional stress and cardiovascular disease are linked has a long history (Brotman, Golden, & Wittstein, 2007), but not until the 1970s did research document an association between cardiovascular disease and a constellation of hostility, high achievement, impatience, and competitiveness (Friedman & Rosenman, 1971). Hostility emerged as the most potent contributor to cardiovascular disease (Williams & Williams, 2006) but was also correlated with other risk factors (e.g., high cholesterol, depression, hypertension) that contribute to mortality and morbidity (Suls & Bunde, 2005). Research has associated depression with vascular changes in the heart and cerebrum (Krishnan, Hays, & Blazer, 1997; Krishnan, 1993), ventricular tachycardia (Carney, Freedland, Rich, Smith, & Jaffe, 1993), decreased R to R variability in the electrocardiogram (Carney et al., 2000), and increased platelet aggregation and hypercoagulability (Kop et al., 2002; Kuijpers, Hamulyak, Strik, Wellens, & Honig, 2002; Laghrissi-Thode, Wagner, Pollock, Johnson, & Finkel, 1997; Pollock, Laghrissi-Thode, & Wagner, 2000; Whyte et al., 2001). The relationship between biological markers and cardiovascular disease may be specific to the type of depression (i.e., "somatic" depression may be more closely associated with biological markers than "cognitive/affective" depression), while the influence of depression on prognosis may be primarily through behavioral factors such as adherence to medical regimens (Ormel & de Jonge, 2011).

Random variation and unknown or unmeasured factors may account for differences across samples in how depression is associated with immunologic parameters, but taken together a general pattern of diminished immunologic function in depression emerges. Recognition of the cytokine link to depression arose from observations of the psychiatric consequences of treatment with interferon (Malek-Ahmadi & Hilsabeck, 2007;

Myint, Schwarz, Steinbusch, & Leonard, 2009). A meta-analysis revealed that depression was associated with lymphopenia and relative neutrophilia; increased CD4/CD8 ratio (T-cell helper to suppressor ratio); increased circulating haptoglobin, IL-6, and PGE_2 (all inflammatory markers); reduced NK cell toxicity ("natural killer" cells involved in viral defense); and reduced lymphoproliferative response to mitogen (Zorrilla et al., 2001). Depression has been associated with increased proinflammatory cytokines (Kop et al., 2002; Musselman et al., 2001) and higher levels of inflammatory markers such as C-reactive protein (CRP; Miller, Stetler, Carney, Freedland, & Banks, 2002). HPA dysregulation may alter immune response, including diminished NK and cytotoxic T-lymphocyte function (Evans et al., 2002) and decreased macrophage function (de Beaurepaire, 2002). Some of the association of depression with inflammatory markers such as CRP and IL-6 may be mediated through the association of depression with health behaviors (physical inactivity, BMI, and smoking; Duivis et al., 2011; Golden et al., 2007).

Studies with a specific focus on susceptibility genes that might underlie the association between depression and cardiovascular disease, diabetes, or cancer are few. In twin models, there was little evidence for a common genetic predisposition to major depression and cardiovascular disease (Kendler et al., 2009). Inference about genetic influence based on twin studies does not identify a specific gene. Nevertheless, few genes purported to be associated with depression have found consistent validation (Lopez-Leon et al., 2008). Uncertainty remains even for the role of polymorphisms of the promoter region of the serotonin transporter gene (Belmaker &Agam, 2008; Risch et al., 2009).

AN INTEGRATED MODEL OF DEPRESSION, STRESS, RESOURCES, AND BEHAVIOR

Mental and physical health must be considered jointly both in research and clinical care of older adults (Katz, 1996). At the same time, attempts to understand the natural history of psychopathology and medical comorbidity should also account for contextual factors such as race, socioeconomic position, and place (and the confluence of these factors). Although genetic factors are more often implicated in early-onset conditions, including early-onset

depression, environmental factors are predominant in the risk, prognosis, and consequences of depression in later life (Katz, 1996). The social environment is both a source of constraints (e.g., stressors) as well as a source of *resources*, that is, opportunities to alleviate stressors (Gibson, 1977). The physical resources available to socially disadvantaged groups that promote health are greatly truncated relative to more advantaged groups (e.g., access to parks and recreation areas), while riskier strategies are highly accessible. For example, socially disadvantaged groups experience considerable limitations in obtaining reasonably priced healthy food and safely engaging in outdoor recreational activities that promote health and prevent disease (Lovasi, Hudson, Guerra & Neckerman, 2009); these same groups have ready access to tobacco and alcohol retailers (LaVeist & Wallace, 2000) and fast food restaurants (Lovasi, Hudson, Guerra & Neckerman, 2009). Strategies to mitigate distress are influenced by a number of contextual factors, including socioeconomic position, the physical environment, cultural norms, race/ethnicity, gender, and age factors (Abdou et al., 2010; Taylor & Stanton, 2007; Umberson, Liu, & Reczek, 2008). Collectively, these contextual factors set the stage for individuals to turn to particular behaviors that alleviate the symptoms of stress in the short term both psychologically and physiologically, while potentially harming long-term health (Jackson, 2002).

Foremost, we acknowledge that a static, two-dimensional figure is an inherently incomplete illustration of the ways in which the pathways described earlier may moderate and/or moderate how depression is related to medical comorbidity, particularly over the life span. Figure 16.2 provides a schematic of how stress, resources, and race intersect with psychiatric and medical comorbidity. This model can be used as a heuristic tool to approach conflicting or inconsistent results across studies that are otherwise difficult to reconcile. It also provides a means of mixing clinical and research paradigms in a cohesive manner.

Stress is an established risk factor for depression (Kessler, 1997); however, the role that stress plays in medical-psychiatric comorbidity has been underexplored. In their seminal study of stress and depression risk, Brown and Harris (1978) identified four broad types of life events related to depression: humiliation, loss, threat, and entrapment (Brown & Harris, 1978). They argued that events characterized by humiliation and loss were more strongly

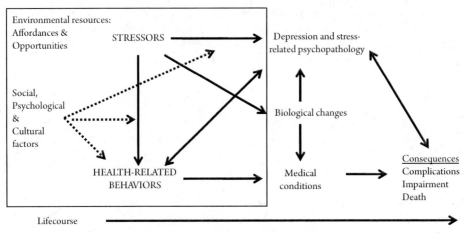

FIGURE 16.2 Conceptual diagram of depression and medical comorbidity.

related to onset of depression than the others. While this study focused primarily on exogenous life events (e.g., divorce, moving, death of a loved one, job loss), it is worth considering how receiving a diagnosis of a chronic medical illness such as diabetes may fit within this typology of events. Clearly there is an element of threat, particularly in the case of a life-threatening diagnosis such as cancer or a heart attack. But there are also aspects of entrapment and humiliation, particularly for diseases that require intense patient self-management and substantial behavior change to adequately control, such as diabetes. For example, a recent qualitative study reported that diabetes patients found it difficult to comply with new meal plans and medication protocols to keep their blood sugar under control, which they reported created additional time pressure and limited their ability to travel and make plans. To deal with this stress, patients reported sometimes engaging in behaviors such as eating high-fat and high-sugar foods, which they referred to as "taking a diabetes break" (Penckofer, Ferrans, Velsor-Friedrich, & Savoy, 2007). Figure 16.2 emphasizes that exposure to stress and coping health behaviors are influenced by environmental resources and social and cultural factors. In particular, due to the confluence of race/ethnicity and socioeconomic position, racial minority status is a critical determining factor in the availability and efficacy of coping resources, in addition to being a critical determinant of the type and degree of stress exposure (e.g., unfair treatment on the basis of race). Certain behaviors are associated with lower risk of medical illness (e.g., social integration and support, physical activity), while others are associated with higher risk (e.g., smoking, poor diet).

Conceptual models can help us reconcile unexpected findings concerning the intersections of depression, medical comorbidity, and race. For example, in the United States, Blacks and Hispanics generally have lower risk of most psychiatric and substance use disorders relative to Whites; however, these groups have substantially higher burden of overall medical morbidity and mortality, particularly for chronic conditions such as type 2 diabetes, cardiovascular disease, and cancer (Jackson, Knight, & Rafferty, 2010; Mezuk et al., 2010). This observation indicates that the relationship between psychiatric conditions and medical morbidity may differ across social groups. In an example from experimental data, the Enhancing Recovery in Coronary Heart Disease (ENRICH-D) Trial, a randomized controlled trial of cognitive-behavioral therapy for depressed patients who had recently had a heart attack, found no overall effect of the intervention on risk of subsequent cardiac events, despite demonstrating a significant reduction in depressive symptoms, relative to usual care (Berkman et al., 2003). However, in a reanalysis of this data investigators reported a significant protective effect of the intervention for White men, but not White women or minority (predominantly Black and Hispanic) men or women (Schneiderman et al., 2004). This finding is particularly unexpected because the intervention was associated with a significant decrease in depressive symptoms for all groups. Gender and race influence the relationship between depression and medical morbidity and should be considered in the design of interventions that account for group differences.

The model also emphasizes the importance of the *life course* in understanding the complexity of the relationships between stress, behavior and psychiatric and medical comorbidity. Over the life course, the relationship between psychiatric and medical conditions may change; turning to diabetes again, depression is predictive of onset of type 2 diabetes (indicating that diabetes is secondary to depression), but among those with diabetes, functional impairment and complications are associated with risk of depression (indicating that depression is secondary to diabetes). These relationships are also dynamic on shorter time scales that accumulate over the course of an illness (e.g., how depressive symptoms influence and are influenced by adherence to self-care regimens, such as regular glucose testing and medication use, as well as preventive health behaviors such as modifying dietary intake). While these relationships are reciprocal, the relative importance of each of these factors varies in predictable ways over the life course. From a clinical standpoint, gaining a comprehensive understanding of the contextual factors and how these factors have accumulated over the life course can inform which intervention efforts may be most effective, and which are likely to fail to achieve long-term benefits.

LINKING CONCEPTUAL AND CLINICAL GUIDEPOSTS

Depression and medical comorbidity remains a rapidly changing and challenging arena of immense importance for public health and for clinical practice. We have only scratched the surface of the complex relationship of depression with medical comorbidity, painting with broad brush strokes the links along psychological, social, behavioral, and biological pathways. We traced the origins of disparities in depression across the arc of the life course to the variations in rates and expression of depression observed in late life. The four pathways act as clinical guideposts: What psychological, social, behavioral, or biological factors are most pressing to address to improve health outcomes? What factors are associated with treatment acceptance and adherence?

Because medical comorbidity can affect depression presentation (Wittink, Barg, & Gallo, 2006), identification (Bogner, Ford, & Gallo, 2006; Crane, Bogner, Rabins, & Gallo, 2006), outcomes (Bogner et al., 2005), and mortality (Bogner, Morales, Post, & Bruce, 2007; Gallo et al., 2007; Gallo, Bogner, Morales, Post, et al., 2005), the challenge is to develop methods and interventions that account

for the context of medical comorbidity. Many older adults do not conceptualize their depression as a medical illness but rather associate their problems with grief, isolation, health concerns, lack of mobility, and lack of resources with the need to "pick yourself up by your own bootstraps" rather than rely on outside help (Switzer et al., 2006). Compared to persons without depression or other psychiatric conditions, persons with comorbid psychiatric disorders and medical conditions such as diabetes and cardiovascular disease may receive a poorer quality of medical care (Mitchell, Malone, & Doebbeling, 2009), though multiple medical conditions do not necessarily signal less depression treatment (Dickinson et al., 2008). The Institute of Medicine has recognized that new models of service delivery are needed that integrate depression and the community (Institute of Medicine, 2008). For these new models to be effective, they must also be informed by a multidisciplinary perspective and reflect the contexts in which individuals live and age.

Disclosures

Dr. Mezuk has no conflicts to disclose. She is funded by NIMH K01-MH093642-A1. She would like to thank Matthew C. Lohman and Scott M. Ratliff for their assistance with creating the figures for this chapter.

Dr. Gallo has no conflicts to disclose. He is funded by NIMH K24MH070407.

REFERENCES

Abdou, C. M., Dunkel, S. C., Jones, F., Rubinov, E., Tsai, S., Jones, L., et al. (2010). Community perspectives: Mixed methods investigation of culture, stress, family, and health in poor communities. *Ethnicity and Disease, 20*, 41–48.

Adam, T. C., & Epel, E. S. (2007). Stress, eating and the reward system. *Physiology and Behavior, 91*, 449–458.

Adams, K.B., Sanders, S., & Auth, E. A. (2004). Loneliness and depression in independent living retirement communities: Risk and resilience factors *Aging and Mental Health, 8*(6), 475–485.

Alexopoulos, G. S., Buckwalter, J. G., Olin, J., Martinez, R., Wainscott, C., & Krishnan, K. R. R. (2002). Comorbidity of late life depression: An opportunity for research on mechanisms and treatment. *Biological Psychiatry, 52*, 543–558.

Ali, S., Stone, M. A., Peters, J. L., Davies, M. J., & Khunti, K. (2006). The prevalence of co-morbid depression in adults with Type 2 diabetes: A systematic review and meta-analysis. *Diabetes Medicine, 23*(11), 1165–1173.

Alpass, F. M., & Neville, S. (2003). Loneliness, health and depression in older males. *Aging and Mental Health, 7*(3), 212–216.

Armario A. (2010). Activation of the hypothalamic-pituitary-adrenal axis by addictive drugs: Different pathways, common outcome. *Trends in Pharmacology Science, 31*(7), 318–325.

Anda, R., Williamson, D., Escobedo, L., Mast, E., Giovino, G., & Remington, P. (1990). Depression and the dynamics of smoking: A national perspective. *Journal of American Medical Association, 264*(12), 1541–1545.

Anda, R., Williamson, D., Jones, D., Macera, C., Eaker, E., Glassman, A., & Marks, J. (1993). Depressed affect, hopelessness, and the risk of ischemic heart disease in a cohort of U.S. adults. *Epidemiology, 4*(4), 285–294.

Anderson, R. J., Freedland, K. E., Clouse, R. E., & Lustman, P. J. (2001). The prevalence of comorbid depression in adults with diabetes: A meta-analysis. *Diabetes Care, 24*(6), 1069–1078.

Andersson, L. (1998). Loneliness research and interventions: A review of the literature. *Aging and Mental Health, 2*(4), 264–274.

Aromaa, A., Raitasalo, R., Reunanen, A., Impivaara, O., Heliovaara, M., Knekt, P., … Maatela, J. (1994). Depression and cardiovascular diseases. *Acta Psychiatrica Scandinavica Supplement, 377*, 77–82.

Atlantis, E., Browning, C., Sims, J., & Kendig, H. (2010). Diabetes incidence associated with depression and antidepressants in the Melbourne Longitudinal Studies on Healthy Ageing (MELSHA). *International Journal of Geriatric Psychiatry, 25*(7), 688–696.

Baer, R. D., Weller, S. C., Garcia de alba Garcia, J., & Salcedo Rocha, A. L. (2004). A comparison of community and physician explanatory models of AIDS in Mexico and the United States. *Medical Anthropology Quarterly, 18*, 3–22.

Bane, C., Hughes, C. M., & McElnay, J. C. (2006). The impact of depressive symptoms and psychosocial factors on medication adherence in cardiovascular disease. *Patient Education Counseling, 60*(2), 187–193.

Barg, F. K., Huss-Ashmore, R., Wittink, M. N., Murray, G. F., Bogner, H. R., & Gallo, J. J. (2006). A mixed methods approach to understand loneliness and depression in older adults. *Journal of Gerontology: Social Sciences, 61*(6), S329–S339.

Bartels, S. J., Coakley, E., Oxman, T. E., Constantino, G., Oslin, D., Chen, H., … Sanchez, H. (2002). Suicidal and death ideation in older primary care patients with depression, anxiety, and at-risk alcohol use. *American Journal of Geriatric Psychiatry, 10*(4), 417–427.

Bartels, S. J. (2004). Caring for the whole person: Integrated health care for older adults with severe mental illness and medical comorbidity. *Journal of the American Geriatrics Society, 52*, S249–S257.

Beck, A. T., Brown, G., Berchick, R. J., Stewart, B. L., & Steer, R. A. (1990). Relationship between hopelessness and ultimate suicide: A replication with psychiatric outpatients. *American Journal of Psychiatry, 147*(2), 190–195.

Beck, A. T., Weissman, A., Lester, D., & Trexler, L. (1974). The measurement of pessimism: the hopelessness scale. *Journal of Consulting and Clinical Psychology, 42*(6), 861–865.

Beevers, C. G., & Miller, I. W. (2004). Perfectionism, cognitive bias, and hopelessness as prospective predictors of suicidal ideation. *Suicide and Life Threatening Behavior, 34*(2), 126–137.

Belmaker, R. H., & Agam, G. (2008). Major depressive disorder. *New England Journal of Medicine, 358*(1), 55–68.

Benjet, C., Wagner, F. A., Borges, G. G., & Medina-Mora, M. E. (2004). The relationship of tobacco smoking with depressive symptomatology in the Third Mexican National Addictions Survey. *Psychological Medicine, 34*, 881–888.

Berkman, L. F. (1995). The role of social relations in health promotion. *Psychosomatic Medicine, 57*, 245–254.

Berkman, L. F., Blumenthal, J., Burg, M., Carney, R. M., Catellier, D., Cowan, M. J., … Schneiderman, N. (2003). Effects of treating depression and low perceived social support on clinical events after myocardial infarction: The Enhancing Recovery in Coronary Heart Disease Patients (ENRICHD) Randomized Trial. *Journal of the American Medical Association, 289*, 3106–3116.

Berkman, L. F., Glass, T., Brissette, I., & Seeman, T. E. (2000). From social integration to health: Durkheim in the new millennium. *Social Science and Medicine, 51*, 843–857.

Black, S. A., Markides, K. S., & Ray, L. A. (2003). Depression predicts increased incidence of adverse health outcomes in older Mexican Americans with type 2 diabetes. *Diabetes Care, 26*(10), 2822–2828.

Bogner, H. R., Dahlberg, B., de Vries, H. F., Cahill, E., & Barg, F. K. (2008). Older patients' views on the relationship between depression and heart disease. *Family Medicine, 40*(9), 652–657.

Bogner, H. R., Morales, K. H., Post, E. P., & Bruce, M. L. (2007). Depression, diabetes, and death: A randomized controlled trial of a depression treatment program for older adults based in

primary care (PROSPECT). *Diabetes Care,*
30(12), 3005–3010.

Bogner, H.R., Cahill, E., Frauenhoffer, C., & Barg,
F. K. (2009). Older primary care patient views
regarding antidepressants: A mixed methods
approach. *Journal of Mental Health, 18*(1), 57–64.

Bogner, H. R., Cary, M. S., Bruce, M. L., Reynolds,
C. F., Mulsant, B., Ten-Have, T., & Alexopoulos,
G. S. (2005). The role of medical comorbidity on
outcomes of major depression in primary care: The
PROSPECT Study. *American Journal of Geriatric
Psychiatry, 13*, 861–868.

Bogner, H. R., Ford, D. E., & Gallo, J. J. (2006). The
role of cardiovascular disease in the identification
and management of depression by primary care
physicians. *American Journal of Geriatric Psychiatry,
14*(1), 71–78.

Boyd, C. M., Darer, J., Boult, C., Fried, L. P., Boult, L.,
& Wu, A. W. (2005). Clinical practice guidelines
and quality of care for older patients with multiple
comorbid diseases: Implications for pay for
performance. *Journal of the American Medical
Assocation, 294*(6), 716–724.

Breslau, J., Aguilar-Gaxiola, S., & Kendler, K. S.
(2006). Specifying race-ethnic differences in risk
for psychiatric diosrder in a USA national sample.
Psychological Medicine, 36, 57–68.

Broadhead, W. E., Blazer, D. G., George, L. K., & Tse,
C. K. (1990). Depression, disability days, and days
lost from work in a prospective epidemiologic
survey. *Journal of the American Medical Association,
264*, 2524–2528.

Brotman, D. J., Golden, S. H., & Wittstein, I. S.
(2007). The cardiovascular toll of stress. *Lancet,
370*(9592), 1089–1100.

Brown, E. S., Varghese, F. P., & McEwen, B. S. (2004).
Association of depression with medical illness:
Does cortisol play a role? *Biological Psychiatry,
55*(1), 1–9.

Brown, G. K., Beck, A. T., Steer, R. A., & Grisham, J.
R. (2000). Risk factors for suicide in psychiatric
outpatients: A 20-year prospective study.
Journal of Consulting and Clinical Psychology, 68,
374–377.

Brown, G. W., Bifulco, A., & Andrews, B. (1990).
Self-esteem and depression. III. Aetiological issues.
*Social Psychiatry and Psychiatric Epidemiology,
25*(5), 235–243.

Brown, G. W., Bifulco, A., Veiel, H. O., & Andrews,
B. (1990). Self-esteem and depression. II. Social
correlates of self-esteem. *Social Psychiatry and
Psychiatric Epidemiology, 25*(5), 225–234.

Brown, G. W., & Harris, T. (1978). *Social origins of
depression: A study of psychiatric disorder in women.*
London: Tavistock.

Burke, H. M., Davis, M. C., Otte, C., & Mohr, D.
C. (2005). Depression and cortisol responses
to psychological stress: A meta-analysis.
Psychoneuroendocrinology, 30(9), 846–856.

Bush, D. E., Ziegelstein, R. C., Tayback, M., Richter,
D., Stevens, S., Zahalsky, H., & Fauerbach, J. A.
(2001). Even minimal symptoms of depression
increase mortality risk after acute myocardial
infarction. *American Journal of Cardiology, 88*(4),
337–341.

Byrne, G. J., & Raphael, B. (1999). Depressive
symptoms and depressive episodes in recently
widowed older men. *International Psychogeriatrics,
11*(1), 67–74.

Callahan, C., Hendrie, H., Nienaber, N., & Tierney,
W. (1996). Suicidal ideation among older primary
care patients. *Journal of the American Geriatrics
Society, 44*, 1205–1209.

Carney, R. M., Freedland, K. E., Rich, M. W., Smith, L.
J., & Jaffe, A. S. (1993). Ventricular tachycardia and
psychiatric depression in patients with coronary
artery disease. *American Journal of Medicine, 95*(1),
23–28.

Carney, R. M., Freedland, K. E., Stein, P. K., Skala,
J. A., Hoffman, P., & Jaffe, A. S. (2000). Change
in heart rate and heart rate variability during
treatment for depression in patients with coronary
heart disease. *Psychosomatic Medicine, 62*(5),
639–647.

Chao, J., Nau, D. P., Aikens, J. E., & Taylor, J. E.
(2005). The mediating role of health beliefs in the
relationship between depressive symptoms and
medication adherence in persons with diabetes.
*Research in Social and Administrative Pharmacy,
1*(4), 508–525.

Chavez, L. R., Hubbell, F. A., McMullin, J. M.,
Martinez, R. G., & Mishra, S. I. (1995).
Structure and meaning in models of breast and
cervical cancer risk factors: A comparison of
perceptions among Latinas, Anglo women, and
physicians. *Medical Anthropology Quarterly, 9*(1),
40–74.

Christakis, N. A., & Fowler, J. H. (2008). The
collective dynamics of smoking in a large social
network. *New England Journal of Medicine, 358*,
2249–2258.

Ciechanowski, P. S., Katon, W. J., & Russo, J. E.
(2000). Depression and diabetes: Impact of
depressive symptoms on adherence, function,
and costs. *Archives of Internal Medicine, 160*(21),
3278–3285.

Clark, P., & Smith, J. (2011). Aging in a cultural
context: cross-national differences in disability and
the moderating role of personal control among
older adults in the United States and England.

Journals of Gerontology Series B, Psychological Sciences Social Sciences, 66, 457–467.

Conner, K. O., Copeland, V. C., Grote, N. K., Koeske, G., Rosen, D., Reynolds, C. F., & Brown, C. (2010). Mental health treatment seeking among older adults with depression: The impact of stigma and race. American Journal of Geriatric Psychiatry, 18, 531–543.

Cooper, L. A., Gonzales, J. J., Gallo, J. J., Rost, K. M., Meredith, L. S., Rubenstein, L. V., ... Quality Improvement for Depression Consortium. (2003). The acceptability of treatment for depression among African-American and white primary care patients. Medical Care, 41, 479–489.

Copeland, J. R. M., Davidson, I. A., Dewey, M. E., Gilmore, C., Larkin, B. A., McWilliam, C., ... Sullivan, C. (1992). Alzheimer's disease, other dementias, depression and pseudodementia prevalence, incidence, and three year outcome in Liverpool. British Journal of Psychiatry, 161, 230–239.

Copeland, J. R. M., Gurland, B. J., Dewey, M. E., Kelleher, M. J., Smith, A. M., & Davidson, I. A. (1987). Is there more depression and neurosis in New York? A comparative community study of the elderly in New York and London using the computer diagnosis AGECAT. British Journal of Psychiatry, 151, 466–473.

Coreil, J., Wilke, J., & Pintado, I. (2004). Cultural models of illness and recovery in breast cancer support groups. Qualitative Health Research, 14(7), 905–923.

Crane, M. K., Bogner, H. R., Rabins, P. V., & Gallo, J. J. (2006). Patient cognitive status and the identification and active management of depression by primary care physicians. Journal of General Internal Medicine, 21(10), 1042–1044.

Dahlberg, B., Barg, F. K., Gallo, J. J., & Wittink, M. N. (2009). Bridging psychiatric and anthropological approaches: The case of "nerves" in the United States. Ethos, 37, 283–313.

Dallman, M. F., Akana, S. F., Laugero, K. D., Gomez, F., Manalo, S., Bell, M. E., & Bhatnagar, S. 2003. A spoonful of sugar: Feedback signals of energy stores and corticosterone regulate responses to chronic stress. Physiology and Behavior, 79, 3–12.

Davidson, K. W., Burg, M. M., Kronish, I. M., Shimbo, D., Dettenborn, L., Mehran, R., ... Rieckmann, N. (2010). Association of anhedonia with recurrent major adverse cardiac events and mortality 1 year after acute coronary syndrome. Archives of General Psychiatry, 67(5), 480–488.

Davis, M. A., Murphy, S. P., & Meuhaus, J. M. (1988). Living arrangements and eating behaviors of older adults in the United States. Journal of Gerontology, 43, S96–S98.

de Beaurepaire, R. (2002). Questions raised by the cytokine hypothesis of depression. Brain, Behavior, and Immunity, 16, 610–617.

de Groot, M., Anderson, R., Freedland, K. E., Clouse, R. E., & Lustman, P. J. (2001). Association of depression and diabetes complications: A meta-analysis. Psychosomatic Medicine, 63(4), 619–630.

De Leon, C. F., Grady, K. L., Eaton, C., Rucker-Whitaker, C., Janssen, I., Calvin, J., & Powell, L. H. (2009). Quality of life in a diverse population of patients with heart failure. Journal of Cardiopulmonary Rehabilitation and Prevention, 29, 171–178.

de Vries, H. F., Northington, G. M., & Bogner, H. R. (2011). Urinary incontinence and new psychological distress among community dwelling older adults. Archives of Gerontology and Geriatrics, 55(1), 49–54.

Dickinson, L. M., Dickinson, W. P., Rost, K., DeGruy, F., Emsermann, C., Froshaug, D., ... Meredith, L. (2008). Clinician burden and depression treatment: Disentangling patient- and clinician-level effects of medical comorbidity. Journal of General Internal Medicine, 23(11), 1763–1769.

DiMatteo, M., Lepper, H., & Croghan, T. (2000). Depression is a risk factor for noncompliance with medical treatment: Meta-analysis of the effects of anxiety and depression on patient adherence. Archives of Internal Medicine, 160(14), 2101–2107.

Duivis, H. E., de Jonge, P., Penninx, B. W., Na, B. Y., Cohen, B. E., & Whooley, M. A. (2011). Depressive symptoms, health behaviors, and subsequent inflammation in patients with coronary heart disease: Prospective findings from the heart and soul study. American Journal of Psychiatry, 168(9), 913–920.

Eaton, W. W. (2002). Epidemiologic evidence on the comorbidity of depression and diabetes. Journal of Psychosomatic Research, 53(4), 903–6.

Eaton, W. W., Anthony, J. C., Gallo, J. J., Cai, G., Tien, A., Romanoski, A., & Lyketsos, C. (1997). Natural history of Diagnostic Interview Schedule / DSM-IV major depression: The Baltimore Epidemiologic Catchment Area follow-up. Archives of General Psychiatry, 54, 993–999.

Eaton, W. W., Armenian, H., Gallo, J. J., Pratt, L., & Ford, D. E. (1996). Depression and risk for onset of type II diabetes. Diabetes Care, 19, 1097–1102.

Eaton, W. W., Kalaydjian, A., Scharfstein, D. O., Mezuk, B., & Ding, Y. (2007). Prevalence and incidence of depressive disorder: The Baltimore

ECA follow-up, 1981–2004. *Acta Psychiatrica Scandinavica, 116*, 182–188.

Eaton, W. W., Shao, H., Nestadt, G., Lee, B. H., Bienvenu, O. J., & Zandi, P. (2008). Population-based study of first onset and chronicity in major depressive disorder. *Archives of General Psychiatry, 65*, 513–520.

Egede, L. E. 2004. Diabetes, major depression, and functional disability among U.S. adults. *Diabetes Care, 27*(2), 421–428.

Egede, L. E., Nietert, P. J., & Zheng, D. (2005). Depression and all-cause and coronary heart disease mortality among adults with and without diabetes. *Diabetes Care, 28*(6), 1339–1345.

Ehlert, U., Gaab, J., & Heinrichs, M. (2001). Psychoneuroendocrinological contributions to the etiology of depression, posttraumatic stress disorder, and stress-related bodily disorders: The role of the hypothalamus-pituitary-adrenal axis. *Biological Psychology, 57*(1–3), 141–152.

Epel, E., Lapidus, R., McEwen, B., & Brownell, K. (2001). Stress may add bite to appetite in women: A laboratory study of stress-induced cortisol and eating behavior. *Psychoneuroendocrinology, 26*(1), 37–49.

Evans, D. L., Ten Have, T. R., Douglas, S. D., Gettes, D. R., Morrison, M., Chiappini, M. S., ... Petitto, J. M. (2002). Association of depression with viral load, CD8 T lymphocytes, and natural killer cells in women with HIV infection. *American Journal of Psychiatry, 159*(10), 1752–1759.

Everson, S. A., Goldberg, D. E., Kaplan, G. A., Cohen, R. D., Pukkala, E., Tuomilehto, J., & Salonen, J. T. (1996). Hopelessness and risk of mortality and incidence of myocardial infarction and cancer. *Psychosomatic Medicine, 58*(2), 113–121.

Everson, S. A., Kaplan, G. A., Goldberg, D. E., Salonen, R., & Salonen, J. T. (1997). Hopelessness and 4-year progression of carotid atherosclerosis. The Kuopio Ischemic Heart Disease Risk Factor Study. *Arteriosclerosis, Thrombosis, and Vascular Biology, 17*(8), 1490–1495.

Ford, D. E., Mead, L. A., Chang, P. P., Cooper-Patrick, L., Wang, N-Y., & Klag, M. J. (1998). Depression is a risk factor for coronary artery disease in men: The Precursors Study. *Archives of Internal Medicine, 158*(13), 1422–1426.

Foster, M. T., Warne, J. P., Ginsberg, A. B., Horneman, H. F., Pecoraro, N. C., Akana, S. F., & Dallman, M. F. (2009). Palatable foods, stress, and energy stores sculpt corticotrophin-releasing factor, adrenocorticotropin, and corticosterone concentrations after restraint. *Endocrinology, 150*, 2325–2333.

Frasure-Smith, N., Lesperance, F., Habra, M., Talajic, M., Khairy, P., Dorian, P., & Roy, D. (2009). Elevated depression symptoms predict long-term cardiovascular mortality in patients with atrial fibrillation and heart failure. *Circulation, 120*(2), 134–40, 3p following 140.

Frasure-Smith, N., Lesperance, F., & Talajic, M. (1993). Depression following myocardial infarction: Impact on 6-month survival. *Journal of the American Medical Association, 270*(15), 1819–1825.

Frasure-Smith, N., Lesperance, F., & Talajic, M. (1995). Depression and 18-month prognosis after myocardial infarction. *Circulation, 91*, 999–1005.

Fried, L. P., Carlson, M. C., Freedman, M., Frick, K. D., Glass, T. A., Hill, J., ... Zeger, S. (2004). A social model for health promotion for an aging population: Initial evidence on the Experience Corps model. *Journal of Urban Health, 81*, 64–78.

Friedman, G. D. (1990). Depression, worry, and the incidence of cancer, letter. *American Journal of Public Health, 80*, 1396–1397.

Friedman, G. D. (1994). Psychiatrically-diagnosed depression and subsequent cancer. *Cancer Epidemiology, 3*, 11–13.

Friedman, M., & Rosenman, R. H. (1971). Type A behavior pattern: Its association with coronary heart disease. *Annals of Clinical Research, 3*(6), 300–312.

Gallo, J. J., Anthony, J. C., & Muthén, B. O. (1994). Age differences in the symptoms of depression: A latent trait analysis. *Journals of Gerontology: Psychological Sciences, 49*, P251–264.

Gallo, J. J., Armenian, H. K., Ford, D. E., Eaton, W. W., & Khachaturian, A. S. (2000). Major depression and cancer: The 13-year-follow-up of the Baltimore Epidemiologic Catchment Area sample (United States). *Cancer Causes and Control, 11*, 1–8.

Gallo, J. J., Bogner, H. R., Morales, K. H., & Ford, D. E. (2005). Patient ethnicity and the identification and active management of depression in late life. *Archives of Internal Medicine, 165*(17), 1962–1968.

Gallo, J. J., Bogner, H. R., Morales, K. H., Post, E. P., Lin, J. Y., & Bruce, M. L. (2007). The effect on mortality of a practice-based depression intervention program for older adults in primary care: A cluster randomized trial. *Annals of Internal Medicine, 146*(10), 689–698.

Gallo, J. J., Bogner, H. R., Morales, K. H., Post, E. P., Ten Have, T., & Bruce, M. L. (2005). Depression, cardiovascular disease, diabetes, and two-year mortality among older, primary-care patients. *American Journal of Geriatric Psychiatry, 13*, 748–755.

Gallo, J. J., Cooper-Patrick, L., & Lesikar, S. (1998). Depressive symptoms of whites and African

Americans aged 60 years and older. *Journal of Gerontology: Psychological Sciences, 53B,* 277–286.

Gallo, J. J., Rabins, P. V., Lyketsos, C. G., Tien, A. Y., & Anthony, J. C. (1997). Depression without sadness: Functional outcomes of nondysphoric depression in later life. *Journal of the American Geriatrics Society, 45,* 570–578.

Gearhardt, A. N., Yokum, S., Orr, P. T., Stice, E., Corbin, W. R., & Brownell, K. D. (2011). Neural correlates of food addiction. *Archives of General Psychiatry, 68*(8), 808–816.

Gibson, J. J. (1977). The theory of affordances. In R. Shaw & J. Bransford (Eds.), *Perceiving, acting and knowing* (pp. 67–82). Hillsdale, NJ: Erlbaum.

Glassman, A. H., Bigger, J. T., Jr., & Gaffney, M. (2009). Psychiatric characteristics associated with long-term mortality among 361 patients having an acute coronary syndrome and major depression: Seven-year follow-up of SADHART participants. *Archives of General Psychiatry, 66*(9), 1022–1029.

Goldberg, D. P., & Hillier, V. F. (1979). A scaled version of the General Health Questionnaire. *Psychological Medicine, 9,* 139–145.

Golden, S. H., Lazo, M., Carnethon, M., Bertoni, A. G., Schreiner, P. J., Diez Roux, A. V., ... Lyketsos, C. (2008). Examining a bidirectional association between depressive symptoms and diabetes. *Journal of the American Medical Association, 299*(23), 2751–2759.

Golden, S. H., Lee, H. B., Schreiner, P. J., Roux, A. D., Fitzpatrick, A. L., Szklo, M., & Lyketsos, C. (2007). Depression and type 2 diabetes mellitus: The multiethnic study of atherosclerosis. *Psychosomatic Medicine, 69*(6), 529–536.

Golding, J. M., Burnam, M. A., Wells, K. B., & Benjamin, B. (1993). Alcohol use, depressive symptoms, and cultural characteristics in two Mexican-American samples. *International Journal of Addiction, 28,* 451–476.

Gonzalez, J. S., Peyrot, M., McCarl, L. A., Collins, E. M., Serpa, L., Mimiaga, M. J., & Safren, S. A. (2008). Depression and diabetes treatment nonadherence: A meta-analysis. *Diabetes Care, 31*(12), 2398–403.

Good, B. J. (1992). Culture and psychopathology. In T. Schwartz, G. M. White, & C. A. Lutz (Eds.), *New directions in psychological anthropology* (pp. 181–205). Cambridge, England: Cambridge University Press.

Gross, A. L., Gallo, J. J., & Eaton, W. W. (2010). Depression and cancer risk: 24 years of follow-up of the Baltimore Epidemiologic Catchment Area sample. *Cancer Causes and Control, 21*(2), 191–199.

Hall, S. M., & Prochaska, J. J. (2009). Treatment of smokers with co-occurring disorders: Emphasis on integration in mental health and addiction treatment settings. *Annual Review of Clinical Psychology, 5,* 409–431.

Hammond, W. P., Mohottige, D., Chantala, K., Hastings, J. F., Neighbors, H. W., & Snowden, L. (2011). Determinants of usual source of care disparities among African American and Caribbean Black men. *Journal of Health Care for the Poor and Underserved, 22,* 157–175.

Hasin, D. S., Stinson, F. S., Ogburn, E., & Grant, B. F. (2007). Prevalence, correlates, disability, and comorbidity of DSM-IV alcohol abuse and dependence in the United States: Results from the National Epidemiologic Survey on Alcohol and Related Conditions. *Archives of General Psychiatry, 64,* 830–842.

Heeren, T. J., van Hemert, A. M., Lagaay, A. M., & Rooymans, H. G. M. (1992). The general population prevalence of non-organic psychiatric disorders in subjects aged 85 years and over. *Psychological Medicine, 22,* 733–738.

Heo, M., Murphy, C. F., Fontaine, K. R., Bruce, M. L., & Alexopolous, G. S. (2008). Population projection of US adults with lifetime experience of depressive disorder by age and sex from 2005 to 2050. *International Journal of Geriatric Psychiatry, 23,* 1266–1270.

Holt-Lunstad, J., Smith, T. B., & Layton, B. (2010). Social relationships and mortality risk: A meta-analytic review. *PloS, 7,* e1000316.

Hong, S. I., & Morrow-Howell, N. (2010). Health outcomes of Experience Corps: A high-commitment volunteer program. *Social Science and Medicine, 71,* 414–420.

Hoptman, M. J., Gunning-Dixon, F. M., Murphy, C. F., Ardekani, B. A., Hrabe, J., Lim, K. O., ... Alexopoulos, G. S. (2009). Blood pressure and white matter integrity in geriatric depression. *Journal of Affective Disorders, 115,* 171–176.

Institute of Medicine. (2008). *Challenges and successes in reducing health disparities: Workshop summary.* Washington, DC: National Academies Press.

Jackson, J. S. (2002). Health and mental health disparities among Black Americans. In M. Hager (Eds.), *Modern psychiatry: Challenges in educating health professionals to meet new needs* (pp. 246–254). New York: Josiah Macy, Jr. Foundation.

Jackson, J. S., & Knight, K. M. (2006). Race and self-regulatory health behaviors: The role of the stress response and the HPA axis in physical and mental health disparities. In K. W. Schaie, & L. Cartensen (Eds.), *Social structures, aging, and self-regulation in the elderly* (pp. 189–207). New York: Springer.

Jackson, J. S., Knight, K. M., & Rafferty, J. A. (2010). Race and unhealthy behaviors: Chronic stress, the HPA axis, and physical and mental health disparities over the life-course. *American Journal of Public Health, 100,* 933–939.

Jansen, A. S. P., Van Nguyen, X., Karpitskiy, V., Mettenleiter, T. C., & Loewy, A. D. (1995). Central command neurons of the sympathetic nervous system: Basis of the fight-or-flight response. *Science, 270,* 644–646.

John, U., Meyer, C., Rumpf, H. J., & Hapke, U. (2004). Smoking, nicotine dependence and psychiatric comorbidity—a population-based study including smoking cessation after three years. *Drug and Alcohol Dependence, 76,* 287–295.

Judd, F., Davis, J., Hodgins, G., Scopelliti, J., Agin, B., & Hulbert, C. (2004). Rural Integrated Primary Care Psychiatry Programme: A systems approach to education, training and service integration. *Australasian Psychiatry, 12*(1), 42–47.

Juurlink, D., Herrmann, N., Szalai, J., Kopp, A., & Redelmeier, D. (2004). Medical illness and the risk of suicide in the elderly. *Archives of Internal Medicine, 164,* 1179–1184.

Kalivas, P. W., & Volkow, N. D. (2005). The neural basis of addiction: A pathology of motivation and choice. *American Journal of Psychiatry, 162*(8), 1403–1413.

Kaplan, G. A., & Reynolds, P. (1988). Depression and cancer mortality and morbidity: Prospective evidence from the Alameda County Study. *Journal of Behavioral Medicine, 11,* 1–13.

Kaplan, M. S., McFarland, B. H., Huguet, N., & Newsom, J. T. (2007). Physical illness, functional limitations, and suicide risk: A population-based study. *American Journal of Orthopsychiatry, 77*(1), 56–60.

Katon, W. J. (2003). Clinical and health services relationships between major depression, depressive symptoms, and general medical illness. *Society of Biological Psychiatry, 54,* 216–226.

Katon, W. J., Rutter, C., Simon, G., Lin, E. H., Ludman, E., Ciechanowski, P., ... Von Korff, M. (2005). The association of comorbid depression with mortality in patients with type 2 diabetes. *Diabetes Care, 28*(11), 2668–2672.

Katon, W., & Schulberg, H. C. (1992). Epidemiology of depression in primary care. *General Hospital Psychiatry, 14,* 237–247.

Katz, I. R. (1996). On the inseparability of mental and physical health in aged persons: Lessons from depression and medical comorbidity. *American Journal of Geriatric Psychiatry, 4,* 1–16.

Kendler, K. S., Gardner, C. O., Fiske, A., & Gatz, M. (2009). Major depression and coronary artery disease in the Swedish twin registry: Phenotypic, genetic, and environmental sources of comorbidity. *Archives of General Psychiatry, 66*(8), 857–863.

Kessler, R. C. (1997). The effects of stressful life events on depression. *Annual Review of Psychology, 48,* 191–214.

Kiecolt-Glaser, J. K. (2010). Stress, food, and inflammation: Psychoneuroimmunology and nutrition at the cutting edge. *Psychosomatic Medicine, 72*(4), 365–369.

Kim, G., DeCoster, J., Chiriboga, D. A., Jang, Y., Allen, R. S., & Parmelee, P. (2011). Associations between self-rated mental health and psychiatric disorders among older adults: Do racial/ethnic differences exist? *American Journal of Geriatric Psychiatry, 19,* 416–422.

Kim, Y. A., Bogner, H. R., Brown, G. K., & Gallo, J. J. (2006). Chronic medical conditions and wishes to die among older primary care patients. *International Journal of Psychiatry in Medicine, 36*(2), 183–198.

Kirschbaum, C., Wust, S., & Strasburger, C. J. (1992). 'Normal' cigarette smoking increases free cortisol in habitual smokers. *Life Sciences, 50*(6), 435–442.

Kleinman, A. (1980). *Patients and healers in the context of culture: An exploration of the borderland between anthropology, medicine, and psychiatry.* Los Angeles: University of California Press.

Kleinman, A. (1988). *Rethinking psychiatry: From cultural category to personal experience.* New York: Free Press.

Knight, B. G., & Sayegh, P. (2010). Cultural values and caregiving: The updated sociocultural stress and coping model. *Journal of Gerontology Series B, Psychological Sciences Social Sciences, 65B,* 5–13.

Kop, W. J., Gottdiener, J. S., Tangen, C. M., Fried, L. P., McBurnie, M. A., Walston, J., ... Tracy, R. P. (2002). Inflammation and coagulation factors in persons > 65 years of age with symptoms of depression but without evidence of myocardial ischemia. *American Journal of Cardiology, 89*(4), 419–424.

Krieger, N. (2004). *Embodying inequality: Epidemiologic perspectives.* Amityville, NY: Baywood.

Krishnan, K. R. R. (1993). Neuroanatomic substrates of depression in the elderly. *Journal of Geriatric Psychiatry and Neurology, 6,* 39–58.

Krishnan, K. R. R., Hays, J. C., & Blazer, D. G. (1997). MRI-defined vascular depression. *American Journal of Psychiatry, 157,* 497–501.

Kubzansky, L. D., Davidson, K. W., & Rozanski, A. (2005). The clinical impact of negative psychological states: Expanding the spectrum of risk for coronary artery disease. *Psychosomatic Medicine, 67*(Suppl 1), S10–S14.

Kuijpers, P. M., Hamulyak, K., Strik, J. J., Wellens, H. J., & Honig, A. (2002). Beta-thromboglobulin and platelet factor 4 levels in post-myocardial infarction patients with major depression. *Psychiatry Research, 109*(2), 207–210.

Kuo, W. H., Gallo, J. J., & Eaton, W. W. (2004). Hopelessness,depression, substance disorder, and suicidality—a 13-year community-based study. *Social Psychiatry and Psychiatric Epidemiology, 39*(6), 497–501.

Laghrissi-Thode, F., Wagner, W. R., Pollock, B. G., Johnson, P. C., & Finkel, M. S. (1997). Elevated platelet factor 4 and beta-thromboglobulin plasma levels in depressed patients with ischemic heart disease. *Biological Psychiatry, 42*(4), 290–295.

LaVeist, T., & Wallace, J. (2000). Helath risk and inequitable distribution of liquor stores in African American neighborhoods. *Social Science and Medicine, 51*(4), 615–617.

Lazarus, R. S., & Folkman, S. (1984a). The stress concept in the life sciences. In *Stress, appraisal and coping* (pp. 1–21). New York: Springer.

Lazarus, R. S., & Folkman, S. (1984b). The concept of coping. In *Stress, appraisal and coping* (pp. 117–139). New York: Springer.

Lesperance, F., Frasure-Smith, N., Talajic, M., & Bourassa, M. G. (2002). Five-year risk of cardiac mortality in relation to initial severity and one-year changes in depression symptoms after myocardial infarction. *Circulation, 105*(9), 1049–1053.

Lett, H. S., Blumenthal, J. A., Babyak, M. A., Catellier, D. J., Carney, R. M., Berkman, L. F.,...Schneiderman, N. (2007). Social support and prognosis in patients at increased psychosocial risk recovering from myocardial infarction. *Health Psychology, 26,* 418–427.

Leventhal, H., Leventhal, E. A., & Contrada, R. J. (1998). Self-regulation, health, and behavior: A perceptual-cognitive approach. *Psychology and Health, 13,* 717–733.

Leventhal, H., Nerenz, D. R., & Steele, D. J. (1984). Illness representations and coping with health threats. In A. Baum, S. E. Taylor, & J. E. Singer (Eds.), *Handbook of psychology and health* (pp. 219–252). Hillsdale, NJ: Erlbaum.

Linkins, R. W., & Comstock, G. W. (1990). Depressed mood and development of cancer. *American Journal of Epidemiology, 132,* 962–972.

Loewe, R., & Freeman, J. (2000). Interpreting diabetes mellitus: Differences between patient and providers models of disease and their implications for clinical practice. *Culture, Medicine and Psychiatry, 24,* 379–401.

Long, M. V., & Martin, P. (2000). Personality, relationship closeness, and loneliness of oldest old adults and their children. *Journals of Gerontology Series B, Psychological Science Social Science, 55*(5), P311–P319.

Lopez-Leon, S., Janssens, A. C., Gonzalez-Zuloeta Ladd, A. M., Del-Favero, J., Claes, S. J., Oostra, B. A., & van Duijn, C. M. (2008). Meta-analyses of genetic studies on major depressive disorder. *Molecular Psychiatry, 13*(8), 772–785.

Lovasi, G., Hutson, M., Guerra, M., Neckerman, K. (2009). Built environments and obesity in disadvantaged populations. *Epidemiologic Reviews, 31,* 7–20.

Luborsky, M. R., & Riley, E. M. (1997). Residents' understanding and experience of depression: Anthropological perspectives. In R. L. Rubinstein & M. P. Lawton (Eds.), *Depression in long term and residential care* (pp. 75–117). New York: Springer.

Lyness, J. M., Niculescu, A., Tu, X., Reynolds, C. F., III, & Caine, E. D. (2006). The relationship of medical comorbidity and depression in older, primary care patients. *Psychosomatics, 47*(5), 435–439.

Maas, J. W., Katz, M. M., Koslow, S. H., Swann, A., Davis, J. M., Berman, N.,...Landis, H. (1994). Adrenomedullary function in depressed patients. *Journal of Psychiatric Research, 28*(4), 357–367.

Malek-Ahmadi, P., & Hilsabeck, R. C. (2007). Neuropsychiatric complications of interferons: Classification, neurochemical bases, and management. *Annals of Clinical Psychiatry, 19*(2), 113–123.

Mantyselka, P., Korniloff, K., Saaristo, T., Koponen, H., Eriksson, J., Puolijoki, H.,...Vanhala, M. 2011. Association of depressive symptoms with impaired glucose regulation, screen-detected, and previously known type 2 diabetes: Findings from the Finnish D2D Survey. *Diabetes Care, 34*(1), 71–76.

Marinelli, M., & Piazza, P. V. (2002). Interaction between glucocorticoid hormones, stress and psychostimulant drugs. *European Journal of Neuroscience, 16*(3), 387–394.

McEwen, B. S. (1998). Protective and damaging effects of stress mediators. *New England Journal of Medicine, 338*(3), 171–179.

McEwen, B. S., & Seeman, T. E. (1999). Protective and damaging effects of mediators of stress: Elaborating and testing the concepts of allostasis and allostatic load. *Annals of the New York Academy of Sciences, 896,* 30–47.

Meeks, T. W., Vahia, I. V., Lavretsky, H., Kulkarni, G., & Jeste, D. V. (2011). A tune in "a minor" can "b major": A review of epidemiology, illness course, and public health implications of subthreshold depression in older adults. *Journal of Affective Disorders, 129*(1–3), 126–142.

Merali, Z., Du, L., Hrdina, P., Palkovits, M., Faludi, G., Poulter, M. O., & Anisman, H. (2004). Dysregulation in the suicide brain: mRNA expression of corticotropin-releasing hormone receptors and GABA(A) receptor subunits in frontal cortical brain region. *Journal of Neuroscience, 24*(6), 1478–1485.

Mezuk, B., Eaton, W. W., Albrecht, S., & Golden, S. H. (2008). Depression and type 2 diabetes over the lifespan: A meta-analysis. *Diabetes Care, 31*(12), 2383–2390.

Mezuk, B., Rafferty, J. A., Kershaw, K. N., Hudson, D., Abdou, C. M., Lee, H., ... Jackson, J. S. (2010). Reconsidering the role of social disadvantage in physical and mental health: Stressful life events, health behaviors, race, and depression. *American Journal of Epidemiology, 172*, 1238–1249.

Miller, G. (2011). Social neuroscience: Why loneliness is hazardous to your health. *Science, 331*, 138–140.

Miller, G., Chen, E., & Cole, S. W. (2009). Health psychology: Developing biologically plausible models linking the social world and physical health. *Annual Review of Psychology, 60*, 501–524.

Miller, G. E., Stetler, C. A., Carney, R. M., Freedland, K. E., & Banks, W. A. (2002). Clinical depression and inflammatory risk markers for coronary heart disease. *American Journal of Cardiology, 90*(12), 1279–1283.

Mitchell, A. J., Malone, D., & Doebbeling, C. C. (2009). Quality of medical care for people with and without comorbid mental illness and substance misuse: Systematic review of comparative studies. *British Journal of Psychiatry, 194*(6), 491–499.

Murray, C. J. L., & Lopez, A. D. (1996). *The global burden of disease: A comprehensive assessment of mortality and disability from diseases, injuries, and risk factors in 1990 and projected to 2020.* Cambridge, MA: Harvard University Press.

Musselman, D. L., Betan, E., Larsen, H., & Phillips, L. S. (2003). Relationship of depression to diabetes types 1 and 2: Epidemiology, biology, and treatment. *Biological Psychiatry, 54*(3), 317–329.

Musselman, D. L., Miller, A. H., Porter, M. R., Manatunga, A., Gao, F., Penna, S., ... Nemeroff, C. B. (2001). Higher than normal plasma interleukin-6 concentrations in cancer patients with depression: Preliminary findings. *American Journal of Psychiatry, 158*(8), 1252–1257.

Myint, A. M., Schwarz, M. J., Steinbusch, H. W., & Leonard, B. E. (2009). Neuropsychiatric disorders related to interferon and interleukins treatment. *Metabolic Brain Disease, 24*(1), 55–68.

Neighbors, H. W., & Jackson, J. S. (1996). Psychosocial problems and help-seeking behavior. In H. W. Neighbors & J. S. Jackson (Eds.), *Mental health in Black America* (pp. 1–13). Thousand Oaks, CA: Sage.

Nestle, M., Wing, R., Birch, L., DiSogra, L., Drewnowski, A., Middleton, S., Sigman-Grant, M., ... Economos, C. (1998). Behavioral and social influences on food choice. *Nutritional Reviews, 56*, 50–64.

Nguyen, H. T., Kitner-Triolo, M., Evans, M. K., & Zonderman, A. B. (2004). Factorial invariance of the CES-D in low socioeconomic status African Americans compared with a nationally representative sample. *Psychiatry Research, 126*, 177–187.

O'Connell, H., Chin, A. V., Cunningham, C., & Lawlor, B. A. (2004). Recent developments: Suicide in older people. *British Medical Journal, 329*(7471), 895–899.

Ormel, J., & de Jonge, P. (2011). Unipolar depression and the progression of coronary artery disease: Toward an integrative model. *Psychotherapy and Psychosomatics, 80*(5), 264–274.

Pedersen, S. S., Denollet, J., Erdman, R. A., Serruys, P. W., & van Domburg, R. T. (2009). Co-occurrence of diabetes and hopelessness predicts adverse prognosis following percutaneous coronary intervention. *Journal of Behavioral Medicine, 32*(3), 294–301.

Penckofer, S., Ferrans, C. E., Velsor-Friedrich, B., & Savoy, S. (2007). The psychological impact of living with diabetes: Women's day-to-day experiences. *Diabetes Educator, 33*, 680–690.

Penninx, B. W., Kritchevsky, S. B., Yaffe, K., Newman, A. B., Simonsick, E. M., Rubin, S., ... Pahor, M. (2003). Inflammatory markers and depressed mood in older persons: Results from the Health, Aging and Body Composition study. *Biological Psychiatry, 54*(5), 566–572.

Penninx, W. J. H., Guralnik, J. M., Pahor, M., Ferrucci, L., Cerhan, J. R., Wallace, R. B., & Havlik, R. J. (1998). Chronically depressed mood and cancer risk in older persons. *Journal of the National Cancer Institute, 90*, 1888–1893.

Persky, V. W., Kempthorne-Rawson, J., & Shekelle, R. B. (1987). Personality and risk of cancer: 20-year follow-up of the Western Electric Study. *Psychosomatic Medicine, 49*, 435–449.

Pinquart, M., & Duberstein, P. R. (2010). Associations of social networks with cancer mortality: A meta-analysis. *Critical Reviews in Oncology/Hematology, 75*, 122–137.

Pinquart, M., & Sorensen, S. (2001). Influences on loneliness in older adults: A meta-analysis. *Basic and Applied Social Psychology, 23*(4), 245–266.

Pollock, B. G., Laghrissi-Thode, F., & Wagner, W. R. (2000). Evaluation of platelet activation in depressed patients with ischemic heart disease after paroxetine or nortriptyline treatment. *Journal of Clinical Psychopharmacology, 20*(2), 137–140.

Polsky, D., Doshi, J. A., Marcus, S., Oslin, D., Rothbard, A., Thomas, N., & Thompson, C. L. (2005). Long-term risk for depressive symptoms after a medical diagnosis. *Archives of Internal Medicine, 165*(11), 1260–1266.

Pratt, L., Ford, D. E., Crum, R. M., Armenian, H. K., Gallo, J. J., & Eaton, W. W. (1996). Depression, psychotropic medication and risk of heart attack: Prospective data from the Baltimore ECA follow-up. *Circulation, 94*, 3123–3129.

Prince, M., Patel, V., Saxena, S., Maj, M., Maselko, J., Phillips, M. R., & Rahman, A. (2007). No health without mental health. *Lancet, 370*(9590), 859–877.

Prochaska, J. J. (2011). Smoking and mental illness—breaking the link. *New England Journal of Medicine, 365*(3), 196–198.

Raue, P. J., Morales, K. H., Post, E. P., Bogner, H. R., Ten-Have, T., & Bruce, M. L. (2010). The wish to die and 5-year mortality in elderly primary care patients. *American Journal of Geriatric Psychiatry, 18*(4), 341–350.

Redd, M., & de Castro, J. M. (1992). Social facilitation of eating: Effects of social instruction on food intake. *Physiology and Behavior, 52*, 749–754.

Risch, N., Herrell, R., Lehner, T., Liang, K. Y., Eaves, L., Hoh, J., . . . Merikangas, K. R. (2009). Interaction between the serotonin transporter gene (5-HTTLPR), stressful life events, and risk of depression. *Journal of the American Medical Association, 301*, 2462–2471.

Rohleder, N., & Kirschbaum, C. (2006). The hypothalamic-pituitary-adrenal (HPA) axis in habitual smokers. *International Journal of Psychophysiology, 59*(3), 236–243.

Rottmann, N., Dalton, S. O., Christensen, J., Frederiksen, K., & Johansen, C. (2010). Self-efficacy, adjustment style and well-being in breast cancer patients: A longitudinal study. *Quality of Life Research, 19*(6), 827–836.

Rubenowitz, E., Waern, M., Wilhelmson, K., & Allebeck, P. (2001). Life events and psychosocial factors in elderly suicides—a case-control study. *Psychological Medicine, 31*(7), 1193–1202.

Rubin, R. R., Ciechanowski, P., Egede, L. E., Lin, E. H., & Lustman, P. J. (2004). Recognizing and treating depression in patients with diabetes. *Current Diabetes Reports, 4*(2), 119–125.

Rustad, J. K., Musselman, D. L., & Nemeroff, C. B. (2011). The relationship of depression and diabetes: Pathophysiological and treatment implications. *Psychoneuroendocrinology, 36*(9), 1276–1286.

Sachs-Ericsson, N., Burns, A. B., Gordon, K. H., Eckel, L. A., Wonderlich, S. A., Crosby, R. D., & Blazer, D. G. (2007). Body mass index and depressive symptoms in older adults: The moderating roles of race, sex, and socioeconomic status. *American Journal of Geriatric Psychiatry, 15*, 815–825.

Sachs-Ericsson, N., Schmidt, N. B., Zvolensky, M. J., Mitchell, M., Collins, N., & Blazer, D. G. (2009). Smoking cessation behavior in older adults by race and gender: The role of health problems and psychological distress. *Nicotine and Tobacco Research, 11*, 433–443.

Saha, S., Freeman, M., Toure, J., Tippens, K. M., Weeks, C., & Ibrahim, S. (2008). Racial and ethnic disparities in the VA health care system: A systematic review. *Journal of General Internal Medicine, 23*, 654–671.

Sapolsky, R. M. (2002). Endocrinology of the stress response. In J. B. Becker, S. M. Breedlove, D. Crews, & M. M. McCarthy (Eds.), *Behavioral endocrinology* (pp. 287–324). Cambridge, MA: MIT Press.

Sayegh, P., & Knight, B. G. (2011). The effects of familism and cultural justification on the mental and physical health of family caretakers. *Journals of Gerontology Series B, Psychological Sciences Social Sciences, 66*, 3–14.

Schneiderman, N., Saab, P. G., Catellier, D. J., Powell, L. H., DeBusk, R. F., Williams, R. B., . . . Kaufmann, P. G. (2004). Psychosocial treatment within sex by ethnicity subgroups in the Enhancing Recovery in Coronary Heart Disease clinical trial. *Psychosomatic Medicine, 66*, 475–483.

Shekelle, R. B., Raynor, W. J., Ostfeld, A. M., Garron, D. C., Bieliauskas, L. A., Liu, S. C., . . . Paul, O. (1981). Psychological depression and 17-year risk of death from cancer. *Psychosomatic Medicine, 43*, 117–125.

Shippee, T. P., Ferraro, K. F., & Thorpe, R. J. (2011). Racial disparity in access to cardiac intensive care over 20 years. *Ethnicity and Health, 16*, 145–165.

Shrestha, L. B., & Heisler, E. J. (2011). The changing demographic profile of the United States. *Congressional Research Service, 7-5700* (RL32701).

Silber, J. H., Rosenbaum, P. R., Even-Shoshan, O., Zhang, X., Bradlow, E. T., Shabbout, M., & Marsh, R. (2003). Length of stay, conditional length of stay, and prolonged stay in pediatric asthma. *Health Services Research, 38*(3), 867–886.

Skoog, I. (1993). The prevalence of psychotic, depressive, and anxiety syndromes in demented and non-demented 85-year olds. *International Journal of Geriatric Psychiatry, 8*, 247–253.

Steptoe, A., Wardle, J., Pollard, T. M., Canaan, L., & Davies, G. J. (1996). Stress, social support, and health-related behavior: A study of smoking, alcohol consumption, and physical exercise. *Journal of Psychosomatic Research, 41*, 171–180.

Suls, J., & Bunde, J. (2005). Anger, anxiety, and depression as risk factors for cardiovascular disease: The problems and implications of overlapping affective dispositions. *Psychological Bulletin, 131*(2), 260–300.

Swartz, K. L., Pratt, L. A., Armenian, H. K., Lee, L. C., & Eaton, W. W. (2000). Mental disorders and the incidence of migraine headaches in a community sample: Results from the Baltimore Epidemiologic Catchment area follow-up study. *Archives of General Psychiatry, 57*(10), 945–50.

Switzer, J., Wittink, M., Karsch, B. B., & Barg, F. K. (2006). "Pull yourself up by your bootstraps": A response to depression in older adults. *Qualitative Health Research, 16*(9), 1207–1216.

Taylor, S. E., & Stanton, A. L. (2007). Coping resources, coping processes, and mental health. *Annual Review of Clinical Psychology, 3*, 377–401.

Tannock, C., & Katona, C. (1995). Minor depression in the aged: Concepts, prevalence, and optimal management. *Drugs and Aging, 6*, 278–292.

Thayer, J. F., Hall, M., Sollers, J. J., III, & Fischer, J. E. (2006). Alcohol use, urinary cortisol, and heart rate variability in apparently healthy men: Evidence for impaired inhibitory control of the HPA axis in heavy drinkers. *International Journal of Psychophysiology, 59*(3), 244–250.

Uhart, M., & Wand, G. S. (2009). Stress, alcohol and drug interaction: An update of human research. *Addiction Biology, 14*(1), 43–64.

Ulrich-Lai, Y. M., Christiansen, A. M., Ostrander, M. M., Jones, A. A., Jones, K. R., Choi, D. C.,... Herman, J. P. (2010). Pleasurable behaviors reduce stress via brain reward pathways. *Proceedings of the National Academy of Sciences USA, 107*, 20529–20534.

Umberson, D., Liu, H., & Reczek, C. (2008). Stress and health behaviors. In: H. Turner, S. Schiemann (Eds.), *Advances in life course research: Stress processes across the life course* (pp. 19–44). Elsevier: Oxford, UK..

US Census Bureau. (2008). *2008 national population projections*. Washington, DC: Author.

van Baarsen, B. (2002). Theories on coping with loss: The impact of social support and self-esteem on adjustment to emotional and social loneliness following a partner's death in later life. *Journals of Gerontology Series B, Psychological Sciences Social Sciences, 57*(1), S33–S42.

Vincent, G. K., & Velkoff, V. A. (2010). The older population in the United States, 2010 to 2050. *Current Population Reports: US Census Bureau,* P25-1138.

Vitaliano, P. P., Murphy, M., Young, H. M., Echeverria, D., & Borson, S. (2011). Does caring for a spouse with dementia promote cognitive decline? A hypothesis and proposed mechanisms. *Journal of the American Geriatrics Society, 59*, 900–908.

Volkow, N. D., & Wise, R. A. (2005). How can drug addiction help us understand obesity? *Nature Neuroscience, 8*(5), 555–560.

Weinberger, M. I., Bruce, M. L., Roth, A. J., Breitbart, W., & Nelson, C. J. (2011). Depression and barriers to mental health care in older cancer patients. *International Journal of Geriatric Psychiatry, 26*(1), 21–26.

Whitfield, K. E., & Hayward, M. D. (2003). The landscape of health disparities among older adults. *Public Policy and Aging Report, 13*, 1–17.

Whitlock, F. A., & Siskind, M. (1979). Depression and cancer: A follow-up study. *Psychological Medicine, 9*, 747–752.

Whooley, M. A., Browner, W. S., & Study of Osteoporotic Fractures Research Group. (1998). Association between depressive symptoms and mortality in older women. *Archives of Internal Medicine, 158*, 2129–2135.

Whyte, E. M., Pollock, B. G., Wagner, W. R., Mulsant, B. H., Ferrell, R. E., Mazumdar, S., & Reynolds, C. F., III. (2001). Influence of serotonin-transporter-linked promoter region polymorphism on platelet activation in geriatric depression. *American Journal of Psychiatry, 158*(12), 2074–2076.

Williams, D. R., González, H. M., Neighbors, H., Nesse, R., Abelson, J. M., Sweetman, J., & Jackson, J. S. (2007). Prevalence and distribution of major depressive disorder in African Americans, Caribbean blacks, and non-Hispanic whites: Results from the National Survey of American Life. *Archives of General Psychiatry, 64*, 305–315.

Williams, L. H., Rutter, C. M., Katon, W. J., Reiber, G. E., Ciechanowski, P., Heckbert, S. R.,... Von Korff, M. (2010). Depression and incident diabetic foot ulcers: A prospective cohort study. *American Journal of Medicine, 123*(8), 748–754 e3.

Williams, L. J., Pasco, J. A., Jacka, F. N., Henry, M. J., Dodd, S., & Berk, M. (2009). Depression and bone metabolism. A review. *Psychotherapy and Psychosomatics*, 78(1), 16–25.

Williams, R. B., & Williams, V. P. (2006). The prevention and treatment of hostility. In M. E. Vollrath (Ed.), *Handbook of personality and health* (pp. 259–275). New York: Wiley.

Wittink, M. N., Barg, F. K., & Gallo, J. J. (2006). Unwritten rules of talking to doctors about depression: Integrating qualitative and quantitative methods. *Annals of Family Medicine*, 4(4), 302–309.

Wittink, M. N., Dahlberg, B., Biruk, C., & Barg, F. K. (2008). How older adults combine medical and experiential notions of depression. *Qualitative Health Research*, 18(9), 1174–1183.

Wittink, M. N., Givens, J. L., Knott, K. A., Coyne, J. C., & Barg, F. K. (2011). Negotiating depression treatment with older adults: Primary care providers' perspectives. *Journal of Mental Health*, 20(5), 429–437.

Wolkowitz, O. M., Epel, E. S., & Mellon, S. (2008). When blue turns to grey: Do stress and depression accelerate cell aging? *World Journal of Biological Psychiatry*, 9(1), 2–5.

Wolkowitz, O. M., Epel, E. S., Reus, V. I., & Mellon, S. H. (2010). Depression gets old fast: Do stress and depression accelerate cell aging? *Depression and Anxiety*, 27(4), 327–338.

Xie, J., Wu, E. W., Xheng, Z. J., Sullivan, P. W., Zhan, L., & Labarthe, D. R. (2008). Patient-reported health status in coronary heart disease in the United States: Age, sex, racial, and ethnic differences. *Circulation*, 118, 491–497.

Xu, J., Kochanek, K. D., Murphy, S. L., & Tejada-Vera, B. (2010). *Deaths: Final data for 2007. National Vital Statistics Reports*. US National Center for Health Statistics, Hyattsville, MD.

Zivin, K., & Kales, H. C. (2008). Adherence to depression treatment in older adults: A narrative review. *Drugs and Aging*, 25(7), 559–571.

Zorrilla, E. P., Luborsky, L., McKay, J. R., Rosenthal, R., Houldin, A., Tax, A., … Schmidt, K. (2001). The relationship of depression and stressors to immunological assays: A meta-analytic review. *Brain, Behavior, and Immunity*, 15(3), 199–226.

17

COMORBID NEUROLOGICAL ILLNESS

Dylan Wint and Jeffrey Cummings

MOOD DISORDERS are the most common behavioral sequelae of neurological conditions. In most neurological diseases, the prevalence of comorbid depression is at least 20%. The elderly are disproportionately affected by neurological disorders such as cerebrovascular disease, dementia, and movement disorders. Thus, the problem of mood disturbances is significantly influenced by neurological disorders in the over-65 age group.

This chapter will address general concepts about diagnosis of mood symptoms in neurological conditions. Cerebrovascular disease, dementias, movement disorders, epilepsy, and brain neoplasms will be discussed. While this is not intended to be a comprehensive treatise on mood disorders in neurological diseases of the elderly, the range of topics will provide a useful framework for approaching most cases.

DEFINING MOOD SYMPTOMS IN NEUROLOGICAL DISORDERS

Perceiving symptoms and signs of mood disorders on a background of severe neurological disease can be difficult. This problem will be addressed in the context of specific diseases later in the chapter. Some general comments are also appropriate. Patients with neurological disease may have impaired ability to report mood disturbances because of degraded recognition, recollection, and/or communication of their emotional states (Chemerinski, Petracca, Sabe, Kremer, & Starkstein, 2001). Accordingly, mental status examination, informant report, and clinical intuition play larger—sometimes even primary—roles in diagnosing mood problems in this population. Subjective descriptions of emotional and neurovegetative status must be carefully investigated with follow-up questions that seek concrete information. For example, a patient who claims his levels of interest and energy are "fine" should be asked to describe how he spends his time during an average day. The patient who says she sleeps well should be asked specifically about what time she goes to sleep, when she wakes up, and how refreshed she is in the morning. Similar inquiries should be directed toward individuals familiar with the patient's daily behavior and function, whose perspectives may be different from the patient's.

Many have encountered the challenge of determining whether to attribute symptoms to a mood disorder or to neurological disease. Incorrectly making these distinctions may result in delayed or improper psychiatric treatment. Fortunately, several investigations have demonstrated that strictly classifying symptoms into neurological or psychological categories (an "etiological" approach) is unnecessary for diagnostic accuracy (Fedoroff, Starkstein, Parikh, Price, & Robinson, 1991; Paradiso, Ohkubo, & Robinson, 1997). An "inclusive" approach—considering all potential depressive symptoms to be mood-related—is sensitive and specific for recognizing depression in neurological diseases (Engedal, Barca, Laks, & Selbaek, 2010; Marsh et al., 2006; Robinson, 2003).

Persistent depression is not an inevitable result of disability or chronic incurable disease. Although depression is common in neurologic diseases, it does not occur in the majority of cases. In fact, careful analyses suggest that worse neurological outcomes may be more likely to *result from*, rather than cause, depression (Chemerinski, Robinson, & Kosier, 2001; Paolucci et al., 1999), highlighting the need for early recognition and effective intervention.

CEREBROVASCULAR DISEASE

Individuals over 65 years old account for more than 70% of the 800,000 strokes that occur each year in the United States. Mood disorders are common after stroke, with depression occurring in 20%–45% and mania in 5% of stroke victims. Poststroke depression (PSD) symptoms usually appear within the first poststroke month but can take longer (Bour et al., 2010). Overt melancholia immediately after stroke, younger age, and severe disability predict the development of depression within a year after a stroke (Carota et al., 2005). The yearly incidence of depression remains as high as 15%–20% for 5 years after stroke, and the prevalence of depression persists at about 30% at 1 year, 3 years, and 5 years after stroke (Ayerbe, Ayis, Rudd, Heuschmann, & Wolfe, 2011). Therefore, vigilant surveillance for depression should continue for at least several years after cerebrovascular events. Transient ischemic attacks also increase the risk of late-life depression in a dose-dependent fashion. This effect is particularly pronounced in individuals who are otherwise at low risk for depression (Luijendijk

et al., 2011). This suggests that stroke and depression have shared risk factors. It also raises the question of whether transient ischemic attacks cause permanent changes that cannot be detected by current neuroimaging techniques.

Studies examining stroke location tend to report increased risk for PSD with left hemisphere strokes, particularly in the frontal lobe and basal ganglia. However, this finding has not been supported in some systematic meta-analyses (Carson et al., 2000; Kouwenhoven, Kirkevold, Engedal, & Kim, 2011). One reason for this inconsistency may be that studies have used varying poststroke intervals to classify PSD. Strokes on the left side may be complicated by depression earlier than strokes on the right, and earlier onset of symptoms predicts continued symptoms a year after the stroke (Kouwenhoven et al., 2011). Thus, studies of the immediate poststroke period might favor detection of left hemisphere strokes, as would studies of 1-year outcomes.

Although not as frequent as depression, mania after stroke is a well-recognized entity (Cummings & Mendez, 1984). Poststroke mania is an extraordinarily lateralized phenomenon, with more than 70% of reported cases being associated with right-sided cerebral lesions (Robinson, Boston, Starkstein, & Price, 1988). Cerebral white matter atrophy, family history of bipolar disorder, and subcortical microvascular ischemic disease are additional risk factors for poststroke mania (Robinson et al., 1988; Starkstein, Pearlson, Boston, & Robinson, 1987). Interestingly, psychomotor agitation and hyperlalia (talkativeness) in poststroke mania are more closely correlated with right hemisphere lesions than are euphoria and irritability, suggesting that mania after right-sided strokes may be defined by a heightened sense of energy, rather than manic affect per se (Braun, Larocque, Daigneault, & Montour-Proulx, 1999). The rightward lateralization of more flagrant manic symptoms may also introduce a bias against detection of mania after left-sided lesions in case-control studies. Cerebellar infarctions are also disproportionately associated with mania (Lauterbach, 1996, 2001; Lauterbach, Harris, & Bina, 2010) and should be considered where other explanations for late-onset bipolar disorder are not evident.

Vascular Depression

The relationship between acute cerebrovascular insults and mood symptoms led naturally to interest in the mood effects of "silent" cerebrovascular disease in older adults. "Vascular depression," a depressive syndrome associated with chronic cerebrovascular disease, may be an entity distinct from either PSD or spontaneous depression (Alexopoulos, Meyers et al., 1997b; Krishnan, Hays, & Blazer, 1997; Steffens & Krishnan, 1998). In addition to higher levels of neurocognitive dysfunction (as might be expected in a population defined by the presence of cerebrovascular disease), authors have suggested that people with vascular depression are less likely to report sad mood and that their symptoms are more resistant to treatment (Alexopoulos, Meyers et al., 1997b; Simpson, Baldwin, Jackson, & Burns, 1998). The possibility that vascular depression may also be a risk factor for dementia is an area of ongoing investigation.

Treatment Considerations

The bulk of the evidence suggests that depression after stroke is effectively and safely treated with standard antidepressants, including tricyclics (Lipsey, Robinson, Pearlson, Rao, & Price, 1984; Robinson et al., 2000), selective serotonin reuptake inhibitors (SSRIs; Wiart, Petit, Joseph, Mazaux, & Barat, 2000), and serotonin-norepinephrine reuptake inhibitors (Rampello et al., 2005). However, some controlled studies have failed to demonstrate any benefits from treatment, possibly because of small sample sizes (Rasmussen et al., 2003). A meta-analysis of PSD treatment studies showed that pharmacologic treatment of PSD is effective, but benefits take at least 3 or 4 weeks to appear (Chen, Guo, Zhan, & Patel, 2006). A full therapeutic trial—8 weeks at an adequate dose—should be undertaken before an antidepressant treatment is deemed ineffective (Trivedi et al., 2006).

Because PSD is common and its consequences are so severe, effective prophylaxis could dramatically improve poststroke recovery. Sertraline given during the first 12 months after stroke markedly reduced the incidence of depression (10% compared to 30% for placebo) in a randomized study (Rasmussen et al., 2003). Similar results were found in a placebo-controlled study of escitalopram (Robinson et al., 2008). Although there have been some studies showing no benefit, pharmacological prophylaxis may be a useful intervention in patients at particularly high risk for PSD (Chen, Patel, Guo, & Zhan, 2007).

Many, if not most, patients with stroke have medical comorbidities. Thoughtfulness in choosing antidepressant medication in these patients is critical. Low-risk nonpharmacological therapies for PSD have also been studied. However, the results have been collectively disappointing and more study is needed to determine the role of such treatments in PSD (Broomfield et al., 2011; Robinson et al., 2008).

DEGENERATIVE DEMENTIAS

Mood disorders are extremely common in dementia, with most studies placing the prevalence of depression in dementia between 20% and 40% (Di Iulio et al., 2010; Lyketsos et al., 2000; Spalletta et al., 2010). Subsyndromal depressive symptoms are even more common than major depression. This high prevalence of mood symptoms may be linked to degenerative changes in neurotransmitter activity and limbic network function. Depression is associated with greater cognitive impairment (Bearden et al., 2006; Paradiso, Duff, Vaidya, Hoth, & Mold, 2010). This may be responsible for "pseudodementia"—cognitive deficits that resolve when depression remits. Recognition of depression in dementia is not always straightforward. Compounding the difficulties inherent in diagnosing psychiatric illness in neurological disorders, atypical depressive symptoms such as agitation, disinhibition, anxiety, irritability, aggression, and psychosis occur more commonly in individuals with dementia (Prado-Jean et al., 2010; Volicer, Van der Steen, & Frijters, 2009). The authors recommend that the emergence of any behavioral symptoms in a patient with dementia should trigger an evaluation for depression.

Apathy in Dementia

Although it is not a mood disorder per se, apathy deserves attention in this context. Apathy is widespread among the neurodegenerative diseases (Starkstein & Leentjens, 2008) and is sometimes conflated with anhedonia because of lack of consensus criteria and imprecise use of the terms in the dementia literature. Some definitions of apathy include "lack of emotional responsivity" (i.e., anhedonia) as a criterion (Starkstein & Leentjens, 2008). Anhedonia and apathy are neither mutually exclusive (Starkstein, Petracca, Chemerinski,

& Kremer, 2001) nor indistinguishable (Levy et al., 1998; Pluck & Brown, 2002; Starkstein, Mayberg, Preziosi et al., 1992a). A helpful way to discriminate between these entities conceptually is to view apathy as a lack of interest in experiencing stimulation, whereas anhedonia is a diminished response to agreeable stimulation that has already occurred. The distinction has important diagnostic and therapeutic implications. Apathy can exist as a core symptom of dementia, particularly Alzheimer's disease (AD) and frontotemporal dementia (FTD), while anhedonia is more likely to be caused by a comorbid depression.

Controlled studies of donepezil (Gauthier et al., 2002; Holmes et al., 2004), metrifonate (Dubois, McKeith, Orgogozo, Collins, & Meulien, 1999; Kaufer, 1998), rivastigmine (McKeith et al., 2000), and galantamine (Erkinjuntti et al., 2002) have found that cholinesterase inhibitors reduce apathy in a variety of dementia syndromes, but a few studies showed no benefit (Drijgers, Aalten, Winogrodzka, Verhey, & Leentjens, 2009). Ginkgo biloba extract EGb 761 may also relieve apathy (Scripnikov, Khomenko, Napryeyenko, & GINDEM-NP Study Group, 2007). Anhedonia and other symptoms of depression require antidepressant treatment.

Alzheimer's Disease

AD is the most common degenerative dementia, occurring in 10% of people over 65 years old. Studies showing elevated rates of cognitive impairment in depressed elders (Devanand et al., 1996) and higher prevalence of depression after development of dementia (Chen, Ganguli, Mulsant, & DeKosky, 1999) suggest that depression can be an early symptom of dementia. Depression may also be a risk factor for AD. Prospective epidemiological studies have demonstrated a dose–response relationship between depressive symptoms in middle age and later onset of cognitive decline (Saczynski et al., 2010; Wilson et al., 2002). The extended interval between depression and dementia onset in these studies makes a strong case for depression as a risk factor, rather than a prodrome, of AD. The data on this question are by no means entirely consistent, with some studies showing no relationship. One explanation for the discrepancies may be that follow-up periods in the positive studies were considerably longer. Study cohorts comprised only of people over 60 years old may overrepresent people who already have some

AD pathology, thereby decreasing the magnitude of between-group differences in rates of progression to dementia.

Depression and AD share many biological features. Among these are hippocampal atrophy (Bowen & Davison, 1980; Hubbard & Anderson, 1985; Sheline, Wang, Gado, Csernansky, & Vannier, 1996), immunological changes, and neuroendocrine abnormalities (Caraci, Copani, Nicoletti, & Drago, 2010; Dowlati et al., 2010; Hashioka, McGeer, Monji, & Kanba, 2009; Plotsky, Owens, & Nemeroff, 1998). These aberrations are plausible contributors to the core features of both diseases. Transient insults to limbic networks during depressive episodes might leave them more vulnerable to damage by AD-associated neuropathology. Alternately, intrusions of AD pathology into limbic structures could produce mood symptoms before cognitive symptoms appear. The underpinnings of the relationship between depression and dementia—like most of what we have learned about each of these illnesses—are likely to be complex (Jorm, 2000). A detailed discussion about the relationship between cognitive impairment and mood disturbances can be found in Chapter 11.

Frontotemporal Dementias

The FTDs are comprised of a group of clinical syndromes (Neary et al., 1998), including behavioral variant FTD, semantic aphasia, and progressive nonfluent aphasia. Many types of pathological changes have been described in FTD, but all eventually cause atrophy and dysfunction of the frontal and temporal lobes (Boeve, 2006). As a result, disturbances of language and social conduct are core features of FTD. The frontal lobes' critical role in behavioral supervision becomes evident in individuals with FTD, who often exhibit mania-like irritability, hyperactivity, and impulsivity. Similarly, deficiencies in motivation and reward responses may cause the FTD patient to display anergia, anhedonia, and disinterest reminiscent of depression (Cummings, 1993). The importance of thorough neurological evaluation in older patients who present with first-time episodes of mood disturbance cannot be overemphasized.

Treatment Considerations

Low starting doses and slow titration should be the overriding principles in pharmacological treatment, as older patients are more sensitive to the side effects of central nervous system–active medications. Practitioners are particularly cautioned regarding medicines with anticholinergic or antihistaminic properties, which are more likely to cause cognitive impairment and excessive sedation in elderly and demented patients. Many tricyclic antidepressants (TCAs) and other antidepressants have such properties and should probably be used for dementia-related depression only after failures of less toxic drugs (Table 17.1; Richelson, 2002, 2003). These concerns are not simply theoretical; many patients suffer unnecessary morbidity because of poor drug selection. In elderly and demented patients, SSRIs may be better tolerated than other types of antidepressants. In patients with dementia, the authors start with a low dose of an SSRI, titrate as tolerated to a therapeutic dose, and allow at least 12 weeks for a full therapeutic trial.

Electroconvulsive therapy may also be of benefit, but it should be administered by an expert in treating this population, because of cognitive risks (Rao & Lyketsos, 2000). Better baseline cognition and the use of antidementia medications may predict better cognitive outcome after a course of electroconvulsive therapy (Hausner, Damian, Sartorius, & Frölich, 2011). Standardized evaluation of cognition and depression symptoms throughout treatment is recommended (Gardner & O'Connor, 2008). A risk/benefit analysis incorporating these data should be performed before each procedure in the treatment course of electroconvulsive therapy. In the authors' experience, patients who experience significant cognitive decline during a course of electroconvulsive therapy benefit from lengthening the intervals between treatments.

DISORDERS OF MOVEMENT

Depression has been recognized and studied in Parkinson's disease (PD) far more extensively than in other movement disorders. However, similar rates of depression are seen across the clinical spectrum of movement disorders (Miller et al., 2007). Some observations about mood disorders in PD are applicable to depression in other movement disorders. About 50% of individuals with PD have clinically significant depressive symptoms (Tandberg, Larsen, Aarsland, & Cummings, 1996), and 17% meet stringent criteria for major depressive disorder (Reijnders, Ehrt, Weber, Aarsland, & Leentjens, 2008). Depression is sometimes evident before the onset of PD motor symptoms (Ishihara & Brayne, 2006), and it is the sole presenting complaint in about 2.5% of PD patients (O'Sullivan et al., 2008). Depression in PD is associated with decreased quality of life and worse cognitive and motor outcomes (Martinez-Martin, Rodriguez-Blazquez, Kurtis, Chaudhuri, & NMSS Validation Group, 2011; Starkstein, Mayberg, Leiguarda, et al., 1992b).

Table 17.1 Antidepressant Receptor Affinity

	MUSCARINIC	ALPHA 1	HISTAMINIC
Tricyclics			
Amitriptyline	++++	+++	+++
Clomipramine	+++	++	+
Desipramine	+	+	+
Doxepin	++	+++	++++
Imipramine	++	+	++
Nortriptyline	++	+	+
Protriptyline	+	+	+
Others			
Mirtazapine			++++
Nefazodone		+++	++
Paroxetine	++		
Sertraline		+	

+ = metabolized by cytochrome.

The rigidity, bradykinesia, and tremor of PD are attributed to degeneration of the substantia nigra *pars compacta* and the ensuing dopamine deficiency, but PD causes widespread brainstem pathology. Among the areas most heavily affected by PD neuropathology are the serotonergic raphe nuclei and noradrenergic locus ceruleus (Jellinger, 1991). Cell losses in these areas likely play a significant role in the pathogenesis of mood disorders in PD (Halliday et al., 1990). Indeed, degeneration of nonnigral brainstem nuclei is more common in PD patients with depression and dementia than in PD patients without behavioral symptoms (Frisina, Haroutunian, & Libow, 2009; Jellinger, 1991).

Despite a wealth of evidence suggesting that depression is a common and important problem in PD, it is underreported by patients and goes unrecognized by their physicians (Shulman, Taback, Rabinstein, & Weiner, 2002). Even when it is detected, depression is often inadequately treated in PD patients (Barone, Goetz, Houben, Koester, Leentjens, Poewe, et al., 2008; Negre-Pages et al., 2010; Weintraub, Moberg, Duda, Katz, & Stern, 2003). There are many possible reasons for these deficiencies. Restricted or sad affect is difficult to evaluate in the hypomimic PD patient. Patients and clinicians often attribute fatigability, anhedonia, insomnia, and anorexia to PD or other age-related conditions (Gotham, Brown, & Marsden, 1986). This difficulty has led to serious consideration about how to properly characterize the problem of depression in PD, a necessary step toward finding its solution. Among the recommendations of an expert working group were interviews of nonpatient informants, more studies of subsyndromal and minor depression in PD, and inclusive approaches to symptom assessment (Marsh et al., 2006).

Although there is a lack of consensus about the ideal definition of depression in PD, lack of clinical effort is the larger contributor to underdiagnosis. Several widely available depression scales are suitable for screening and rating depression symptoms in PD (Schrag et al., 2007). The lack of a PD-specific scale does not preclude diagnosis, management, or research into this important clinical syndrome. Clinicians dealing with PD patients must proactively ask about depression and have a low threshold for diagnosing and treating it (Chen, Kales, et al., 2007; Marsh et al., 2006).

Mania is not common in PD. However, disorders of impulse control associated with PD medications have been observed for decades and can affect more than 10% of PD patients (Ceravolo, Frosini, Rossi, & Bonuccelli, 2010; Ryback & Schwab, 1971). This may be a result of mesolimbic overstimulation and is more common with dopamine agonists than other anti-PD drugs (Voon et al., 2010; Weintraub et al., 2010). Pathological gambling, sexual disorders, compulsive eating, and shopping sprees have been documented. The authors have observed patients in whom hyperactivity, pressured speech, and increased goal-directed activity appear only during medication peaks.

Mania has also occurred with deep brain stimulation (DBS) of the globus pallidus and subthalamic nucleus in patients with PD (Chopra et al., 2011; Kulisevsky et al., 2002; Miyawaki, Perlmutter, Tröster, Videen, & Koller, 2000). Although the biological underpinnings of this phenomenon are not clearly understood, compelling evidence suggests that stimulation of the ventral substantia nigra plays an important role (Ulla et al., 2011). Preoperative psychopathology of the patient may also increase the likelihood of mood symptoms after DBS (Schneider et al., 2010).

Treatment Considerations

Motor and mood symptoms in PD are often closely related (Solla et al., 2011). In fact, some PD patients experience clear worsening of depression and anxiety during their motor "off" periods. Patients should be specifically queried about correlations between mood symptoms and medication timing or motor symptoms (Marsh et al., 2006). Optimizing motor function can significantly ameliorate mood symptoms, so this should be the first step in addressing PD-related depression (Imamura, Okayasu, & Nagatsu, 2010).

If depressive symptoms are clearly independent of motor fluctuations, then treatment with standard antidepressants is warranted. Both TCAs and SSRIs are effective, with some studies suggesting a faster and more robust response with TCAs (Devos et al., 2008; Lemke et al., 2004; Menza et al., 2009). However, the anticholinergic and antiadrenergic effects of TCAs warrant cautious use in older individuals with PD, who may have underlying autonomic dysfunction. Adverse reactions are often uncomfortable (constipation, dry mouth, drowsiness) and sometimes dangerous (fecal impaction, orthostatic hypotension, dysrhythmias).

The use of dopamine agonists (pramipexole, bromocriptine, possibly ropinirole) to treat depressive symptoms in PD even when motor symptoms are well controlled has increasing support and some positive controlled studies (Barone et al., 2006, 2010; Jouvent et al., 1983). However, there is inconsistency between various studies and the antidepressant efficacy of these agents is still in question (Leentjens, 2011). The effect of anti-PD medicines on depression may be limited to dopamine agonists, as levodopa, amantadine, and trihexiphenidyl fail to improve depression in PD (Cummings, 1992). The monoamine oxidase inhibitor selegiline may ameliorate depression independent of its effects on motor symptoms (Bodkin & Amsterdam, 2002; Steur & Ballering, 1997).

Bupropion, which exerts its antidepressant effect by augmenting dopaminergic and noradrenergic neurotransmission, has been suggested as an ideal treatment for depression in PD (Raskin & Durst, 2010). Bupropion has been effective in treating PD patients with otherwise intractable depression (Zaluska & Dyduch, 2011), but there are no controlled studies supporting the superiority of bupropion over other antidepressants. Atomoxetine, a selective norepinephrine reuptake inhibitor, failed to relieve depression in a placebo-controlled trial (Weintraub et al., 2010).

Electroconvulsive therapy has long been recognized as an effective treatment for depression associated with PD, and it can also improve motor symptoms (Burke, Peterson, & Rubin, 1988; Yudofsky, 1979). Cognitive-behavioral therapy was effective in a randomized controlled trial (Dobkin et al., 2011). Other nonpharmacological interventions, including transcranial magnetic stimulation and other psychotherapies, are promising but require further investigation (Epstein et al., 2007; Farabaugh et al., 2010; Miyasaki et al., 2006; Pal, Nagy, Aschermann, Balazs, & Kovacs, 2010; Sproesser, Viana, Quagliato, & de Souza, 2010).

Successful treatment of PD-related impulse control disorders is usually accomplished by reducing the dose of dopamine replacement medication, particularly dopamine agonists (Ceravolo, Frosini, Rossi, & Bonuccelli, 2009). If that is ineffective, standard antimanic treatments may be helpful. However, lithium and divalproex can exacerbate Parkinsonian movement symptoms (Van Gerpen, 2002). Atypical antipsychotics, all of which possess some dopamine-blocking capacity, must also be used with caution. Quetiapine and clozapine have the lowest propensity for dopamine blockade (Richelson & Souder, 2000).

Huntington's Disease

Huntington's disease (HD) is associated with complex neurobehavioral features that often arise before motor symptoms appear. So important are the psychiatric symptoms in HD that some have advocated classifying it as a psychiatric disorder with associated motor features. Depressive disorders occur in about 40% of HD patients (Caine & Shoulson, 1983; Folstein, Abbott, Chase, Jensen, & Folstein, 1983), and the prevalence of depression is especially high in those older than 50 (Schoenfeld et al., 1984). Potential contributors to depression in HD include awareness of the disease's relentlessness and incurability, changes in basal ganglia physiology, or frontal lobe dysfunction (Mayberg et al., 1992; Paulsen et al., 2005). The authors have also observed depression associated with guilt about burdening loved ones or transmitting the disease to a child. Systematic studies of treatment are lacking, but there are reports of success with a variety of interventions, including antidepressant medications and electroconvulsive therapy (Naarding, Kremer, & Zitman, 2001).

Tetrabenazine, the only FDA-approved treatment for HD, is associated with high rates of depression (Jankovic & Orman, 1988). Tetrabenazine-linked depression may be ameliorated by reducing the dose (Jankovic & Beach, 1997). It has also been successfully treated with the noradrenaline reuptake inhibitor reboxetine (Schreiber, Krieg, & Eichhorn, 1999). Tetrabenazine should generally be avoided in depressed patients.

Clinically significant manic symptoms have also been described in HD, but mania occurs in less than 10% of HD patients (Mendez, 1994). As it is an unusual symptom of a rare disease, mania in HD has not been well studied. Valproic acid can be useful for treating impulsivity and other manic symptoms, but the authors and others have observed development of additional movement symptoms, particularly parkinsonism and tremor (Grove, Quintanilla, & DeVaney, 2000; Salazar, Tschopp, Calandra, & Micheli, 2008). Some have found lithium to be ineffective and poorly tolerated in individuals with mania and HD (Rosenblatt & Leroi, 2000). However, some of the authors' patients have benefited from lithium administration.

Huntington noted "that form of insanity which leads to suicide, is marked" in his original description of the disease (Huntington, 1872). Between 2% and 6% of deaths in HD occur by suicide, at least four times as many as in the general population (Farrer, 1986; Schoenfeld et al., 1984). Suicide is also more common in HD than in most other chronic debilitating diseases (Harris & Barraclough, 1994). In individuals at genetic risk for HD, rates of suicidal ideation are elevated even before motor symptoms appear and rise as neurological abnormalities become increasingly severe (Paulsen, Hoth, Nehl, & Stierman, 2005). Increased suicide in HD may be driven by the same forces that cause depression. Impulsivity caused by frontal-subcortical dysfunction probably also plays a role.

MULTIPLE SCLEROSIS

The stereotypical picture of a multiple sclerosis (MS) patient is that of an adult in her 30s or 40s, but there are many elderly who suffer from MS, including the 5%–10% of MS patients whose first symptoms appear after age 50 (Noseworthy, Paty, Wonnacott, Feasby, & Ebers, 1983). Although methodological issues have been raised (Minden & Schiffer, 1990), investigators have consistently found the lifetime prevalence of depression in MS to be higher than in other chronic diseases, usually exceeding 40% (Minden, Orav, & Reich, 1987; Sadovnick et al., 1996). In 20% of older-onset MS patients, a major depressive episode is diagnosed within the 2 years preceding the first motor symptoms (Polliack, Barak, & Achiron, 2001). Mood symptoms in MS have a major impact on quality of life (Janardhan & Bakshi, 2002; Lobentanz et al., 2004). Rates of suicidal ideation are far greater than those in the general population (Bronnum-Hansen, Stenager, Nylev Stenager, & Koch-Henriksen, 2005; Sadovnick, Eisen, Ebers, & Paty, 1991; Stenager et al., 1992) and suicide attempts are more common than in other disabling neurological diseases (Giannini et al., 2010). Completed suicide is an all-too-common outcome of depression in MS (Paparrigopoulos, Ferentinos, Kouzoupis, Koutsis, & Papadimitriou, 2010; Sadovnick et al., 1991).

There are myriad potential causes of depression in MS. Focal cerebral lesions are an obvious candidate. The presence of visible cerebral lesions (as opposed to disease limited to the spinal cord) was associated with higher rates of depression in one study (Rabins et al., 1986). This X-ray computed tomography–based study could not determine the effect of brainstem lesions. The relationship between specific cerebral locations and depression has also been evaluated; left hemisphere (Feinstein et al., 2004; Pujol, Bello, Deus, Martí-Vilalta, & Capdevila, 1997) and right frontal (Zorzon et al., 2001) involvement appears to increase depression risk. Concerns have been raised about interferons as exacerbating factors in depression and suicide. While some data suggested a causative link (Jacobs et al., 2000; Klapper 1994), large methodologically sound studies have failed to support initial findings (Feinstein, 2000; Feinstein, O'Connor, & Feinstein, 2002; Patten & Metz, 2002). High-dose corticosteroids used for acute management of MS exacerbations can cause emotional and neuropsychological changes that resemble depression (Antonijevic & Steiger, 2003; Dresler et al., 2010), but steroid treatment in MS does not seem to cause major depressive episodes. Depression and suicide in MS are clearly associated with the disease, but not its treatment.

The first placebo-controlled study addressing treatment concluded that desipramine was effective but poorly tolerated in MS patients (Schiffer & Wineman, 1990). Case reports have supported the use of monoamine oxidase inhibitors and SSRIs (Siegert & Abernethy, 2005). Small controlled and uncontrolled studies have advocated sertraline, cognitive-behavioral therapy, paroxetine, and electroconvulsive therapy for depression in MS (Ehde et al., 2008; Krystal & Coffey, 1997; Larcombe & Wilson, 1984; Mohr, Boudewyn, Goodkin, Bostrom, & Epstein, 2001). A rigorous reanalysis of some treatment studies suggested that the reported effects were not as clinically significant as they first appeared (Koch, Glazenborg, Uyttenboogaart, Mostert, & De Keyser, 2011). The high rates of depression and suicide in MS demand much more investigation of their treatments than has been undertaken thus far (Koch et al., 2011).

Mania is more common in MS than in the general population and other chronic conditions (Joffe, Lippert, Gray, Sawa, & Horvath, 1987; Schiffer, Wineman, & Weitkamp, 1986). Mania in MS can be effectively treated with standard bipolar medications. Although mania can be seen with glucocorticoid treatment, steroids are clearly not the main cause of this phenomenon. Strategies that have been used successfully by the authors to treat steroid-associated mania include shortening the steroid course, lowering the dose, or adding divalproex or lithium. In a few patients who have repeatedly demonstrated susceptibility to steroid-associated mania, divalproex 500–1,500 mg per night during the steroid course has prevented further episodes. Lithium and gabapentin have been used with reported success by other groups (Falk, Mahnke, & Poskanzer, 1979; Ginsberg & Sussman, 2001).

EPILEPSY

Epilepsy can occur at any age, but incidence rates rise sharply in the over-65 age group, and more than one third of epilepsy cases are in seniors (Hauser, Annegers, & Kurland, 1991). Depression occurs in 30%–40% of individuals with epilepsy (Ettinger, Reed, Cramer, & Epilepsy Impact Project Group, 2004). In some patients, depression has no relationship to seizure frequency. Others experience depressive episodes as strictly pre-, intra-, or postictal phenomena. "Forced normalization" refers to exacerbation of depression when a patient becomes seizure-free (Schmitz, 2005). Depression in epilepsy is well recognized by neurologists but often ignored (Gilliam et al., 2004; Paradiso, Hermann, Blumer, Davies, & Robinson, 2001).

A variety of factors play important roles in epilepsy-related depression. Seizure foci in the temporal lobe, a major node in the limbic network, are associated with higher rates of depression. The importance of limbic network dysfunction as an explanation for depression in epilepsy is further highlighted by the fact that frontal lobe dysfunction increases the risk of depression in temporal lobe epilepsy (Schmitz, 2005).

Antiepileptic drugs (AEDs) may also contribute to depression. Barbiturates, more than other AEDs, have a well-characterized tendency to cause depression (Lopez-Gomez et al., 2005; Robertson, Trimble, & Townsend, 1987). Vigabatrin is also associated with treatment-emergent depression, with prevalence rates between 3% and 12% (Levinson & Devinsky, 1999; Thomas, Trimble, Schmitz, & Ring, 1996). Up to 10% of individuals who take topiramate experience psychomotor slowing and inattentiveness, emotional lability, or depression (Martin et al., 1999; Mula, Trimble, Lhatoo, & Sander, 2003). Treatment with levetiracetam, felbamate, zonisamide, and tiagabine have lower (2%–5%), but significant, associations with depression. Other antiepileptics confer minimal, if any, additional risk (Mula & Sander, 2007).

A 2008 United States Food and Drug Administration (FDA) analysis of 199 placebo-controlled trials found that suicidal thoughts or behavior occurred in 0.43% of subjects taking AEDs, compared to 0.24% of placebo-treated subjects (Administration, 2008).

Later that year, the FDA required manufacturers of AEDs to include in their prescribing information a warning that use of these drugs can increase the risk of suicidal thoughts and behaviors. There is continuing controversy about the interpretation of the FDA's findings (Arana, Wentworth, Ayuso-Mateos, & Arellano, 2010; Pompili & Baldessarini, 2010). What is clear, however, is the need to actively and persistently monitor for suicidality in patients with epilepsy.

Many standard pharmacological and nonpharmacological treatments are effective for treating depression in epilepsy, but safety and tolerability are harder to negotiate in this population than most. The antidepressants bupropion, clomipramine, amoxapine, and maprotiline can dramatically lower seizure threshold at therapeutic doses and are to be used with caution (if at all) in patients with epilepsy (Kanner, 2008). However, the small tendency of all antidepressants to increase the risk of convulsions may not be clinically important (Noe, Locke, & Sirven, 2011). A large meta-analysis of Phase II and Phase III trials showed that seizure risk decreased in depressed patients treated with antidepressants (except bupropion) versus placebo (Alper, Schwartz, Kolts, & Khan, 2007). Studies of citalopram, reboxetine, mirtazapine, and sertraline have suggested that these drugs are safe and effective in treating depression in individuals with epilepsy (Kuhn et al., 2003; Specchio et al., 2004).

Many antidepressants and AEDs are pharmacokinetically complicated. Inhibition or induction of cytochrome P450 enzymes and serum protein displacement can lead to unexpected toxicity or lack of efficacy. Table 17.2 summarizes some of the more important pharmacokinetic properties of antiepileptics and antidepressants (Kanner, 2008; Spina, Santoro, & D'Arrigo, 2008). There may also be not yet described drug–drug interactions involving processes such as gastrointestinal absorption and transport across the blood–brain barrier.

Mania does not seem to be particularly common in epilepsy except in two circumstances. Postictal mania is associated with temporal lobe seizure foci. Transient mania may be seen after seizure surgery, especially right temporal lobectomies (Carran, O'Connor, Bilker, & Sperling et al., 2003). Mania may appear to be less common in epilepsy because many AEDs, including valproic acid, carbamazepine, lamotrigine, and phenytoin have been associated with antimanic activity.

Table 17.2 Cytochrome P450 Interactions of Antiepileptic Drugs and Antidepressants

	CYP1A2	CYP2C9	CYP2C19	CYP2D6	CYP3A4
Antiepileptics					
Carbamazepine	+++	+++	+++		+++
Felbamate			– –		
Oxcarbazepine			– –		+
Phenobarbital	+++	+++	+++		+++
Phenytoin	+++	+++	+++		+++
Primidone	+++	+++	+++		+++
Topiramate			– –		+
Valproic acid		– –			
Antidepressants					
Bupropion				–	
Duloxetine				–	
Fluoxetine		– –		– –	
Fluvoxamine		– –	– –		
Nefazodone				– –	
Paroxetine				– –	
Substrates					
Amitriptyline	■		■	■	■
Citalopram			■	■	■
Clomipramine	■		■	■	■
Desipramine				■	
Duloxetine	■			■	
Escitalopram			■	■	■
Fluoxetine			■	■	
Fluvoxamine	■			■	
Imipramine			■	■	■
Mirtazapine	■			■	■
Nefazodone					■
Nortriptyline				■	
Paroxetine				■	
Phenobarbital		■	■		
Phenytoin		■	■		
Sertraline				■	■
Valproic acid		■			
Venlafaxine				■	■

+ = increases rate of activity; – = decreases rate of activity.
Kanner, 2008; Spina, Santoro et al., 2008
■ = metabolized by cytochrome

CEREBRAL NEOPLASMS

The incidence of primary brain tumors rises after age 55 (Brown, Schrot, Bauer, & Letendre, 2009). The age of peak incidence of glioblastoma, astrocytoma, and oligodendroglioma is after 60 years of age (Wrensch, Minn, Chew, Bondy, & Berger, 2002). Brain tumors combine the devastating effects of both oncologic and neurologic disease (Weitzner, 1999). Pituitary tumors, which add endocrinological dysfunction to this potent mix, may be associated with especially high rates of depression (Kelly, 1996). Overall, more than one in four patients with primary brain tumors—up to three times the rates of tumors in other sites—meet criteria for major depressive disorder, and more than 50% report at least one depressive symptom (Wellisch, Kaleita, Freeman, Cloughesy, & Goldman, 2002). Depression has adverse consequences for neurological performance, daily functioning, and survival of brain tumor patients (Gathinji et al., 2009; Litofsky et al., 2004; Mainio, Hakko, Niemelä, Koivukangas, & Räsänen, 2005).

Treatment of depression in brain tumors has not been rigorously examined (Litofsky & Resnick, 2009; Rooney & Grant, 2010). One consistent finding, however, is that even when depression is recognized by health care providers, the majority of patients initially go without treatment (Arnold et al., 2008; Litofsky et al., 2004; Litofsky & Resnick, 2009). A recent meta-analysis was unable to instantiate any controlled studies of pharmacological treatment of depression in individuals with cerebral neoplasms (Rooney & Grant, 2010). Antidepressant studies that included patients with brain tumors either measured depression incidentally or were not specific to brain neoplasms (Morrow et al., 2003; Moss, Simpson, Pelletier, & Forsyth, 2006). Thus, their findings cannot be generally applied to patients with depression associated with primary central nervous system neoplasms. The authors use standard antidepressant treatments for patients with depression and brain tumors. Because of its propensity to lower seizure threshold, bupropion is used cautiously with cortically based tumors. Presence of a space-occupying lesion has traditionally been considered a relative contraindication to electroconvulsive therapy, and the authors recommend consultation with a neurosurgeon before using electroconvulsive therapy in patients with brain tumors. There is strong anecdotal evidence that electroconvulsive therapy can be used safely in individuals with small, solitary intracranial masses that lack significant mass effect. In patients with large, multiple, or highly edematous neoplasms, electroconvulsive therapy should be a last resort (Rasmussen, Perry, Sutor, & Moore, 2007).

CONCLUSIONS

The problem of mood disorders in the elderly is complicated by the high rates of neurological disease in this age group. While this problem is widely recognized by clinicians, and repeatedly documented in the literature, mood disorders in the elderly with neurological illnesses remain underdiagnosed and undertreated. Some of the reasons include failure of clinicians to distinguish mood symptoms from symptoms of primary illness, the tendency of patients and doctors to misattribute mood problems to reactions to physical illness, and the relative absence of controlled observational and treatment studies. This important area merits further investigation, as it may illuminate mechanisms of cognitive and behavioral function and dysfunction. More important, elderly patients with neurological disorders and mood dysfunction deserve better evaluation and treatment than are found in the inadequate state of the art.

Disclosures

Dr. Wint has no disclosures to report.

Dr. Cummings has consulted for the following pharmaceutical and device companies: Abbott, Anavex, Astellas, Avanir, Bayer, Bristol Myers Squibb, Elan, EnVivo, ExonHit, Genentech, Janssen, Lundbeck, Medavante, Medivation, Merck, Neurokos, Novartis, Pfizer, Prana, QR Pharma, Sonexa, Takeda, Toyama, and UBC.

REFERENCES

Alexopoulos, G. S., Meyers, B. S., Young, R. C., Campbell, S., Silbersweig, D., & Charlson, M. (1997a). 'Vascular depression' hypothesis. *Archives of General Psychiatry, 54*(10), 915–922.

Alexopoulos, G. S., Meyers, B. S., Young, R. C., Kakuma, T., Silbersweig, D., & Charlson, M. (1997b). Clinically defined vascular depression. *American Journal of Psychiatry 154*(4), 562–565.

Alper, K., Schwartz, K. A., Kolts, R. L., & Khan, A. (2007). Seizure incidence in psychopharmacological clinical trials: An analysis of Food and Drug Administration (FDA) summary basis of approval reports. *Biological Psychiatry, 62*(4), 345–354.

Antonijevic, I. A., & Steiger, A. (2003). Depression-like changes of the sleep-EEG during high dose corticosteroid treatment in patients with multiple sclerosis. *Psychoneuroendocrinology, 28*(6), 780–795.

Arana, A., Wentworth, C. E., Ayuso-Mateos, J. L., & Arellano, F. M. (2010). Suicide-related events in patients treated with antiepileptic drugs. *New England Journal of Medicine, 363*(6), 542–551.

Arnold, S. D., Forman, L. M., Brigidi, B. D., Carter, K. E., Schweitzer, H. A., Quinn, H. E.,…Raynor, R. H. (2008). Evaluation and characterization of generalized anxiety and depression in patients with primary brain tumors. *Neuro-Oncology, 10*(2), 171–181.

Ayerbe, L., Ayis, S., Rudd, A. G., Heuschmann, P. U., & Wolfe, C. D. (2011). Natural history, predictors, and associations of depression 5 years after stroke: The South London stroke register. *Stroke, 42*(7), 1907–1911.

Barone, P., Goetz, C., Houben, J. J., Koester, J., Leentjens, A. F., Poewe, W., et al. (2008). PRODEST—Depressive symptoms in Parkinson's disease: Effect of antidepressant treatment on symptom items of depression. *Neurology, 70*(11), A287–A287.

Barone, P., Poewe, W., Albrecht, S., Debieuvre, C., Massey, D., Rascol, O.,…Weintraub, D. (2010). Pramipexole for the treatment of depressive symptoms in patients with Parkinson's disease: A randomised, double-blind, placebo-controlled trial. *Lancet Neurology, 9*(6), 573–580.

Barone, P., Scarzella, L., Marconi, R., Antonini, A., Morgante, L., Bracco, F.,…Depression/Parkinson Italian Study Group. (2006). Pramipexole versus sertraline in the treatment of depression in Parkinson's disease: A national multicenter parallel-group randomized study. *Journal of Neurology, 253*(5), 601–607.

Bearden, C. E., Glahn, D. C., Monkul, E. S., Barrett, J., Najt, P., Villarreal, V., & Soares, J. C. (2006). Patterns of memory impairment in bipolar disorder and unipolar major depression. *Psychiatry Research, 142*(2–3), 139–150.

Bodkin, J. A., & Amsterdam, J. D. (2002). Transdermal selegiline in major depression: A double-blind, placebo-controlled, parallel-group study in outpatients. *American Journal of Psychiatry, 159*(11), 1869–1875.

Boeve, B. F. (2006). A review of the non-Alzheimer dementias. *Journal of Clinical Psychiatry, 67*(12), 1985–2001; discussion 1983–1984.

Bour, A., Rasquin, S., Aben, I., Boreas, A., Limburg, M., & Verhey, F. (2010). A one-year follow-up study into the course of depression after stroke. *Journal of Nutrition, Health, and Aging, 14*(6), 488–493.

Bowen, D. M., & Davison, A. N. (1980). Biochemical changes in the cholinergic system of the ageing brain and in senile dementia. *Psychological Medicine, 10*(2), 315–319.

Braun, C. M., Larocque, C., Daigneault, S., & Montour-Proulx, I. (1999). Mania, pseudomania, depression, and pseudodepression resulting from focal unilateral cortical lesions. *Neuropsychiatry, Neuropsychology, and Behavioral Neurology, 12*(1), 35–51.

Bronnum-Hansen, H., Stenager, E., Nylev Stenager, E., & Koch-Henriksen, N. (2005). Suicide among Danes with multiple sclerosis. *Journal of Neurology, Neurosurgery, and Psychiatry, 76*(10), 1457–1459.

Broomfield, N. M., Laidlaw, K., Hickabottom, E., Murray, M. F., Pendrey, R., Whittick, J. E., & Gillespie, D. C. (2011). Post-stroke depression: The case for augmented, individually tailored cognitive behavioural therapy. *Clinical Psychology and Psychotherapy, 18*(3), 202–217.

Brown, M., Schrot, R., Bauer, K., & Letendre, D. (2009). Incidence of first primary central nervous system tumors in California, 2001–2005. *Journal of Neurooncology, 94*(2), 249–261.

Burke, W. J., Peterson, J., & Rubin, E. H (1988). Electroconvulsive therapy in the treatment of combined depression and Parkinson's disease. *Psychosomatics, 29*(3), 341–346.

Caine, E. D., & Shoulson, I. (1983). Psychiatric syndromes in Huntington's disease. *American Journal of Psychiatry, 140*(6), 728–733.

Caraci, F., Copani, A., Nicoletti, F., & Drago, F. (2010). Depression and Alzheimer's disease: neurobiological links and common pharmacological targets. *European Journal of Pharmacology, 626*(1), 64–71.

Carota, A., Berney, A., Aybek, S., Iaria, G., Staub, F., Ghika-Schmid, F., & Bogousslavsky, J. (2005). A prospective study of predictors of poststroke depression. *Neurology, 64*(3), 428–433.

Carran, M. A., Kohler, C. G., O'Connor, M. J., Bilker, W. B., & Sperling, M. R. (2003). Mania following temporal lobectomy. *Neurology, 61*(6), 770–774.

Carson, A. J., MacHale, S., Allen, K., Lawrie, S. M., Dennis, M., House, A., & Sharpe, M. (2000). Depression after stroke and lesion location: A systematic review. *Lancet, 356*(9224), 122–126.

Ceravolo, R., Frosini, D., Rossi, C., & Bonuccelli, U (2009). Impulse control disorders in Parkinson's disease: Definition, epidemiology, risk factors, neurobiology and management. *Parkinsonism and Related Disorders, 15*(Suppl 4), S111–115.

Ceravolo, R., Frosini, D., Rossi, C., & Bonuccelli, U. (2010). Spectrum of addictions in Parkinson's disease: From dopamine dysregulation syndrome to impulse control disorders. *Journal of Neurology, 257*(Suppl 2), S276–283.

Chemerinski, E., Petracca, G., Sabe, L., Kremer, J., & Starkstein, S. E. (2001). The specificity of depressive symptoms in patients with Alzheimer's disease. *American Journal of Psychiatry, 158*(1), 68–72.

Chemerinski, E., Robinson, R. G., & Kosier, J. T (2001). Improved recovery in activities of daily living associated with remission of poststroke depression. *Stroke, 32*(1), 113–117.

Chen, P., Ganguli, M., Mulsant, B. H., & DeKosky, S. T (1999). The temporal relationship between depressive symptoms and dementia: A community-based prospective study. *Archives of General Psychiatry, 56*(3), 261–266.

Chen, P., Kales, H. C., Weintraub, D., Blow, F. C., Jiang, L., & Mellow, A. M. (2007). Antidepressant treatment of veterans with Parkinson's disease and depression: Analysis of a national sample. *Journal of Geriatric Psychiatry and Neurology, 20*(3), 161–165.

Chen, Y., Guo, J. J., Zhan, S., & Patel, N. C (2006). Treatment effects of antidepressants in patients with post-stroke depression: A meta-analysis. *Annals of Pharmacotherapy, 40*(12), 2115–2122.

Chen, Y., Patel, N. C., Guo, J. J., & Zhan, S (2007). Antidepressant prophylaxis for poststroke depression: A meta-analysis. *International Clinical Psychopharmacology, 22*(3), 159–166.

Chopra, A., Tye, S. J., Lee, K. H., Matsumoto, J., Klassen, B., Adams, A. C., … Frye, M. A. (2011). Voltage-dependent mania after subthalamic nucleus deep brain stimulation in Parkinson's disease: A case report. *Biological Psychiatry, 70*(2), e5–7.

Cummings, J. L. (1992). Depression and Parkinson's disease: A review. *American Journal of Psychiatry, 149*(4), 443–454.

Cummings, J. L. (1993). Frontal-subcortical circuits and human behavior. *Archives of Neurology, 50*(8), 873–880.

Cummings, J. L., & Mendez, M. F. (1984). Secondary mania with focal cerebrovascular lesions. *American Journal of Psychiatry, 141*(9), 1084–1087.

Devanand, D. P., Sano, M., Tang, M. X., Taylor, S., Gurland, B. J., Wilder, D., … Mayeux, R. (1996). Depressed mood and the incidence of Alzheimer's disease in the elderly living in the community. *Archives of General Psychiatry, 53*(2), 175–182.

Devos, D., Dujardin, K., Poirot, I., Moreau, C., Cottencin, O., Thomas, P., … Defebvre, L. (2008). Comparison of desipramine and citalopram treatments for depression in Parkinson's disease: A double-blind, randomized, placebo-controlled study. *Movement Disorders, 23*(6), 850–857.

Di Iulio, F., Palmer, K., Blundo, C., Casini, A. R., Gianni, W., Caltagirone, C., & Spalletta, G. (2010). Occurrence of neuropsychiatric symptoms and psychiatric disorders in mild Alzheimer's disease and mild cognitive impairment subtypes. *International Psychogeriatrics, 22*(4), 629–640.

Dobkin, R. D., Menza, M., Allen, L. A., Gara, M. A., Mark, M. H., Tiu, J., … Friedman, J. (2011). Cognitive-behavioral therapy for depression in Parkinson's disease: A randomized, controlled trial. *American Journal of Psychiatry, 168*(10), 1066–1074.

Dowlati, Y., Herrmann, N., Swardfager, W., Liu, H., Sham, L., Reim, E. K., & Lanctôt, K. L. (2010). A meta-analysis of cytokines in major depression. *Biological Psychiatry, 67*(5), 446–457.

Dresler, M., Genzel, L., Kluge, M., Schüssler, P., Weber, F., Rosenhagen, M., & Steiger, A. (2010). Off-line memory consolidation impairments in multiple sclerosis patients receiving high-dose corticosteroid treatment mirror consolidation impairments in depression. *Psychoneuroendocrinology, 35*(8), 1194–1202.

Drijgers, R. L., Aalten, P., Winogrodzka, A., Verhey, F. R., & Leentjens, A. F. (2009). Pharmacological treatment of apathy in neurodegenerative diseases: A systematic review. *Dementia and Geriatric Cognitive Disorders, 28*(1), 13–22.

Dubois, B., McKeith, I., Orgogozo, J. M., Collins, O., & Meulien, D. (1999). A multicentre, randomized, double-blind, placebo-controlled study to evaluate the efficacy, tolerability and safety of two doses of metrifonate in patients with mild-to-moderate Alzheimer's disease: The MALT study. *International Journal of Geriatric Psychiatry, 14*(11), 973–982.

Ehde, D. M., Kraft, G. H., Chwastiak, L., Sullivan, M. D., Gibbons, L. E., Bombardier, C. H., & Wadhwani, R. (2008). Efficacy of paroxetine in treating major depressive disorder in persons with multiple sclerosis. *General Hospital Psychiatry, 30*(1), 40–48.

Engedal, K., Barca, M. L., Laks, J., & Selbaek, G. (2010). Depression in Alzheimer's disease: specificity of depressive symptoms using three different clinical criteria. *International Journal of Geriatric Psychiatry, 26*(9), 944–951.

Epstein, C. M., Evatt, M. L., Funk, A., Girard-Siqueira, L., Lupei, N., Slaughter, L., … DeLong, M. R.

(2007). An open study of repetitive transcranial magnetic stimulation in treatment-resistant depression with Parkinson's disease. *Clinical Neurophysiology, 118*(10), 2189–2194.

Erkinjuntti, T., Kurz, A., Gauthier, S., Bullock, R., Lilienfeld, S., & Damaraju, C. V. (2002). Efficacy of galantamine in probable vascular dementia and Alzheimer's disease combined with cerebrovascular disease: A randomised trial. *Lancet, 359*(9314), 1283–1290.

Ettinger, A., Reed, M., Cramer, J., & Epilepsy Impact Project Group. (2004). Depression and comorbidity in community-based patients with epilepsy or asthma. *Neurology, 63*(6), 1008–1014.

Falk, W. E., Mahnke, M. W., & Poskanzer, D. C. (1979). Lithium prophylaxis of corticotropin-induced psychosis. *Journal of the American Medical Association, 241*(10), 1011–1012.

Farabaugh, A., Locascio, J. J., Yap, L., Growdon, J., Fava, M., Crawford, C., ... Alpert, J. E. (2010). Cognitive-behavioral therapy for patients with Parkinson's disease and comorbid major depressive disorder. *Psychosomatics, 51*(2), 124–129.

Farrer, L. A. (1986). Suicide and attempted suicide in Huntington disease: Implications for preclinical testing of persons at risk. *American Journal of Medical Genetics, 24*(2), 305–311.

Fedoroff, J. P., Starkstein, S. E., Parikh, R. M., Price, T. R., & Robinson, R. G. (1991). Are depressive symptoms nonspecific in patients with acute stroke? *American Journal of Psychiatry, 148*(9), 1172–1176.

Feinstein, A. (2000). Multiple sclerosis, disease modifying treatments and depression: A critical methodological review. *Multiple Sclerosis, 6*(5), 343–348.

Feinstein, A., O'Connor, P., & Feinstein, K. (2002). Multiple sclerosis, interferon beta-1b and depression A prospective investigation. *Journal of Neurology, 249*(7), 815–820.

Feinstein, A., Roy, P., Lobaugh, N., Feinstein, K., O'Connor, P., & Black, S. (2004). Structural brain abnormalities in multiple sclerosis patients with major depression. *Neurology, 62*(4), 586–590.

Folstein, S., Abbott, M. H., Chase, G. A., Jensen, B. A., & Folstein, M. F. (1983). The association of affective disorder with Huntington's disease in a case series and in families. *Psychological Medicine, 13*(3), 537–542.

Frisina, P. G., Haroutunian, V., & Libow, L. S. (2009). The neuropathological basis for depression in Parkinson's disease. *Parkinsonism and Related Disorders, 15*(2), 144–148.

Gardner, B. K., & O'Connor, D. W. (2008). A review of the cognitive effects of electroconvulsive therapy in older adults. *Journal of ECT, 24*(1), 68–80.

Gathinji, M., McGirt, M. J., Attenello, F. J., Chaichana, K. L., Than, K., Olivi, A., ... Quinones-Hinojosa, A. (2009). Association of preoperative depression and survival after resection of malignant brain astrocytoma. *Surgery and Neurology, 71*(3), 299–303.

Gauthier, S., Feldman, H., Hecker, J., Vellas, B., Ames, D., Subbiah, P., ... Donepezil MSAD Study Investigators Group. (2002). Efficacy of donepezil on behavioral symptoms in patients with moderate to severe Alzheimer's disease. *International Psychogeriatrics, 14*(4), 389–404.

Giannini, M. J., Bergmark, B., Kreshover, S., Elias, E., Plummer, C., & O'Keefe, E. (2010). Understanding suicide and disability through three major disabling conditions: Intellectual disability, spinal cord injury, and multiple sclerosis. *Disability Health Journal, 3*(2), 74–78.

Gilliam, F. G., Santos, J., Vahle, V., Carter, J., Brown, K., & Hecimovic, H. (2004). Depression in epilepsy: Ignoring clinical expression of neuronal network dysfunction? *Epilepsia, 45*(Suppl 2), 28–33.

Ginsberg, D. L., & Sussman, N. (2001). Gabapentin as prophylaxis against steroid-induced mania. *Canadian Journal of Psychiatry, 46*(5), 455–456.

Gotham, A. M., Brown, R. G., & Marsden, C. D. (1986). Depression in Parkinson's disease: A quantitative and qualitative analysis. *Journal of Neurology, Neurosurgery, and Psychiatry, 49*(4), 381–389.

Grove, V. E., Jr., Quintanilla, J., & DeVaney, G. T. (2000). Improvement of Huntington's disease with olanzapine and valproate. *New England Journal of Medicine 343*(13), 973–974.

Halliday, G. M., Li, Y. W., Blumbergs, P. C., Joh, T. H., Cotton, R. G., Howe, P. R., ... Geffen, L. B. (1990). Neuropathology of immunohistochemically identified brainstem neurons in Parkinson's disease. *Annals of Neurology, 27*(4), 373–385.

Harris, E. C., & Barraclough, B. M. (1994). Suicide as an outcome for medical disorders. *Medicine (Baltimore), 73*(6), 281–296.

Hashioka, S., McGeer, P. L., Monji, A., & Kanba, S. (2009). Anti-inflammatory effects of antidepressants: Possibilities for preventives against Alzheimer's disease. *Central Nervous System Agents Medical Chemistry, 9*(1), 12–19.

Hauser, W. A., Annegers, J. F., & Kurland, L. T. (1991). Prevalence of epilepsy in Rochester, Minnesota: 1940–1980. *Epilepsia, 32*(4), 429–445.

Hausner, L., Damian, M., Sartorius, A., & Frölich, L. (2011). Efficacy and cognitive side effects of electroconvulsive therapy (ECT) in depressed elderly inpatients with coexisting mild cognitive impairment or dementia. *Journal of Clinical Psychiatry*, 72(1), 91–97.

Holmes, C., Wilkinson, D., Dean, C., Vethanayagam, S., Olivieri, S., Langley, A., ... Damms, J. (2004). The efficacy of donepezil in the treatment of neuropsychiatric symptoms in Alzheimer disease. *Neurology*, 63(2), 214–219.

Hubbard, B. M., & Anderson, J. M. (1985). Age-related variations in the neuron content of the cerebral cortex in senile dementia of Alzheimer type. *Neuropathology and Applied Neurobiology*, 11(5), 369–382.

Huntington, G. (1872). On chorea. *Medical and Surgical Reporter*, 26(5), 317–321.

Imamura, K., Okayasu, N., & Nagatsu, T. (2010). The relationship between depression and regional cerebral blood flow in Parkinson's disease and the effect of selegiline treatment. *Acta Neurologica Scandinavica*, 126(3), 210–218.

Ishihara, L., & Brayne, C. (2006). A systematic review of depression and mental illness preceding Parkinson's disease. *Acta Neurologica Scandinavica*, 113(4), 211–220.

Jacobs, L. D., Beck, R. W., Simon, J. H., Kinkel, R. P., Brownscheidle, C. M., Murray, T. J., ... Sandrock, A. W. (2000). Intramuscular interferon beta-1a therapy initiated during a first demyelinating event in multiple sclerosis. CHAMPS Study Group. *New England Journal of Medicine*, 343(13), 898–904.

Janardhan, V., & Bakshi, R. (2002). Quality of life in patients with multiple sclerosis: The impact of fatigue and depression. *Journal of Neurological Science*, 205(1), 51–58.

Jankovic, J., & Beach, J. (1997). Long-term effects of tetrabenazine in hyperkinetic movement disorders. *Neurology*, 48(2), 358–362.

Jankovic, J., & Orman, J. (1988). Tetrabenazine therapy of dystonia, chorea, tics, and other dyskinesias. *Neurology*, 38(3), 391–394.

Jellinger, K. A. (1991). Pathology of Parkinson's disease. Changes other than the nigrostriatal pathway. *Molecular and Chemical Neuropathology*, 14(3), 153–197.

Joffe, R. T., Lippert, G. P., Gray, T. A., Sawa, G., & Horvath, Z. (1987). Mood disorder and multiple sclerosis. *Archives of Neurology*, 44(4), 376–378.

Jorm, A. F. (2000). Is depression a risk factor for dementia or cognitive decline? A review. *Gerontology*, 46(4), 219–227.

Jouvent, R., Abensour, P., Bonnet, A. M., Widlocher, D., Agid, Y., & Lhermitte, F. (1983). Antiparkinsonian and antidepressant effects of high doses of bromocriptine. An independent

comparison. *Journal of Affective Disorders*, 5(2), 141–145.

Kanner, A. M. (2008). The use of psychotropic drugs in epilepsy: What every neurologist should know. *Seminars in Neurology*, 28(3), 379–388.

Kaufer, D. (1998). Beyond the cholinergic hypothesis: The effect of metrifonate and other cholinesterase inhibitors on neuropsychiatric symptoms in Alzheimer's disease. *Dementia and Geriatric Cognitive Disorders*, 9(Suppl 2), 8–14.

Kelly, W. F. (1996). Psychiatric aspects of Cushing's syndrome. *QJM*, 89(7), 543–551.

Klapper, J. A. (1994). Interferon beta treatment of multiple sclerosis. *Neurology*, 44(1), 188; author reply 188–190.

Koch, M. W., Glazenborg, A., Uyttenboogaart, M., Mostert, J., & De Keyser, J. (2011). Pharmacologic treatment of depression in multiple sclerosis. *Cochrane Database of Systematic Reviews*, 2, CD007295.

Kouwenhoven, S. E., Kirkevold, M., Engedal, K., & Kim, H. S. (2011). Depression in acute stroke: prevalence, dominant symptoms and associated factors. A systematic literature review. *Disability and Rehabilitation*, 33(7), 539–556.

Krishnan, K. R., Hays, J. C., & Blazer, D. G. (1997). MRI-defined vascular depression. *American Journal of Psychiatry*, 154(4), 497–501:

Krystal, A. D., & Coffey, C. E. (1997). Neuropsychiatric considerations in the use of electroconvulsive therapy. *Journal of Neuropsychiatry and Clinical Neuroscience*, 9(2), 283–292.

Kuhn, K. U., Quednow, B. B., Thiel, M., Falkai, P., Maier, W., & Elger, C. E. (2003). Antidepressive treatment in patients with temporal lobe epilepsy and major depression: A prospective study with three different antidepressants. *Epilepsy and Behavior*, 4(6), 674–679.

Kulisevsky, J., Berthier, M. L., Gironell, A., Pascual-Sedano, B., Molet, J., & Parés, P. (2002). Mania following deep brain stimulation for Parkinson's disease. *Neurology*, 59(9), 1421–1424.

Larcombe, N. A., & Wilson, P. H. (1984). An evaluation of cognitive-behaviour therapy for depression in patients with multiple sclerosis. *British Journal of Psychiatry*, 145, 366–371.

Lauterbach, E. C. (1996). Bipolar disorders, dystonia, and compulsion after dysfunction of the cerebellum, dentatorubrothalamic tract, and substantia nigra. *Biological Psychiatry*, 40(8), 726–730.

Lauterbach, E. C. (2001). Cerebellar-subcortical circuits and mania in cerebellar disease. *Journal of Neuropsychiatry and Clinical Neuroscience*, 13(1), 112.

Lauterbach, E. C., Harris, J. B., & Bina, W. F., III. (2010). Mood and neurobehavioral correlates of cerebellar lesions. *Cognitive and Behavioral Neurology*, 23(2), 63–73.

Leentjens, A. F. (2011). The role of dopamine agonists in the treatment of depression in patients with Parkinson's disease: A systematic review. *Drugs*, 71(3), 273–286.

Lemke, M. R., Fuchs, G., Gemende, I., Herting, B., Oehlwein, C., Reichmann, H.,…Volkmann, J. (2004). Depression and Parkinson's disease. *Journal of Neurology*, 251, 24–27.

Levinson, D. F., & Devinsky, O. (1999). Psychiatric adverse events during vigabatrin therapy. *Neurology*, 53(7), 1503–1511.

Levy, M. L., Cummings, J. L., Fairbanks, L. A., Masterman, D., Miller, B. L., Craig, A. H.,…Litvan, I. (1998). Apathy is not depression. *Journal of Neuropsychiatry and Clinical Neuroscience*, 10(3), 314–319.

Lipsey, J. R., Robinson, R. G., Pearlson, G. D., Rao, K., & Price, T. R. (1984). Nortriptyline treatment of post-stroke depression: A double-blind study. *Lancet*, 1(8372), 297–300.

Litofsky, N. S., Farace, E., Anderson, F. Jr., Meyers, C. A., Huang, W., Laws, E. R. Jr., & Glioma Outcomes Project Investigators. (2004). Depression in patients with high-grade glioma: Results of the Glioma Outcomes Project. *Neurosurgery*, 54(2), 358–366; discussion 366–357.

Litofsky, N. S., & Resnick, A. G. (2009). The relationships between depression and brain tumors. *Journal of Neurooncology*, 94(2), 153–161.

Lobentanz, I. S., Asenbaum, S., Vass, K., Sauter, C., Klösch, G., Kollegger, H.,…Zeitlhofer, J. (2004). Factors influencing quality of life in multiple sclerosis patients: Disability, depressive mood, fatigue and sleep quality. *Acta Neurologica Scandinavica*, 110(1), 6–13.

Lopez-Gomez, M., Ramirez-Bermudez, J., Campillo, C., Sosa, A. L., Espinola, M., & Ruiz, I. (2005). Primidone is associated with interictal depression in patients with epilepsy. *Epilepsy and Behavior*, 6(3), 413–416.

Luijendijk, H. J., Stricker, B. H., Wieberdink, R. G., Koudstaal, P. J., Hofman, A., Breteler, M. M., & Tiemeier, H. (2011). Transient ischemic attack and incident depression. *Stroke*, 42(7), 1857–1861.

Lyketsos, C. G., Steinberg, M., Tschanz, J. T., Norton, M. C., Steffens, D. C., & Breitner, J. C. (2000). Mental and behavioral disturbances in dementia: Findings from the Cache County Study on Memory in Aging. *American Journal of Psychiatry*, 157(5), 708–714.

Mainio, A., Hakko, H., Niemelä, A., Koivukangas, J., & Räsänen, P. (2005). Depression and functional outcome in patients with brain tumors: A population-based 1-year follow-up study. *Journal of Neurosurgery*, 103(5), 841–847.

Marsh, L., McDonald, W. M., Cummings, J., Ravina, B., & NINDS/NIMH Work Group on Depression and Parkinson's Disease. (2006). Provisional diagnostic criteria for depression in Parkinson's disease: Report of an NINDS/NIMH Work Group. *Movement Disorders*, 21(2), 148–158.

Martin, R., Kuzniecky, R., Ho, S., Hetherington, H., Pan, J., Sinclair, K.,…Faught, E. (1999). Cognitive effects of topiramate, gabapentin, and lamotrigine in healthy young adults. *Neurology*, 52(2), 321–327.

Martinez-Martin, P., Rodriguez-Blazquez, C., Kurtis, M. M., Chaudhuri, K. R., & NMSS Validation Group. (2011). The impact of non-motor symptoms on health-related quality of life of patients with Parkinson's disease. *Movement Disorders*, 26(3), 399–406.

Mayberg, H. S., Starkstein, S. E., Peyser, C. E., Brandt, J., Dannals, R. F., & Folstein, S. E. (1992). Paralimbic frontal lobe hypometabolism in depression associated with Huntington's disease. *Neurology*, 42(9), 1791–1797.

McKeith, I., Del Ser, T., Spano, P., Emre, M., Wesnes, K., Anand, R.,…Spiegel, R. (2000). Efficacy of rivastigmine in dementia with Lewy bodies: A randomised, double-blind, placebo-controlled international study. *Lancet*, 356(9247), 2031–2036.

Mendez, M. F. (1994). Huntington's disease: Update and review of neuropsychiatric aspects. *International Journal of Psychiatry in Medicine*, 24(3), 189–208.

Menza, M., Dobkin, R. D., Marin, H., Mark, M. H., Gara, M., Buyske, S.,…Dicke, A. (2009). A controlled trial of antidepressants in patients with Parkinson disease and depression. *Neurology*, 72(10), 886–892.

Miller, K. M., Okun, M. S., Fernandez, H. F., Jacobson, C. E., IV, Rodriguez, R. L., & Bowers, D. (2007). Depression symptoms in movement disorders: Comparing Parkinson's disease, dystonia, and essential tremor. *Movement Disorders*, 22(5), 666–672.

Minden, S. L., Orav, J., & Reich, P. (1987). Depression in multiple sclerosis. *General Hospital Psychiatry*, 9(6), 426–434.

Minden, S. L., & Schiffer, R. B. (1990). Affective disorders in multiple sclerosis. Review and recommendations for clinical research. *Archives of Neurology*, 47(1), 98–104.

Miyasaki, J. M., Shannon, K., Voon, V., Ravina, B., Kleiner-Fisman, G., Anderson, K.,…Quality

Standards Subcommittee of the American Academy of Neurology. (2006). Practice Parameter: Evaluation and treatment of depression, psychosis, and dementia in Parkinson disease (an evidence-based review), report of the Quality Standards Subcommittee of the American Academy of Neurology. *Neurology, 66*(7), 996–1002.

Miyawaki, E., Perlmutter, J. S., Tröster, A. I., Videen, T. O., & Koller, W. C. (2000). The behavioral complications of pallidal stimulation: A case report. *Brain and Cognition, 42*(3), 417–434.

Mohr, D. C., Boudewyn, A. C., Goodkin, D. E., Bostrom, A., & Epstein, L. (2001). Comparative outcomes for individual cognitive-behavior therapy, supportive-expressive group psychotherapy, and sertraline for the treatment of depression in multiple sclerosis. *Journal of Consulting and Clinical Psychology, 69*(6), 942–949.

Morrow, G. R., Hickok, J. T., Roscoe, J. A., Raubertas, R. F., Andrews, P. L., Flynn, P. J., . . . University of Rochester Cancer Center Community Clinical Oncology Program. (2003). Differential effects of paroxetine on fatigue and depression: A randomized, double-blind trial from the University of Rochester Cancer Center Community Clinical Oncology Program. *Journal of Clinical Oncology, 21*(24), 4635–4641.

Moss, E. L., Simpson, J. S., Pelletier, G., & Forsyth, P. (2006). An open-label study of the effects of bupropion SR on fatigue, depression and quality of life of mixed-site cancer patients and their partners. *Psychooncology, 15*(3), 259–267.

Mula, M., & Sander, J. W. (2007). Negative effects of antiepileptic drugs on mood in patients with epilepsy. *Drug Safety, 30*(7), 555–567.

Mula, M., Trimble, M. R., Lhatoo, S. D., & Sander, J. W. (2003). Topiramate and psychiatric adverse events in patients with epilepsy. *Epilepsia, 44*(5), 659–663.

Naarding, P., Kremer, H. P., & Zitman, F. G. (2001). Huntington's disease: A review of the literature on prevalence and treatment of neuropsychiatric phenomena. *European Psychiatry, 16*(8), 439–445.

Neary, D., Snowden, J. S., Gustafson, L., Passant, U., Stuss, D., Black, S., . . . Benson, D. F. (1998). Frontotemporal lobar degeneration: A consensus on clinical diagnostic criteria. *Neurology, 51*(6), 1546–1554.

Negre-Pages, L., Grandjean, H., Lapeyre-Mestre, M., Montastruc, J. L., Fourrier, A., Lépine, J. P., . . . DoPaMiP Study Group. (2010). Anxious and depressive symptoms in Parkinson's disease: The French cross-sectional DoPaMiP study. *Movement Disorders, 25*(2), 157–166.

Noe, K. H., Locke, D. E., & Sirven, J. I. (2011). Treatment of depression in patients with epilepsy. *Current Treatment Options in Neurology, 13*(4), 371–379.

Noseworthy, J., Paty, D., Wonnacott, T., Feasby, T., & Ebers, G. (1983). Multiple sclerosis after age 50. *Neurology, 33*(12), 1537–1544.

O'Sullivan, S. S., Williams, D. R., Gallagher, D. A., Massey, L. A., Silveira-Moriyama, L., & Lees, A. J. (2008). Nonmotor symptoms as presenting complaints in Parkinson's disease: A clinicopathological study. *Movement Disorders, 23*(1), 101–106.

Pal, E., Nagy, F., Aschermann, Z., Balazs, E., & Kovacs, N. (2010). The impact of left prefrontal repetitive transcranial magnetic stimulation on depression in Parkinson's disease: A randomized, double-blind, placebo-controlled study. *Movement Disorders, 25*(14), 2311–2317.

Paolucci, S., Antonucci, G., Pratesi, L., Traballesi, M., Grasso, M. G., & Lubich, S. (1999). Poststroke depression and its role in rehabilitation of inpatients. *Archives of Physical Medicine and Rehabilitation, 80*(9), 985–990.

Paparrigopoulos, T., Ferentinos, P., Kouzoupis, A., Koutsis, G., & Papadimitriou, G. N. (2010). The neuropsychiatry of multiple sclerosis: Focus on disorders of mood, affect and behaviour. *International Review of Psychiatry, 22*(1), 14–21.

Paradiso, S., Duff, K., Vaidya, J. G., Hoth, A., & Mold, J. W. (2010). Cognitive and daily functioning in older adults with vegetative symptoms of depression. *International Journal of Geriatric Psychiatry, 25*(6), 569–577.

Paradiso, S., Hermann, B. P., Blumer, D., Davies, K., & Robinson, R. G. (2001). Impact of depressed mood on neuropsychological status in temporal lobe epilepsy. *Journal of Neurology, Neurosurgery, and Psychiatry, 70*(2), 180–185.

Paradiso, S., Ohkubo, T., & Robinson, R. G. (1997). Vegetative and psychological symptoms associated with depressed mood over the first two years after stroke. *International Journal of Psychiatry in Medicine, 27*(2), 137–157.

Patten, S. B., & Metz, L. M. (2002). Interferon beta1a and depression in secondary progressive MS: Data from the SPECTRIMS Trial. *Neurology, 59*(5), 744–746.

Paulsen, J. S., Hoth, K. F., Nehl, C., & Stierman, L. (2005). Critical periods of suicide risk in Huntington's disease. *American Journal of Psychiatry, 162*(4), 725–731.

Paulsen, J. S., Nehl, C., Hoth, K. F., Kanz, J. E., Benjamin, M., Conybeare, R., . . . Turner, B. (2005). Depression and stages of Huntington's disease.

Journal of Neuropsychiatry and Clinical Neuroscience, 17(4), 496–502.

Plotsky, P. M., Owens, M. J., & Nemeroff, C. B. (1998). Psychoneuroendocrinology of depression. Hypothalamic-pituitary-adrenal axis. *Psychiatric Clinics of North America, 21*(2), 293–307.

Pluck, G. C., & Brown, R. G. (2002). Apathy in Parkinson's disease. *Journal of Neurology, Neurosurgery, and Psychiatry, 73*(6), 636–642.

Polliack, M. L., Barak, Y., & Achiron, A. (2001). Late-onset multiple sclerosis. *Journal of the American Geriatrics Society, 49*(2), 168–171.

Pompili, M., & Baldessarini, R. J. (2010). Epilepsy: Risk of suicidal behavior with antiepileptic drugs. *Nature Reviews Neurology, 6*(12), 651–653.

Prado-Jean, A., Couratier, P., Druet-Cabanac, M., Nubukpo, P., Bernard-Bourzeix, L., Thomas, P.,...Clément, J. P. (2010). Specific psychological and behavioral symptoms of depression in patients with dementia. *International Journal of Geriatric Psychiatry, 25*(10), 1065–1072.

Pujol, J., Bello, J., Deus, J., Martí-Vilalta, J. L., & Capdevila, A. (1997). Lesions in the left arcuate fasciculus region and depressive symptoms in multiple sclerosis. *Neurology, 49*(4), 1105–1110.

Rabins, P. V., Brooks, B. R., O'Donnell, P., Pearlson, G. D., Moberg, P., Jubelt, B.,...Folstein, M. F. (1986). Structural brain correlates of emotional disorder in multiple sclerosis. *Brain, 109*(Pt 4), 585–597.

Rampello, L., Alvano, A., Chiechio, S., Raffaele, R., Vecchio, I., & Malaguarnera, M. (2005). An evaluation of efficacy and safety of reboxetine in elderly patients affected by "retarded" post-stroke depression. A random, placebo-controlled study. *Archives of Gerontology and Geriatrics, 40*(3), 275–285.

Rao, V., & Lyketsos, C. G. (2000). The benefits and risks of ECT for patients with primary dementia who also suffer from depression. *International Journal of Geriatric Psychiatry, 15*(8), 729–735.

Raskin, S., & Durst, R. (2010). Bupropion as the treatment of choice in depression associated with Parkinson's disease and it's various treatments. *Medical Hypotheses, 75*(6), 544–546.

Rasmussen, A., Lunde, M., Poulsen, D. L., Sørensen, K., Qvitzau, S., & Bech, P. (2003). A double-blind, placebo-controlled study of sertraline in the prevention of depression in stroke patients. *Psychosomatics, 44*(3), 216–221.

Rasmussen, K. G., Perry, C. L., Sutor, B., & Moore, K. M. (2007). ECT in patients with intracranial masses. *Journal of Neuropsychiatry and Clinical Neuroscience, 19*(2), 191–193.

Reijnders, J. S., Ehrt, U., Weber, W. E., Aarsland, D., & Leentjens, A. F. (2008). A systematic review of prevalence studies of depression in Parkinson's disease. *Movement Disorders, 23*(2), 183–189; quiz 313.

Richelson, E. (2002). The clinical relevance of antidepressant interaction with neurotransmitter transporters and receptors. *Psychopharmacology Bulletin, 36*(4), 133–150.

Richelson, E. (2003). Interactions of antidepressants with neurotransmitter transporters and receptors and their clinical relevance. *Journal of Clinical Psychiatry, 64*(Suppl 13), 5–12.

Richelson, E., & Souder, T. (2000). Binding of antipsychotic drugs to human brain receptors focus on newer generation compounds. *Life Sciences, 68*(1), 29–39.

Robertson, M. M., Trimble, M. R., & Townsend, H. R. (1987). Phenomenology of depression in epilepsy. *Epilepsia, 28*(4), 364–372.

Robinson, R. G. (2003). Poststroke depression: Prevalence, diagnosis, treatment, and disease progression. *Biological Psychiatry, 54*(3), 376–387.

Robinson, R. G., Boston, J. D., Starkstein, S. E., & Price, T. R. (1988). Comparison of mania and depression after brain injury: Causal factors. *American Journal of Psychiatry, 145*(2), 172–178.

Robinson, R. G., Jorge, R. E., Moser, D. J., Acion, L., Solodkin, A., Small, S. L.,...Arndt, S. (2008). Escitalopram and problem-solving therapy for prevention of poststroke depression: A randomized controlled trial. *Journal of the American Medical Association, 299*(20), 2391–2400.

Robinson, R. G., Schultz, S. K., Castillo, C., Kopel, T., Kosier, J. T., Newman, R. M.,...Starkstein, S. E. (2000). Nortriptyline versus fluoxetine in the treatment of depression and in short-term recovery after stroke: A placebo-controlled, double-blind study. *American Journal of Psychiatry, 157*(3), 351–359.

Rooney, A., & Grant, R. (2010). Pharmacological treatment of depression in patients with a primary brain tumour. *Cochrane Database of Systematic Reviews, 3*, CD006932.

Rosenblatt, A., & Leroi, I. (2000). Neuropsychiatry of Huntington's disease and other basal ganglia disorders. *Psychosomatics, 41*(1), 24–30.

Ryback, R. S., & Schwab, R. S. (1971). Manic response to levodopa therapy. Report of a case. *New England Journal of Medicine, 285*(14), 788–789.

Saczynski, J. S., Beiser, A., Seshadri, S., Auerbach, S., Wolf, P. A., & Au, R. (2010). Depressive symptoms and risk of dementia: The Framingham Heart Study. *Neurology, 75*(1), 35–41.

Sadovnick, A. D., Eisen, K., Ebers, G. C., & Paty, D. W. (1991). Cause of death in patients attending multiple sclerosis clinics. *Neurology, 41*(8), 1193–1196.

Sadovnick, A. D., Remick, R. A., Allen, J., Swartz, E., Yee, I. M., Eisen, K.,…Paty, D. W. (1996). Depression and multiple sclerosis. *Neurology, 46*(3), 628–632.

Salazar, Z., Tschopp, L., Calandra, C., & Micheli, F. (2008). Pisa syndrome and parkinsonism secondary to valproic acid in Huntington's disease. *Movement Disorders, 23*(16), 2430–2431.

Schiffer, R. B., & Wineman, N. M. (1990). Antidepressant pharmacotherapy of depression associated with multiple sclerosis. *American Journal of Psychiatry, 147*(11), 1493–1497.

Schiffer, R. B., Wineman, N. M., & Weitkamp, L. R. (1986). Association between bipolar affective disorder and multiple sclerosis. *American Journal of Psychiatry, 143*(1), 94–95.

Schmitz, B. (2005). Depression and mania in patients with epilepsy. *Epilepsia, 46*(Suppl 4), 45–49.

Schneider, F., Reske, M., Finkelmeyer, A., Wojtecki, L., Timmermann, L., Brosig, T.,…Schnitzler, A. (2010). Predicting acute affective symptoms after deep brain stimulation surgery in Parkinson's disease. *Stereotactic and Functional Neurosurg, 88*(6), 367–373.

Schoenfeld, M., Myers, R. H., Cupples, L. A., Berkman, B., Sax, D. S., & Clark, E. (1984). Increased rate of suicide among patients with Huntington's disease. *Journal of Neurology, Neurosurgery, and Psychiatry, 47*(12), 1283–1287.

Schrag, A., Barone, P., Brown, R. G., Leentjens, A. F., McDonald, W. M., Starkstein, S.,…Goetz, C. G. (2007). Depression rating scales in Parkinson's disease: Critique and recommendations. *Movement Disorders, 22*(8), 1077–1092.

Schreiber, W., Krieg, J. C., & Eichhorn, T. (1999). Reversal of tetrabenazine induced depression by selective noradrenaline (norepinephrine) reuptake inhibition. *Journal of Neurology, Neurosurgery, and Psychiatry, 67*(4), 550.

Scripnikov, A., Khomenko, A., Napryeyenko, O., & GINDEM-NP Study Group. (2007). Effects of Ginkgo biloba extract EGb 761 on neuropsychiatric symptoms of dementia: Findings from a randomised controlled trial. *Wiener Medizinische Wochenschrift, 157*(13–14), 295–300.

Sheline, Y. I., Wang, P. W., Gado, M. H., Csernansky, J. G., & Vannier, M. W. (1996). Hippocampal atrophy in recurrent major depression. *Proceedings of the National Academy of Sciences USA, 93*(9), 3908–3913.

Shulman, L. M., Taback, R. L., Rabinstein, A. A., & Weiner, W. J. (2002). Non-recognition of depression and other non-motor symptoms in Parkinson's disease. *Parkinsonism and Related Disorders, 8*(3), 193–197.

Siegert, R. J., & Abernethy, D. A. (2005). Depression in multiple sclerosis: A review. *Journal of Neurology, Neurosurgery, and Psychiatry, 76*(4), 469–475.

Simpson, S., Baldwin, R. C., Jackson, A., & Burns, A. S. (1998). Is subcortical disease associated with a poor response to antidepressants? Neurological, neuropsychological and neuroradiological findings in late-life depression. *Psychological Medicine 28*(5), 1015–1026.

Solla, P., Cannas, A., Floris, G. L., Orofino, G., Costantino, E., Boi, A., Serra, C.,…Marrosu, F. (2011). Behavioral, neuropsychiatric and cognitive disorders in Parkinson's disease patients with and without motor complications. *Progress in Neuropsychopharmacology and Biological Psychiatry, 35*(4), 1009–1013.

Spalletta, G., Musicco, M., Padovani, A., Rozzini, L., Perri, R., Fadda, L.,…Palmer, K. (2010). Neuropsychiatric symptoms and syndromes in a large cohort of newly diagnosed, untreated patients with Alzheimer disease. *American Journal of Geriatric Psychiatry, 18*(11), 1026–1035.

Specchio, L. M., Iudice, A., Specchio, N., La Neve, A., Spinelli, A., Galli, R.,…Murri, L. (2004). Citalopram as treatment of depression in patients with epilepsy. *Clinical Neuropharmacology, 27*(3), 133–136.

Spina, E., Santoro, V., & D'Arrigo, C. (2008). Clinically relevant pharmacokinetic drug interactions with second-generation antidepressants: An update. *Clinical Therapy, 30*(7), 1206–1227.

Sproesser, E., Viana, M. A., Quagliato, E. M., & de Souza, E. A. (2010). The effect of psychotherapy in patients with PD: A controlled study. *Parkinsonism and Related Disorders, 16*(4), 298–300.

Starkstein, S. E., & Leentjens, A. F. (2008). The nosological position of apathy in clinical practice. *Journal of Neurology, Neurosurgery, and Psychiatry, 79*(10), 1088–1092.

Starkstein, S. E., Mayberg, H. S., Leiguarda, R., Preziosi, T. J., & Robinson, R. G. (1992). A prospective longitudinal study of depression, cognitive decline, and physical impairments in patients with Parkinson's disease. *Journal of Neurology, Neurosurgery, and Psychiatry, 55*(5), 377–382.

Starkstein, S. E., Mayberg, H. S., Preziosi, T. J., Andrezejewski, P., Leiguarda, R., & Robinson, R. G. (1992). Reliability, validity, and clinical correlates of apathy in Parkinson's disease. *Journal of Neuropsychiatry and Clinical Neuroscience, 4*(2), 134–139.

Starkstein, S. E., Pearlson, G. D., Boston, J., & Robinson, R. G. (1987). Mania after brain injury. A controlled study of causative factors. *Archives of Neurology*, 44(10), 1069–1073.

Starkstein, S. E., Petracca, G., Chemerinski, E., & Kremer, J. (2001). Syndromic validity of apathy in Alzheimer's disease. *American Journal of Psychiatry*, 158(6), 872–877.

Steffens, D. C., & Krishnan, K. R. (1998). Structural neuroimaging and mood disorders: Recent findings, implications for classification, and future directions. *Biological Psychiatry*, 43(10), 705–712.

Stenager, E. N., Stenager, E., Koch-Henriksen, N., Brønnum-Hansen, H., Hyllested, K., Jensen, K., & Bille-Brahe, U. (1992). Suicide and multiple sclerosis: An epidemiological investigation. *Journal of Neurology, Neurosurgery, and Psychiatry*, 55(7), 542–545.

Steur, E. N., & Ballering, L. A. (1997). Moclobemide and selegeline in the treatment of depression in Parkinson's disease. *Journal of Neurology, Neurosurgery, and Psychiatry*, 63(4), 547.

Tandberg, E., Larsen, J. P., Aarsland, D., & Cummings, J. L. (1996). The occurrence of depression in Parkinson's disease. A community-based study. *Archives of Neurology*, 53(2), 175–179.

Thomas, L., Trimble, M., Schmitz, B., & Ring, H. (1996). Vigabatrin and behaviour disorders: A retrospective survey. *Epilepsy Research*, 25(1), 21–27.

Trivedi, M. H., Rush, A. J., Wisniewski, S. R., Nierenberg, A. A., Warden, D., Ritz, L., ... STAR*D Study Team. (2006). Evaluation of outcomes with citalopram for depression using measurement-based care in STAR*D: Implications for clinical practice. *American Journal of Psychiatry*, 163(1), 28–40.

Ulla, M., Thobois, S., Llorca, P. M., Derost, P., Lemaire, J. J., Chereau-Boudet, I., ... Durif, F. (2011). Contact dependent reproducible hypomania induced by deep brain stimulation in Parkinson's disease: Clinical, anatomical and functional imaging study. *Journal of Neurology, Neurosurgery, and Psychiatry*, 82(6), 607–614.

US Department of Health and Human Services Food and Drug Administration (2008). *Statistical review and evaluation: Antiepileptic drugs and suicidality.* http://www.fda.gov/downloads/Drugs/DrugSafety/PostmarketDrugSafetyInformationfor PatientsandProviders/UCM192556.pdf.

Van Gerpen, J. A. (2002). Drug-induced parkinsonism. *Neurologist*, 8(6), 363–370.

Volicer, L., Van der Steen, J. T., & Frijters, D. H. (2009). Modifiable factors related to abusive behaviors in nursing home residents with dementia. *Journal of the American Medical Directors Association*, 10(9), 617–622.

Voon, V., Reynolds, B., Brezing, C., Gallea, C., Skaljic, M., Ekanayake, V., ... Hallett, M. (2010). Impulsive choice and response in dopamine agonist-related impulse control behaviors. *Psychopharmacology (Berlin)*, 207(4), 645–659.

Weintraub, D., Koester, J., Potenza, M. N., Siderowf, A. D., Stacy, M., Voon, V., ... Lang, A. E. (2010). Impulse control disorders in Parkinson disease: A cross-sectional study of 3090 patients. *Archives of Neurology*, 67(5), 589–595.

Weintraub, D., Mavandadi, S., Mamikonyan, E., Siderowf, A. D., Duda, J. E., Hurtig, H. I., ... Stern, M. B. (2010). Atomoxetine for depression and other neuropsychiatric symptoms in Parkinson disease. *Neurology*, 75(5), 448–455.

Weintraub, D., Moberg, P. J., Duda, J. E., Katz, I. R., & Stern, M. B. (2003). Recognition and treatment of depression in Parkinson's disease. *Journal of Geriatric Psychiatry and Neurology*, 16(3), 178–183.

Weitzner, M. A. (1999). Psychosocial and neuropsychiatric aspects of patients with primary brain tumors. *Cancer Investigations*, 17(4), 285–291; discussion 296–287.

Wellisch, D. K., Kaleita, T. A., Freeman, D., Cloughesy, T., & Goldman, J. (2002). Predicting major depression in brain tumor patients. *Psychooncology*, 11(3), 230–238.

Wiart, L., Petit, H., Joseph, P. A., Mazaux, J. M., & Barat, M. (2000). Fluoxetine in early poststroke depression: A double-blind placebo-controlled study. *Stroke*, 31(8), 1829–1832.

Wilson, R. S., Barnes, L. L., Mendes de Leon, C. F., Aggarwal, N. T., Schneider, J. S., Bach, J., ... Bennett, D. A. (2002). Depressive symptoms, cognitive decline, and risk of AD in older persons. *Neurology*, 59(3), 364–370.

Wrensch, M., Minn, Y., Chew, T., Bondy, M., & Berger, M. S. (2002). Epidemiology of primary brain tumors: Current concepts and review of the literature. *Neuro-Oncology*, 4(4), 278–299.

Yudofsky, S. C. (1979). Parkinson's disease, depression, and electroconvulsive therapy: A clinical and neurobiologic synthesis. *Comprehensive Psychiatry*, 20(6), 579–581.

Zaluska, M., & Dyduch, A. (2011). Bupropion in the treatment of depression in Parkinson's disease. *International Psychogeriatrics*, 23(2), 325–327.

Zorzon, M., de Masi, R., Nasuelli, D., Ukmar, M., Mucelli, R. P., Cazzato, G., ... Zivadinov, R. (2001). Depression and anxiety in multiple sclerosis. A clinical and MRI study in 95 subjects. *Journal of Neurology*, 248(5), 416–421.

18

SUBSTANCE ABUSE COMORBIDITY

David W. Oslin and Amy Helstrom

WHILE EPIDEMIOLOGICAL research suggests that overall rates of alcohol and illicit drug use begin to decline with age, individuals who abuse alcohol and other substances in late life may be at increased risk of a number of negative physical and mental health outcomes that are often exacerbated with advancing age, such as cognitive decline, increased risk of suicide, and compromised immune function. Added to this concern, shifting demographic changes and cohort trends in the population suggest that the prevalence of substance misuse in later life may be increasing. Most notable among demographic changes is the aging of the baby boom generation, which is both a significantly large cohort and a group that poses significant challenges with higher rates of reported illicit drugs and alcohol misuse than previous cohorts (Koenig, George, & Schneider, 1994). One estimate projects that by 2020, the number of older adults needing treatment for drug and alcohol problems will rise to approximately 4 million, a three-fold increase from 1.7 million in 2000 (Blank, 2009).

Because of its pattern of underdetection, drug and alcohol problems in the elderly have been described as "insidious" and as an "invisible epidemic" (Blow, 1998; Gage & Melillo, 2011). Other substances misused by older adults are sometimes similarly overlooked but nonetheless are associated with adverse health consequences. Tobacco use is the leading cause of preventable mortality among the elderly and two thirds of smoking deaths in the United States per year involve people over age 60 (Ossip-Klein, Pearson, McIntosh, & Orleans, 1999). Other types of substance use, abuse, and dependence are also associated with significant adverse outcomes among older adults. Substance use disorders are associated with numerous health and social problems and increases the risk of hospitalization, nursing home placement, and death among older adults (Mokdad et al., 2004; Moore, Whiteman, & Ward, 2007). Moreover, the level of alcohol and substance use that may be significantly problematic among younger cohorts (e.g., heavy drinking) may be associated with more serious health risks among the elderly (Oslin, 2000).

Complicating the picture of substance misuse in later life is the frequent co-occurrence of comorbid mood disorders (Blazer & Koenig, 1993). Not only is depression frequently comorbid with alcohol misuse and substance use, but the presence of substance use and misuse can often negatively impact the course and recovery of depression. Conversely, depression has also been shown to adversely affect recovery from substance use and impact health behavior changes, such as smoking cessation.

This chapter will focus on the intersection between the use and abuse of addictive substances and the presence and course of depressive disorders. Although older adults engage in substance use of many types just as do younger adults (e.g., Boeri, Sterk, & Elifson, 2008), emphasis will be placed on those substances that the authors believe most significantly impact older adults' health, including alcohol, cigarettes, and benzodiazepines.

DEFINING COMORBIDITY

Because the terms "comorbidity" and "dual diagnosis" have been used to refer to a variety of interactions of diseases, the use of these terms can be confusing. Most often comorbidity is used to describe the co-occurrence of two diseases. For example, a patient who presents with both alcoholism and depression would be considered to be experiencing comorbid diagnoses. At the other end of the spectrum, comorbidity has been used to imply any lifetime correlation between two disorders even when the disorders occur at different times in a person's life. For example, an older adult with current symptoms of a depressive disorder that has a past history of alcohol dependence but does not currently drink would be considered to experience comorbid disorders. In this case, the past history of alcohol dependence may be important in predicting treatment outcomes for the depressive disorder and may influence the choices for treatment. Comorbidity has also been defined more narrowly as two or more disorders that interact to produce an effect not seen by either disorder alone. While all of these definitions are valid and acceptable, in an effort to present information from a variety of research studies, this chapter will include the spectrum of definitions of comorbidity.

DEFINING MISUSE, ABUSE, AND DEPENDENCE

Older adults pose special concerns when developing alcohol consumption guidelines. Compared with younger people, older adults have an increased sensitivity to alcohol as well as over-the-counter and prescription medications. There is an age-related decrease in lean body mass and total body water in relation to total fat volume, and the resultant decrease in total body volume increases the serum concentration of alcohol and other mood-altering chemicals in the body. Central nervous system sensitivity to alcohol also increases with age and interactions between medication and alcohol is a particular concern in this age group. For some patients, any alcohol use, coupled with the use of specific over-the-counter or prescription medications, can be problematic (Oslin, 2000).

Because of these issues, alcohol use recommendations for older adults are generally lower than those set for adults under age 65. The National Institute on Alcohol Abuse and Alcoholism (NIAAA) recommends that persons age 65 and older consume no more than one standard drink/day or seven standard drinks/week (NIAAA, 2003). In addition, older adults should consume no more than four standard drinks on any drinking day. These drinking limit recommendations are consistent with data regarding the relationship between heavy consumption and alcohol-related problems within this age group (Moos, Brennan, Schutte, & Moos, 2004). These recommendations are also consistent with the current evidence for a beneficial health effect of low-risk drinking (Klatsky & Armstrong, 1993).

THE PREVALENCE OF ADDICTIONS IN LATE LIFE

Alcohol

Alcohol consumption by older adults differs significantly from that of middle-aged and younger adults, and it is important to consider age and cohort effects when identifying and treating alcohol misuse (e.g., Moore et al., 2005). While many abstain, current prevalence estimates suggest that 40%–52% of older adults drink and that 10%–22% of older adults drink daily (e.g., Barry, Blow et al., 1998; National Center for Health Statistics, 2003; Sacco, Bucholz,

& Spitznagel, 2009). A significant number of these older adults drink alcohol beyond the levels recommended by US national guidelines and recommendations (e.g., Breslow & Smothers, 2004). Recent studies have addressed concern regarding cohort changes related to alcohol use among older adults. While the prevalence of alcohol dependence among older adults is still lower than among younger groups, it is rising among healthy older adults who were raised during a time of greater drug and alcohol use. For example, in a study that spanned 20 years, between 10% and 30% of participants still engaged in high-risk drinking and/or experienced drinking problems at 20-year follow-up when they were 75–85 years old (Moos, Schutte, Brennan, & Moos, 2010). There is also evidence to suggest that binge drinking (i.e., four or more drinks for women and five or more drinks for men on one occasion) among older adults is particularly frequent. In a recent survey of US adults aged 18 and over in 48 states, the frequency of binge drinking was highest among individuals aged 65 and over (Kanny, Liu, & Brewer, 2012).

Tobacco

Research conducted over the past 50 years, including many large-scale epidemiological studies, has produced overwhelming evidence that smoking is harmful at any age. Cigarette smoking accounts for greater than 400,000 deaths annually in the United States and is considered the most significant cause of preventable morbidity and mortality (Centers for Disease Control and Prevention [CDC], 2005). It has been well documented that smoking increases risks of respiratory and nonrespiratory cancers, cardiovascular disease, cerebrovascular disease, nonmalignant respiratory disease (e.g., chronic obstructive pulmonary disease), as well as other nonmalignant diseases, such as ulcer and osteoporosis (Hays, Dale, Hurt, & Croghan, 1998; Rapuri, Gallahger, & Smith, 2007). Among older adults, smoking prevalence is lower than among younger adults with an estimated smoking prevalence rate of 8.3% among individuals >65 years of age compared to 22.2% for individuals <64 years (CDC, 2007). However, older adults are half as likely to attempt to quit smoking as young adults. With the number of older adults increasing due to population changes, the number of older adult smokers could increase significantly even if the proportion of smokers remains largely unchanged.

Benzodiazepines and Other Substances

It is estimated that the number of adults aged 50 years and over will double by the year 2020 (Han, Gfroerer, Colliver, & Penne, 2008). The general belief is that older adults who engage in substance abuse represent only younger addicts grown old with few older adults initiating drug use in their later years. However, substance use, including prescription medication misuse, is still a significant concern among older adults. For example, a study among an elder-specific drug program in a veteran population found that one quarter of patients had either a primary drug abuse problem or a concurrent drug and alcohol problem (Schonfeld et al., 2000). Population-based studies estimate that the current proportion of older adults who abuse substances is 2.8% (Han et al., 2008).

A common problem with the elderly is the misuse of prescription and over-the-counter medications. This includes the misuse of substances such as sedative/hypnotics, narcotic, and nonnarcotic analgesics, diet aids, decongestants, and a wide variety of other over-the-counter medications. Benzodiazepines have historically been among the most commonly prescribed medications in the United States. The prevalence of benzodiazepine use increases with age, and the elderly are more likely to take benzodiazepines chronically (De Wilde et al., 2007; Holroyd & Duryee, 1997).

A study by Blazer and colleagues suggests that the rate of benzodiazepine use has been consistent over recent decades with 10%–15% of elderly actively taking benzodiazepines (Blazer, Hybels, Simonsick, & Hanlon, 2000). Benzodiazepines are often inappropriately prescribed for illnesses such as depression, psychosis, and chronic insomnia (Simon, VonKorff, Barlow, Pabiniak, & Wagner, 1996; Straand & Rokstad, 1997). Unfortunately, these same disorders can obscure detection of substance use disorders in the elderly. McInnes and Powell (1994) interviewed substance use among 640 elderly patients admitted to inpatient hospitals and compared interview results to physician diagnosis and disposition. Results indicated that medical staff only identified 25% of problem users (including benzodiazepines, tobacco, and alcohol) among this sample and only considered 10% of problem users for referral for drug or alcohol treatment.

In summary, the use and abuse of alcohol, cigarettes, and benzodiazepines are common in late life. The impact of late-life addictions will continue to grow as the population of older adults increases. Cohort changes may also influence the magnitude of late-life addictions since the baby boom generation, who are now entering late life, grew up during a time when alcohol and drug use was more acceptable compared to prior generations. This may be even more significant for older women as evidenced by the increased use of cigarettes associated with increases in cancer rates over the last several decades. There is strong speculation that similar increases are occurring in alcohol and drug dependence in women and that these rates will continue to increase over the next several decades.

CO-OCCURRENCE OF LATE-LIFE DEPRESSION AND USE OF ADDICTIVE SUBSTANCES

Older adults experiencing emotional and social problems such as depression, bereavement, and social isolation may be at greater risk for substance abuse (Reid, Boutros, O'Connor, Cadariu, & Concato, 2002). Several studies that have examined the co-occurrence of depression and substance abuse and dependence have included older adults. The National Comorbidity Study, which was designed to explore the epidemiology of various comorbid conditions, indicated that alcoholism and depression were the most common comorbid conditions across the life span (Kessler et al., 1996). Other studies, including the Epidemiologic Catchment Area (ECA) study, have found alcoholism presents 1.6 times more often in depressed than nondepressed subjects (Helzer & Pryzbeck, 1988; Kessler et al., 1996). Risky alcohol use among older adults may be part of a larger pattern of health risk that is tied to substance abuse. For example, a recent study of drinkers age 60 and over identified that having major depression along with being the child of an alcoholic and being a current smoker was associated with increased risk of being a high-risk drinker (Sacco et al., 2009). This same study also noted that being either a former or current smoker increased participants' risk of being a moderate risk drinker.

Smoking and depression have also been shown to co-occur at higher rates than would be expected if they were unrelated disorders. For instance, In a study of over 90,000 women aged 63 and older, depressive symptoms were related to smoking status such that, in comparison to nonsmokers, with each one unit increase in depressive symptoms was related to a 19% increase in light smoking and a 28% increase in heavy smoking. In other studies with both male and female elderly participants (e.g., Green, Polen, & Brody, 2003), depression was shown to be related to a greater risk of smoking.

Relatively few studies have examined the impact of benzodiazepine use in the elderly. In a retrospective study of elderly patients in Canada, the authors estimated that, based on prescription information for over 63,000 patients, 30.8% received benzodiazepine for more than 30 days and 12.9% received a long-acting benzodiapepine (Tamblyn et al., 1994). In another study in the U.S., using cross-sectional analyses of nursing home residents, 13% of residents took benzodiazepines and 42% of those had no appropriate indication for the medication (Stevenson et al., 2010).

THE CONSEQUENCES OF COMORBIDITY

Overall, the interaction between depression and comorbid substance abuse is complex. Findings suggest a strong interaction between depression and substance abuse in some patients and weaker interactions in others. Significant depressive symptoms can precede (primary or independent depression), occur simultaneously with (indeterminate), or develop as a consequence of (reactive or secondary depression) significant alcohol use. Clinically, making a diagnosis of primary depression would lead to treatment plans to address both disorders concurrently, whereas determining a diagnosis of secondary depression would suggest treating the addiction while watchfully waiting for the resolution of the depressive symptoms. Making a distinction between these diagnoses places an emphasis on the temporal relationship of the depression symptoms and periods of abstinence. Thus, depression that either precedes the onset of substance use or occurs during a prolonged period of abstinence is considered primary depression or independent depression. Correspondingly, depression that develops as a consequence of substance use is considered reactive or secondary depression.

These distinctions between primary and secondary disorders are very difficult to make reliably, and there are likely other factors that are important in the understanding of the interaction, including environmental factors, personality traits, genetic factors,

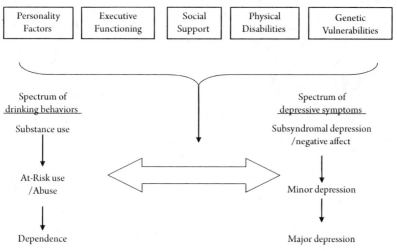

```
Personality        Executive        Social        Physical        Genetic
  Factors         Functioning      Support       Disabilities   Vulnerabilities
```

Spectrum of   Spectrum of
drinking behaviors   depressive symptoms

Substance use   Subsyndromal depression
                                               /negative affect

At-Risk use   Minor depression
/Abuse

Dependence   Major depression

FIGURE 18.1 Complex interactions between substance use and depressive symptoms.

and social supports. Figure 18.1 represents one conceptual model for understanding the reciprocal interaction of these problems. Given the weight of evidence suggesting these problems do interact to produce greater disability, it stands to reason that focusing treatment in a way to address both problems would be beneficial to patients.

Alcohol

Alcohol misuse may have a complicated relationship with mood disorders and research has produced somewhat mixed results about this relationship. Oslin and colleagues conducted a longitudinal descriptive study of middle age and older adults who have recently received a DUI charge (Oslin, O'Brien, & Katz, 1999). The results from the study demonstrated greater self-rated disability among older subjects who are suffering from concurrent alcohol dependence and major depression compared to subjects with either alcohol abuse or dependence alone. Among those with current major depression, at 1-year assessment participants continued to show greater dysfunction in several areas after accounting for the baseline level of disability. These results suggest a low rate of spontaneous recovery and a need for disease-specific interventions among those subjects with comorbid major depression.

Depressed adults with alcohol dependence have been shown to have a more complicated clinical course of depression with an increased risk of suicide, more social dysfunction than nondepressed alcohol-dependent adults, and worse prognosis

(Blixen, McDougall, & Suen, 1997; Hanna & Grant, 1997; Schuckit, Tipp et al., 1997). They also tend to seek more treatment and utilize more health services than those without alcohol problems (Fortney, Booth, & Curran, 1999). The distinction between primary and secondary alcoholism has implications for understanding the consequences of the comorbidity. Some research suggests that people with primary major depression with comorbid alcoholism have more severe symptoms, are less likely to show improvement of depressive symptoms, and have a greater chance for suicide compared to subjects with secondary depression (Schuckit, Tipp et al., 1997; Tsuang, Cowley, Ries, Dunner, & Roy-Byrne, 1995). Thus, it is entirely possible that the consequences of comorbid depression, including long-term outcomes, are worse in primary depressed patients compared to patients with secondary depression. The significance of these treatment outcome differences among older adults is unclear. It is speculated that because of the lower prevalence of alcohol dependence and the modest prevalence of depressive disorders, primary depression may be more common in late life.

Smoking

In the general population, compared to nonsmokers, individuals who smoke have higher rates of psychological distress than nonsmokers (e.g., Hughes & Brandon, 2003). This cross-sectional relationship holds true for older adults, with smokers demonstrating higher rates of depressive symptoms as well as anxiety symptoms and general psychological distress compared to nonsmokers (Honda, 2005; Lam et al., 2004). Both cross-sectional and longitudinal studies have identified a complex relationship between depressive symptoms and smoking, and it is generally agreed that depressive symptoms are a barrier to smoking reduction and cessation (e.g., Breslau, Novak, & Kessler, 2004). Kenney and colleagues (2009) examined 442 late-middle-aged smokers across a 10-year period and found that the presence of depressive disorder negatively impacts smoking cessation among older adults who smoke. Findings suggested that depressive symptoms predicted a lower likelihood of smoking cessation. Additionally, for individuals who were concurrently drinking at baseline, the relationship between depression and smoking cessation may be strengthened, contributing toward the challenge of quitting smoking.

The effects of smoking on the treatment of late-life depression have been addressed in relatively few of the studies conducted on the treatment of late-life depression. Patten and colleagues compared hospitalized smokers with a primary mood disorder with a matched sample of depressed nonsmokers (Patten et al., 2001). Although smoking did not predict overall worse treatment outcomes, smoking was associated with less improvement in certain symptoms such as fatigue. In another study, the presence of depression did not appear to impact the success of smoking cessation (Keuthen et al., 2000; Vazquez & Becona, 1999). Results from a prospective study (Sachs-Ericsson et al., 2009) of over 4,000 participants suggest that a subgroup of older smokers (i.e., those with higher levels of psychological distress and health problems) may be more likely to quit smoking than older smokers with fewer such problems. Conversely, the study identified another subgroup of older smokers reporting fairly good health and lower levels of distress who are less likely to quit smoking. The authors suggest that those patients may particularly benefit from interventions targeting increasing motivation for change. While it is clear that more research needs to be done in this area, taken together these findings suggest that it may be important to address comorbid smoking in the treatment of depression.

Benzodiazepines and Other Substances

The consequences of using benzodiazepines in the context of depression has evolved over the years from a recognition that benzodiazepines alone are a poor choice for treatment of depression to questions regarding the risks and benefits of benzodiazepine use as an adjunct to an antidepressant. There is clear evidence that benzodiazepines can increase the risks for falls and may impair cognition in older adults (Hemmelgarn, Suissa, Huang, Boivin, & Pinard, 1997; Newman, Enright et al., 1997; Ried, Johnson, & Gettman, 1998). These findings have been most consistent with longer acting benzodiazepines and with higher doses. The risks are also most apparent with chronic use rather than short-term use (<3 months). A review of randomized controlled trials of depression management, mostly in younger adults, indicates that patients may have greater improvement and less attrition with the use of benzodiazepines in addition to an antidepressant (Furukawa, Streiner, & Young, 2001). The reviewed studies were conducted over short time periods (<8 weeks) and did not address the long-term risks or benefits of benzodiazepine use. Given that most older adults take benzodiazepines chronically, it is not clear that the short-term studies are a clear indication of the risks associated with benzodiazepine use.

TREATMENT CONSIDERATIONS

Relatively few studies have examined programs specifically addressing alcohol and substance use among elderly patients (Gage & Melillo, 2011). As noted earlier, since for some older patients, comorbidities that may not be as relevant for younger cohorts of substance users may present additional challenges in helping older patients move toward sobriety, data about such specialized programs are needed. There are a limited number of studies that address the treatment of patients who present with comorbid substance use and depression in part due to exclusion of patients with comorbid substance use from clinical trials. However, new data are being added that add to our understanding of optimum treatment for this comorbid presentation.

Alcohol

Mason and colleagues conducted a placebo-controlled study of desipramine in patients with alcoholism with and without major depression (Mason, Kocsis et al., 1996). In this study, all of the depressed subjects had a diagnosis of secondary major depression, and the sample size was small with 10 to 15 subjects in each group. Despite this, there was a significant drug effect on reducing depressive symptoms in the desipramine-treated group compared to the placebo-treated group. There was no effect on the number of subjects who relapsed but a significant effect in increasing the time to relapse. In a third study, Cornelius and colleagues evaluated subjects with primary major depression and comorbid alcoholism (Cornelius et al., 1997). Patients were randomly assigned to placebo or fluoxetine. Fluoxetine significantly improved depressive symptoms over the 12 weeks. This study also found a drug effect for a reduction in total alcohol consumption, although there was no information regarding the number of subjects who achieved full remission from both illnesses. In a fourth study, Roy-Byrne and colleagues (2000) examined nefazadone as monotherapy in treating primary depression complicated by alcoholism. This study demonstrated an antidepressant effect but no effect on drinking outcomes. Nunes and Levin (2004) conducted a meta-analysis examining the efficacy of antidepressant medications for treatment of combined depression and substance use disorders. The authors identified 44 placebo-controlled clinical trials and included 14 for their analysis (N = 848). Results identified an effect size of 0.38 (CI = 0.18–0.58), suggesting a modest benefit to patients with combined depression and substance use disorder.

While these studies have begun to shed light on the treatment of comorbid depression and alcoholism, they have not addressed treatment of older adults specifically. In the absence of empirical data, specific treatment recommendations for older adults with comorbid substance abuse are derived from a consensus development process that reviewed existing data to develop treatment guidelines (Blow, 1998). Once significant substance use and any associated problems have been identified, it is important to note that the older persons with a substance use problem often present with a variety of treatment needs. It is therefore important to have an array of services available for older adults that can be tailored to these individual needs and have the flexibility to adapt to changing needs over time. The spectrum of alcohol interventions for older adults ranges from minimal advice or brief structured interventions for at-risk or problem drinkers to formalized alcoholism treatment for drinkers who meet criteria for abuse and/or dependence. The array of formalized treatment options available includes various psychotherapeutic options, educational tools, rehabilitative and residential models, and psychopharmacological treatments. An example of how this tailoring of needs is important is the contrast between the at-risk drinker or benzodiazepine user and the severely dependent patient. It is unlikely that the at-risk user will need the intensity of services necessary to be as successful as in the severely dependent patient. Indeed, requiring the at-risk drinker to attend a mandatory set of services may be more detrimental to his or her outcome than helpful. The use of brief interventions and individual therapy focused on alcohol use can also easily be incorporated into the context of the treatment of depression without necessitating a referral to a specialty addiction service.

The assessment of any substance abuser starts with a thorough history and a physical and laboratory examination. In addition to quantifying the frequency and quantity of use, assessing the presence of substance-specific problems should be considered part of routine practice. For older adults who drink, instruments such as the Alcohol Use Disorders Test (AUDIT; Bush, Kivlahan, McDonell, Fihn, & Bradley, 1998), shown in Figure 18.2, Moore, Hays, Reuben, & Beck, 2000; Saunders, Aasland, Babor, de la Fuente, & Grant, 1993). Included in the initial assessment is the patient's potential to suffer acute withdrawal. Severe withdrawal such as that from alcohol use can be life threatening and warrants careful attention. Patients with severe symptoms of dependency or withdrawal potential and patients with significant medical or psychiatric comorbidity may require inpatient hospitalization for acute stabilization prior to implementing an outpatient management strategy.

Traditionally, outpatient substance abuse treatment has been reserved for specialized clinics focused only on substance abuse. It is becoming increasingly apparent that this model is inadequate in addressing the broader public health demand and there is a need to involve a variety of clinicians and clinical settings in delivering substance abuse treatment. This is particularly important in older adults with concurrent depression who rarely seek specialized addiction services. The traditional addiction clinic is focused on supportive group psychotherapy and encouragement to attend regular self-help group meetings such as Alcoholics Anonymous (AA), Alcoholics Victorious, Rational Recovery, or Narcotics Anonymous. For older adults, peer-specific group activities are considered superior to mixed-age group activities. Individual psychosocial support is also very effective in the treatment of late-life alcoholism (Oslin, Pettinati,

How often did you have a drink containing alcohol in the past year?

———	Never	(0 parts)
———	Monthly or less	(1 parts)
———	Two to four times a month	(2 parts)
———	Two to three times per week	(3 parts)
———	Four or more times a week	(4 parts)

If you answered 'never' score questions 2 and 3 as zero

How many drinks did you have on a typical day when you were drinking in the past year?

———	1 or 2	(0 parts)
———	3 or 4	(1 parts)
———	5 or 6	(2 parts)
———	7 to 9	(3 parts)
———	10 or more	(4 parts)

How often did you have six or more drinks on one occasion in the past year?

———	Never	(0 parts)
———	Less than monthly	(1 parts)
———	Monthly	(2 parts)
———	Weekly	(3 parts)
———	Daily or almost daily	(4 parts)

Possible range=0–12. For older adults, a score of 3 or more is considered positive.

FIGURE 18.2 Alcohol Use Disorders Identification Test-C (AUDIT-C) Alcohol Screening. Possible range 0–12. For older adults, a score of 3 or more is considered positive.

Source. Adapted from Bush, K., Kivlahan, D.R., McDonell, M. B., et al. (1998). The AUDIT Alcohol Consumption Questions (AUDIT-C): An effective brief screening test for problem drinking. *Archives of Internal Medicine,* 158, 1789–1795. Copyright © 1998, American Medical Association. All rights reserved. Adapted with permission.

& Volpicelli, 2002). Outpatient rehabilitation, in addition to focusing on active addiction issues, usually needs to address issues of time management. Abstinence reduces the time spent in maintaining the substance use disorder. The management of this time, which is often the greater part of a patient's day, is critical to the prognosis of treatment. Use of resources such as day programs and senior centers can be beneficial especially in cognitively impaired patients. Social services such as financial support are

often needed to stabilize the patient in early recovery. Supervised living arrangements such as halfway houses, group homes, nursing homes and residing with relatives should also be considered.

Low-intensity, brief interventions have been suggested as cost-effective and practical techniques that can be used as an initial approach to at-risk and problem drinkers in primary care settings or for those patients followed in a mental health clinic with low levels of drinking. Treatment manuals for at-risk drinking specifically designed for older adults have been published (Barry, Oslin et al., 2001). Brief intervention studies have been conducted in a wide range of health care settings, ranging from hospitals and primary health care locations to mental health clinics. Two brief alcohol intervention trials with older adults specifically (Barry, Blow et al., 1998; Fleming, Manwell, Barry, Adams, & Stauffacher, 1999) were designed as randomized clinical brief intervention trials to reduce hazardous drinking with older adults using advice protocols in primary care settings. These studies have shown that older adults can be engaged in brief intervention protocols, the protocols are acceptable in this population, and there is a substantial reduction in drinking among the at-risk drinkers receiving the interventions compared to a control group.

The use of medications to support abstinence may be of benefit, but it is not well studied. No research to date has addressed pharmacological treatment of older age alcoholics, although studies are under way using naltrexone, as well as various antidepressants, including the serotonin-specific reuptake inhibitors (SSRIs). Some of the general principles used in treating younger patients should be applied to older drinkers as well. For example, benzodiazepines are important in the treatment of alcohol detoxification, but they have no clinical place in maintaining long-term abstinence because of their abuse potential and the potential for fostering further alcohol or benzodiazepine abuse. Disulfiram may benefit some well-motivated patients, but cardiac and hepatic disease limits the use of this agent in the older alcoholic.

Of special interest to mental health providers are the effects of moderate or at-risk alcohol consumption treatment response for other mental health disorders such as depression. In a study of 74 elderly participants who met criteria for a depressive disorder and alcohol dependence, participants were randomly assigned to 12 weeks of naltrexone or placebo with all participants also receiving sertraline (Oslin, 2005). At follow-up, 42% of participants had a remission in their depression and no drinking relapse, suggesting that addressing both depression and alcohol misuse concurrently may be beneficial.

A promising area of research regarding treatment for older adults with depression, anxiety, or alcohol misuse suggests that an integrated model of care may be helpful for treating older adults (Bartels et al., 2004). In a study of almost 25,000 patients across 10 sites, the authors identified that 71% of patients engaged in treatment in an integrated model (i.e., co-located primary care and mental health) compared with 49% in an enhanced referral model (i.e., facilitated scheduling). The authors report that older primary care patients were more likely to accept collaborative mental health treatment within primary care than in mental health specialty clinics. Additional research regarding the modalities of care that most effectively deliver treatment to older patients with comorbid alcohol or other substance use and depression will be helpful in targeting services for this population.

DETOXIFICATION AND WITHDRAWAL

Alcohol withdrawal symptoms commonly occur in patients who stop drinking or markedly cut down their drinking after regular heavy use. During hospitalizations, patients may be particularly vulnerable to alcohol or benzodiazepine withdrawal if the clinical team is unaware of the use of these substances. Alcohol withdrawal can range from mild and almost unnoticeable symptoms to severe and life-threatening ones. The classical set of symptoms associated with alcohol withdrawal includes autonomic hyperactivity (increased pulse rate, increased blood pressure, and increased temperature), restlessness, disturbed sleep, anxiety, nausea, and tremor. More severe withdrawal can be manifested by auditory, visual, or tactile hallucinations, delirium, seizures, and coma. Other substances of abuse such as benzodiazepines, opioids, and cocaine have distinct withdrawal symptoms that are also potentially life threatening. Elderly patients have been shown to have a longer duration of withdrawal symptoms, and withdrawal has the potential for complicating other medical and psychiatric illnesses. However, there is no evidence to suggest that older patients are more prone to alcohol withdrawal or need longer treatment for withdrawal symptoms (Brower, Mudd, Blow, Young, & Hill, 1994).

Highlighted by the potential for life-threatening complications, clinicians caring for patients who abuse substances need to have a fundamental understanding of withdrawal symptoms and the potential complications. All clinicians should demonstrate knowledge of the most common withdrawal symptoms and the anticipated time course of the symptoms. In addition, all clinicians should be able to complete a standardized assessment of withdrawal such as the Clinical Institute Withdrawal from Alcohol-version A, revised (Sullivan, Skora, Schneiderman, Naranjo, & Sellers, 1989). Those clinicians in settings in which withdrawal management or treatment is available need also to be competent in providing detoxification management. This includes the use of benzodiazepines for the management of alcohol withdrawal.

Smoking

Smoking cessation is beneficial at any age, and individuals who have smoked for decades can benefit substantially from abstaining from cigarette smoking (Center for Disease and Control and Prevention [CDC], 2005). The health benefits of cessation for older adults are unequivocal and often quite dramatic and include reducing the risk of heart disease and stroke. Other benefits for older adults who quit include significant and rapid improvements in circulation and pulmonary perfusion, increased mobility, improved physical function, and reduction in osteoporosis and hip fracture (e.g., Hermanson, Omenn, Kronmal, & Gersh, 1988). Older adults who stop smoking may also benefit from less cognitive decline and brain atrophy following smoking cessation (Almeida et al., 2011).

Smoking cessation may be negatively impacted by a number of age-related factors. Cognitive changes related to age might be associated with additional challenges in quitting smoking. A recent study suggested that age-related deficits in cognitive functioning were associated with decreased likelihood of a successful quit attempt (Brega, Grigsby, Kooken, Hamman, & Baxter, 2008). Motivation to quit smoking may vary among older adults due to a number of factors, including psychological distress and physical health. A recent study (Sachs-Ericsson et al., 2009) examined subgroups of older adult smokers both cross-sectionally and prospectively and found that baseline psychological distress and health problems were associated with greater likelihood of smoking cessation 3 years later. A subgroup of older smokers with fairly good health and lower levels of distress were less likely to quit smoking. These findings suggest that treatment programs for older adult smokers may need to tailor interventions to boost motivation for smokers with fewer health problems and psychological distress. Smoking cessation treatments have not typically been designed with the older adult in mind and, in general, research surrounding the development of effective interventions for smoking cessation for older adults is very limited.

Benzodiazepines

Addressing inappropriate use and misuse of medications relies on physicians and pharmacists to monitor medication use carefully, avoiding dangerous combinations of drugs, medications with a high potential for side effects, and ineffective or unnecessary medications. A practical approach to monitoring psychoactive medication use would be to reevaluate use every 3 to 6 months. Only patients with a documented response to the treatment should continue on to maintenance treatment. Patients without a response or partial response should be reevaluated to consider the appropriate diagnosis and further care. This consideration is also a point in which a consultation with a specialty geriatric mental health provider could be advantageous.

Research regarding the use of benzodiazepines among the elderly underscores the importance of using these medications with caution. In a mixed quantitative/qualitative study, the authors examined elderly benzodiazepine users' willingness to taper or discontinue benzodiazepine use (Cook, Biyanova, Thompson, & Coyne, 2007). Anxiety sensitivity and frequency of daily benzodiazepine use were negatively related to participants' willingness to taper or discontinue. Since results from this study suggest that higher daily benzodiazepine use was related to greater refusal to attempt withdrawal, close attention to initiation or increase of benzodiazepines this population may be particularly important.

SUMMARY

As older adults live longer and as generational changes occur, there are individuals in this age group who will be abusing alcohol and other substances than ever before. Given the co-occurrence of depression with substance use, this comorbid presentation will be seen increasingly often by clinicians who treat older adults, making this a growing public health issue. As a complicating factor in the treatment of depression, it is also clear that alcohol, cigarettes, and possibly benzodiazepines can play a significant barrier to positive treatment outcomes. Thus, it seems imperative that mental health providers be able to recognize these issues and make the management of substance use problems a part of the treatment plan for depression.

As few older adults with substance abuse problems seek help from addiction services, it can also be argued that the focus of identification and initial management of addiction problems in late life be addressed by mental health professionals. Often older adults find insurance forms, paperwork, and referrals to be complex, and these logistic issues may severely limit patient access to formal care. This is particularly true of older adults with addiction problems who must cope with these logistic barriers as well as substantial personal barriers in the way of shame and stigma. As older patients with comorbid depression and substance use are more likely to seek help for their depression, mental health professionals may be particularly poised to manage older patients with comorbid substance abuse, although all behavioral health providers should be trained in the management of depression and substance abuse. Mental health providers embedded within primary care may play a key role in both increasing access and treatment engagement for older patients with depression and comorbid substance use.

Disclosures

Dr. Oslin has no conflicts to disclose. All of his research is funded by Veterans research and NIH. Dr. Helstrom has no conflicts to disclose. All of her research funding is funded by Veterans Affairs research (Center for the Evaluation of PACT; CEPACT and VISN 4 Competitive Pilot Project Award).

REFERENCES

American Psychiatric Association. (1994). *Diagnostic and statistical manual of mental disorders* (4th ed.). Washington, DC: Author.

Almeida, O. P., Garrido, G. J., Alfonso, H., Hulse, G., Lautenschlager, N. T., Hankey, G. J., & Flicker, L. (2011). 24-month effect of smoking cessation on cognitive function and brain structure in later life. *Neuroimage, 55*, 1480–1489.

Barry, K. L., Blow, F. C., (1998). Elder-specific brief alcohol intervention: 3-month outcomes. Alcoholism. *Clinical and Experimental Research, 22*, 32 A.

Barry, K. L., Blow, F., & Oslin, D. W. (2001). *Prevention and management of alcohol problems in older adults.* New York: Springer Publishing.

Bartels, S. J., Coakley, E. H., Zubritsky, C., Ware, J. H., Miles, K. M., Arean, P. A., ... Levkoff, S. E. (2004). Improving access to geriatric mental health services: A randomized trial comparing treatment engagement with integrate versus enhanced referral care for depression, anxiety, and at-risk alcohol use. *American Journal of Psychiatry, 161*, 1455–1462.

Cook, J. M., Biyanova, T., Thompson, R., & Coyne, J. C. (2007). Older primary care patients' willingness to consider discontinuation of chronic benzodiazepines. *General Hospital Psychiatry, 29*, 396–401.

Blank, K. (2009). *Older adults and substance abuse: New data highlight concerns.* Washington, DC: US Department of Health and Human Services, Substance Abuse and Mental Health Services Administration.

Blazer, D., Hybels, C., Simonsick, E., & Hanlon, J. T. (2000). Sedative, hypnotic, and antianxiety medication use in an aging cohort over ten years: A racial comparison. *Journal of the American Geriatrics Society, 48*, 1073–1079.

Blazer, D. G., & Koenig, H. G. (1993). Mood disorders. In E. W. Busse & D. G. Blazer (Eds.), *The American Psychiatric Association textbook of geriatric psychiatry* (pp. 235–263). Washington, DC: American Psychiatric Association Press.

Blixen, C. E., McDougall, G. J., & Suen, L. J. (1997). Dual diagnosis in elders discharged from a psychiatric hospital. *International Journal of Geriatric Psychiatry, 12*, 307–313.

Blow, F. (1998). *Substance abuse among older adults. Treatment Improvement Protocol. C. f. S. A. Treatment.* Washington DC: US Government Printing Office.

Boeri, M. W., Sterk, C. E., & Elifson, K. W. (2008). Reconceptualizing early and late onset: A life course analysis of older heroin users. *Gerontologist, 48*, 637–645.

Brega, A., Grigsby, J., Kooken, R., Hamman, R., & Baxter, J. (2008). The impact of executive cognitive functioning on rates of smoking cessation in the San Luis Valley Health and Aging Study. *Age and Ageing, 37*, 521–525.

Breslau, N., Novak, S. P., & Kessler, R.C. (2004). Psychiatric disorders and stages of smoking. *Biological Psychiatry, 55*, 69–76.

Breslow, R. A. & Smothers, B. (2004). Drinking pattersn of older Americans: national health interview surveys, 1997–2001. *Journal of Studies on Alcohol, 65*, 232–240.

Brower, K. J., Mudd, S., Blow, F. C., Young, J. P., & Hill, E. M. (1994). Severity and treatment of alcohol withdrawal in elderly versus younger patients. *Alcoholism: Clinical and Experimental Research, 18*, 196–201.

Bush, K., Kivlahan, D. R., McDonell, M. B., Fihn, S. D., & Bradley, K. A. (1998). The AUDIT alcohol consumption questions (AUDIT-C): An effective brief screening test for problem drinking. Ambulatory Care Quality Improvement Project (ACQUIP). Alcohol Use Disorders Identification Test. *Archives of Internal Medicine, 158*, 1789–1795.

Centers for Disease Control and Prevention (CDC). (2005). Annual smoking: Attributable mortality, years of potential life lost, and productivity losses– United States, 1997–2001. *Morbidity and Mortality Weekly Review, 54*, 625–628.

Cornelius, J. R., Salloum, I. M., Ehler, J. G., Jarrett, P. J., Cornelius, M. D., Perel, J. M., ... Black, A. (1997). Fluoxetine in depressed alcoholics: A double-blind, placebo-controlled trial. *Archives of General Psychiatry, 54*, 700–705.

De Wilde, S., Carey, I. M., Harris, T., Richrds, N., Victor, C., Hilton, S. R., & Cook, D. G. (2007). Trends in potentially inappropriate prescribing amongst older IK primary care patients. *Pharmacoepidemiologic Drug Safety, 16*, 658–667.

Fleming, M., Manwell, L., Barry, K. L., Adams, W., & Stauffacher, E. A. (1999). Brief physician advice for alcohol problems in older adults: A randomized community-based trial. *Journal of Family Practice, 48*, 378–384.

Fortney, J. C., Booth, B. M., & Curran, G. M. (1999). Do patients with alcohol dependence use more services? A comparative analysis with other chronic disorders. *Alcoholism: Clinical and Experimental Research, 23*, 127–133.

Furukawa, T. A., Streiner, D. L., & Young, L. T. (2001). Is antidepressant-benzodiazepine combination therapy clinically more useful? A meta-analytic study. *Journal of Affective Disorders, 65*, 173–177.

Gage, S., & Melillo, K. D. (2011). Substance abuse in older adults. *Journal of Gerontological Nursing, 37*, 8–11.

Green, C. A., Polen, M. R., & Brody, K. K. (2003). Depression, functional status, treatment for psychiatric problems, and the health-related practices of elderly HMO members. *American Journal of Health Promotion, 17*, 269–275.

Han, B., Gfroerer, J. C., Colliver, J. D., & Penne, M. A. (2008). Substance use disorder among older adults in the United States in 2020. *Addiction, 104,* 88–96.

Hanna, E. Z., & Grant, B. F. (1997). Gender differences in DSM-IV alcohol use disorders and major depression as distributed in the general population: Clinical implications. *Comprehensive Psychiatry, 38,* 202–212.

Hays, J., Dale, L., Hurt, R. D., & Croghan, I. T. (1998). Trends in smoking-related diseases: Why smoking cessation is still the best medicine. *Postgraduate Medicine, 104,* 56–71.

Helzer, J. E., & Pryzbeck, T. R. (1988). The co-occurrence of alcoholism with other psychiatric disorders in the general population and its impact on treatment. *Journal of Studies on Alcohol, 49,* 219–224.

Hemmelgarn, B., Suissa, S., Huang, A., Boivin, J. F., & Pinard, G. (1997). Benzodiazepine use and the risk of motor vehicle crash in the elderly. *Journal of the American Medical Association, 278,* 27–31.

Hermanson, B., Omenn, G., Kronmal, R. A., & Gersh, B. J. (1988). Beneficial six-year outcome of smoking cessation in older men and women with coronary artery disease. *New England Journal of Medicine, 319,* 1365–1369.

Hodgins, D. C., el-Guebaly, N., Armstrong, S., & Dufour, M. (1999). Implications of depression on outcome from alcohol dependence: A 3-year prospective follow-up. *Alcoholism: Clinical and Experimental Research, 23,* 151–157.

Holahan, C. K., Holahan, C. J., Powers, D. A., Hayes, R. B., Marti, C. N., & Ockene, J. K. (2011). Depressive symptoms and smoking in middle-aged and older women. *Nicotine & Tobacco Research, 13,* 722–731.

Holroyd, S., & Duryee, J (1997). Substance use disorders in a geriatric psychiatry outpatient clinic: Prevalence and epidemiologic characteristics. *Journal of Nervous and Mental Disease, 185,* 627–632.

Honda, K. (2005). Psychosocial correlates of smoking cessation among elderly ever-smokers in the United States. *Addictive Behaviors, 30,* 375–381.

Hughes, J. R., & Brandon, T. (2003). A softer view of hardening. *Nicotine and Tobacco Research, 5,* 961–962.

Kanny, D., Liu, Y., & Brewer, R. D. (2012). Vital signs: Binge drinking prevalence, frequency, and intensity among adults–United States, 2010. *Morbidity and Mortality Weekly Report, 61,* 14–19.

Kenney, B. A., Holahon, C. J., Holahan, C. K., Brennan, P. L., Schutte, K. K., & Moos, R. H. (2009). Depressive symptoms, drinking problems, and smoking cessation in older smokers. *Addictive Behaviors, 34,* 548–553.

Kessler, R. C., Nelson, C. B., McGonagle, K. A., Liu, J., Swartz, M., & Blazer, D. G. (1996). Comorbidity of DSM III R major depressive disorder in the general population: Results from the US national comorbidity survey. *British Journal of Psychiatry, 168*(Suppl 30), 17–30.

Keuthen, N. J., Niaura, R. S., Borrelli, B., Goldstein, M., DePue, J., Murphy, C., ... Abrams, D. (2000).Comorbidity, smoking behavior and treatment outcome. *Psychotherapy and Psychosomatics, 69,* 244–50.

Klatsky, A. L., & Armstrong, A. (1993). Alcohol use, other traits and risk of unnatural death: A prospective study. *Alcohol: Clinical and Experimental Research, 17,* 1156–1162.

Koenig, H. G., George, L. K., & Schneider, R. (1994). Mental health care for older adults in the year 2020: A dangerous and avoided topic. *Gerontologist, 34,* 674–679.

Lam, T., Li, Z., Ho, S., Chan, W., Ho, K., Li, M., & Leung, G. M. (2004). Smoking and depressive symptoms in Chinese elderly in Hong Kong. *Acta Psychiatrica Scandinavica, 110,* 195–200.

Mason, B. J., Kocsis, J. H., Ritvo, E. C., & Cutler, R. B. (1996). A double-blind, placebo-controlled trial of desipramine for primary alcohol dependence stratified on the presence or absence of major depression. *Journal of the American Medical Association, 275,* 761–767.

McInnes, E., & Powell, J. (1994). Drug and alcohol referrals: are elderly substance abuse diagnoses and referrals being missed? *British Medical Journal, 308,* 444–446.

Mokdad, A. H., Marks, J. S., Stroup, D. F., & Gerberding, J. L. (2004). Actual causes of death in the United States, 2000. *Journal of the American Medical Association, 291,* 1238–45.

Moore, A. A., Hays, R. D., Reuben, D. B., & Beck, J. C. (2000). Using a criterion standard to validate the Alcohol-Related Problems Survey (ARPS): A screening measure to identify harmful and hazardous drinking in older persons. *Aging (Milano), 12,* 221–7.

Moore, A. A., Gould, R., Reuben, D. B., Greendale, G. A., Carter, M. K., Zhou, K., & Karlamangla, A. (2005). Longitudinal patterns and predictors of alcohol consumption in the United States. *American Journal of Public Health, 95,* 458–464.

Moore, A. A., Whiteman, E. J., & Ward, K. T. (2007). Risks of combined alcohol/medication use in older adults. *American Journal of Geriatric Pharmacotherapy, 5,* 64–74.

falseMoos, R. H., Brennan, P. L., Schutte, K., & Moos, B. S. (2004). High-risk alcohol consumption and late-life alcohol problems. *American Journal of Public Health*, 1985–1991.

Moos, R. H., Schutte, K. K., Brennan, P. L., & Moos, B. S. (2010). Late-life and life history predictors of older adults of high-risk alcohol consumption and drinking problems. *Drug and Alcohol Dependence, 108*, 13–20.

National Center for Health Statistics. (2003). *2001–2002 National Health and Nutrition Examination Survey (NHANES)*. Washington, DC: U.S. Government Printing Office.

National Institute on Alcohol Abuse and Alcoholism (NIAAA). (2003) Helping patients with alcohol problems: A health practitioner's guide. NIH pub. No. 03-3769. Bethesda, MD: Author.

Newman, A., Enright, P., Manolio, T. A., Haponik, E. F., & Wahl, P. W. (1997). Sleep disturbances, psyhcosocial correlates, and cardiovascular disease in 5201 older adults: The cardiovascular health study. *Journal of the American Geriatrics Society, 45*, 1–7.

Nunes, E. V., & Levin, F. R. (2004). Treatment of depression in patients with alcohol or other drug dependence. *Journal of the American Medical Association, 291*, 1887–1896.

Oslin, D. W. (2000). Alcohol use in late life: Disability and comorbidity. *Journal of Geriatric Psychiatry and Neurology, 13*, 134–140.

Oslin, D. W. (2005). Treatment of late-life depression complicated by alcohol dependence. *American Journal of Geriatric Psychiatry, 13*, 491–500.

Oslin, D. W., O'Brien, C. P., & Katz, I. R. (1999). The disabling nature of comorbid depression among older DUI recipients. *American Journal on Addictions, 8*, 128–135.

Oslin, D. W., Pettinati, H., & Volpicelli, J. R. (2002). Alcoholism treatment adherence: Older age predicts better adherence and drinking outcomes. *American Journal of Geriatric Psychiatry, 10*, 740–747.

Ossip-Klein, D. J., Pearson, T. A., McIntosh, S., & Orleans, C. T. (1999). Smoking is a geriatric health issue. *Nicotine and Tobacco Research, 1*, 299–300.

Patten, C. A., Gillin, J. C., Golshan, S., Wolter, T. D., Rapaport, M., & Kelsoe, J. (2001). Relationship of mood disturbance to cigarette smoking status among 252 patients with a current mood disorder. *Journal of Clinical Psychiatry, 62*, 319–324.

Rapuri, P. B., Gallagher, J. C., & Smith, L. M. (2007). Smoking as a risk factor for decreased physical performance in elderly women. *Journals of Gerontology Series A, Biological Sciences and Medical Sciences, 62*, 93–99.

Reid, M. C., Boutros, N. N., O'Connor, P. G., Cadariu, A., & Concato, J. (2002). The health-related effects of alcohol use in older persons: A systematic review. *Substance Abuse, 23*, 146–64.

Ried, L. D., Johnson, R. E., & Gettman, D. A. (1998). Benzodiazepine exposure and functional status in older people. *Journal of the American Geriatric Society, 46*, 71–76.

Roy-Byrne, P. P., Pages, K. P., Russo, J. E., Jaffe, C., Blume, A. W., Kingsley, E., … Ries, R. K. (2000). Nefazodone treatment of major depression in alcohol-dependent patients: A double-blind, placebo-controlled trial. *Journal of Clinical Psychopharmacology, 20*, 129–136.

Sacco, P., Bucholz, K. K., & Spitznagel, E. L. (2009). Alcohol use among older adults in the national epidemiologic survey on alcohol and related conditions: A latent class analysis. *Journal of Studies on Alcohol and Drugs, 70*, 829–838.

Sachs-Ericsson, N., Schmidt, N. B., Avolensky, M. J., Mitchell, M., Collins, N., & Blazer, D. (2009). Smoking cessation behavior in older adults by race and gender: The role of health problems and psychological distress. *Nicotine and Tobacco Research, 11*, 433–443.

Saunders, J. B., Aasland, O. G., Babor, T. F., de la Fuente, J. R., & Grant, M. (1993). Development of the alcohol-use disorders identification test (AUDIT)–WHO collaborative project on early detection of persons with harmful alcohol-consumption. *Addiction, 88*, 791–804.

Schonfeld, L., Dupree, L. W., Dickson-Duhrmann, E., Royer, C. M., McDermott, C. H., … Jarvik, L. F. (2000). Cognitive-behavioral treatment of older veterans with substance abuse problems. *Journal of Geriatric Psychiatry and Neurology, 13*, 124–129.

Schuckit, M. A., Tipp, J. E., Bergman, M., Reich, W., Hesselbrock, V. M., & Smith, T. L. (1997). Comparison of induced and independent major depressive disorders in 2,945 alcoholics. *American Journal of Psychiatry, 154*, 948–957.

Schweizer, E., Case, W. G., & Rickels, K. (1989). Benzodiazepine dependence and withdrawal in elderly patients. *American Journal of Psychiatry, 146*, 529–31.

Simon, G., VonKorff, M., Barlow, W., Pabiniak, C., & Wagner, E. (1996). Predictors of chronic benzodiazepine use in a health maintenance organization sample. *Journal of Clinical Epidemiology, 49*, 1067–1073.

Speer, D., & Bates, K (1992). Comorbid mental and substance disorders among older psychiatric patients. *Journal of the American Geriatric Society, 40,* 886–890.

Stevenson, D. G., Decker, S. L., Dwyer, L. L., Huskamp, H. A., Grabowski, D. C., Metzger, E. D., & Mitchell, S. L. (2010). Antipsychotic and benzodiazepine use among nursing home residents: Findings from the 2004 national nursing home survey. *American Journal of Geriatric Psychiatry, 18,* 1078–1092.

Straand, J., & Rokstad, K. (1997). General practitioners' prescribing patterns of benzodiazepine hypnotics: Are elderly patients at particular risk for overprescribing? A report from the More & Romsdal Prescription Study. *Scandinavian Journal of Primary Health Care, 15,* 16–21.

Sullivan, J. T., Sykora, K., Schneiderman, J., Naranjo, C. A., & Sellers, E. M. (1989). Assessment of alcohol withdrawal: The revised clinical institute withdrawal. *British Journal of Addiction, 84,* 1353–1357.

Tamblyn, R. M., McLeod, P. J., Abrahamowicz, M., Monette, J., Gayton, D. C., Berson, L., Dauphinee, D., Grad, R. M., Huang, A. R., Isaac, L. M., Schnarch, B. S., & Snell, L. S. (1994). Questionable prescribing for elderly patients in Quebec. *CMAJ , 150,* 1801–1809.

Tsuang, D., Cowley, D., Ries, R., Dunner, D. L., & Roy-Byrne, P. P. (1995). The effects of substance use disorder on the clinical presentation of anxiety and depression in an outpatient psychiatric clinic. *Journal of Clinical Psychiatry, 56,* 549–555.

United States Department of Health and Human Services. (1990). *The health benefits of smoking cessation.* Washington, DC: US Government Printing Office.

Vazquez, F. L., & Becona, E. (1999). Depression and smoking in a smoking cessation programme. *Journal of Affective Disorders, 55,* 125–132.

19

COMORBID PAIN DISORDERS

Jordan F. Karp and Jonathan McGovern

WHILE PAIN management is not traditionally the domain of psychiatry, a growing body of literature supports a complex and bidirectional relationship between psychiatric illness and psychosocial distress and the experience of pain. The perception of pain is universal yet idiosyncratic—inherently colored by individual biopsychosocial factors such as personality; coping skills; and cognitive, interpersonal, and emotional responses to painful stimuli (Farrell & Gibson, 2004; Parmelee, 2005). In this context, it is hardly surprising to find a robust overlap of psychiatric and pain disorders reported in the literature. Therefore, it is not only prudent but *essential* for mental health practitioners to understand the assessment and treatment of persistent pain in the context of psychiatric illness, especially in late life, given the high prevalence of painful conditions in late life.

Between 2000 and 2010, the US Census data showed an enormous 31.5% increase in the 45- to 64-year-old demographic and a 15.1% increase in the number of people over the age of 65 (US Census Bureau, 2011). These two age groups comprise the fastest growing segments in the United States—growth largely driven by the baby boomer cohort, who, in 2011, began to cross the threshold into the elderly population (defined as 65 years and older; AGS Panel on Persistent Pain in Older Persons, 2002). Unfortunately, many find the "golden years" of retirement to be fraught with painful medical conditions. While the point prevalence of acute pain is similar in adults of all ages (Crook, Rideout, & Browne, 1984), the prevalence of persistent pain increases with age (Helme & Gibson, 2001). Therefore, in the coming years, clinicians in the United States should expect to see a greater number of patients presenting with pain complaints, as the American population shifts toward a greater proportion of older adults. It is therefore imperative for both geriatric and general mental health practitioners to become proficient in the assessment and treatment of pain in the elderly patient. This chapter will discuss the epidemiology of comorbid pain disorders in older adults, biopsychosocial differences in pain perception and reporting in late life, and the role of mental health professionals in the assessment and treatment of pain in the elderly.

EPIDEMIOLOGICAL CONSIDERATIONS IN THE MEASUREMENT OF PAIN IN OLDER ADULTS

Pain is an intrinsically subjective experience, which complicates its measurement—a fact underscored by the discrepancy in the reported prevalence of persistent pain in the literature. Direct comparison of prevalence statistics is difficult in part due to the variability between studies in the location and type of pain assessed as well as the measures used for assessment (Farrell & Gibson, 2004). The necessary reliance on self-report, which is considered to be the gold standard of pain measurement (AGS Panel on Persistent Pain in Older Persons, 2002), adds another layer of complexity. As Jones and Macfarlane point out, it is not the epidemiology of pain per se that is studied but the reporting of pain (Jones & Macfarlane, 2005). This becomes a salient issue in cognitively impaired (Herr, Bjoro, & Decker, 2006; Krulewitch et al., 2000) and nonverbal (Bjoro & Herr, 2008) older adults, in whom pain is frequently undetected due to a lack of appropriate measures.

Attitudes of both patients and clinicians are also thought to underlie the underreporting and inadequate treatment of pain in the elderly. Patients may be hesitant to report pain due to the erroneous belief that pain is a normal and unavoidable part of aging (Gignac et al., 2006; Weiner & Rudy, 2002; Yates, Dewar, & Fentiman, 1995). In addition, a 2001 study found that people over the age of 60 were more reluctant to report pain and were less likely to describe an abnormal sensation as painful compared with younger adults (Yong, Gibson, Horne, & Helme, 2001). This stoicism was most pronounced in patients 80 years and older, likely contributing to the common observation that the prevalence of pain increases with age until around 70 years and then appears to plateau or decrease (Helme & Gibson, 2001). Patient reticence must not be understood as an excuse to blame the patient for inadequate pain management but as an important consideration for the geriatric clinician. Physicians and nurses are less likely to communicate with older patients about their level of pain (de Rond, de Wit, van Dam, &

Muller, 2000), which undoubtedly contributes to the elevated risk of receiving inadequate pain assessment and treatment compared with younger adults (Chodosh et al., 2004).

Despite the challenges in estimating its prevalence, the data show persistent pain to be commonplace in the lives of many older adults. The American Geriatrics Society reports that between 25% and 50% of community-dwelling elders experience persistent pain that interferes with daily life, while 45%–80% of nursing home residents have untreated or undertreated pain (AGS Panel on Persistent Pain in Older Persons, 2002). A 1996 study found that greater than 60% of community-dwelling adults over the age of 65 reported taking one or more analgesics (Hanlon, Fillenbaum, Studenski, Ziqubu-Page, & Wall, 1996). People over 65 years old are more likely to have persistent pain that interferes with daily activities (Thomas, Peat, Harris, Wilkie, & Croft, 2004), placing them at an elevated risk for psychosocial comorbidities, including depression, anxiety, social isolation, limited mobility, sleep disturbance, increased health care utilization (AGS Panel on Persistent Pain in Older Persons, 2002), and suicide (Voaklander, Rowe, Dryden, Pahal, Saar, & Kelly, 2008).

THE DEPRESSION-PAIN SYNDROME

It is becoming increasingly evident that the coexistence of persistent pain and depression cannot be explained by a simple cause and effect model, but that these conditions overlap in a relationship of mutual exacerbation. To emphasize the frequency of coincidence as well as the intersection of biology, neurochemistry, and response to treatment, others have used the label "depression-pain syndrome" (Bair, Robinson, Katon, & Kroenke, 2003; Lindsay & Wyckoff, 1981). In a comprehensive literature review, Fishbain et al. found the presence, duration, and severity of pain, as well as the number of pain sites, to be consistently associated with severity of depression (Fishbain, Cutler, Rosomoff, & Rosomoff, 1997). While this review included, but was not restricted to, studies of pain and depression in the elderly, similar studies have replicated this result in samples of older adults (Casten, Parmelee, Kleban, Lawton, & Katz, 1995; Parmelee, Katz, & Lawton, 1991; Williamson & Schulz, 1992), even when adjusting for medical comorbidity. While the temporal relationship of comorbid pain and depression has yet to be fully elucidated, there is evidence that pain at any time in life is a risk for depression in late life, and that depression is also a risk for developing pain (Reid, Williams, Concato, Tinetti, & Gill, 2003).

DEFINITION AND PATHOGENESIS OF CHRONIC NONMALIGNANT PAIN

Chronic pain is defined as pain that persists beyond the expected time of healing, or more than 3 to 6 months. The nervous system is responsible for the perception of pain. While a number of disorders may cause chronic pain, generally speaking there are two types of conditions that underlie its pathogenesis: nociceptive and neuropathic. *Nociceptive pain* is associated with tissue damage and a normal nervous system (e.g., pain associated with osteoarthritis or myofascial pain), while *neuropathic pain* is associated with physiological nervous system dysfunction (e.g., diabetic neuropathy, postherpetic neuralgia). Not infrequently in late life, these two types of pain coexist. Low back pain in older adults is an example of a painful condition often resulting from both nociceptive and neuropathic pain (Weiner, 2007).

THE EFFECT OF AGE ON PAIN PERCEPTION

Age-associated changes in pain processing have several biological correlates. For example, the density of both myelinated and unmyelinated peripheral fibers has been found to decrease with age (Ochoa & Mair, 1989; Rafalowska, Drac, & Rosinska, 1976). In contrast, the number of both myelinated and unmyelinated sensory fibers that show signs of neurodegeneration or damage increases with advanced age. This may be associated with slowing of peripheral nerve conduction velocity (Drac, Babiuch, & Wisniewska, 1991; Kakigi, 1987). Impairment in the early warning functions of nociceptive A-delta fibers has also been observed (Gibson & Farrell, 2004). Interpreting the observations about age on pain threshold is complex. For example, it has been reported that somatosensory thresholds for non-noxious stimuli increase with age, whereas pressure pain thresholds have been reported to both increase and decrease, and heat pain thresholds may show no age-related changes (Gibson & Farrell, 2004).

Threshold and tolerance of experimentally induced ischemic pain is significantly less in older than in younger adults (Edwards & Fillingim, 2001). Apart from an enhanced temporal summation of heat pain and electrical pain (Farrell & Gibson, 2007), pain summation may not be critically affected by age (Lautenbacher, Kunz, Strate, Nielsen, & Arendt-Nielsen, 2005). However, recent work has suggested that the nociceptive system of older subjects may indeed have a reduced capacity to down-regulate subsequent to sensitization (Farrell & Gibson, 2007). Changes in significant neurotransmitters and both age-related and more severe neurodegenerative brain changes, described in the next section, may account for these pain responses.

SIGNIFICANT NEUROTRANSMITTERS

In addition to modulating mood, anxiety, and cognition, serotonin, norepinephrine, γ-aminobutyric acid (GABA), glutamate, and acetylcholine are involved in nociceptive pathways. Modulating levels of these neurotransmitters with reuptake and enzyme inhibitors can enhance analgesia (Godfrey, 1996). Indeed, tricyclic antidepressants and serotonin norepinephrine reuptake inhibitors have been observed to offer relief from persistent pain for some patients. This may be due to an increase in the duration and concentration of neurotransmitters in synapses associated with central pain regulation (Sorkin & Wallace, 1999).

The midbrain, pons, and medulla, especially around the cerebral aqueduct (i.e., the periaqueductal gray matter) (Berne & Levy, 1998) are involved in top-down or supraspinal analgesia (for further reading on the gate control theory of pain regulation and descending inhibition, the reader is referred to the seminal paper by Melzack and Wall (1965). These areas of the central nervous system facilitate descending inhibition and decrease the "amount" of nociceptive information reaching the cerebral cortex. These areas of the brain are rich in endogenous opioids and opioid receptors, and they also give rise to fiber tracts that project to the dorsal horn of the spinal cord, where serotonin, norepinephrine, and acetylcholine are released. These tracts inhibit nociceptive input from afferents and/or output by nociceptive second-order neurons. These neurotransmitters, especially serotonin, result in inhibition of dorsal horn nociceptive structures, which is mediated by the activation of opioid-releasing interneurons. The spinal actions of norepinephrine on the dorsal horn nociceptive mechanisms are mediated by α-2 receptors and are inhibitory (Strassman, 2002).

AGE-ASSOCIATED BRAIN CHANGES

Age-related changes within the nervous system (e.g., peripheral nociceptors, spinal cord, and brain) may affect the pain experience in older adults. In the brains of most older adults, some evidence of pathological changes are evident (Bennett et al., 2006; Hulette et al., 1998). Alterations in brain morphology (loss of cortical volume, senile neuritic plaques, neurofibrillary tangles) are associated with decrements in neuropsychological performance, even in the absence of clinical dementia (Cook et al., 2002; Zimmerman et al., 2006). It is unknown whether these nonclinical brain changes, which affect the frontal cortex, anterior cingulate cortex, insular cortex, and hypothalamus (regions associated with the motivational-affective experience of pain and with descending inhibition, also known as the medial pain system), make pain more bothersome and/or interfere with the effect of analgesics. Functionally, neuronal death and gliosis may directly interrupt neuronal tracts involved in descending inhibition, especially those involved with the periaqueductal gray, locus coeruleus, and nucleus raphe magnus—areas rich in opioid and monoamine receptors (Zhang, Tang, Yuan, & Jia, 1997; Zhuo & Gebhart, 1990).

There is evidence of a progressive age-related loss of serotonergic and noradrenergic neurons in the dorsal horn (Iwata et al., 2002; Ko, King, Gordon, & Crisp, 1997). Within the limbic system, there is a decline in the concentration and turnover of catecholamines (Becker & Cohen, 1984), GABA (Spokes, 1979), and opioid receptors (Amenta, Zaccheo, & Collier, 1991) and a reduction in serotonin receptor density (Kakiuchi, 2000), particularly within the anterior cingulate and prefrontal cortex—brain areas involved in descending inhibition (Sheline, Mintun, Moerlein, & Snyder, 2002). The cerebral cortex displays similar age-dependent reductions in dopamine, noradrenaline, GABA, and acetylcholine neurotransmission (DeKosky, Scheff, & Markesbery, 1985; Gottfries, 1980; Grote, Moses, Robins, Hudgens, & Croninger, 1974; McGeer & McGeer, 1976; Robinson, 1975; Rogers & Bloom, 1985; White et al., 1977) and a reduction in the density of serotonin (Marcusson, Morgan, Winblad, & Finch, 1984; Wong et al., 1984) and glutamate receptors (Segovia, Del Arco, Prieto, & Mora, 2001). Age-related changes in glutamate and GABA are also noticeable in the prefrontal cortex and may result in abnormal pain summation (Grachev, Swarnkar, Szeverenyi, Ramachandran, & Apkarian, 2001). The neurochemicals necessary for pain modulation may not be sufficiently available in older adults, which may lead to central sensitization, lower pain threshold, and persistent pain (Karp, Shega, Morone, & Weiner, 2008).

Alzheimer's disease (AD) primarily affects the medial pain system (Rub, Del Tredici, Del Turco, & Braak, 2002), with corresponding effects on the motivational–affective, cognitive–evaluative, and autonomic–neuroendocrine components of pain. The lateral pain system, involved with the sensory-discriminative elements of pain, only becomes involved relatively late in the disease (Scherder, 2000). Patients with AD may have less affective response to pain (Scherder, Bouma, Borkent, & Rahman, 1999) while maintaining a comparable pain threshold to cognitively intact patients (Benedetti et al., 1999). Support also exists for similar and exaggerated affective pain responses in AD. Porter and colleagues (Porter et al., 1996) demonstrated exaggerated facial expressions in response to venipuncture in older adults with AD when compared with cognitively intact older adults. One functional magnetic resonance imaging study demonstrated activation of the medial and lateral pain pathways in both AD and control subjects and comparable unpleasantness ratings in response to mechanical pressure stimuli (Cole et al., 2006). Those with AD demonstrated greater amplitude and duration of pain-related activity in sensory, affective, and cognitive processing regions, interpreted as greater attention to noxious stimuli. For a discussion of the impact of other types of dementia on pain processing, the reader is referred to a review by Scherder and colleagues (Scherder, Sergeant, & Swaab, 2003).

PSYCHIATRIC CONDITIONS AND COMORBID PAIN

As described earlier, there is overlap between areas of the brain involved in psychiatric conditions and in persistent pain. The prefrontal cortex, anterior cingulate, limbic system, reward circuits, and midbrain loci such as the locus coerulus and raphe nucleus are frequently dysregulated in mood and anxiety as well as pain conditions. In addition to a linked biology, impaired coping mechanisms are often observed in both affective and chronic pain states. For example, passive coping skills, an external locus of control, low self-efficacy, and high learned helplessness are often present in both affective and pain conditions (Turk & Rudy, 1988). The similar biology and psychology help explain the reciprocity between these conditions.

Somatoform Disorders

Somatoform disorders are a group of psychiatric conditions that cause unexplained physical symptoms. They include somatization disorder (involving multisystem physical symptoms), undifferentiated somatoform disorder (fewer symptoms than somatization disorder), conversion disorder (voluntary motor or sensory function symptoms), pain disorder (pain with strong psychological involvement), hypochondriasis (fear of having a life-threatening illness or condition), and somatoform disorder not otherwise specified (used when criteria are not clearly met for one of the other somatoform disorders) (Oyama, Paltoo, & Greengold, 2007). Up to 50% of primary care patients present with physical symptoms that cannot be explained by a general medical condition. The unexplained symptoms of somatoform disorders, especially when they involve pain, often lead to general health anxiety; frequent or recurrent and excessive preoccupation with unexplained physical symptoms; inaccurate or exaggerated beliefs about somatic symptoms; difficult encounters with the health care system; disproportionate disability; displays of strong, often negative emotions toward the physician or office staff; unrealistic expectations; and, occasionally, resistance to or noncompliance with diagnostic or treatment efforts. These behaviors may result in more frequent office visits, unnecessary laboratory or imaging tests, or costly and potentially dangerous invasive procedures (Barsky, Orav, & Bates, 2005; Hiller, Fichter, & Rief, 2003; Oyama, Paltoo, & Greengold, 2007). The following example illustrates a case of an older patient with a somatoform disorder focused on pain symptoms.

LC is a 71-year-old divorced woman who is a retired nurse. She has lived with chronic low back pain for the past 12 years since she fell on ice and fractured her coccyx. Since then she has undergone a laminectomy and fusion because her surgeon noted arthritic changes in her back during one of her many spinal MRIs. LC is preoccupied with her back pain and feels it is disabling, despite being high functioning in many aspects of her life. She is active with her grandchildren, participates in volunteer work at her church, and enjoys bingo with her friends. However, she frequently visits neurosurgeons, orthopedic surgeons, chiropractors, pain medicine specialists, and naturopathic clinicians in an effort to treat lingering low back pain. Her description of her pain alternates between *la belle indifference* and tearful descriptions of how her life is ruined by the pain. LC endorses high levels of anxiety and is fearful of "injuring" her back with any exercise or rehabilitation, articulating that she is concerned that movement may cause irreparable injury to her back, resulting in paralysis. When she becomes more anxious about family or finances, she notices that she tenses her shoulders and back, and this behavior makes her back ache more. She also experiences alternation between constipation, diarrhea, and abdominal bloating and frequent genitourinary symptoms, in particular urinary frequency and pelvic discomfort without objective evidence of pathology. In addition to these symptoms, she often experiences paresthesias in her arms and hands, worse when she is stressed or tired. When these symptoms flare, she feels they are best treated with higher doses of ibuprofen and Vicodin, despite being informed that anxiety may be making her pain symptoms worse. She has been resistant to participating in an interdisciplinary pain management program because she wants a "cure" for her pain, not to learn "how to manage it," and is offended that some of her physicians think that the "pain is all in my head."

LC is an example of a case frequently observed in primary care, the emergency department, pain clinics, and ultimately at the psychiatrist or psychologist's office. While not depressed, LC has a preoccupation with medically unexplained symptoms and pain in her back that has led to surgeries, high levels of health service utilization, exposure to medications with potentially dangerous side effects, and a worsening of general health and conditioning because of her concerns that activity will damage her back. We frequently observe high levels of somatic preoccupation in anxious older adults after they have experienced an injury or illness. High levels of fear avoidance, minimal insight into other contributors to her pain (like anxiety), an external locus of control, and low self-efficacy (that she can manage her pain on her own) are frequently present in older patients with somatoform disorders—especially pain of unclear etiology.

Affective Disorders

Depression and anxiety are frequently comorbid with pain. Depressed and anxious patients often complain of more "aches and pains" than nondepressed and nonanxious counterparts. However, depressed and anxious older adults are at increased risk of developing a painful condition such as arthritis, headache, low back pain, pelvic pain, chest pain, and fibromyalgia than patients without emotional problems. For example, in a survey of community-dwelling older adults, the presence of depressive symptoms was observed to be a strong, independent, and highly prevalent risk factor for the occurrence of disabling back pain (Reid et al., 2003). In another study of necessary and discretionary activities in older adults with knee osteoarthritis, the authors reported that at baseline, the relationships of depression with functional disability and activity limitation were wholly mediated by pain. In contrast, activity participation was independently linked with depression, even controlling for health and demographic variables. A 1-year follow-up revealed that depressive symptoms increased with increasing health problems, and with reduction in activity participation over time (Parmelee, Harralson, Smith, & Schumacher, 2007). In a study of nursing home residents, it was observed that depressed individuals were more likely to have pain, regardless of the presence of cognitive impairment. Multiple regression revealed that depressed affect was predicted by more pain, a greater number of medical diagnoses, and poor quality of the social network (Cohen-Mansfield & Marx, 1983). These findings are consistent with our clinical work in community-dwelling seniors; pain is often associated with high levels of medical comorbidity and social isolation. We view this as "pain homeostenosis" (Karp et al., 2008). In other words, the older organism has a compromised ability to maintain a low-pain state because of other medical and psychosocial problems.

Substance Use

The rates of alcohol and substance misuse are greater among patients with pain than in pain-free individuals. In a study of older adults defined as either problem drinkers or non-problem drinkers, at baseline, older problem drinkers reported more severe pain, more disruption of daily activities due to pain, and more frequent use of alcohol to manage pain than did older non-problem drinkers. More pain was associated with more use of alcohol to manage pain; this relationship was stronger among older adults with drinking problems than among those without drinking problems (Brennan, Schutte, & Moos, 2005). While alcohol was the most frequently reported primary substance of abuse for all substance abuse treatment admissions aged 50 or older (US Department of Health and Human Services, 2005), misuse of benzodiazepines and especially opioid analgesics is concerning for older adults living with pain. While this misuse may represent undertreatment of pain or an attempt to reduce comorbid emotional distress, these drugs may also be misused for their euphoric or mood-altering properties. In addition to being illegal, this behavior carries the risk of overdose and diversion.

Disordered Sleep

A survey of 1,765 Australian residents found pain to be the most significant predictor of poor sleep (Moffitt, Kalucy, Kalucy, Baum, & Cooke, 1991). Common sense indicates that it is difficult to initiate and maintain sleep in the presence of a painful stimulus such as low back pain or diabetic neuropathic pain. Thus, sleep disturbance in the context of pain may be attributed to the pain itself. However, evidence from animal models and human investigations indicates a complex relationship between pain and sleep disturbance (Aaron et al., 1996; Landis, Levine, & Robinson, 1989). In one study of 100 individuals referred to a multidisciplinary outpatient chronic pain clinic, 70% reported "poor" sleep while another 20% reported "fair" sleep. Poor sleepers were differentiated from better sleepers by fewer hours of sleep, more hours spent reclining during the day, more disability, and greater ratings of pain intensity. Additionally, those who reported greater sleep disturbances endorsed significantly higher levels of depression and anxiety. Wittig et al. suggest that pain tolerance decreases with lack of sleep and may partially account for increased pain perception (Wittig, Zorick, Blumer, Heilbronn, & Roth, 1982). Given that, in old age, the majority experiences structural changes in sleep while the minority expresses complaints of unsatisfactory sleep quality, it is reasonable to conclude that age-related change per se is not a sufficient condition for the development of insomnia. Rather, the experimental and epidemiological evidence clearly points to the existence of health, situational, and psychological factors that are strongly associated with the onset and/or maintenance of disturbed sleep. Because these factors may occur in combination and are often superimposed upon sleep already compromised by ontogenetic changes, it follows that sleep problems in later life are frequently multifactorial in origin. Depression and/or pain are prime examples of health and psychological factors that contribute to the experience of nonrestorative sleep.

ASSESSMENT

According to McCaffery (1968), "pain is whatever the patient says it is." However, to be assured that pain is being assessed effectively, clinicians need to ask about its presence. Waiting for patients to self-report pain when it might not be their chief complaint can lead to underdiagnosis and subsequent undertreatment. Additionally, many older adults may be reticent to discuss pain with clinicians for a variety of reasons; commonly encountered barriers to communicating about pain include cognitive or verbal impairment, misconceptions about the normality of pain in late life, fears about the consequences of using opioid analgesics, and increased stoicism (Martin, Williams, Hadjistavropoulos, Hadjistavropoulos, & MacLean, 2005). Additionally, older patients may be reluctant to report pain due to fears that it may indicate a new disease process which may require additional diagnostic tests or hospitalizations (Catananti & Gambassi, 2007).

Despite these difficulties, a brief pain assessment can be easily integrated into the standard psychiatric evaluation of the geriatric patient and, in light of the well-established consequences of persistent pain for psychosocial well-being, may even be viewed as a crucial element of the patient interview. Many dimensions of pain have been suggested for inclusion in assessment and can be placed in one of six categories: (1) location; (2) intensity or severity; (3) type or quality (description); (4) duration; (5) factors that relieve or aggravate; and (6) effect of pain on function (AGS Panel on Chronic Pain in Older Persons, 2002; Ferrell, Stein, & Beck, 2000). Table 19.1 lists probes to elicit this information.

Herr and colleagues have explored the preferences of older patients for a variety of unidimensional pain measures and the psychometrics of these

measures (e.g., correlation among measures, stability across repeated assessments) (Taylor, Harris, Epps, & Herr, 2005). They compared the Faces Pain Scale (FPS), the Verbal Descriptor Scale (VDS), the Numeric Rating Scale (NRS), and the Iowa Pain Thermometer (IPT) for assessing pain in cognitively impaired and cognitively intact older adults. Concurrent validity of the VDS, NRS, and IPT was supported with Spearman rank correlation coefficients ranging from .78 to .86 in the cognitively impaired group. The FPS, however, demonstrated weak correlations with other scales when used with the impaired group, ranging from .48 to .53. In the cognitively intact group, strong correlations ranging from .96 to .97 were found among all of the scales. Test-retest reliability at a 2-week interval was acceptable in the cognitively intact group (Spearman rank correlations ranged from .67 to .85) and unacceptable for most scales in the cognitively impaired group (correlations ranged from .26 to .67). When asked about scale preference, both the cognitively impaired and the intact groups preferred the IPT and the VDS. This work suggests that both cognitively impaired as well as cognitively intact older adults can utilize unidimensional pain measures, but repeated assessments among cognitively impaired older adults may not provide reliable data.

For patients with limited verbal communication skills, such as those with severe dementia or an aphasic disorder, observed behaviors may be the only key to assessing pain. Kunz et al. (2007) studied the facial expression of pain in dementia patients experiencing mechanically induced pain, contrasting their observations with similar expressions in normals of similar age experiencing the same painful stimulation. Subjects underwent repeated trials with a pressure algometer applied to right and left forearms at two intensities. To score event-related facial expressions, they videotaped faces under varying experimental conditions and analyzed the recordings using the Facial Action Coding System (FACS) (Simon, Craig, Gosselin, Belin, & Rainville, 2008). Kunz et al. (Kunz, Scharmann, Hemmeter, Schepelmann, & Lautenbacher, 2007) observed that the demented patients displayed higher frequencies and higher intensities of facial responses during painful stimulation. Facial expression appeared to be less socially inhibited in demented patients than normals, indicating that nociception and pain reflect just as validly in the facial expressions of dementia patients as in the facial expressions of normals. The findings of Kunz et al. (2007) suggest that facial expression is less socially

Table 19.1 Assessment of Pain

DIMENSION	PROMPTS TO ELICIT THIS INFORMATION
Location	Where do you hurt? Point to where you hurt. Does the pain radiate? Do you hurt anywhere else? Do you often feel like you hurt all over?
Intensity/severity	On a scale of 0–10, with "0" being no pain and "10" being the worst pain imaginable, how would you rate your current level of pain? Now how would you rate your average pain over the past week? Is your pain different with activity versus when you are resting? Tell me about that.
Type or quality (description)	What is the pain like? Is it aching, stabbing, burning, throbbing, or heavy? Is it worse in the morning, during the day with activity, or worse at night, like when you are in bed.
Duration	How long have you been experiencing this pain? Was there an event that caused the pain (i.e., motor vehicle accident, herpes zoster, progressing arthritis) or did the pain start suddenly?
Factors that aggravate or alleviate pain	What makes the pain worse? Does activity or exercise, heat, cold, fatigue, stress, anxiety, make your pain worse. How do you cope with the pain? How do you get through the day? Do you use medications (and if so, how much and what kind and who prescribes them), relaxation, pacing activities, rest, prayer, distraction, heat or cold, or some other coping method?
Effect of Pain on Function	How has pain affected your life? How does pain affect your sleep? Are you unable to take care of your home and/or have you given up certain activities like travel because of your pain?

inhibited in demented patients and therefore an even better indicator of pain than it is in cognitively normal people, who tend to conform facial expression to the social context. In another study comparing cognitively impaired individuals with cognitively normal older adults undergoing gingival injection of local anesthetic, changes in facial expression proved to be the most useful measure overall in identifying pain in both cognitively intact and cognitively impaired older patients, and it was more sensitive in the cognitively impaired patients (Hsu, Shuman, Hamamoto, Hodges, & Feldt, 2007).

There are several promising operationalized behavioral assessments of pain in demented patients. For this chapter, we have selected the Pain Assessment in Advanced Dementia (PAINAD) (Warden, Hurley, & Volicer, 2003) scale because of its good psychometrics and ease of use. The PAINAD measure has good internal consistency with a one-factor solution, is highly correlated with another measure of distress in Alzheimer's disease (the Discomfort Scale—Dementia of Alzheimer Type [DS-DAT]), and there is evidence of significant change in scores before and after receiving a pain medication. The five items of the PAINAD (each scored from 0 to 2, with higher scores indicating more pain) address the following: (1) breathing independent of vocalization; (2) negative vocalization; (3) facial expression; (4) body language; and (5) consolability.

GENERAL APPROACH TO TREATMENT—THE ROLE OF THE GERIATRIC PSYCHIATRIST

According to Weiner (2007), to afford an optimal response to therapy, the practitioner must keep three general principles in mind and communicate them to their older patients in order to establish reasonable treatment expectations:

- Chronic pain is a syndrome with many potential contributors, all of which require treatment to afford an optimal clinical outcome.
- Chronic pain is treatable but not curable; improvement is the rule, not the exception.
- It is often possible to improve functional ability to a greater extent than the severity of pain is reduced.

Psychiatrists treating older adults with comorbid pain conditions should be well versed in the precise language of chronic pain syndromes; understand the stepped-care and often multidisciplinary approach to pain management; be familiar with the different classes, usual formulations, and risks associated with analgesic medications; and be knowledgeable about pain management resources in their community. These recommendations are consistent with a recent report describing the need for more pain education during psychiatric residency because (1) the neuroanatomical and functional overlap between pain and emotion/reward/motivation brain circuitry suggests integration and mutual modulation of these systems; (2) psychiatric disorders are commonly associated with alterations in pain processing, whereas chronic pain may impair emotional and neurocognitive functioning; and (3) given its stressful nature, pain may serve as a functional probe for unraveling pathophysiological mechanisms inherent in psychiatric morbidity (Elman, Zubieta, & Borsook, 2011).

During the initial psychiatric evaluation, active medical problems should be ascertained. If not spontaneously offered, patients should be asked about problems with arthritis. Osteoarthritis most commonly affects the knee, hip, and hand (Bijlsma, Berenbaum, & Lafeber, 2011). Inquiring about frequent low back pain (the most common site of musculoskeletal pain in late life (Bressler, Keyes, Rochon, & Badley, 1999) may also elicit useful information about a disorder that is associated with tremendous functional limitations (Morone et al., 2009). If diabetes is included as an active medical problem, patients should be asked about neuropathic symptoms, especially in their hands or feet. Patients may experience both sensory loss (numbness) and/or painful neuropathy (often described as "burning," "tingling," "stabbing," or an "electrical pain") (Tesfaye et al., 2011). Neuropathic symptoms are often worse in the evening and at night, while the symptoms of arthritis are often worse in the morning subsequent to relative immobility of joints during the night. If patients describe a plethora of medically unexplained symptoms such as paresthesias, bowel or bladder dysfunction, mental "fogginess," fatigue, and sleep disturbance, clinicians should inquire about symptoms consistent with fibromyalgia. We have found that a simple screen for fibromyalgia is to ask, "Do you often feel like you hurt all over?" (Arnold, Clauw, McCarberg, & FibroCollaborative, 2011).

If geriatric psychiatrists are not comfortable with performing a fibromyalgia tender point examination (Wolfe et al., 1990), assessing symptoms outlined by Pope and Hudson (Pope & Hudson, 1991) may be a reasonable substitute and guide to treatment. The criteria proposed by Pope and Hudson for fibromyalgia are listed in Table 19.2. These broad categories of painful conditions—nociceptive (e.g., arthritis), neuropathic (e.g., diabetic peripheral neuropathic pain), and idiopathic (e.g., fibromyalgia, or pain associated with depression)—help the psychiatrist working with older adults to plan treatment and communicate more effectively with other physicians and across disciplines such as rehabilitation specialists. Attending to painful conditions, to which many patients attribute disability and associated emotional symptoms (e.g., irritability, poor sleep, demoralization), can strengthen rapport between patients and their psychiatrist.

If a painful condition is diagnosed comorbid with a psychiatric disorder, clinicians may approach both disorders with a unified approach. There are several caveats for successful treatment when pain and psychiatric conditions such as depression or anxiety are comorbid. The first is that there is no one-sized-fits-all treatment. Patients require an individualized approach for both psychiatric as well as pain conditions. Patients and physicians need to work as partners in developing and implementing a

Table 19.2 Pope and Hudson Criteria for Fibromyalgia

Widespread pain > 3 months duration

Pain at > 11 of 18 tender points **OR:**

> 4 of 6 of the following symptoms

1. Generalized fatigue
2. Headaches
3. Sleep disturbance (hypersomnia or insomnia)
4. Neuropsychiatric complaints (one or more of the following: forgetfulness, excessive irritability, confusion, difficulty thinking, inability to concentrate, depression)
5. Numbness, tingling sensations
6. Symptoms of irritable bowel syndrome (periodically altered bowel habits with lower abdominal pain or distension relieved or aggravated by bowel movements; no blood)

successful treatment. The second caveat is that expectations for improvement should be established early in treatment. If a patient says that her average pain severity is a 9/10 over the past 2 weeks, the physician should ask the patient what would be a reasonable amount of pain she can live with. If the patient responds that she imagines she can comfortably live at an average pain severity of 4/10, the patient should be further pressed to qualify what that "4" means. Does it mean she won't have to take a narcotic analgesic every 6 hours but only on an as-needed basis? Does it mean she will be able to successfully walk 1 mile/day without disabling pain? Does it mean she will be able to sleep soundly throughout the night, unawakened by back pain when she changes positions? Clarifying expectations for and goals of treatment allows the patient/physician dyad a common language of pain and disability that is tailored specifically for that patient. A third and critical caveat for successful treatment is that psychiatric, psychosocial, and medical comorbidity must be diagnosed and treated. As mentioned earlier, pain homeostenosis is the inability of the organism (in this case, the patient) to maintain a pain-free (or low-pain) state because of these comorbidities. This concept is consistent with the field of geriatric medicine, in which the aging organism is compromised by numerous problems that reduce physiological reserve. When (1) medical comorbidity such as hypertension, diabetes, or loss of vision or hearing; (2) psychiatric comorbidity such as anxiety, insomnia, or substance misuse; and (3) psychosocial problems such as loneliness, poverty, and social isolation increase "pain homeostenosis," patients have less descending inhibition of pain and reduced ability to engage in effective treatments such as maintaining an analgesic regimen or participating in physical therapy.

Pharmacologic Treatment

Figure 19.1 illustrates our stepped-care approach for depressed older adults living with pain. We support a parsimonious approach in which (1) depression, (2) anxiety, (3) insomnia or fatigue, and (4) cognitive impairment are addressed simultaneous to pain management. The serotonin norepinephrine reuptake inhibitors (SNRIs), including duloxetine and milnacipran, are the only antidepressants currently approved for the treatment of pain conditions. Currently, duloxetine is approved for the treatment of diabetic peripheral neuropathic pain (DPNP) and fibromyalgia. Over 52 weeks of follow-up for the treatment of DPNP, patients receiving duloxetine experienced outcomes similar to, or significantly better than, that of routine care on most measures of tolerability, diabetic complications, and quality of life (Wernicke et al., 2006). Numerous studies have described the safe and effective use of duloxetine in older adults up to 120 mg/day (Karp et al., 2009; Raskin et al., 2008). Milnacipran is approved for the treatment of fibromyalgia in the United States (Arnold, Gendreau, Palmer, Gendreau, & Wang, 2010). It has been used as an antidepressant in Europe and Asia for many years. Venlafaxine is another SNRI that is more inhibitory of norepinephrine at doses greater than 150 mg/day (Muth et al., 1986). While not approved for the treatment of any painful conditions, several reports have described its efficacy and safety in older adults and in patients living with neuropathic and nociceptive

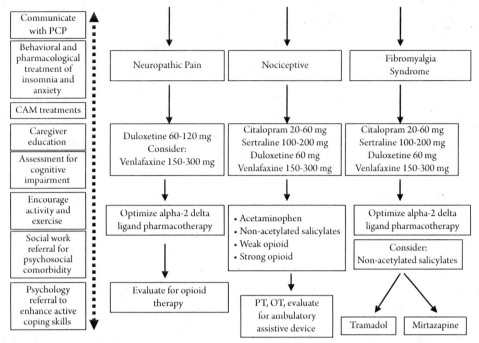

FIGURE 19.1 The multidisciplinary approach to managing older adults with coexisting depression and pain should be guided by the type of pain and should include the principles and recommendations described in the boxes to the left of the dashed-line vertical arrow.

pain conditions (Rowbotham, Goli, Kunz, & Lei, 2004; Sullivan, Bentley, Fan, & Gardner, 2009).

The tricyclic antidepressants have long been used for their analgesic properties. In addition to inhibiting norepinephrine and serotonin reuptake, they also inhibit calcium channels in the periphery. This calcium channel inhibition is hypothesized to enhance analgesia (Antkiewicz-Michaluk, Romanska, Michaluk, & Vetulani, 1991). For example, the tricyclic amitriptyline has been shown to reduce brain activation during pain in the perigenual (limbic) anterior cingulate cortex and parietal association cortex in patients with irritable bowel syndrome when exposed to stress (Morgan, Pickens, Gautam, Kessler, & Mertz, 2005). While most research on tricyclics for pain—in particular, neuropathic pain—has focused on imipramine and amitryptyline, in general we restrict the use of tricyclics in late life to nortriptyline because of its lower anticholinergic burden (Chew et al., 2008). Our rule of thumb for all patients over 50 for whom we prescribe a tricyclic is to obtain an electrocardiogram prior to initiating treatment. Often, analgesia can be achieved with low doses of tricyclics, in the range of 10–50 mg/day. When prescribing

nortriptyline for neuropathic pain or fibromyalgia, we generally start at 10 mg at night, increasing the dose by 10 mg/week. Improvement in pain and sleep is often observed at doses no greater than 25 mg/day. The risk of cardiac conduction abnormality (in particular, prolongation of the QT interval) is increased when tricyclics are co-prescribed with methadone, so caution should be exercised when these medications are combined. Co-prescription of most SSRIs (in particular, fluoxetine, sertraline, paroxetine, venlafaxine, and duloxetine) may increase levels of tricyclic medications contributing to tricyclic toxicity (e.g., dry mouth, urinary retention, constipation, sedation, cardiotoxicity). All psychiatric and analgesic medications carry the risk of side effects. Table 19.3 lists common neuropsychiatric side effects associated with frequently prescribed analgesic medications.

Nonpharmacologic Treatment

As stated earlier, management of pain, especially when comorbid with affective, anxiety, and somatoform disorders, requires an individualized approach that is often multimodal. The goal of psychosocial

Table 19.3 Possible Neuropsychiatric Side Effects of Analgesic Medications

Corticosteroids	• Delirium • Dementia • Depression • Mania • Mood lability • Psychosis
Nonsteroidal Antiinflammatory Drugs	• Depression/anxiety • Impaired concentration • Hypertension (if severe and sustained, may cause mental status changes) • Meningitis (especially in patients with systemic lupus erythematosis)
Opioids	• Delirium • Depression/anxiety • Sedation/somnolence • Irritability • Non-restorative sleep
Tricyclic Antidepressants	• Sedation • Confusion (often related to anticholinergic burden) • Delirium • Insomnia
Alpha-2 Delta Ligands	• Sedation/somnolence • Delirium

interventions for patients living with pain and psychiatric comorbidity is to reduce learned helplessness, improve self-efficacy for managing symptoms and stress, and behavioral activation. These principles are based on both the successful Stanford Self-Management Program (Lorig, 2003; Lorig & Holman, 1993; Von Korff & Moore, 2001) and on cognitive-behavioral therapy (Keefe, 1996; Kerns, Otis, & Marcus, 2001; Reid, Otis, Barry, & Kerns, 2003). The general goals of both approaches are for patients to learn to modify their behavior through the use and discussion of behavioral plans and problem-solving techniques to sustain behavioral change. Briefly, the Stanford Self-Management Program teaches patients about chronic pain, including triggers and flare-ups; how to cope with fear and other negative emotions; and strategies for physical activity, muscle relaxation, deep breathing, distraction, sleep hygiene, and working with clinicians and their families (Keefe, 1996). The basic principles of cognitive-behavioral therapy for pain management are described in Table 19.4.

CONCLUSION

Given the linked neurobiology between pain and psychiatric conditions; overlapping treatments; and similar effects on functioning, disability, physical health, caregiver burden, medical comorbidity, and mortality, psychiatrists must attend to both conditions to optimize the care of these complex patients. Knowledge about the pathophysiology, diagnosis, and treatment of common pain conditions in late life will improve interdisciplinary communication, guide treatment planning, and enhance patient outcomes. We acknowledge that most late-life psychiatrists will not assume primary responsibility for the management of pain conditions in late life. However, knowing how to precisely communicate with primary care, pain medicine, psychology, and rehabilitation colleagues about diagnosis, symptoms, links between pain and psychiatric disorders, and treatment options, will increase the chance that pain and functional disability, problems that interfere with the efficacy of treatment of comorbid psychiatric conditions, are effectively managed.

Table 19.4 Principles of CBT for Older Adults Living with Pain

- Provision of a treatment rationale that helps patients understand that cognitions and behavior can affect the pain experience.
- Teaching patients that they play a role in controlling their pain.
- Progressive muscle relaxation and deep breathing techniques to decrease muscle tension, reduce anxiety and emotional distress, and distract the patient from pain.
- Pleasant activity scheduling and teaching patients to pace activity are used to help patients increase their level and range of activities.
- Cognitive restructuring to help patients identify and challenge catastrophic thoughts about pain and replace them with more adaptive thoughts consistent with active coping.
- Improved problem solving by following the outline of Problem Solving Therapy
  - Precisely Identify the problem
  - Create a goal
  - Brainstorm possible solutions
  - Generate Pros and Cons for each possible solution
  - Select the most thoughtful solution
  - Create an action plan
  - Follow-up on the action plan at the next visit to assess progress and troubleshoot solutions to practical challenges.
- Inclusion of caregivers to educate them about chronic pain
- Teaching patients how to more effectively utilize pain medications and self-management remedies like hot and cold.
- Relapse prevention to manage stress and pain flares.

Disclosures

Dr. Karp receives research support in the form of medication supplies from Pfizer and Reckitt Benckiser. He is a stock owner of Corcept. He receives or has received research funding from the NIH, RAND, and the Brain and Behavior Research Foundation.

Mr. McGovern has nothing to disclose.

REFERENCES

Aaron, L. A., Bradley, L. A., Alarcon, G. S., Alexander, R. W., Triana-Alexander, M., Martin, M. Y., & Alberts, K. R. (1996). Psychiatric diagnoses in patients with fibromyalgia are related to health care-seeking behavior rather than to illness. *Arthritis and Rheumatism, 39*, 436–445.

AGS Panel on Persistent Pain in Older Persons. (2002). The management of persistent pain in older persons. *Journal of the American Geriatrics Society, 50*, S205–S224.

Amenta, F., Zaccheo, D., & Collier, W. L. (1991). Neurotransmitters, neuroreceptors and aging. *Mechanisms of Ageing and Development, 61*, 249–273.

Antkiewicz-Michaluk, L., Romanska, I., Michaluk, J., Vetulani, J. (1991). Role of calcium channels in effects of antidepressant drugs on responsiveness to pain. *Psychopharmacology, 105*, 269–274.

Arnold, L. M., Clauw, D. J., McCarberg, B. H., & FibroCollaborative. (2011). Improving the recognition and diagnosis of fibromyalgia. *Mayo Clinic Proceedings, 86*, 457–464.

Arnold, L. M., Gendreau, R. M., Palmer, R. H., Gendreau, J. F., & Wang, Y. (2010). Efficacy and safety of milnacipran 100 mg/day in patients with fibromyalgia: Results of a randomized, double-blind, placebo-controlled trial. *Arthritis and Rheumatism, 62*, 2745–2756.

Bair, M. J., Robinson, R. L., Katon, W., & Kroenke, K. (2003). Depression and pain comorbidity: A literature review. *Archives of Internal Medicine, 163*, 2433–2445.

Barsky, A. J., Orav, E. J., & Bates, D. W. (2005). Somatization increases medical utilization and costs independent of psychiatric and medical comorbidity. *Archives of General Psychiatry, 62*, 903–910.

Becker, P. M., & Cohen, H. J. (1984). The functional approach to the care of the elderly: A conceptual framework. *Journal of the American Geriatrics Society, 32*, 923–929.

Benedetti, F., Vighetti, S., Ricco, C., Lagna, E., Bergamasco, B., Pinessi, L., & Rainero, I. (1999). Pain threshold and tolerance in Alzheimer's disease. *Pain, 80*, 377–382.

Bennett, D. A., Schneider, J. A., Arvanitakis, Z., Kelly, J. F., Aggarwal, N. T., Shah, R. C., & Wilson, R. S. (2006). Neuropathology of older persons without cognitive impairment from two community-based studies. *Neurology, 66*, 1837–1844.

Berne, R., & Levy, M. (1998). *Physiology*. St. Louis, MO: Mosby.

Bijlsma, J. W., Berenbaum, F., & Lafeber, F. P. (2011). Osteoarthritis: An update with relevance for clinical practice. *Lancet, 377*, 2115–2126.

Bjoro, K., & Herr, K. (2008). Assessment of pain in the nonverbal or cognitively impaired older adult. *Clinical Geriatric Medicine, 24*, 237–262, vi.

Brennan, P. L., Schutte, K. K., & Moos, R. H. (2005). Pain and use of alcohol to manage pain: Prevalence and 3-year outcomes among older problem and non-problem drinkers. *Addiction, 100*, 777–786.

Bressler, H. B., Keyes, W. J., Rochon, P. A., & Badley, E. (1999). The prevalence of low back pain in the elderly. A systematic review of the literature. *Spine, 24*, 1813–1819.

Catananti, C., & Gambassi, G. (2010). Pain assessment in the elderly. *Surgical Oncology, 19*, 140–148.

Casten, R. J., Parmelee, P. A., Kleban, M. H., Lawton, M. P., & Katz, I. R. (1995). The relationships among anxiety, depression, and pain in a geriatric institutionalized sample. *Pain, 61*, 271–276.

Chew, M. L., Mulsant, B. H., Pollock, B. G., Lehman, M. E., Greenspan, A., Mahmoud, R. A.,...Gharabawi, G. (2008). Anticholinergic activity of 107 medications commonly used by older adults. *Journal of the American Geriatrics Society, 56*, 1333–1341.

Chodosh, J., Solomon, D. H., Roth, C. P., Chang, J. T., MacLean, C. H., Ferrell, B. A.,...Wenger, N. S. The quality of medical care provided to vulnerable older patients with chronic pain. *Journal of the American Geriatrics Society, 52*, 756–761.

Cohen-Mansfield, J., & Marx, M. S. (1993). Pain and depression in the nursing home: Corroborating results. *Journal of Gerontology, 48*, P96–P97.

Cole, L. J., Farrell, M. J., Duff, E. P., Barber, J. B., Egan, G. F., & Gibson, S. J. (2006). Pain sensitivity and fMRI pain-related brain activity in Alzheimer's disease. *Brain, 129*, 2957–2965.

Cook, I. A., Leuchter, A. F., Morgan, M. L., Conlee, E. W., David, S., Lufkin, R.,...Rosenberg-Thompson, S. (2002). Cognitive and physiologic correlates of subclinical structural brain disease in elderly healthy control subjects. *Archives of Neurology, 59*, 1612–1620.

Crook, J., Rideout, E., & Browne, G. (1984). The prevalence of pain complaints in a general population. *Pain, 18*, 299–314.

DeKosky, S. T., Scheff, S. W., & Markesbery, W. R. (1985). Laminar organization of cholinergic circuits in human frontal cortex in Alzheimer's disease and aging. *Neurology, 35*, 1425–1431.

de Rond, M. E., de Wit, R., van Dam, F. S., & Muller, M. J. (2000). A pain monitoring program for nurses: Effects on communication, assessment and documentation of patients' pain. *Journal of Pain Symptom Management, 20*, 424–439.

Edwards, R. R., & Fillingim, R. B. (2001). Age-associated differences in responses to noxious stimuli. *Journals of Gerontology Series A, Biological Sciences and Medical Sciences, 56*, M180–M185.

Drac, H., Babiuch, M., & Wisniewska, W. (1991). Morphological and biochemical changes in peripheral nerves with aging. *Neuropatologia Polska, 29*, 49–67.

Elman, I., Zubieta, J-K., & Borsook, D. (2011). The missing P in psychiatric training: Why it is important to teach pain to psychiatrists. *Archives of General Psychiatry, 68*, 12–20.

Farrell, M. J., & Gibson, S. J. (2004). Psychosocial aspects of pain in older people. In R. H. Dworkin & W. S. Breitbart (Eds.), *Psychosocial aspects of pain: A handbook for health care providers* (pp. 495–518). Seattle, WA: IASP Press.

Farrell, M., & Gibson, S. (2007). Age interacts with stimulus frequency in the temporal summation of pain. *Pain Medicine, 8*, 514–520.

Ferrell, B. A., Stein, W. M., & Beck, J. C. (2000). The Geriatric Pain Measure: Validity, reliability and factor analysis. *Journal of the American Geriatrics Society, 48*, 1669–1673.

Fishbain, D. A., Cutler, R., Rosomoff, H. L., & Rosomoff, R. S. (1997). Chronic pain-associated depression: Antecedent or consequence of chronic pain? A review. *Clinical Journal of Pain, 13*, 116–137.

Gibson, S. J., & Farrell, M. (2004). A review of age differences in the neurophysiology of nociception and the perceptual experience of pain. *Clinical Journal of Pain, 20*, 227–239.

Gignac, M. A., Davis, A. M., Hawker, G., Wright, J. G., Mahomed, N., Fortin, P. R., & Badley, E. M. (2006). "What do you expect? You're just getting older": A comparison of perceived osteoarthritis-related and aging-related health experiences in middle- and older-age adults. *Arthritis & Rheumatism*, 55, 905–912.

Godfrey, R. G. (1996). A guide to the understanding and use of tricyclic antidepressants in the overall management of fibromyalgia and other chronic pain syndromes. *Archives of Internal Medicine*, 156, 1047–1052.

Gottfries, C. (1980). Amine metabolism in normal ageing and in dementia disorders. In P. Roberts (Ed.), *Biochemistry of dementia* (pp. 213–239). New York: Wiley.

Grote, S. S., Moses, S. G., Robins, E., Hudgens, R. W., & Croninger, A. B. (1974). A study of selected catecholamine metabolizing enzymes: A comparison of depressive suicides and alcoholic suicides with controls. *Journal of Neurochemistry*, 23, 791–802.

Grachev, I. D., Swarnkar, A., Szeverenyi, N. M., Ramachandran, T. S., & Apkarian, A. V. (2001). Aging alters the multichemical networking profile of the human brain: An in vivo (1)H-MRS study of young versus middle-aged subjects. *Journal of Neurochemistry*, 77, 292–303.

Hanlon, J. T., Fillenbaum, G. G., Studenski, S. A., Ziqubu-Page, T., & Wall, W. E., Jr. (1996). Factors associated with suboptimal analgesic use in community-dwelling elderly. *Annals of Pharmacotherapy*, 30, 739–744.

Hiller, W., Fichter, M. M., & Rief, W. (2003). A controlled treatment study of somatoform disorders including analysis of healthcare utilization and cost-effectiveness. *Journal of Psychosomatic Research*, 54, 369–380.

Helme, R. D., & Gibson, S. J. The epidemiology of pain in elderly people. *Clinical Geriatric Medicine*, 17, 417–431, v.

Herr, K., Bjoro, K., & Decker, S. (2006). Tools for assessment of pain in nonverbal older adults with dementia: A state-of-the-science review. *Journal of Pain Symptom Management*, 31, 170–192.

Hsu, K. T., Shuman, S. K., Hamamoto, D. T., Hodges, J. S., & Feldt, K. S. (2007). The application of facial expressions to the assessment of orofacial pain in cognitively impaired older adults. *Journal of the American Dental Association*, 138, 963–969; quiz 1021–1022.

Hulette, C. M., Welsh-Bohmer, K. A., Murray, M. G., Saunders, A. M., Mash, D. C., & McIntyre, L. M. (1998). Neuropathological and neuropsychological changes in "normal" aging: Evidence for preclinical Alzheimer disease in cognitively normal individuals. *Journal of Neuropathology and Experimental Neurology*, 57, 1168–1174.

Iwata, K., Fukuoka, T., Kondo, E., Tsuboi, Y., Tashiro, A., Noguchi, K.,...Kanda, K. (2002). Plastic changes in nociceptive transmission of the rat spinal cord with advancing age. *Journal of Neurophysiology*, 87, 1086–1093.

Jones, G. T., & Macfarlane, G. J. (2005). Epidemiology of pain in older persons. In S. J. Gibson & D. K. Weiner (Eds.), *Pain in older persons* (pp. 3–22). Seattle, WA: IASP Press.

Kakigi, R. (1987). The effect of aging on somatosensory evoked potentials following stimulation of the posterior tibial nerve in man. *Electroencephalography and Clinical Neurophysiology*, 68, 277–286.

Kakiuchi, T., Nishiyama, S., Sato, K., Ohba, H., Nakanishi, S., & Tsukada, H. (2000). Age-related reduction of [11C]MDL100,907 binding to central 5-HT(2A) receptors: PET study in the conscious monkey brain. *Brain Research*, 883, 135–142.

Karp, J. F., Shega, J. W., Morone, N. E., & Weiner, D. K. (2008). Advances in understanding the mechanisms and management of persistent pain in older adults. *British Journal of Anaesthesia*, 101, 111–120.

Karp, J., Weiner, D., Dew, M., Begley, A., Miller, M., & Reynolds, C. (2009). Duloxetine and care management treatment of older adults with comorbid major depressive disorder and chronic low back pain: Results of an open-label pilot study. *International Journal of Geriatric Psychiatry*, 25, 633–642.

Keefe, F. (1996). Cognitive behavioral therapy for managing pain. *Clinical Psychologist*, 49, 4–5.

Kerns, R. D., Otis, J. D., & Marcus, K. S. (2001). Cognitive-behavioral therapy for chronic pain in the elderly. *Clinics in Geriatric Medicine*, 17, 503–523.

Ko, M. L., King, M. A., Gordon, T. L., & Crisp, T. (1997). The effects of aging on spinal neurochemistry in the rat. *Brain Research Bulletin*, 42, 95–98.

Krulewitch, H., London, M. R., Skakel, V. J., Lundstedt, G. J., Thomason, H., & Brummel-Smith, K. (2000). Assessment of pain in cognitively impaired older adults: A comparison of pain assessment tools and their use by nonprofessional caregivers. *Journal of the American Geriatrics Society*, 48, 1607–1611.

Kunz, M., Scharmann, S., Hemmeter, U., Schepelmann, K., & Lautenbacher, S. (2007). The facial expression of pain in patients with dementia. *Pain*, 133, 221–228.

Landis, C. A., Levine, J. D., & Robinson, C. R. (1989). Decreased slow-wave and paradoxical sleep in a rat chronic pain model. *Sleep*, 12, 167–177.

Lautenbacher, S., Kunz, M., Strate, P., Nielsen, J., &
Arendt-Nielsen, L. (2005). Age effects on pain
thresholds, temporal summation and spatial
summation of heat and pressure pain. *Pain, 115*,
410–418.

Lindsay, P. G., & Wyckoff, M. (1981). The
depression-pain syndrome and its response to
antidepressants. *Psychosomatics, 22*, 571–573,
576–577.

Lorig, K. (2003). Self-management education: more
than a nice extra. *Medical Care, 41*, 699–701.

Lorig, K., & Holman, H. (1993). Arthritis
self-management studies: A twelve-year review.
Health Education Quarterly, 20, 17–28.

Marcusson, J. O., Morgan, D. G., Winblad, B., & Finch,
C. E. (1984). Serotonin-2 binding sites in human
frontal cortex and hippocampus. Selective loss of
S-2A sites with age. *Brain Research, 311*, 51–56.

Martin, R., Williams, J., Hadjistavropoulos, T.,
Hadjistavropoulos, H. D., & MacLean, M.
(2005). A qualitative investigation of seniors'
and caregivers' views on pain assessment and
management. *Canadian Journal of Nursing
Research, 37*, 142–164.

McCaffery, M. (1968). Nursing practice theories
related to cognition, bodily pain, and man-
environment interactions (p. 95). Los Angeles,
CA: University of California at Los Angeles
Students' Store.

Melzack, R., & Wall, P. (1965). Pain mechanisms: A
new theory. *Science, 150*, 971–979.

McGeer, E., & McGeer, P. (1976). Neurotransmitter
metabolism in the ageing brain. In R. Terry & S.
Gershon (Eds.), *Neurobiology of aging* (pp. 389–
401). New York: Raven Press.

Moffitt, P. F., Kalucy, E. C., Kalucy, R. S., Baum, F. E.,
& Cooke, R. D. (1991). Sleep difficulties, pain and
other correlates. *Journal of Internal Medicine, 230*,
245–249.

Morgan, V., Pickens, D., Gautam, S., Kessler, R., &
Mertz, H. (2005). Amitriptyline reduces rectal
pain related activation of the anterior cingulate
cortex in patients with irritable bowel syndrome.
Gut, 54, 601–607.

Morone, N., Karp, J., Lynch, C., Bost, J., El Khoudary,
S., & Weiner, D. (2009). Impact of chronic
musculoskeletal pathology on older adults: A
study of differences between knee OA and low
back pain. *Pain Medicine, 10*, 693–701.

Muth, E. A., Haskins, J. T., Moyer, J. A., Husbands,
G. E., Nielsen, S. T., & Sigg, E. B. (1986).
Antidepressant biochemical profile of the
novel bicyclic compound Wy-45,030, an ethyl
cyclohexanol derivative. *Biochemical Pharmacology,
35*, 4493–4497.

Ochoa, J., & Mair, W. G. (1969). The normal
sural nerve in man. II. Changes in the axons
and Schwann cells due to ageing. *Acta
Neuropathologica, 13*, 217–239.

Oyama, O., Paltoo, C., & Greengold, J. (2007).
Somatoform disorders. *American Family Physician,
76*, 1333–1338.

Parmelee, P. A. (2005). Measuring mood and
psychosocial function associated with pain in late
life. In S. J. Gibson & D. K. Weiner (Eds.), *Pain in
older persons* (pp. 175–202). Seattle, WA: IASP
Press.

Parmelee, P. A., Harralson, T. L., Smith, L. A., &
Schumacher, H. R. (2007). Necessary and
discretionary activities in knee osteoarthritis: Do
they mediate the pain-depression relationship?
Pain Medicine, 8, 449–461.

Parmelee, P. A., Katz, I. R., & Lawton, M. P. (1991).
The relation of pain to depression among
institutionalized aged. *Journal of Gerontology, 46*,
P15–P21.

Pope, H. G., Jr., & Hudson, J. I. (1991). A
supplemental interview for forms of "affective
spectrum disorder". *International Journal of
Psychiatry in Medicine, 21*, 205–232.

Porter, F. L., Malhotra, K. M., Wolf, C. M., Morris, J.
C., Miller, J. P., & Smith, M. C. (1996). Dementia
and response to pain in the elderly. *Pain, 68*,
413–421.

Rafalowska, J., Drac, H., & Rosinska, K. (1976).
Histological and electrophysiological changes of
the lower motor neuron with aging. *Polish Medical
Sciences and History Bulletin, 15*, 271–280.

Raskin, J., Wiltse, C. G., Dinkel, J. J., Walker, D. J.,
Desaiah, D., & Katona, C. (2008). Safety and
tolerability of duloxetine at 60 mg once daily in
elderly patients with major depressive disorder.
Journal of Clinical Psychopharmacology, 28, 32–38.

Reid, M. C., Otis, J., Barry, L. C., & Kerns, R. D.
(2003). Cognitive-behavioral therapy for chronic
low back pain in older persons: A preliminary
study. *Pain Medicine, 4*, 223–230.

Reid, M. C., Williams, C. S., Concato, J., Tinetti, M.
E., & Gill, T. M. (2003). Depressive symptoms
as a risk factor for disabling back pain in
community-dwelling older persons. *Journal of the
American Geriatrics Society, 51*, 1710–1717.

Robinson, D. (1975). Changes in MAO and
monoamines with human development. *Federal
Proceedings, 34*, 103–107.

Rogers, J., & Bloom, F. (1985). Neurotransmitter
metabolism and function in the aging nervous
system. In C. E. Finch (Ed.), *Handbook of the
biology of aging* (pp. 645–662). New York: Van
Nostrand Reinhold.

Rowbotham, M., Goli, V., Kunz, N., & Lei, D. (2004). Venlafaxine extended release in the treatment of painful diabetic neuropathy: A double-blind, placebo-controlled study. *Pain, 110*, 697–706.

Rub, U., Del Tredici, K., Del Turco, D., & Braak, H. (2002). The intralaminar nuclei assigned to the medial pain system and other components of this system are early and progressively affected by the Alzheimer's disease-related cytoskeletal pathology. *Journal of Chemical Neuroanatomy, 23*, 279–290.

Scherder, E. J. (2000). Low use of analgesics in Alzheimer's disease: Possible mechanisms. *Psychiatry, 63*, 1–12.

Scherder, E., Bouma, A., Borkent, M., & Rahman, O. (1999). Alzheimer patients report less pain intensity and pain affect than non-demented elderly. *Psychiatry, 62*, 265–272.

Scherder, E. J. A., Sergeant, J. A., & Swaab, D. F. (2003). Pain processing in dementia and its relation to neuropathology. *Lancet Neurology, 2*, 677–686.

Segovia, G., Del Arco, A., Prieto, L., & Mora, F. (2001). Glutamate-glutamine cycle and aging in striatum of the awake rat: Effects of a glutamate transporter blocker. *Neurochemical Research, 26*, 37–41.

Sheline, Y. I., Mintun, M. A., Moerlein, S. M., & Snyder, A. Z. (2002). Greater loss of 5-HT(2A) receptors in midlife than in late life. *American Journal of Psychiatry, 159*, 430–435.

Simon, D., Craig, K. D., Gosselin, F., Belin, P., & Rainville, P. (2008). Recognition and discrimination of prototypical dynamic expressions of pain and emotions. *Pain, 135*, 55–64.

Sorkin, L. S., & Wallace, M. S. (1999). Acute pain mechanisms. *Surgical Clinics of North America, 79*, 213–229.

Spokes, E. G. (1979). An analysis of factors influencing measurements of dopamine, noradrenaline, glutamate decarboxylase and choline acetylase in human post-mortem brain tissue. *Brain, 102*, 333–346.

Strassman, A. (2002). Neurotransmitters. In C. Warfield & H. Fausett (Eds.), *Manual of pain management* (pp. 15–18). Philadelphia, PA: Lippincott, Williams, and Wilkins.

Sullivan, M., Bentley, S., Fan, M. Y., Gardner, G. (2009). A single-blind placebo run-in study of venlafaxine XR for activity-limiting osteoarthritis pain. *Pain Medicine, 10*, 806–812.

Taylor, L. J., Harris, J., Epps, C. D., & Herr, K. (2005). Psychometric evaluation of selected pain intensity scales for use with cognitively impaired and cognitively intact older adults. *Rehabilitation Nursing, 30*, 55–61.

Tesfaye, S., Vileikyte, L., Rayman, G., Sindrup, S., Perkins, B., Baconja, M., et al. (2011). Painful diabetic peripheral neuropathy: Consensus recommendations on diagnosis, assessment and management. Diabetes/metabolism research and reviews. *Diabetes/Metabolism Research and Reviews*. ePub, ahead of print.

Thomas, E., Peat, G., Harris, L., Wilkie, R., & Croft, P. R. (2004). The prevalence of pain and pain interference in a general population of older adults: Cross-sectional findings from the North Staffordshire Osteoarthritis Project (NorStOP). *Pain, 110*, 361–368.

Turk, D. C., & Rudy, T. E. (1988). Toward an empirically derived taxonomy of chronic pain patients: Integration of psychological assessment data. *Journal of Consulting and Clinical Psychology, 56*, 233–238.

US Census Bureau. (2011). *2010 census summary file 1: 2010 census of population and housing.* Washington, DC: Office of the Census.

US Department of Health and Human Services. (2005). *The DASIS Report: Older adults in substance abuse treatment, 2005.* Washington, DC: Government Printing Office.

Voaklander, D. C., Rowe, B. H., Dryden, D. M., Pahal, J., Saar, P., & Kelly, K. D. (2008). Medical illness, medication use and suicide in seniors: a population-based case-control study. *Journal of Epidemiology and Community Health, 62*, 138–146.

Von Korff, M., & Moore, J. C. (2001). Stepped care for back pain: activating approaches for primary care. *Annals of Internal Medicine, 134*, 911–917.

Warden, V., Hurley, A. C., & Volicer, L. (2003). Development and psychometric evaluation of the Pain Assessment in Advanced Dementia (PAINAD) scale. *Journal of the American Medical Directors Association, 4*, 9–15.

Weiner, D. K. (2007). Office management of chronic pain in the elderly. *American Journal of Medicine, 120*, 306–315.

Weiner, D. K., & Rudy, T. E. (2002). Attitudinal barriers to effective treatment of persistent pain in nursing home residents. *Journal of the American Geriatrics Society, 50*, 2035–2040.

Wernicke, J. F., Pritchett, Y. L., D'Souza, D. N., Waninger, A., Tran, P., Iyengar, S., & Raskin, J. (2006). A randomized controlled trial of duloxetine in diabetic peripheral neuropathic pain. *Neurology, 67*, 1411–1420.

White, P., Hiley, C. R., Goodhardt, M. J., Carrasco, L. H., Keet, J. P., Williams, I. E., & Bowen, D. M.

(1977). Neocortical cholinergic neurons in elderly people. *Lancet, 1,* 668–671.

Williamson, G. M., & Schulz, R. (1992). Pain, activity restriction, and symptoms of depression among community-residing elderly adults. *Journal of Gerontology, 47,* P367–P372.

Wittig, R. M., Zorick, F. J., Blumer, D., Heilbronn, M., & Roth, T. (1982). Disturbed sleep in patients complaining of chronic pain. *Journal of Nervous and Mental Disease, 170,* 429–431.

Wolfe, F., Smythe, H. A., Yunus, M. B., Bennett, R. M., Bombardier, C., Goldenberg, D. L., ... Clark, P. (1990). The American College of Rheumatology 1990 Criteria for the Classification of Fibromyalgia. Report of the Multicenter Criteria Committee. *Arthritis and Rheumatism, 33,* 160–172.

Wong, D. F., Wagner, H. N., Jr., Dannals, R. F., Links, J. M., Frost, J. J., Ravert, H. T., ... Douglass, K. H. (1984). Effects of age on dopamine and serotonin receptors measured by positron tomography in the living human brain. *Science, 226,* 1393–1396.

Yates, P., Dewar, A., & Fentiman, B. (1995). Pain: The views of elderly people living in long-term residential care settings. *Journal of Advanced Nursing, 21,* 667–674.

Yong, H. H., Gibson, S. J., Horne, D. J., & Helme, R. D. (2001). Development of a pain attitudes questionnaire to assess stoicism and cautiousness for possible age differences. *Journals of Gerontology Series B, Psychological Science Social Science, 56,* P279–P284.

Zhang, S., Tang, J. S., Yuan, B., & Jia, H. (1997). Involvement of the frontal ventrolateral orbital cortex in descending inhibition of nociception mediated by the periaqueductal gray in rats. *Neuroscience Letters, 224,* 142–146.

Zhuo, M., & Gebhart, G. F. (1990). Spinal cholinergic and monoaminergic receptors mediate descending inhibition from the nuclei reticularis gigantocellularis and gigantocellularis pars alpha in the rat. *Brain Research, 535,* 67–78.

Zimmerman, M. E., Brickman, A. M., Paul, R. H., Grieve, S. M., Tate, D. F., Gunstad, J., ... Gordon, E. (2006). The relationship between frontal gray matter volume and cognition varies across the healthy adult lifespan. *American Journal of Geriatric Psychiatry, 14,* 823–833.

20

BIDIRECTIONAL RELATIONSHIPS BETWEEN SLEEP, INSOMNIA, AND DEPRESSION

Chiara Baglioni, Mathias Berger, and Dieter Riemann

EVEN IN ancient times, it was known that people suffering from melancholia also experience troubled sleep. Philosophers and physicians like Plato or Hippocrates (see R. Burton, *The Anatomy of Melancholy*; first published in 1621) noted that patients afflicted with melancholia complained about sleep disturbances, including problems falling asleep, maintaining sleep, or waking up too early in the morning. It was the founder of modern psychiatry, Kraepelin (1909), who at the turn of the 20th century coined the term *endogenous depression* and noted, based on his clinical observations, that different types of depression may be accompanied by specific forms of sleep disturbances. In his nosology, problems falling asleep (prolonged sleep latency) were assumed to be typical for neurotic (psychological) depression, whereas early morning awakening and sleep maintenance problems were proposed to be tightly linked to the so-called endogenous (assumed to be a biological form) subtype of depression. Polysomnographic research in psychopathology, which started in the 1960s, initially focused on these sleep continuity disturbances, but it was quickly discovered that distinct alterations of the REM sleep pattern occur in depressed patients. Whereas in healthy subjects the latency to REM sleep, that is, the interval from sleep onset to the occurrence of the first REM period, may vary from 70 to 90 minutes, it was observed that in many depressed patients REM latency was shortened to 50 minutes or in extreme cases even to an interval below 20 minutes (so-called sleep-onset REM periods, or SOREMP). The group of Kupfer and colleagues in Pittsburgh, who were the first to systematically study these phenomena, postulated that shortened REM latency may be a marker of primary/melancholic/endogenous depression compared to the secondary or neurotic/nonendogenous forms (Kupfer, 1976; Kupfer & Foster, 1972). More intensive work from this (Kupfer, Reynolds, Grochocinski, Ulrich, & McEachran, 1986) and other groups (e.g., Berger, Doerr, Lund, Bronisch, & von Zerssen, 1982; Berger & Riemann, 1993; Lauer, Riemann, Wiegand, & Berger, 1991; Riemann, Hohagen, Bahro, & Berger,

• 347

1994a) indicated, however, that a short REM latency is not a specific marker for the biological forms of depression but may also occur in nonendogenous subtypes. Apart from shortened REM latency, in depressed patients also an increased amount of REM sleep, a prolongation of the first REM period, and an increased number of eye movements during REM periods (i.e., increased REM density) was noted. Furthermore, the clinically well-known alterations of sleep continuity were confirmed by polysomnography and a reduction of slow-wave sleep was noted in affective disorders. Figure 20.1 shows an example (single case) from our own investigations highlighting polysomnographically captured sleep changes in a severely depressed patient compared to a healthy sleeper.

The issue of the specificity of sleep markers for depressive disorders was put to an empirical test by a meta-analysis of the polysomnographic literature (Benca, Obermeyer, Thisted, & Gillin, 1992). This analysis revealed that alterations of REM sleep like shortened REM latency do indeed occur more frequently in depression than in any other psychopathological condition. However, it was also noted that a shortened REM latency may occur to a lesser degree also in patients with borderline personality disorder, alcohol dependency, eating disorders, or other psychopathological conditions. The same unspecific results were demonstrated for slow-wave

sleep distribution and sleep continuity measures like sleep onset latency or the wake time after sleep onset (WASO). Nevertheless, when summarizing the findings, it became clear that the combined occurrence of changes in sleep continuity, a reduction of slow-wave sleep, and REM sleep disinhibition are most prominent in patients suffering from a depressive disorder.

MECHANISMS INVOLVED IN THE RELATIONSHIP BETWEEN SLEEP AND DEPRESSION

Theories of Sleep Regulation in Depression

THE CHOLINERGIC-AMINERGIC HYPOTHESIS

The so-called reciprocal interaction model of non-REM and REM sleep regulation as postulated by Hobson et al. (1975) had a huge influence on theories trying to explain REM sleep abnormalities in depressed patients (McCarley, 1982). According to this model, cholinergic neurons in the brainstem trigger and maintain REM sleep, whereas noradrenergic and serotonergic neurons are active during non-REM sleep. These groups of neurons do reciprocally inhibit and stimulate each other, thus

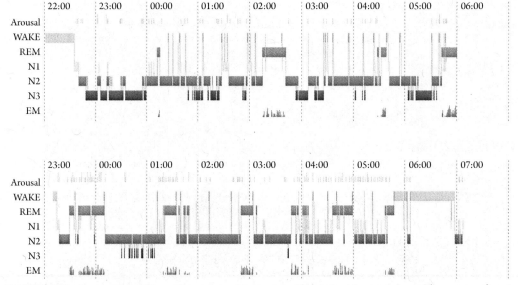

FIGURE 20.1. Comparison of the polysomnographic sleep profile of a healthy good sleeper (upper panel) and a severely depressed patient (lower panel). REM: rapid eye movements sleep; N1: NREM sleep, stage 1; N2: NREM sleep, stage 2; N3: NREM sleep, deep sleep; EM: eye movements (See color insert).

explaining the alternation of non-REM and REM sleep. This model fitted well with the earlier postulated cholinergic-aminergic neurotransmitter imbalance hypothesis of depression (Janowsky, El-Yousef, Davis, & Sekerke, 1972).

A huge body of evidence tested whether cholinomimetics (either cholinesterase inhibitors or muscarinic agonists) have an impact on REM sleep regulation in healthy subjects. Our own group (overview: Riemann et al., 1994b, 1996) was able to show that in healthy subjects different types of drugs like physostigmine, galantamine, RS 86, SDZ 210–086, and tacrine were able to shorten REM latency by about 20 minutes and to decrease slow-wave sleep. This effect was even more pronounced, when administering cholinergic drugs to patients with depression. Gillin and colleagues and our group (e.g., Berger, Riemann, Höchli, & Spiegel, 1989; Gillin, Sutton, & Ruiz, 1991; Riemann & Berger, 1992; Riemann et al., 1994c) were able to demonstrate clearly that additional cholinergic stimulation enhanced the difference in REM latency between healthy subjects and patients with depression, also compared to other psychopathological conditions like eating disorders or schizophrenia.

The relevance of the reciprocal interaction model of non-REM/ REM sleep regulation for the pathophysiology of depression is based on work demonstrating that neuronal centers involved in the regulation of REM sleep are also linked to higher brain areas (e.g., limbic system). Locus ceruleus and dorsal raphe are the decisive parts of the central nervous system's monoaminergic neuronal system. REM sleep generating cholinergic neurons is linked to cholinergic neuronal populations in higher brain areas (e.g., Hobson, Lydic, & Baghdoyan, 1986). Thus, REM sleep dysregulation may serve as a window to neurochemical processes that are involved in the regulation of affect. Positron emission tomography studies (e.g., Nofzinger et al., 2004) of sleep in depression further supported this view and gave evidence for the close links between altered REM sleep and increased anterior paralimbic activation, reflecting emotional dysfunction in depression.

CHRONOBIOLOGICAL MODELS

A well-known approach to explain alterations of sleep in depression based on chronobiological principles is the two-process model of sleep regulation proposed by Borbély and coworkers (Borbély, 1982; Borbély & Wirz-Justice, 1982). In short, this model (see Fig. 20.2) acknowledges the importance of circadian rhythms (process C) for the understanding of sleep-wake behavior in humans and animals, which is influenced by the light-dark cycle as primary Zeitgeber. Process S reflects sleep pressure and is under homeostatic control. Process S can be measured through slow-wave activity (SWA) during sleep. SWA is dependent on prior wakefulness:

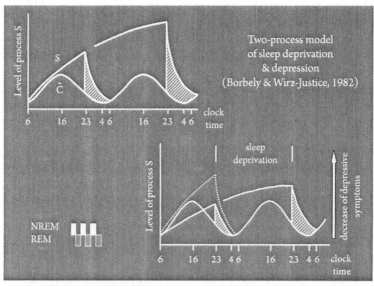

FIGURE 20.2. The two-process model of sleep, sleep deprivation and depression according to Borbély and Wirz-Justice, 1982 (modified from Borbély and Wirz-Justice, 1982).

Longer periods of wake time lead to increased SWA and vice versa. Borbély and Wirz-Justice (1982) used this model to explain REM sleep disinhibition, reduced slow-wave sleep, and the effects of sleep deprivation on depressed mood. It was hypothesized that REM sleep in depression occurs earlier as a consequence of reduced SWA. The antidepressive effects of sleep deprivation were explained by suggesting that prolonged wakefulness corrects a supposedly deficient process in depression. Kupfer et al. (1990) proposed that rather than SWA or delta power over the whole night to be reduced that the "delta ratio" (the ratio of delta sleep in the first to the second non-REM cycle) is reduced in depression. In healthy subjects, usually a decrease of delta sleep from the first to the second non-REM period is shown, whereas no such decline or even an increase was noted in depressive patients.

Germain and Kupfer (2008) elegantly summarized chronobiologically inspired theories about sleep and depression relationships. Earlier studies pointed to a phase advance or a desynchronization of biological rhythms in depression. Circadian hypotheses of depression included the phase-shift hypothesis (Lewy, Sack, Miller, & Hoban, 1987), the internal phase coincidence model (e.g., Borbély & Wirz-Justice, 1982), or the social rhythm model (Ehlers, Kupfer, Frank, & Monk, 1993). At present, intensive research is devoted to the molecular genetic basis of circadian rhythmicity and altered circadian rhythms in depression.

Insomnia and Depression

INSOMNIA AND EMOTIONS

Whereas former research aimed at identifying specific markers for depression or its subtypes, a shift of paradigm occurred targeting the role of insomnia as an independent factor. The psychophysiological mechanisms underlying the relationship between insomnia and depression are, however, not yet well understood. Both insomnia and depression are characterized by high levels of arousal. Neurobiological and sleep electroencephalography (EEG) studies suggest that hyperarousal compared to the norm could be a psychophysiological mediator of the relationship between the two disorders. Recently, it was proposed that another factor underlying the close link between sleep disturbances and depression might be emotion dysregulation (Baglioni, Spiegelhalder, Lombardo, & Riemann, 2010).

Recent experimental data suggest that poor sleepers and people with insomnia report more negative emotions both in general and close to sleep time as compared to good sleepers (e.g., Buysse et al., 2007; McCrae et al., 2008; Ong, Cardé, Gross, & Manber, 2011). The role of positive emotions, instead, is still unclear and needs further investigation. The relationship between emotions and sleep quality has been specifically evaluated in the elderly population. Berry and Webb (1983, 1985) used polysomnography recordings and showed that increased sleep efficiency and total sleep time were associated with positive affect states as measured by mood scales in elderly women. Additionally, increased wake time after sleep onset was related to negative affective states. McCrae et al. (2008) evaluated 14 days of sleep diaries, actigraphy recordings, and morning self-report of positive and negative affective states in 103 participants aged over 60 years old with no severe psychiatric condition or other sleep disorder than insomnia, and no intake of medications. Results showed that self-reported good sleep quality and diminished wake time were associated with increased positive affective states. Self-reported bad sleep quality and heightened wake time was, instead, associated with increased negative and decreased positive affective states.

Although the relationship between emotions and insomnia is becoming a focus of interest for sleep researchers, only very few studies by now have evaluated the physiological correlates of emotional processes in insomnia. It is suggested that insomnia is initially characterized by a specific alteration of the arousal system (i.e., hyperarousal; overview: Riemann et al., 2010). When the disorder becomes chronic with a systematic worsening of the daytime consequences and quality of life, the emotional system, which is closely connected with the arousal system, is subjected to changes. This sequence could explain why people with insomnia are at a higher risk for developing depression as compared to good sleepers.

META-ANALYSIS—INSOMNIA AS A PREDICTOR OF DEPRESSION

Historically, insomnia has been conceptualized as a symptom of psychopathology, especially in relation to mood disorders (overview: Riemann, Berger, & Voderholzer, 2001). More recently, insomnia is reconsidered as an independent diagnostic entity. Specifically in relation to depression, insomnia may often exist many years before the first onset of an episode of depression, and it does not necessarily remit after successful treatment of depression. Ford and Kamerow (1989) were the first to stress that insomnia symptoms might represent a possible predictor of depression. Since then, more than 40 studies have been published evaluating the predictor question (overview: Baglioni et al., 2010; Riemann, 2009). Our group has recently published a meta-analysis of longitudinal epidemiological studies investigating the causal link between insomnia and depression (Baglioni et al., 2011). Longitudinal studies published between 1980 (date of the publication of the *DSM-III*) and 2010 were identified by literature search using PUBMED, MEDLINE, PsycINFO, and PsycArticles and performed for all languages. The 21 studies (short references are provided in Fig. 20.3; for complete references see Baglioni et al., 2011) selected for meta-analytic computations (according to strict quality criteria) had a mean sample size at follow-up of 3,200 participants with a mean age of 46 years (SD = 22.4). The mean percentage of women in the studies was 55% (SD = 4.5). On average, the follow-up assessment was conducted after 71 months (SD = 96.0 months) equaling almost 6 years.

Incidence of depression at follow-up in people with insomniac symptoms was 13.1%, while it was 4.0% in people without sleep difficulties. Considering that an incidence rate of 9.9% has been reported for depression in the general population (Murphy et al., 2002), it is interesting to notice that (a) the incidence is increased in patients with insomnia and (b) the incidence is extremely reduced in a group without any experience of sleep difficulties. The logarithms of the odds ratios and their confidence intervals were used for meta-analytic calculations (for details, see Baglioni et al., 2011). The summarized odd ratios determined by applying the "fixed-effects meta-analytic model" was of 2.1 (CI: 1.9–2.4). A graphic representation of the meta-analytic computation is reported in Figure 20.3.

Classifying the studies according to age, we considered three groups: working-age group, elderly group (>60), and a children and adolescent group. The same meta-analytic calculations were applied to each one of these three age groups. Studies with mixed-age participants (i.e., studies recruiting participants aged 18 years or older) were not considered for age-group calculations. The elderly group was heterogeneous (Q-value = 8.8; df(Q) = 5; p = 0.1; and I2 = 43.1); however, this heterogeneity was explained by studies that considered clinical samples and not the general population as the other studies (Brabbins et al., 1993; Hein et al., 2003; Perlis et al., 2006; for full references, see Baglioni et al., 2011).

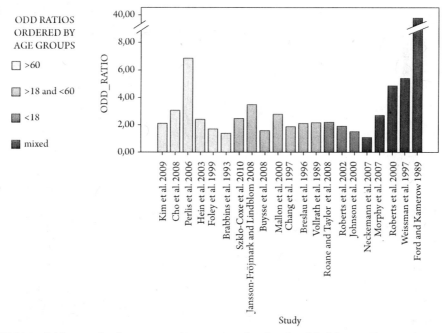

FIGURE 20.3. Odds ratios for depression with insomnia at baseline (modified from Baglioni et al., 2011).

Once we excluded data from these studies, we found nonheterogeneity between studies in all three age groups. The summarizing odds ratios for these three age groups were, respectively, 1.9 (CI: 1.6–2.3) for the elderly group; 2.1 (CI: 1.7–2.6) for the working-age group; and 2.0 (CI: 1.5–2.7) for the children and adolescents group.

Sleep Continuity and Architecture in Depression

JUST SHORTENED REM LATENCY?

Sleep research in depression in the 1970s and 1980s largely concentrated on REM latency and other REM sleep parameters (including REM sleep percentage, duration of the first REM period, and eye movement density of REM sleep) as the primary variables of interest. Several studies compared primary versus secondary depression, psychotic versus nonpsychotic depression, and unipolar versus bipolar depression and also looked at sleep in manic patients. This work (summarized in Riemann et al., 2001) revealed that some specificity of REM sleep abnormalities may hold true for the more severe or more biologically influenced depressive subtypes; it became, however, also clear that by exactly age- and gender-matching subgroups, differences between subgroups of depression disappeared or were weakened.

AGE AND GENDER INFLUENCES ON SLEEP AND DEPRESSION

Several research groups took a closer look at the impact of age and gender on sleep in depression. For age, for example in our own work (Lauer et al., 1991; Riemann et al., 1994a), we were able to show that most of the sleep parameters investigated in healthy controls and patients with depression vary with age to a considerable amount. REM latency became increasingly shortened over an age range from 18 to 65 years. Studies beyond that age showed that this difference becomes even more pronounced in late-life depression (Dykierek et al., 1998; Reynolds, Kupfer, Houck, & Hoch, 1988).

An important line of research in elderly subjects included the comparison of aged good sleepers, old-age depression, and dementia of the Alzheimer type. Clinically, sometimes the exact differential diagnosis between old-age depression and dementia of the Alzheimer type is very difficult because of an overlap of symptoms regarding either cognitive dysfunctions and/or depressed mood. Reynolds et al. (1988) were able to show that especially parameters of REM sleep are very helpful to differentiate Alzheimer dementia from old-age depression. Whereas in old-age depression the abnormalities of REM sleep become even more pronounced, in dementia of the Alzheimer type only rarely is a disinhibition of REM sleep encountered. On the contrary, patients later being diagnosed as definitely suffering from Alzheimer's disease mainly displayed a decrease in REM sleep percentage and prolonged REM sleep latencies compared to the norm. Interestingly, also total sleep deprivation (see later) as a therapeutic method in depression revealed strong differences between old-age depression and patients suffering from Alzheimer dementia; whereas a distinct effect on mood with a rather sudden improvement was noticed in old-age depression, no such effect occurs in Alzheimer dementia following total sleep deprivation.

A more differentiated line of research looking at aged subjects was pursued by Reynolds and coworkers, who investigated sleep in elderly subjects suffering from bereavement due to death of the spouse (Monk, Germain, & Reynolds, 2008; Reynolds et al., 1992, 1993). It was shown that the presence of major depression in this population was accompanied by marked changes in sleep encompassing disturbed sleep continuity and REM sleep abnormalities. Interestingly, subjects showing fairly unperturbed sleep patterns following bereavement longitudinally coped better with the loss of the spouse, thus indicating resilience typical for successful aging. Monk et al. (2008) suggested that specific cognitive-behavioral interventions (CBT-I) for sleep problems in the elderly, especially the bereaved, may help patients recover from this stressful type of situation and even have a better long-term outcome. This applies especially for brief types of intervention (Buysse et al., 2011). Monk et al. (2008) point out that though there are a variety of hypnotic drugs for insomniac complaints, concerns about nocturnal falls, side effects, and associated cognitive impairment strongly favor nonpharmacological treatment approaches in this age group. Besides age effects, gender differences were also investigated in the study of sleep in depression. Reynolds and colleagues (1990) found that male depressive subjects displayed significantly decreased slow-wave sleep compared to female depressives. Similar results have been shown for healthy sleepers (Williams et al.,

1974). Armitage and colleagues (1995) additionally showed that spectral analysis of the sleep EEG revealed increased fast frequencies (beta activity) in female compared to male depressed patients.

Overall, recent evidence (e.g., Dew et al., 2003) from longitudinal studies indicates that parameters of sleep (for example, prolonged sleep latency) in healthy elderly populations can be predictive of increased mortality in the next years. Identification and proper treatment of a sleep complaint, be it insomnia or an organic pathology, may significantly improve well-being, enhance quality of life, and decrease mortality in the elderly. As in younger patients, any complaint of insomnia should be carefully evaluated as part of the clinical anamnesis, including the use of sleep questionnaires, sleep diaries, sometimes actigraphy or even polysomnography, when a specific pathology like periodic leg movements or disturbed nocturnal breathing (i.e., sleep apnea) is suspected.

TREATMENTS AND CLINICAL RECOMMENDATIONS

The Effect of Antidepressant Treatments on Sleep

A large body of evidence has shown that many antidepressant substances (overviews: Buysse, 2011; Peterson & Benca, 2011; Riemann et al., 2001) demonstrate strong and acute REM suppressing effects of these substances. This applies for the classical tricyclic antidepressants, such as amitriptyline, clomipramine, desipramine, or imipramine, as well for the tetracyclic mianserin and selective 5-HT reuptake inhibitors such as fluoxetine or newer antidepressants like venlafaxine. MAO inhibitors like phenelzine, tranylcypromine, or brofaromine have a strong REM sleep–suppressing effect as well. Exceptions to this rule were noted for trimipramine (Wiegand, Berger, Zulley, & von Zerssen, 1986), trazodone (Ware & Pittard, 1990), and newer drugs like nefazodone (Wiegand, Galanakis, & Schreiner, 2004) or mirtazapine (Winokur et al., 2000), which do not suppress REM sleep. An intriguing hypothesis had postulated that REM sleep suppression may be a sine qua non of effective antidepressants (Vogel, Vogel, McAbee, & Thurmond, 1980). The work on substances like trimipramine, trazodone, nefazodone, or mirtazapine seriously puts this hypothesis in doubt.

Beyond the effects on REM sleep, antidepressants may have a variety of effects on sleep continuity and on REM sleep. Sedating antidepressants like doxepine, amitriptyline, trimipramine, trazodone, or mirtazapine (overview: Buysse, 2011) usually have a positive impact on variables of sleep continuity and especially sleep maintenance. Activating selective serotonine reuptake inhibitors, on the other hand, may even worsen insomnia in depressed patients (overview: Peterson & Benca, 2011). Encouraging work for the treatment of late-life depression with respect to sleep problems has been reported for nortriptyline (Reynolds, Alexopoulos, Katz, & Lebowitz, 2001).

General caution with respect to elderly depressed patients is warranted concerning pharmacological treatment options (due to known side effects) because of the increased morbidity and altered hepatic and renal function in this population.

Sleep-Wake Manipulations

SLEEP DEPRIVATION THERAPY

Wu and Bunney (1990), from a meta-analysis of sleep deprivation studies in depressed patients concluded that 50% to 60% of depressed patients display a rapid, but only transient improvement of mood after sleep deprivation therapy. As 80% of unmedicated sleep deprivation responders relapse after the next night of sleep or even a brief nap, the clinical usefulness of this therapy seems limited. From a research point of view, however, sleep deprivation therapy offers the opportunity to correlate swift changes in mood with simultaneous changes of biological variables (overview: Wirz-Justice & van den Hoofdakker, 1999). A positive diurnal variation (DV) of mood with a spontaneous improvement toward the afternoon and evening hours is predictive for a positive response to sleep deprivation therapy (overview: van den Hoofdakker, 1997). Riemann et al. (1991) showed that besides a positive DV, shortened REM latency predicted a positive response to sleep deprivation. It was observed that sleep deprivation responders, compared to nonresponders, showed a prolongation of REM latency after sleep deprivation (e.g., Riemann & Berger, 1990). Work by Reynolds and colleagues (e.g., 1997, 2005) suggested that sleep deprivation therapy is also a valuable treatment option in old-age depression.

The mechanism of action of sleep deprivation is still unclear. Positron emission tomography revealed that depressed sleep deprivation responders had an elevated glucose metabolism in the cingulate gyrus prior to the intervention normalizing after sleep deprivation (e.g., Wu et al., 1992; Smith et al., 1999). Corroborating evidence performing single photon emission computed tomography prior to and after following sleep deprivation was reported (e.g., Ebert, Feistel, Barocka, & Kaschka, 1994; Volk et al., 1997). Signal transduction in the gyrus cinguli is dominated by cholinergic neurotransmission (Wu et al., 1992), which is involved in REM sleep regulation.

Besides chronobiological models for sleep deprivation effects, neurochemical hypotheses are discussed. Ebert and Berger (1998) noted similarities between the rapid onset of mood changes following sleep deprivation and the effects of psychostimulants. More recent models emphasize the importance of the inhibitory neuromodulator adenosine, which is widely accepted to be a key player in sleep regulation (overview: Porkka-Heiskanen, Strecker, & McCarley, 1999).

SELECTIVE DEPRIVATION OF REM SLEEP

Based on the observation of REM sleep suppression following the administration of many effective antidepressants, the question arose whether this pharmacological effect may be a "conditio sine qua non" or even the basic underlying mechanism of action of antidepressant treatments. Vogel and colleagues (Vogel et al., 1980) tested this hypothesis by depriving REM sleep without pharmacological intervention by selective nocturnal awakenings over a period of 3 weeks in endogenously depressed patients. This experimental therapy led to a 50% reduction of the percentage of REM sleep and exhibited an antidepressive treatment response comparable to that of imipramine. A control group of patients was deprived of non-REM sleep by selective awakenings and did not show any clinical improvement. Only one study (Grözinger, 2000) attempted to replicate the findings of Vogel and colleagues with a methodologically improved design. Selective REM sleep deprivation was compared to the same amount of well-balanced awakenings leading to non-REM sleep deprivation in depressed inpatients. In accordance with the data of Vogel, REM deprivation induced an antidepressant effect. The non-REM deprivation group, however, exhibited an even stronger antidepressant effect, raising more doubts about the necessity of REM sleep suppression as an important mechanism of antidepressant action.

SLEEP DEPRIVATION COMBINED WITH SLEEP PHASE ADVANCE

A sophisticated strategy to study the impact of sleep on depressed mood is the "nap paradigm" after successful sleep deprivation. Even very brief periods of sleep during the sleep deprivation periods reverse the positive effects of the procedure (e.g., Knowles et al., 1979). Our own work (Riemann, Wiegand, Lauer, & Berger, 1993; Wiegand, Berger, Zulley, Lauer, & von Zerssen, 1987; Wiegand, Riemann, Schreiber, Lauer, & Berger, 1993) showed that the depressiogenic effect of naps was independent of the occurrence of REM sleep (vs. non-REM sleep) but displayed a circadian rhythm: Whereas afternoon naps had almost no effect on mood after successful sleep deprivation, morning naps more frequently led to a relapse to depressed mood. Based on the results of these nap studies and earlier findings showing that partial sleep deprivation in the second but not in the first half of the night has antidepressive effects (overview: Wehr, 1990), we postulated, based on the "internal coincidence model" (Wehr & Wirz-Justice, 1981), that sleep exerts a depressiogenic effect only within a critical time zone in the early morning hours. Based on the assumption that the avoidance of sleep during the early morning hours is crucial for the sleep deprivation effect, a combined sleep deprivation and sleep phase advance protocol was developed. Depressed patients who responded positively to one night of sleep deprivation were kept on a phase advance schedule allowing them to sleep from 5.00 p.m. until midnight after the sleep deprivation night. The advanced sleep phase was then shifted to the normal phase position within 1 week. It was shown in several studies that this combined sleep deprivation and sleep phase advance therapy was able to maintain the positive effect of sleep deprivation in about 60%–75% of the sleep deprivation responders (e.g., Berger et al., 1997; Riemann et al., 1999), compared to a 40% response rate in a control condition ("phase delay"). In our studies the positive effects of this procedure on mood were independent of age when including an age range from 18 to 70 years.

Effects of Psychotherapy

PSYCHOTHERAPY FOR DEPRESSION: THE ROLE OF SLEEP

Work with interpersonal therapy (IPT) and cognitive-behavioral therapy (CBT) for depression indicated that these approaches work better in depressed patients with relatively unperturbed sleep profiles (e.g., Thase et al., 1997). These studies in depressed patients with normal and abnormal sleep profiles (judged on the basis of sleep efficiency, REM density, and REM latency) demonstrated that the treatment response to IPT was significantly worse in the group with abnormal sleep profiles. The authors concluded from their studies that the abnormal sleep profiles reflect a more marked disturbance of central nervous system arousal that is in need of pharmacotherapy and may not be adequately treated by psychotherapy alone.

PSYCHOTHERAPY FOR INSOMNIA: EFFECTS ON DEPRESSIVE SYMPTOMS

Treatment of Insomnia—Outcome on Depression

The inclusion of protocols directed to reduce sleep difficulties and related cognitive and emotional aspects to the routine of psychological therapy of depression seems to lead to better outcomes and to diminish the risk for recurrent depression. Some recent studies showed that adding cognitive-behavior therapy for insomnia (CBT-I) is efficacious in patients with both symptoms of insomnia and depression. Taylor et al. (2007) published a pilot study evaluating the efficacy of CBT-I in a sample of 10 patients with both depression and insomnia. Results showed that psychological treatment for insomnia was efficacious not only for sleep symptoms but also had an ameliorating effect for depressive symptoms. Consistently with these results, Manber et al. (2008) found that CBT-I in 30 patients with both symptoms of insomnia and depression is efficacious and guarantees a better treatment outcome in this population than standard antidepressive treatment alone. In 2009, Edinger et al. (2009) published a randomized controlled trial in which people with primary insomnia (N = 40) and insomnia comorbid with mixed psychiatric disorders (N = 41) were assigned to CBT-I or sleep hygiene interventions. Results showed that CBT-I was equally efficacious for primary and comorbid insomnia. These findings suggest that psychological treatment for insomnia should be included in the standard treatment for depression. Specifically with respect to the elderly population, it was also reported that untreated insomnia within an adult and elderly population with comorbid major depression is associated with higher depression-related and overall direct costs compared to major depression without insomnia (Asche, Joish, Camacho, & Drake, 2010).

Prevention of Depression by Insomnia Treatment

There is a recent interest in developing new treatment algorithms directed to administer psychological treatment of insomnia which is easy accessible to the general population or through general practitioners. These interventions aim at preventing the development of chronic symptoms of insomnia, and consequently to put a halt to a sequential process which gradually reduces the quality of life and ends in the development of depressive symptoms. One approach suggested is the "stepped-care model" (e.g., Espie et al., 2007). This model offers a generic approach to care management by delivering low-intensity treatments to a wide number of individuals. In case of treatment failure, individuals can step forward to next levels that are characterized by more specialized programs and care deliverers. The first level would work as a prevention program for individuals at risk, while the superior levels would correspond to CBT-I delivered by a trained psychologist. At the first level, one possible method is to deliver CBT-I in primary care through structured protocols administered by unspecialized professionals. Espie et al. (2007) found that trained and supervised nurses can successfully deliver CBT-I in primary care routine of general medicine practice. CBT-I was organized in a structured protocol divided in five sessions comprising sleep information, sleep hygiene and relaxation, sleep scheduling, cognitive approaches, and developing a strong and natural sleep pattern. Another possible first-level alternative to disseminate CBT-I protocols in primary care and reach a large number of individuals is the use of the Internet. A meta-analysis of six randomized controlled trials (Cheng & Dizon, 2012) evaluating the efficacy of CBT-I delivered through the Internet has indicated a significant improvement in the treatment groups with respect to sleep quality, sleep efficiency, number of awakenings, and sleep-onset latency. However, no significant effect was found with respect to other sleep variables, as total sleep time, wake after sleep onset, and total time spent in bed. Moreover, some studies have reported significant effects on cognitive variables, for example on dysfunctional beliefs about sleep and pre-sleep mental activity, and on daytime consequences (Ritterband et al., 2009; Ström, Pettersson, & Andersson, 2004; Vincent & Lewycky, 2009). An Internet-based

CBT-I program may be an effective tool to reach people who are not willing or do not have the possibility to go to a psychotherapist. However, it might be possible that Internet interventions work better with younger adults or working people. In the case of the elderly population, an improvement of consideration of insomnia symptoms in primary care routine could be more adequate and better received by the patients.

INSOMNIA AS A TRANSDIAGNOSTIC FACTOR IN PSYCHIATRY

The *Diagnostic and Statistical Manual of Mental Disorders*, fourth edition, text revision (*DSM-IV-TR*; APA, 2000) lists sleep disturbance as a symptom of many psychiatric disorders, for example, major depression, bipolar disorder, posttraumatic stress disorder, generalized anxiety disorder, separation anxiety disorders, and alcohol withdrawal. Moreover, there are many other psychiatric disorders for which sleep disturbances are not listed as a symptom but are included in the clinical presentation. Alison Harvey (2008, 2009; Harvey, Murray, Chandler, & Soehner, 2011) noticed that, as such, sleep disturbances qualify as a transdiagnostic process in the context of psychiatric disorders. A transdiagnostic process signifies a process that is common across various psychiatric disorders. However, insomnia is not only a descriptive transdiagnostic process, which would simple mean a phenomenon that occurs in most psychiatric disorders. The data from the longitudinal studies evaluating the causal relationship between insomnia and depression have shown that insomnia is not just a consequence or an epiphenomenon of psychopathology, but it is a mechanism contributing to the development and maintenance of most psychiatric disorders. A mechanistically transdiagnostic process can operate at different levels: biological, psychological and emotional, social and contextual. Data consistent with the transdiagnostic hypothesis refer to the reciprocal relationship between insomnia and emotion regulation; genes known to be important in the generation and regulation of circadian rhythms that have been linked to a range of psychiatric disorders; and the interplay between sleep/circadian biology and neurotransmitter systems known to be important across a range of psychiatric disorders, as the dopamine and the serotonin systems (see also Wulff, Gatti, Wettstein, & Foster, 2010).

The transdiagnostic prospective has fascinating advantages and relevant clinical implications. Advantages refer to a point of view that does not focus on a specific disorder but instead on mechanisms that are common to different disorders. It has been evidenced that it is rare that a mental illness occurs by itself, as it is generally the case that psychiatric disorders are comorbid (Harvey, 2008). Consequently, a perspective focused on the understanding of shared psychological and neurobiological mechanisms, such as insomnia, signals a change of perspective in the interpretation of psychopathology. Clinical implications need also to be considered. If insomnia is a mechanistically transdiagnostic process in psychopathology, then a transdiagnostic intervention for insomnia or sleep disturbances could increase the efficacy of the treatment of psychiatric disorders. In other words, including sleep therapy protocols in standardized primary care protocols for other psychiatric disorders could enhance the outcome and represent a useful general health intervention. Brief behavioral treatment protocols (overview: Buysse et al., 2011) may be ideally suited to fill this gap.

Disclosures

No conflicts to disclose. Dr. Baglioni is funded by the Federal Ministry of Education and Research of Germany (Bundesministerium für Bildung und Forschung [BMBF], project INSCAI).

Prof. Berger and Prof. Riemann have no conflicts to disclose.

REFERENCES

Armitage, R., Hudson, A., Trivedi, M., & Rush, A. J. (1995). Sex differences in the distribution of EEG frequencies during sleep: Unipolar depressed outpatients. *Journal of Affective Disorders, 34,* 121–129.

Asche, C. V., Joish, V. N., Camacho, F., & Drake, C. L. (2010). The direct costs of untreated comorbid insomnia in a managed care population with major depressive disorder. *Current Medical Research and Opinion 26,* 1843–1853.

Baglioni, C., Battagliese, G., Feige, B., Spiegelhalder, K., Nissen, C., Voderholzer, U.,…Riemann, D. (2011). Insomnia as a predictor of depression: A meta-analytic evaluation of longitudinal epidemiological studies. *Journal of Affective Disorders, 135,* 10–19.

Baglioni, C., Spiegelhalder, K., Lombardo, C., & Riemann, D. (2010). Sleep and emotions: A focus on insomnia. *Sleep Medicine Review, 14*, 227–238.

Benca, R. M., Obermeyer, W. H., Thisted, R. A., & Gillin, J. C. (1992). Sleep and psychiatric disorders: A meta-analysis. *Archives of General Psychiatry, 49*, 651–668.

Berger, M., Doerr, P., Lund, R., Bronisch, T., & von Zerssen, D. (1982). Neuroendocrinological and neurophysiological studies in major depressive disorders: Are there biological markers for the endogenous subtype? *Biological Psychiatry, 17*, 1217–1242.

Berger, M., & Riemann, D. (1993). Symposium: Normal and abnormal REM sleep regulation: REM sleep in depression—an overview. *Journal of Sleep Research, 2*, 211–223.

Berger, M., Riemann, D., Höchli, D., & Spiegel, R. (1989). The cholinergic REM-sleep-induction test with RS 86: State- or traitmarker of depression? *Archives of General Psychiatry, 46*, 421–428.

Berger, M., Vollmann, J., Hohagen, F., König, A., Lohner, H., Voderholzer, U., & Riemann, D. (1997). Sleep deprivation combined with consecutive sleep phase advance as a fast-acting therapy in depression: An open pilot trial in medicated and unmedicated patients. *American Journal of Psychiatry, 154*, 870–872.

Berry, D. T. R., & Webb, W. B. (1983). State measures and sleep stages. *Psychological Reports, 52*, 807–812.

Berry, D. T. R., & Webb, W. B. (1985). Mood and sleep in aging women. *Journal of Personal and Social Psychology, 49*, 1724–1727.

Borbély, A. A. (1982). A two process model of sleep regulation. *Human Neurobiology, 1*, 195–204.

Borbély, A. A., & Wirz-Justice, A. (1982). Sleep, sleep deprivation and depression. *Human Neurobiology, 1*, 205–210.

Burton, R. (1621). *The anatomy of melancholy.* Oxford: H. Cripps.

Buysse, D. J. (2011). Clinical pharmacology of other drugs used as hypnotics. In M. H. Kryger, T. Roth, & W. C. Dement (Eds.), *Principles and practice of sleep medicine* (5th ed., pp. 492–509). Elsevier Saunders, St. Louis, MO.

Buysse, D. J., Germain, A., Moul, D. E., Franzen, P. L., Brar, L. K., Fletcher, M. E.,…Monk, T. H. (2011). Efficacy of brief behavioural treatment for chronic insomnia in older adults. *Archives of Internal Medicine, 171*, 887–895.

Buysse, D. J., Thompson, W., Scott, J., Franzen, P. L., Germain, A., Hall, M.,…Kupfer, D. J. (2007). Daytime symptoms in primary insomnia: A prospective analysis using ecological momentary assessment. *Sleep Medicine, 8*, 198–208.

Cheng, S. K., & Dizon, J. (2012). Computerized cognitive-behaviour therapy for insomnia: A systematic review and meta-analysis. *Pscyotherapy and Psychosomatics, 81*, 206–212.

Dew, M. A., Hoch, C. C., Buysse, D. J., Monk, T. H., Begley, A. E., Houck, P. R.,…Reynolds, C. F., III. (2003). Healthy older adults' sleep predicts all-cause mortality at 4 to 19 years of follow-up. *Psychosomatic Medicine, 65*, 63–73.

Dykierek, P., Stadtmüller, G., Schramm, P., Bahro, M., van Calker, D., Braus, D. F.,…Riemann, D. (1998). The value of REM sleep parameters in differentiating Alzheimer's disease from old-age depression and normal aging. *Journal of Psychiatric Research, 32*, 1–9.

Ebert, D., & Berger, M. (1998). Neurobiological similarities in antidepressant sleep deprivation and psychostimulant use: A psychostimulant theory of antidepressant sleep deprivation. *Psychopharmacology, 140*, 1–10.

Ebert, D., Feistel, H., Barocka, A., & Kaschka, W. (1994). Increased limbic blood flow and total sleep deprivation in major depression with melancholia. *Psychiatric Research: Neuroimaging, 55*, 101–111.

Edinger, J. D., Olsen, M. K., Stechuchak, K. M., Means, M. K., Lineberger, M. D., Kirby, A., & Carney, C. E. (2009). Cognitive behavioral therapy for patients with primary insomnia or insomnia associated predominantly with mixed psychiatric disorders: A randomized controlled trial. *Sleep, 32*, 499–510.

Ehlers, C. L., Kupfer, D. J., Frank, E., & Monk, T. H. (1993). Biological rhythms and depression: The role of zeitgebers and zeitstoreres. *Depression, 1*, 285–293.

Espie, C. A., MacMahon, K. M. A., Kelly, H. L., Broomfield, N. M., Douglas, N. J., Engleman, H. M.,…Wilson, P. (2007). Randomized clinical effectiveness trial of nurse-administered small-group cognitive behaviour therapy for persistent insomnia in general practice. *Sleep, 30*, 574–584.

Ford, D. E., & Kamerow, D. B. (1989). Epidemiologic study of sleep disturbances and psychiatric disorders: An opportunity for prevention? *Journal of the American Medical Association, 262*, 1479–1484.

Germain, A., & Kupfer, D. J. (2008). Circadian rhythm disturbances in depression. *Human Psychopharmacology, 23*, 571–585.

Gillin, J. C., Sutton, L., & Ruiz, C. (1991). The cholinergic REM induction test with arecholine in depression. *Archives of General Psychiatry, 48*, 264–270.

Grözinger, M. (2000). *Auswirkungen von REM-Schlafentzug und anderen Weckparadigmen auf den ultradianen Schlafzyklus und die Symptomatik depressiver Patienten.* Unveröffentlichte Habilitationsschrift, Medizinische Fakultät der Universität Mainz.

Harvey, A. G. (2008). Insomnia, psychiatric disorders, and the transdiagnostic perspective. *Current Directions in Psychological Science, 17,* 299–303.

Harvey, A. G. (2009). A transdiagnostic approach to treating sleep disturbance in psychiatric disorders. *Cognitive Behavioral Therapy, 38,* 35–42.

Harvey, A. G., Murray, G., Chandler, R. A., & Soehner, A. (2011). Sleep disturbance as transdiagnostic: Consideration of neurobiological mechanisms. *Clinical Psychology Review, 31,* 225–235.

Hobson, J. A., Lydic, R., & Baghdoyan, H. A. (1986). Evolving concepts of sleep cycle generation: From brain centers to neuronal populations. *Behavioral and Brain Sciences, 9,* 371–448.

Hobson, J. A., McCarley, R. W., & Wyzinski, P. W. (1975). Sleep cycle oscillation: Reciprocal discharge by two brainstem neuronal groups. *Science, 189,* 55–58.

Janowsky, D. S., El-Yousef, M. K., Davis, J. M., & Sekerke, H. J. (1972). A cholinergic-adre-nergic hypothesis of mania and depression. *Lancet, 2,* 632–635.

Knowles, J. B., Southmayd, S. E., Delva, N., MacLean, A. W., Cairns, J., & Letemendia, F. J. (1979). Five variations of sleep deprivation in a depressed woman. *British Journal of Psychiatry, 135,* 403–410.

Kraepelin, E. (1909). *Psychiatrie.* Leipzig, Germany: J.A. Barth.

Kupfer, D. J. (1976). REM latency: A psychobiologic marker for primary depressive disease. *Biological Psychiatry, 11,* 159–174.

Kupfer, D. J., & Foster, F. G. (1972). Interval between onset of sleep and rapid eye movement sleep as an indicator of depression. *Lancet, 2,* 648–649.

Kupfer, D. J., Frank, E., McEachran, A., & Grochocinski, V. I. (1990). Delta sleep ratio. *Archives of General Psychiatry, 47,* 1100–1105.

Kupfer, D. J., Reynolds, C. F., Grochocinski, V. J., Ulrich, R. F., & McEachran, A. B. (1986). Aspects of short REM latency in affective states: A revisit. *Psychiatry Research, 19,* 29–39.

Lauer, C. J., Riemann, D., Wiegand, M., & Berger, M. (1991). From early to late adulthood: Changes in EEG sleep of depressed patients and healthy volunteers. *Biological Psychiatry, 29,* 979–993.

Lewy, A. J., Sack, R. L., Miller, L. S., & Hoban, T. M. (1987). Antidepressant and circadian phase-shifting effects of light. *Science, 235,* 352–354.

Manber, R., Edinger, J. D., Gress, J. L., San Pedro-Salcedo, M. G., Kuo, T. F., & Kalista, T. (2008). Cognitive behavioral therapy for insomnia enhances depression outcome in patients with comorbid major depressive disorder and insomnia. *Sleep, 31,* 489–495.

McCarley, R. W. (1982). REM sleep and depression: Common neurobiological control mechanisms. *American Journal of Psychiatry, 139,* 565–570.

McCrae, C. S., McNamara, J. P., Rowe, M. A., Dzjerzewski, J. M., Dirk, J., Marsiske, M., & Craggs, J. G. (2008). Sleep and affect in older adults: Using multilevel modelling to examine daily associations. *Journal of Sleep Research, 17,* 42–53.

Monk, T. H., Germain, A., & Reynolds, C.F., III. (2008). Sleep disturbance in bereavement. *Psychiatry Annals, 38,* 671–675.

Murphy, J. M., Nierenberg, A. A., Laird, N. M., Monson, R. R., Sobol, A. M., & Leighton, A. H. (2002). Incidence of major depression: Prediction from subthreshold categories in the Stirling County Study. *Journal of Affective Disorders, 68,* 251–259.

Nofzinger, E. A., Buysse, D. J., Germain, A., Carter, C., Luna, B., Price, J. C., ... Kupfer, D. J. (2004). Increased activation of anterior paralimbic and executive cortex from waking to rapid eye movement sleep in depression. *Archives of General Psychiatry, 61,* 695–702.

Ong, J. C., Cardé, N. B., Gross, J. J., & Manber, R. (2011). A two-dimensional approach to assessing affective states in good and poor sleepers. *Journal of Sleep Research, 20,* 606–10.

Peterson, M. J., & Benca, R. M. (2011). Mood disorders. In M. H. Kryger T. Roth & W. C. Dement (Eds.), *Principles and practice of sleep medicine* (5th ed., pp. 1488–1500). Elsevier Saunders. St. Louis, MO.

Porkka-Heiskanen, T., Strecker, R. E., & McCarley, R. W. (1999). Brain site-specificity of extracellular adenosine concentration changes during sleep deprivation and spontaneous sleep: An in vivo microdialysis study. *Neuroscience, 99,* 507–517.

Reynolds, C.F., III. (1997). Treatment of major depression in later life: A life cycle perspective. *Psychiatric Quarterly, 68,* 221–246.

Reynolds, C. F., III, Alexopoulos, G. S., Katz, I. R., & Lebowitz, B. D. (2001). Chronic depression in the elderly: Approaches for prevention. *Drugs and Aging, 18,* 507–514.

Reynolds, C. F., III, Hoch, C. C., Buysse, D. J., Houck, P. R., Schlernitzauer, M., ... Kupfer, D. J. (1992). Electroencephalographic sleep in spousal bereavement and bereavement-related depression of late life. *Biological Psychiatry, 31*, 69–82.

Reynolds, C.F., III, Hoch, C. C., Buysse, D. J., Houck, P. R., Schlernitzauer, M., Pasternak, R. E., ... Kupfer, D. J. (1993). Sleep after spousal bereavement: A study of recovery from stress. *Biological Psychiatry, 34*, 791–797.

Reynolds, C. F., III, Kupfer, D. J., Houck, P. R., & Hoch, C. C. (1988). Discrimination of elderly depressed and demented patients by electroencephalographic sleep data. *Archives of General Psychiatry, 45*, 258–262.

Reynolds, C. F., III, Kupfer, D. J., Thase, M. E., Frank, E., Jarret, D. B., Coble, P. A., ... Houck, P. R. (1990). Sleep, gender, and depression: An analysis of gender effects on the electroencephalographic sleep of 302 depressed outpatients. *Biological Psychiatry, 28*, 673–684.

Reynolds, C. F., III, Smith, G. S., Dew, M. A., Mulsant, B. H., Miller, M. D., Schlernitzauer, M., ... Pollock, B. G. (2005). Accelerating symptom-reduction in late-life depression. *American Journal of Geriatric Psychiatry, 13*, 353–358.

Ricmann, D. (2009). Does effective management of sleep disorders reduce depressive symptoms and the risk of depression? *Drugs, 69*, 43–64.

Riemann, D., & Berger, M. (1990). The effects of total sleep deprivation and subsequent treatment with clomipramine on depressive symptoms and sleep electroencephalography in patients with a major depressive disorder. *Acta Psychiatrica Scandinavica, 81*, 24–31.

Riemann, D., & Berger, M. (1992). Sleep, age, depression and the chrolinergic REM induction test with RS 86. *Progress in Neuropsychopharmacology and Biological Psychiatry, 16*, 311–316.

Riemann, D., Berger, M., & Voderholzer, U. (2001). Sleep and depression—results from psychobiological studies: An overview. *Biological Psychology, 57*, 67–103.

Riemann, D., Hohagen, F., Bahro, M., & Berger, M. (1994a). Sleep in depression: The influence of age, gender and diagnostic subtype on baseline sleep and the chrolinergic REM induction test with RS 86. *European Archives of Psychiatry and Clinical Neuroscience, 243*, 279–290.

Riemann, D., Hohagen, F., Bahro, M., Lis, S., Stadtmüller, G., Gann, H., & Berger, M. (1994b). Cholinergic neurotransmission, REM sleep and depression. *Journal of Psychosomatic Research, 38*, 15–25.

Riemann, D., Hohagen, F., Gann, H., Olbrich, R., Wark, H. J., Bohus, M., ... Berger, M. (1994c). The REM sleep response to cholinergic stimulation:

Indicator of muscarinic supersensitivity in schizophrenia? *Journal of Psychiatry Research, 218*, 195–210.

Riemann, D., König, A., Hohagen, F., Kiemen, A., Voderholzer, U., Backhaus, J., ... Berger, M. (1999). How to preserve the antidepressive effect of sleep deprivation: A comparison of sleep phase advance and sleep phase delay. *European Archives of Psychiatry and Clinical Neuroscience, 249*, 231–237.

Riemann, D., Lis, S., Fritsch-Montero, R., Meier, T., Krieger, S., Hohagen, F., & Berger, M. (1996). Effect of tetrahydroaminoacridine on sleep in healthy subjects. *Biological Psychiatry, 39*, 796–802.

Riemann, D., Spiegelhalder, K., Feige, B., Voderholzer, U., Berger, M., Perlis, M., & Nissen, C. (2010). The hyperarousal model of insomnia: A review of the concept and ist evidence. *Sleep Medicine Review, 14*, 19–31.

Riemann, D., Wiegand, M., & Berger, M. (1991). Are there predictors for sleep deprivation response? *Biological Psychiatry, 29*, 707–710.

Riemann, D., Wiegand, M., Lauer, C. J., & Berger, M. (1993). Naps after total sleep deprivation in depressed patients: Are they depressiogenic? *Psychiatry Research, 49*, 109–120.

Ritterband, L. M., Thorndike, F. P., Gonder-Frederick, L. A., Magee, J. C., Bailey, E. T., Saylor, D. K., & Morin, C. M. (2009). Efficacy of an internet-based behavioral intervention for adults with insomnia. *Archives of General Psychiatry, 66*, 692–698.

Smith, G. S., Reynolds, C. F., III, Pollock, B., Derbyshire, S., Nofzinger, E., Dew, M. A., ... Kupfer, D. J. (1999). Cerebral glucose metabolic res-ponse to combined sleep deprivation and antidepressant treatment in geriatric depression. *American Journal of Psychiatry, 156*, 683–689.

Ström, L., Pettersson, R., & Andersson, G. (2004). Internet-based treatment for insomnia: A controlled evaluation. *Journal of Consulting and Clinical Psycholgy, 72*, 113–120.

Taylor, D. J., Lichstein, K. L., Weinstock, J., Sanford, S., & Temple, J. R. (2007). A pilot study of cognitive-behavioral therapy of insomnia in people with mild depression. *Behavior Therapy, 38*, 49–57.

Thase, M. E., Buysse, D. J., Frank, E., Cherry, C. R., Cornes, C. L., Mallinger, A. G., & Kupfer, D. J. (1997). Which depressed patients will respond to Interpersonal Psychotherapy? The role of abnormal EEG sleep profiles. *American Journal of Psychiatry, 154*, 502–509.

Van den Hoofdakker, R. H. (1997). Total sleep deprivation: Clinical and theoretical aspects. In A. Honig, H.M. Van Praag (Eds.), *Depression* (pp. 563–589). London: Wiley.

Vincent, N., & Lewycky, S. (2009). Logging on for better sleep: RCT of the effectiveness of online treatment for insomnia. *Sleep, 32,* 807–815.

Vogel, G. W., Vogel, F., McAbee, R. S., & Thurmond, A. J. (1980). Improvement of depression by REM sleep deprivation. *Archives of General Psychiatry, 37,* 247–253.

Volk, S., Kaendler, S., Hertel, A., Maul, F. D., Manoocheri, R., Weber, R., ... Hör, G. (1997). Can response to partial sleep deprivation in depressed patients be predicted by regional changes of cerebral blood flow? *Psychiatry Research: Neuroimmunology, 75,* 67–74.

Ware, J. C., & Pittard, J. T. (1990). Increased deep sleep after trazodone use: A double-blind placebo-controlled study in healthy young adults. *Journal of Clinical Psychiatry, 51,* 18–22.

Wehr, T. A. (1990). Manipulations of sleep and phototherapy: Non-pharma-cological alternatives in the treatment of depression. *Clinical Neuropharmacology, 13,* 554–865.

Wehr, T. A., & Wirz-Justice, A. (1981). Internal coincidence model for sleep deprivation and depression. In W. P. Koella (Ed.), *Sleep* (pp. 26–33). Basel, Switzerland: Karger.

Wiegand, M., Berger, M., Zulley, J., & von Zerssen, D. (1986). The effect of trimipramine on sleep in patients with major depressive disorder. *Pharmacopsychiatry, 19,* 198–199.

Wiegand, M., Berger, M., Zulley, J., Lauer, C.J., & von Zerssen, D. (1987). The influence of daytime naps on the therapeutic effect of sleep deprivation. *Biological Psychiatry, 22,* 389–392.

Wiegand, M., Galanakis, P., & Schreiner, R. (2004). Nefazodone in primary insomnia: An open pilot study. *Progress in Neuropsychopharmacology and Biological Psychiatry, 28,* 1071–1078.

Wiegand, M., Riemann, D., Schreiber, W., Lauer, C. J., & Berger, M. (1993). Morning and afternoon naps in depressed patients after total sleep deprivation: Sleep structure and impact on mood. *Biological Psychiatry, 33,* 467–476.

Winokur, A., Sateia, M. J., Hayes, J. B., Bayles-Dazet, W., MacDonald, M. M., & Gary, K. A. (2000). Acute effects of mirtazapine on sleep continuity and sleep architecture in depressed patients: A pilot study. *Biological Psychiatry, 48,* 75–78.

Wirz-Justice, A., & van den Hoofdakker, R. (1999). Sleep deprivation in depression: What do we know, where do we go? *Biological Psychiatry, 46,* 445–453.

Wu, J. C., & Bunney, W. E. (1990). The biological basis of an antidepressant reponse to sleep deprivation and relapse: Review and hypothesis. *American Journal of Psychiatry, 147,* 14–21.

Wu, J. C., Gillin, J. C., Buchsbaum, M. S., Hershey, T., Johnson, J. C., & Bunney, W. E. (1992). Effect of sleep deprivation on brain metabolism of depressed patients. *American Journal of Psychiatry, 149,* 538–543.

Wulff, K., Gatti, S., Wettstein, J. G., & Foster, R. G. (2010). Sleep and circadian rhythm disruption in psychiatric and neurodegenerative disease. *Nature Reviews, 11,* 1–11.

SECTION 3

TREATMENT AND PREVENTION

21

USE OF ADJUNCTIVE THERAPY IN OLDER DEPRESSED ADULTS WHO ARE RESISTANT TO ANTIDEPRESSANT TREATMENT

J. Craig Nelson

DEPRESSION IS a common disorder in older adults that not only causes suffering but increases the risk of suicide, increases disability, and decreases quality of life (Blazer, Hughes, & George, 1987; Bondareff et al., 2000; Bruce, Seeman, Merrill, & Blazer, 1994; Conwell, 2004). Depression appears to have a bidirectional association with various medical disorders such that one increases the risk of the other. In some instances, for example, heart disease and stroke, the presence of depression appears to aggravate the course of the medical illness, including increasing the risk of death (Bruce, Leaf, Rozal, Florio, & Hoff, 1994; Pratt et al., 1996; Pulska, Pahkala, Laippalla, & Kivela, 1998; Simonsick, Wallace, Blazer, & Berkman, 1995; Whooley et al., 1998).

Antidepressants have been the mainstay of treatment for older depressed adults in both specialty and primary care settings. However, there are limitations to their use. The action of antidepressants is delayed and takes weeks to achieve a full effect, and often they are not effective. As a consequence

various strategies have developed to either speed up response or improve efficacy. One of these strategies is to add a second agent to the first. The use of two marketed antidepressants has been described as combined treatment. The use of a second agent that is not a marketed antidepressant has usually been described as augmentation; however, recently the FDA has recommended the use of the term "adjunctive" rather than "augmentation" to avoid the implication that the second agent has a synergistic effect. The term "adjunctive" would include synergistic effects and additive antidepressant effects of the second agent. In this chapter, adjunctive therapy will be used broadly to refer to both combinations of two antidepressants and the addition of a nonapproved antidepressant agent to an antidepressant.

USE OF ADJUNCTIVE TREATMENTS

Adjunctive treatments in depression have been used with different aims. They have been given at the beginning of treatment to either speed up response or achieve greater efficacy at the end of the first trial (enhancement), or they have been used to achieve remission in patients who have failed initial antidepressant treatment.

Acceleration Trials

In nongeriatric samples, various agents have been added at the beginning of treatment to speed up response. Agents with placebo-controlled evidence supporting rapid effects include lithium (Crossly & Bauer, 2007), thyroid (Altshuler et al., 2001), and pindolol (Portella et al., 2011). None of these agents have been tested in late-life depression to accelerate response. The only placebo-controlled acceleration trial in elderly depressed adults was reported by Lavretsky et al. (2006). The study was undertaken based on a prior open-label trial (Lavretsky, Kim, Kumar, & Reynolds, 2003). The controlled trial was a small (N = 16) proof of concept study in which methylphenidate or placebo was added to citalopram. Methylphenidate (MPD) was started at 2.5 mg twice a day and citalopram at 20 mg a day. MPD was increased to 5 mg twice a day after 3 days. In patients not showing initial response, MPD could be increased up to 20 mg/day and citalopram up to 40 mg. (Since the study was published, the FDA has recommended that doses of citalopram above 20 mg not be used in older adults because of the risk of prolonged cardiac conduction.) The mean dose of MPD achieved was 15 mg/day. Those receiving the stimulant did respond more quickly. At 3 weeks, 5 of the 10 receiving MPD and citalopram responded versus none of the citalopram plus placebo patients. At 8 weeks, response rates 4/10 versus 2/6 were not significantly different but more in the adjunctive group remitted (4/10 vs. 0/6). Three patients in the MPD adjunctive group discontinued because of side effects, but none was severe. No changes in blood pressure or heart rate were noted. The speed of response in this study was not dramatic, but for safety reasons methylphenidate was started at a low dose and increased slowly. This may have attenuated the effects. In contrast, in the 1970s the "dextroamphetamine test" was explored as a method to predict later treatment response to norepinephrine tricyclic agents (Fawcett & Siomopoulos, 1971). While the aim of the test failed to be demonstrated, about 50% of patients receiving dextroamphetamine 5 mg three times a day had substantial improvement within the first 48 hours. In the late-life depression study, the dosing schedule was much more cautious.

This strategy still deserves further study, but in older patients the potential benefits of rapid effects may be offset by the need for cautious dosing to assure safety.

In nongeriatric samples antidepressant combinations also have been employed from the beginning of treatment to enhance final outcome. Enhanced response at the end of the trial has been reported in mixed-age samples for the combination of fluoxetine and desipramine (Nelson et al., 2004), and the combination of mirtazapine with selective serotonin reuptake inhibitors (SSRIs) and serotonin–norepinephrine reuptake inhibitors (SNRIs; Blier et al., 2009, 2010). Recently the COMED study failed to find an advantage for antidepressant combinations (escitalopram and bupropion, mirtazapine and venlafaxine) given at the beginning of treatment (Rush et al., 2011). It seems likely, however, that the advantage of combination therapy may be more obvious in patients who have already failed treatment with the first treatment. To my knowledge, no controlled study of combination treatment given at the beginning of treatment has been reported in late-life depression.

USE OF ADJUNCTIVE TREATMENTS IN ANTIDEPRESSANT-RESISTANT DEPRESSION

Antidepressant-Resistant Depression

While several antidepressants and psychotherapies have been shown to be effective in late-life depression, a substantial percentage of patients do not respond. In a recent meta-analysis of placebo-controlled studies of second-generation antidepressants in patients 60 years and older with major depressive disorder (MDD), the pooled response rate on antidepressants was 44.4% and the remission rate was 32.6% (Nelson, Delucchi, & Schneider, 2008). Rates of response and remission were higher in the longer duration trials, but even in those 10- and 12-week trials, the mean pooled rate of response was 55% and the mean pooled remission rate was 37.9%. Even with this "best estimate" 45% of the patients failed to respond and 62% failed to remit with a single antidepressant. These rates come from industry-sponsored antidepressant trials in which patients with comorbid psychiatric disorders were often excluded. Had these trials included patients with comorbid psychiatric disorders, rates of response and remission would likely have been even lower.

Two large trials in primary care suggest that rates of response and remission are no higher in that setting. In the IMPACT study, a large study of 1,801 depressed patients aged 60 years or older, the remission rate with usual care peaked at 6 months and was 16.7% (Unützer et al., 2002). The PROSPECT study also examined treatment of depression in a primary care setting (Alexopoulos et al., 2005). The remission rates in patients with major depression receiving usual care was 16% at 4 months. In both the IMPACT and PROSPECT study, the care management intervention improved outcome; however, at 6 and 4 months, respectively, remission rates were 30% and 33%. These outcomes and the meta-analysis cited earlier suggest that approximately two thirds of elderly depressed patients will fail to achieve remission with the first treatment trial. Treatment resistance to the first trial is the norm, not the exception.

In the subsequent discussion of adjunctive treatments, given the paucity of data, treatment resistance will be defined very liberally as failure to respond to at least one antidepressant with adequate dose and duration defined by the author of the study. It is noted that sometimes 4 weeks was considered an adequate prior trial, and many might consider that inadequate. In addition, treatment resistance will be limited to *antidepressant* treatment resistance because failure to respond to psychotherapy or electroconvulsive therapy (ECT) may be different in terms of predicting response to subsequent drug treatment.

Use of Antidepressant Combinations for Antidepressant Treatment Resistance

To my knowledge, *no controlled trials of antidepressant combinations have been performed in older adults with depression*. In the nongeriatric literature, combinations of fluoxetine and desipramine, and mirtazapine with SSRIs or venlafaxine have been shown to be more effective than monotherapy (Blier et al., 2009, 2010; Carpenter, Yasmin, & Price, 2002; Nelson et al., 2004). Only one of these studies limited the sample to antidepressant treatment-resistant patients (Carpenter et al., 2002). In the other trials about half of the patients included were treatment resistant. Open trials suggest that combining bupropion and an SSRI may improve efficacy, and

bupropion-SSRI combinations have been popular in nongeriatric practice (Fredman et al., 2000). While the use of adjunctive bupropion in STAR*D appeared to be effective in antidepressant-resistant depression, this was an open trial (Trivedi, Fava, et al., 2006). In that trial, adjunctive bupropion was more effective than buspirone on some secondary outcomes. Mirtazapine has been a popular agent in geriatric patients because of its secondary effects (sedation and stimulation of appetite). In placebo-controlled monotherapy trials, bupropion and mirtazapine have been shown to be effective in older patients (aged 65 and older or 55 and older, respectively) (Halikas, 1995; Hewett et al., 2010). Thus, if a patient has failed an initial SSRI, adding bupropion or mirtazapine may increase efficacy regardless of whether there is any synergistic effect.

Use of Adjunctive Agents for Antidepressant Treatment Resistance

To my knowledge and review, *no prospective controlled adjunctive trials have been performed in older adults with depression*, but clinicians treating older patients often are forced to rely on evidence from mixed-age samples. A recent comprehensive review of adjunctive and combination trials in mixed-age samples may be useful (Connolly & Thase, 2011). Recently a review of the existing literature on treatment of resistant depression in adults 55 years and older was published (Cooper et al., 2011). The authors limited their search to trials that required evidence of prior treatment. They found 14 published reports, of which five reports described switching to monotherapy with another antidepressant and nine described adjunctive or combination strategies. Given the paucity of data, I reviewed a broader spectrum of studies.

LITHIUM

In mixed-age adults, adjunctive lithium has been studied in 11 placebo-controlled trials reviewed or reported elsewhere (Crossley & Bauer, 2007; Joffe, Sokolov, & Levitt, 2006). A meta-analysis of 10 trials found a large effect of treatment (Crossley & Bauer, 2007). However, most of the studies were small (fewer than 36 patients); lithium was often added after fairly brief periods of the initial treatment (5 weeks or less); and most trials added lithium to tricyclics. One recent small trial that added lithium to second-generation antidepressants failed to find an advantage of lithium over placebo (Joffe et al., 2006). The only trial that attempted to establish antidepressant treatment resistance found no effect of lithium augmentation in mixed-age patients (Nierenberg et al., 2003).

While there are no controlled acute phase studies of adjunctive lithium in elderly depressed patients, six open-label trials have been reported (Table 21.1) (Finch & Katona, 1989; Flint & Rifat, 1994; Kok, Vink, Heeren, & Nolen, 2007; Lafferman, Solomon, & Ruskin, 1988; van Marwijk et al., 1990; Zimmer, Rosen, Thornton, Perel, & Reynolds, 1991). A few additional studies reported the use of adjunctive lithium but did not report outcome specifically for lithium (Dew et al., 2007; Flint & Rifat, 1998), or they included patients from a prior publication (Kok, Nolen, & Heeren, 2009). Response rates, usually defined as "complete response," ranged from 20% to 55% with a pooled mean of 34.4%; however, four of the trials required only 4 weeks of prior treatment and, as Zimmer et al. (1991) noted, after 4 weeks many patients continue to improve. It is very difficult to conclude in an open trial that the rate of improvement exceeds that expected with time. Three of the trials observed serious side effects. In one a "stroke-like" syndrome was observed. In the largest trial, 12 episodes of neurotoxicity were observed in 10 patients. In each case, toxicity resolved with discontinuation of lithium.

Lithium is the only combination or adjunctive agent that has controlled data supporting its use to prevent relapse. Bauer et al. (2000) randomized 29 mixed-age patients who had responded to adjunctive lithium to either continue on lithium or switch to placebo. Over the next 4 months, 7 of 15 patients receiving placebo relapsed versus none of the 14 patients continuing on lithium. The most informative study of lithium in the elderly was conducted by Wilkinson et al. (2002). The authors conducted a 2-year, double-blind, relapse prevention study in 49 unipolar depressed patients aged 65 years or older (mean age: 76 years) who had responded to initial antidepressant treatment (amitriptyline, N = 13; lofepramine, N = 7; various SSRIs, N = 26; and venlafaxine, N = 3). A unique aspect of the design is that lithium was not required during the acute phase of treatment. Patients were then randomized to adjunctive lithium or placebo in addition to their antidepressant. During the first 6 months, 4 of 24 patients on placebo and 0 of 25 on lithium relapsed ($X^2 = 4.5, p = .05$). After 2 years, 8 of 24 patients on placebo and 1 of 25 on lithium had relapsed ($X^2 =$

5.7, $p = .01$). The mean lithium dose was 348 mg/d (range: 200–400) and the mean serum level was 0.43 mmol/L. While lithium helped to prevent relapse, it did not significantly affect the level of depressive symptoms present on the Montgomery Asberg Depression Rating Scale (MADRS; Montgomery & Asberg, 1979). Low-dose lithium was tolerated fairly well. Four patients on lithium discontinued due to adverse events versus three on placebo. The study suggested that even in patients not selected as responding to adjunctive lithium, lithium offered prophylactic benefit.

While relatively more studies of lithium have been reported in older adults, lithium remains a difficult drug to use in this age group. Decreased renal clearance with aging, various medications, and salt restriction can increase lithium serum levels. A recent study found greater variability of brain lithium levels, lack of predictable brain levels based on serum levels, and an association of frontal lobe dysfunction with lithium levels in older patients, all of which complicate its use (Forester et al., 2009). When these factors are combined with the narrow therapeutic index of lithium, this agent becomes the most difficult psychotropic agent to administer in the elderly. As noted earlier, neurotoxicity with delirium can occur. While this is reversible and fairly easily managed in a psychiatric inpatient setting, it can be quite frightening to patients, family, and staff in other settings.

THYROID

Adjunctive triiodothyronine (T3) is another older strategy. There are no controlled trials of adjunctive T3 in older depressed adults. In mixed-aged samples, T3 has been used to accelerate response, been given at the beginning of treatment to enhance response, or used in treatment-resistant patients. The acceleration or enhancement trials found mixed results but some supporting evidence (Altshuler et al., 2001; Cooper et al., 2011). Aronson et al., (1996) reviewed the trials of T3 in antidepressant-resistant patients (all trials augmented tricyclics) and performed a meta-analysis of the placebo-controlled trials. While the meta-analysis was not significant, the design of these trials varied greatly. The best designed trial (a parallel randomized placebo-controlled trial) did find thyroid more effective and comparable to adjunctive lithium (Joffe, Singer, Levitt, & MacDonald, 1993). In the only controlled study of T3 in patients resistant to second-generation antidepressants,

Table 21.1 Adjunctive Lithium Trials in Late-Life Depression

STUDY	N	AGE	DIAGNOSIS	DURATION PRIOR RX	DESIGN	DURATION LITHIUM	LITHIUM SERUM TARGET	RESPONSE	AES
Lafferman et al., 1988	14	61–82	13 of 14 with MDD	4 weeks	Open, retrospective series	3 weeks	0.8–1.2	7 complete 3 partial	4 discontinued due to AEs, one case of neurotoxicity (a stroke-like syndrome)
Finch & Katona, 1989	9	65–83	ICD9 296, N = 7; ICD9 300, N = 2; 5 psychotic	Not specified; failed ≥ one trial	Open, retrospective series	Not given, followed up to 20 months	No target given, levels obtained 0.43–0.86	5 "good" response, 1 partial	2 discontinued due to AEs, including reduced renal function; 1 dose reduced due to lithium toxicity
Van Marwijk et al., 1990	51	64–88	42 unipolar, 9 bipolar; 41 of 51 MDD	4 weeks, cyclic ADs (47 of 51)	Open, chart review	Not given	0.4–0.8	18 complete 15 partial 18 nonresponse	10 severe AEs (neurotoxicity); 4 cases of hypothyroidism
Zimmer et al., 1991	15	59–89	MDD; 3 psychotic; 2 bipolar	4 weeks, nortriptyline	Open, prospective series	3 weeks	0.3–1.0	3 complete 7 partial 5 nonresponse	Minimal AEs
Flint & Rifat, 1994	21	64–88	Unipolar MDD	6 weeks, various ADs	Open, prospective	2 weeks	0.5–1.0	5 complete 3 partial 13 non response	10 dose reduction due to neuromuscular or neurologic side effects
Kok et al., 2007	15	≥60, mean 73.6	MDD; 7 psychotic	4 weeks; 3 venlafaxine 12 nortriptyline	Open, randomized	6 weeks	0.6–1.2	5 remission 7 response	No discontinuations due to AEs

AD, antidepressant; AE, adverse events; MDD, major depressive disorder.

Table 21.2 Adjunctive Atypical Antipsychotic Trials in Late-Life Depression

STUDY	N	AGE	DIAGNOSIS	DURATION PRIOR RX	DESIGN	DRUG AND DOSE	OUTCOME	DISCONTINUATIONS DUE TO ADVERSE EVENTS
Acute phase trials								
Rutherford et al., 2007	20	≥50; mean, 63	MDD unipolar, nonpsychotic	6 weeks escitalopram (15) or other SSRI	6 weeks Open-label prospective trial	Aripiprazole 5–15 mg/day, Modal dose 10 mg	10 of 20 achieved HDRS ≤ 10	3 discontinued due to adverse events
Sheffrin et al., 2009	24	≥65; mean, 74	MDD unipolar, nonpsychotic	16 weeks escitalopram and 12 weeks SNRI	12 weeks Open-label prospective trial	Aripiprazole 2.5–15 mg/day, Mean dose 9 mg	12 of 24 achieved HDRS ≤ 10	2 discontinued due to adverse events
Steffens et al., 2011	409	≥50; mean, 56	MDD unipolar, nonpsychotic	1–3 trials by history; 8-week prospective trial	6 weeks Double-blind Placebo-controlled	Aripiprazole 5–15 mg/day, Modal dose 10 mg	Response rates: 39.7% vs. 24.4%, $p < .001$ Remission rates: 32.5% vs. 17.1%, $p < .001$	12 (5.7%) discontinued due to adverse events
Alexopoulos et al., 2008	93	≥55; mean, 63	MDD unipolar, nonpsychotic	6 weeks citalopram 20–40	4–6 weeks Open label	Risperidone 0.25–1.0 mg/day Mean modal dose 0.7 mg	Remission (HDRS ≤ 7) 63/93 (67.7%)	Not stated
Relapse prevention trial								
Alexopoulos et al., 2008	63	≥55; mean, 62.5	MDD unipolar, nonpsychotic		24 weeks Double-blind, placebo-controlled relapse prevention	Risperidone 0.25–1.0 mg/day Mean modal dose 0.8 mg Citalopram 39 mg/day	Median time to relapse 105 vs. 57, $p = .07$ Relapse rates: 56% vs. 65%, $p = $ n.s.	2 /32 (6%) discontinued due to adverse events

AD, antidepressant; HDRS, Hamilton Depression Rating Scale; MDD, major depressive disorder; SNRI, serotonin–norepinephrine reuptake inhibitor; SSRI, selective serotonin reuptake inhibitor.

neither T3 nor lithium was more effective than placebo (Joffe et al., 2006); however, this small trial included only 36 patients who were randomized to four different treatment groups. In the randomized STAR*D open-label comparison trial of lithium and T3, T3 was much better tolerated than lithium but not significantly more effective (Nierenberg et al., 2006). To my knowledge, there are no studies of adjunctive T3 in treatment-resistant, late-life depression.

ATYPICAL AGENTS

The use of conventional antipsychotic agents, reviewed elsewhere (Nelson, 1987), has a long history. Antipsychotic agents were used in nonpsychotic depression both as monotherapy and adjunctive therapy. The use of the conventional agents in nonpsychotic depressed patients declined rapidly as the risk of tardive dyskinesia became recognized. In 1999, Ostroff and Nelson reported a series of cases successfully treated with adjunctive risperidone in patients failing an SSRI. This was followed in 2001 by the first placebo-controlled trial of the olanzapine-fluoxetine combination (Shelton et al., 2001). Currently 16 controlled trials of atypical agents, including risperidone, olanzapine, quetiapine, and aripiprazole, have been performed in a total of 3,480 patients. A meta-analysis of these agents found the differences in response and remission to drug and placebo were significant (Nelson & Papakostas, 2009). Overall, the number needed to treat for response was 9. Each of the agents was significantly superior to adjunctive placebo.

No prospective placebo-controlled studies of the atypicals have been performed in late-life depression. An open-label adjunctive aripiprazole study of 20 patients with major depression aged 50 and older (mean age 63), who had failed to remit with a 6-week trial of an SSRI, was reported by Rutherford et al. (2007). Fifteen of the 20 were treated by the authors with escitalopram up to 20 mg, and five others had been treated with other SSRIs. Aripiprazole was started at 5 mg/day and increased by 5 mg every 2 weeks up to a maximum of 15 mg/day (final modal dose = 10 mg). Ten of the 20 patients remitted on the Hamilton Depression Rating Scale (HDRS) ≤ 10 (Hamilton, 1960). Three patients discontinued due to adverse effects (two for intolerable anxiety and one for a rash). Sheffrin et al. (2009) reported a careful systematic open-label study of 24 clearly antidepressant treatment-resistant patients aged 65

years or older. Patients were required to have failed up to *16 weeks* of escitalopram followed by duloxetine or venlafaxine for 12 weeks. Aripiprazole was started at 2.5 mg and increased by that amount weekly based on response and tolerance up to a maximum of 15 mg. The mean final dose was 9.0 mg/day. Twelve of 24 patients achieved remission (HDRS ≤ 10). Two patients withdrew due to side effects (sedation or akathisia). In this study, 6 of 24 patients experienced mild or transient akathisia, and 74% experienced at least mild restlessness. The latter was more common at higher doses and usually resolved with dose decrease.

The largest study of an adjunctive atypical was reported by Steffens et al. (2011). This was a secondary analysis of the pooled data from three similar 6-week prospective placebo-controlled trials. In the pooled data, 409 patients were aged 50 years and older. All had unipolar major depression and had failed 1–3 historical antidepressant trials and one prospective 8-week trial of an SSRI or venlafaxine. Patients were then randomized to adjunctive aripiprazole or placebo. Aripiprazole was started at 5 mg/day, increased to 10 mg after 1 week, and then dose could be adjusted up to 15 mg/day. The mean final dose was 9.9 mg/day. Eighty-eight percent of the patients on aripiprazole or placebo completed the study. Both response rates (39.7 vs. 24.4%) and remission rates (32.5 vs. 17.1%) were significantly higher on aripiprazole than placebo. The number needed to treat was 7 for both response and remission. Outcome in three subgroups aged 50–54, 55–60, and 61–67 was relatively similar. There was no indication of a decline in efficacy in the oldest group. In the pooled dataset, 679 patients were 49 years or younger. These patients also had a significantly higher remission rate than placebo, 26.9% versus 16.4%, but the remission rate on drug was somewhat lower than in the older patients. The NNT for remission (10) in the younger patients was higher than in the older patients (NNT = 7). Of interest, the rate of akathisia was lower in the older patients than in younger patients (17.1% vs. 26.0%).

There are few data regarding long-term use of atypical agents. Alexopoulos et al. (2008) published a secondary analysis of the adjunctive risperidone relapse prevention study. This is the only controlled relapse prevention study published for an atypical agent in late-life depression. All patients were initially started on citalopram. Nonresponders received adjunctive risperidone. Patients then entered a

24-week, double-blind trial in which the SSRI was continued but patients were randomized to stay on risperidone or switch to placebo. Of the 101 older patients who completed the citalopram trial, an unusually high number of patients, 93, failed the trial. Of the 93, 63 patients achieved remission when risperidone was added to citalopram and entered the controlled trial. The median time to relapse with adjunctive risperidone was 105 days versus 57 days in the placebo group ($p = .07$). Relapse rates were 56% (18 of 32) and 65% (20 of 31). Mean modal doses were 0.7 mg/day for risperidone and 39.3 mg/day for citalopram. Although the findings were not significant, the study was underpowered, particularly for the analysis of the older subgroup. During the double-blind phase the only side effect reported in more than two patients was headache, which occurred in three risperidone patients. Mean weight gain was 0.9 kg during the adjunctive phase and 0.8 kg in the risperidone group versus –0.3 kg in the placebo group during the double-blind phase.

The risk of tardive dyskinesia (TD) in older patients treated with antipsychotics has been a concern since Jeste et al. (1995) reported a substantially higher rate of TD during treatment with conventional antipsychotics (26% at 1 year; 52% at 2 years). A rate of 4% per year was previously reported in younger patients (Tardive Dyskinesia Task Force Report, 1980). Because of this, there was concern about rates of TD during long-term treatment with atypical antipsychotics in older patients with nonpsychotic depression. This concern was heightened by a reported TD rate of 8.5% during a 12-week trial of olanzapine alone or combined with sertraline in psychotic depression (Meyers et al., 2009). Meyers subsequently indicated that this rate was based on a change in the AIMS score, that treatment was seldom discontinued in these patients, and he questioned whether clinicians in the trial thought the rating was clinically meaningful (personal communication, 2009). Other reports have not noted such high rates. In 560 patients who received adjunctive olanzapine during a 76-week, open-label trial, no cases of TD were observed (Corya et al., 2003). In the risperidone relapse prevention study cited earlier, mean AIMS scores declined during the open adjunctive phase (0.7 to 0.5) and during the continuation phase (0.6 to 0.3) in the risperidone group (Alexopoulos et al., 2008). In a 52-week, open-label extension trial of adjunctive aripiprazole in depression, an annualized TD rate of 0.7% was observed (Berman et al., 2008). In these latter atypical extension trials, TD was absent or the rate was quite low and different from that observed in the olanzapine psychotic depression trial. It appears likely that the high rate reported in the psychotic depression trial is not representative of clinically observed TD.

STIMULANTS

Although the controlled studies of adjunctive stimulant agents in depression are quite limited, some investigators have suggested these agents might be especially useful in older adults (Murray & Cassem, 1998; Wittenborn, 1980). Although placebo-controlled monotherapy trials of stimulant drugs in mixed-age adults, reviewed elsewhere (Satel & Nelson, 1989) were disappointing, four of five monotherapy trials in geriatric patients performed between 1956 and 1975 reported positive results, especially in terms of effects on apathy, mood, and motor retardation (Darvil & Woolley, 1959; Dube, Osgood, & Notkin, 1956; Holliday & Joffe, 1965; Kaplitz, 1975; Landman, Preisig, & Perlmann, 1958). These studies, however, were of limited value because diagnoses were poorly defined, many patients appeared to have dementia or brain disease, and it is doubtful these patients had a primary depressive disorder.

Two large series of 66 and 198 cases from the Massachusetts General Hospital consultation service (Masand, Pickett, & Murray, 1991; Woods, Tesar, Murray, & Cassem, 1986) suggested the value of adjunctive dextroamphetamine and methylphenidate in medically ill depressed patients. The mean age in the two samples was 72 and 65 years, respectively. Fifty to 70% of the patients in the two series had a marked or moderate response to one of these stimulants. Usually the effect was seen in 48 hours. The mean doses of dextroamphetamine were 12 mg/d and 9 mg/d (range: 2.5 mg to 30 mg) in the two samples. The mean doses of methylphenidate were 13.5 and 11 mg/d (range: 5–30 mg/d) in the two samples. Ten percent of the patients discontinued treatment because of side effects. The most common were agitation, confusion, nervousness, hypomania, and delusions.

Two relatively recent placebo-controlled studies have been reported. Wallace (1995) described a cross-over trial in 16 medically ill patients with a mean age of 72 years. Patients received methylphenidate up to 20 mg/day or placebo for 4 days and were then crossed over to the other agent. The authors found a significant effect for both methylphenidate and order of administration. During the first 4 days both drug and placebo reduced depression scores. During the second 4 days only methylphenidate reduced depressive symptoms. A second placebo-controlled, 2-week trial was reported by Wagner and Rabkin (2000). Although this study included men aged 18–65, all had medical illness (advanced human immunodeficiency virus.) Patients were randomized to dextroamphetamine or placebo and titrated up to a dose of 40 mg/day. The most common dose was 30 mg/d. Patients receiving dextroamphetamine were significantly more likely to respond.

Stimulants have also been used as adjunctive therapy; however, none of the studies have focused on elderly patients. Five open studies, reviewed previously (Ayd & Zohar, 1987; Nelson, 1997), reported successful attempts to add either dextroamphetamine or methylphenidate to tricyclic (TCA) or monoamine oxidase inhibitor antidepressants. In the largest of these studies, Fawcett et al. (1991) found that 25 of 32 patients who had failed prior treatments responded to the stimulant and many maintained the response for several months. Stimulants have also been used with second-generation antidepressants. Two case series with seven and five cases, respectively, have been reported with positive results (Masand, Anand, & Tanquary, 1998; Stoll, Srinvasan, Diamond, Workum, & Cole, 1996). In 2006, Patkar et al. reported a placebo-controlled trial of methylphenidate (18–54 mg/day) in 60 mixed-age patients who had failed to respond to an antidepressant trial. Although response and remission rates favored the stimulant, the differences were not significant. Ravindran et al. (2008) reported a 5-week, placebo-controlled adjunctive trial of osmotic release methylphenidate in 145 mixed-age patients with MDD who had failed 1–3 trials of antidepressants. At 5 days and 14 days, change on the MADRS was significantly greater with MPD than placebo, but at days 21 to 35 and endpoint it was not. Change on scales for apathy and fatigue did indicate a significant advantage for the drug. In 2011 Trivedi reported the findings of a controlled trial of adjunctive lisdexamfetamine in 246 patients aged 18–55 with MDD. Patients began an 8-week course of escitalopram up to 20 mg/day. Those with at least residual symptoms (HAMD score ≥ 4, N = 177) were randomized to adjunctive lisdexamfetamine (20 mg/d up to 50 mg/d) or placebo. The primary outcome, change on the MADRS scale in nonremitting patients (MADRS >10), was significant ($p = .09$) after 6 weeks of treatment using an a priori defined probability level of 0.1 for signal detection. Active drug was not more effective than placebo in remitting patients with residual symptoms. One interpretation of this study is that it may be difficult to detect significant differences in symptom change in patients with mild symptoms. Alternatively, these three latter trials (Patkar et al., 2006; Ravindran et al., 2008; Trivedi et al., 2011) failed to show clear evidence of efficacy of stimulants in treatment-resistant depression.

In the studies of dextroamphetamine and MPD the most common side effects were behavioral symptoms, including agitation, nervousness, and irritability. Suspiciousness, hypomania, and delusions, while less common, did occur. Cardiovascular effects, however, were uncommon. In the study of MPD in 145 MDD patients, mean pulse increased by 1.3 beats per minute (bpm) in the MPD group and mean systolic blood pressure by 1.1 mm Hg. There were no electrocardiogram (ECG) abnormalities noted. In the lisdexamfetamine study mean pulse rate increased by 4.8 bpm on the ECG and mean systolic pressure rose 2.3 mmHg. It should be remembered, however, that the stimulant drugs, like many of the adjunctive agents, have not been studied in large safety trials in older depressed subjects. As a consequence, our knowledge of less common potential safety issues is limited.

MODAFINIL

Adjunctive modafinil has also been studied in mixed-age depressed patients. Two similar trials were conducted in depressed patients who had a partial response to SSRI treatment and had residual sleepiness or fatigue (DeBattista et al., 2003; Fava, Thase, & DeBattista, 2005). In the first, modafinil 100 to 400 mg/d was added to the SSRI for 6 weeks. In the second trial, modafinil 200 mg/d was given for 8 weeks. In both studies modafinil reduced sleepiness and fatigue but significantly reduced depressive symptoms only in the second trial.

Two enhancement trials were reported for modafinil in mixed-age patients; that is, patients were started on modafinil or placebo with an antidepressant at the beginning of treatment. In the first (Dunlop et al., 2007), a 6-week trial of modafinil 200 mg/day in 73 MDD patients with sleepiness or fatigue, modafinil failed to improve sleepiness on the Epworth Sleepiness Scale but did improve hypersomnia on the 31-item HDRS scale. The HDRS total score was significantly better in the modafinil group at some time points during the trial but not at endpoint. Abolfazli et al. (2011) reported a placebo-controlled 6-week trial in 46 mixed-age MDD patients who were randomly assigned to a 6-week trial of fluoxetine 40 mg with either modafinil 400 mg/d or placebo added at the beginning of treatment. Modafinil was significantly more effective than placebo. In all of these trials, few side effects were reported.

None of the prior modafinil trials were conducted in late-life depression, but controlled trials of modafinil monotherapy have been performed in relatively older medically ill depressed patients, for example, cancer patients (N = 631; mean age, 60 years) (Jean-Pierre et al., 2010) and ALS patients (N = 32; mean age, 58 years) (Rabkin et al., 2009). In both trials, fatigue was the primary target symptom. Patients were not selected for depression, but depression scales were employed. In both studies, modafinil had a significant effect on fatigue, but the depressive symptoms did not show significant change.

PINDOLOL AND BUSPIRONE

Pindolol and buspirone have both been explored as adjunctive agents for use with SSRIs. While the evidence suggests pindolol may accelerate response, studies to date have found no evidence of efficacy in antidepressant-resistant depression (Moreno, Gelenberg, Bachar, & Delgado, 1997; Perez, Soler, Puigdemont, Alvarez, & Artigas, 1999). Two controlled trials of adjunctive buspirone after either 4 or 6 weeks of antidepressant therapy, respectively (Appelberg et al., 2001; Landen, Björling, Agren, & Fahlén, 1998), and one open-label randomized trial at the beginning of treatment (Onder & Tural, 2003) found no significant effect of adjunctive buspirone.

Hormone Therapy

Because levels of estrogen and testosterone decline in older adults, it is reasonable to wonder whether replacement therapy or adjunctive treatment would facilitate antidepressant response. In two retrospective analyses, Schneider et al. (1997, 2001) found that women who were receiving hormone replacement therapy (HRT) during treatment with fluoxetine or sertraline were more likely to respond to the SSRI than those who did not. Randomization,

however, was not stratified for HRT, so that other factors associated with HRT such as quality of medical care or socioeconomic status, may account for the differences in outcome. A few prospective trials have been conducted to explore this question. None of the studies of depressed women limited selection to late-life patients, but samples were generally older.

Two monotherapy trials were disappointing. An 8-week randomized trial of estradiol versus placebo in 83 postmenopausal women with depressive disorders found no difference in percent change on the Hamilton scale (Morrison et al., 2004). An open, random-assignment, 8-week trial of estrogen plus progesterone versus escitalopram in 32 peri- and postmenopausal women found escitalopram much more effective for full remission of depression (75% vs. 25%) (Soares et al., 2006). These studies suggest estrogen is not an effective *monotherapy* for depression in postmenopausal women.

A small controlled adjunctive study randomized perimenopausal women to conjugated estrogen (N = 11) or placebo (N = 6) for a 6-week trial (Morgan et al., 2005). The subjects had MDD, a partial response to an antidepressant, and perimenopausal symptoms. Change on the HDRS was greater in the group receiving estrogen; however, a perimenopausal sample may be less relevant to late-life women. Two augmentation trials in postmenopausal women have been performed. Rasgon et al. (2002) studied 22 women with MDD who were postmenopausal and ranged in age from 41 to 65 (mean age, 55). Onset of MDD was within the past month and none had received prior antidepressant treatment. Sertraline was started at 50 mg and then raised to 100 mg for the remainder of the 10-week trial. The subjects were randomized to receive double-blind transdermal estradiol or a placebo patch. Both groups improved with time, but there was no advantage for treatment with estradiol. A larger trial was reported by Dias et al. (2006). Seventy-two patients with MDD, a MADRS score >19, and verified menopausal status were included. In this double-blind, 24-week study, all women received venlfaxine 75 mg to 225 mg. They were randomized to receive adjunctive estrogen 0.625 mg plus medroxyprogesterone 2.5 mg plus methyltestosterone 2.5 mg, or estrogen plus medroxyprogesterone, or methyltestosterone only, or no hormone therapy. Appropriate placebos were employed for each of the hormones. Only the group receiving methyltestosterone alone had better outcomes than the group receiving venlafaxine and placebo.

These two studies suggest that adjunctive estrogen with an antidepressant in depressed postmenopausal women is not effective. In addition, given concerns about the hazards of HRT, the routine use of adjunctive hormones in depression would not be recommended. These data, however, do not rule out the possibility that there are individuals who might benefit from adjunctive hormone therapy. In particular, the value of adjunctive estrogen might be more apparent in treatment-resistant patients. For example, in the Rasgon study, onset of depression had been within the past month and patients were treatment naïve. Sertraline appeared quite effective regardless of adjunctive estrogen. The value of adjunctive estrogen is in part supported by a report by Stewart and colleagues (2004), who examined a group of middle-aged women before and after the report of the Women's Health Initiative. After the report, HRT was frequently discontinued and 11 women reported onset of depression, within a mean of 3 weeks of terminating HRT. Eight of these women were receiving antidepressants. Reinstitution of HRT was effective in 4 of 7 patients. These findings suggest HRT may have an adjunctive effect, especially in women who have not responded to an antidepressant alone.

To my knowledge, the only study of HRT in elderly women and its effects on mood was reported by Almeida et al. (2006). One hundred and fifteen women, 70 years and older were randomized to estradiol or placebo for a 20-week study period. Patients were rated with the Beck Depression Scale but were not selected for depression at entry. Estradiol was not associated with improvement in cognition, depression, or quality of life.

TESTOSTERONE

In the past decade 10 randomized controlled studies of testosterone have been reported. Six of these were monotherapy trials usually in hypogonadal men (Rabkin, Wagner, McElhiney, Rabkin, & Lin, 2004; Rabkin, Wagner, & Rabkin, 2000; Seidman, Spatz, Rizzo, & Roose, 2001; Seidman et al., 2009; Seidman & Roose, 2006; Shores, Kivlahan, Sadak, Li, & Matsumoto, 2009). Testosterone was administered in an injectable formulation or as a gel. Two of the monotherapy studies included men with MDD; the other four had various depressive diagnoses. Two trials, one in dysthymia (N = 23) and one in

"non-MDD" depression (N = 33), found a significant effect (Seidman et al., 2009; Shores et al., 2009); four trials found no difference between testosterone and placebo. In these trials all patients improved.

Four adjunctive testosterone trials have been reported (Orengo, Fullerton, & Kunik, 2005; Pope, Cohane, Kanayama, Siegel, & Hudson, 2003; Pope et al., 2010; Seidman & Roose, 2005). Numbers of subjects were 22, 26, 18, and 100, respectively. Three of the trials limited the sample to MDD. The mean age in three samples was 46, 49, and 50. One trial selected men 50 and older. All required failure to respond to at least one adequate antidepressant trial. Patients included were those with low or borderline testosterone serum levels, and some studies required that prostate-specific antigen (PSA) levels be within a normal range. One of the four trials (N = 22) found a significant effect for testosterone compared with placebo (Pope et al., 2003). The other three, including the largest study (N = 100) (Pope et al., 2010), did not find a significant difference between testosterone and placebo. Pope et al. (2010) suggested that some men do show a marked effect of testosterone but that currently it is not possible to identify them before treatment. In the aforementioned studies few subjects reported significant side effects. However, as some authors noted, the numbers of subjects studied and the relatively short period of treatment does not allow for assessment of the long-term safety of testosterone administration. There has been concern that administration of testosterone might increase the risk of prostate cancer (Kanayama, Amiaz, Seidman, & Pope, 2007); however, in a 30-month trial of testosterone for contraception in 1,045 Chinese men, PSA levels remained within a normal range during the study (Gu et al., 2009).

Cognitive Enhancing Agents

Because late-life depression is often associated with cognitive deficits and may be an early expression of early vascular disease or Alzheimer's disease, the possibility of using cognitive enhancing drugs for adjunctive treatment of depression would seem logical. Holzheimer et al. (2008) investigated this strategy using galantamine. Thirty-eight nondemented adults aged 50 years or older with MDD were randomized to receive galantamine or placebo for 24 weeks in addition to an antidepressant. Prior antidepressants, if present, were discontinued. All patients started venlafaxine XR, which could be advanced up to 225 mg/day. If patients did not improve or could not tolerate venlafaxine, they could be switched to citalopram. Galantamine was started at 4 mg bid and then increased to 8 mg bid. Both groups improved and galantamine was not superior to placebo. The 12-week discontinuation rate, 53% versus 16%, was significantly higher on drug than placebo, but discontinuation due to adverse events did not differ. Although this was not a study of treatment-resistant depression, the mean number of prior antidepressants received was two.

MEMANTINE

Lenze and colleagues (2011) reported a 12-week randomized controlled trial of memantine monotherapy for 35 patients aged 60 and older who displayed depressive symptoms or apathy after disabling medical events that resulted in their admission to a nursing home. Both groups improved, but there were no differences between the treatment groups.

DONEPEZIL

Reynolds et al. (2011) reported a 2-year study of adjunctive donepezil in 130 previously depressed subjects 65 years and older who had been successfully treated with an antidepressant. The sample included 73 subjects with normal cognition and 57 with mild cognitive impairment (MCI). Subjects were then randomized to receive donepezil or placebo with their antidepressant. Adjunctive donepezil did result in small but significant improvement in global cognitive function at 1 year, but this difference was not apparent at 2 years. A post-hoc analysis revealed that among subjects with MCI, significantly fewer subjects on donepezil progressed to dementia over the 2 years, 3 of 30 subjects on donepezil versus 9 of 27 subjects on placebo. However, recurrence of depression was significantly *more frequent* in the donepezil group than in those receiving placebo, 44% on drug versus 12% on placebo (log-rank test, $p = .03$). In the cognitively normal group, the difference in recurrence, 30% versus 22%, was small and not significant. In summary, this study found little effect of adjunctive donepezil in cognitively intact subjects. In MCI subjects donepezil appeared to reduce conversion to dementia (NNT = 5) but increased the risk of depression recurrence (NNH = 4). This latter finding, while post hoc, may be consistent with the cholinergic hypothesis of depression

proposed by Janowsky et al. (1972) years ago and consistent with the recent report that scopolamine, an *anti*-cholinergic agent, has antidepressant effects (Drevets & Furey, 2010). While adjunctive donepezil is not commonly used to prevent depression, it is used in older depressed patients to improve cognition. The findings of this study indicate that potential advantages for cognition need to be weighed against the potential hazard of increasing risk of depression recurrence.

NUTRITIONAL SUPPLEMENTS

Decreased appetite is a common symptom in older depressed adults. Weight loss can be profound. Dehydration can result in hospital admission. It is reasonable to wonder whether nutritional disturbances might develop, aggravate depression, and interfere with antidepressant treatment in older adults. Omega-3 fatty acids, SAMe, and folic acid have all been employed as adjunctive treatments. Omega-3 fatty acid, recently reviewed (Sublette, Ellis, Geant, & Mann, 2011), has been most frequently studied. A variety of disorders—unipolar depression, bipolar depression, perinatal depression, childhood depression, and depression with medical disorders—have been studied. Eight placebo-controlled trials of adjunctive omega-3 with antidepressants in unipolar adult (mixed-age) depression have been performed with trials ranging in size from 16 to 122 for a total number of 442 individuals included. The samples vary with respect to treatment resistance and vary in their findings. A recent meta-analysis found that a critical feature was the proportion of eicosapentaenoic acid (EPA) versus docosahexaenoic acid (DHA) in the supplement (Sublette et al., 2011). In trials using supplements with more than 60% EPA, a significant effect of omega-3 was found. Supplements with less than 60% were not effective. The meta-analysis included studies of various types. If limited to placebo-controlled contrasts of antidepressant with adjunctive omega-3 in unipolar depression, of the seven contrasts using >60% EPA, six found a positive effect. The three contrasts with <60% EPA were all negative.

SAMe has been explored as monotherapy in depression and reviewed previously (Bressa, 1994). In an analysis of six mixed-age, placebo-controlled trials, Bressa (1994) found SAMe significantly more effective than placebo. Recently a trial of SAMe in well-described, antidepressant treatment-resistant, mixed-age unipolar major depression has been reported with positive results (Papakostas, Mischoulon, Shyu, Alpert, & Fava, 2010). The age range was 18 to 80 years. The target dose of SAMe was 800 mg b.i.d. Fifty-one percent of patients receiving SAMe responded versus 21% of placebo patients. Adjunctive folic acid has also been employed. Coppen and Bailey (2000) reported a study of 127 depressed subjects (mean age, 42 years) treated with fluoxetine and either adjunctive folic acid 500 μg/day or placebo. These patients had a "new" episode and apparently were not treatment resistant. Women receiving folate had a better response than those receiving placebo. The difference in men was not significant.

In summary, the use of nutritional supplements would appear to be a fruitful area of study in older patients. In mixed-age samples, the efficacy of adjunctive omega-3 rich in EPA appears to be fairly well supported, adjunctive SAMe appears effective in resistant depression in one sample, and folic acid may have efficacy in women. None of these strategies has been explored in late-life depression, even though the relative mild adverse event profiles would argue for their use. Alternatively there is little evidence or experience comparing the magnitude of the effect of these supplements with more traditional treatments for depression.

NOVEL TREATMENTS

There are a few other novel adjunctive treatments for depression. Depression is associated with activation of pro-inflammatory cytokines (van West & Maes, 1999). Certain features of "sickness behavior" such as fatigue and lack of drive may be associated with elevated cytokines (Dantzer, 2006), and these symptoms are often present in depression. Some investigators have reasoned *that inhibition of cyclooxygenase-2* might reduce prostaglandin E_2 synthesis and might be helpful in depression. An open-label trial found adjunctive acetylsalicylic acid (ASA), which inhibits COX-2, appeared to enhance response rates in 24 depressed patients who had failed at least 4 weeks of antidepressant therapy (Mendlewicz et al., 2006). Two controlled trials of the COX-2 inhibitor celecoxib have been performed in mixed-age samples (Akhondzadeh et al., 2009; Muller et al., 2006). Both were 6-week, placebo-controlled adjunctive trials of celecoxib 400 mg/day in MDD patients. Celecoxib was added to reboxetine in the first trial and fluoxetine in the second. Each trial included 40 patients. Neither

study limited selection to antidepressant-resistant patients. Adjunctive celecoxib was more effective than placebo in both trials. Remission rates were 45% with adjunctive therapy and 20% with placebo in the first trial and 35% and 5% for drug and placebo in the second. A third 6-week controlled trial examined celecoxib in depressed or mixed-state bipolar patients but failed to show a significant effect (Nery et al., 2008). While the trials in unipolar depression are encouraging, another recent study found that commonly used anti-inflammatory drugs antagonized antidepressant-induced behaviors in rodents and that a post-hoc analysis of patients in STAR*D revealed that patients who received anti-inflammatory agents were less likely to remit than those who did not receive such agents (Warner-Schmidt, Vanover, Chen, Marshall, & Greengard, 2011). The latter study, however, was not able to control for the condition for which anti-inflammatory agents were given and others have found that depressed patients with pain are less likely to remit than those without pain (Leuchter et al., 2010).

A recent study compared effects of celecoxib or naproxen versus placebo on depressive symptoms in the ADAPT study (Fields, Drye, Vaidya, & Lyketsos, 2011). This is of particular interest because participants in the study were 70 years or older. This was a primary prevention trial in which the investigators examined the effect of the use of anti-inflammatory agents, celecoxib 200 mg twice a day or naproxen 220 mg twice a day versus placebo on the risk of developing Alzheimer's dementia. Patients were cognitively normal at baseline. During the trial, depressive symptoms were measured on the Geriatric Depression Scale (GDS; Yesavage et al., 1982) at baseline and then yearly thereafter. A total of 2,311 subjects were randomized, of whom 449 had a GDS score of >5 indicating probably depression. Neither celecoxib nor naproxen had an effect on symptoms of depression. It is first noteworthy that this was a monotherapy trial of the two agents rather than adjunctive therapy. In addition, 75% to 80% of those with depression had relatively low scores, that is, 6–10 on the GDS, and traditional antidepressants have not been shown to be superior to placebo in mild depression. While these data suggest no protective effect of NSAIDs on depressive symptoms, they do not address the question of whether NSAIDs would be useful as adjunctive therapy or monotherapy in older patients with moderate to severe major depression.

Nimodipine has also been examined as an adjunct. Nimodipine is a calcium channel blocker that protects neurons from elevated levels of intracellular calcium and has been used to reduce the frequency and severity of ischemic events. It was hypothesized it might be useful in late-life MDD associated with vascular disease for acute symptoms and to prevent relapse. Taragano and associates have conducted two double-blind, controlled trials of adjunctive nimodipine in Argentina (2001, 2005). The first trial, at four sites, included 84 patients with MDD (mean age, 68.7), who also met criteria for vascular depression (Alexopoulos et al., 1997). All were treated with an antidepressant and in addition were randomized to either nimodipine 90 mg/day or vitamin C. Depression was rated with the Hamilton scale over a 300-day period. Acute outcome was assessed at 60 days and relapse over the next 240 days. At 60 days, both groups showed substantial improvement, but the nimodipine group showed significantly greater symptom improvement and significantly higher remission rates (45% vs. 25%) but not response rates (68% vs. 56%). Among the responders, 8 of 25 controls and 2 of 27 on nimodipine experienced a recurrence between days 120 and 300 (X^2 test, $p = .06$). The second trial, at three sites, included 101 patients with MDD and vascular depression (mean age, 69.9) who were treated for a two month acute phase and a 6-month relapse prevention phase. All patients received fluoxetine and in addition were randomized to nimodipine 30 mg t.i.d. or placebo. Patients on nimodipine had greater symptom reduction and higher rates of remission (54% vs. 27%) at 61 days. Among the remitters, fewer patients on nimodipine relapsed (1 of 27 vs. 5 of 14) between days 122 and 244.

The use of opiates in depression has a long history, although interest in these agents for depression waned with the introduction of the tricyclic and monoamine oxidase inhibitors. Interest was rekindled by the introduction of opioid partial agonist and mixed agonist-antagonist agents such as *buprenorphine* in part because of their reduced liability for abuse and dependence. Two small trials of buprenorphine have been performed. In 1982, Emrich et al. administered buprenorphine to 10 patients with major depression using a double-blind design. Patients started on placebo, then buprenorphine 0.2 mg twice a day was substituted for placebo and given for 5 to 8 days and then placebo was readministered. Ratings performed every 2 days indicated significant improvement relative to placebo.

The second study was an open-label design also in 10 patients with major depression, but in this case patients had failed prior trials of antidepressants from at least two drug classes (Bodkin, Zornberg, Lukas, & Cole, 1995). Three patients were unable to tolerate the drug and dropped out. Seven completed 4 to 6 weeks of treatment and of these, four remitted and two were moderately improved. The mean final dose was 1.26 mg/day.

The trials of celecoxib, nimodipine, and buprenorphine are quite interesting. An agent useful in vascular depression might be especially valuable given the apparent lack of efficacy found for citalopram in a post-hoc analysis of MDD patients over 74 years of age with executive dysfunction in the "old-old" study (Sneed et al., 2010). The anti-inflammatory agents and calcium channel blockers might have value for other medical conditions common in older depressed patients. Buprenorphine might be useful for management of substance abuse and comorbid depression. Another advantage of these agents is that they have been used for other indications in sizable numbers of patients and their safety and tolerability issues are well known. Although clinical experience with these agents in depression is limited, they suggest new mechanisms to explore.

SEQUENTIAL USE OF TREATMENTS IN PRACTICE

While the meta-analysis of antidepressant efficacy in late-life depression and the findings of the IMPACT and PROSPECT trials suggest rather modest outcomes with single antidepressant trials, studies of sequential trials in older depressed adults are more encouraging. Whyte et al. (2004) described response to three successive augmentation trials with bupropion, nortriptyline, or lithium in depressed subjects aged 69 or older with unipolar nonpsychotic major depression. Patients receiving augmentation had failed to respond to paroxetine with interpersonal psychotherapy (IPT). During the first augmentation trial 24 of 53 (45%) patients responded. Five of 16 patients receiving a second trial responded. Three of seven patients responded to a third trial. Thus, after three trials, 32 of the 53 (60%) patients responded. There were 32 adverse events that led to discontinuation of treatment. The number and percent of patients discontinuing due to adverse events were 21/42 (50%) for bupropion, 4/17 (24%) for nortriptyline, and 7/17 (41%) for lithium. Dew et al. (2007) from the same group noted that patients who required adjunctive treatment after prior inadequate response responded more slowly than patients receiving initial treatment. Kok et al. (2009) described a group of 81 patients aged 60 years or older who began treatment in a double-blind comparison trial of venlafaxine and nortriptyline. Among patients who failed to achieve remission, 32 patients were offered a series of 51 subsequent trials—switch from venlafaxine to nortriptyline, lithium augmentation, switch to phenelzine, or ECT. Fourteen of 22 (64%) remitted with adjunctive lithium, 6 of 15 (40%) remitted with a switch to a TCA (either nortriptyline or clomipramine N = 1), 0 of 8 remitted with phenelzine, and 3 of 5 (60%) remitted with ECT. From the beginning of the double-blind trial, 78 of 81 (96.3%) responded and 68/81 (84%) remitted during 3 years of sequential treatments. These two series of patients suggest that if patients can remain in treatment, a favorable outcome can be obtained in a high percentage of patients.

AN ALGORITHM FOR TREATMENT

At the outset, the use of the term "algorithm" seems optimistic if it implies that a series of successive treatments can be determined based on empirical evidence. We have good evidence that several antidepressants are effective as initial treatment in patients with major depression over the age of 60 years. There are no prospective random-assignment, placebo-controlled studies of adjunctive therapies in older adults who failed the first treatment. There is no controlled evidence whether any adjunctive agent is more effective than another. Adverse event and safety data come mainly from open-label data or case series rather than head-to-head trials.

As a consequence of these limitations, geriatric mental health clinicians still rely heavily on the findings of trials conducted in nongeriatric samples. Admittedly, studies conducted in mixed-age patients with major depression are likely to apply to patients with major depression in the 60- to 75-year age range. As age increases, medical illness, concomitant medical treatments, and disability resulting from medical illness increase, making the application of findings in younger patients more difficult. In addition, as patients age, the incidence of vascular disease and Alzheimer's disease increases, and these disorders appear to influence response to treatment. Ideally, treatment recommendations for depressed elders would be based on studies of those

patients, but lacking the data, we still rely on studies of younger patients.

If a patient fails initial antidepressant treatment, or even before that treatment, there are a number of nonpharmacologic issues that should be considered. Recent reviews indicate that psychotherapy is an effective treatment in older adults (Mackin & Arean, 2005). Cognitive-behavioral therapy appears best established. Interpersonal psychotherapy appears useful in older adults when combined with antidepressant therapy. The recent study of problem-solving therapy in older depressed adults with executive dysfunction provides solid evidence of efficacy for that treatment (Arean et al., 2010). Ideally, predictors of response to drug treatment or psychotherapy would guide treatment, but these predictors are lacking in elderly patients. The issue is often settled by the patient's preference.

There are other factors to consider. Has the medical examination of the patient been adequate? A discussion of medical disorders that may contribute to depression is beyond the scope of this chapter (see Chapter 16), but it should always be considered. Are there basic needs that are not being met? The STAR*D trial found that low income, being unemployed, and low educational status all contribute to poor outcome of antidepressant treatment (Trivedi, Rush, et al., 2006). An interesting study of elders with major social problems found case management that addressed social problems was as or more effective than cognitive-behavioral therapy during the first year of treatment (Arean et al., 2005). Upcoming events that are viewed as adverse or unwanted can interfere with recovery from depression. For example, during a trial of elders with MDD, we observed several patients who were in the hospital anticipating transfer to a nursing home for the first time with very negative expectations (Nelson, Mazure, & Jatlow, 1995). These patients otherwise had the attributes of other patients with MDD and were being treated with therapeutic plasma levels of desipramine. None of these patients responded to treatment. Follow-up of these patients revealed that all but one patient recovered during the weeks after nursing home placement without change in their medication. Unfortunately, there may be other negatively anticipated events or circumstances that are difficult to change, for example, a diagnosis of a progressive malignancy.

When a clinician encounters a patient who has failed the initial treatment, the first question is whether treatment was adequate. An algorithm for the PROSPECT study (Mulsant et al., 2001) provides guidelines for dosage. While it makes sense to follow the adage "Start low and go slow," a common mistake is to be too cautious and never achieve an adequate dose. The issue of trial length remains unclear. A comparison of response in younger and older patients (Reynolds et al., 1996) found final response to be similar but that older patients responded more slowly during the initial weeks of treatment. Slower dose adjustment may in part contribute. STAR*D found that among patients who remitted, half did so during the second 6 weeks of a 12-week trial (Trivedi et al., 2006). The meta-analysis of antidepressants described earlier also found better rates of response and remission in 10- and 12-week trials (Nelson et al., 2008). Taking these data into account, it is reasonable and usually feasible to complete a longer trial, for example, 12 weeks, if the patient is showing signs of progressive improvement. The value of a longer trial comes into question when the patient has minimal response. Sackeim and colleagues (2006) examined remission in patients from two similar 12-week trials of antidepressants. They found that at 6 weeks patients who demonstrated minimal change (e.g., less than 25% improvement) were not likely to remit at 12 weeks. They questioned the recommendation of long trials for everyone and noted the drawbacks of prolonged exposure to ineffective treatment. Mulsant et al. (2006) in an elderly sample of 472 patients with MDD found that patients with less than 30% improvement after 4 weeks had a substantially lower chance of response after 12 weeks. In mixed-age and older subjects, evidence is mounting that minimal change after 4 to 6 weeks of treatment predicts poor outcome at 12 weeks. Taking this into account, one cannot simply say that a 6, 8, or 12-week trial is best or recommended. Certainly if minimal change has occurred at 6 weeks, change is recommended. But the length of the trial may need to be adjusted to allow for dose adjustment.

Perhaps the most neglected aspect of the assessment of a prior failed treatment is assessment of adherence (Zivin & Kales, 2008). Patients can be asked about adherence in a nonthreatening way. "Normalizing" the behavior is helpful. For example, one can ask, "It is fairly common for patients to miss doses of medication. How many times did you miss a dose in the past week?" Education about depression and its treatment as well as addressing barriers to treatment will help to improve adherence.

Adherence is related to clinical management. The efficacy of all of our antidepressant treatments is based on trials in which patients are seen frequently. Typically patients are seen weekly for the first month and then every other week. Because depressed patients are likely to be pessimistic or even hopeless, reassurance and encouragement are critical. In placebo-controlled trials, placebo and clinical management account for about 75% of the response (Nelson et al., 2008). Clinicians cannot assume that the response rates obtained in clinical trials will be obtained in clinical practice if patients are seen infrequently.

Once it is determined that the patient has had an adequate antidepressant trial and has failed to achieve remission, the clinician has several choices. The algorithm for the PROSPECT study recommended adjunctive treatment for patients who achieved a partial response. The idea is to maintain the improvement that has been made and build on it. There is not universal agreement on what constitutes "partial response." The literature on prediction of lack of response or remission at the end of treatment has usually defined minimal response as less than 25% or 30% improvement. Thus, 25% improvement up to remission defines partial response. Because this range of improvement is broad, the clinician is faced with two different clinical circumstances. Some patients, while improved, will still be fairly depressed, and the aim of adjunctive treatment will be global improvement of the depression. Alternatively, there will be patients who are close to remission but have specific residual symptoms. These patients may benefit from therapy targeted toward specific symptoms.

Adjunctive Therapy for Partial Responders Who Remain Moderately Depressed

Adjunctive treatment could take the form of adding a second antidepressant or adding another agent not approved for use as an antidepressant. The clinician and the patient will need to weigh the likely efficacy of adjunctive therapy against its potential to cause side effects or safety issues. One advantage of adding an approved antidepressant is that these agents have shown efficacy during monotherapy. Thus, even if there is no synergistic effect, the second agent may be effective. Potential combination agents with an SSRI—bupropion, mirtazapine, and nortriptyline—have all shown efficacy in late-life depression (Halikas, 1995; Hewett et al., 2010; Katz, Simpson, Curlik, Parmelee, & Muhly, 1990). Of these agents, the efficacy of the combination of mirtazapine and SSRIs is best supported in mixed-age samples, and clinical experience suggests mirtazapine is a useful drug in older patients. Although some data suggest nortriptyline is fairly well tolerated (Whyte et al., 2004), safety issues make it a second choice. There are no controlled trials of adjunctive bupropion therapy in younger or older patients with treatment-resistant depression, but this has been a popular strategy based on the difference in its mechanism of action, and STAR*D provides some support for efficacy. Although there are no comparison trials of these agents during adjunctive treatment that address differential efficacy, even if there were slight differences, it would still be likely that the choice of the agent will be based on secondary effects. Mirtazapine is more sedating and may increase appetite early in treatment. Bupropion is the least sedating antidepressant and also least likely to increase appetite or weight.

The atypical antipsychotic agents are now the best established adjunctive therapy in mixed-age patients based on strength of the evidence. In older patients, aripiprazole has been reported to be effective in antidepressant treatment-resistant depression in two open trials and one secondary analysis of a large controlled trial (N = 409)

sample. While aripiprazole has been best studied in older depressed patients, the lack of evidence for the other agents in older patients does not mean they are necessarily less effective. All of the atypical agents have the advantage of having fairly rapid effects. Much of the improvement occurs in the first 2 weeks; thus, the clinician will know fairly quickly if the drug is going to work. These advantages will need to be weighed against potential side effects and safety issues. While the acute phase tolerability of the atypical agents is not much different from other antidepressants, the atypicals do carry safety issues of metabolic syndrome, and the relatively uncommon risks of neuroleptic malignant syndrome and tardive dyskinesia that are not associated with other antidepressants or adjunctive agents.

Based on the considerations of efficacy, side effects, and clinical experience with these agents, for adjunctive treatment for partial responders who remain moderately depressed, adjunctive mirtazapine, bupropion, or an atypical agent, particularly aripiprazole, would be Category 1 agents (see Table 21.3).

Although the efficacy of adjunctive lithium in older patients is supported by six open-label studies and lithium is the only adjunctive strategy with two long-term randomized controlled trials (one in older patients), lithium is difficult to use and is potentially toxic. The PROSPECT algorithm (2001) placed lithium lower in the algorithm because it is less well

Table 21.3 Guideline for Adjunctive Treatment of Late-Life Depression in Patients With Partial Response (e.g., greater than 25% improvement but less than remission)

	RATIONALE	ADJUNCTIVE AGENTS
Category 1	Agents with evidence of efficacy in older adults either as monotherapy* or as adjunctive agents	Mirtazapine, bupropion, atypical antipsychotic (particularly aripiprazole)[†]
Category 2	Similar to Category 1 but with greater toxicity, safety, or complexity of administration	Lithium, nortriptyline
Category 3	Agents with evidence of efficacy in mixed-age patients or considerable experience in older adults, or better tolerability	Dextroamphetamine, methylphenidate, omega-3, SAMe; (marginal) thyroid

*Agents with evidence of efficacy as monotherapy are likely to have additive effects regardless of whether there is a synergistic effect. This is in part the difference between adjunctive treatment and "augmentation."
[†]Aripiprazole is singled out as the only atypical agent with evidence of efficacy from a secondary analysis of placebo-controlled data in older adults.

tolerated. I would agree but for slightly different reasons. When carefully adjusted, lithium is fairly well tolerated; however, in older subjects careful adjustment of lithium can be quite complicated. Its use in the elderly should be restricted to experts familiar with lithium. As a consequence, adjunctive lithium is a Category 2 adjunctive agent. For similar reasons, complicated administration and safety issues, nortriptyline is a Category 2 agent.

A number of agents comprise Category 3. These agents have some evidence of efficacy in mixed-age patients, some experience in older patients has been reported and/or they are relatively well tolerated and easily administered. Stimulant agents—dextroamphetamine and methylphenidate, omega-3 (several positive adjunctive trials in mixed-age patients and good tolerability), and SAMe (a single well-described controlled trial in treatment-resistant, mixed-age patients and good tolerability)—would be included in this Category 3. Inclusion of adjunctive thyroid in Category 3 is marginal. The meta-analysis of controlled trials in mixed-age patients was negative. In the only positive placebo-controlled trial, patients were receiving tricyclic agents, and treatment resistance was not established. In addition, there is essentially no published experience with T3 in older depressed patients. Controlled trials of adjunctive buspirone, pindolol, galantamine, estrogen, and testosterone indicate lack of efficacy. Adjunctive use of donepezil for prophylaxis in previously depressed older adults with MCI may increase risk of depressive relapse.

Adjunctive Treatment of Specific Residual Symptoms

In patients who have responded but not remitted and have prominent residual symptoms, agents that target specific symptoms may be selected. In some cases, agents that are approved for use for specific symptoms, for example, antianxiety agents, may be useful even if not specifically studied in depressed patients (Menza, Marin, & Opper, 2003). Hypnotic agents can improve sleep disturbance. Evidence with eszopiclone (Fava, 2006) and trazodone (Nierenberg, Adler, Peselow, Zornberg, & Rosenthal, 1994; Nierenberg, Cole, & Glass, 1992) suggest these agents may help sleep and improve depression. Modafinil appears to reduce drowsiness and fatigue in depressed patients with a partial response to SSRIs (Fava et al., 2007). Dextroamphetamine

and methylphenidate have also been used for this purpose without controlled supporting data.

Treatment of anxious residual symptoms may be more challenging. As Salzman (2004) has noted, treatment of anxiety in late life has been woefully understudied. SSRIs have been considered the treatment of choice for several anxiety disorders and in older patients (Flint, 2005); yet in depressed patients with residual symptoms, the patient is usually receiving an SSRI or SNRI. If the patient were taking bupropion, adding an SSRI for residual anxiety might make logical sense. Aripiprazole has been reported to be effective for both anxious and nonanxious, mixed-age depressed patients (Trivedi et al., 2008), and a growing literature describes the use of atypical antipsychotics in anxiety disorders (Vulink, Figee, & Denys, 2011). Reports of their use for residual anxiety in depressed patients are limited to open-label studies in mixed-age patients. While buspirone has not been effective for adjunctive treatment of depression (see earlier), its efficacy for anxiety symptoms suggests it might be considered for residual symptoms. Benzodiazepines have been used in depressed patients with anxiety, although these agents can pose problems in the elderly. They can contribute to gait disturbance and falls (Landi et al., 2005), although this problem plagues other psychotropic agents. Withdrawal of benzodiazepines in elderly patients can be quite difficult. Finally, amnestic problems can develop during benzodiazepine use (Chavant, Favrelière, Lafay-Chebassier, Plazanet, & Pérault-Pochat, 2011) and older patients may be more vulnerable to these effects. These memory deficits may be subtle, develop gradually, and either go undetected or be mistaken for dementia. Pregabalin has emerged as another potential treatment for anxiety symptoms. Several placebo-controlled trials in mixed-age patients with generalized anxiety disorder indicate efficacy that appears comparable to that of the antidepressant drugs (Baldwin, Woods, Lawson, & Taylor, 2011). A single, placebo-controlled, 8-week trial (N = 273) found evidence of efficacy in generalized anxiety disorder patients 65 years and older (Montgomery, Chatamra, Pauer, Whalen, & Baldinetti, 2008). Doses in the study ranged from 150 to 600 mg/day. Pregabalin appeared well tolerated; the discontinuation rate for adverse events was similar for drug and placebo (10.7% vs. 9.4%). A meta-analysis of fixed dose studies found the optimal dose in mixed-age generalized anxiety disorder patients to be from 200 to 450 mg/day. In this analysis doses of 150 mg/day were less effective, and doses of 600 mg/day did not increase efficacy (Bech, 2007). To my knowledge, augmentation trials of pregabalin in depression have not been reported; however, given the apparent advantageous side effect profile, this might be a useful agent for residual symptoms of anxiety.

Adjunctive Treatment for Patients With Minimal Initial Response

Most algorithms and guidelines suggest that patients showing minimal response to the first antidepressant should be switched to another agent (APA Guideline for Major Depression, 2010; Mulsant et al., 2001). This is based on logical and practical considerations. First, since little improvement occurred, there is little to lose by stopping the first agent. Second, monotherapy with a second agent may be better tolerated and more easily adjusted than adjunctive therapy, especially in an older patient. And finally monotherapy may be less costly and reduce risk of drug interactions. However, there is little empirical evidence addressing the question of efficacy in minimal responders. We recently performed a secondary analysis of adjunctive aripiprazole in 746 depressed patients who had less than 25% improvement during the initial antidepressant trial (Nelson et al., 2012). The actual drug effect (based on the drug-placebo difference in response rates) was large in this group, NNT = 6. Similar to the results in the full sample, most of the change occurred in the first 2 weeks. It is unclear if these rapid effects were simply the result of aripiprazole itself or if initial antidepressant treatment, though ineffective clinically, resulted in neurochemical changes that "primed the pump." To my knowledge, this study is the first to examine response to an adjunctive agent in patients with minimal response to initial treatment. Given the limited data, it is not possible to make broad recommendations for the use of adjunctive treatments in minimal responders. The potential value of atypical antipsychotics, and aripiprazole in particular, might be kept in mind especially because of the rapid effects. It might be worth noting that the first report of adjunctive atypical use found rapid effects when risperidone was given to fairly severely depressed patients, most of whom had shown *minimal response* to the initial antidepressant and were being evaluated for ECT (Ostroff & Nelson, 1999).

SUMMARY

Several adjunctive treatments appear to be useful in older depressed adults as they are in mixed-age patients. They are helpful in those with partial response to initial treatment, and selected agents may be useful for specific residual symptoms. Evidence for the use of atypical agents in minimal responders to initial treatment is preliminary. While resistance to initial antidepressant treatment is common in older depressed adults, studies of sequential trials suggest relatively high remission rates if patients and clinicians are persistent.

Disclosures
During the past 12 months, Dr. Nelson has served as a consultant to Bristol Myers Squibb, Cenestra Health, Corcept, Eli Lilly, Forest, Lundbeck, Medtronic, Merck, Mylan Specialty, Otsuka, Pfizer, Sunovion, and Theracos; he has served on advisory boards for Avanir, Bristol Myers Squibb, and Eli Lilly; he has received lecture honoraria from Otsuka Asia but is not on a US Speakers Bureau; he receives research support from NIMH and HRSA.

REFERENCES

Abolfazli, R., Hosseini, M., Ghanizadeh, A., Ghaleiha, A., Tabrizi, M., Raznahan, M.,...Akhondzadeh, S. (2011). Double-blind randomized parallel-group clinical trial of efficacy of the combination fluoxetine plus modafinil versus fluoxetine plus placebo in the treatment of major depression. *Depression and Anxiety, 28*(4), 297–302.

Akhondzadeh, S., Jafari, S., Raisi, F., Nasehi, A. A., Ghoreishi, A., Salehi, B.,...Kamalipour, A. (2009). Clinical trial of adjunctive celecoxib treatment in patients with major depression: A double blind and placebo controlled trial. *Depression and Anxiety, 26*(7), 607–611.

Alexopoulos, G. S., Canuso, C. M., Gharabawi, G. M., Bossie, C. A., Greenspan, A., Turkoz, I., & Reynolds, C. F., III. (2008). Placebo-controlled study of relapse prevention with risperidone augmentation in older patients with resistant depression. *American Journal of Geriatric Psychiatry, 16*(1), 21–30.

Alexopoulos, G. S., Katz, I. R., Bruce, M. L., Heo, M., Ten Have, T., Raue, P.,...PROSPECT Group. (2005). Remission in depressed geriatric primary care patients: A report from the PROSPECT study. *American Journal of Psychiatry, 162*(4), 718–724.

Alexopoulos, G. S., Meyers, B. S., Young, R. C., Campbell, S., Silbersweig, D., & Charlson, M. (1997). `Vascular depression' hypothesis. *Archive of General Psychiatry, 54,* 915–922.

Almeida, O. P., Lautenschlager, N. T., Vasikaran, S., Leedman, P., Gelavis, A., & Flicker, L. (2006). A 20-week randomized controlled trial of estradiol replacement therapy for women aged 70 years and older: Effect on mood, cognition and quality of life. *Neurobiology of Aging, 27*(1), 141–149.

Altshuler, L. L., Bauer, M., Frye, M. A., Gitlin, M. J., Mintz, J., Szuba, M. P., . . . Whybrow, P. C. (2001). Does thyroid supplementation accelerate tricyclic antidepressant response? A review and meta-analysis of the literature. *American Journal of Psychiatry, 158*(10), 1617–1622.

American Psychiatric Association. (2010). Practice guideline for the treatment of patients with major depressive disorder. *American Journal of Psychiatry, 167,* A34.

Appelberg, B. G., Syvälahti, E. K., Koskinen, T. E., Mehtonen, O. P., Muhonen, T. T., & Naukkarinen, H. H. (2001). Patients with severe depression may benefit from buspirone augmentation of selective serotonin reuptake inhibitors: Results from a placebo-controlled, randomized, double-blind, placebo wash-in study. *Journal of Clinical Psychiatry, 62*(6), 448–452.

Areán, P. A., Gum, A., McCulloch, C. E., Bostrom, A., Gallagher-Thompson, D., & Thompson, L. (2005). Treatment of depression in low-income older adults. *Psychology and Aging, 20*(4), 601–609.

Areán, P. A., Raue, P., Mackin, R. S., Kanellopoulos, D., McCulloch, C., & Alexopoulos, G. S. (2010). Problem-solving therapy and supportive therapy in older adults with major depression and executive dysfunction. *American Journal of Psychiatry, 167*(11), 1391–1398.

Aronson, R., Offman, H. J., Joffe, R. T., & Naylor, C. D. (1996). Triiodothyronine augmentation in the treatment of refractory depression. A meta-analysis. *Archives of General Psychiatry, 53*(9), 842–848.

Ayd, F., & Zohar, J. (1987). Psychostimulant (amphetamine or methylphenidate) therapy for chronic and treatment-resistant depression. In J Zohar & R. H. Belmaker (Eds.), *Treating resistant depression* (pp. 343–355). New York: PMA Publishing.

Baldwin, D., Woods, R., Lawson, R., & Taylor, D. (20110> Efficacy of drug treatments for generalised anxiety disorder: Systematic review and meta-analysis. *British Medical Journal. 342,* d1199.

Bauer, M., Bschor, T., Kunz, D., Berghöfer, A., Ströhle, A., & Müller-Oerlinghausen, B.(2000). Double-blind, placebo-controlled trial of the use of lithium to augment antidepressant medication in continuation treatment of unipolar major depression. *American Journal of Psychiatry, 157*(9), 1429–1435.

Bech, P. (2007). Dose-response relationship of pregabalin in patients with generalized anxiety disorder. A pooled analysis of four placebo-controlled trials. *Pharmacopsychiatry, 40*(4), 163–168.

Berman, R. M., Hazel, J., Swanink, R., McQuade, R. D., Carson, W. H., & Marcus, R. N. (2008, May 3–6). *Long term safety and tolerability of open-label aripiprazole augmentation of antidepressant therapy in major depressive disorder (Study CN138–164).* Paper presented at the 161st Annual Meeting of the American Psychiatric Association, Washington, DC.

Blazer, D., Hughes, D. C., & George, L. K. (1987). The epidemiology of depression in an elderly community population. *Gerontologist, 27,* 281–287.

Blier, P., Gobbi, G., Turcotte, J. E., de Montigny, C., Boucher, N., Hébert, C., & Debonnel, G. (2009). Mirtazapine and paroxetine in major depression: A comparison of monotherapy versus their combination from treatment initiation. *European Neuropsychopharmacology, 19*(7), 457–465.

Blier, P., Ward, H. E., Tremblay, P., Laberge, L., Hébert, C., & Bergeron, R. (2010). Combination of antidepressant medications from treatment initiation for major depressive disorder: A double-blind randomized study. *American Journal of Psychiatry, 167*(3), 281–288.

Bodkin, J. A., Zornberg, G. L., Lukas, S. E., & Cole, J. O. (1995). Buprenorphine treatment of refractory depression. *Journal of Clinical Psychopharmacology, 15*(1), 49–57.

Bondareff, W., Alpert, M., Friedhoff, A. J., Richter, E. M., Clary, C. M., & Batzar, E. (2000). Comparison of sertraline and nortriptyline in the treatment of major depressive disorder in late life. *American Journal of Psychiatry, 157,* 729–736.

Bressa, G. M. (1994). S-adenosyl-l-methionine (SAMe) as antidepressant: Meta-analysis of clinical studies. *Acta Neurologica Scandinavica Supplement, 154,* 7–14

Bruce, M. L., Leaf, P. J., Rozal, G. P., Florio, L., & Hoff, R. A. (1994). Psychiatric status and 9-year mortality data in the New Haven Epidemiologic

Catchment Area Study. *American Journal of Psychiatry, 151*(5), 716–721.

Bruce, M. L., Seeman, T. E., Merrill, S. S., & Blazer, D. G. (1994). The impact of depressive symptomatology on physical disability: MacArthur Studies of Successful Aging. *American Journal of Public Health, 84*, 1796–1799.

Carpenter, L. L., Yasmin, S., & Price, L. H. (2002). A double-blind, placebo-controlled study of antidepressant augmentation with mirtazapine. *Biological Psychiatry, 51*(2), 183–188.

Chavant, F., Favrelière, S., Lafay-Chebassier, C., Plazanet, C., & Pérault-Pochat, M. C. (2011). Memory disorders associated with consumption of drugs: Updating through a case/noncase study in the French PharmacoVigilance Database. *British Journal of Clinical Pharmacology, 72*(6), 898–904.

Connolly, K. R., & Thase, M. E. (2011)If at first you don't succeed: A review of the evidence for antidepressant augmentation, combination, and switching strategies. *Drugs, 71*(1), 43–64.

Conwell, Y. (2004). Suicide. In S. P. Roose & H. A. Sackeim (Eds.), *Late life depression* (pp. 95–114). Oxford, England: Oxford University Press.

Cooper, C., Katona, C., Lyketsos, K., Blazer, D., Brodaty, H., Rabins, P.,...Livingston, G. (2011). A systematic review of treatments for refractory depression in older people. *American Journal of Psychiatry, 168*(7), 681–688.

Coppen, A., & Bailey, J. (2000). Enhancement of the antidepressant action of fluoxetine by folic acid: A randomised, placebo controlled trial. *Journal of Affective Disorders, 60*(2), 121–130.

Corya, S. A., Andersen, S. W., Detke, H. C., Kelly, L. S., Van Campen, L. E., Sanger, T. M.,...Dubé, S. (2003). Long-term antidepressant efficacy and safety of olanzapine/fluoxetine combination: A 76-week open-label study. *Journal of Clinical Psychiatry, 64*, 1349–1356.

Crossley, N. A., & Bauer, M. (2007). Acceleration and augmentation of antidepressants with lithium for depressive disorders: Two meta-analyses of randomized, placebo-controlled trials. *Journal of Clinical Psychiatry, 68*, 935–940.

Dantzer, R. (2006). Cytokine, sickness behavior, and depression. *Neurologic Clinics, 24*(3), 441–460.

Darvill, F. T., & Woolley, S. (1959). Double-blind evaluation of methylphenidate hydrochloride. *Journal of the American Medical Association, 169*, 1739–1741.

DeBattista, C., Doghramji, K., Menza, M. A., Rosenthal, M. H., Fieve, R. R., & Modafinil in Depression Study Group. (2003). Adjunct modafinil for the short-term treatment of fatigue and sleepiness in patients with major

depressive disorder: A preliminary double-blind, placebo-controlled study. *Journal of Clinical Psychiatry, 64*(9), 1057–1064.

Dew, M. A., Whyte, E. M., Lenze, E. J., Houck, P. R., Mulsant, B. H., Pollock, B. G.,...Reynolds, C. F., III. (2007). Recovery from major depression inolder adults receiving augmentation of antidepressant pharmacotherapy. *American Journal of Psychiatry, 164*, 892–899.

Dias, R. S., Kerr-Corrêa, F., Moreno, R. A., Trinca, L. A., Pontes, A., Halbe, H. W.,...Dalben, I. S. (2006). Efficacy of hormone therapy with and without methyltestosterone augmentation of venlafaxine in the treatment of postmenopausal depression: A double-blind controlled pilot study. *Menopause, 13*(2), 202–211.

Drevets, W. C., & Furey, M. L. (2010). Replication of scopolamine's antidepressant efficacy in major depressive disorder: A randomized, placebo-controlled clinical trial. *Biological Psychiatry, 67*(5), 432–438.

Dube, A. H., Osgood, C. K., & Notkin, H. (1956). The effects of an analeptic (Ritalin), an ataraxic (reserpine) and a placebo in senile states. *Journal of Chronic Disorders, 5*, 220–234.

Dunlop, B. W., Crits-Christoph, P., Evans, D. L., Hirschowitz, J., Solvason, H. B., Rickels, K.,...Ninan, P. T. (2007). Coadministration of modafinil and a selective serotonin reuptake inhibitor from the initiation of treatment of major depressive disorder with fatigue and sleepiness: A double-blind, placebo-controlled study. *Journal of Clinical Psychopharmacology, 27*(6), 614–619.

Emrich, H. M., Vogt, P., & Herz, A. (1982). Possible antidepressive effects of opioids: Action of buprenorphine. *Annals of the New York Academy of Sciences, 398*, 108–112.

Fava, M., Thase, M. E., & DeBattista, C. (2005). A multicenter, placebo-controlled study of modafinil augmentation in partial responders to selective serotonin reuptake inhibitors with persistent fatigue and sleepiness. *Journal of Clinical Psychiatry, 66*(1), 85–93.

Fava, M., Thase, M. E., DeBattista, C., Doghramji, K., Arora, S., & Hughes, R. J. (2007). Modafinil augmentation of selective serotonin reuptake inhibitor therapy in MDD partial responders with persistent fatigue and sleepiness. *Annals of Clinical Psychiatry, 19*(3), 153–159.

Fava, M., McCall, W. V., Krystal, A., Wessel, T., Rubens, R., Caron, J.,...Roth, T. (2006). Eszopiclone co-administered with fluoxetine in patients with insomnia coexisting with major depressive disorder. *Biological Psychiatry, 59*(11), 1052–1060.

Fawcett, J., Kravitz, H. M., Zajecka, J. M., & Schaff, M. R. (1991). CNS stimulant potentiation of monoamine oxidase inhibitors in treatment-refractory depression. *Journal of Clinical Psychopharmacology, 11*, 127–132.

Fawcett, J., & Siomopoulos, V. (1971). Dexamphetamine response as a possible predictor of improvement with tricyclic therapy in depression. *Archives of General Psychiatry, 25*, 247–255.

Fields, C., Drye, L., Vaidya, V., & Lyketsos, C., for the ADAPT Research Group. (2011). Celecoxib or Naproxen treatment does not benefit depressive symptoms in persons age 70 and older: Findings from a randomized controlled trial. *American Journal of Geriatric Psychiatry*, ePub ahead of print.

Finch, E. J. L., & Katona, C. L. E. (1989). Lithium augmentation in the treatment of refractory depression in old age. *International Journal of Geriatric Psychiatry, 4*, 41–46.

Flint, A. J. (2005). Generalised anxiety disorder in elderly patients : Epidemiology, diagnosis and treatment options. *Drugs and Aging, 22*(2), 101–114.

Flint, A. J., & Rifat, S. L. (1994). A prospective study of lithium augmentation in antidepressant-resistant geriatric depression. *Journal of Clinical Psychopharmacology, 14*(5), 353–356.

Forester, B. P., Streeter, C. C., Berlow, Y. A., Tian, H., Wardrop, M., Finn, C. T., ... Moore, C. M. (2009). Brain lithium levels and effects on cognition and mood in geriatric bipolar disorder: A lithium-7 magnetic resonance spectroscopy study. *American Journal of Geriatric Psychiatry, 17*(1), 13–23.

Fredman, S. J., Fava, M., Kienke, A. S., White, C. N., Nierenberg, A. A., & Rosenbaum, J. F. (2000). Partial response, nonresponse, and relapse with selective serotonin reuptake inhibitors in major depression: A survey of current "next-step" practices. *Journal of Clinical Psychiatry, 61*(6), 403–408.

Gu, Y., Liang, X., Wu, W., Song, S., Cheng, L., Bo, L., ... Yao, K. (2009). Multicenter contraceptive efficacy trial of injectable testosterone undecanoate in Chinese men. *Journal of Clinical Endocrinology and Metabolism, 94*(6), 1910–1915.

Halikas, J. A. (1995). Org 3770 (mirtazapine) versus trazodone: A placebo controlled trial in depressed elderly patients. *Human Psychopharmacology, 10*(Suppl 2), S125–S133.

Hamilton, M. (1960). A rating scale for depression. *Journal of Neurology, Neurosurgery, and Psychiatry, 23*, 56–61.

Hewett, K., Chrzanowski, W., Jokinen, R., Felgentreff, R., Shrivastava, R. K., Gee, M. D., ... Modell, J. G. (2010). Double-blind, placebo-controlled evaluation of extended-release bupropion in elderly patients with major depressive disorder. *Journal of Psychopharmacology, 24*(4), 521–529

Holliday, A. R., & Joffe, J. R. (1965). A controlled evaluation of protriptyline compared to placebo and to methylphenidate (abstr). *Journal of New Drugs, 5*, 257–258.

Holtzheimer, P. E., III, Meeks, T. W., Kelley, M. E., Mufti, M., Young, R., McWhorter, K., ... McDonald, W. M. (2008). A double blind, placebo-controlled pilot study of galantamine augmentation of antidepressant treatment in older adults with major depression. *International Journal of Geriatric Psychiatry, 23*(6), 625–631.

Janowsky, D. S., el-Yousef, M. K., Davis, J. M., & Sekerke, H. J. (1972). A cholinergic-adrenergic hypothesis of mania and depression. *Lancet, 2*(7778), 632–635.

Jean-Pierre, P., Morrow, G. R., Roscoe, J. A., Heckler, C., Mohile, S., Janelsins, M., ... Hopkins, J. O. (2010). A phase 3 randomized, placebo-controlled, double-blind, clinical trial of the effect of modafinil on cancer-related fatigue among 631 patients receiving chemotherapy: A University of Rochester Cancer Center Community Clinical Oncology Program Research base study. *Cancer, 116*(14), 3513–3520.

Jeste, D. V., Caligiuri, M. P., Paulsen, J. S., Heaton, R. K., Lacro, J. P., Harris, M. J., ... McAdams, L. A. (1995). Risk of tardive dyskinesia in older patients. A prospective longitudinal study of 266 outpatients. *Archives of General Psychiatry, 52*(9), 756–765.

Joffe, R. T., Singer, W., Levitt, A. J., & MacDonald, C. (1993). A placebo-controlled comparison of lithium and triiodothyronine augmentation of tricyclic antidepressants in unipolar refractory depression. *Archives of General Psychiatry, 50*, 387–393.

Joffe, R. T., Sokolov, S. T., & Levitt, A. J. (2006). Lithium and triiodothyronine augmentation of antidepressants. *Canadian Journal of Psychiatry, 51*(12), 791–793.

Kanayama, G., Amiaz, R., Seidman, S., & Pope, H. G., Jr. (2007). Testosterone supplementation for depressed men: Current research and suggested treatment guidelines. *Experimental and Clinical Psychopharmacology, 15*(6), 529–538.

Kaplitz, S. (1975). Withdrawn, apathetic geriatric patients responsive to methylphenidate. *Journal of the American Geriatrics Society, 23*, 271–276.

Katz, I. R., Simpson, G. M., Curlik, S. M., Parmelee, P. A., & Muhly, C. (1990). Pharmacologic treatment of major depression for elderly patients in residential care settings. *Journal of Clinical Psychiatry, 51*(Suppl), 41–47; discussion 48.

Kok, R. M., Nolen, W. A., & Heeren, T. J. (2009). Outcome of late-life depression after 3 years of sequential treatment. *Acta Psychiatrica Scandinavica, 119*, 274–281.

Kok, R. M., Vink, D., Heeren, T. J., & Nolen, W. A. (2007). Lithium augmentation compared with phenelzine in treatment-resistant depression in the elderly: An open, randomized, controlled trial. *Journal of Clinical Psychiatry, 68*(8), 1177–1185.

Lafferman, J., Solomon, K., & Ruskin, P. (1988). Lithium augmentation for treatment-resistant depression in the elderly. *Journal of Geriatric Psychiatry and Neurology, 1*(1), 49–52.

Landén, M., Björling, G., Agren, H., & Fahlén, T. (1998). A randomized, double-blind, placebo-controlled trial of buspirone in combination with an SSRI in patients with treatment-refractory depression. *Journal of Clinical Psychiatry, 59*(12), 664–668.

Landi, F., Onder, G., Cesari, M., Barillaro, C., Russo, A., Bernabei, R., & Silver Network Home Care Study Group. (2005). Psychotropic medications and risk for falls among community-dwelling frail older people: An observational study. *Journals of Gerontology Series A, Biological Science Medical Science, 60*(5), 622–626.

Landman, M. E., Preisig, R., & Perlmann, M. (1958). A practical mood stimulant. *Journal of the Medical Society of New Jersey, 55*, 55–58.

Lavretsky, H., Kim, M. D., Kumar, A., & Reynolds, C. F., III. (2003). Combined treatment with methylphenidate and citalopram for accelerated response in the elderly: An open trial. *Journal of Clinical Psychiatry, 64*(12), 1410–1414.

Lavretsky, H., Park, S., Siddarth, P., Kumar, A., & Reynolds, C. F., III. (2006). Methylphenidate-enhanced antidepressant response to citalopram in the elderly: A double-blind, placebo-controlled pilot trial. *American Journal of Geriatric Psychiatry, 14*(2), 181–185.

Lenze, E. J., Skidmore, E. R., Begley, A. E., Newcomer, J. W., Butters, M. A., & Whyte, E. M. (2011). Memantine for late-life depression and apathy after a disabling medical event: A 12-week, double-blind placebo-controlled pilot study. *International Journal of Geriatric Psychiatry, 27*(9), 974–980.

Leuchter, A. F., Husain, M. M., Cook, I. A., Trivedi, M. H., Wisniewski, S. R., Gilmer, W. S.,...Rush, A. J. (2010). Painful physical symptoms and treatment outcome in major depressive disorder: A STAR*D (Sequenced Treatment Alternatives to Relieve Depression) report. *Psychology in Medicine, 40*(2), 239–251.

Mackin, R. S., & Areán, P. A. (2005). Evidence-based psychotherapeutic interventions for geriatric depression. *Psychiatric Clinics of North America, 28*(4), 805–820.

Masand, P., Anand, V. S., & Tanquary, J. F. (1998). Psychostimulant augmentation of second generation antidepressants: A case series. *Depression and Anxiety, 7*, 89–91.

Masand, P., Pickett, P., & Murray, G. B. (1991). Psychostimulants for secondary depression in medical illness. *Psychosomatics, 32*, 203–208.

Mendlewicz, J., Kriwin, P., Oswald, P., Souery, D., Alboni, S., & Brunello, N. (2006). Shortened onset of action of antidepressants in major depression using acetylsalicylic acid augmentation: A pilot open-label study. *International Clinical Psychopharmacology, 21*(4), 227–231.

Menza, M., Marin, H., & Opper, R. S. (2003). Residual symptoms in depression: can treatment be symptom-specific? *Journal of Clinical Psychiatry, 64*(5), 516–523.

Meyers, B. S., Flint, A. J., Rothschild, A. J., Mulsant, B. H., Whyte, E. M., Peasley-Miklus, C.,...STOP-PD Group. (2009). A double-blind randomized controlled trial of Olanzapine plus Sertraline vs Olanzapine plus placebo for psychotic depression: The study of pharmacotherapy of psychotic depression (STOP-PD). *Archives of General Psychiatry, 66*(8), 838–847.

Montgomery, S. A., & Asberg, M. (1979). A new depression scale designed to be sensitive to change. *British Journal of Psychiatry, 134*, 382–389

Moreno, F. A., Gelenberg, A. J., Bachar, K., & Delgado, P. L. (1997). Pindolol augmentation of treatment-resistant depressed patients. *Journal of Clinical Psychiatry, 58*(10), 437–439.

Morrison, M. F., Kallan, M. J., Ten Have, T., Katz, I., Tweedy, K., & Battistini, M. (2004). Lack of efficacy of estradiol for depression in postmenopausal women: A randomized, controlled trial. *Biological Psychiatry, 55*(4), 406–412.

Montgomery, S., Chatamra, K., Pauer, L., Whalen, E., & Baldinetti, F. (2008). Efficacy and safety of pregabalin in elderly people with generalised anxiety disorder. *British Journal of Psychiatry, 193*(5), 389–394.

Müller, N., Schwarz, M. J., Dehning, S., Douhe, A., Cerovecki, A., Goldstein-Müller, B.,...Riedel, M. (2006). The cyclooxygenase-2 inhibitor celecoxib has therapeutic effects in major depression:

Results of a double-blind, randomized, placebo controlled, add-on pilot study to reboxetine. *Molecular Psychiatry, 11*(7), 680–684.

Mulsant, B. H., Alexopoulos, G. S., Reynolds, C. F., Katz, I. R., Abrams, R., Oslin, D.,...PROSPECT Study Group. (2001). Pharmacological treatment of depression in older primary care patients: The PROSPECT algorithm. *International Journal of Geriatric Psychiatry, 16*, 585–592.

Murray, G. B., & Cassem, E. (1998). Use of stimulants in depressed patients with medical illness. In J. C. Nelson (Ed.), *Geriatric psychopharmacology* (pp. 245–257). New York: Marcel Dekker.

Nelson, J. C. (1987). The use of antipsychotic drugs in the treatment of depression. In J. Zohar & R. H. Belmaker (Eds.), *Treating resistant depression* (pp. 131–146). New York: PMA.

Nelson, J. C. (1997). Augmentation strategies for treatment of unipolar major depression. In A. J. Rush (Ed.), *Mood disorders, systematic medication management, modern problems of pharmacopsychiatry* (Vol 25., pp. 34–55). Basel, Switzerland: Karger.

Nelson, J. C., Delucchi, K., & Schneider, L. S. (2008). The efficacy of second generation antidepressants in late life depression: A meta-analysis. *American Journal of Geriatric Psychiatry, 16*, 558–567.

Nelson, J. C., Mazure, C. M., & Jatlow, P. I. (1995). Desipramine treatment of major depression in patients over 75 years of age. *Journal of Clinical Psychopharmacology, 15*, 99–105.

Nelson, J. C., & Papakostas, G. (2009). Atypical antipsychotic augmentation in major depressive disorder: A meta-analysis of placebo-controlled random assignment trials. *American Journal of Psychiatry, 166*(9), 980–991.

Nelson, J. C., Thase, M. E., Bellocchio, E. E., Rollin, L. M., Eudicone, J. M., McQuade. R. D.,...Baker, R. A. (2012). Efficacy of adjunctive aripiprazole in patients with major depressive disorder who showed minimal response to initial antidepressant therapy. *International Clinical Psychopharmacology, 27*(3), 125–133.

Nery, F. G., Monkul, E. S., Hatch, J. P., Fonseca, M., Zunta-Soares, G. B., Frey, B. N.,...Soares, J. C. (2008). Celecoxib as an adjunct in the treatment of depressive or mixed episodes of bipolar disorder: A double-blind, randomized, placebo-controlled study. *Human Psychopharmacology, 23*(2), 87–94.

Nierenberg, A. A., Adler, L. A., Peselow, E., Zornberg, G., & Rosenthal, M. (1994). Trazodone for antidepressant-associated insomnia. *American Journal of Psychiatry, 151*(7), 1069–1072.

Nierenberg, A. A., Cole, J. O., & Glass, L. (1992). Possible trazodone potentiation of fluoxetine: A case series. *Journal of Clinical Psychiatry, 53*(3), 83–85.

Nierenberg, A. A., Fava, M., Trivedi, M. H., Wisniewski, S. R., Thase, M. E., McGrath, P. J.,...Rush, A. J. (2006). A comparison of lithium and T(3) augmentation following two failed medication treatments for depression: A STAR*D report. *American Journal of Psychiatry, 163*(9), 1519–1530.

Nierenberg, A. A., Papakostas, G. I., Petersen, T., Montoya, H. D., Worthington, J. J., Tedlow, J.,...Fava, M. (2003). Lithium augmentation of nortriptyline for subjects resistant to multiple antidepressants. *Journal of Clinical Psychopharmacology, 23*(1), 92–95.

Onder, E., & Tural, U. (2003). Faster response in depressive patients treated with fluoxetine alone than in combination with buspirone. *Journal of Affective Disorders, 76*(1–3), 223–227.

Orengo, C. A., Fullerton, L., & Kunik, M. E. (2005). Safety and efficacy of testosterone gel 1% augmentation in depressed men with partial response to antidepressant therapy. *Journal of Geriatric Psychiatry and Neurology, 18*(1), 20–24.

Ostroff, R. B., & Nelson, J. C. (1999). Risperidone augmentation of selective serotonin reuptake inhibitors in major depression. *Journal of Clinical Psychiatry, 60*, 256–259.

Papakostas, G. I., Mischoulon, D., Shyu, I., Alpert, J. E., & Fava, M. (2010). S-adenosyl methionine (SAMe) augmentation of serotonin reuptake inhibitors for antidepressant nonresponders with major depressive disorder: A double-blind, randomized clinical trial. *American Journal of Psychiatry, 167*(8), 942–948.

Patkar, A. A., Masand, P. S., Pae, C. U., Peindl, K., Hooper-Wood, C., Mannelli, P., & Ciccone, P. (2006). A randomized, double-blind, placebo-controlled trial of augmentation with an extended release formulation of methylphenidate in outpatients with treatment-resistant depression. *Journal of Clinical Psychopharmacology, 26*(6), 653–656.

Pérez, V., Soler, J., Puigdemont, D., Alvarez, E., & Artigas, F. (1999). A double-blind, randomized, placebo-controlled trial of pindolol augmentation in depressive patients resistant to serotonin reuptake inhibitors. Grup de Recerca en Trastorns Afectius. *Archives of General Psychiatry, 56*(4), 375–379.

Pope, H. G., Jr., Amiaz, R., Brennan, B. P., Orr, G., Weiser, M., Kelly, J. F.,...Seidman, S. N. (2010). Parallel-group placebo-controlled trial of testosterone gel in men with major depressive disorder displaying an incomplete response to standard antidepressant treatment. *Journal of Clinical Psychopharmacology, 30*(2), 126–134.

Pope, H. G., Jr., Cohane, G. H., Kanayama, G., Siegel, A. J., & Hudson, J. I. (2003). Testosterone gel supplementation for men with refractory depression: A randomized, placebo-controlled trial. *American Journal of Psychiatry, 160*(1), 105–111.

Portella, M. J., de Diego-Adeliño, J., Ballesteros, J., Puigdemont, D., Oller, S., Santos, B., ... Pérez, V. (2011). Can we really accelerate and enhance the selective serotonin reuptake inhibitor antidepressant effect: A randomized clinical trial and a meta-analysis of pindolol in nonresistant depression. *Journal of Clinical Psychiatry, 72*(7), 962–969.

Pratt, L. A., Ford, D. E., Crum, R. M., Armenian, H. K., Gallo, J. J., & Eaton, W. W. (1996). Depression, psychotropic medication, and risk of myocardial infarction: Prospective data from the Baltimore ECA follow-up. *Circulation, 94*, 3123–3129.

Pulska, T., Pahkala, K., Laippalla, P., & Kivela, S. L. (1998). Major depression as a predictor of premature deaths in elderly people in Finland: A community study. *Acta Psychiatrica Scandinavica, 97*(6), 408–411.

Rabkin, J. G., Gordon, P. H., McElhiney, M., Rabkin, R., Chew, S., & Mitsumoto, H. (2009). Modafinil treatment of fatigue in patients with ALS: A placebo-controlled study. *Muscle and Nerve, 39*(3), 297–303.

Rabkin, J. G., Wagner, G. J., McElhiney, M. C., Rabkin, R., & Lin, S. H. (2004). Testosterone versus fluoxetine for depression and fatigue in HIV/AIDS: A placebo-controlled trial. *Journal of Clinical Psychopharmacology, 24*(4), 379–385.

Rabkin, J. G., Wagner, G. J., & Rabkin, R. (2000). A double-blind, placebo-controlled trial of testosterone therapy for HIV-positive men with hypogonadal symptoms. *Archives of General Psychiatry, 57*(2), 141–147.

Rasgon, N. L., Altshuler, L. L., Fairbanks, L. A., Dunkin, J. J., Davtyan, C., Elman, S., & Rapkin, A. J. (2002). Estrogen replacement therapy in the treatment of major depressive disorder in perimenopausal women. *Journal of Clinical Psychiatry, 63*(Suppl 7), 45–48.

Ravindran, A. V., Kennedy, S. H., O'Donovan, M. C., Fallu, A., Camacho, F., & Binder, C. E. (2008). Osmotic-release oral system methylphenidate augmentation of antidepressant monotherapy in major depressive disorder: Results of a double-blind, randomized, placebo-controlled trial. *Journal of Clinical Psychiatry, 69*(1), 87–94.

Reynolds, C. F., Butters, M. A., Lopez, O., Pollock, B. G., Dew, M. A., Mulsant, B. H., ... DeKosky, S. T. (2011). Maintenance treatment of depression in old age: A randomized, double-blind, placebo-controlled evaluation of the efficacy and safety of donepezil combined with antidepressant pharmacotherapy. *Archives of General Psychiatry, 68*(1), 51–60.

Reynolds, C. F., Frank, E., Kupfer, D. J., Thase, M. E., Perel, J. M., Mazumdar, S., & Houck, P. R. (1996). Treatment outcome in recurrent major depression: a post hoc comparison of elderly ("young old") and midlife patients. *American Journal of Psychiatry, 153*(10), 1288–1292.

Rush, A. J., Trivedi, M. H., Stewart, J. W., Nierenberg, A. A., Fava, M., Kurian, B. T., ... Wisniewski, S. R. (2011). Combining medications to enhance depression outcomes (CO-MED), acute and long-term outcomes of a single-blind randomized study. *American Journal of Psychiatry, 168*(7), 689–701.

Rutherford, B., Sneed, J., Miyazaki, M., Eisenstadt, R., Devanand, D., Sackeim, H., & Roose, S. (2007). An open trial of aripiprazole augmentation for SSRI nonremitters with late-life depression. *International Journal of Geriatric Psychiatry, 22*(10), 986–991.

Sackeim, H. A., Roose, S. P., & Lavori, P. W. (2006). Determining the duration of antidepressant treatment: Application of signal detection methodology and the need for duration adaptive designs (DAD). *Biological Psychiatry, 59*(6), 483–492.

Salzman, C. (2004). Late-life anxiety disorders. *Psychopharmacol Bulletin, 38*(1), 25–30.

Satel, S. L., & Nelson, J. C. (1989). Stimulants in the treatment of depression: a critical overview. *Journal of Clinical Psychiatry, 50*, 241–249.

Schneider, L. S., Small, G. W., & Clary, C. M. (2001). Estrogen replacement therapy and antidepressant response to sertraline in older depressed women. *American Journal of Geriatric Psychiatry, 9*, 393–399.

Schneider, L. S., Small, G. W., Hamilton, S. H., Bystritsky, A., Nemeroff, C. B., & Meyers, B. S. (1997). Estrogen replacement and response to fluoxetine in a multicenter geriatric depression trial. Fluoxetine Collaborative Study Group. *American Journal of Geriatric Psychiatry, 5*, 97–106.

Seidman, S. N., Miyazaki, M., & Roose, S. P. (2005). Intramuscular testosterone supplementation to selective serotonin reuptake inhibitor in treatment-resistant depressed men: Randomized placebo-controlled clinical trial. *Journal of Clinical Psychopharmacology*, 25(6), 584–588.

Seidman, S. N., Orr, G., Raviv, G., Levi, R., Roose, S. P., Kravitz, E., ... Weiser, M. (2009). Effects of testosterone replacement in middle-aged men with dysthymia: A randomized, placebo-controlled clinical trial. *Journal of Clinical Psychopharmacology*, 29(3), 216–221.

Seidman, S. N., & Roose, S. P. The sexual effects of testosterone replacement in depressed men: Randomized, placebo-controlled clinical trial. *Journal of Sex and Marital Therapy*, 32(3), 267–273.

Seidman, S. N., Spatz, E., Rizzo, C., & Roose, S. P. (2001). Testosterone replacement therapy for hypogonadal men with major depressive disorder: A randomized, placebo-controlled clinical trial. *Journal of Clinical Psychiatry*, 62(6), 406–412.

Sheffrin, M., Driscoll, H. P., Lenze, E. J., Mulsant, B. H., Pollock, B. G., Miller, M. D., ... Reynolds, C. F., III. (2009). Getting to remission: Use of aripiprazole for incomplete response in late-life depression. *Journal of Clinical Psychiatry*, 70(2), 208–213.

Shelton, R. C., Tollefson, G. D., Tohen, M., Stahl, S., Gannon, K. S., Jacobs, T. G., ... Meltzer, H. Y. (2001). A novel augmentation strategy for treating resistant major depression. *American Journal of Psychiatry*, 158, 131–134.

Shores, M. M., Kivlahan, D. R., Sadak, T. I., Li, E. J., & Matsumoto, A. M. (2009). A randomized, double-blind, placebo-controlled study of testosterone treatment in hypogonadal older men with subthreshold depression (dysthymia or minor depression). *Journal of Clinical Psychiatry*, 70(7), 1009–1016.

Simonsick, E. M., Wallace, R. B., Blazer, D. G., & Berkman, L. F. (1995). Depressive symptomatology and hypertension-associated morbidity and mortality in older adults. *Psychosomatic Medicine*, 57, 427–435.

Soares, C. N., Arsenio, H., Joffe, H., Bankier, B., Cassano, P., Petrillo, L. F., & Cohen, L. S. (2006). Escitalopram versus ethinyl estradiol and norethindrone acetate for symptomatic peri- and postmenopausal women: Impact on depression, vasomotor symptoms, sleep, and quality of life. *Menopause*, 13(5), 780–786.

Steffens, D. C., Nelson, J. C., Eudicone, J. M., Andersson, C., Yang, H., Tran, Q. V., ... Berman, R. M. (2011). Efficacy and safety of adjunctive aripiprazole in major depressive disorder in older patients: A pooled subpopulation analysis. *International Journal of Geriatric Psychiatry*, 26(6), 564–572.

Stewart, D. E., Rolfe, D. E., & Robertson, E. (2004). Depression, estrogen, and the Women's Health Initiative. *Psychosomatics*, 45(5), 445–447.

Stoll, A. L., Srinvasan, S. P., Diamond, L., Workum, S. B., & Cole, J. O. (1996). Methylphenidate augmentation of serotonin selective reuptake inhibitors: A case series. *Journal of Clinical Psychiatry*, 57, 72–76.

Sublette, M. E., Ellis, S. P., Geant, A. L., & Mann, J. J. (2011). Meta-analysis of the effects of eicosapentaenoic acid (EPA) in clinical trials in depression. *Journal of Clinical Psychiatry*, 72(12), 1577–1584.

Taragano, F. E., Allegri, R., Vicario, A., Bagnatti, P., & Lyketsos, C. G. (2001). A double blind, randomized clinical trial assessing the efficacy and safety of augmenting standard antidepressant therapy with nimodipine in the treatment of "vascular depression". *International Journal of Geriatric Psychiatry*, 16(3), 254–260.

Taragano, F. E., Bagnatti, P., & Allegri, R. F. (2005). A double-blind, randomized clinical trial to assess the augmentation with nimodipine of antidepressant therapy in the treatment of "vascular depression". *International Psychogeriatrics*, 17(3), 487–498.

Tardive dyskinesia: summary of a Task Force Report of the American Psychiatric Association. By the Task Force on Late Neurological Effects of Antipsychotic Drugs. (1980). *American Journal of Psychiatry*, 137(10), 1163–1172.

Trivedi, M. H., Cutler, A. J., Richards, C., Lasser, R., Geibel B., Gao J, Sambunaris A., Patkar A. (2011, May 14–18). *Efficacy and safety of lisdexamfetamine dimesylate as augmentation therapy in adults with major depressive disorder treated with an antidepressant.* Paper presented at the Annual Meeting of the American Psychiatric Association, Honolulu HI.

Trivedi, M. H., Fava, M., Wisniewski, S. R., Thase, M. E., Quitkin, F., Warden, D., ... STAR*D Study Team. (2006). Medication augmentation after the failure of SSRIs for depression. *New England Journal of Medicine*, 354(12), 1243–1252.

Trivedi, M. H., Rush, A. J., Wisniewski, S. R., Nierenberg, A. A., Warden, D., Ritz, L., ... STAR*D Study Team. (2006). Evaluation of outcomes with citalopram for depression using measurement-based care in STAR*D: Implications for clinical practice. *American Journal of Psychiatry*, 163(1), 28–40.

Trivedi, M. H., Thase, M. E., Fava, M., Nelson, C. J., Yang, H., Qi, Y., ... Berman, R. M. (2008). Adjunctive aripiprazole in major depressive disorder: Analysis of efficacy and safety in patients with anxious and atypical features. *Journal of Clinical Psychiatry, 69*(12), 1928–1936.

Unützer, J., Katon, W., Callahan, C. M., Williams, J. W. Jr,, Hunkeler, E., Harpole, L.,...IMPACT Investigators. (2002). Improving mood-promoting access to collaborative treatment. Collaborative care management of late-life depression in the primary care setting: A randomized controlled trial. *Journal of the American Medical Association, 288*(22), 2836–2845.

van Marwijk, H. W., Bekker, F. M., Nolen, W. A., Jansen, P. A., van Nieuwkerk, J. F., & Hop, W. C. (1990). Lithium augmentation in geriatric depression. *Journal of Affective Disorders. 20*(4), 217–223.

van West, D., & Maes, M. (1999). Activation of the inflammatory response system: A new look at the etiopathogenesis of major depression. *Neuroendocrinology Letters, 20*(1/2), 11–17

Vulink, N. C., Figee, M., & Denys, D. (2011). Review of atypical antipsychotics in anxiety. *European Neuropsychopharmacology, 21*(6), 429–449.

Warner-Schmidt, J. L., Vanover, K. E., Chen, E. Y., Marshall, J. J., & Greengard, P. (2011). Antidepressant effects of selective serotonin reuptake inhibitors (SSRIs) are attenuated by antiinflammatory drugs in mice and humans. *Proceedings of the National Academy of Sciences USA, 108*(22), 9262–9267.

Wittenborn, J. R. (1980). Antidepressant use of amphetamines and other psychostimulants. *Modern Problems in Pharmacopsychiatry, 18*, 178–195.

Whyte, E. M., Basinski, J., Farhi, P., Dew, M. A., Begley, A., Mulsant, B. H., & Reynolds, C. F. (2004). Geriatric depression treatment in nonresponders to selective serotonin reuptake inhibitors. *Journal of Clinical Psychiatry, 65*, 1634–1641.

Wilkinson, D., Holmes, C., Woolford, J., Stammers, S., & North, J. (2002). Prophylactic therapy with lithium in elderly patients with unipolar major depression. *International Journal of Geriatric Psychiatry, 17*(7), 619–622.

Whooley, M. A., & Browner, W. S. (1998). Association between depressive symptoms and mortality in older women. Study of Osteoporotic Fractures Research Group. *Archives of Internal Medicine, 158*(19), 2129–2135.

Woods, S. W., Tesar, G. E., Murray, G. B., & Cassem, N. H. (1986). Psychostimulant treatment of depressive disorders secondary to medical illness. *Journal of Clinical Psychiatry, 47*, 12–15.

Yesavage, J. A., Brink, T. L., Rose, T. L., Lum, O., Huang, V., Adey, M., & Leirer, V. O. (1982–1983). Development and validation of a geriatric depression screening scale: A preliminary report. *Journal of Psychiatric Research, 17*(1), 37–49.

Zimmer, B., Rosen, J., Thornton, J. E., Perel, J. M., & Reynolds, C. F., III. (1991). Adjunctive lithium carbonate in nortriptyline-resistant elderly depressed patients. *Journal of Clinical Psychopharmacology, 11*(4), 254–256.

Zivin, K., & Kales, H. C. (2008). Adherence to depression treatment in older adults: A narrative review. *Drugs and Aging, 25*(7), 559–571.

22

PSYCHOTHERAPY

Patricia A. Areán

PSYCHOTHERAPY IS a term used to describe behavioral interventions that address the symptoms and psychosocial causes or consequences of mental illness. There are several forms of psychotherapy; some focus on intentional relationship building between a trained psychotherapist and a patient to address the psychosocial problems the patient is grappling with; others focus on teaching patients methods for solving psychosocial problems. Even though there are several types of psychotherapy, many have been found to be effective in treating mood disorders in late life, and three in particular are evidence-based treatments for late-life mood disorders. An *evidence-based treatment (EBT)* is any intervention that has been studied scientifically and found to be effective in treating a target disorder (Norcross & Wampold, 2011). The EBTs for late-life depression are cognitive-behavioral therapy (CBT), interpersonal therapy (IPT), and problem-solving treatment (PST; Mackin & Areàn, 2005). Each section of this chapter will briefly describe the evidence base for each EBT as a stand-alone treatment and in

combination with medication management, and it will provide a brief overview of how to perform the intervention. The next section will describe how the interventions have been adapted for older adults, and the chapter concludes with directions for future research and practice.

PSYCHOTHERAPY AS A PREFERRED TREATMENT MODALITY IN LATE-LIFE DEPRESSION

Although the evidence base for psychotherapy indicates that it is as good as other interventions for mild to moderate depression, one of the important features of psychotherapy in late life is that it tends to be a preferred mode of treatment by most older adults, in particular ethnic minority elderly. Although there are limitations in the preference literature in terms of accuracy of stated preferences, nearly all the studies done to measure older patient preferences have found that when offered a choice between medications and counseling, preference studies indicate that between 50% and 75% of older adults of all ethnicities will prefer counseling (Cooper-Patrick et al., 1997; Gallagher-Thompson, Solano, Coon, & Areàn, 2003; Gum et al., 2006; Gum, Iser, & Petkus, 2010; Hodges et al., 2009; Mohlman, 2011; Raue, Schulberg, Heo, Klimstra, & Bruce, 2009; Raue, Weinberger, Sirey, Meyers, & Bruce, 2011). Despite this preference, very few older adults have access to high-quality psychotherapy and have limited resources to utilize it well. Most older adults are reluctant to access mental health services, where psychotherapy tends to be offered.

COGNITIVE-BEHAVIORAL THERAPY

Intervention Theory and Overview

Cognitive-behavioral therapy (CBT) has the largest evidence base of the three EBTs for late-life depression (Kiosses, Leon, & Areàn, 2011) and is the only EBT for late-life generalized anxiety disorders (Thorp et al., 2009). Existing late-life depression CBT manuals focus on a combination of cognitive restructuring and behavioral activation. The theory behind CBT for late-life depression states that older people become depressed either because they lack adequate coping skills to manage the challenges of aging (increased medical illness, increased social isolation, decreased social position, increased caregiver burden), develop a pessimistic view of the world and their role in it, and as a result become less active socially (Thompson, Gallagher, & Breckenridge, 1987). CBT attempts to address symptoms and consequences of depression through teaching people as set of skills for mood regulation and engagement in pleasant activities. CBT consists of 12–16 weekly sessions, either in a group format or as an individual therapy. Each skill set is presented in modules. The first module focuses on teaching patients *how to monitor their mood* on a daily basis and *how to recognize social and environmental triggers for negative emotion*. In this module patients are given a simple daily mood rating, usually a scale of 0–9, with zero representing the most depressed they have felt and 9 the happiest they have felt. Patients track their mood on a daily basis and also note events that occurred during the day that may have contributed to their mood, be it positive or negative. The therapist and patient review patterns in mood during the week and work together to identify social and environmental circumstances that influence mood. The next module then focuses

on *identifying patterns in how patients interpret their environment and social interactions negatively*; research shows that people with depression exhibit a strong negativity bias, in that they attend to threat and negative cues more than they do positive cues (Fales et al., 2008; Poulsen, Luu, Crane, Quiring, & Tucker, 2009). This particular module focuses on identifying the negative social cues that patients attend to and helping them refocus their attention on all relevant social cues, both positive and negative. These exercises allow patients to reinterpret social cues to allow patients to consider alternative ways of interacting or solving problems, by attending to all the important information available, not just the negative information. The final module focuses on *social and behavioral activation*. People with depression tend to withdraw from pleasurable activities, either because they do not anticipate enjoying the activity or because they lack energy to engage in the activity (Gallo & Rabins, 1999); this is a common presentation for older adults with late-life depression (Gallo & Rabins, 1999). This module helps patients identify all the activities they have stopped engaging in because of depression, reengaging in the easiest activities first and then working up the list of activities until patients can reengage in all activities.

Evidence Base

The evidence base for CBT is positive for general depressive disorders (Barrowclough et al., 2001; Gallagher, 1985; Mackin & Areàn, 2005). It has been found to be effective for treating depression in older primary care patients (Laidlaw et al., 2008; Serfaty et al., 2009), for older adults who have a marginal response to antidepressants (Wilkinson et al., 2009), in patients with heart disease (Strachowski et al., 2008), and older patients suffering from caregiver distress (Gallagher, 1985). It does not appear to be very effective, however, for low-income older adults unless coupled with clinical case management (P. A. Areàn, Gum, et al., 2005). Meta-analyses find that there is no real advantage for CBT over other types of therapies, although it is better than no treatment (Peng, Huang, Chen, & Lu, 2009); older people tend to have better outcomes with CBT, potentially due to better attendance to therapy (Walker & Clarke, 2001).

Pros and Cons

There are several advantages for CBT as a psychotherapy for late life beyond its evidence base. First,

CBT is a brief intervention that can be used in a variety of settings, including primary care medicine (Laidlaw et al., 2008), and there is evidence that it can be effective over the telephone with disabled adults (Mohr, Hart, & Vella, 2007) and older adults (F. Scogin et al., 2007). Additionally, CBT for late-life depression has been translated into Spanish and Chinese, although there are no studies of the efficacy of CBT for late-life depression in these languages. Because the focus of CBT is on current problems and functioning, the intervention may have broader appeal to patients who are reluctant to engage in psychological therapies, and the brevity of the intervention may also be appealing to patients who are concerned about cost of treatment and the time commitment needed to benefit from psychotherapy. In fact, one study has shown that one-session CBT can be a very effective intervention for older adults with depression (Kunik et al., 2001). The challenge of CBT is that it requires highly skilled clinicians to administer, and there is research to show that CBT is difficult to learn by clinicians who are most likely to work with older adults (e.g., aging service providers), and even when trained, the long-term fidelity to CBT tends to diminish over time without ongoing access to technical assistance and supervision (Aarons, Fettes, Flores, & Sommerfeld, 2009; Aarons, Sommerfeld, Hecht, Silovsky, & Chaffin, 2009; Hamblen, Norris, Gibson, & Lee, 2010).

PROBLEM-SOLVING TREATMENT

Intervention Overview

PST is a newer, learning-based behavioral intervention that is similar to CBT but has distilled the elements of CBT to focus specifically on solving psychosocial problems patients feel are contributing to their depression (P. A. Areàn et al., 1993). The theory behind PST states that depression is a function of repeated and failed attempts to solve problems, which leads to patients feeling hopeless and helpless in the face of psychosocial stress. As a result, patients withdraw socially in an attempt to avoid new problems. Patients experience difficulties solving problems either because the problem they are faced with is particularly challenging or because patients have never learned to be effective problem solvers. PST theorists also propose that all psychotherapies teach people to be better problem solvers implicitly; as such, a more direct approach to managing depression is through explicit instruction

in how to solve problems (Nezu & Perri, 1989). PST is specifically relevant to late-life depression. The intervention directly addresses new problems that patients may not have encountered before, but it allows the therapist to draw from older patients' life experience to address the problem at hand. PST has not been greatly modified for older adults, with the exception of PST versions for cognitive impairments. PST for older adults who have comorbid cognitive impairments generally uses a great number of sessions and to the degree possible includes family members in the action plans developed (Kiosses, Teri, Velligan, & Alexopoulos, 2011). PST has also been modified for homebound older adults and low-income elderly, combining clinical case management with PST (P. A. Areàn, Mackin, et al., 2010). Although these modifications are not specific to older adults, Rovner et al. modified PST for people with vision impairment; the modification includes using tape recorders to remind patients of the PST steps and as a means to record the outcome of action plans (Rovner, Casten, Hegel, Leiby, & Tasman, 2007). Although the data on the effectiveness of tele–mental health PST has not been published (Hegel et al., 2010), currently there are studies investigating the effects of PST on late-life depression via telephone, Skype, and Internet technologies.

PST teaches a seven-step process to solve problems, such as the need for increased social engagement, relationship problems, mood management, and basic health problems. The treatment is divided into three stages: (1) psychoeducation about depression and patient activation (session 1), (2) problem-solving skill acquisition (sessions 2–5), which begins with creating a list of problems and goals that will be the focus of treatment, selecting one problem, focusing on and defining the problem clearly, setting an achievable goal, creating a list of potential ways of reaching the goal, choosing among goal-directed options for solving the problem, creating an action plan, and evaluating the plan once it is implemented; and (3) relapse prevention (session 6), which includes a discussion of how to use the PST process for future problems. While the main goal of treatment is to teach these skills to patients and help them overcome depression, the process includes a collaborative therapeutic stance, clinician ability to engage and motivate the patient to focus on problems rather than avoid them, and support of the patient in his or her recovery from depression.

Evidence Base

Over the last 10 years, PST has established a substantial evidence base. It has (1) documented evidence as a depression treatment in research and the community (Alexopoulos et al., 2011; P. Areàn, Hegel, Vannoy, Fan, & Unuzter, 2008; Cuijpers, van Straten, & Warmerdam, 2007); (2) it is effective for patients across the life span (P. A. Areàn, Raue, et al., 2010; Hegel, et al., 2010) and across service settings (Rovner, Casten, Hegel, & Tasman, 2006); and (3) it is a simple, brief intervention that can be learned and implemented by a variety of community providers (e.g., social workers, case managers) (Kiosses, Areàn, Teri, & Alexopoulos, 2010; Tasman & Rovner, 2004; Unutzer et al., 2001). PST is particularly effective for patients who exhibit a form of late-life depression that is associated with a poor response to antidepressant medication (Alexopoulos et al., 2011; P. A. Areàn, Raue, et al., 2010).

Pros and Cons

The major advantage of PST is its simplicity, brevity, and an existing training program for providers from any discipline. The intervention fits nicely into primary care medicine (P. A. Areàn, Ayalon, et al., 2005; Unutzer et al., 2001) and aging services (Ciechanowski et al., 2004) and can effect rapid results in these settings; one study found that older primary care patients demonstrate substantial results within four sessions of PST (P. Areàn et al., 2008). Although a well-developed training network exists for community providers from all backgrounds (http://pstnetwork.ucsf.edu and www.impact-uw.edu), the training can often be more onerous than many agencies are willing to support (3 months of ongoing expert supervision of clinicians in training), and the long-term effects of this training on provider behavior are unknown; additionally, the less experience the clinician in training has in brief structured therapies, the harder it is for the clinician to learn PST (Hegel, Dietrich, Seville, & Jordan, 2004).

INTERPERSONAL THERAPY

Intervention Overview

IPT is a time-limited intervention to help patients overcome interpersonal problems through discussion and skill development to manage interpersonal problems effectively. The IPT theory of depression proposes that interpersonal issues are often the primary cause of depression, and there are four basic interpersonal conflicts: (1) grief after the loss of a loved one; (2) conflict in significant relationships; (3) difficulties adapting to changes in relationships or life circumstances; and (4) difficulties stemming from social isolation (Frank, Kupfer, Wagner, McEachran, & Cornes, 1991). For older adults in particular, problems related to grief and difficulties adapting to changes in life circumstances (e.g., retirement, disability) are a primary focus of the intervention (Taylor et al., 1999). IPT is also an effective preventative intervention in older adults at risk for developing major depression (Cuijpers, van Straten, Andersson, & van Oppen, 2008).

IPT is divided into three phases: acute treatment, maintenance, and relapse prevention. Early acute phase sessions focus on discussion of the depression diagnosis, assessment of patients' major interpersonal problem areas, and agreeing on a treatment plan to address the problem areas. Subsequent phases focus on current interpersonal problems (rather than exploration of past relationships) and strategies to resolve the interpersonal problem area. In older adults, it is most common to work on grief and adaptation. Problems with grief tend to be delayed or distorted grief reactions that are beyond what would normally be expected for the typical grief reaction. The therapist works with the older patient to facilitate grieving, coping with difficult emotions related to loss, and working toward finding new relationships and activities that can help to resolve feelings of loss. For adaptation (also referred to as role transition), IPT helps the patient accept the loss of the old role by discussing feelings related to the transition, and eventually to support the new role the older person will be moving toward (Frank et al., 1991). During maintenance phase, the therapist and patient discuss gains made through treatment, identify areas of more work that the patient can do on his or her own, and discuss feelings related to treatment termination. Once the patient has responded to treatment, the maintenance phase generally consists of once-a-month check-in, and if the patient has had a chronic recurrent course of depression, IPT includes additional twice-a-year check-ins to ensure treatment gains are maintained.

Evidence Base

Although the evidence base for IPT in the general adult population is extensive, the research on late-life depression is small, and most of the larger studies have focused on relapse prevention (P. A. Areàn & Cook, 2002). While there are promising findings with regard to acute response to IPT in older adults with depression (Miller et al., 2001; Miller, Frank, Cornes, Houck, & Reynolds, 2003; Reynolds et al., 1999), as a prevention intervention, it is not as helpful for older adults who have experienced chronic recurrent depression (Carreira et al., 2008; Reynolds et al., 2010). IPT for older adults has mostly been studied in psychiatric medical centers, and although there are recent studies of IPT in primary medicine in younger adults (Grigoriadis & Ravitz, 2007; Krupnick et al., 2008; Van Voorhees et al., 2007), there has only been one such study for older adults (Post, Miller, & Schulberg, 2008), and the specific effects of IPT have not been evaluated (Bruce et al., 2004).

Pros and Cons

There are a number of advantages for IPT that make it an appealing intervention for older adults. The focus on age-specific issues, such as grief and role transition, can be particularly helpful for a variety of problems older adults face (loss, retirement, changes in health status, moving). This age-specific focus may make IPT particularly appealing to older adults who may be reluctant to use structured learning-based approaches. Additionally, like all adult populations, older adults may benefit from different types of treatment at different points in the time course of coping with caregiving issues or disability. A study comparing CBT to a brief dynamic treatment suggests that for caregiving issues (which would be a role transition), people having to cope with the pain associated with a new diagnosis and what that means for a couple's future respond better to a more interpersonally focused intervention, whereas people who have moved past the loss of the relationship benefit best with strategic methods for coping with practical problems associated with caregiving (Gallagher & Thompson, 1983).

The main disadvantage of IPT for late-life depression is that the effects of this intervention in settings other than psychiatry clinics, using non–mental health clinicians, is unknown. It is not clear whether the typical community provider can provide IPT well and with long-term fidelity, nor is it clear that IPT is suited for aging service settings. More research on the application of IPT in nontraditional mental health settings is needed.

OTHER PSYCHOTHERAPIES: REMINISCENCE, SUPPORTIVE, AND FAMILY THERAPIES

Although CBT, IPT, and PST are the leading EBPs for late-life depression, other psychotherapies have been used in practice with older adults with depression. Early in the history of geriatric psychotherapy research, reminiscence therapy was a popular intervention; from a theoretical perspective, it made sense that older adults, who actively engage in the life review process, would benefit from an intervention that helped patients review life events, focus on what can be learned from those events, and how to apply that knowledge to coping with current events (Karel & Hinrichsen, 2000). Since the first study of reminiscence in late-life depression was conducted (Goldwasser, Auerbach, & Harkins, 1987), the intervention has undergone a number of modifications, including integration with CBT. The combined reminiscence and CBT intervention is referred to as life review, and it incorporates cognitive-behavioral interventions into the reminiscence process. As a patient discusses past events with the therapist, the therapists uses cognitive restructuring techniques to help the patient reframe negative life events (Cappeliez & Robitaille, 2010). Although a meta-analysis indicated that life review and reminiscence therapies are effective alternatives for treating late-life depression, particularly in early phases of the mental illness (Bohlmeijer, Valenkamp, Westerhof, Smit, & Cuijpers, 2005), the authors of the meta-analysis also indicated that there are too few randomized clinical trials to draw firm conclusions about its efficacy (Bohlmeijer, Smit, & Cuijpers, 2003).

Supportive therapy is also in wide use in community practices serving older adults. Supportive therapy was originally developed as a placebo control for psychotherapy trials, and while it has benefits for major depression, meta-analyses disagree as to its comparative effectiveness to CBT, IPT, or PST. One meta-analysis found that CBT was no better than supportive therapy for treating depression (Tolin, 2010), while another found supportive therapy to be somewhat less effective than other therapies (Cuijpers et al., 2008). In older adults, research has shown supportive therapy to be a powerful intervention, no less effective than CBT (P. A. Areàn & Cook, 2002), but somewhat less effective than PST (Alexopoulos, Raue, Kanellopoulos, Mackin, & Areàn, 2008).

Table 22–1 Comparison of Psychotherapies for Late-Life Depression

PSYCHOTHERAPY	THEORY	PROS	CONS
Cognitive Behavioral	Late-life depression is a function of a lack adequate coping skills to manage the challenges of aging, a pessimistic view of the world and their role in it, and social isolation.	• Large evidence-base; • Brief intervention; • In Spanish and Chinese • Present focus may be more appealing • Telephone and primary care versions.	• Need skilled providers.
Problem Solving	Late-life depression is due to repeated, failed attempts to solve problems, hopelessness and helpless in the face of psychosocial stress. Patients experience difficulties solving problems either because the problem they are faced with is particularly challenging or because patients have never learned to be effective problem solvers.	• Brief • Simple structure • Any provider can do PST • Can be done in any care setting, or home care • Can be done over the telephone or via Skype • Available in Chinese, Japanese and Spanish	• Training program may be too onerous for typical clinician.
Interpersonal	Interpersonal Issues Are The Primary Cause Of Depression, In Particular 1) Grief After The Loss Of A Loved One; 2) Conflict In Significant Relationships; 3) Difficulties Adapting To Changes In Relationships Or Life Circumstances; And 4) Difficulties Stemming From Social Isolation.	• Age Specific Focus • Loner Treatment Frame • Can Be Given In Primary Care	• Skill Set/ Experience Needed By Provider Is Unknown.

There has been far less research on the treatment of depression in late life using couples or family interventions. Most studies involving family intervention focus on managing the co-occurrence of depression and cognitive impairment/dementia; in these studies, the interventions themselves do no impact on depression symptoms of the patient but do tend to alleviate depression experienced by the family caring for the patient (Ayalon, Gum, Feliciano, & Areàn, 2006). Two recent studies focused on PST augmented with family intervention for patients with mild to moderate cognitive impairment found the combination of these interventions to be effective in reducing depression (Gellis & Bruce, 2010; Kiosses, Teri, et al., 2011), but neither study can provide information about the relative impact adding the family intervention has over and above the effects of PST on late-life depression (V. M. Wilkins, Kiosses, & Ravdin, 2010).

ADAPTING PSYCHOTHERAPY FOR LATE-LIFE POPULATIONS

CBT, PST, and IPT are effective interventions for late-life depression and require very little in the way of modification for special populations. Most modifications of these treatments involve increasing acceptability of the treatment in certain cultures and accommodating physical and cognitive impairments.

Culture

Most cultural modifications of psychotherapies for older adults focus on how to make the therapy more accessible to people of different cultures by adapting the framework and presentation of the therapy. Framework adaptations include translating the treatment into language that is consistent with cultural values, beliefs, and practices (Bernal & Domenech Rodriguez, 2009). A number of models for adapting psychotherapies exist, including Bernal's ecological validity framework (Bernal, Bonilla, & Bellido, 1995), in which treatment manuals are modified not only by language but by including relevant metaphors to explain therapeutic concepts and use of different delivery methods (for instance, the use of story boards for Mexican immigrants to explain CBT); the cultural accommodation model (CAM; Leong, 2006), which is a three-step process that begins with identifying cultural gaps in

the psychotherapy, followed by investigation into research to fill in any cultural gaps and a final step that tests the culturally accommodated intervention; and finally, the formative method for adapting psychotherapy (FMAP; Hwang, 2009), which is a community-based approach that involves mental health providers and consumer stakeholders in the modification.

CBT has been culturally modified for depressed older adults and caregivers using the Bernal model (Gallagher-Thompson et al., 2003; Gallagher-Thompson et al., 2010), and PST has been adapted for older Chinese (Chu, Huynh, & Areàn, 2011), African American (P. A. Areàn, Mackin, et al., 2010), and Hispanic immigrants using the FMAP model. While IPT has been adapted for Hispanic women (Grote et al., 2009), there is no published literature on its adaptation in older minorities. Most of the adaptations include the use of multimedia to illustrate therapeutic principles of the treatment (Gallagher-Thompson et al., 2010) (e.g., DVD soap opera type illustrations of therapeutic strategies), the inclusion of family members in treatment planning (P. A. Areàn, Mackin, et al., 2010), less reliance on forms and written educational materials when the patient's educational level is lower than high school (van der Waerden, Hoefnagels, & Hosman, 2011) (e.g., use of conversation to walk patients through procedures), and a shift from an equal and collaborative therapeutic style between therapist and patient to a benign authoritative style (Chu et al., 2011) (e.g., emphasizing a doctor–patient relationship).

Disability

The biggest complicating factor of psychotherapy for older adults, particularly those who are disabled, is the need to work with a therapist on a weekly basis. Many older adults see this requirement as a burden if they have to come to a psychiatric clinic to receive services; some older adults do not drive because of disability, making a 1-hour visit to a therapist at times a 3-hour ordeal; even if the intervention is provided in primary care medicine, regular and frequent face-to-face visits can be complicated. Additionally, those with visual impairments may have difficulty with interventions like CBT and PST that are structured around the use of written forms.

Tele–mental health approaches can be helpful in overcoming the barriers associated with transportation/mobility. CBT and PST have been adapted to account for transportation limitations. CBT for rural older adults consists of one face-to-face visit, followed by the use of in-home educational materials and follow-up telephone calls to support the use of CBT strategies (Floyd et al., 2006; Floyd, Scogin, McKendree-Smith, Floyd, & Rokke, 2004; Kaufman, Scogin, Burgio, Morthland, & Ford, 2007; F. Scogin, Jamison, & Davis, 1990; F. Scogin, Jamison, & Gochneaur, 1989; F. R. Scogin, Hanson, & Welsh, 2003) and has been found to be an effective alternative to in-person intensive CBT (F. Scogin, et al., 2007). PST has been adapted to be provided over the telephone and via Skype technologies, although neither administration has an existing evidence base. PST can be delivered in the patient's home, and while this minimizes patient burdens and barriers to care, the cost of providers to go to one's home increases (P. A. Areàn, Mackin, et al., 2010).

Technology can also help with barriers associated with visual and hearing impairment. As stated previously, PST has been adapted for visually impaired adults by using recording devises to remind patients of the PST steps and for recording mood and action plan outcomes (Rovner et al., 2007). CBT has been adapted for people with hearing impairments and includes the use of hearing aides and visual cues to illustrate therapeutic principles (Tisdelle & St Lawrence, 1986). Mobility in general can be an issue for interventions that include engagement in pleasant activities (CBT and PST); in these interventions, pleasant activity work focuses on increasing low physical demand, pleasant activities (talking to family members over Skype) and developing action plans that include methods for overcoming physical limitations that interfere with engaging in activities outside the home (e.g., using paratransit to get to church).

Cognitive Impairment

As many as 30% of older adults with depression suffer from some form of mild cognitive impairment. Although many people have speculated that these impairments would interfere with the process of psychotherapy (C. H. Wilkins, Mathews, & Sheline, 2009), actual data are mixed, with some studies finding no influence of impairments on psychotherapy outcomes (P. A. Areàn, Raue, et al., 2010), while others find effects for memory impairment specifically (McDougall, 1999). It is important to match modifications of therapy to type of cognitive impairment (Alexopoulos, Raue, & Areàn, 2003). For instance, people exhibiting impairments

in executive functions tend to present with disorganization, difficulty starting tasks, and difficulty with solving problems. Previous research has found that patients with this presentation do quite well in structured, problem-focused therapies, such as PST (P. A. Areàn, Raue, et al., 2010). Patients with memory impairments may do best with interventions that rely on mood induction and life review strategies that support the illustration of therapeutic techniques, or recall pleasant memories as a means of modulating affect; CBT has been adapted for people with memory impairments by including life review strategies (Peng et al., 2009; Pinquart, Duberstein, & Lyness, 2007).

CONCLUSION AND FUTURE DIRECTIONS

Psychotherapy for late-life mood disorders has gained momentum over the past few decades, and while there are still fewer studies of psychotherapy in late life than there are for medication interventions, the evidence base is strong, and it is widely acknowledged that these interventions are useful first-line treatments for late-life depression (Charney et al., 2003). The future direction for psychotherapy in late-life mood disorders is likely to focus on three key questions: What are the moderators of psychotherapy outcomes? Is technology a viable option for treating late-life depression? What are the methods needed for training professionals who are most likely to encounter an older adults with depression in evidence-based treatments?

Understanding the Key Elements

Although psychotherapy is a viable treatment option for older adults, there are likely to be considerable variations in response to treatment that could inform how clinicians make choices in treating older adults with this type of intervention. Of particular note is the potential impact that cognitive functions may have on treatment outcomes. For decades it has been assumed that age-related cognitive decline could have an impact on the ability of older adults to benefit from psychotherapies, particularly those that rely on learning new behaviors (Gaitz, 1985). However, recent evidence suggests that mild cognitive impairments that are either associated with age or with depression may not have a significant impact on response to any psychotherapy, and for some patients, psychotherapy may provide a compensatory framework for these deficits. As an example, Areàn, Raue, et al. (2010) and Alexopoulos et al. (2011) demonstrated that PST was particularly helpful for patients with mild executive dysfunction but also noted that supportive therapy had a significant impact on outcomes as well. As of this writing, there has been no other study of cognition and its impact on psychotherapy, or the potential role that psychotherapy could have in targeting specific symptoms of depression. The PST for late-life depression study is the first step in an important line of inquiry that could result in important information related to the role psychotherapy could have in treating different presentations of late-life depression.

An additional area of investigation is the role that nonspecific therapeutic factors may have in the treatment of depression in certain populations of older adults. One of the interesting outcomes of psychotherapy research is that when comparing two psychotherapies for depression in late life, there is rarely a difference between active treatments (an exception to this is the PST study of executive dysfunction). Areàn et al. (P. A. Areàn, Gum, et al., 2005) and Gum et al. (Gum, Areàn, & Bostrom, 2007) have found that case management (e.g., a combination of supportive therapy and linkage to social services) in low-income populations is a very powerful intervention. This may suggest that depression in late life that is due to social adversity (e.g., poverty, urban stress, social isolation) may respond best to interventions that specifically link patients to social interventions than to address the sociological causes of depression. Additionally, the psychotherapy field has for years debated the importance of support in the treatment of depression; while supportive therapies in general are found to be less effective than active interventions such as CBT or IPT (Cuijpers, van Straten, Bohlmeijer, Hollon, & Andersson, 2010), in older adults the impact of simple support or clinical management is rather powerful (P. A. Areàn, Raue, et al., 2010). Mental health research funders have recently announced interest in studying the impact of nonspecific factors.

Maximizing Fidelity to Treatment

One of the biggest challenges faced by the psychotherapy field is the implementation of evidence-based psychotherapies for late-life depression. Older people with depression are identified in non–mental health settings by providers who do not have the background necessary to provide most

psychotherapies (Choi, 2009; Snowden, Steinman, & Frederick, 2008; Steinman et al., 2007). Generally, to ensure that providers adequately offer psychotherapy to older adults, a number of processes should be in place. Services for older adults have to be invested in the support of evidence-based psychotherapy. Several studies of behavioral interventions for mental illnesses have shown that even after intensive training in these interventions, providers demonstrate substantial drift in their fidelity to the treatment model, which may compromise the effects of treatment (Ammerman et al., 2007; Baer et al., 2007; Barlow, Levitt, & Bufka, 1999). Solutions to therapist drift include ongoing access to technical assistance from experts in the intervention (Mancini et al., 2009) and ongoing quality assurance assessment of therapist quality (W. Cross, Matthieu, Cerel, & Knox, 2007; W. Cross, West, et al., 2011; W. Cross & Wyman, 2006; W. W. Cross, 2011). Although research on the best methods for maintaining fidelity is still under development, research on adult learning methods suggest that the best methods for training new clinical behaviors in novice clinicians is to first train the clinician in the basic aspects of the intervention; in psychotherapy with older adults these skills would include basic communication strategies, how to direct the flow of discussion without the older person feeling unheard or dismissed, and how to talk about depression in a way that will minimize and address problems related to stigma. After the basics are in place, treatment-specific strategies can be learned. When research therapists are trained in a new intervention, the training typically consists of observation-based feedback, whereby the therapist videotapes therapy sessions and an expert provides guidance and feedback on the case. While this method works well in research, it is more complicated to train clinicians using this method in community settings (e.g., HIPAA concerns). For this reason, some psychotherapy centers, such as the PST network (http://pstnetwork.ucsf.edu), are beginning to rely on a combination of live patient review and standardized patient role-plays. Standardized patients are actors who are trained in a basic script but are also trained to respond to the clinician in training based on how the clinician conducts the interview. The standardized patient participates in giving feedback to the clinician in training. Standardized patients have been in use in medical schools for over a decade, with positive results in training early career physicians in how to conduct medical interviews and exams, and in training educators in suicide detection among adolescents (Bourgeois et al., 2008; W. F. Cross et al., 2011). This method could serve as a means of providing initial experience in psychotherapy and would maximize the chance that when a clinician conducts her first psychotherapy session, she will be able to deliver the intervention effectively. This method can also be used in quality assurance of long-term fidelity to the treatment in question.

Another approach to managing long-term fidelity has been to develop computerized versions of the intervention and training staff in how to use the program with the patient in the room. These methods have been applied to CBT and PST, with very positive effects (Craske et al., 2009). The advantages with this method of psychotherapy implementation are that provider training is simplified and both clinician and patient are likely to use a truly evidence-based treatment.

SUMMARY

Psychotherapy for late-life depression is a viable and effective intervention. Most older adults profess a preference for these treatments, and existing treatments have the potential for being targeted to specific presentations of depression. Although training providers in services where older adults are most likely to receive treatment is a challenge, there are models for provider training that could make these interventions more accessible to the general public. Future research in psychotherapy for late-life depression should focus on treatment matching based on clinical characteristics and differential causes of depression.

Disclosure
Dr. Areàn has no conflicts to disclose. She is funded by NIMH, MIMHHD, and NIDA only. Grant support: NIMH: K24 MH074717, R01 MH075900, R24 MH077192, T32 MH018261, R01 DK061937, and R01 MD007019.

REFERENCES

Aarons, G. A., Fettes, D. L., Flores, L. E., Jr., & Sommerfeld, D. H. (2009). Evidence-based practice implementation and staff emotional exhaustion in children's services. [Research Support, N.I.H., Extramural]. *Behaviour Research and Therapy, 47*(11), 954–960.

Aarons, G. A., Sommerfeld, D. H., Hecht, D. B., Silovsky, J. F., & Chaffin, M. J. (2009). The impact of evidence-based practice implementation and fidelity monitoring on staff turnover: Evidence for a protective effect. [Research Support, N.I.H., Extramural]. *Journal of consulting and clinical psychology, 77*(2), 270–280.

Alexopoulos, G. S., Raue, P., & Areàn, P. (2003). Problem-solving therapy versus supportive therapy in geriatric major depression with executive dysfunction. [Clinical Trial Randomized Controlled Trial Research Support, Non-US Government Research Support, US Government, P.H.S.]. *American Journal of Geriatric Psychiatry, 11*(1), 46–52.

Alexopoulos, G. S., Raue, P. J., Kanellopoulos, D., Mackin, S., & Areàn, P. A. (2008). Problem solving therapy for the depression-executive dysfunction syndrome of late life. [Case Reports Research Support, N.I.H., Extramural Research Support, Non-US Government Research Support, US Government, P.H.S. Review]. *International Journal of Geriatric Psychiatry, 23*(8), 782–788.

Alexopoulos, G. S., Raue, P. J., Kiosses, D. N., Mackin, R. S., Kanellopoulos, D., McCulloch, C., & Areàn, P. A. (2011). Problem-solving therapy and supportive therapy in older adults with major depression and executive dysfunction: effect on disability. [Comparative Study Randomized Controlled Trial Research Support, N.I.H., Extramural Research Support, Non-US Government]. *Archives of General Psychiatry, 68*(1), 33–41.

Ammerman, R. T., Putnam, F. W., Kopke, J. E., Gannon, T. A., Short, J. A., Van Ginkel, J. B., ... Spector, A. R. (2007). Development and implementation of a quality assurance infrastructure in a multisite home visitation program in Ohio and Kentucky. *Journal of Prevention and Intervention in the Community, 34*(1–2), 89–107.

Areàn, P., Hegel, M., Vannoy, S., Fan, M. Y., & Unuzter, J. (2008). Effectiveness of problem-solving therapy for older, primary care patients with depression: results from the IMPACT project. [Comparative Study Multicenter Study Research Support, Non-US Government]. *Gerontologist, 48*(3), 311–323.

Areàn, P. A., Ayalon, L., Hunkeler, E., Lin, E. H., Tang, L., Harpole, L., ... Unutzer, J. (2005). Improving depression care for older, minority patients in primary care. [Clinical Trial Multicenter Study Randomized Controlled Trial Research Support, Non-US Government]. *Medical Care, 43*(4), 381–390.

Areàn, P. A., & Cook, B. L. (2002). Psychotherapy and combined psychotherapy/pharmacotherapy for late life depression. *Biological Psychiatry, 52*(3), 293–303.

Areàn, P. A., Gum, A., McCulloch, C. E., Bostrom, A., Gallagher-Thompson, D., & Thompson, L. (2005). Treatment of depression in low-income older adults. [Comparative Study Randomized Controlled Trial Research Support, N.I.H., Extramural]. *Psychology and Aging, 20*(4), 601–609.

Areàn, P. A., Mackin, S., Vargas-Dwyer, E., Raue, P., Sirey, J. A., Kanellopolos, D., & Alexopoulos, G. S. (2010). Treating depression in disabled, low-income elderly: A conceptual model and recommendations for care. [Review]. *International Journal of Geriatric Psychiatry, 25*(8), 765–769.

Areàn, P. A., Perri, M. G., Nezu, A. M., Schein, R. L., Christopher, F., & Joseph, T. X. (1993). Comparative effectiveness of social problem-solving therapy and reminiscence therapy as treatments for depression in older adults. [Clinical Trial Comparative Study Randomized Controlled Trial]. *Journal of Consulting and Clinical Psychology, 61*(6), 1003–1010.

Areàn, P. A., Raue, P., Mackin, R. S., Kanellopoulos, D., McCulloch, C., & Alexopoulos, G. S. (2010). Problem-solving therapy and supportive therapy in older adults with major depression and executive dysfunction. [Comparative Study Multicenter Study Randomized Controlled Trial Research Support, N.I.H., Extramural Research Support, Non-US Government]. *American Journal of Psychiatry, 167*(11), 1391–1398.

Ayalon, L., Gum, A. M., Feliciano, L., & Areàn, P. A. (2006). Effectiveness of nonpharmacological interventions for the management of neuropsychiatric symptoms in patients with dementia: A systematic review. [Review]. *Archives of Internal Medicine, 166*(20), 2182–2188.

Baer, J. S., Ball, S. A., Campbell, B. K., Miele, G. M., Schoener, E. P., & Tracy, K. (2007). Training and fidelity monitoring of behavioral interventions in multi-site addictions research. [Research Support, N.I.H., Extramural Review]. *Drug and Alcohol Dependence, 87*(2–3), 107–118.

Barlow, D. H., Levitt, J. T., & Bufka, L. F. (1999). The dissemination of empirically supported treatments: A view to the future. [Review]. *Behaviour Research and Therapy, 37*(Suppl 1), S147–162.

Barrowclough, C., King, P., Colville, J., Russell, E., Burns, A., & Tarrier, N. (2001). A randomized trial of the effectiveness of cognitive-behavioral therapy and supportive counseling for anxiety symptoms in older adults. [Clinical Trial Randomized Controlled Trial Research Support, Non-US Government]. *Journal of Consulting and Clinical Psychology, 69*(5), 756–762.

Bernal, G., Bonilla, J., & Bellido, C. (1995). Ecological validity and cultural sensitivity for outcome research: Issues for the cultural adaptation and development of psychosocial treatments with Hispanics. *Journal of Abnormal Child Psychology, 23*(1), 67–82.

Bernal, G., & Domenech Rodriguez, M. M. (2009). Advances in Latino family research: Cultural adaptations of evidence-based interventions. [Research Support, N.I.H., Extramural]. *Family process, 48*(2), 169–178.

Bohlmeijer, E., Smit, F., & Cuijpers, P. (2003). Effects of reminiscence and life review on late-life depression: A meta-analysis. [Meta-Analysis]. *International Journal of Geriatric Psychiatry, 18*(12), 1088–1094.

Bohlmeijer, E., Valenkamp, M., Westerhof, G., Smit, F., & Cuijpers, P. (2005). Creative reminiscence as an early intervention for depression: Results of a pilot project. [Clinical Trial]. *Aging and Mental Health, 9*(4), 302–304.

Bourgeois, J. A., Ton, H., Onate, J., McCarthy, T., Stevenson, F. T., Servis, M. E., & Wilkes, M. S. (2008). The doctoring curriculum at the University of California, Davis School Of Medicine: Leadership and participant roles for psychiatry faculty. *Academic Psychiatry, 32*(3), 249–254.

Bruce, M. L., Ten Have, T. R., Reynolds, C. F., III, Katz, II, Schulberg, H. C., Mulsant, B. H., ... Alexopoulos, G. S. (2004). Reducing suicidal ideation and depressive symptoms in depressed older primary care patients: A randomized controlled trial. [Clinical Trial Multicenter Study Randomized Controlled Trial Research Support, Non-US Government Research Support, US Government, P.H.S.]. *Journal of the American Medical Association, 291*(9), 1081–1091.

Cappeliez, P., & Robitaille, A. (2010). Coping mediates the relationships between reminiscence and psychological well-being among older adults. [Research Support, Non-US Government]. *Aging and Mental Health, 14*(7), 807–818.

Carreira, K., Miller, M. D., Frank, E., Houck, P. R., Morse, J. Q., Dew, M. A., ... Reynolds, C. F., III. (2008). A controlled evaluation of monthly maintenance interpersonal psychotherapy in late-life depression with varying levels of cognitive function. [Randomized Controlled Trial Research Support, N.I.H., Extramural Research Support, Non-US Government]. *International Journal of Geriatric Psychiatry, 23*(11), 1110–1113.

Charney, D. S., Reynolds, C. F., III, Lewis, L., Lebowitz, B. D., Sunderland, T., Alexopoulos, G. S., ... Young, R. C. (2003). Depression and Bipolar Support Alliance consensus statement on the unmet needs in diagnosis and treatment of mood disorders in late life. [Consensus Development Conference Consensus Development Conference, NIH Research Support, Non-US Government Research Support, US Government, P.H.S. Review]. *Archives of General Psychiatry, 60*(7), 664–672.

Choi, N. G. (2009). The integration of social and psychologic services to improve low-income homebound older adults' access to depression treatment. *Family and Community Health, 32*(1 Suppl), S27–35.

Chu, J. P., Huynh, L., & Areàn, P. (2011). Cultural adaptation of evidence-based practice utilizing an iterative stakeholder process and theoretical framework: Problem solving therapy for Chinese older adults. *International Journal of Geriatric Psychiatry*. doi: 10.1002/gps.2698

Ciechanowski, P., Wagner, E., Schmaling, K., Schwartz, S., Williams, B., Diehr, P., ... LoGerfo, J. (2004). Community-integrated home-based depression treatment in older adults: a randomized controlled trial. [Clinical Trial Randomized Controlled Trial Research Support, US Government, P.H.S.]. *Journal of the American Medical Association, 291*(13), 1569–1577.

Cooper-Patrick, L., Powe, N. R., Jenckes, M. W., Gonzales, J. J., Levine, D. M., & Ford, D. E. (1997). Identification of patient attitudes and preferences regarding treatment of depression. [Clinical Trial Comparative Study Research Support, Non-US Government Research Support, US Government, P.H.S.]. *Journal of General Internal Medicine, 12*(7), 431–438.

Craske, M. G., Roy-Byrne, P. P., Stein, M. B., Sullivan, G., Sherbourne, C., & Bystritsky, A. (2009). Treatment for anxiety disorders: Efficacy to effectiveness to implementation. [Research Support, N.I.H., Extramural]. *Behaviour Research and Therapy, 47*(11), 931–937.

Cross, W., Matthieu, M. M., Cerel, J., & Knox, K. L. (2007). Proximate outcomes of gatekeeper training for suicide prevention in the workplace. [Clinical Trial Research Support, N.I.H., Extramural]. *Suicide and Life-Threatening Behavior, 37*(6), 659–670.

Cross, W., West, J., Wyman, P., Schmeelk-Cone, K., Teisi, M., & Tu, X. (2011). *A closer look at implementer fidelity: Are we measuring what we intend to measure?* Paper presented at the 20th Annual Conference of the Society for Prevention Research, Washington, May 29–June 1, 2012 DC.

Cross, W., & Wyman, P. A. (2006). Training and motivational factors as predictors of job satisfaction and anticipated job retention among implementers of a school-based prevention program. [Multicenter Study Research Support, US Government, P.H.S.]. *Journal of Primary Prevention, 27*(2), 195–215.

Cross, W. F., Seaburn, D., Gibbs, D., Schmeelk-Cone, K., White, A. M., & Caine, E. D. (2011). Does practice make perfect? A randomized control trial of behavioral rehearsal on suicide prevention gatekeeper skills. [Comparative Study Randomized Controlled Trial Research Support, American Recovery and Reinvestment Act Research Support, N.I.H., Extramural]. *Journal of Primary Prevention, 32*(3–4), 195–211.

Cross, W. F., & West, J. C. (2011). Examining implementer fidelity: Conceptualizing and measuring adherence and competence. *Journal of Children's Services, 6*(1), 18–33.

Cuijpers, P., van Straten, A., Andersson, G., & van Oppen, P. (2008). Psychotherapy for depression in adults: A meta-analysis of comparative outcome studies. [Meta-Analysis]. *Journal of Consulting and Clinical Psychology, 76*(6), 909–922.

Cuijpers, P., van Straten, A., Bohlmeijer, E., Hollon, S. D., & Andersson, G. (2010). The effects of psychotherapy for adult depression are overestimated: A meta-analysis of study quality and effect size. [Meta-Analysis]. *Psychological Medicine, 40*(2), 211–223.

Cuijpers, P., van Straten, A., & Warmerdam, L. (2007). Problem solving therapies for depression: A meta-analysis. [Meta-Analysis]. *European Psychiatry, 22*(1), 9–15.

Fales, C. L., Barch, D. M., Rundle, M. M., Mintun, M. A., Snyder, A. Z., Cohen, J. D., ... Sheline, Y. I. (2008). Altered emotional interference processing in affective and cognitive-control brain circuitry in major depression. [Research Support, N.I.H., Extramural]. *Biological Psychiatry, 63*(4), 377–384.

Floyd, M., Rohen, N., Shackelford, J. A., Hubbard, K. L., Parnell, M. B., Scogin, F., & Coates, A. (2006). Two-year follow-up of bibliotherapy and individual cognitive therapy for depressed older adults. [Comparative Study Controlled Clinical Trial]. *Behavior Modification, 30*(3), 281–294.

Floyd, M., Scogin, F., McKendree-Smith, N. L., Floyd, D. L., & Rokke, P. D. (2004). Cognitive therapy for depression: A comparison of individual psychotherapy and bibliotherapy for depressed older adults. *Behavior Modification, 28*(2), 297–318.

Frank, E., Kupfer, D. J., Wagner, E. F., McEachran, A. B., & Cornes, C. (1991). Efficacy of interpersonal psychotherapy as a maintenance treatment of recurrent depression. Contributing factors. [Clinical Trial Randomized Controlled Trial Research Support, Non-US Government Research Support, US Government, P.H.S.]. *Archives of General Psychiatry, 48*(12), 1053–1059.

Gaitz, C. M. (1985). The diagnosis and treatment of mental illness in late life. *Community Mental Health Journal, 21*(2), 119–130.

Gallagher, D. E. (1985). Intervention strategies to assist caregivers of frail elders: Current research status and future research directions. [Research Support, US Government, P.H.S. Review]. *Annual Review of Gerontology and Geriatrics, 5*, 249–282.

Gallagher, D. E., & Thompson, L. W. (1983). Effectiveness of psychotherapy for both endogenous and nonendogenous depression in older adult outpatients. [Comparative Study Research Support, US Government, P.H.S.]. *Journal of Gerontology, 38*(6), 707–712.

Gallagher-Thompson, D., Coon, D. W., Solano, N., Ambler, C., Rabinowitz, Y., & Thompson, L. W. (2003). Change in indices of distress among Latino and Anglo female caregivers of elderly relatives with dementia: Site-specific results from the REACH national collaborative study. [Clinical Trial Comparative Study Randomized Controlled Trial Research Support, US Government, P.H.S.]. *Gerontologist, 43*(4), 580–591.

Gallagher-Thompson, D., Solano, N., Coon, D., & Areàn, P. (2003). Recruitment and retention of latino dementia family caregivers in intervention research: Issues to face, lessons to learn. [Research Support, US Government, P.H.S. Review]. *Gerontologist, 43*(1), 45–51.

Gallagher-Thompson, D., Wang, P. C., Liu, W., Cheung, V., Peng, R., China, D., & Thompson, L. W. (2010). Effectiveness of a psychoeducational skill training DVD program to reduce stress in Chinese American dementia caregivers: Results of a preliminary study. [Randomized Controlled Trial Research Support, Non-US Government]. *Aging and Mental Health, 14*(3), 263–273.

Gallo, J. J., & Rabins, P. V. (1999). Depression without sadness: Alternative presentations of depression in late life. [Review]. *American Family Physician, 60*(3), 820–826.

Gellis, Z. D., & Bruce, M. L. (2010). Problem solving therapy for subthreshold depression in home healthcare patients with cardiovascular disease. [Randomized Controlled Trial Research Support, N.I.H., Extramural]. *American Journal of Geriatric Psychiatry, 18*(6), 464–474.

Goldwasser, A. N., Auerbach, S. M., & Harkins, S. W. (1987). Cognitive, affective, and behavioral effects of reminiscence group therapy on demented elderly. *International Journal of Aging and Human Development, 25*(3), 209–222.

Grigoriadis, S., & Ravitz, P. (2007). An approach to interpersonal psychotherapy for postpartum depression: Focusing on interpersonal changes. [Case Reports Review]. *Canadian Family Physician/Medecin de Famille Canadien, 53*(9), 1469–1475.

Grote, N. K., Swartz, H. A., Geibel, S. L., Zuckoff, A., Houck, P. R., & Frank, E. (2009). A randomized controlled trial of culturally relevant, brief interpersonal psychotherapy for perinatal depression. [Randomized Controlled Trial Research Support, N.I.H., Extramural Research Support, Non-US Government]. *Psychiatric Services, 60*(3), 313–321.

Gum, A. M., Areàn, P. A., & Bostrom, A. (2007). Low-income depressed older adults with psychiatric comorbidity: Secondary analyses of response to psychotherapy and case management. [Comparative Study Randomized Controlled Trial Research Support, N.I.H., Extramural]. *International Journal of Geriatric Psychiatry, 22*(2), 124–130.

Gum, A. M., Areàn, P. A., Hunkeler, E., Tang, L., Katon, W., Hitchcock, P., ... Unutzer, J. (2006). Depression treatment preferences in older primary care patients. [Multicenter Study Randomized Controlled Trial Research Support, Non-US Government]. *Gerontologist, 46*(1), 14–22.

Gum, A. M., Iser, L., & Petkus, A. (2010). Behavioral health service utilization and preferences of older adults receiving home-based aging services. [Research Support, Non-US Government]. *American Journal of Geriatric Psychiatry, 18*(6), 491–501.

Hamblen, J. L., Norris, F. H., Gibson, L., & Lee, L. (2010). Training community therapists to deliver cognitive behavioral therapy in the aftermath of disaster. [Research Support, Non-US Government]. *International Journal of Emergency Mental Health, 12*(1), 33–40.

Hegel, M. T., Dietrich, A. J., Seville, J. L., & Jordan, C. B. (2004). Training residents in problem-solving treatment of depression: A pilot feasibility and impact study. [Evaluation Studies Research Support, US Government, P.H.S.]. *Family Medicine, 36*(3), 204–208.

Hegel, M. T., Lyons, K. D., Hull, J. G., Kaufman, P., Urquhart, L., Li, Z., & Ahles, T. A. (2010). Feasibility study of a randomized controlled trial of a telephone-delivered problem-solving-occupational therapy intervention to reduce participation restrictions in rural breast cancer survivors undergoing chemotherapy. *Psycho-oncology.* doi: 10.1002/pon.1830

Hodges, L., Butcher, I., Kleiboer, A., McHugh, G., Murray, G., Walker, J., ... Sharpe, M. (2009). Patient and general practitioner preferences for the treatment of depression in patients with cancer: How, who, and where? [Research Support, Non-US Government]. *Journal of Psychosomatic Research*, 67(5), 399–402.

Hwang, W-C. (2009). The Formative Method for Adapting Psychotherapy (FMAP): A community-based development approach to culturally adapting therapy. *Professional Psychology: Research and Practice*, 40(4), 369–377.

Karel, M. J., & Hinrichsen, G. (2000). Treatment of depression in late life: Psychotherapeutic interventions. [Review]. *Clinical Psychology Review*, 20(6), 707–729.

Kaufman, A. V., Scogin, F. R., Burgio, L. D., Morthland, M. P., & Ford, B. K. (2007). Providing mental health services to older people living in rural communities. [Research Support, N.I.H., Extramural]. *Journal of Gerontological Social Work*, 48(3–4), 349–365.

Kiosses, D. N., Areàn, P. A., Teri, L., & Alexopoulos, G. S. (2010). Home-delivered problem adaptation therapy (PATH) for depressed, cognitively impaired, disabled elders: A preliminary study. [Randomized Controlled Trial Research Support, N.I.H., Extramural Research Support, Non-US Government]. *American Journal of Geriatric Psychiatry*, 18(11), 988–998.

Kiosses, D. N., Leon, A. C., & Areàn, P. A. (2011). Psychosocial interventions for late-life major depression: Evidence-based treatments, predictors of treatment outcomes, and moderators of treatment effects. *Psychiatric Clinics of North America*, 34(2), 377–401, viii.

Kiosses, D. N., Teri, L., Velligan, D. I., & Alexopoulos, G. S. (2011). A home-delivered intervention for depressed, cognitively impaired, disabled elders. [Case Reports Research Support, N.I.H., Extramural Research Support, Non-US Government]. *International Journal of Geriatric Psychiatry*, 26(3), 256–262.

Krupnick, J. L., Green, B. L., Stockton, P., Miranda, J., Krause, E., & Mete, M. (2008). Group interpersonal psychotherapy for low-income women with posttraumatic stress disorder. [Randomized Controlled Trial Research Support, N.I.H., Extramural]. *Psychotherapy Research*, 18(5), 497–507.

Kunik, M. E., Braun, U., Stanley, M. A., Wristers, K., Molinari, V., Stoebner, D., & Orengo, C. A. (2001). One session cognitive behavioural therapy for elderly patients with chronic obstructive pulmonary disease. [Clinical Trial Evaluation Studies Randomized Controlled Trial Research Support, Non-US Government Research Support, US Government, Non-P.H.S. Research Support, US Government, P.H.S.]. *Psychological Medicine*, 31(4), 717–723.

Laidlaw, K., Davidson, K., Toner, H., Jackson, G., Clark, S., Law, J., ... Cross, S. (2008). A randomised controlled trial of cognitive behaviour therapy vs treatment as usual in the treatment of mild to moderate late life depression. [Comparative Study Randomized Controlled Trial Research Support, Non-US Government]. *International Journal of Geriatric Psychiatry*, 23(8), 843–850.

Leong, F. T., & Lee, S-H. (2006). A cultural accommodation model for cross-cultural psychotherapy: Illustrated with the case of Asian Americans. *Psychotherapy*, 43(4), 410–423.

Mackin, R. S., & Areàn, P. A. (2005). Evidence-based psychotherapeutic interventions for geriatric depression. [Review]. *Psychiatric Clinics of North America*, 28(4), 805–820, vii–viii.

Mancini, P., Bosco, E., D'Agosta, L., Traisci, G., Nicastri, M., Capelli, G., ... Filipo, R. (2009). Implementation of perceptual channels in children implanted with a HiRes 90K device. *Acta Oto-Laryngologica*, 129(12), 1442–1450.

McDougall, G. J., Jr. (1999). Cognitive interventions among older adults. [Review]. *Annual Review of Nursing Research*, 17, 219–240.

Miller, M. D., Cornes, C., Frank, E., Ehrenpreis, L., Silberman, R., Schlernitzauer, M. A., ... Reynolds, C. F., III. (2001). Interpersonal psychotherapy for late-life depression: past, present, and future. [Research Support, US Government, P.H.S.]. *Journal of Psychotherapy Practice and Research*, 10(4), 231–238.

Miller, M. D., Frank, E., Cornes, C., Houck, P. R., & Reynolds, C. F., III. (2003). The value of maintenance interpersonal psychotherapy (IPT) in older adults with different IPT foci. [Clinical Trial Randomized Controlled Trial Research Support, US Government, P.H.S.]. *American Journal of Geriatric Psychiatry*, 11(1), 97–102.

Mohlman, J. (2011). A community based survey of older adults' preferences for treatment of anxiety. *Psychology and Aging.* doi: 10.1037/a0023126

Mohr, D. C., Hart, S., & Vella, L. (2007). Reduction in disability in a randomized controlled trial of telephone-administered cognitive-behavioral therapy. [Evaluation Studies Randomized Controlled Trial Research Support, N.I.H., Extramural]. *Health Psychology, 26*(5), 554–563.

Nezu, A. M., & Perri, M. G. (1989). Social problem-solving therapy for unipolar depression: An initial dismantling investigation. [Clinical Trial Randomized Controlled Trial]. *Journal of Consulting and Clinical Psychology, 57*(3), 408–413.

Norcross, J. C., & Wampold, B. E. (2011). Evidence-based therapy relationships: Research conclusions and clinical practices. *Psychotherapy, 48*(1), 98–102.

Peng, X. D., Huang, C. Q., Chen, L. J., & Lu, Z. C. (2009). Cognitive behavioural therapy and reminiscence techniques for the treatment of depression in the elderly: a systematic review. [Meta-Analysis Review]. *Journal of International Medical Research, 37*(4), 975–982.

Pinquart, M., Duberstein, P. R., & Lyness, J. M. (2007). Effects of psychotherapy and other behavioral interventions on clinically depressed older adults: A meta-analysis. [Meta-Analysis]. *Aging and Mental Health, 11*(6), 645–657.

Post, E. P., Miller, M. D., & Schulberg, H. C. (2008). Using interpersonal psychotherapy (IPT) to treat depression in older primary care patients. *Geriatrics, 63*(3), 18–28.

Poulsen, C., Luu, P., Crane, S. M., Quiring, J., & Tucker, D. M. (2009). Frontolimbic activity and cognitive bias in major depression. *Journal of Abnormal Psychology, 118*(3), 494–506.

Raue, P. J., Schulberg, H. C., Heo, M., Klimstra, S., & Bruce, M. L. (2009). Patients' depression treatment preferences and initiation, adherence, and outcome: A randomized primary care study. [Randomized Controlled Trial Research Support, N.I.H., Extramural Research Support, Non-US Government]. *Psychiatric Services, 60*(3), 337–343.

Raue, P. J., Weinberger, M. I., Sirey, J. A., Meyers, B. S., & Bruce, M. L. (2011). Preferences for depression treatment among elderly home health care patients. [Research Support, N.I.H., Extramural]. *Psychiatric Services, 62*(5), 532–537.

Reynolds, C. F., III, Dew, M. A., Martire, L. M., Miller, M. D., Cyranowski, J. M., Lenze, E., ... Frank, E. (2010). Treating depression to remission in older adults: A controlled evaluation of combined escitalopram with interpersonal psychotherapy versus escitalopram with depression care management. [Randomized Controlled Trial Research Support, N.I.H., Extramural]. *International Journal of Geriatric Psychiatry, 25*(11), 1134–1141.

Reynolds, C. F., 3rd, Frank, E., Perel, J. M., Imber, S. D., Cornes, C., Miller, M. D., ... Kupfer,

D. J. (1999). Nortriptyline and interpersonal psychotherapy as maintenance therapies for recurrent major depression: A randomized controlled trial in patients older than 59 years. [Clinical Trial Randomized Controlled Trial Research Support, US Government, P.H.S.]. *Journal of the American Medical Association, 281*(1), 39–45.

Rovner, B. W., Casten, R. J., Hegel, M. T., Leiby, B. E., & Tasman, W. S. (2007). Preventing depression in age-related macular degeneration. [Randomized Controlled Trial Research Support, N.I.H., Extramural Research Support, Non-US Government]. *Archives of General Psychiatry, 64*(8), 886–892.

Rovner, B. W., Casten, R. J., Hegel, M. T., & Tasman, W. S. (2006). Minimal depression and vision function in age-related macular degeneration. [Randomized Controlled Trial Research Support, N.I.H., Extramural Research Support, Non-US Government]. *Ophthalmology, 113*(10), 1743–1747.

Scogin, F., Jamison, C., & Davis, N. (1990). Two-year follow-up of bibliotherapy for depression in older adults. *Journal of Consulting and Clinical Psychology, 58*(5), 665–667.

Scogin, F., Jamison, C., & Gochneaur, K. (1989). Comparative efficacy of cognitive and behavioral bibliotherapy for mildly and moderately depressed older adults. [Clinical Trial Comparative Study Randomized Controlled Trial Research Support, Non-US Government]. *Journal of Consulting and Clinical Psychology, 57*(3), 403–407.

Scogin, F., Morthland, M., Kaufman, A., Burgio, L., Chaplin, W., & Kong, G. (2007). Improving quality of life in diverse rural older adults: A randomized trial of a psychological treatment. [Randomized Controlled Trial Research Support, N.I.H., Extramural]. *Psychology and Aging, 22*(4), 657–665.

Scogin, F. R., Hanson, A., & Welsh, D. (2003). Self-administered treatment in stepped-care models of depression treatment. *Journal of Clinical Psychology, 59*(3), 341–349.

Serfaty, M. A., Haworth, D., Blanchard, M., Buszewicz, M., Murad, S., & King, M. (2009). Clinical effectiveness of individual cognitive behavioral therapy for depressed older people in primary care: A randomized controlled trial. [Comparative Study Randomized Controlled Trial Research Support, Non-US Government]. *Archives of General Psychiatry, 66*(12), 1332–1340.

Snowden, M., Steinman, L., & Frederick, J. (2008). Treating depression in older adults: Challenges to implementing the recommendations of an expert panel. [Research Support, US Government, P.H.S. Review]. *Preventing Chronic Disease, 5*(1), A26.

Steinman, L. E., Frederick, J. T., Prohaska, T., Satariano, W. A., Dornberg-Lee, S., Fisher, R.,...Snowden, M. (2007). Recommendations for treating depression in community-based older adults. [Consensus Development Conference Research Support, US Government, P.H.S.]. *American Journal of Preventive Medicine, 33*(3), 175–181.

Strachowski, D., Khaylis, A., Conrad, A., Neri, E., Spiegel, D., & Taylor, C. B. (2008). The effects of cognitive behavior therapy on depression in older patients with cardiovascular risk. [Research Support, N.I.H., Extramural]. *Depression and Anxiety, 25*(8), E1–10.

Tasman, W., & Rovner, B. (2004). Age-related macular degeneration: Treating the whole patient. [Editorial]. *Archives of Ophthalmology, 122*(4), 648–649.

Taylor, M. P., Reynolds, C. F., III, Frank, E., Cornes, C., Miller, M. D., Stack, J. A.,...Kupfer, D. J. (1999). Which elderly depressed patients remain well on maintenance interpersonal psychotherapy alone? Report from the Pittsburgh study of maintenance therapies in late-life depression. [Clinical Trial Randomized Controlled Trial Research Support, US Government, P.H.S.]. *Depression and Anxiety, 10*(2), 55–60.

Thompson, L. W., Gallagher, D., & Breckenridge, J. S. (1987). Comparative effectiveness of psychotherapies for depressed elders. [Research Support, US Government, P.H.S.]. *Journal of Consulting and Clinical Psychology, 55*(3), 385–390.

Thorp, S. R., Ayers, C. R., Nuevo, R., Stoddard, J. A., Sorrell, J. T., & Wetherell, J. L. (2009). Meta-analysis comparing different behavioral treatments for late-life anxiety. [Comparative Study Evaluation Studies Meta-Analysis Research Support, N.I.H., Extramural]. *American Journal of Geriatric Psychiatry, 17*(2), 105–115.

Tisdelle, D. A., & St Lawrence, J. S. (1986). Social skills training to enhance the interpersonal adjustment of a speech and hearing impaired adult. [Case Reports]. *Journal of Communication Disorders, 19*(3), 197–207.

Tolin, D. F. (2010). Is cognitive-behavioral therapy more effective than other therapies? A meta-analytic review. [Comparative Study Meta-Analysis Research Support, N.I.H.,

Extramural Research Support, Non-US Government]. *Clinical Psychology Review, 30*(6), 710–720.

Unutzer, J., Katon, W., Williams, J. W., Jr., Callahan, C. M., Harpole, L., Hunkeler, E. M.,...Langston, C. A. (2001). Improving primary care for depression in late life: The design of a multicenter randomized trial. [Clinical Trial Multicenter Study Randomized Controlled Trial Research Support, Non-US Government]. *Medical Care, 39*(8), 785–799.

van der Waerden, J. E., Hoefnagels, C., & Hosman, C. M. (2011). Psychosocial preventive interventions to reduce depressive symptoms in low-SES women at risk: A meta-analysis. [Meta-Analysis Research Support, Non-US Government Review]. *Journal of Affective Disorders, 128*(1–2), 10–23.

Van Voorhees, B. W., Ellis, J. M., Gollan, J. K., Bell, C. C., Stuart, S. S., Fogel, J.,...Ford, D. E. (2007). Development and process evaluation of a primary care internet-based intervention to prevent depression in emerging adults. *Primary Care Companion to the Journal of Clinical Psychiatry, 9*(5), 346–355.

Walker, D. A., & Clarke, M. (2001). Cognitive behavioural psychotherapy: A comparison between younger and older adults in two inner city mental health teams. [Comparative Study]. *Aging and Mental Health, 5*(2), 197–199.

Wilkins, C. H., Mathews, J., & Sheline, Y. I. (2009). Late life depression with cognitive impairment: Evaluation and treatment. [Research Support, N.I.H., Extramural Research Support, Non-US Government Review]. *Clinical Interventions in Aging, 4*, 51–57.

Wilkins, V. M., Kiosses, D., & Ravdin, L. D. (2010). Late-life depression with comorbid cognitive impairment and disability: Nonpharmacological interventions. [Research Support, N.I.H., Extramural Review]. *Clinical Interventions in Aging, 5*, 323–331.

Wilkinson, P., Alder, N., Juszczak, E., Matthews, H., Merritt, C., Montgomery, H.,...Jacoby, R. (2009). A pilot randomised controlled trial of a brief cognitive behavioural group intervention to reduce recurrence rates in late life depression. [Randomized Controlled Trial Research Support, Non-US Government]. *International Journal of Geriatric Psychiatry, 24*(1), 68–75.

23

ELECTROCONVULSIVE THERAPY AND NEUROMODULATION IN THE TREATMENT OF LATE-LIFE MOOD DISORDERS

William M. McDonald and Arshya Vahabzadeh

SINCE ELECTROCONVULSIVE therapy (ECT) was first introduced by the Italians Cerletti and Bini in 1938, ECT has been recognized as one of the most effective treatments for severe mood disorders (Abrams, 1992). Increasingly ECT has been used in the treatment of elderly mood disorders (Kramer, 1985), and research in ECT over the last 70 years has informed the field as to the optimal techniques, parameters, and indications for the use of ECT in elders (Greenberg & Kellner, 2005).

While many psychotherapeutic and psychopharmacological treatments for depression exist, older individuals suffering from late-life depression need special consideration. Age-related physiological changes and medical comorbidity complicate psychopharmacological treatment. Older individuals are more likely to be sensitive to, and develop side effects from, antidepressant medication (Katz, Simpson, Curlik, Parmelee, & Muhly, 1990; Mark et al., 2011) and ECT is generally well tolerated by elders (Damm et al., 2010).

In comparison to other modalities, ECT has many potential advantages. ECT has been shown to be particularly effective in treating depression in older individuals (O'Connor et al., 2001; Tew et al., 1999). Patients often have a rapid response and side effects are typically minor and transient (Damm et al., 2010). The safety profile of ECT includes one of the lowest mortality rates of any procedure performed under a general anesthetic (Abrams, 1997). In light of the advantages of using ECT for late-life depression, some authors have questioned why ECT is not considered earlier in the treatment algorithm (Beale & Kellner, 2000; Roose & Sackeim, 2004).

Several barriers interfere with the availability and use of ECT in the elderly. ECT availability is determined by factors such as physician and mental health worker attitudes toward the procedure (Berg, 2009; Latey & Fahy, 1985; Sackeim Devanand, & Nobler, 1995), which vary widely (Janicak, Mask, Trimakas, & Gibbons, 1985). There remains considerable stigma associated with ECT with negative media depictions and images of the less refined past practices predominating (van der Wurff, Stek, Hoogendijk, & Beekman, 2004). Interestingly, it appears that older individuals hold fewer misconceptions regarding ECT than their younger counterparts (Dowman, Patel, & Rajput, 2005) and the use of ECT in geriatric patients in the United States actually increased from 1987 to 1992, the last time practice patterns were systematically assessed (Rosenbach, Hermann, & Dorwart, 1997).

This chapter will explore the indications, side effects, and practical considerations of using ECT for late-life depression. Additionally, the authors will outline other emerging neuromodulatory techniques such as transcranial magnetic stimulation and deep brain stimulation in the treatment of late-life mood disorders.

MECHANISM OF ANTIDEPRESSANT ACTION

Despite the robust evidence outlining the effectiveness of ECT in the treatment of depression, the exact mechanism by which ECT acts as an antidepressant is not entirely clear. Psychological, psychodynamic, and biological theories have all been postulated as being responsible for its antidepressant action. Although ECT has some biomarkers in common with antidepressant treatment, other biomarkers associated with antidepressant response such as the increase in brain-derived neurotropic factor (BDNF) (Fernandes et al., 2009) or the length of the serotonin transporter gene (Rasmussen & Black, 2009) have not been correlated with response to ECT. It would seem likely that ECT may have a unique mechanism of action particularly given the response to ECT in depressed patients who have failed multiple antidepressant trials.

Most recent theories have focused on the wide-ranging impact of ECT on the neurophysiological system. ECT is known to affect almost all neurotransmitters, a multitude of hormonal systems, and neurogenesis (Merkl, Heuser, & Bajbouj, 2009). This widespread effect makes identifying exactly which changes are responsible for its antidepressant effect a difficult task.

The anticonvulsant hypothesis is one of the most widely accepted theories. It attributes the antidepressant effect of ECT to its anticonvulsant action. During a course of ECT an increase in the seizure threshold, a decrease in seizure duration,

and alterations in cerebral blood flow are all documented (Sackeim, 1999).

Neurotransmitter changes, including changes in gamma-aminobutyric acid (GABA) and an endogenous opioid type substance, have been proposed as being integral to the anticonvulsant hypothesis (Sackeim, Decina, Prohovnik, Malitz, & Resor, 1983). Changes in GABA-ergic transmission following electroconvulsive stimulation have been demonstrated in both human and animal models (Sanacora et al., 2003; Sartorius, Mahlstedt, Vollmayr, Henn, & Ende, 2007). Sanacora et al. demonstrated a doubling of GABA-ergic activity in the occipital cortex of depressed human patients following ECT, with previous research having already highlighted hypoactivity of GABA in the occipital cortex of depressed individuals (Sanacora et al., 1999, 2003).

Experiments in animals have suggested that an opioid type substance and changes in opioid receptor density may be responsible for the anticonvulsant effect (Holaday, Tortella, Meyerhoff, Belenky, & Hitzemann, 1986; Tortella & Long, 1985). Tortella et al. demonstrated that the observed anticonvulsant effect could be transmitted from an electroconvulsively stimulated rat to a nonstimulated rat through cerebrospinal fluid. The study also observed how this effect could be antagonized with the opiate receptor antagonist, naltrexone (Tortella & Long, 1985, 1988). In contrast to animal studies, use of naltrexone in humans has not demonstrated any change in seizure duration (Prudic, Fitzsimons, Nobler, & Sackeim, 1999).

ECT may also normalize deficits in glutaminergic transmission (Pfleiderer et al., 2003); these deficits have been demonstrated in the anterior cingulate cortex and prefrontal areas of individuals with depression (Capizzano, Jorge, Acion, & Robinson, 2007). The increase in glutaminergic transmission as a result of ECT has been reported to correlate to improvements in depression symptom scales (Zhang et al., 2012).

ELECTROCONVULSIVE THERAPY FOR LATE-LIFE DEPRESSION

ECT is a primary somatic treatment in geriatric mood disorders, particularly when the patient is treatment resistant or intolerant to pharmacotherapy. Ensuring prompt diagnosis and treatment is crucial in minimizing the morbidity and mortality of late-life mood disorder and considering the specific risk factors, including the increased risk of suicide in the depressed elderly (Conwell & Brent, 1995). ECT has been shown to be an effective treatment for late-life depression (O'Connor et al., 2001; Tew et al., 1999).

O'Connor et al. investigated the remission rates of 253 patients with unipolar and bipolar depression who were treated with bitemporal ECT (O'Connor et al., 2001). The highest remission rates were seen in the 45–64 years group and over 65 years age group (89.8% and 90%, respectively). Remission rates for the patients less than 45 years old were significantly lower (70%). Tew et al. had similar findings in patients older than 75 years who were given a course of ECT for major depression. Remission rates were highest in patients 60–74 years old and over 75 years old (73% and 67%, respectively). Patients under the age of 59 years had a significantly lower response to ECT (54%) (Tew et al., 1999).

Suicidal Ideation

Lack of recognition of the risk of suicide among the elderly depressed is a major issue in the clinical care of the depressed elders (Conwell et al., 1998). Suicide in the elderly is of significant concern given that they use more lethal means and communicate their suicidal intent less commonly than their younger counterparts. The American Psychiatric Association guidelines for the treatment of elderly depression support the utility of ECT as a fast and effective treatment in reducing suicidal ideation (Weiner, 2001).

Early reports by Prudic and Sackeim (1999) noted the effectiveness of ECT in treating suicidal patients.Two more recent studies have demonstrated the effectiveness in treating suicidal ideation with ECT (Kellner et al., 2005; Patel, Patel, Hardy, Benzies, & Tare, 2006). Kellner et al. demonstrated that depressed patients who were administered ECT had a more rapid reduction in suicidal ideation. Patients over 50 years old were the subgroup with the most rapid cessation of suicidal ideation (Kellner et al., 2005). After a course of bitemporal ECT, the absence of suicidal ideation was noted in 89% of patients over 50 years, but only 76% of patients less than 50 years of age. Kellner et al. found a significant relationship between resolution of expressed suicidal intent and age ($p < .03$).

Psychotic Features

Patients with late-life depression are more likely to demonstrate comorbid psychotic features (Brodaty et al., 1997). Psychotic depression has been noted to be particularly resistant to pharmacological treatment (Meyers et al., 2001). In contrast, ECT appears to be especially effective in treating depression with psychotic features (Birkenhager, Pluijms, & Lucius, 2003; Petrides et al., 2001). Petrides et al. compared the rates of remission in 253 depressed patients with and without psychotic features. Most patients met criteria for nonpsychotic depression (nonpsychotic, $n = 176$ vs. psychotic, $n = 77$). Study completers had an overall remission rate of 87% and patients with psychotic depression had a significantly higher remission rate than patients without comorbid psychosis prior to receiving ECT (95% and 83%, respectively, $p < .01$). Patients diagnosed with psychotic depression also demonstrated a faster remission of symptoms compared to their nonpsychotic counterparts (Petrides et al., 2001).

ELECTROCONVULSIVE THERAPY FOR LATE-LIFE BIPOLAR DISORDER

In adult patients, ECT is effective in the treatment of acute mania in the patients with bipolar disorder. A review by Mukerjee et al. found that 80% of patients diagnosed with acute mania responded significantly or underwent remission following use of ECT (Mukherjee, Sackeim, & Schnur, 1994). This response rate is all the more impressive since a considerable proportion of the patients in this review had demonstrated resistance to pharmacotherapy. Unilateral ECT has also been demonstrated to be effective in the treatment of mania which did not respond to pharmacotherapy (Robinson, Penzner, Arkow, Kahn, & Berman, 2011). However, there are no randomized clinical trials comparing pharmacotherapy to ECT in the elderly, and the clinical guidance for the use of ECT in older patients with mania is based on extrapolation from studies in younger adults and published case studies (Blazer & Steffens, 2009; McDonald & Nemeroff, 1996).

ECT has also been demonstrated to be effective in the treatment of mixed affective states (Devanand et al., 2000). In a nonrandomized trial of 130 patients with unipolar, bipolar I, and bipolar II depression, Medda et al. (Medda, Perugi, Zanello, Ciuffa, & Cassano, 2009) found an excellent remission rate for depressive symptoms in all groups (70.5% for unipolar, 56.7% for bipolar II, and 65.3% for bipolar I), with significant residual manic and psychotic symptoms in the bipolar patients. In the subgroup of bipolar I patients with depression or mixed states, Medda et al. found that both groups responded to ECT, although the patients diagnosed in a mixed state had more residual agitation and psychosis after a course of ECT (Medda et al., 2010).

Ciapparelli et al. evaluated 23 medication-nonresponsive patients diagnosed with mixed mania and bipolar depression (Ciapparelli et al., 2001). Patients in both groups had a significant decrease in depressive and psychotic symptoms; however, the response in the mixed mania group was more rapid and associated with a greater reduction in suicidal ideation. In contrast to patients with unipolar depression (e.g., Petrides et al., 2001), response to ECT was not influenced by the presence of delusions.

The data for the efficacy of ECT in older patients with bipolar depression are limited to patients who have failed multiple medications or are unable to tolerate pharmacotherapy (Aziz, Lorberg, & Tampi, 2006). Nevertheless, ECT has been shown to be effective in both the depressed and mixed bipolar patients with late-life depression. Compared to older unipolar patients, elders with bipolar depression have an equivalent response rate and a faster rate of response (Daly et al., 2001).

Little et al. (2004) reported on a cases series of patients over 65 years old with bipolar depression who were treated with ECT. They found ECT to be clinically effective in treating bipolar depression; however, their report was limited by a small sample size (n = 5).

ELECTROCONVULSIVE THERAPY IN NEUROPSYCHIATRIC DISORDERS

There is considerable support in the literature for the fact that older patients who are pharmacotherapy treatment resistant have more neuroanatomic brain changes and are more likely to be administered ECT (Coffey, Figiel, Djang, Saunders, & Weiner, 1989, Coffey, Figiel, Djang, & Weiner, 1990; Steffens et al., 2001). There is also evidence that neuroanatomic changes are associated with ECT-induced delirium (Figiel, Coffey, Djang, Hoffman, & Doraiswamy, 1990).

There are little data beyond case reports that ECT is effective in treating agitated dementia (Bang, Price, Prentice, & Campbell, 2008; Burgut

& Kellner, 2010; Burgut, Popeo, & Kellner, 2010; Fazzari et al., 2009; Katagai, Yasui-Furukori, Kikuchi, & Kaneko, 2007; Sutor & Rasmussen, 2008; Wu, Prentice, & Campbell, 2010). Case reports also support the use of ECT in demented patients with comorbid affective disorder (Fisman, Rabheru, & Sharma, 2001; McDonald & Thompson 2001; Rao & Lyketsos 2000; Suzuki, Takano, & Matsuoka, 2009; Takahashi, Mizukami, Yasuno, & Asada, 2009; Weintraub & Lippmann, 2001).

Treating patients with dementia can be challenging given the potential for cognitive side effects, yet patients with dementia can be safely and effectively treated with ECT. In a consecutive case series of 43 elderly depressed patients with no cognitive impairment (NCI), mild cognitive impairment (MCI), or dementia, Hausner et al. (Hausner, Damian, Sartorius, & Frölich, 2011) found that all three groups had a good response to a course of ECT and that ECT was well tolerated in spite of preexisting cognitive impairment. Overall the pre-ECT Mini Mental Status Examination (MMSE) score was the most significant predictor of cognitive decline 6 weeks post ECT with a trend toward significance at 6 months. In fact, at 6 months the NCI and MCI groups showed an improvement over baseline using the MMSE, and the dementia group remained stable. Although encouraging, these results should be interpreted with caution as the MMSE is a crude indicator of global cognitive function and would not assess more subtle problems with autobiographical memory or other subtypes of cognitive dysfunction associated with ECT.

Psychiatric comorbidity is common among people with Parkinson's disease (PD). Depression is the most commonly associated psychiatric condition and can affect over 40% of patients with PD (Cummings & Masterman, 1999; McDonald, Holtzheimer, & Byrd, 2006). ECT is an effective treatment for PD with comorbid depression and has been associated with an improvement in both depressive symptoms and also parkinsonian motor symptoms (Moellentine et al., 1998). Motor symptom improvement precedes the improvement in depressive symptoms (Cummings, 1992). Improvement in motor symptoms may be related to increased dopaminergic activity, release, and synthesis as a result of ECT (Fall, Ekman, Granérus, Thorell, & Wålinder, 1995). ECT has also been reported to be effective in treating drug-induced parkinsonism, which had not responded to typical treatment options (Baez & Avery, 2011).

Moellentine et al. conducted a study examining the effectiveness of ECT in psychiatric conditions among people diagnosed with PD and comorbid depression and anxiety. Despite a small number of participants ($n = 25$), they demonstrated significant improvements in both depressive and anxiety symptoms. Global assessment of functioning was also reported as being significantly improved as a result of a course of ECT (Moellentine et al., 1998).

THE STIGMA OF ELECTROCONVULSIVE THERAPY

Stigma surrounding the use of ECT is substantial and has been described as being the biggest barrier to the public acceptance of this treatment modality (Dowman et al., 2005). Misconceptions and stigma surrounding ECT has been attributed to a multitude of factors. Negative depictions in film and news media, the efforts of coalitions lobbying against ECT, and resources on the Internet have all been identified as sources of stigma. Patients, their families, and the public have all been identified as having significant misconceptions regarding ECT (Kerr, McGrath, O'Kearney, & Price, 1982; McFarquhar & Thompson, 2008; Payne & Prudic, 2009).

European research into public attitudes toward ECT suggests less than 2% of the public are in favor of ECT treatment, while more than 50% believe it to be harmful. Kerr et al. sampled attitudes toward ECT by visitors to a general psychiatric hospital. Over 60% of visitors expressed feelings of fear or dread toward electroconvulsive therapy (Kerr et al., 1982). A majority of these visitors (60.7%) felt ECT was inhumane, with a similar percentage having expressed major concern regarding fear of pain with the procedure. Previous research highlighted additional concerns among patients who were concerned with the potential for brain damage, memory loss, and personality change with ECT (Malcolm, 1989).

While there is evidence that older individuals may hold fewer misconceptions regarding ECT than their younger counterparts, international data on their attitudes are concerning (Bustin et al., 2008; Dowman et al., 2005; Lauber, Nordt, Falcato, & Rössler, 2005). Bustin et al. conducted an attitudinal-based study involving 75 elderly patients across Argentina, the United Kingdom, and Canada (Bustin et al., 2008). While knowledge about ECT was better in Canada and the United Kingdom in comparison to Argentina, this did not lead to a significant difference in overall attitudes toward ECT. Disappointingly, only a minority of participants felt ECT was safe in patients over the age of 65 years (24%) and only a small percentage of participants felt that ECT was more effective than medications (15%). The majority of patients stated they would also decline treatment with ECT if it were recommended to them.

The principal role of the psychiatrist is to ensure that our patients are well informed about the effectiveness and safety profile of ECT. Active involvement of older individuals in decision making is particularly important. Older individuals have a greater desire to be actively involved in decision making in psychiatric settings compared to younger individuals (O'Neal et al., 2008). Often when older individuals are treated, the close friends and families may have an important role in the decision-making process. Therefore, it is important that all persons who are involved in the decision-making process are given sufficient, accurate, and understandable information regarding ECT.

METHODOLOGY OF ELECTROCONVULSIVE THERAPY

Electrode Placement

There are two primary electrode placements used in ECT: bitemporal and unilateral placements. Bitemporal (BT) ECT involves positioning of electrodes on each temple and may also be referred to as bilateral ECT. BT ECT is the standard to which the efficacy and side effects of other electrode placements are compared. BT ECT has been recognized as being the placement of choice in clinical situations that necessitate rapid psychiatric stabilization (Kellner et al., 2010).

Unfortunately, the cognitive side effects of BT ECT have remained a significant concern, especially in older individuals with comorbid neuropsychiatric disease (Flint & Gagnon, 2002). An attempt to minimize these cognitive side effects has resulted in the increasing use of right unilateral ECT. This involves placement of electrodes on the right temple and in the vertex position (the point which crossects a line drawn between external auditory canals and a line running vertically down the posterior aspect of the skull).

Right unilateral (RUL) ECT potentially avoids the detrimental effects on the dominant language

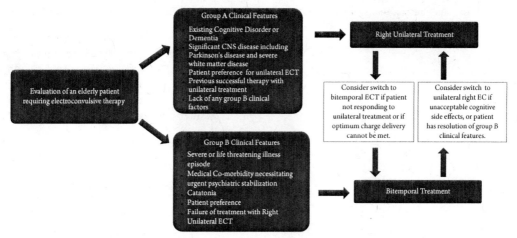

FIGURE 23.1 Algorithmic approach to electroconvulsive therapy (ECT) electrode placement in elderly individuals. CNS, central nervous system.

areas typically found in the left hemisphere. While originally the efficacy of RUL ECT appeared lower than BT ECT, this finding was due in part to the underdosing of stimulus charge. Recent data demonstrate that using high-dose RUL ECT (six times the seizure threshold) demonstrate efficacy similar to BT ECT dosed at 1.5–2.5 times seizure threshold (Kellner et al., 2010; McCall, Reboussin, Weiner, & Sackeim, 2000; Sackeim, Decina, Kanzler, Kerr, & Malitz, 1987; Sackeim et al., 1986; Sackeim et al., 2000).

Modern ECT practice supports the technique of dosing ECT according to the individual patient's seizure threshold. The seizure threshold is determined by a number of factors, including skull thickness, concomitant medication, gender (males > females), and type of treatment (BT ECT has higher seizure threshold than RUL ECT), but the most important factor is the age of the subject (older aged patients have a higher seizure threshold than matched younger patients) (Petrides et al., 2009). The fact that age is one of the most important determinants in seizure threshold is the background for the oft used half-age method in determining the dose of BTECT (Petrides et al., 2009). The half-age method states that the machine should be set for percentage output in millicoulombs (mCs) equal to the patients age divided by two (e.g., a 50-year-old would be treated a 25% of the total output of the machine).

Using the seizure titration method, the cognitive side effects of ECT would be minimized because the patient is administered the lowest effective dose of ECT. In fact, the dose at which ECT is administered above the seizure threshold is the most significant

determinant of the cognitive side effects of ECT (McCall et al., 2000; Quante et al., 2011). And although BT ECT has been shown to have more cognitive side effects than RUL ECT (O'Connor, Gardner, Eppingstall, & Tofler, 2010; Sackeim et al., 2007, 2008), a recent randomized controlled trial supports the fact efficacy of RUL ECT at 6 times the seizure threshold is equivalent to BT ECT at 1.5 times seizure in respect to efficacy and cognitive side effects (Kellner et al., 2010).

A treatment algorithm is outlined in Figure 23.1. This treatment algorithm assumes that older patients will start with RUL ECT unless there are significant severity factors, including catatonia or life-threatening psychiatric symptoms (e.g., severe suicidal ideation, refusal to eat). BT ECT has been shown to work faster in decreasing symptoms and suicidal ideation (Kellner et al., 2005) so speed of response should be considered in choosing electrode placement. Another factor to be considered is previous response to RUL ECT.

Bifrontal (BF) ECT was not included in this algorithm. BF ECT is potentially as effective as BT ECT with fewer cognitive side effects since it avoids direct stimulation of the temporal lobes. The most recent randomized trial of BF ECT shows that it has no advantage over BT ECT in terms of efficacy or cognitive side effects (Kellner et al., 2010). However, this study was not focused on the elderly. Future research is needed to determine the role of BF ECT in this algorithm.

At the present time the most reasonable approach to stimulus dosing would be to use brief-pulse RUL ECT dosed at least six times the seizure threshold for patients meeting Group A clinical features. It should be noted that brief-pulse RUL ECT has been shown to have a slower speed of response than longer pulse width RUL ECT (.3 msec versus 1.0 msec) (Sienaert, Vansteelandt, Demyttenaere, & Peuskens, 2009). If speed of response is a major clinical factor, then using a longer pulse width RUL or BT ECT would be appropriate.

Given the data that higher dose RUL (>6 times the seizure threshold) is more effective using RUL ECT (McCall, Farah et al., 1995), the dose of RUL ECT should be increased after perhaps the fourth treatment if there is no response to RUL ECT. The clinician should balance the fact that the efficacy of RUL ECT increases with increased dose above seizure threshold, although the cognitive side effects also increase (McCall, Farah et al., 1995).

If the patient meets Group B clinical features or shows no response to RUL, he or she should be administered BT ECT at 1.5 times the seizure threshold. Given the data on the lack of efficacy of brief-pulse BT ECT (Sackeim et al., 2008), patients treated with BT should be treated at longer pulse widths (i.e., 1.0 msec or longer). Patients who do not respond to 1.5 times the seizure threshold should be increased to at least 2.5 times the seizure threshold. Consideration should be given to allowing the patient a week or two between switching from RUL to BT ECT to decrease the potential for cumulative cognitive side effects.

Another approach was outlined by Kellner as a modal approach to dosing ECT (Kellner, 2001). Kellner argues that patients, including older patients, should be treated with high-dose RUL ECT or BT ECT based on the half-age method. This approach certainly has merit and is easy to implement, although it does not take into account the possibility that clinical factors (e.g., the use of concomitant anticonvulsant medications) that could artificially raise the seizure threshold and the half-age method could underestimate the dose of ECT needed.

Nevertheless, the extant data would support the use of seizure titration (either by a half-age estimate or using a seizure titration method) particularly when implementing BT ECT as a way to decrease the potential for cognitive side effects in the elderly. Other means for decreasing cognitive side effects are to administer ECT twice a week rather than three times a week (McAllister, Perri, Jordan, Rauscher, & Sattin, 1987; Shapira, Tubi, & Lerer, 2000), and twice a week ECT should be considered for elderly patients.

Pretreatment Medical Assessment

Comprehensive medical assessment is essential prior to ECT, especially considering the increasing medical morbidity present in older adults. The assessment process is best undertaken through a coordinated approach by both psychiatrist and anesthesiologist. Assessment priorities are to identify and manage conditions that may elevate the risk of complications with ECT and the accompanying anesthesia. A detailed medical history and examination are integral to this assessment process (American Psychiatric Association, 2001). A detailed neurological examination is recommended, and special attention must be paid to both cardiac and respiratory comorbidity. Basic laboratory testing should also be undertaken, including a complete blood count and electrolyte studies. A chest X-ray may also be necessary in patients with significant pulmonary disease or cardiac failure. Consideration of spinal X-rays may be appropriate in those with spinal pathology or a strong history of back pain. Routine electrocardiogram has also been recommended in those above 50 years of age (Tess & Smetana, 2009). Brain imaging is not recommended as routine unless a brain abnormality is suspected or positive neurological signs are encountered (American Psychiatric Association, 2001).

The American Psychiatric Association's 2001 consensus statement identified no absolute contraindications to ECT treatment (American Psychiatric Association, 2001). ECT maintains an impressive safety profile and remains one of the lowest risk treatment procedures involving general anesthesia with a mortality rate as low as 0.002% (Abrams, 1997).

There are several conditions that increase the likelihood of complications with ECT therapy. These are outlined in Table 23.1 and include the presence of unstable cardiac conditions and intracranial lesions.

CARDIOVASCULAR DISEASE

While most cardiovascular complications are transient, they remain key causes of the mortality and morbidity associated with ECT (Magid, Lapid, Sampson, & Mueller, 2005). The presence of preexisting cardiac disease predisposes to the development of both transient and longer lasting cardiovascular complications following administration of ECT (Zielinski et al., 1993). During the

Table 23.1. Conditions increasing risk of complications in ECT

- Recent Myocardial Infarction
- Unstable Cardiac Disease
- Intracranial Mass or Aneurysm
- Ischemic or Hemorrhagic Stroke
- Severe pulmonary disease
- American Society of Anesthesiology physical status
- classification level 4 or 5*

*Level 4: patients with severe systemic disease that is a constant threat to life and moribund patients Level 5: moribund patients who are not expected to survive without the operation.

administration of ECT, marked cardiovascular and hemodynamic changes are noted.

Increased sympathetic nervous system tone with accompanying catecholamine release occurs after a transient initial parasympathetic response. The sympathetic response typically lasts 10 minutes, and in adults over 50 years of age, systolic blood pressure and heart rate can rise by 29% and 58%, respectively (Takada et al., 2005). When assessing patients who have a significant cardiac history, the opinion of a cardiologist is recommended.

At present, there are no guidelines in existence that stratify cardiovascular risk prior to ECT. Tess and Smetana have suggested that ECT should be considered as a low-risk procedure as defined by American College of Cardiology and the American Heart Association (Fleisher et al., 2007; Tess & Smetana, 2009). Consultation with a cardiologist with expertise in ECT would be useful in patients who have cardiac failure, previous myocardial infarction, arrhythmia, uncontrolled hypertension, and valvular heart disease since these patients have been identified as a high-risk group (e.g., diabetic patients) (Gerring & Shields, 1982).

Myocardial infarction is a recognized complication of ECT, and the presence of a recent myocardial infarction is a relative contraindication to the use of ECT (Lopez-Gomez, Sanchez-Corral, Cobo, Jara, & Esplugas, 1999). Myocardial tissue that has been damaged and weakened due to infarction will be under increased stress during sympathetically driven hypertension and tachycardia observed following ECT. Fatal outcomes associated with recent myocardial infarction, although rare, have included ventricular arrhythmias and cardiac rupture

(Abrams, 1992; Ali & Tidmarsh, 1997). A decision to proceed with ECT in older adults with a recent myocardial infarction must consider patient preference, individual circumstances, cardiology recommendations, and the urgency of ECT.

Hypertension is commonly encountered in older individuals. Hypertension should be stabilized prior to ECT. Patients who are currently controlled on their antihypertensive medication should continue to receive it during ECT. Beta-blockers have been demonstrated to attenuate cardiovascular response following ECT administration (van den Broek et al., 2008).

ECT can be safely used in patients with pacemakers and implantable cardioverter defibrillators (ICDs) (Davis et al., 2009; Dolenc, Barnes, Hayes, & Rasmussen, 2004). Cardiology or internal medicine consult should be sought in these cases as the devices require pre- and posttherapy interrogation. ICD devices should be deactivated prior to commencement of ECT (Dolenc et al., 2004). ECT is unlikely to affect pacemakers due to high tissue resistance and high voltage circuits in pacemakers (Abrams, 2002).

ECT has also been used safely in people with atrial fibrillation. ECT can, however, cause the heart to revert to sinus rhythm, therefore raising the possibility of embolization (Petrides & Fink, 1996). In light of this, anticoagulation should be continued to minimize this risk (Petrides & Fink, 1996).

There has been recent evidence demonstrating the relative safety of ECT in individuals with a prolonged QTc (Pullen, Rasmussen, Angstman, Rivera, & Mueller, 2011). While a statistical association between prolonged QTc and a cardiac event requiring intervention was noted, serious complications remained rare. The research supports the judicious use of ECT even in patients with a QTc of 500 milliseconds or longer given adequate medical assessment and monitoring.

NEUROLOGICAL DISEASE

Seizures are believed to cause a transient increase in intracranial pressure (Maltbie et al., 1980). This is believed to occur as a result of increased cerebral blood flow and metabolism (Ingvar, 1986; Maltbie et al., 1980). The accompanying increased carbon dioxide production, decreased pH, and systemic hypertension are believed to be responsible for causing a 300% increase in cerebral blood flow (Ingvar, 1986).

The presence of an intracranial mass is a relative contraindication to the use of ECT (American Psychiatric Association, 2001). Some factors may increase the risk of complications, which include surrounding edema, mass effect, or raised intracranial pressure. Neuroimaging is advised alongside consultation with neurology or neurosurgery. There have, however, been several reports of uncomplicated ECT in people with intracranial masses (Kohler & Burock, 2001; McKinney, Beale, & Kellner, 1998; Rasmussen, Perry, Sutor, & Moore, 2007). It has been suggested that if there is a solitary mass that lacks edema, mass effect, or increased intracranial pressure, then the risk of complications is unlikely to be elevated (Rasmussen et al., 2007).

The presence of an intracranial mass warrants daily neurological examination if a course of ECT is undertaken, with prompt access to neuroimaging and neurosurgical consultation if focal neurological signs develop (Rasmussen et al., 2007). The removal of an intracranial mass may sometimes be followed by a postoperative placement of a metallic skull plate. The use of ECT with a modified technique of electrode placement has been successfully documented in patients with metallic skull plates (Ling, Manepalli, & Grossberg, 2010; Madan & Anderson, 2001).

Intracranial vascular lesions are also a relative contraindication to ECT with concerns regarding the risk of rupture following rapid increases in cerebral blood flow (American Psychiatric Association, 2001). Although there is a paucity of studies with vascular lesions and ECT, several reports have shown no mortality when intraprocedural blood pressure is controlled (Najjar & Guttmacher, 1998; Zahedi, Yang, O'Hanlon, Tanev, & Shea, 2006).

ECT has also been successfully used in people who have had a stroke. Two small studies have reported on ECT treatment in poststroke depression cases.

The two studies consisted of 14 and 20 people diagnosed with poststroke depression and underwent treatment with ECT. Improvement in depressive symptoms was observed in the majority of patients, 12 and 19 cases, respectively (Currier, Murray, & Welch, 1992; Murray, Shea, & Conn, 1986). In both samples there were no instances of exacerbation of stroke or worsening of neurological function.

A third study by Martin et al. noted no significant side effects to ECT among 14 older individuals with a history of a cerebrovascular accident (Martin, Figiel, Mattingly, Zorumski, & Jarvis, 1992). Four individuals in the study had experienced a stroke less than 1 month prior to commencement of ECT.

Despite this limited evidence base suggesting ECT is safe to use among those with a history of stroke, a couple of case reports have identified stroke as being a potential complication of treatment with ECT (Bruce, Henry, & Greer, 2006; Lee, 2006). This combined with the lack of double-blind, randomized controlled trials into the use of ECT in poststroke patients suggests a need for caution and further research. It has been suggested that waiting at least 1 month following stroke may be a way of minimizing risk, and this is in keeping with stroke guidelines for individuals undergoing noncardiac surgery (Tess & Smetana, 2009). The guidelines are generally that patients should wait at least 6 months post stroke, particularly in patients in whom the stroke was hemorrhagic and the cerebrovascular system was more severely compromised.

PULMONARY DISEASE

Chronic obstructive pulmonary disease (COPD) and asthma are prevalent among older individuals. There is, however, a paucity of literature focusing on the risk associated with such conditions in individuals treated with ECT.

Limited evidence appears to suggest that with adequate treatment and control of symptoms, the use of ECT in people with asthma and COPD is safe and effective (Mueller, Schak, Barnes, & Rasmussen, 2006; Schak, Mueller, Barnes, & Rasmussen, 2008). Mueller et al. studied the safety of ECT use among patients with asthma. In their study 12% of patients developed an exacerbation of their asthma following ECT treatment. In these cases the exacerbation was subsequently controlled with standard asthma medications and the patients all subsequently completed their courses of ECT (Mueller et al., 2006). It is recommended that during an acute exacerbation of COPD or asthma, ECT should be postponed until the condition is controlled. Exceptionally, ECT may proceed if the condition was life threatening, and the rapid administration of ECT was critical.

The use of theophylline may be encountered in patients with COPD or asthma. Theophylline has been linked to the development of status epilepticus in patients receiving ECT and should be tapered and discontinued if possible prior to treatment (Devanand, Decina, Sackeim, & Prudic, 1988).

The administration of ECT has also been associated, albeit rarely, with the development of pulmonary edema (Bryson, Popeo, & Kellner, 2012). While a literature review demonstrated only eight cases, the potentially serious nature of clinically significant pulmonary edema warrants attention. ECT has been associated with both cardiogenic and negative-pressure pulmonary edema. Negative pressure pulmonary edema is believed to be precipitated by inadequate muscular paralysis, which allows the patient to take a substantial inspiratory effort despite a closed glottis or obstructed airway. Male gender and an athletic build may be additional risk factors for the development of this type of pulmonary edema as a result of an individual's enhanced ability to generate a large inspiratory effort. Prevention may be best achieved by ensuring adequate neuromuscular blockade (Myers, Gopalka, Glick, Goldman, & Dinwiddie, 2007).

ANESTHETIC AGENTS

An ideal anesthetic agent in ECT would not alter seizure duration or threshold, have a rapid onset, maintain a brief duration of action, and demonstrate a robust safety profile. A variety of different agents are used for anesthesia in ECT, including propofol, methohexital, thiopental, and etomidate. Methohexital is generally considered the first-line anesthetic agent for ECT. Methohexital has an established safety record, is short acting, and is inexpensive. The typical stating dose is in the range of .75–1.0 mg/ kg with dosage adjustments made after the first treatment.

Thiopental is another short-acting barbiturate that has been used for ECT anesthesia. A relative disadvantage to using thiopental is the concern that, compared to methohexital, thiopental may be associated with significantly more hemodynamic instability (Zaidi & Khan, 2000).

In recent years, propofol is being used more commonly in ECT anesthesia. Propofol has a number of potential advantages over the short-acting barbiturates and etomidate. Propofol has been shown to decrease hemodynamic changes associated with ECT (Gazdag, Kocsis, Tolna, & Iványi, 2004; Geretsegger et al., 2007), including a reduced risk of cardiac arrhythmias (Hooten & Rasmussen, 2008). Propofol has also been linked to faster recovery times and decreased confusion immediately post ECT compared to other agents (Butterfield, Graf, Macleod, Ries, & Zis, 2004; Geretsegger et al.,

2007). One potential downside to using propofol is the concern that propofol is associated with a reduction in the seizure duration and need for increased seizure charge (Eranti, Mogg, Pluck, Landau, & McLoughlin, 2009). The result, particularly in older adults with increased baseline seizure thresholds, could be missed seizures, although there is no evidence that using propofol resulted in either a reduction in seizure quality or in the therapeutic response to ECT (Eranti et al., 2009; Gazdag et al., 2004). Propofol is dosed in the range of 0.75–1.5 mg/kg. Propofol can cause pain on injection, and some patients may require the addition of a very small dose of lidocaine in the i.v. Lidocaine also has anticonvulsant properties and so should be used judiciously in these patients.

Etomidate has also been used for ECT anesthesia and has some advantages. Etomidate is associated with longer seizure times than the barbiturates and propofol (Gazdag et al., 2004) and is useful in patients with missed or aborted seizures. Etomidate is also less likely to cause hypotension and is useful in patients with unstable medical conditions such as congestive heart failure. However, geriatric patients with hypertension have had cardiac depression following etomidate administration and should be monitored closely. Etomidate is associated with an increased recovery time, and patients are more likely to complain of headaches and nausea in recovery. Etomidate is also associated with myoclonic movements and venous pain when given i.v. The usual dose of etomidate is 0.15–0.30 mg/kg.

Ketamine (2–3 mg/kg) has also been used in patients with missed or aborted seizures, although ketamine's potential side effects include altered states of consciousness and hallucinations immediately after ECT. Interestingly, compared to methohexital, ketamine is associated with increased midictal EEG slow-wave amplitude (suggesting improved seizure quality) and a faster time to reorientation (Krystal et al., 2003). Recent data on the efficacy of ketamine in the treatment of severe mood disorders (Diazgranados, Ibrahim et al., 2010a,b; Ibrahim et al., 2011; Zarate et al., 2010) may add further support for the use of ketamine in ECT.

Another strategy to increase the seizure length and lower the seizure threshold has been to add the narcotic anesthetics remifentanil or alfentanil to the primary anesthetic agent (e.g., methohexital) (Andersen, Arsland, & Holst-Larsen, 2001; Locala et al., 2005; Porter, Booth, Gray, & Frampton, 2008; Vishne, Aronov, Amiaz, Etchin, & Grunhaus, 2005).

For example, Andersen et al. compared 0.75 mg/kg of methohexital to a combination of 0.5 mg/ kg of methohexital and 1.0 mg/ kg of remifentanil. They found that the mean motor seizure duration was significantly longer with methohexital-remifentanil combination than with methohexitalalone, whereas recovery time, time to spontaneous breathing, and peak postictal hemodynamic changes were similar (Andersen et al., 2001).

In addition to the anesthetic agents, anticholinergic agents are given prior to ECT to block the vagally mediated bradyarrhythmias and asystole that can occur immediately after the onset of the seizure. Either atropine, 0.4–0.8 mg i.v. (or 0.3–0.6 mg i.m.) or glycopyrrolate, 0.2–0.4 mg i.v. or i.m., is given a few minutes prior to the seizure (i.v.) or a couple of hours prior to ECT (i.m.). Intravenous anticholinergic agents are typically used as they are more efficient at blocking the increased vagal tone, although i.m. anticholinergics given 2–3 hours prior to the treatment are more effective at decreasing secretions. Glycopyrrolate is less efficient than atropine at crossing the blood–brain barrier and therefore would potentially cause fewer cognitive side effects. However, studies have shown no significant differences in the effects of the two drugs on cognition (Kelway, Simpson, Smith, & Halsall, 1986; Sommer, Satlin, Friedman, & Cole, 1989) and in one study glycopyrrolate resulted in significantly more cardiac arrhythmias, nausea and vomiting, and episodes of bradycardia than atropine (Kramer, Allen, & Friedman, 1986).

Succinylcholine (0.5–1.0 mg/kg) is used as the primary nondepolarizing muscle relaxant and administered soon after the anesthetic agent when the patient is unconscious. Succinylcholine should be avoided in patients who have a known pseudo-cholinesterase deficiency, cholinesterase inhibition (secondary to medications used to treat glaucoma or exposure to organophosphate pesticides), hypercalcemia, severe neuromuscular disease or injury (such as quadriplegia, amyotrophic lateral sclerosis, muscular dystrophy), severe osteoporosis, severe muscular rigidity, widespread burns (due to the potential for potassium release that could lead to significant hyperkalemia during the seizure), or personal or family history of malignant hyperthermia (American Psychiatric Association, 2001). Nondepolarizing muscle relaxants such asrocuronium (0.45–0.6 mg/kg) can be used instead of succinylcholine, although they are associated with longer recovery times (Bailine, Petrides, Doft, &

Lui, 2003; Ding & White, 2002; Geretsegger et al., 2007; Hooten & Rasmussen, 2008; Milne, Kenny, & Schraag, 2003; Mitchell, Torda, Hickie, & Burke, 1991; Nishikawa, Higuchi, Kawagishi, Shimodate, & Yamakage, 2011).

The Electroconvulsive Therapy Consent Process

The ECT consent process in the elderly can be complicated by underlying cognitive problems that make it difficult for an individual to understand both the risks and benefits of the procedure. Lapid et al. (Lapid, Rummans, Pankratz, & Appelbaum, 2004) found that the depressed elderly as a group had adequate decisional capacities to consent to ECT. Compared to younger patients, the depressed elderly showed greater improvement in decisional capacity with education. The elderly should be questioned specifically to determine that they understood the risks and benefits of the procedure.

The elderly often have the court or a guardian signing informed consent as their power of attorney. The specific law regarding who can function as a medical power of attorney is state specific. The hospital attorney should be contacted to determine a specific process for ECT consent and the consent should be a part of the bylaws related to ECT for the hospital.

The recommendations from the APA Task Force for ECT (American Psychiatric Association, 2001) have a sample consent form. This consent is an excellent guide to ECT services in making certain they include all of the necessary elements for a proper consent.

Side Effects of Electroconvulsive Therapy

MUSCLE SORENESS, HEADACHES, AND NAUSEA

Common ECT side effects include muscle soreness, particularly in the neck and shoulders, which usually decreases as the treatment course progresses. Muscle soreness can be managed using enteric coated aspirin, acetaminophen, or 15 mg of ketorolac pretreatment i.v. Ketorolac can be difficult for older patients to tolerate, particularly those with compromised renal function.

Patients, particularly those with a history of migraines, may also develop a headache after ECT.

Migraine headaches can be managed by using intranasal sumatriptan or other migraine medication 10–15 minutes prior to ECT.

Nausea can be managed using routine antiemetics such as promethazine. More severe nausea may require the use of intravenous odansetron.

In some cases, changing the anesthetic medication may be useful in treating the headaches and nausea post ECT. Propofol generally has fewer post anesthesia emergent side effects, whereas etomidate is associated with more headaches and nausea in the recovery room post ECT (Stadtland, Erfurth, Ruta, & Michael, 2002). However, propofol is also associated with decreasing the ECT seizure time, and etomidate may prolong seizure time compared to the standard anesthetic agent, methohexital (Freeman, 2009). Therefore, changing the anesthetic agent could potentially change the total seizure time.

COGNITIVE SIDE EFFECTS

ECT is associated with cognitive side effects, including reduced concentration, disorientation, impaired attention, anterograde and retrograde memory loss, and retrograde memory loss of autobiographic facts (Lisanby, Maddox, Prudic, Devanand, & Sackeim, 2000). Bilateral electrode placement is associated with more memory dysfunction than right unilateral electrode placement (Lisanby et al., 2000; Sackeim et al., 1993), although one recent study found no significant differences in electrode placements and cognitive problems (Kellner et al., 2010). Other predictors of longer term cognitive deficits, including autobiographical memory problems, are pre-ECT global cognitive impairment (Hausner et al., 2011; Sobin et al., 1995) and postictal confusion (Sobin et al., 1995).

Unipolar and bipolar disorder are also associated with ECT-related cognitive side effects, including verbal learning and memory deficits, particularly in the elderly (Hausner et al., 2011). MacQueen et al. evaluated patients who had received ECT at least 6 months before memory assessment and another group with bipolar disorder that were matched on a number of clinical variables, including past illness burden, but had never received ECT (MacQueen, Parkin, Marriott, Bégin, & Hasey, 2007). They found that bipolar patients who had received ECT more than 6 months prior to memory testing were more impaired on a variety of learning and memory tests than patients with no past ECT.

There is some evidence that acetylcholinesterase inhibitors (ACHE-I) given during ECT may improve long-term outcomes in patients with dementia (Hausner et al., 2011). Physostigmine (a cholinergic agonist) can reverse the memory problems associated with ECT (Levin, Elizur, & Korczyn, 1987) and nondemented patients receiving concomitant ACHE-I's demonstrated improved performance on delayed memory and abstract reasoning following ECT and recovered more rapidly in personal memory (Matthews et al., 2008; Prakash, Kotwal, & Prabhu, 2006). However, many of these studies are preliminary and none of these strategies are recommended for clinical practice.

Increasing age does not necessarily increase the risk of cognitive side effects from ECT. Cognitive side effects are increased due to increasing neurological dysfunction from conditions such as cerebrovascular disease, Parkinson's disease, and dementia, which, of course, are often associated with increasing age (Flint & Gagnon, 2002).

While BT ECT has been shown to be more effective and demonstrate a more rapid antidepressant action compared to RUL ECT, it has been linked to greater cognitive side effects (UK ECT Review Group, 2003). BT ECT is particularly useful in a setting where a delay in treatment response would be particularly harmful to the patient.

Practically, the use of RUL ECT over BT ECT in the initial treatment course is reasonable in patients with underlying neurological dysfunction, including Alzheimer's dementia and Parkinson's disease. Patients who do not respond to RUL ECT, despite optimized treatment parameters, can be switched to BT ECT using a dose titration method. Also increasing the treatment interval to twice a week instead of three times a week can lessen confusion during the course of ECT and is as effective as treating three times a week (McAllister et al., 1987; Shapira et al., 2000).

POSTICTAL AGITATION

Postictal agitation (PIA) should be managed aggressively in the elderly as it can lead to serious injury in both the staff and patient. Some medications may increase the risk of PIA, including both lithium (El-Mallakh, 1987) and carbidopa (Nymeyer & Grossberg, 1997), but generally it is difficult to predict which patients will have PIA.

If PIA does occur and i.v. access is available, a small dose of midazolam or additional methohexital can be used. Intravenous haloperidol is not recommended because of the association with *torsades de pointe* (Greene, McDonald, Duggan, & Cooper, 2000). If there is no i.v. access, then intramuscular atypical antipsychotics are effective in many patients. Our group has found that the addition of the dissolvable atypical antipsychotic medication such as olanzapine orrisperidone 5–10 minutes prior to ECT can be very effective and does not require administration of any additional liquids.

CONTINUATION AND MAINTENANCE OF ELECTROCONVULSIVE THERAPY

The prevention of relapse and recurrence of a depressive episode is an essential part of follow-up care. It is important to recognize that up to 84% of patients who present for ECT, if left untreated, will relapse within 6 months of achieving remission of their depression with ECT (Sackeim et al., 2001). Geriatric depression, particularly if the onset is late in life, has an increased rate of recurrence after an initial response to somatic treatment (Mitchell & Subramaniam, 2005). Both pharmacotherapy and ECT have been used in an attempt to reduce this high relapse rate.

The use of pharmacotherapy to prevent relapse following remission with ECT has been termed *continuation pharmacotherapy* (C-Pharm). There is evidence to suggest that C-Pharm can reduce relapse rates, especially when a combination of medications is used (Kellner et al., 2006; Sackeim et al., 2001). Sackheim et al. demonstrated that the use of nortriptyline alone and also in combination with lithium was superior to placebo in reducing relapse following ECT treatment. The study also demonstrated that the combination of nortriptyline and lithium was superior in reducing relapse compared to nortriptylinemonotherapy (relapse rates being 39% and 60%, respectively) (Sackeim et al., 2001). Of course, the combination of lithium and nortriptyline can be difficult for older patients to tolerate.

The high relapse rates after a course of ECT despite use of C-Pharm has prompted the use of continuation and maintenance ECT to decrease the likelihood of relapse. Continuation ECT is defined as ECT that is given during the 6 month time period following the resolution of the treated depressive episode. ECT given after this 6-month period is referred to as maintenance ECT (American Psychiatric Association, 2001). In this chapter the term *continuation ECT* is used as an umbrella term for both continuation and maintenance ECT.

Kellner et al. demonstrated that continuation ECT is as effective as a combination of nortripyline and lithium in preventing relapse of depression (Kellner et al., 2006). While the study was not specifically limited to older individuals, the mean age was 57.2 years. A total of 201 patients were randomized to either receive continuation ECT or C-Pharm. Continuation ECT was given according to a fixed schedule of bilateral ECT. Specifically ECT was given weekly for 4 weeks, biweekly for 8 weeks, and then monthly for 2 months. Outcome was determined by use of the Hamilton Rating Scale for Depression 24 Item with two consecutive ratings above 16 with a minimum increase of 10 points from baseline being indicative of relapse. Both relapse rates and dropout rates between continuation ECT and C-Pharm groups were not statistically significant. Relapse rates were 37.1% for the continuation ECT group and 31.6% for the C-Pharm group. The majority of relapses in both groups occurred within 6 weeks of continuation therapy.

While Kellner et al. studied all age groups, smaller studies have specifically focused on continuation ECT in older individuals. Navarro et al. conducted a small, randomized, single-blind trial focusing on continuation ECT and C-Pharm among older individuals with psychotic depression in remission following ECT (Navarro et al., 2008). Treatment groups were split with 17 patients receiving nortriptyline monotherapy and 16 patients receiving nortriptyline/ECT combination therapy. While four patients in the nortriptyline monotherapy group relapsed over the following 24 months, relapse was only seen in one patient in the nortriptyline/ECT combination therapy group. There use of a combination of nortripyline/ECT as opposed to nortriptyline monotherapy was associated with less risk of relapse and a longer time until relapse ($p = .009$). Serra et al. had reported similar findings in another small, single-blind randomized control trial (Serra et al., 2006).

Despite this evidence, many questions remain regarding the optimum schedule and length of continuation ECT. A recent systematic review of the efficacy and safety of continuation ECT noted a lack of methodologically rigorous studies (van Schaik et al., 2012). In particular, research in older individuals in areas regarding cognition, comorbid medical disorders, and electrode placement remain largely unaddressed. There are a limited number of randomized control trials, and a high relapse rate persists in all of the reported trials. It has been suggested that the use of a symptom titrated and flexibly scheduled ECT regimen may perhaps be more beneficial, although evidence supporting this is currently limited (Lisanby et al., 2008).

NEUROMODULATION

Transcranial Magnetic Stimulation

TMS is a noninvasive treatment that generates rapidly changing electromagnetic fields to induce localized intracerebral electrical currents. Transcranial magnetic stimulation was approved by the FDA in 2008 for the treatment of major depressive disorder. TMS has been used for a variety of other psychiatric conditions, including schizophrenia, posttraumatic stress disorder, and obsessive-compulsive disorder; however, its use in these conditions is preliminary (Aleman, Sommer, & Kahn, 2007; Alonso et al., 2001; Grisaru, Amir, Cohen, & Kaplan, 1998). Of particular relevance to older individuals, TMS has also been used in both stroke rehabilitation (Chang et al., 2010; Weiduschat et al., 2011) and in the treatment of Parkinson's disease (Khedr, Farweez, & Islam, 2003). TMS has shown promise as an effective antidepressant treatment, although it may be less effective than ECT (Eranti et al., 2007). In contrast to ECT and deep brain stimulation (DBS), TMS differentiates itself by being nonconvulsive and noninvasive, respectively.

TMS is administered through an applicator, which contains a coil that is typically placed on an area of scalp, which overlies the area of the cerebral cortex that is being stimulated. The passage of a brief current in the coil results in a transient magnetic field, which produces an electric current with focal neuronal depolarization in the targeted brain region. TMS is believed to be able to activate cortical neurons at depths as deep as 1.5–3 cm (Rossi, Hallett, Rossini, Pascual-Leone, & Safety of TMS Consensus Group, 2009). The frequency of the administered TMS is also thought to be of therapeutic importance. High-frequency TMS is believed to be cortically activating, while lower frequencies are thought to suppress cortical activity (Kimbrell et al., 1999; Pascual-Leone, Valls-Sole, Wassermann, & Hallett, 1994; Wassermann, Wedegaertner, Ziemann, George, & Chen, 1998). When TMS is repeatedly administered during a treatment session, it is

referred to as repetitive TMS (rTMS) (Schlaepfer, George, Mayberg, & WFSBP Task Force on Brain Stimulation, 2010).

There is increasing evidence to suggest that TMS is an effective treatment of depression. O'Reardon et al. conducted a double-blind multisite study involving 301 depressed patients randomized to active TMS or sham TMS (O'Reardon et al., 2007). TMS was administered five times a week. Symptom change was monitored with the primary outcome being the Montgomery–Asberg Depression Rating Scale (MADRS) and secondary outcome being both the 17- and 24-Hamilton Depression Rating Scale. Response rates were significant at 4 and 6 weeks on all three rating scales. Remission rates were also significantly increased with the use of active TMS. Remission rates as defined by MADRS at 6 weeks were 14.2% for active TMS compared to 5.2% for sham TMS. Active TMS was extremely well tolerated with a dropout rate due to side effects being 4.5%. Side effects were generally minor and transient with the most commonly experienced side effects being muscle twitching (20.6%), application site pain and discomfort (35.8% and 10.9%). Nonresponders in this trial were subsequently enrolled in an open-label extension study conducted by Avery et al. (2008). This study demonstrated that an additional 6 weeks of TMS treatment resulted in symptoms response in 42.4% of patients with remission being achieved in 20%. These results suggest that prolonged use of TMS may be associated with increased therapeutic benefit. More recent research has produced similar positive findings in the general population (George et al., 2010).

In sharp contrast to ECT, older age is a predictor of a reduced antidepressant effect for TMS (Figiel et al., 1998; Fregni et al., 2006; Nahas, Li et al., 2004). TMS in the elderly demonstrated minimal or no benefit in the treatment of depressive symptoms in the elderly in some early studies (Manes et al., 2001; Mosimann et al., 2004). Many early studies involving TMS had small sample sizes, suboptimal TMS treatment parameters, and used estimated applicator positioning as opposed to higher accuracy neuroimaging aided positioning. Regardless, because of the negative findings in the elderly, the two major randomized clinical trials in TMS (George et al., 2010; O'Reardon et al., 2007) excluded patients greater than 70 years of age.

It remains unclear why older individuals have reduced antidepressant effect from TMS. It has been suggested that age-related atrophy of the frontal cortex may increase the distance between applicator coil on the scalp and cerebral cortex, a distance that has been correlated with the antidepressant effect of TMS (Fregni et al., 2006; Mosimann et al., 2002; Mosimann et al., 2004). Nahas et al. demonstrated that TMS could have significant antidepressant effect in older individuals when TMS intensity was adjusted for the degree of prefrontal atrophy (Nahas et al., 2004).

Jorge et al. studied the response of older individuals with vascular depression to treatment with TMS. Participants had a mean age exceeding 60 years of age (Jorge, Moser, Acion, & Robinson, 2008). The study consisted of two separate experiments; each experiment compared a set active TMS regime with sham TMS. Stimulation site identification was accurately determined through the use of neuroimaging. Individuals younger than 65 years were noted to have a better antidepressant response to active TMS ($p = .01$). Interestingly the study also noted that lower volumes of left and right frontal gray matter were associated with a worse antidepressant response to active TMS.

Older individuals with depression may also respond more slowly to antidepressants when compared their younger counterparts (Reynolds et al., 1996; Salzman 1999), although these findings are disputed (Whyte et al., 2004). This potentially slower response to antidepressants may extend to TMS. The short treatment durations in studies may obscure a delayed responsiveness to TMS in older individuals with depression.

In 2008 the Food and Drug Administration (FDA) approved the use of TMS in "the treatment of Major Depressive Disorder in adult patients who have failed to achieve satisfactory improvement from one prior antidepressant medication at or above the minimal effective dose and duration in the current episode." Further research is needed to clarify the optimal parameters for TMS in the treatment of depression in older individuals. Recent emerging research gives cause of optimism for the future role of TMS as an alternative to antidepressant medications and ECT in older depressed individuals.

Other Neuromodulation Devices

Other neuromodulation devices also hold some promise in the treatment of depression, although they have not specifically targeted the elderly. Vagal nerve stimulation (VNS) stimulates the vagal nerve, which has afferent fibers that connect to the nucleus of the solitary tract, which in turn projects connections to other locations in the central nervous system that are felt to be responsible for the mood effects of the treatments (Nemeroff et al., 2006). VNS was approved in 2005 by the FDA for the treatment of resistant depression. The approval was controversial and based on naturalistic follow-up data rather than a rigorous randomized clinical trial (George et al., 2005; Rush, Marangell et al., 2005; Rush, Sackeim et al., 2005). The procedure to implant the device is an outpatient operative procedure and is expensive and potentially has more inherent risks in an elderly population. The device also has to be programmed by a clinician with special training. Insurance companies, including Medicare, have been slow to approve payment for the procedure or the follow-up programming.

Magnetic seizure therapy (MST) is a promising alternative to ECT in the elderly. MST is a novel brain stimulation method using transcranial magnetic stimulation at convulsive parameters in order to induce therapeutic seizures under general anesthesia. Unlike the subconvulsive therapies, VNS and TMS, MST induces a seizure at the same setting used for electroconvulsive therapy (ECT). In contrast to ECT-induced seizures, the MST seizures are more localized (Cycowicz, Luber, Spellman, & Lisanby, 2008, Cycowicz, Luber, Spellman, & Lisanby, 2009) and cause fewer cognitive side effects (Kirov et al., 2008; Spellman et al., 2008) with similar efficacy in depression to ECT (Kosel, Frick, Lisanby, Fisch, & Schlaepfer, 2003). Although MST is still investigational, this side effect profile is promising in potentially serving as an alternative to some patients who cannot tolerate the cognitive side effects of ECT.

Deep brain stimulation (DBS) is an additional subconvulsive stimulus with efficacy in treatment-resistant depression. DBS targets subcortical neurons and was originally developed to treat the motor symptoms of Parkinson's disease (Rascol, Lozano, Stern, & Poewe, 2011). Researchers in depression have more recently applied this technique to the treatment of resistant mood disorders by targeting areas in the anterior cingulated, ventral striatum, and nucleus accumbens (Conca, Di Pauli, Hinterhuber, & Kapfhammer, 2011; Hirschfeld, 2011;Vieta & Colom, 2011). The early results of these investigational trials are promising, but the role of DBS in treatment-resistant depression is unclear and will need further study.

FUTURE DIRECTIONS AND SUMMARY

ECT is one of the most important somatic treatments in psychiatry. The modern practice of ECT has proven to be a safe and effective treatment for affective disorders, particularly when the disorder is resistant to medication. Older individuals appear to have greater responsiveness to treatment with ECT compared to their younger peers. However, their higher medical comorbidity and risk of cognitive side effects require careful pretreatment medical assessment and monitoring.

Future research will continue to develop and refine both ECT and new neuromodulatory treatments. At present, there are two important multicenter National Institute of Mental Health sponsored studies in progress that are evaluating methods to effectively prevent relapse after an acute course of ECT. The Prolonging Remission in Depressed Elderly (PRIDE) study will determine whether medications alone or medications (venlafaxine and lithium) and ECT work best to prevent depressive relapse and to improve quality of life for older people with severe mood disorders. The maintenance studies to date randomized patients to ECT alone or medication alone, and this study will evaluate the common practice of medication plus ECT versus ECT alone in continuation treatment.

The Symptom-Titrated, Algorithm-Based Longitudinal ECT (STABLE) study is a novel approach to individualize the continuation ECT schedule. A criticism of the trials evaluating the effectiveness of continuation ECT is that the trials have implemented a rigid treatment schedule. In STABLE, a treatment algorithm based on symptoms will adapt the ECT schedule to symptom fluctuations to prevent overtreatment of those who do not need it and to recapture response in those who might have otherwise relapsed with a rigid dosing schedule.

The establishment of the optimal parameters for ECT in the elderly, and in particular right unilateral placement, may help to further improve the clinical practice of ECT. Future research should examine the efficacy of the ultrabrief pulse width treatments in RUL and BT ECT. These pulse widths have the potential for delivering a more efficient stimulus with lower energy and fewer cognitive side effects. The role of bifrontal ECT should also be evaluated in the treatment algorithm for geriatric depression.

With refinements in the safety of ECT, the elderly with neuropsychiatric disease (e.g., PD, AD, post stroke) can be treated with few medical complications. Future research is needed to determine the effectiveness of recent advancements in ECT methodology in decreasing the potential for cognitive side effects in depressed elderly patients with and without neuropsychiatric disease. Ultrabrief pulse ECT, bifrontal ECT, modifications to the anesthetic medication regimen, and adjunctive medications should be evaluated further to decrease the cognitive side effects in the elderly.

There is also a need for research on the effectiveness of ECT in treating the nonaffective symptoms of neuropsychiatric disease. Increasingly patients with AD and other neurodegenerative diseases are being referred to ECT to treat generalized symptoms of agitation. Unfortunately the research supporting this practice is limited to a single small retrospective chart review (Ujkaj et al., 2012) and case reports (e.g., Sutor & Rasmussen, 2008).

Although there are little data to support this practice beyond case reports, there are few other treatment options for agitated patients with dementia when medications have failed. If ECT can be shown to be effective to treat specific symptoms of dementia, this could be a needed and important treatment. However, given the advanced age and often frail medical condition of these patients, they are difficult to treat and should not be exposed to the risks of anesthesia and ECT without evidence for therapeutic efficacy.

The neuromodulation treatments are particularly interesting in the elderly. Neuromodulation provides a potential to treat resistant patients with few cognitive side effects. Neuromodulation also has the potential to circumvent the disrupted circuits in geriatric depression and target the underlying neurobiology. It will continue to be explored, with some targeted to achieving remission in ECT-resistant patients. Other neuromodulatory therapies are being developed to become as effective as ECT while minimizing cognitive side effects or mitigating the need for general anesthesia.

More recently we have been able to further identify the anatomical correlates of mood disorders. Recognition of the role of areas like the anterior cingulate gyrus in the etiologic role of depression is leading to more targeted interventions such as that witness in DBS. In the meantime, ECT continues to remain an important and highly effective treatment modality in late-life mood disorders and will continue to do so for the considerable future.

Disclosures

Dr. Arshya Vahabzadeh has no conflicts to disclose.

Dr. McDonald has the following disclosures: 1. He was PI on an NIMH grant (R01 MH069886–01). The investigators on this grant were given TMS devices for no cost from Neuronetics. Emory University employs Dr. McDonald and also holds a patent for a TMS device that is marketed by Neuronetics. 2. He is PI on a multicenter study sponsored by the Stanley Foundation investigating transcranial direct stimulation (tDCS) with tDCS machines donated by Soterix. 3. He is PI on a multicenter grant sponsored by CervelNeurotech investigating a new transcranial magnetic stimulation device. 4. He is the chair of the Task Force for ECT and Neuromodulation on the APA's Committee for Research and Quality. 5. He has a contract with Oxford University Press to coedit a book, *Clinical Guide to Transcranial Magnetic Stimulation in the Treatment of Depression,* and could receive royalties from this book.

REFERENCES

Abrams, R. (1992). *Electroconvulsive therapy* (2nd ed.). New York: Oxford University Press.

Abrams, R. (1997). The mortality rate with ECT. *Convulsive Therapy, 13*(3), 125–127.

Abrams, R. (2002). *Electroconvulsive therapy.* Oxford, England and New York: Oxford Unversity Press.

Aleman, A., Sommer, I. E., & Kahn, R. S. (2007). Efficacy of slow repetitive transcranial magnetic stimulation in the treatment of resistant auditory hallucinations in schizophrenia: A meta-analysis. *Journal of Clinical Psychiatry, 68*(3), 416–421.

Ali, P. B., & Tidmarsh, M. D. (1997). Cardiac rupture during electroconvulsive therapy. *Anaesthesia, 52*(9), 884–886.

Alonso, P., Pujol, J., Cardoner, N., Benlloch, L., Deus, J., Menchón, J. M., ... Vallejo, J. (2001). Right prefrontal repetitive transcranial magnetic stimulation in obsessive-compulsive disorder: A double-blind, placebo-controlled study. *American Journal of Psychiatry, 158*(7), 1143–1145.

American Psychiatric Association. (2001). *The practice of electroconvulsive therapy: recommendations for treatment, training and privileging. Task Force Report on ECT.* Washington, DC: Author.

Andersen, F. A., Arsland, D., & Holst-Larsen, H. (2001). Effects of combined methohexitone-remifentanil anaesthesia in electroconvulsive therapy. *Acta Anaesthesiologica Sandinavica, 45*(7), 830–833.

Avery, D. H., Isenberg, K. E., Sampson, S. M., Janicak, P. G., Lisanby, S. H., Maixner, D. F., ... George, M. S. (2008). Transcranial magnetic stimulation in the acute treatment of major depressive disorder: Clinical response in an open-label extension trial. *Journal of Clinical Psychiatry, 69*(3), 441–451.

Aziz, R., Lorberg, B., & Tampi, R. R. (2006). Treatments for late-life bipolar disorder. *American Journal of Geriatric Pharmacotherapy, 4*(4), 347–364.

Baez, M. A., & Avery, J. (2011). Improvement in drug-induced parkinsonism with electroconvulsive therapy. *American Journal of Geriatric Pharmacotherapy, 9*(3), 190–193.

Bailine, S. H., Petrides, G., Doft, M., & Lui, G. (2003). Indications for the use of propofol in electroconvulsive therapy. *Journal of ECT, 19*(3), 129–132.

Bang, J., Price, D., Prentice, G., & Campbell, J. (2008). ECT treatment for two cases of dementia-related pathological yelling. *Journal of Neuropsychiatry and Clinical Neurosciences, 20*(3), 379–380.

Beale, M. D., & Kellner, C. H. (2000). ECT in treatment algorithms: No need to save the best for last. *Journal of ECT, 16*(1), 1–2.

Berg, J. E. (2009). Electroconvulsive treatment—more than electricity?: An odyssey of facilities. *Journal of ECT, 25*(4), 250–255.

Birkenhager, T. K., Pluijms, E. M., & Lucius, S. A. (2003). ECT response in delusional versus non-delusional depressed inpatients. *Journal of Affective Disorders, 74*(2), 191–195.

Blazer, D. G., & Steffens, D. C. (2009). *The American Psychiatric Publishing textbook of geriatric psychiatry.* Washington, DC: American Psychiatric Publishing.

Brodaty, H., Luscombe, G., Parker, G., Wilhelm, K., Hickie, I., Austin, M. P., & Mitchell, P. (1997). Increased rate of psychosis and psychomotor change in depression with age. *Psychological Medicine, 27*(5), 1205–1213.

Bruce, B. B., Henry, M. E., & Greer, D. M. (2006). Ischemic stroke after electroconvulsive therapy. *Journal of ECT, 22*(2), 150–152.

Bryson, E. O., Popeo, D. M., & Kellner, C. H. (2012). Electroconvulsive therapy (ECT) after pulmonary edema. *Journal of ECT, 28*(2), e25–e26.

Burgut, F. T., & Kellner, C. H. (2010). Electroconvulsive therapy (ECT) for dementia with Lewy bodies. *Medical Hypotheses, 75*(2), 139–140.

Burgut, F. T., Popeo, D., & Kellner, C. H. (2010). ECT for agitation in dementia: Is it appropriate? *Medical Hypotheses, 75*(1), 5–6.

Bustin, J., Rapoport, M. J., Krishna, M., Matusevich, D., Finkelsztein, C., Strejilevich, S., & Anderson, D. (2008). Are patients' attitudes towards and knowledge of electroconvulsive therapy transcultural? A multi-national pilot study. *International Journal of Geriatric Psychiatry, 23*(5), 497–503.

Butterfield, N. N., Graf, P., Macleod, B. A., Ries, C. R., & Zis, A. P. (2004). Propofol reduces cognitive impairment after electroconvulsive therapy. *Journal of ECT, 20*(1), 3–9.

Capizzano, A. A., Jorge, R. E., Acion, L. C., & Robinson, R. G. (2007). In vivo proton magnetic resonance spectroscopy in patients with mood disorders: A technically oriented review. *Journal of Magnetic Resonance Imaging, 26*(6), 1378–1389.

Chang, W. H., Kim, Y. H., Bang, O. Y., Kim, S. T., Park, Y. H., & Lee, P. K. (2010). Long-term effects of rTMS on motor recovery in patients after subacute stroke. *Journal of Rehabilitation Medicine, 42*(8), 758–764.

Ciapparelli, A., Dell'Osso, L., Tundo, A., Pini, S., Chiavacci, M. C., Di Sacco, I., & Cassano, G. B. (2001). Electroconvulsive therapy in medication-nonresponsive patients with mixed mania and bipolar depression. *Journal of Clinical Psychiatry, 62*(7), 552–555.

Coffey, C. E., Figiel, G. S., Djang, W. T., Saunders, W. B., & Weiner, R. D. (1989). White matter hyperintensity on magnetic resonance imaging: Clinical and neuroanatomic correlates in the depressed elderly. *Journal of Neuropsychiatry and Clinical Neurosciences, 1*(2), 135–144.

Coffey, C. E., Figiel, G. S., Djang, W. T., & Weiner, R. D. (1990). Subcortical hyperintensity on magnetic resonance imaging: A comparison of normal and depressed elderly subjects. *American Journal of Psychiatry, 147*(2), 187–189.

Conca, A., Di Pauli, J., Hinterhuber, H., & Kapfhammer, H. P. (2011). [Deep brain stimulation: a review on current research]. *Neuropsychiatrie : Klinik, Diagnostik, Therapie und Rehabilitation : Organ der Gesellschaft Österreichischer Nervenärzte und Psychiater, 25*(1), 1–8.

Conwell, Y., & Brent, D. (1995). Suicide and aging. I: Patterns of psychiatric diagnosis. *International Journal of Psychogeriatrics, 7*(2), 149–164.

Conwell, Y., Duberstein, P. R., Cox, C., Herrmann, J., Forbes, N., & Caine, E. D. (1998). Age differences in behaviors leading to completed suicide. *American Journal of Geriatric Psychiatry, 6*(2), 122–126.

Cummings, J. L. (1992). Depression and Parkinson's disease: A review. *American Journal of Psychiatry, 149*(4), 443–454.

Cummings, J. L., & Masterman, D. L. (1999). Depression in patients with Parkinson's disease. *International Journal of Geriatric Psychiatry, 14*(9), 711–718.

Currier, M. B., Murray, G. B., & Welch, C. C. (1992). Electroconvulsive therapy for post-stroke depressed geriatric patients. *Journal of Neuropsychiatry and Clinical Neurosciences, 4*(2), 140–144.

Cycowicz, Y. M., Luber, B., Spellman, T., & Lisanby, S. H. (2008). Differential neurophysiological effects of magnetic seizure therapy (MST) and electroconvulsive shock (ECS) in non-human primates. *Clinical EEG and Neuroscience, 39*(3), 144–149.

Cycowicz, Y. M., Luber, B., Spellman, T., & Lisanby, S. H. (2009). Neurophysiological characterization of high-dose magnetic seizure therapy: Comparisons with electroconvulsive shock and cognitive outcomes. *Journal of ECT, 25*(3), 157–164.

Daly, J. J., Prudic, J., Devanand, D. P., Nobler, M. S., Lisanby, S. H., Peyser, S., Sackeim, H. A. (2001). ECT in bipolar and unipolar depression: Differences in speed of response. *Bipolar Disorders, 3*(2), 95–104.

Damm, J., Eser, D., Schüle, C., Obermeier, M., Möller, H. J., Rupprecht, R., & Baghai, T. C. (2010). Influence of age on effectiveness and tolerability of electroconvulsive therapy. *Journal of ECT, 26*(4), 282–288.

Davis, A., Zisselman, M., Simmons, T., McCall, W. V., McCafferty, J., & Rosenquist, P. B. (2009). Electroconvulsive therapy in the setting of implantable cardioverter-defibrillators. *Journal of ECT, 25*(3), 198–201.

Devanand, D. P., Decina, P., Sackeim, H. A., & Prudic, J. (1988). Status epilepticus following ECT in a patient receiving theophylline. *Journal of Clinical Psychopharmacology, 8*(2), 153.

Devanand, D. P., Polanco, P., Cruz, R., Shah, S., Paykina, N., Singh, K., & Majors, L. (2000). The efficacy of ECT in mixed affective states. *Journal of ECT, 16*(1), 32–37.

Diazgranados, N., Ibrahim, L., Brutsche, N. E., Newberg, A., Kronstein, P., Khalife, S., … Zarate, C. A., Jr. (2010). A randomized add-on trial of an N-methyl-D-aspartate antagonist in treatment-resistant bipolar depression. *Archives of General Psychiatry, 67*(8), 793–802.

Diazgranados, N., Ibrahim, L. A., Brutsche, N. E., Ameli, R., Henter, I. D., Luckenbaugh, D. A., … Zarate, C. A., Jr. (2010). Rapid resolution of suicidal ideation after a single infusion of an N-methyl-D-aspartate antagonist in patients with treatment-resistant major depressive disorder. *Journal of Clinical Psychiatry, 71*(12), 1605–1611.

Ding, Z., & White, P. F. (2002). Anesthesia for electroconvulsive therapy. *Anesthesia and Analgesia, 94*(5), 1351–1364.

Dolenc, T. J., Barnes, R. D., Hayes, D. L., & Rasmussen, K. G. (2004). Electroconvulsive therapy in patients with cardiac pacemakers and implantable cardioverter defibrillators. *Pacing and Clinical Electrophysiology, 27*(9), 1257–1263.

Dowman, J., Patel, A., & Rajput, K. (2005). Electroconvulsive therapy: Attitudes and misconceptions. *Journal of ECT, 21*(2), 84–87.

El-Mallakh, R. S. (1987). Lithium and ECT Interaction. *Convulsive Therapy, 3*(4), 309.

Eranti, S., Mogg, A., Pluck, G., Landau, S., Purvis, R., Brown, R. G., ... McLoughlin, D. M. (2007). A randomized, controlled trial with 6-month follow-up of repetitive transcranial magnetic stimulation and electroconvulsive therapy for severe depression. *American Journal of Psychiatry, 164*(1), 73–81.

Eranti, S. V., Mogg, A. J., Pluck, G. C., Landau, S., & McLoughlin, D. M. (2009). Methohexitone, propofol and etomidate in electroconvulsive therapy for depression: A naturalistic comparison study. *Journal of Affective Disorders, 113*(1–2), 165–171.

Fall, P. A., Ekman, R., Granérus, A. K., Thorell, L. H., & Wålinder, J. (1995). ECT in Parkinson's disease. Changes in motor symptoms, monoamine metabolites and neuropeptides. *Journal of Neural Transmission, 10*(2–3), 129–140.

Fazzari, G., Benzoni, O., Sangaletti, A., Bonera, F., Nassini, S., Mazzarini, L., ... Girardi, P. (2009). Improvement of cognition in a patient with Cotard's delusions and frontotemporal atrophy receiving electroconvulsive therapy (ECT) for depression. *International Journal of Psychogeriatrics, 21*(3), 600–603.

Fernandes, B., Gama, C. S., Massuda, R., Torres, M., Camargo, D., Kunz, M., ... Inês Lobato M. (2009). Serum brain-derived neurotrophic factor (BDNF) is not associated with response to electroconvulsive therapy (ECT), a pilot study in drug resistant depressed patients. *Neuroscience Letters, 453*(3), 195–198.

Figiel, G. S., Coffey, C. E., Djang, W. T., Hoffman, G., Jr., & Doraiswamy, P. M. (1990). Brain magnetic resonance imaging findings in ECT-induced delirium. *Journal of Neuropsychiatry and Clinical Neurosciences, 2*(1), 53–58.

Figiel, G. S., Epstein, C., McDonald, W. M., Amazon-Leece, J., Figiel, L., Saldivia, A., & Glover, S. (1998). The use of rapid-rate transcranial magnetic stimulation (rTMS) in refractory depressed patients. *Journal of Neuropsychiatry and Clinical Neurosciences, 10*(1), 20–25.

Fisman, M., Rabheru, K., & Sharma, V. (2001). Response to ECT in depressed, demented patients; possible role of apolipoprotein E(4) as response marker. *International Journal of Geriatric Psychiatry, 16*(9), 919–920.

Fleisher, L. A., Beckman, J. A., Brown, K. A., Calkins, H., Chaikof, E. L., Fleischmann, K. E., ... Society for Vascular Surgery, (2007). ACC/AHA 2007 guidelines on perioperative cardiovascular evaluation and care for noncardiac surgery: A report of the American College of Cardiology/ American Heart Association Task Force on Practice Guidelines (Writing Committee to Revise the 2002 Guidelines on Perioperative Cardiovascular Evaluation for Noncardiac Surgery) developed in collaboration with the American Society of Echocardiography, American Society of Nuclear Cardiology, Heart Rhythm Society, Society of Cardiovascular Anesthesiologists, Society for Cardiovascular Angiography and Interventions, Society for Vascular Medicine and Biology, and Society for Vascular Surgery. *Journal of the American College of Cardiology, 50*(17), e159–241.

Flint, A. J., & Gagnon, N. (2002). Effective use of electroconvulsive therapy in late-life depression. *Candian Journal of Psychiatry, 47*(8), 734–741.

Freeman, S. A. (2009). Post-electroconvulsive therapy agitation with etomidate. *Journal of ECT, 25*(2), 133–134.

Fregni, F., Marcolin, M. A., Myczkowski, M., Amiaz, R., Hasey, G., Rumi, D. O., ... Pascual-Leone, A. (2006). Predictors of antidepressant response in clinical trials of transcranial magnetic stimulation. *International Journal of Neuropsychopharmacology, 9*(6), 641–654.

Gazdag, G., Kocsis, N., Tolna, J., & Iványi, Z. (2004). Etomidate versus propofol for electroconvulsive therapy in patients with schizophrenia. *Journal of ECT, 20*(4), 225–229.

George, M. S., Lisanby, S. H., Avery, D., McDonald, W. M., Durkalski, V., Pavlicova, M., ... Sackeim, H. A. (2010). Daily left prefrontal transcranial magnetic stimulation therapy for major depressive disorder: A sham-controlled randomized trial. *Archives of General Psychiatry, 67*(5), 507–516.

George, M. S., Rush, A. J., Marangell, L. B., Sackeim, H. A., Brannan, S. K., Davis, S. M., ... Goodnick, P. (2005). A one-year comparison of vagus nerve stimulation with treatment as usual for treatment-resistant depression. *Biological Psychiatry, 58*(5), 364–373.

Geretsegger, C., Nickel, M., Judendorfer, B., Rochowanski, E., Novak, E., & Aichhorn, W. (2007). Propofol and methohexital as anesthetic agents for electroconvulsive therapy: A randomized, double-blind comparison of electroconvulsive therapy seizure quality, therapeutic efficacy, and cognitive performance. *Journal of ECT, 23*(4), 239–243.

Gerring, J. P., & Shields, H. M. (1982). The identification and management of patients with a high risk for cardiac arrhythmias during modified ECT. *Journal of Clinical Psychiatry, 43*(4), 140–143.

Greenberg, R. M., & Kellner, C. H. (2005). Electroconvulsive therapy: A selected review. *American Journal of Geriatr Psychiatry, 13*(4), 268–281.

Greene, Y. M., McDonald, W. M., Duggan, J., & Cooper, R. (2000). Ventricular ectopy associated with low-dose intravenous haloperidol and electroconvulsive therapy. *Journal of ECT, 16*(3), 309–311.

Grisaru, N., Amir, M., Cohen, H., & Kaplan, Z. (1998). Effect of transcranial magnetic stimulation in posttraumatic stress disorder: A preliminary study. *Biological Psychiatry, 44*(1), 52–55.

Hausner, L., Damian, M., Sartorius, A., & Frölich, L. (2011). Efficacy and cognitive side effects of electroconvulsive therapy (ECT) in depressed elderly inpatients with coexisting mild cognitive impairment or dementia. *Journal of Clinical Psychiatry, 72*(1), 91–97.

Hirschfeld, R. M. (2011). Deep brain stimulation for treatment-resistant depression. *American Journal of Psychiatry, 168*(5), 455–456.

Holaday, J. W., Tortella, F. C., Meyerhoff, J. L., Belenky, G. L., & Hitzemann, R. J. (1986). Electroconvulsive shock activates endogenous opioid systems: Behavioral and biochemical correlates. *Annals of the New York Academy of Sciences, 467*, 249–255.

Hooten, W. M., & Rasmussen, K. G., Jr. (2008). Effects of general anesthetic agents in adults receiving electroconvulsive therapy: A systematic review. *Journal of ECT, 24*(3), 208–223.

Ibrahim, L., Diazgranados, N., Luckenbaugh, D. A., Machado-Vieira, R., Baumann, J., Mallinger, A. G., & Zarate, C. A., Jr. (2011). Rapid decrease in depressive symptoms with an N-methyl-d-aspartate antagonist in ECT-resistant major depression. *Progress in Neuropsychopharmacology and Biological Psychiatry, 35*(4), 1155–1159.

Ingvar, M. (1986). Cerebral blood flow and metabolic rate during seizures. Relationship to epileptic brain damage. *Annals of the New York Academy of Sciences, 462*, 194–206.

Janicak, P. G., Mask, J., Trimakas, K. A., & Gibbons, R. (1985). ECT: An assessment of mental health professionals' knowledge and attitudes. *Journal of Clinical Psychiatry, 46*(7), 262–266.

Jorge, R. E., Moser, D. J., Acion, L., & Robinson, R. G. (2008). Treatment of vascular depression using repetitive transcranial magnetic stimulation. *Archives of General Psychiatry, 65*(3), 268–276.

Katagai, H., Yasui-Furukori, N., Kikuchi, A., & Kaneko, S. (2007). Effective electroconvulsive therapy in a 92-year-old dementia patient with psychotic feature. *Psychiatry and Clinical Neurosciences, 61*(5), 568–570.

Katz, I. R., Simpson, G. M., Curlik, S. M., Parmelee, P. A., & Muhly, C. (1990). Pharmacologic treatment of major depression for elderly patients in residential care settings. *Journal of Clinical Psychiatry, 51*(Suppl), 41–47; discussion 48.

Kellner, C. H. (2001). Towards the modal ECT treatment. *Journal of ECT, 17*(1), 1–2.

Kellner, C. H., Fink, M., Knapp, R., Petrides, G., Husain, M., Rummans, T., ... Malur, C. (2005). Relief of expressed suicidal intent by ECT: A consortium for research in ECT study. *American Journal of Psychiatry, 162*(5), 977–982.

Kellner, C. H., Knapp, R., Husain, M. M., Rasmussen, K., Sampson, S., Cullum, M., ... Petrides, G. (2010). Bifrontal, bitemporal and right unilateral electrode placement in ECT: Randomised trial. *British Journal of Psychiatry, 196*, 226–234.

Kellner, C. H., Knapp, R. G., Petrides, G., Rummans, T. A., Husain, M. M., Rasmussen, K., ... Fink, M. (2006). Continuation electroconvulsive therapy vs pharmacotherapy for relapse prevention in major depression: A multisite study from the Consortium for Research in Electroconvulsive Therapy (CORE). *Archives of General Psychiatry, 63*(12), 1337–1344.

Kelway, B., Simpson, K. H., Smith, R. J., & Halsall, P. J. (1986). Effects of atropine and glycopyrrolate on cognitive function following anaesthesia and electroconvulsive therapy (ECT). *International Clinical Psychopharmacology, 1*(4), 296–302.

Kerr, R. A., McGrath, J. J., O'Kearney, R. T., & Price, J. (1982). ECT: Misconceptions and attitudes. *Australia New Zealand Journal of Psychiatry, 16*(1), 43–49.

Khedr, E. M., Farweez, H. M., & Islam, H. (2003). Therapeutic effect of repetitive transcranial magnetic stimulation on motor function in Parkinson's disease patients. *European Journal of Neurology, 10*(5), 567–572.

Kimbrell, T. A., Little, J. T., Dunn, R. T., Frye, M. A., Greenberg, B. D., Wassermann, E. M.,...Post, R. M. (1999). Frequency dependence of antidepressant response to left prefrontal repetitive transcranial magnetic stimulation (rTMS) as a function of baseline cerebral glucose metabolism. *Biological Psychiatry, 46*(12), 1603–1613.

Kirov, G., Ebmeier, K. P., Scott, A. I., Atkins, M., Khalid, N., Carrick, L.,...Lisanby SH. (2008). Quick recovery of orientation after magnetic seizure therapy for major depressive disorder. *British Journal of Psychiatry, 193*(2), 152–155.

Kohler, C. G., & Burock, M. (2001). ECT for psychotic depression associated with a brain tumor. *American Journal of Psychiatry, 158*(12), 2089.

Kosel, M., Frick, C., Lisanby, S. H., Fisch, H. U., & Schlaepfer, T. E. (2003). Magnetic seizure therapy improves mood in refractory major depression. *Neuropsychopharmacology, 28*(11), 2045–2048.

Kramer, B. A. (1985). Use of ECT in California, 1977–1983. *American Journal of Psychiatry, 142*(10), 1190–1192.

Kramer, B. A., Allen, R. E., & Friedman, B. (1986). Atropine and glycopyrrolate as ECT preanesthesia. *Journal of Clinical Psychiatry, 47*(4), 199–200.

Krystal, A. D., Weiner, R. D., Dean, M. D., Lindahl, V. H., Tramontozzi, L. A., III, Falcone, G., & Coffey, C. E. (2003). Comparison of seizure duration, ictal EEG, and cognitive effects of ketamine and methohexital anesthesia with ECT. *Journal of Neuropsychiatry and Clinical Neurosciences, 15*(1), 27–34.

Lapid, M. I., Rummans, T. A., Pankratz, V. S., & Appelbaum, P. S. (2004). Decisional capacity of depressed elderly to consent to electroconvulsive therapy. *Journal of Geriatric Psychiatry and Neurology, 17*(1), 42–46.

Latey, R. H., & Fahy, T. J. (1985). Electroconvulsive therapy in the Republic of Ireland 1982: A summary of findings. *British Journal of Psychiatry, 147*: 438–439.

Lauber, C., Nordt, C., Falcato, L., & Rössler, W. (2005). Can a seizure help? The public's attitude toward electroconvulsive therapy. *Psychiatry Research, 134*(2), 205–209.

Lee, K. (2006). Acute embolic stroke after electroconvulsive therapy. *Journal of ECT, 22*(1), 67–69.

Levin, Y., Elizur, A., & Korczyn, A. D. (1987). Physostigmine improves ECT-induced memory disturbances. *Neurology, 37*(5), 871–875.

Ling, T., III, Manepalli, J., & Grossberg, G. (2010). Electroconvulsive therapy in the presence of a metallic skull plate after meningioma resection. *Journal of ECT, 26*(2), 136–138.

Lisanby, S. H., Maddox, J. H., Prudic, J., Devanand, D. P., & Sackeim, H. A. (2000). The effects of electroconvulsive therapy on memory of autobiographical and public events. *Archives of General Psychiatry, 57*(6), 581–590.

Lisanby, S. H., Sampson, S., Husain, M. M., Petrides, G., Knapp, R. G., McCall, V.,...Kellner, C. H. (2008). Toward individualized post-electroconvulsive therapy care: Piloting the Symptom-Titrated, Algorithm-Based Longitudinal ECT (STABLE) intervention. *Journal of ECT, 24*(3), 179–182.

Little, J. D., Atkins, M. R., Munday, J., Lyall, G., Greene, D., Chubb, G., & Orr, M. (2004). Bifrontal electroconvulsive therapy in the elderly: A 2-year retrospective. *Journal of ECT, 20*(3), 139–141.

Locala, J. A., Irefin, S. A., Malone, D., Cywinski, J. B., Samuel, S. W., & Naugle, R. (2005). The comparative hemodynamic effects of methohexital and remifentanil in electroconvulsive therapy. *Journal of ECT, 21*(1), 12–15.

Lopez-Gomez, D., Sanchez-Corral, M. A., Cobo, J. V., Jara, F., & Esplugas, E. (1999). [Myocardial infarction after electroconvulsive therapy]. *Revista española de cardiología, 52*(7), 536.

MacQueen, G., Parkin, C., Marriott, M., Bégin, H., & Hasey, G. (2007). The long-term impact of treatment with electroconvulsive therapy on discrete memory systems in patients with bipolar disorder. *Journal of Psychiatry and Neuroscience, 32*(4), 241–249.

Madan, S., & Anderson, K. (2001). ECT for a patient with a metallic skull plate. *Journal of ECT, 17*(4), 289–291.

Magid, M., Lapid, M. I., Sampson, S. M., & Mueller, P. S. (2005). Use of electroconvulsive therapy in a patient 10 days after myocardial infarction. *Journal of ECT, 21*(3), 182–185.

Malcolm, K. (1989). Patients' perceptions and knowledge of electroconvulsive therapy. *Psychiatric Bulletin, 13*, 161–165.

Maltbie, A. A., Wingfield, M. S., Volow, M. R., Weiner, R. D., Sullivan, J. L., & Cavenar, J. O., Jr. (1980). Electroconvulsive therapy in the presence of brain tumor. Case reports and an evaluation of risk. *Journal of Nervous and Mental Disease, 168*(7), 400–405.

Manes, F., Jorge, R., Morcuende, M., Yamada, T., Paradiso, S., & Robinson, R. G. (2001). A controlled study of repetitive transcranial magnetic stimulation as a treatment of depression in the elderly. *International Journal of Psychogeriatrics, 13*(2), 225–231.

Mark, T. L. J., Vijay, N., Hay, J. W., Sheehan, D. V., Johnston, S. S., & Cao, Z. (2011). Antidepressant use in geriatric populations: The burden of side effects and interactions and their impact on adherence and costs. *American Journal of Geriatric Psychiatry, 19*(3), 211–221.

Martin, M., Figiel, G., Mattingly, G., Zorumski, C. F., & Jarvis, M. R. (1992). ECT-induced interictal delirium in patients with a history of a CVA. *Journal of Geriatric Psychiatry and Neurology, 5*(3), 149–155.

Matthews, J. D., Blais, M., Park, L., Welch, C., Baity, M., Murakami, J., ... Fava, M. (2008). The impact of galantamine on cognition and mood during electroconvulsive therapy: A pilot study. *Journal of Psychiatric Research, 42*(7), 526–531.

McAllister, D. A., Perri, M. G., Jordan, R. C., Rauscher, F. P., & Sattin, A. (1987). Effects of ECT given two vs. three times weekly. *Psychiatry Research, 21*(1), 63–69.

McCall, W. V., Farah, B. A., (1995). Comparison of the efficacy of titrated moderate-dose and fixed, high-dose right unilateral ECT in elderly patients. *American Journal of Geriatric Psychiatry, 3*, 317–324.

McCall, W. V., Reboussin, D. M., Weiner, R. D., & Sackeim, H. A. (2000). Titrated moderately suprathreshold vs fixed high-dose right unilateral electroconvulsive therapy: acute antidepressant and cognitive effects. *Archives of General Psychiatry, 57*(5), 438–444.

McDonald, W. M., Holtzheimer, P. E., III, & Byrd, E. H. (2006). The diagnosis and treatment of depression in Parkinson's disease. *Current Treatment Options in Neurology, 8*(3), 245–255.

McDonald, W. M., & Nemeroff, C. B. (1996). The diagnosis and treatment of mania in the elderly. *Bulletin of the Menninger Clinic, 60*(2), 174–196.

McDonald, W. M., & Thompson, T. R. (2001). Treatment of mania in dementia with electroconvulsive therapy. *Psychopharmacology Bulletin, 35*(2), 72–82.

McFarquhar, T. F., & Thompson, J. (2008). Knowledge and attitudes regarding electroconvulsive therapy among medical students and the general public. *Journal of ECT, 24*(4), 244–253.

McKinney, P. A., Beale, M. D., & Kellner, C. H. (1998). Electroconvulsive therapy in a patient with a cerebellar meningioma. *Journal of ECT, 14*(1), 49–52.

Medda, P., Perugi, G., Zanello, S., Ciuffa, M., & Cassano, G. B. (2009). Response to ECT in bipolar I, bipolar II and unipolar depression. *Journal of Affective Disorders, 118*(1–3), 55–59.

Medda, P., Perugi, G., Zanello, S., Ciuffa, M., Rizzato, S., & Cassano, G. B. (2010). Comparative

response to electroconvulsive therapy in medication-resistant bipolar I patients with depression and mixed state. *Journal of ECT, 26*(2), 82–86.

Merkl, A., Heuser, I., & Bajbouj, M. (2009). Antidepressant electroconvulsive therapy: Mechanism of action, recent advances and limitations. *Experimental Neurology, 219*(1), 20–26.

Meyers, B. S., Klimstra, S. A., Gabriele, M., Hamilton, M., Kakuma, T., Tirumalasetti, F., & Alexopoulos, G. S. (2001). Continuation treatment of delusional depression in older adults. *American Journal of Geriatr Psychiatry, 9*(4), 415–422.

Milne, S. E., Kenny, G. N., & Schraag, S. (2003). Propofol sparing effect of remifentanil using closed-loop anaesthesia. *British Journal of Anaesthesia, 90*(5), 623–629.

Mitchell, A. J., & Subramaniam, H. (2005). Prognosis of depression in old age compared to middle age: A systematic review of comparative studies. *American Journal of Psychiatry, 162*(9), 1588–1601.

Mitchell, P., Torda, T., Hickie, I., & Burke, C. (1991). Propofol as an anaesthetic agent for ECT: Effect on outcome and length of course. *Australia New Zealand Journal of Psychiatry, 25*(2), 255–261.

Moellentine, C., Rummans, T., Ahlskog, J. E., Harmsen, W. S., Suman, V. J., O'Connor, M. K., ... Pileggi, T. (1998). Effectiveness of ECT in patients with parkinsonism. *Journal of Neuropsychiatry and Clinical Neurosciences, 10*(2), 187–193.

Mosimann, U. P., Marre, S. C., Werlen, S., Schmitt, W., Hess, C. W., Fisch, H. U., & Schlaepfer, T. E. (2002). Antidepressant effects of repetitive transcranial magnetic stimulation in the elderly: Correlation between effect size and coil-cortex distance. *Archives of General Psychiatry, 59*(6), 560–561.

Mosimann, U. P., Schmitt, W., Greenberg, B. D., Kosel, M., Müri, R. M., Berkhoff, M., ... Schlaepfer, T. E. (2004). Repetitive transcranial magnetic stimulation: A putative add-on treatment for major depression in elderly patients. *Psychiatry Research, 126*(2), 123–133.

Mueller, P. S., Schak, K. M., Barnes, R. D., & Rasmussen, K. G. (2006). Safety of electroconvulsive therapy in patients with asthma. *Netherlands Journal of Medicine, 64*(11), 417–421.

Mukherjee, S., Sackeim, H. A., & Schnur, D. B. (1994). Electroconvulsive therapy of acute manic episodes: A review of 50 years' experience. *American Journal of Psychiatry, 151*(2), 169–176.

Murray, G. B., Shea, V., & Conn, D. K. (1986). Electroconvulsive therapy for poststroke depression. *Journal of Clinical Psychiatry, 47*(5), 258–260.

Myers, C. L., Gopalka, A., Glick, D., Goldman, M. B., & Dinwiddie, S. H. (2007). A case of negative-pressure pulmonary edema after electroconvulsive therapy. *Journal of ECT, 23*(4), 281–283.

Nahas, Z., Li, X., Kozel, F. A., Mirzki, D., Memon, M., Miller, K., George, M. S. (2004). Safety and benefits of distance-adjusted prefrontal transcranial magnetic stimulation in depressed patients 55–75 years of age: A pilot study. *Depress and Anxiety, 19*(4), 249–256.

Najjar, F., & Guttmacher, L. B. (1998). ECT in the presence of intracranial aneurysm. *Journal of ECT, 14*(4), 266–271.

Navarro, V., Gasto, C., Torres, X., Masana, G., Penadés, R., Guarch, J., Catalán, R. (2008). Continuation/maintenance treatment with nortriptyline versus combined nortriptyline and ECT in late-life psychotic depression: A two-year randomized study. *American Journal of Geriatric Psychiatry, 16*(6), 498–505.

Nemeroff, C. B., Mayberg, H. S., Krahl, S. E., McNamara, J., Frazer, A., Henry, T. R.,...Brannan, S. K. (2006). VNS therapy in treatment-resistant depression: Clinical evidence and putative neurobiological mechanisms. *Neuropsychopharmacology, 31*(7), 1345–1355.

Nishikawa, K., Higuchi, M., Kawagishi, T., Shimodate, Y., & Yamakage, M. (2011). Effect of divided supplementation of remifentanil on seizure duration and hemodynamic responses during electroconvulsive therapy under propofol anesthesia. *Journal of Anesthesia, 25*(1), 29–33.

Nymeyer, L., & Grossberg, G. T. (1997). Delirium in a 75-year-old woman receiving ECT and levodopa. *Convulsive Therapy, 13*(2), 114–116.

O'Connor, D. W., Gardner, B., Eppingstall, B., & Tofler, D. (2010). Cognition in elderly patients receiving unilateral and bilateral electroconvulsive therapy: A prospective, naturalistic comparison. *Journal of Affective Disorders, 124*(3), 235–240.

O'Connor, M. K., Knapp, R., Husain, M., Rummans, T. A., Petrides, G., Smith, G.,...Kellner, C. (2001). The influence of age on the response of major depression to electroconvulsive therapy: A C.O.R.E. Report. *American Journal of Geriatric Psychiatry, 9*(4), 382–390.

O'Neal, E. L., Adams, J. R., McHugo, G. J., Van Citters, A. D., Drake, R. E., & Bartels, S. J. (2008). Preferences of older and younger adults with serious mental illness for involvement in decision-making in medical and psychiatric settings. *American Journal of Geriatr Psychiatry, 16*(10), 826–833.

O'Reardon, J. P., Solvason, H. B., Janicak, P. G., Sampson, S., Isenberg, K. E., Nahas, Z.,...Sackeim, H. A. (2007). Efficacy and safety of transcranial magnetic stimulation in the acute treatment of major depression: A multisite randomized controlled trial. *Biological Psychiatry, 62*(11), 1208–1216.

Pascual-Leone, A., Valls-Sole, J., Wassermann, E. M., & Hallett, M. (1994). Responses to rapid-rate transcranial magnetic stimulation of the human motor cortex. *Brain, 117*(Pt 4), 847–858.

Patel, M., Patel, S., Hardy, D. W., Benzies, B. J., & Tare, V. (2006). Should electroconvulsive therapy be an early consideration for suicidal patients? *Journal of ECT, 22*(2), 113–115.

Payne, N. A., & Prudic, J. (2009). Electroconvulsive therapy: Part II: A biopsychosocial perspective. *Journal of Psychiatric Practice, 15*(5), 369–390.

Petrides, G., Braga, R. J., Fink, M., Mueller, M., Knapp, R., Husain, M.,...CORE (Consortium for Research in ECT) Group. (2009). Seizure threshold in a large sample: Implications for stimulus dosing strategies in bilateral electroconvulsive therapy: A report from CORE. *Journal of ECT, 25*(4), 232–237.

Petrides, G., & Fink, M. (1996). Atrial fibrillation, anticoagulation, and electroconvulsive therapy. *Convulsive Therapy, 12*(2), 91–98.

Petrides, G., Fink, M., Husain, M. M., Knapp, R. G., Rush, A. J., Mueller, M.,...Kellner, C. H. (2001). ECT remission rates in psychotic versus nonpsychotic depressed patients: A report from CORE. *Journal of ECT, 17*(4), 244–253.

Pfleiderer, B., Michael, N., Erfurth, A., Ohrmann, P., Hohmann, U., Wolgast, M.,...Heindel, W. (2003). Effective electroconvulsive therapy reverses glutamate/glutamine deficit in the left anterior cingulum of unipolar depressed patients. *Psychiatry Research, 122*(3), 185–192.

Porter, R., Booth, D., Gray, H., & Frampton, C. (2008). Effects of the addition of remifentanil to propofol anesthesia on seizure length and postictal suppression index in electroconvulsive therapy. *Journal of ECT, 24*(3), 203–207.

Prakash, J., Kotwal, A., & Prabhu, H. (2006). Therapeutic and prophylactic utility of the memory-enhancing drug donepezil hydrochloride on cognition of patients undergoing electroconvulsive therapy: A randomized controlled trial. *Journal of ECT, 22*(3), 163–168.

Prudic, J., Fitzsimons, L., Nobler, M. S., & Sackeim, H. A. (1999). Naloxone in the prevention of the adverse cognitive effects of ECT: A within-subject, placebo controlled study. *Neuropsychopharmacology, 21*(2), 285–293.

Prudic, J., & Sackeim, H. A. (1999). Electroconvulsive therapy and suicide risk. *Journal of Clinical Psychiatry, 60*(Suppl 2), 104–110; discussion 111–106.

Pullen, S. J., Rasmussen, K. G., Angstman, E. R., Rivera, F., & Mueller, P. S. (2011). The safety of electroconvulsive therapy in patients with prolonged QTc intervals on the electrocardiogram. *Journal of ECT, 27*(3), 192–200.

Quante, A., Luborzewski, A., Brakemeier, E. L., Merkl, A., Danker-Hopfe, H., & Bajbouj, M. (2011). Effects of 3 different stimulus intensities of ultrabrief stimuli in right unilateral electroconvulsive therapy in major depression: A randomized, double-blind pilot study. *Journal of Psychiatric Research, 45*(2), 174–178.

Rao, V., & Lyketsos, C. G. (2000). The benefits and risks of ECT for patients with primary dementia who also suffer from depression. *International Journal of Geriatric Psychiatry, 15*(8), 729–735.

Rascol, O., Lozano, A., Stern, M., & Poewe, W. (2011). Milestones in Parkinson's disease therapeutics. *Movement Disorders, 26*(6), 1072–1082.

Rasmussen, K. G., & Black, J. L. (2009). Serotonin transporter gene status and electroconvulsive therapy outcomes: A retrospective analysis of 83 patients. *Journal of Clinical Psychiatry, 70*(1), 92–94.

Rasmussen, K. G., Perry, C. L., Sutor, B., & Moore, K. M. (2007). ECT in patients with intracranial masses. *Journal of Neuropsychiatry and Clinical Neurosciences, 19*(2), 191–193.

Reynolds, C. F., III, Frank, E., Kupfer, D. J., Thase, M. E., Perel, J. M., Mazumdar, S., & Houck, P. R. (1996). Treatment outcome in recurrent major depression: A post hoc comparison of elderly (young old) and midlife patients. *American Journal of Psychiatry, 153*(10), 1288–1292.

Robinson, L. A., Penzner, J. B., Arkow, S., Kahn, D. A., & Berman, J. A. (2011). Electroconvulsive therapy for the treatment of refractory mania. *Journal of Psychiatric Practice, 17*(1), 61–66.

Roose, S. P., & Sackeim, H. A. (2004). *Late-life depression.* New York: Oxford University Press.

Rosenbach, M. L., Hermann, R. C., & Dorwart, R. A. (1997). Use of electroconvulsive therapy in the Medicare population between 1987 and 1992. *Psychiatric Services, 48*(12), 1537–1542.

Rossi, S., Hallett, M., Rossini, P. M., Pascual-Leone, A., & Safety of TMS Consensus Group. (2009). Safety, ethical considerations, and application guidelines for the use of transcranial magnetic stimulation in clinical practice and research. *Clinical Neurophysiology, 120*(12), 2008–2039.

Rush, A. J., Marangell, L. B., Sackeim, H. A., George, M. S., Brannan, S. K., Davis, S. M., … Cooke RG. (2005). Vagus nerve stimulation for treatment-resistant depression: A randomized, controlled acute phase trial. *Biological Psychiatry, 58*(5), 347–354.

Rush, A. J., Sackeim, H. A., Marangell, L. B., George, M. S., Brannan, S. K., Davis, S. M., … Barry, J. J. (2005). Effects of 12 months of vagus nerve stimulation in treatment-resistant depression: A naturalistic study. *Biological Psychiatry, 58*(5), 355–363.

Sackeim, H. A. (1999). The anticonvulsant hypothesis of the mechanisms of action of ECT: Current status. *Journal of ECT, 15*(1), 5–26.

Sackeim, H. A., Decina, P., Kanzler, M., Kerr, B., & Malitz, S. (1987). Effects of electrode placement on the efficacy of titrated, low-dose ECT. *American Journal of Psychiatry, 144*(11), 1449–1455.

Sackeim, H. A., Decina, P., Prohovnik, I., Malitz, S., & Resor, S. R. (1983). Anticonvulsant and antidepressant properties of electroconvulsive therapy: A proposed mechanism of action. *Biological Psychiatry, 18*(11), 1301–1310.

Sackeim, H. A., Decina, P., Prohovnik, I., Portnoy, S., Kanzler, M., & Malitz, S. (1986). Dosage, seizure threshold, and the antidepressant efficacy of electroconvulsive therapy. *Annals of the New York Academy of Sciences, 462,* 398–410.

Sackeim H.A., Devanand D.P., Nobler M.S. Electroconvulsive therapy. In: Bloom F.E., Kupfer D.J., eds. *Psychopharmacology: The Fourth Generation of Progress.* New York, NY: Raven Press, Ltd; 1995:1123–1141.

Sackeim, H. A., Haskett, R. F., Mulsant, B. H., Thase, M. E., Mann, J. J., Pettinati, H. M., … Prudic, J. (2001). Continuation pharmacotherapy in the prevention of relapse following electroconvulsive therapy: A randomized controlled trial. *Journal of the American Medical Association, 285*(10), 1299–1307.

Sackeim, H. A., Prudic, J., Devanand, D. P., Kiersky, J. E., Fitzsimons, L., Moody, B. J., … Settembrino, J. M. (1993). Effects of stimulus intensity and electrode placement on the efficacy and cognitive effects of electroconvulsive therapy. *New England Journal of Medicine, 328*(12), 839–846.

Sackeim, H. A., Prudic, J., Devanand, D. P., Nobler, M. S., Lisanby, S. H., Peyser, S., … Clark, J. (2000). A prospective, randomized, double-blind comparison of bilateral and right unilateral electroconvulsive therapy at different stimulus intensities. *Archives of General Psychiatry*, 57(5), 425–434.

Sackeim, H. A., Prudic, J., Fuller, R., Keilp, J., Lavori, P. W., & Olfson, M. (2007). The cognitive effects of electroconvulsive therapy in community settings. *Neuropsychopharmacology*, 32(1), 244–254.

Sackeim, H. A., Prudic, J., Nobler, M. S., Fitzsimons, L., Lisanby, S. H., Payne, N., ...Devanand, D. P. (2008). Effects of pulse width and electrode placement on the efficacy and cognitive effects of electroconvulsive therapy. *Brain Stimulation*, 1(2), 71–83.

Salzman, C. (1999). Practical considerations for the treatment of depression in elderly and very elderly long-term care patients. *Journal of Clinical Psychiatry*, 60(Suppl 20), 30–33.

Sanacora, G., Mason, G. F., Rothman, D. L., Behar, K. L., Hyder, F., Petroff, O. A., ...Krystal, J. H. (1999). Reduced cortical gamma-aminobutyric acid levels in depressed patients determined by proton magnetic resonance spectroscopy. *Archives of General Psychiatry*, 56(11), 1043–1047.

Sanacora, G., Mason, G. F., Rothman, D. L., Hyder, F., Ciarcia, J. J., Ostroff, R. B., ...Krystal, J. H. (2003). Increased cortical GABA concentrations in depressed patients receiving ECT. *American Journal of Psychiatry*, 160(3), 577–579.

Sartorius, A., Mahlstedt, M. M., Vollmayr, B., Henn, F. A., & Ende, G. (2007). Elevated spectroscopic glutamate/gamma-amino butyric acid in rats bred for learned helplessness. *Neuroreport*, 18(14), 1469–1473.

Schak, K. M., Mueller, P. S., Barnes, R. D., & Rasmussen, K. G. (2008). The safety of ECT in patients with chronic obstructive pulmonary disease. *Psychosomatics*, 49(3), 208–211.

Schlaepfer, T. E., George, M. S., Mayberg, H., & WFSBP Task Force on Brain Stimulation. (2010). WFSBP Guidelines on Brain Stimulation Treatments in Psychiatry. *World Journal of Biological Psychiatry*, 11(1), 2–18.

Serra, M., Gasto, C., Navarro, V., Torres, X., Blanch, J., & Masana, G. (2006). [Maintenance electroconvulsive therapy in elderly psychotic unipolar depression]. *Medicina Clinica (Barc)*, 126(13), 491–492.

Shapira, B., Tubi, N., & Lerer, B. (2000). Balancing speed of response to ECT in major depression and adverse cognitive effects: Role of treatment schedule. *Journal of ECT*, 16(2), 97–109.

Sienaert, P., Vansteelandt, K., Demyttenaere, K., & Peuskens, J. (2009). Ultra-brief pulse ECT in bipolar and unipolar depressive disorder: Differences in speed of response. *Bipolar Disorder*, 11(4), 418–424.

Sobin, C., Sackeim, H. A., Prudic, J., Devanand, D. P., Moody, B. J., & McElhiney, M. C. (1995). Predictors of retrograde amnesia following ECT. *American Journal of Psychiatry*, 152(7), 995–1001.

Sommer, B. R., Satlin, A., Friedman, L., & Cole, J. O. (1989). Glycopyrrolate versus atropine in post-ECT amnesia in the elderly. *Journal of Geriatric Psychiatry and Neurology*, 2(1), 18–21.

Spellman, T., McClintock, S. M., Terrace, H., Luber, B., Husain, M. M., & Lisanby, S. H. (2008). Differential effects of high-dose magnetic seizure therapy and electroconvulsive shock on cognitive function. *Biological Psychiatry*, 63(12), 1163–1170.

Stadtland, C., Erfurth, A., Ruta, U., & Michael, N. (2002). A switch from propofol to etomidate during an ECT course increases EEG and motor seizure duration. *Journal of ECT*, 18(1), 22–25.

Steffens, D. C., Conway, C. R., Dombeck, C. B., Wagner, H. R., Tupler, L. A., & Weiner, R. D. (2001). Severity of subcortical gray matter hyperintensity predicts ECT response in geriatric depression. *Journal of ECT*, 17(1), 45–49.

Sutor, B., & Rasmussen, K. G. (2008). Electroconvulsive therapy for agitation in Alzheimer disease: A case series. *Journal of ECT*, 24(3), 239–241.

Suzuki, K., Takano, T., & Matsuoka, H. (2009). A case of catatonia resembling frontotemporal dementia and resolved with electroconvulsive therapy. *World Journal of Biological Psychiatry*, 10(3), 245–247.

Takada, J. Y., Solimene, M. C., da Luz, P. L., Grupi, C. J., Giorgi, D. M., Rigonatti, S. P., ...Ramires, J. A. (2005). Assessment of the cardiovascular effects of electroconvulsive therapy in individuals older than 50 years. *Brazilian Journal of Medical and Biological Research*, 38(9), 1349–1357.

Takahashi, S., Mizukami, K., Yasuno, F., & Asada, T. (2009). Depression associated with dementia with Lewy bodies (DLB) and the effect of somatotherapy. *Psychogeriatrics*, 9(2), 56–61.

Tess, A. V., & Smetana, G. W. (2009). Medical evaluation of patients undergoing electroconvulsive therapy. *New England Journal of Medicine*, 360(14), 1437–1444.

Tew, J. D., Jr., Mulsant, B. H., Haskett, R. F., Prudic, J., Thase, M. E., Crowe, R. R., ...Sackeim, H. A. (1999). Acute efficacy of ECT in the treatment of major depression in the old-old. *American Journal of Psychiatry*, 156(12), 1865–1870.

Tortella, F. C., & Long, J. B. (1985). Endogenous anticonvulsant substance in rat cerebrospinal fluid after a generalized seizure. *Science*, 228(4703), 1106–1108.

Tortella, F. C., & Long, J. B. (1988). Characterization of opioid peptide-like anticonvulsant activity in rat cerebrospinal fluid. *Brain Research, 456*(1), 139–146.

Ujkaj, M., Davidoff, D. A., Seiner, S. J., Ellison, J. M., Harper, D. G., & Forester, B. P. (2012). Safety and efficacy of electroconvulsive therapy for the treatment of agitation and aggression in patients with dementia. *American Journal of Geriatric Psychiatry, 20*(1), 61–72.

UK ECT Review Group. 2003. Efficacy and safety of electroconvulsive therapy in depressive disorders: A systematic review and meta-analysis. *Lancet, 361*(9360), 799–808.

van den Broek, W. W., Groenland, T. H., Mulder, P. G., Kusuma, A., Birkenhäger, T. K., Pluijms, E. M., & Bruijn, J. A. (2008). [Beta-blockers and electroconvulsive therapy: a review]. *Tijdschrift voor Psychiatrie, 50*(4), 205–215.

van der Wurff, F. B., Stek, M. L., Hoogendijk, W. J., & Beekman, A. T. (2004). Discrepancy between opinion and attitude on the practice of ECT by psychiatrists specializing in old age in the Netherlands. *Journal of ECT, 20*(1), 37–41.

van Schaik, A. M., Comijs, H. C., Sonnenberg, C. M., Beekman, A. T., Sienaert, P., & Stek, M. L. (2012). Efficacy and safety of continuation and maintenance electroconvulsive therapy in depressed elderly patients: A systematic review. *American Journal of Geriatric Psychiatry, 20*(1), 5–17.

Vieta, E., & Colom, F. (2011). Therapeutic options in treatment-resistant depression. *Annals of Medicine, 43*(7), 512–530.

Vishne, T., Aronov, S., Amiaz, R., Etchin, A., & Grunhaus, L. (2005). Remifentanil supplementation of propofol during electroconvulsive therapy: Effect on seizure duration and cardiovascular stability. *Journal of ECT, 21*(4), 235–238.

Wassermann, E. M., Wedegaertner, F. R., Ziemann, U., George, M. S., & Chen, R. (1998). Crossed reduction of human motor cortex excitability by 1-Hz transcranial magnetic stimulation. *Neuroscience Letters, 250*(3), 141–144.

Weiduschat, N., Thiel, A., Rubi-Fessen, I., Hartmann, A., Kessler, J., Merl, P.,...Heiss, W. D. (2011). Effects of repetitive transcranial magnetic stimulation in aphasic stroke: A randomized controlled pilot study. *Stroke, 42*(2), 409–415.

Weiner, R. D. (Ed.). (2001). *The practice of electroconvulsive therapy: Recommendations for treatment, training, and privileging.* Washington, DC: American Psychiatric Association.

Weintraub, D., & Lippmann, S. B. (2001). ECT for major depression and mania with advanced dementia. *Journal of ECT, 17*(1), 65–67.

Whyte, E. M., Dew, M. A., Gildengers, A., Lenze, E. J., Bharucha, A., Mulsant, B. H., & Reynolds, C. F. (2004). Time course of response to antidepressants in late-life major depression: Therapeutic implications. *Drugs and Aging, 21*(8), 531–554.

Wu, Q., Prentice, G., & Campbell, J. J. (2010). ECT treatment for two cases of dementia-related aggressive behavior. *Journal of Neuropsychiatry and Clinical Neuroscience, 22*(2), E10–11.

Zahedi, S., Yang, C., O'Hanlon, D., Tanev, K., & Shea, W. P. (2006). Electroconvulsive therapy and venous angiomas: Two case reports and review of the literature. *Journal of ECT, 22*(3), 228–230.

Zaidi, N. A., & Khan, F. A. (2000). Comparison of thiopentone sodium and propofol for electro convulsive therapy (ECT). *Journal of the Pakistan Medical Association, 50*(2), 60–63.

Zarate, C., Jr., Machado-Vieira, R., Henter, I., Ibrahim, L., Diazgranados, N., & Salvadore, G. (2010). Glutamatergic modulators: The future of treating mood disorders? *Harvard Review of Psychiatry, 18*(5), 293–303.

Zhang, J., Narr, K. L., Woods, R. P., Phillips, O. R., Alger, J. R., & Espinoza, R. T. (2012). Glutamate normalization with ECT treatment response in major depression. *Molecular Psychiatry*, doi: 10.1038/mp.2012.46. ePub ahead of print.

Zielinski, R. J., Roose, S. P., Devanand, D. P., Woodring, S., & Sackeim, H. A. (1993). Cardiovascular complications of ECT in depressed patients with cardiac disease. *American Journal of Psychiatry, 150*(6), 904–909.

24

COMPLEMENTARY AND ALTERNATIVE MEDICINE APPROACHES FOR TREATMENT AND PREVENTION OF LATE-LIFE MOOD DISORDERS

David Merrill, Martha Payne, and Helen Lavretsky

THERE IS currently extensive use of complementary and alternative medicine (CAM) in the United States, both to sustain well-being and to treat a wide variety of physical and mental disorders. The most recent comprehensive assessment of CAM use in the United States, conducted as part of the 2007 National Health Interview Survey (NHIS), found that roughly 40% of US adults had used at least one CAM therapy within the past year (Barnes, Bloom, & Nahin, 2008). In addition, it is known that Americans make more visits to CAM providers each year than to primary care physicians and spend at least as much money on out-of-pocket expenses for CAM services as they do for all conventional physician services combined (Eisenberg et al., 1998).

Approximately 10% of all CAM visits are initiated specifically to address a psychiatric condition (Simon et al., 2004). Similarly, roughly 10% of adults with a self-identified mental condition report going to CAM practitioners, and half of those visits are made specifically to address the mental health condition (Druss & Rosenheck, 2000). Treatment of depression and anxiety is one of the most common reasons for use of CAM, with over half of depressed and anxious individuals using CAM therapies, often in addition to conventional treatments (Kessler et al., 2001). The use of CAM for treatment of mood and anxiety disorders includes acupuncture, deep breathing exercises, massage therapy, meditation, naturopathy, and yoga (Barnes et al., 2008).

An estimated 33%–88% of older adults may be using CAM therapies (Barnes et al., 2008; Ness, Cirillo, Weir, Nisly, & Wallace, 2005), including those with late-life depression and bipolar disorder (Keaton et al., 2009). With aging baby boomers expected to accelerate use of CAM among older adults in the coming years, the importance of mental health professionals having a working knowledge of CAM techniques intended to address late-life mood disorders becomes increasingly clear. The purpose of this chapter is to review the efficacy and safety of some CAM approaches relevant to late-life mood disorders in older adults.

COMPLEMENTARY AND ALTERNATIVE MEDICINE: DEFINITION AND DOMAINS

CAM therapies are defined by the National Center for Complementary and Alternative Medicine (NCCAM) as "a group of diverse medical and health care systems, practices, and products that are not generally considered part of conventional medicine" (NCCAM-NIH Website, 2010), with "conventional" medicine being defined as the approaches used by clinicians in the routine daily practice of Western or allopathic medicine that are within the currently accepted standard of care. Given the multiple potential applications of singular CAM approaches, the domains of CAM overlap, and moreover, continue to evolve over time as CAM therapies receive greater study and application across multiple settings. NCCAM has helped define and describe the major domains of CAM (NCCAM-NIH Website, 2010)—domains that were similarly adapted into several major groups for

the 2007 NHIS (Barnes et al., 2008), as described in Table 24.1.

STUDIES OF COMPLEMENTARY AND ALTERNATIVE MEDICINE USE IN LATE-LIFE MOOD DISORDERS

Studies examining CAM therapies for the treatment and prevention of late-life mood disorders are limited. A relatively recent review of randomized controlled trials (RCTs) of CAM for older adults found 33 trials of sufficient quality to include in the review, and a number of these studies were focused on addressing sleep and anxiety rather than mood disorders (Meeks, Wetherell, Irwin, Redwine, & Jeste, 2007). Of the 33 included trials, most had methodological limitations and while 67% had positive outcomes, the positive studies were, on average, of lower methodological quality than the negative reports.

In contrast, there have been a number of recent reviews and guidelines published based on the relatively larger but still limited number of RCTs testing CAM therapies for treatment of both depression and bipolar disorder in younger and middle-aged adults

Table 24.1 Complementary and Alternative Medicine Domains and Examples

DOMAIN	EXAMPLES	COMMENTS
Biologically based therapies	Herbal (botanical) medicines, vitamins, nonvitamin/nonmineral natural products (e.g., omega-3 fatty acids)	18% of US adults use nonvitamin/nonmineral natural products
Mind-body medicine	Biofeedback, meditation techniques, yoga, Tai chi, energy therapies (e.g., light therapy, Qi gong, and healing touch), exercise	Focuses on interactions between brain, mind, body, and behavior to affect physical function and promote health
Manipulative and body-based practices	Chiropractic spinal manipulation, massage therapies, movement therapies (e.g., Pilates)	Focuses on structure and functional systems of the body, including bones and joints, soft tissues, circulatory and lymphatic systems
Alternative medical systems	Acupuncture, Ayurveda, homeopathy/naturopathy, and traditional healers (e.g., Native American healers)	Focuses on achieving optimal health and well-being
Other complementary and alternative practices	Spirituality, pastoral care, and expressive therapies	Approaches not formally categorized

(Andreescu, Mulsant, & Emanuel, 2008; Freeman et al., 2010; Sarris, Kavanagh, & Byrne, 2010; van der Watt, Laugharne, & Janca, 2008). As such, this evidence base will be included in this discussion of potential CAM therapies for treatment of mood disorders in older adults. Overall, the conclusion of a 2010 report published by an American Psychiatric Association Task Force charged with reviewing the available evidence base for CAM approaches in adults was that several approaches have promising preliminary results from various trials (Freeman et al., 2010). However, task force participants went on to state that each CAM approach needs separate evaluation in larger and more rigorous controlled studies prior to being recommended confidently as specific treatments.

Nonetheless, given current widespread use of CAM, there is an urgent need for greater awareness about CAM approaches among mental health care providers, especially with the known underreporting of CAM use by patients to conventional practitioners (Simon et al., 2004). Next, we review CAM therapies of potential relevance for use in the treatment and prevention of late-life mood disorders summarized in Table 24.2.

BIOLOGICALLY BASED THERAPIES AND NATURAL PRODUCTS

Omega-3 Fatty Acids

One of the most widely used CAM therapies is dietary supplementation with omega-3 polyunsaturated fatty acids. Of the 18% of the US population who reported use of nonvitamin, nonmineral natural products in the 2007 NHIS survey, over 37% reported using fish oil or omega-3 fatty acids within the past 30 days (Barnes et al., 2008). The omega-3 fatty acids, comprising a subtype of polyunsaturated fatty acids, include alpha-linolenic acid (ALA) and its derivatives eicosapentaenoic acid (EPA) and docosahexanoic acid (DHA). ALA is an essential fatty acid, meaning that it cannot be produced by the body and therefore must be consumed in the diet. In humans, the conversion of ALA to EPA, and further to DHA, is very inefficient, indicating that dietary intake of EPA and DHA may be beneficial. Omega-3 fatty acids are necessary for normal human development and cellular function throughout the life span. These functions include roles in membrane fluidity, serotonin metabolism, cellular regulation, protection

from oxidative stress, and anti-inflammatory effects (Sinclair, Begg, Mathai, & Weisinger, 2007), which may be beneficial for depression through both neuronal and vascular mechanisms.

EPA and DHA, long chain marine fatty acids, are primarily found in cold-water fish and seafood (e.g., salmon and scallops), and algae, while ALA is found in cold-adapted plants and nuts (e.g., flaxseed and walnuts). All of these omega-3s are found in fortified foods and dietary supplements (including algal, fish, and flaxseed oils). In contrast, omega-6 fatty acids, another subtype of polyunsaturated fatty acids, are ubiquitous in the diet as they are found in commonly used vegetable oils from heat-adapted plants such as peanut, safflower, canola, and sunflower.

Deficiencies and/or imbalances in omega-3s are hypothesized to underlie multiple health conditions. The typical Western diet is high in the pro-inflammatory omega-6 fatty acids but relatively low in omega-3 fatty acids, intake of which is correlated with reduced production of pro-inflammatory cytokines (Galli & Calder, 2009). This imbalance is related to increased incidence of diseases mediated by high chronic inflammation, including heart disease, asthma, inflammatory bowel disease, and rheumatoid arthritis. When combined with increased adiposity, this imbalance is related to increased levels of depression (Shelton & Miller, 2010). Many older individuals have a subtype of late-life depression characterized by vascular brain changes (Krishnan, Hays, & Blazer, 1997), which may lend themselves to influence by omega-3 consumption. Deficiencies in omega-3 fatty acids may also lead to disruption of neuronal membrane structure and function, leading to dysfunctional suppression of neuronal transmission and increased recurrence of bipolar episodes (Stoll et al., 1999).

Observational studies have noted the connection between omega-3 consumption and a variety of health conditions, including depression. Lower levels of fish consumption correlate with higher rates of depression and suicidal ideations (Hibbeln, 1998; Tanskanen et al., 2001; Timonen et al., 2004). On aggregate, a number of studies have shown lowered levels of omega-3 fatty acids in depressed patients (Lin, Huang, & Su, 2010); however, it is not clear whether levels reflect dietary inadequacy or an underlying dysregulation of fatty acid metabolism in depression (Maes et al., 1999). Also of note, the majority of these studies were conducted in nonelderly populations.

Table 24.2 Complementary and Alternative Medicine Interventions for the Treatment of Late-Life Mood Disorders

MODE OF INTERVENTION	POSTULATED MECHANISM OF ACTION	DEPRESSION	MAIN ADVERSE EFFECTS AND DRUG INTERACTIONS
St. John's wort	Monoamine oxidase inhibition and reduced monoamine reuptake	Close to 40 RCTs; mixed results with some positive and some failed trials as compared to placebo or to an active control	Mania, serotonergic syndrome, photosensitivity, multiple drug interactions with HIV protease inhibitors, warfarin, digoxin, oral contraceptives, anticonvulsants
Omega-3 fatty acids (fish oil)	Mood stabilization, neuroprotection, reduction in amyloid production	Several RCTs are mixed or negative in the effect on mood and well-being	Fishy aftertaste, gastrointestinal distress, increased effect of warfarin and NSAIDs
SAMe	Cofactor in neurotransmitter synthesis, methylation homocysteine to methionine	Several RCTs; parenteral SAMe is superior to placebo	Mania, gastrointestinal distress, headache; interaction with SSRIs
Folate and B12	Cofactor in neurotransmitter synthesis, methylation homocysteine to methionine, precursor to SAMe	Folic acid is an effective adjunct	Mania induction, interaction with SSRIs
Gingko biloba	Scavenging free radical; lowering oxidative stress; reducing neural damages; increased blood flow to the brain	Several RCTs in postmenopausal women, and for sexual side effects of antidepressants—mixed results	Increased bleeding time, allergic reactions
Ayurveda	Indian treatment system with the use of herbs, diet, and lifestyle to achieve balance in cognition and well-being	Few studies suggestive of positive effect	Consistent with above side effect of herbals
Acupuncture	Balancing energy flow through the meridians in the body	Small RCTs with poor controls, randomization and blinding and inconclusive results	Needle phobia, bleeding

(*Continued*)

Table 24.2 (Continued)

MODE OF INTERVENTION	POSTULATED MECHANISM OF ACTION	DEPRESSION	MAIN ADVERSE EFFECTS AND DRUG INTERACTIONS
Yoga	Postures, breath, meditation—rebalancing the mind-body connections	Reduces depression and enhances well-being in a few studies	Possible injury
Spirituality	Lowers stress and enhances cognition via church attendance and prayer	Improves depression in practitioners	Limited acceptability
Exercise	Improved cardiovascular function, release of endorphins, increased energy, mental stimulation	Improved mood and wellbeing, especially in minor depression	Possible injury
Expressive therapies (art, music, dance)	Allows expression of emotional and cognitive facets of self	Improves mood, stress reduction	Possible injury

AD, Alzheimer's disease; NSAIDs, nonsteroidal anti-inflammatory drugs; RCT, randomized controlled trial; SAMe, S-adenosyl-L-methionine; SSRI, selective serotonin reuptake inhibitor; VAD, vascular dementia.

Source: Adapted from Lavretsky, H. (2009). The use of complementary and alternative medicine for treatment of late-life neuropsychiatric disorders. *Aging Health*, 5(1), 61–78.

Several recent reviews and meta-analyses on the use of omega-3 fatty acids to treat depression in adult populations have recently been published, with the included studies differing between reports. One such comprehensive review found that actual diagnosis of depression predicted a more robust response to omega-3 supplementation compared to simply having depressive symptoms, lending support to the hypothesis of omega-3 fatty acid supplementation benefitting individuals diagnosed with depression (Appleton, Rogers, & Ness, 2010). Dose ranges of omega-3 fatty acid supplementation for depression and bipolar disorder have varied in clinical trials, with amounts and ratios of DHA and EPA differing between trials. There is some evidence that EPA, rather than DHA, is mediating the potential benefits of omega-3 fatty acid supplementation in cases of depression (Martins, 2009). In addition to dose and type of omega-3 supplementation, study differences may be due to baseline omega-3 intake levels, effect of supplementation upon omega-6 intakes, medication use, and heterogeneity of depression.

The number of published studies on omega-3 fatty acid use in late-life mood disorders is limited. A small ($n = 46$) recent double-blind, placebo-controlled study in depressed females living in an Italian nursing home found that omega-3 fatty acid supplementation (1.67 g of EPA and 0.83 g of DHA) significantly improved depressive symptoms and quality of life as measured by the geriatric depression scale (GDS) and Short-Form 36-Item Health Survey (SF-36), respectively (Rondanelli et al., 2011). This report lends support to the idea that omega-3 fatty acids may have a role in the treatment of late-life neuropsychiatric disorders; however, additional larger, well-designed, randomized controlled studies focusing on older adults are needed before their use can be recommended confidently to patients and their families. Lastly, in addition to efficacy for depression, there remain concerns about safety and sustainability related to consumption of marine foods and oils. A significant portion of seafood as well as some fish oil dietary supplements has heavy metal contamination with methyl mercury (Hughner, Maher, & Childs, 2008). Additionally, there are sustainability and environmental concerns related to overfishing and commercial aquaculture.

S-Adenosyl-L-Methionine

Prescribed in Europe for nearly 40 years and introduced in the United States as an over-the-counter supplement in 1999, S-adenosyl-L-methionine (SAMe) is a naturally occurring compound normally synthesized in the body from the amino acid L-methionine as part of a multistep metabolic pathway involving folic acid and vitamin B-12 (Mischoulon & Fava, 2002; Papakostas, 2009). SAMe is the sole methyl donor in the nervous system, necessary as a cofactor for the rate-limiting steps of serotonin, norepinephrine, and dopamine synthesis (Paul, McDonnell, & Kelly, 2004). Cerebrospinal fluid levels of SAMe have been shown to be decreased in severely depressed patients and these levels rise in response to treatment with the supplement (Bottiglieri et al., 1990). Given its role in intracellular metabolism and the observed changes in SAMe level during depression, SAMe has been developed and studied for its potential use as an antidepressant.

Initial oral formulations of SAMe were relatively unstable, necessitating parenteral (intravenous or intramuscular) administration of SAMe for clinical use. However, the more recent development of stable oral forms of SAMe has allowed for more widespread testing and use of this compound. Small open trials of SAMe use in depressed patients initially found promising results, prompting a number of larger controlled trials. Independent meta-analyses of these trials have found that SAMe treatment yields results superior to placebo and equivalent to several tricyclic antidepressants, including clomipramine, amitriptyline, and imipramine (Bressa, 1994; Hardy et al., 2003).

An open trial showed potential for SAMe as an augmentation strategy in patients with incomplete responses to selective serotonin reuptake inhibitors or venlafaxine (Alpert et al., 2004). A recently published small 6-week double-blind RCT of SAMe versus placebo found that HAM-D response and remission rates were significantly higher for the SAMe group (36% and 26%) than placebo (18% and 12%), while side effect profiles did not differ significantly (Papakostas, Mischoulon, Shyu, Alpert,

& Fava, 2010). The parenteral dose range in clinical trials of SAMe has been between 15 and 1,000 mg/day, with most trials delivering 100–200 mg/day to subjects. Oral doses have ranged from 400 to 1,600 mg/day, with most trials dosing between 800 and 1,600 mg/day (Mischoulon & Fava, 2002). SAMe is generally well tolerated, with common side effects including mild insomnia, decreased appetite, constipation, nausea, dry mouth, sweating, dizziness, and nervousness. Increased anxiety, mania, or hypomania has been reported in patients with bipolar depression (Carney, Chary, Bottiglieri, Reynolds, & Toone, 1987). As such, bipolar patients should not take SAMe without concomitant administration of mood stabilizers coupled with close clinical monitoring for development of switching into a manic or hypomanic state.

Overall, SAMe appears to have adequate safety and efficacy as a treatment of depression; however, there is currently a dearth of evidence regarding use of SAMe in late-life depression. For all ages, further controlled studies are warranted as a considerable amount of the current evidence for younger adults comes from small or open-label trials. More trials are also needed for oral forms of SAMe, as initial data stem largely from subjects given parenteral forms of SAMe (Papakostas, 2009). An additional consideration for use of SAMe has been cost, with 200–400 mg tablets typically costing approximately $1 per tablet as of the printing of this chapter. While this price is expected to drop in the coming years, it currently remains an obstacle for patients unable to afford high out-of-pocket expenses.

St. John's Wort (*Hypericum perforatum*)

St. John's wort (*Hypericum perforatum*) is a wildflower found throughout the world that has been used for medicinal purposes for thousands of years. Various standardized extracts of this natural dietary supplement having been studied more recently. St. John's wort is prescribed widely in Europe for the treatment of depression, particularly in Germany, where there have been a number of large positive trials comparing St. John's wort to placebo and standard antidepressants. While also available in the United States as an over-the-counter supplement, excitement over St. John's wort has been tempered by highly publicized negative clinical trials and associated reviews (Hypericum Depression Trial Study Group, 2002; Shelton, 2009; Shelton et al., 2001).

Despite these negative findings, a recently updated systematic review of the evidence base for use of St. John's wort in depression for adults suggests that St. John's wort is superior to placebo and similarly effective as standard antidepressants for mild to moderate depression (Linde et al., 2008). The review comments on the differences observed between European versus US trials; however, the etiology of this difference is not explained and remains poorly understood.

In older adults, the available evidence base for use of St. John's wort for treatment of depression is limited. A small ($n = 149$) randomized double-blind study comparing St. John's wort (800 mg of extract LoHyp-57) and fluoxetine (20 mg) found equivalent efficacy of these agents in reducing Hamilton Depression Scale (HAM-D) scores over 6 weeks for mild to moderate depression in a mostly female sample of older adults (Harrer, Schmidt, Kuhn, & Biller, 1999). In this small trial, the proportion of subjects experiencing adverse events were similar for both St. John's wort ($n = 12$) and fluoxetine ($n = 17$).

Clinical trials have used various divided doses of St. John's wort totaling between 600 mg to 1,800 mg daily, with the most common dose being 300 mg three times daily. The flower or leaf extract preparations available on the market vary considerably in their pharmaceutical quality. Common side effects from St. John's wort include dry mouth, dizziness, diarrhea, nausea, increased sensitivity to sunlight, and fatigue. There is some evidence that St. John's wort may be better tolerated than older selective serotonin reuptake inhibitors (SSRIs) such as paroxetine (Kasper et al., 2010); however, head-to-head comparisons have not been completed with newer SSRIs, which typically have a lower incidence of side effects.

St. John's wort is relatively well tolerated and safe when used alone; however, when taken in combination with other medications, patients and clinicians need to be aware of a number of potentially dangerous drug–drug interactions (Izzo & Ernst, 2009). St. John's wort is known for its monoamine oxidase inhibition and also for affecting the cytochrome P-450 (CYP) liver enzyme system. In particular, St. John's wort induces CYP 3A/3A4, which can lead to altered levels of anticonvulsant, antibiotic, and oral contraceptive medications. Among a number of other drug–drug interactions, a recent experimental study found that St. John's wort significantly decreases the concentration and effectiveness of oxycodone when given to patients with chronic pain (Nieminen et al., 2010).

In summary, for older adults who would rather not take conventional Western medications, St. John's wort can be considered as an alternative natural remedy for mild-to-moderate depression. However, the ideal patient will be free of comorbid medical conditions and all patients using St. John's wort should be informed about potential side effects and drug–drug interactions, as such interactions can have serious, even potentially lethal, consequences.

MIND-BODY MEDICINE

Mindful Physical Exercise

Mind-body medicine encompasses a number of CAM therapies, including a group of techniques collectively known as mindful physical exercise (e.g., Qigong, yoga, and Tai Chi). Mindful physical exercise has become an increasingly utilized approach for improving psychological well-being and is defined as "physical exercise executed with a profound inwardly directed contemplative focus" (Forge, 2005). As such, mindful physical exercise contains the following key elements: (1) a noncompetitive, nonjudgmental meditative component; (2) mental focus on muscular movement and proprioceptive awareness combined with a low to moderate level of muscular activity; (3) centered breathing; (4) a focus on anatomic alignment (i.e., spine, trunk, and pelvis) and proper physical form; and (5) energy-centric awareness of individual flow of intrinsic energy, vital life force, qi, and so on. Mindful exercise interventions have shown promise in addressing depressive symptoms in older adults. For example, a study of 82 older adult participants with depression randomized to either 16 weeks of Qigong practice or newspaper reading groups found that Qigong participants showed significantly greater improvements in mood, self-efficacy, and personal well-being (Tsang, Fung, Chan, Lee, & Chan, 2006).

Yoga

Widely practiced in India and beyond, yoga is an ancient multifaceted approach to health that involves multiple postures, breathing techniques, and meditation to balance the body's energy centers. Practice of yoga typically benefits from instruction by expert instructors and requires the dedication by participants to multiple weekly sessions and continual use for maximal benefit.

Prior review of published RCTs of yoga for depression in adults revealed that while all trials found benefit of the approach, trial methodologies have generally been weak with lack of blinding, short duration of the intervention, variable outcome measures, limited information about subjects, randomization procedures, compliance, and dropout rates (Pilkington, Kirkwood, Rampes, & Richardson, 2005). Comparative studies of yoga have likewise been limited, with one trial demonstrating that yoga was as effective as tricyclic antidepressants (Janakiramaiah et al., 2000) and another trial showing that yoga may provide benefit as an augmentation strategy for antidepressant treatment (Sharma, Das, Mondal, Goswampi, & Gandhi, 2005). Yoga is commonly used in combination with other treatments for depression, anxiety, and stress-related disorders.

Data on use of yoga for anxiety and depression in older adults are more limited; however, one significant study of 69 older adults in India did compare the impact of yoga to Ayurveda or a waitlist control condition on sleep and depressive symptoms (Krishnamurthy & Telles, 2007; Manjunath & Telles, 2005). Participants in the yoga group practiced physical postures, relaxation techniques, regulated breathing, devotional songs, and attended lectures for over 7 hours a week during the course of the 6-month trial. Practice of yoga significantly impacted quality of sleep and level of depressive symptoms when compared to the two control conditions, neither of which demonstrated significant effects. In particular, depressive symptoms, as measured by the short form of the Geriatric Depression Scale, decreased in the yoga group from a baseline average of 10.6 to 8.1 by 3 months and 6.7 by 6 months. The average time to fall asleep decreased in the yoga group by 10 minutes, while total number of hours slept increased by 60 minutes and resulted in a greater feeling of being rested after 6 months.

In summary, both alternative and more integrative approaches combining conventional therapies with complementary use of yoga show promise for improving outcomes in geriatric depression. Response to yoga in older adults with bipolar disorder has not yet been examined.

Tai Chi

The practice of the Chinese marital art Tai Chi has been reported to benefit a wide variety of health conditions. A recent systematic review found significant effects of Tai Chi on depression and anxiety, but caution was urged as a number of the reviewed studies had methodological limitations (Wang et al., 2009). In older adults, a 6-month RCT was completed in previously sedentary participants to assess the impact of three times/week Tai Chi on sleep in comparison to a stretching exercise group (Li et al., 2004). The study found that the Tai Chi group participants reported significantly improved sleep latency and greater total sleep duration when compared to the control group. While the study was not completed in a depressed population, these findings suggest a benefit of this approach for sedentary older adults struggling with sleep issues as part of their mood disturbance. Furthermore, with the appropriate accommodation for participants with physical limitations, Tai Chi can be used in a variety of settings and, for example, has been shown to improve components of physical and mental health quality of life in nursing home residents (Lee, Lee, & Woo, 2010).

CONVENTIONAL PHYSICAL EXERCISE

Conventional physical exercise has received considerable attention for its potential role in treatment of depression, based initially on results of observational studies. A large (N = 6,828) cross-sectional study of men and women ages 20–88 years old found that aerobic fitness and physical activity levels as measured by a maximal treadmill test and self-report, respectively, significantly related to both degree of depressive symptoms and emotional well-being (Galper, Trivedi, Barlow, Dunn, & Kampert, 2006). Interestingly, these relationships occurred in a graded, dose-dependent fashion, with progressively higher levels of fitness associated with increasingly lower levels of depressive symptoms and higher degrees of self-reported well-being. For physical activity levels, a similar dose–response relationship was observed; however, the greatest benefit was seen at between 11–19 miles per week of walking, jogging, or running. In older adults, the large (N = 1,947) 5-year observational Alameda County Study found that greater baseline levels of physical activity were protective against the subsequent development of depression in older adults (Strawbridge, Deleger, Roberts, & Kaplan, 2002). Similarly, an 8-year longitudinal study of older adults observed that age-related decreases in the intensity of exercise over time increased the risk of depressive symptoms at the conclusion of the study (Lampinen, Heikkinen, & Ruoppila, 2000), while having three or more chronic medical conditions and a decreased ability to perform activities of daily living were also associated with more depression over time.

Several reviews and meta-analyses have been completed demonstrating the effects of exercise on depressive symptoms across a wide variety of populations and using an equally varied set of approaches to increase physical activity of study participants. Exercise has generally been shown to exert positive effects on overall mood and well-being, and in addition, to prevent relapse of depressive symptoms for subjects who maintain activity levels. However, the majority of RCTs examining the effects of exercise on depressive symptoms have been methodologically limited, with an inadequacy of randomization, insufficient blinding, failure to use intention to treat analyses, and use of self-reported measures of depression. A recently updated Cochrane review and meta-analysis of exercise for depression examined 25 trials and concluded that, when only methodologically sound trials were included for review, exercise effects on depression diminish in magnitude and actually lose statistical significance (Mead et al., 2009). Review and meta-analysis of trials completed in older adults have revealed that, similar to trials of younger adults, the strength of conclusions drawn from positive trials of exercise interventions for depression in older adults is limited by the methodological shortcomings of completed studies (Sjosten & Kivela, 2006).

Still, a relatively large number of RCTs have targeted increasing exercise behaviors in younger and older adults with depression through structured exercise interventions and shown positive results. As stated earlier, many of the studies have had methodological limitations, including relatively small sample sizes and a focus on short-term rather than long-term effects of exercise on mood. The Depression Outcomes Study of Exercise (DOSE) found that aerobic exercise of sufficient intensity to meet public health recommendations for physical activity (i.e., greater than 150 minutes per week) significantly reduced depressive symptoms as measured on the HAM-D when compared to either lower intensity aerobic exercise or flexibility training (47% reduction vs. 30% for each of the control conditions, $p = .01$; Dunn, Trivedi, Burks, Rantz, & Pomeroy, 2005). Interestingly, total amount of exercise per week, rather than frequency of sessions, appeared to be the significant factor in determining the positive effect on mood, an effect that was observed regardless of age or gender in the population studied.

A recent study in adults diagnosed with major depressive disorder found that 16 weeks of exercise was equivalent to standard antidepressant therapy with sertraline 50–200 mg daily (Blumenthal et al., 2007). Both supervised group exercise and home-based exercise programs were equally efficacious in decreasing depressive symptoms to the point of remission, which was the primary outcome measure of the study. Neither exercise nor antidepressant therapy treatment achieved results superior to placebo effects, largely due to a high placebo response rate in the study, which the authors suggested resulted from nonspecific factors such as patient expectations, ongoing symptom monitoring, and greater attention due to study involvement. Preliminary examination of adjunctive use of exercise for depression has been completed in adults and been found to be beneficial in reducing depressive symptoms; a larger, well-designed trial is ongoing and aims to address the methodological limitations of the prior studies noted earlier (Trivedi et al., 2006a, 2006b).

The effects of aerobic exercise in depressed adults age 50 and older were examined and compared to either monotherapy with sertraline as a standard antidepressant or a combination of both approaches (Blumenthal et al., 1999). The study found that after 16 weeks, all three groups demonstrated equivalent significant reductions in depressive symptoms as measured by scores on the HDS and the Beck Depression Inventory. Furthermore, a 10-month follow-up study showed that participants in the exercise group who had improved to the point of remission during the initial study showed lower rates of relapse than those taking antidepressants, and independent continuation of exercising related to a reduced probability of being depressed at the end of the trial (Babyak et al., 2000). Another study of exercise for older adults found that 10 weeks of weight-bearing exercises classes provided as an adjunctive treatment significantly lessened depressive symptoms in a group of older adults who had not responded to antidepressant therapy alone when compared to a health education course (Mather et al., 2002).

The effectiveness of a number of lifestyle interventions, including those promoting increases in conventional physical exercise, has been recently reviewed (Jepson, Harris, Platt, & Tannahill, 2010). Studies have found that structured interventions can increase physical activity levels in children, adolescents, adults, and older adults. Review of the effectiveness of physical activity interventions in older adults (>50 years old) included 38 studies utilizing 57 interventions categorized as home-based, group-based, or educational in nature (van der Bij, Laurant, & Wensing, 2002). Overall, interventions were relatively successful in initiating increased levels of physical activity in the short run; however, maintenance of these gains was diminished over time and there was not convincing evidence that behavioral reinforcement strategies were beneficial. Another review of exercise interventions found that while many older adults increase physical activity levels in response to a wide variety of interventions, the amount of increase is seldom enough to convincingly impact health outcomes in a positive manner (Conn, Minor, Burks, Rantz, & Pomeroy, 2003).

In summary, preliminary evidence points to exercise as having a significant potential to lessen symptoms in depressed older adults, and furthermore, to prevent relapse of depression and/or development of depressive symptoms in older adults experiencing acute stressors associated with aging (Harris, Cronkite, & Moos, 2006). Given the multitude of potential general health benefits of exercise, including impacts on cardiovascular, muscular, and bone health, clinicians can feel comfortable recommending appropriately supervised increases in physical activity. The physical activity readiness questionnaire (PAR-Q) is a validated measure that can be used to screen individuals for health conditions which would prevent a safe initiation of a new physical activity program prior to referral to their primary care physician to address potentially harmful underlying health risks. Once ready to proceed, older adults can be referred to community centers that provide exercise services of interest.

Mindfulness Meditation

Mindfulness-based approaches to stress reduction may help individuals become more emotionally aware, and they have been shown to reduce anxiety and dysphoria in healthy and clinical populations of younger adults (Grossman, Niemann, Schmidt, & Walach, 2004). A recently published review of the effect of mindfulness meditation on cellular aging suggests that mindfulness meditation techniques shift cognitive appraisals from threat to challenge,

decrease ruminative thought, reduce stress arousal, and directly increase positive arousal states that affect telomerase activity and telomere length, thereby improving longevity (Epel, Daubenmier, Moskowitz, Folkman, & Blackburn, 2009). Another recently published study documented the effects of intensive meditation training in the participants of the Buddhist retreat on telomerase activity with higher activity post retreat compared to the waitlist control (Jacobs et al., 2011). The results implicate a potential effect of meditation on biological aging. The authors suggested that potential mediators of the effect were positive cognition such as perceived control (of life circumstances) versus emotional negativity and neuroticism. Currently, there is only preliminary evidence that the use of mind-body techniques, such as meditation, can be useful in preventing diseases of aging. Future studies should address this potential.

ALTERNATIVE MEDICAL SYSTEMS

Acupuncture

Acupuncture is the Chinese practice of inserting needles into the body at specific points to manipulate the body's flow of energy to balance the endocrine system regulating heart rate, body temperature, and potentially, emotional changes. Prior reviews of RCTs using acupuncture to treat depression have found some evidence for benefit; however, the majority of included studies have been of relatively low quality with placebo acupuncture treatment at times yielding similar results to treatment acupuncture (Leo & Ligot, 2007). Cochrane database review of studies examining acupuncture for depression found insufficient evidence to determine the efficacy of acupuncture in comparison to standard antidepressants, sham acupuncture, or waitlist controls (Smith, Hay, & Macpherson, 2010). Most recently, a RCT comparing electroacupuncture to control acupuncture in 53 subjects diagnosed with mild to moderate major depression found significant but similar improvements in depressive symptoms for both techniques (Andreescu, Glick, Emeremni, Houck, & Mulsant, 2011).

In older adults, the literature is limited, with a pilot study of acupuncture for depression in older adults finding positive effects on measures of mood and well-being (Williams & Graham, 2006). A Chinese study of 101 adults with "post-wind stroke depression," a traditional Chinese medicine diagnosis, found that "mind-refreshing antidepressive" acupuncture was as effective as low-dose doxepin plus routine acupuncture and more effective than routine acupuncture alone (Li et al., 1994). In conclusion, while acupuncture has been used in clinics to assist people with a number of ailments, including anxiety and depression, evidence currently remains limited and further large, well-designed studies are needed in this area.

Ayurveda

Ayurveda, which translates to "the science of life" and has been described as "knowledge of how to live," is a complete natural health care system that began in India over 5,000 years ago and has been used within the context of mental health and aging for memory enhancement and anxiety reduction. Promoting immune system function through anti-inflammatory remedies, Ayurveda is widely used contemporarily in India as a system of primary health care. With its emphasis on developing an individualized regimen for patients, which includes dietary, meditation, herbal, and other components, interest in Ayurveda is growing worldwide to treat a number of maladies, including depression. Through yoga and/or transcendental meditation techniques, Ayurveda promotes lifestyle change and education about how to release stress and tension. Furthermore, Ayurveda is geared toward treating chronic disorders associated with the aging process, and promising preliminary results related to use of Ayurveda have been found in studies of depression, anxiety, sleep disorders, hypertension, diabetes mellitus, Parkinson's disease, and Alzheimer's disease (Sharma, Chandola, Singh, & Basisht, 2007).

OTHER COMPLEMENTARY AND ALTERNATIVE MEDICINE PRACTICES

Religion and Spirituality

Religious and spiritual practices are common among older adults, and the level of involvement in such activities has been shown to correlate with lower levels of depressive symptoms (Husaini, Blasi, & Miller, 1999). While some have hypothesized that the positive impact of religion on mood lies simply in increased socialization, religious coping has been shown to impact level of depressive symptoms

independent of the socialization effects of religion (Bosworth, Park, McQuoid, Hays, & Steffens, 2003). Beyond simply holding religious beliefs, a threshold of active involvement in faith-based activities, such as greater than weekly church attendance, may be necessary for the protective effect of religiosity on depression (Norton et al., 2008).

Incorporating an assessment of spiritual and religious practices into standard clinical encounters may positively impact the ability of clinicians to detect depressive symptoms and provide treatments viewed as more congruent with patient beliefs. Such concepts were demonstrated in a study of older African American participants, many of whom described depression as stemming from a "loss of faith," where incorporation of faith and spiritual/religious activities would lead to greater levels of patient empowerment and improved possibility of positive outcomes from conventional medical treatments (Wittink, Joo, Lewis, & Barg, 2009). Indeed, bringing appropriate elements of religious beliefs into cognitive-behavioral therapy practices has been shown to accelerate the response to psychotherapy (Paukert et al., 2009).

In summary, clinicians asking about and reinforcing positively held spiritual and religious beliefs appears to be an effective complementary strategy to routine psychotherapy and psychopharmacological management of late-life mood symptoms.

Expressive Therapies

Engagement in the creative arts holds potential as a positive coping strategy for dealing with the otherwise potentially depressive changes associated with normal aging such as retirement, lack of purpose, and social isolation (Flood & Phillips, 2007). Although formal study of such activities is limited, psychological and neurobiological theories of aging support the notion that enriching activities will have a beneficial effect on overall physical and mental health. For example, older adults enrolled into a 12-month structured chorale program reported significant improvements in overall physical health, better morale, less loneliness, and a trend toward increased overall activities (Cohen et al., 2006).

A multimodal program including components of rhythm and dance, physical and outdoor exercising, and multiple seminars on creativity, philosophy, and communication demonstrated significant impacts on multiple outcome measures (Cohen, 2005). The 75 older adults enrolled in this 4-month program participated in multiple individual and group sessions held throughout each week of the study. Formal testing revealed that subjects reported an improved sense of purpose in life, fewer depressive symptoms, and lowered levels of hypochondriasis. These gains were maintained when reassessed 6 months post intervention. Thus, such interventions hold potential for older adults to experientially integrate the emotional, physical, and cognitive aspects of self that are at risk of fragmentation and decline with aging.

SUMMARY

Late-life mood disorders are among the most common reasons for using complementary and alternative therapies in older adults. The amount of rigorous scientific data to support the efficacy of complementary therapies in the treatment of depression and bipolar disorder is extremely limited in adults and often times essentially nonexistent in older adults. There is a need for further research involving larger, well-designed RCTs to determine the efficacy of complementary and alternative therapies in the treatment of mood disorders during late life. The ultimate goal is development of effective, well-tolerated, and safe treatment approaches for these serious and disabling conditions.

Disclosures:

Dr. Merrill has no disclosures to report.

Dr. Payne has no disclosures to report.

Dr. Lavretsky reports that she is a consultant or paid advisory board member for Dey Phrama, and Lilly, Inc., and that she has received research grants from Forest Research Institute and from the Alzheimer's Research and Prevention Foundation.

Funding: This work was supported by the American Federation for Aging Research, The John A. Hartford Foundation, and the Centers of Excellence National Program for Dr. Merrill; the NIH grants MH077650, MH086481, and AT003480 to Dr. Lavretsky; and K12-HD043446 to Dr. Payne.

REFERENCES

Alpert, J. E., Papakostas, G., Mischoulon, D., Worthington, J. J., III, Petersen, T., Mahal, Y., ... Fava, M. (2004). S-adenosyl-L-methionine (SAMe) as an adjunct for resistant major depressive disorder: An open trial following partial or nonresponse to selective serotonin reuptake inhibitors or venlafaxine. *Journal of Clinical Psychopharmacology, 24*(6), 661–664.

Andreescu, C., Glick, R. M., Emeremni, C. A., Houck, P. R., & Mulsant, B. H. (2011). Acupuncture for the treatment of major depressive disorder: A randomized controlled trial. *Journal of Clinical Psychiatry, 72*(8), 1129–1135.

Andreescu, C., Mulsant, B. H., & Emanuel, J. E. (2008). Complementary and alternative medicine in the treatment of bipolar disorder—a review of the evidence. *Journal of Affective Disorders 110*(1–2), 16–26.

Appleton, K. M., Rogers, P. J., & Ness, A. R. (2010). Updated systematic review and meta-analysis of the effects of n-3 long-chain polyunsaturated fatty acids on depressed mood. *American Journal of Clinical Nutrition, 91*(3), 757–770.

Babyak, M., Blumenthal, J. A., Herman, S., Khatri, P., Doraiswamy, M., Moore, K., ... Krishnan, K. R. (2000). Exercise treatment for major depression: Maintenance of therapeutic benefit at 10 months. *Psychosomatic Medicine, 62*(5), 633–638.

Barnes, P. M., Bloom, B., & Nahin, R. L. (2008). Complementary and alternative medicine use among adults and children: United States, 2007. *National Health Statistics Reports, *(12), 1–23.

Blumenthal, J. A., Babyak, M. A., Doraiswamy, P. M., Watkins, L., Hoffman, B. M., Barbour, K. A., ... Sherwood, A. (2007). Exercise and pharmacotherapy in the treatment of major depressive disorder. *Psychosomatic Medicine, 69*(7), 587–596.

Blumenthal, J. A., Babyak, M. A., Moore, K. A., Craighead, W. E., Herman, S., Khatri, P., ... Krishnan, K. R. (1999). Effects of exercise training on older patients with major depression. *Archives of Internal Medicine, 159*(19), 2349–2356.

Bosworth, H. B., Park, K. S., McQuoid, D. R., Hays, J. C., & Steffens, D. C. (2003). The impact of religious practice and religious coping on geriatric depression. *International Journal of Geriatric Psychiatry, 18*(10), 905–914.

Bottiglieri, T., Godfrey, P., Flynn, T., Carney, M. W., Toone, B. K., & Reynolds, E. H. (1990). Cerebrospinal fluid S-adenosylmethionine in depression and dementia: Effects of treatment with parenteral and oral S-adenosylmethionine. *Journal of Neurology, Neurosurgery, and Psychiatry, 53*(12), 1096–1098.

Bressa, G. M. (1994). S-adenosyl-l-methionine (SAMe) as antidepressant: Meta-analysis of clinical studies. *Acta Neurologica Scandinavica Supplementum, 154,* 7–14.

Carney, M. W., Chary, T. K., Bottiglieri, T., Reynolds, E. H., & Toone, B. K. (1987). Switch mechanism in affective illness and oral S-adenosylmethionine (SAM). *British Journal of Psychiatry, 150*, 724–725.

Cohen, G. (2005). *The mature mind: The positive power of the aging brain*. New York: Basic Books.

Cohen, G. D., Perlstein, S., Chapline, J., Kelly, J., Firth, K. M., & Simmens, S. (2006). The impact of professionally conducted cultural programs on the physical health, mental health, and social functioning of older adults. *Gerontologist, 46*(6), 726–734.

Conn, V. S., Minor, M. A., Burks, K. J., Rantz, M. J., & Pomeroy, S. H. (2003). Integrative review of physical activity intervention research with aging adults. *Journal of the American Geriatrics Society, 51*(8), 1159–1168.

Druss, B. G., & Rosenheck, R. A. (2000). Use of practitioner-based complementary therapies by persons reporting mental conditions in the United States. *Archives of General Psychiatry 57*(7), 708–714.

Dunn, A. L., Trivedi, M. H., Burks, K. J., Rantz, M. J., & Pomeroy, S. H. (2005). Exercise treatment for depression: Efficacy and dose response. *American Journal of Preventive Medicine, 28*(1), 1–8.

Eisenberg, D. M., Davis, R. B., Ettner, S. L., Appel, S., Wilkey, S., Van Rompay, M., & Kessler, R. C. (1998). Trends in alternative medicine use in the United States, 1990–1997: Results of a follow-up national survey. *Journal of American Medical Association, 280*(18), 1569–1575.

Epel, E., Daubenmier, J., Moskowitz, J. T., Folkman, S., & Blackburn, E. (2009). Can meditation slow rate of cellular aging? Cognitive stress, mindfulness, and telomeres. *Annals of the New York Academy of Sciences, 1172*, 34–53.

Flood, M., & Phillips, K. D. (2007). Creativity in older adults: A plethora of possibilities. *Issues in Mental Health Nursing, 28*(4), 389–411.

Forge, R. L. (2005). Aligning mind and body: Exploring the disciplines of mindful exercise. *ACSM's Health and Fitness Journal, 9*(5), 7–14.

Freeman, M. P., Fava, M., Lake, J., Trivedi, M. H., Wisner, K. L., & Mischoulon, D. (2010). Complementary and alternative medicine in major depressive disorder: The American Psychiatric Association Task Force report. *Journal of Clinical Psychiatry, 71*(6), 669–681.

Galli, C., & Calder, P. C. (2009). Effects of fat and fatty acid intake on inflammatory and immune responses: A critical review. *Annals of Nutrition and Metabolism, 55*(1–3), 123–139.

Galper, D. I., Trivedi, M. H., Barlow, C. E., Dunn, A. L., & Kampert, J. B. (2006). Inverse association between physical inactivity and mental health in men and women. *Medicine and Science in Sports and Exercise, 38*(1), 173–178.

Grossman, P., Niemann, L., Schmidt, S., & Walach, H. (2004). Mindfulness-based stress reduction and health benefits. A meta-analysis. *Journal of Psychosomatic Research, 57*(1), 35–43.

Hardy, M., Coulter, I., Morton, S. C., Favreau, J., Venuturupalli, S., Chiappelli, F., … Shekelle, P. (2003). S-adenosyl-L-methionine for treatment of depression, osteoarthritis, and liver disease. *Evidence Report/Technology Assessment (Summary),* (64), 1–3.

Harrer, G., Schmidt, U., Kuhn, U., & Biller, A. (1999). Comparison of equivalence between the St. John's wort extract LoHyp-57 and fluoxetine. *Arzneimittel-Forschung, 49*(4), 289–296.

Harris, A. H., Cronkite, R., & Moos, R. (2006). Physical activity, exercise coping, and depression in a 10-year cohort study of depressed patients. *Journal of Affective Disorders, 93*(1–3), 79–85.

Hibbeln, J. R. (1998). Fish consumption and major depression. *Lancet, 351*(9110), 1213.

Hughner, R. S., Maher, J. K., & Childs, N. M. (2008). Review of food policy and consumer issues of mercury in fish. *Journal of the American College of Nutrition, 27*(2), 185–194.

Husaini, B. A., Blasi, A. J., & Miller, O. (1999). Does public and private religiosity have a moderating effect on depression? A bi-racial study of elders in the American South. *International Journal of Aging and Human Development, 48*(1), 63–72.

Hypericum Depression Trial Study Group. (2002). Effect of Hypericum perforatum (St John's wort) in major depressive disorder: A randomized controlled trial. *Journal of American Medical Association, 287*(14), 1807–1814.

Izzo, A. A., & Ernst, E. (2009). Interactions between herbal medicines and prescribed drugs: An updated systematic review. *Drugs, 69*(13), 1777–1798.

Jacobs, T. L., Epel, E. S., Lin, J., Blackburn, E. H., Wolkowitz, O. M., Bridwell, D. A., … Saron, C. D. (2011). Intensive meditation training, immune cell telomerase activity, and psychological mediators. *Psychoneuroendocrinology, 36*(5), 664–681.

Janakiramaiah, N., Gangadhar, B. N., Naga Venkatesha Murthy, P. J., Harish, M. G., Subbakrishna, D. K., & Vedamurthachar, A. (2000). Antidepressant efficacy of Sudarshan Kriya Yoga (SKY) in melancholia: A randomized comparison with electroconvulsive therapy (ECT) and imipramine. *Journal of Affective Disorders, 57*(1–3), 255–259.

Jepson, R. G., Harris, F. M., Platt, S., & Tannahill, C. (2010). The effectiveness of interventions to change six health behaviours: A review of reviews. *BMC Public Health, 10*, 538.

Kasper, S., Gastpar, M., Möller, H. J., Müller, W. E., Volz, H. P., Dienel, A., & Kieser, M. (2010). Better tolerability of St. John's wort extract WS 5570 compared to treatment with SSRIs: A reanalysis of data from controlled clinical trials in acute major depression. *International Clinical Psychopharmacology*, 25(4), 204–213.

Keaton, D., Lamkin, N., Cassidy, K. A., Meyer, W. J., Ignacio, R. V., Aulakh, L., … Sajatovic, M. (2009). Utilization of herbal and nutritional compounds among older adults with bipolar disorder and with major depression. *International Journal of Geriatric Psychiatry*, 24(10), 1087–1093.

Kessler, R. C., Soukup, J., Davis, R. B., Foster, D. F., Wilkey, S. A., Van Rompay, M. I., & Eisenberg, D. M. (2001). The use of complementary and alternative therapies to treat anxiety and depression in the United States. *American Journal of Psychiatry*, 158(2), 289–294.

Krishnamurthy, M. N., & Telles, S. (2007). Assessing depression following two ancient Indian interventions: Effects of yoga and ayurveda on older adults in a residential home. *Journal of Gerontological Nursing*, 33(2), 17–23.

Krishnan, K. R., Hays, J. C., & Blazer, D. G. (1997). MRI-defined vascular depression. *American Journal of Psychiatry*, 154(4), 497–501.

Lampinen, P., Heikkinen, R. L., & Ruoppila, I. (2000). Changes in intensity of physical exercise as predictors of depressive symptoms among older adults: An eight-year follow-up. *Preventive Medicine*, 30(5), 371–380.

Lee, L. Y., Lee, D. T., & Woo, J. (2010). The psychosocial effect of Tai Chi on nursing home residents. *Journal of Clinical Nursing*, 19(7–8), 927–938.

Leo, R. J., & Ligot, J. S., Jr. (2007). A systematic review of randomized controlled trials of acupuncture in the treatment of depression. *Journal of Affective Disorders*, 97(1–3), 13–22.

Li, C. D., Huang, Y., Li, Y. K., Hu, K. M., & Jiang, Z. Y. . (1994). Treating post-stroke depression with mind-refreshing antidepressive acupuncture therapy: A clinical study of 21 cases. *International Journal of Clinical Acupuncture*, 5(4), 389–393.

Li, F., Fisher, K. J., Harmer, P., Irbe, D., Tearse, R. G., & Weimer, C. (2004). Tai chi and self-rated quality of sleep and daytime sleepiness in older adults: A randomized controlled trial. *Journal of the American Geriatrics Society*, 52(6), 892–900.

Lin, P. Y., Huang, S. Y., & Su, K. P. (2010). A meta-analytic review of polyunsaturated fatty acid compositions in patients with depression. *Biological Psychiatry*, 68(2), 140–147.

Linde, K., Berner, M. M., & Kriston L. (2008). St John's wort for major depression. *Cochrane Database of Systematic Reviews*, 4, CD000448.

Maes, M., Christophe, A., Delanghe, J., Altamura, C., Neels, H., & Meltzer, H. Y. (1999). Lowered omega3 polyunsaturated fatty acids in serum phospholipids and cholesteryl esters of depressed patients. *Psychiatry Research*, 85(3), 275–291.

Manjunath, N. K., & Telles, S. (2005). Influence of yoga and ayurveda on self-rated sleep in a geriatric population. *Indian Journal of Medical Research*, 121(5), 683–690.

Martins, J. G. (2009). EPA but not DHA appears to be responsible for the efficacy of omega-3 long chain polyunsaturated fatty acid supplementation in depression: Evidence from a meta-analysis of randomized controlled trials. *Journal of the American College of Nutrition*, 28(5), 525–542.

Mather, A. S., Rodriguez, C., Guthrie, M. F., McHarg, A. M., Reid, I. C., & McMurdo, M. E. (2002). Effects of exercise on depressive symptoms in older adults with poorly responsive depressive disorder: Randomised controlled trial. *British Journal of Psychiatry*, 180, 411–415.

Mead, G. E., Morley, W., Campbell, P., Greig, C. A., McMurdo, M., & Lawlor, D. A. (2009). Exercise for depression. *Cochrane Database of Systematic Reviews*, (3), CD004366.

Meeks, T. W., Wetherell, J. L., Irwin, M. R., Redwine, L. S., & Jeste, D. V. (2007). Complementary and alternative treatments for late-life depression, anxiety, and sleep disturbance: A review of randomized controlled trials. *Journal of Clinical Psychiatry*, 68(10), 1461–1471.

Mischoulon, D., & Fava, M. (2002). Role of S-adenosyl-L-methionine in the treatment of depression: A review of the evidence. *American Journal of Clinical Nutrition*, 76(5), 1158S-1161S.

NCCAM-NIH Website (2010). What is Complementary and Alternative Medicine? (2010). http://nccam.nih.gov/health/whatiscam. Accessed 10/09/2012, National Center for Complementary and Alternative Medicine—National Institutes of Health.

Ness, J., Cirillo, D. J., Weir, D. R., Nisly, N. L., & Wallace, R. B.. (2005). Use of complementary medicine in older Americans: Results from the Health and Retirement Study. *Gerontologist*, 45(4), 516–524.

Nieminen, T. H., Hagelberg, N. M., Saari, T. I., Neuvonen, M., Laine, K., Neuvonen, P. J., & Olkkola, K. T. (2010). St John's wort greatly reduces the concentrations of oral oxycodone. *European Journal of Pain*, 14(8), 854–859.

Norton, M. C., Singh, A., Skoog, I., Corcoran, C., Tschanz, J. T., Zandi, P. P., ... Cache County Investigators. (2008). Church attendance and new episodes of major depression in a community study of older adults: The Cache County Study. *Journals of Gerontology Series B, Psychological Science Social Science, 63*(3), P129–137.

Papakostas, G. I. (2009). Evidence for S-adenosyl-L-methionine (SAM-e) for the treatment of major depressive disorder. *Journal of Clinical Psychiatry, 70*(Suppl 5), 18–22.

Papakostas, G. I., Mischoulon, D., Shyu, I., Alpert, J. E., & Fava, M. (2010). S-adenosyl methionine (SAMe) augmentation of serotonin reuptake inhibitors for antidepressant nonresponders with major depressive disorder: A double-blind, randomized clinical trial. *American Journal of Psychiatry, 167*(8), 942–948.

Paukert, A. L., Phillips, L., Cully, J. A., Loboprabhu, S. M., Lomax, J. W., & Stanley, M. A. (2009). Integration of religion into cognitive-behavioral therapy for geriatric anxiety and depression. *Journal of Psychiatric Practice, 15*(2), 103–112.

Paul, R. T., McDonnell, A. P., & Kelly, C. B. (2004). Folic acid: Neurochemistry, metabolism and relationship to depression. *Human Psychopharmacology, 19*(7), 477–488.

Pilkington, K., Kirkwood, G., Rampes, H., & Richardson, J. (2005). Yoga for depression: The research evidence. *Journal of Affective Disorders, 89*(1–3), 13–24.

Rondanelli, M., Giacosa, A., Comstock, G. W., Hoffman, S. C., Norkus, E. P., & Fried, L. P. (2011). Long chain omega 3 polyunsaturated fatty acids supplementation in the treatment of elderly depression: Effects on depressive symptoms, on phospholipids fatty acids profile and on health-related quality of life. *Journal of Nutrition, Health and Aging, 15*(1), 37–44.

Sarris, J., Kavanagh, D. J., & Byrne, G. (2010). Adjuvant use of nutritional and herbal medicines with antidepressants, mood stabilizers and benzodiazepines. *Journal of Psychiatric Research, 44*(1), 32–41.

Sharma, H., Chandola, H. M., Singh, G., & Basisht, G. (2007). Utilization of Ayurveda in health care: An approach for prevention, health promotion, and treatment of disease. Part 1—Ayurveda, the science of life. *Journal of Alternative and Complementary Medicine, 13*(9), 1011–1019.

Sharma, V. K., Das, S., Mondal, S., Goswampi, U., & Gandhi, A. (2005). Effect of Sahaj Yoga on depressive disorders. *Indian Journal of Physiology and Pharmacology, 49*(4), 462–468.

Shelton, R. C. (2009). St John's wort (Hypericum perforatum) in major depression. *Journal of Clinical Psychiatry, 70*(Suppl 5), 23–27.

Shelton, R. C., Keller, M. B., Gelenberg, A., Dunner, D. L., Hirschfeld, R., Thase, M. E., ... Halbreich, U. (2001). Effectiveness of St John's wort in major depression: A randomized controlled trial. *Journal of the American Medical Association, 285*(15), 1978–1986.

Shelton, R. C., & Miller, A. H. (2010). Eating ourselves to death (and despair), the contribution of adiposity and inflammation to depression. *Progress in Neurobiology, 91*(4), 275–299.

Simon, G. E., Cherkin, D. C., Sherman, K. J., Eisenberg, D. M., Deyo, R. A., & Davis, R. B. (2004). Mental health visits to complementary and alternative medicine providers. *General Hospital Psychiatry, 26*(3), 171–177.

Sinclair, A. J., Begg, D., Mathai, M., & Weisinger, R. S. (2007). Omega 3 fatty acids and the brain: Review of studies in depression. *Asia Pacifici Journal of Clinical Nutrition, 16*(Suppl 1), 391–397.

Sjosten, N., & Kivela, S. L. (2006). The effects of physical exercise on depressive symptoms among the aged: A systematic review. *International Journal of Geriatric Psychiatry, 21*(5), 410–418.

Smith, C. A., Hay, P. P., & Macpherson, H. (2010). Acupuncture for depression. *Cochrane Database of Systematic Reviews, 1*, CD004046.

Stoll, A. L., Severus, W. E., Freeman, M. P., Rueter, S., Zboyan, H. A., Diamond, E., ... Marangell, L. B. (1999). Omega 3 fatty acids in bipolar disorder: A preliminary double-blind, placebo-controlled trial. *Archives of General Psychiatry, 56*(5), 407–412.

Strawbridge, W. J., Deleger, S., Roberts, R. E., & Kaplan, G. A. (2002). Physical activity reduces the risk of subsequent depression for older adults. *American Journal of Epidemiology, 156*(4), 328–334.

Tanskanen, A., Hibbeln, J. R., Hintikka, J., Haatainen, K., Honkalampi, K., & Viinamäki, H. (2001). Fish consumption, depression, and suicidality in a general population. *Archives of General Psychiatry, 58*(5), 512–513.

Timonen, M., Horrobin, D., Jokelainen, J., Laitinen, J., Herva, A., & Räsänen, P. (2004). Fish consumption and depression: The Northern Finland 1966 birth cohort study. *Journal of Affective Disorders, 82*(3), 447–452.

Trivedi, M. H., Greer, T. L., Grannemann, B. D., Chambliss, H. O., & Jordan, A. N. (2006a). Exercise as an augmentation strategy for treatment of major depression. *Journal of Psychiatric Practice, 12*(4), 205–213.

Trivedi, M. H., Greer, T. L., Grannemann, B. D., Church, T. S., Galper, D. I., Sunderajan, P., ... Carmody, T. I. (2006b). TREAD: TReatment with Exercise Augmentation for Depression: Study rationale and design. *Clinical Trials*, 3(3), 291–305.

Tsang, H. W., Fung, K. M., Chan, A. S., Lee, G., & Chan, F. (2006). Effect of a qigong exercise programme on elderly with depression. *International Journal of Geriatric Psychiatry*, 21(9), 890–897.

van der Bij, A. K., Laurant, M. G., & Wensing, M. (2002). Effectiveness of physical activity interventions for older adults: A review. *American Journal of Preventive Medicine*, 22(2), 120–133.

van der Watt, G., Laugharne, J., & Janca, A. (2008). Complementary and alternative medicine in the treatment of anxiety and depression. *Current Opinion in Psychiatry*, 21(1), 37–42.

Wang, W. C., Zhang, A. L., Rasmussen, B., Lin, L. W., Dunning, T., Kang, S. W., ... Lo, S. K. (2009). The effect of Tai Chi on psychosocial well-being: A systematic review of randomized controlled trials. *Journal of Acupuncture and Meridian Studies*, 2(3), 171–181.

Williams, J., & Graham, C. (2006). Acupuncture for older adults with depression-a pilot study to assess acceptability and feasibility. *International Journal of Geriatric Psychiatry*, 21(6), 599–600.

Wittink, M. N., Joo, J. H., Lewis, L. M., & Barg, F. K. (2009). Losing faith and using faith: Older African Americans discuss spirituality, religious activities, and depression. *Journal of General Internal Medicine*, 24(3), 402–407.

25

PREVENTION OF DEPRESSION IN LATER LIFE

A DEVELOPMENTAL PERSPECTIVE

Aartjan T. F. Beekman, Pim Cuijpers, and Filip Smit

THROUGHOUT HEALTH care, everything we do is aimed toward prevention. This ranges form preventing the onset of disease in those who are well, through preventing chronicity, disability, and other consequences of disease in those who are ill, to preventing relapses in those who have recovered. Mrazek and Haggerty (1994) have defined and delineated the various types of prevention that are involved in different phases of development of disease. Inspired by their pioneering work, Figure 25.1 brings together a schematized developmental history of disease and the corresponding types of preventative action that would be appropriate in each stage (Beekman, 2004).

Universal prevention targets the whole population and aims to help reinforce resilience or prevent health risks. Selective prevention is restricted to those who are exposed to known risk factors for disease. The aim is to prevent the onset of disease efficiently, by focusing on those who are known to be at high risk. Depending on how common the risk factor is, this involves far fewer people than the whole population. However, depending on how easy it is to

screen out those who are exposed to a risk factor, this involves more or less cumbersome and expensive screening procedures. Indicated prevention is aimed at people who exhibit some signs or symptoms of the disorder but in whom there is no fully developed disease as yet. The terminology used to describe the symptoms of those involved in indicated prevention varies from subclinical or subthreshold symptoms, to prodromal symptoms. The people involved are on the brink of developing a full-blown disease and may be deemed at ultra-high risk or even in the early stages of the disorder. In terms of the number of people involved, this again involves far fewer people than the stage before (selective prevention), but again it may involve cumbersome or expensive screening procedures. Universal, selective, and indicated prevention share their aim of preventing the onset of full-fledged disease and are sometimes collectively named primary prevention. This chapter will focus on primary prevention of late-life depression, recognizing that it is part of a larger repertoire of interventions.

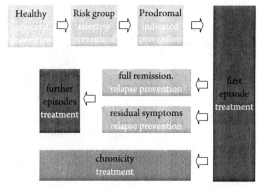

FIGURE 25.1 Developmental stages of mental disorder and corresponding preventive interventions (Beekman, 2004).

Prevention aims to interfere with the natural history or development of disease. In other areas of medicine the developmental history of disease is the starting point of diagnosis and treatment. In oncology, decades of clinical and scientific work have brought about a well-developed staging model of cancer (see Dighe et al., 2010; Hariharan et al., 2010 Paesmans et al., 2010; Xing et al., 2011 for some recent examples). The bottom-line idea behind this has been that early detection and treatment is the only way to prevent the disease from developing beyond the point at which treatment may be helpful. In most cancers there is a window of opportunity for treatments that work very well in patients who are detected early, but which lose their effectiveness later in the development of the cancer. Although this has not been proven in psychiatry, it is extremely likely that a similar line of reasoning would apply to most psychiatric disorders. Using this line of thinking, McGorry (2007) has convincingly argued for a staging approach to psychosis. The idea here is, similar to what has been achieved in oncology, to detect and treat psychosis as early as possible, hopefully thereby reducing the damage to both the patient and the community. The idea of staging psychiatric illness with the aim to prevent damage to the patient and to society is slowly finding its way in our field and has inspired the writing of the current chapter. Although staging is not yet well developed in psychiatric disorders, the models proposed have consistently included the stages summarized in Figure 25.1 (Fava & Kelner, 1993). As was described, these stages map onto different types of preventive intervention.

The next paragraphs will discuss (1) a staging and profiling model of late-life depression, (2) the corresponding types of preventative intervention that would be appropriate in the early stages of development of late-life depression, (3) the evidence of studies that have tested the effectiveness of such preventative interventions for late-life depression, and (4) the public health, economic, and ethical implications this may have.

STAGING AND PROFILING LATE-LIFE DEPRESSION

The dominant diagnostic guidelines in psychiatry (*ICD* and *DSM*) were designed with the principal aim to provide a universal language to reliably describe and classify psychopathology. Although successful, the resulting diagnoses are insufficiently sensitive to the stage of development, the etiology, or the prognosis of psychiatric disorders and are not sufficiently helpful in selecting appropriate treatment. Depression is a prime example of this.

Figure 25.2 summarizes prospective data of a large cohort of adult patients with major depressive disorder (MDD). The people under study were derived from a representative community survey in the Netherlands and were selected to include only recent-onset episodes of *DSM-IV* MDD (Spijker et al., 2003). The survival curve steeply declines over the first months, demonstrating that many patients

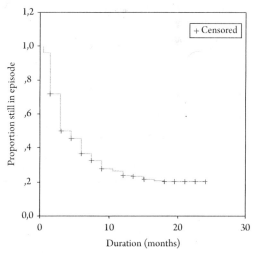

FIGURE 25.2 Survival curve of a cohort ($n = 250$) with newly originated (first or recurrent) major depressive episodes in the general population; +, censored cases (Spijker et al., 2003).

recover quickly. In more exact numbers, the median time to recovery was 3 months. Mostly this occurred without treatment. This would suggest that MDD, in many patients, is a self-limiting condition. However, the survival curve flattens out after the first 6–9 months. After the first year, very few people recover. When expressed in numbers, 20% of those diagnosed at baseline had not recovered after 1 year and were unlikely to recover any time soon after that. Evidently, the same diagnosis (MDD) may be indicative of both a self-limiting disorder and a chronic disease. For both clinical and research purposes, a diagnosis that is more sensitive to the prognosis would be desirable. A first step would be to adopt a simple staging model for depression, such as has been proposed for other psychiatric disorders (Fava, 1993; Hetrick et al., 2008).

Figure 25.3 also summarizes prospective data of a large cohort of patients diagnosed with MDD. These data were derived from a study among older (65+) patients of general practitioners in the Netherlands, who were recruited through screening (Licht-Strunk et al., 2009). Comparing the survival curves, it is striking that the prognosis is worse. The median time to recovery was 18 months, which is six times as long as what was found among the younger adults in the community. After 1 year, only 35% of the patients had recovered, compared with 80% in the younger community sample. However, after this first year the curve did not flatten out and people kept recovering. After 3 years, 68% had recovered and at the end of the study most patients had reached recovery. This suggests that the outcome may be similar in the long run, but that it takes a lot longer for older people to recover than it takes among younger people. A direct comparison is unfair because of methodological differences between the two studies involved, but the two sets of data do suggest that the natural history of depression may differ considerably by age. Is this plausible? Are there reasons one might have predicted this, or, better, are there factors that may explain this? Probably yes. Looking at the known risk factors to develop depression, later life presents people with a very different set of potential risks than earlier in life. This involves both the more biological domains of risk (such as neurodegeneration, cardiovascular and cerebrovascular risk, HPA-axis changes, and inflammatory markers), the interpersonal domain (loss of loved ones and loss of functioning and roles), and psychological changes (less cognitive and emotional reserve capacity). Indeed, among older people several "new" subtypes of depression have been described, which are deemed to be especially common in later life. Examples are vascular depression (Alexopoulos et al., 1997), metabolic depression (Lamers et al., 2010; Vogelzangs et al., 2011), and amyloid associated depression (Sun et al., 2008). In all the papers describing these putative subtypes of depression, reference is made to the idea that their prognosis would be different (usually worse) and that treatment would be different (usually directed not only at the depressive symptom but also involving the underlying etiology).

It appears that both the etiology and the prognosis of depression may differ for older when compared to younger adults and that this may be explained by the biological and psychosocial changes accompanying aging. This is described here for two reasons. The first is that a simple staging model of depression becomes much more informative when it is supplemented with data on factors that may predict whether transitions between the stages are more or less likely. This is what is meant with the word profiling: a profile of risk factors that predict transitions. The second point is that depression is a complex disorder at any age, but that this complexity increases in later life. A staging and profiling model for affective disorders would be especially helpful for geriatric psychiatry. Conversely, the development of such a model may benefit especially from research carried out among older patients.

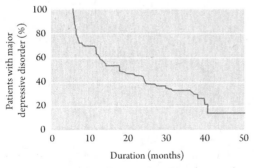

FIGURE 25.3 Survival curve of a cohort ($n = 204$) of older patients with major depressive disorder recruited from general practitioners' practices in the Netherlands (Licht-Strunk et al., 2009).

PREVENTATIVE INTERVENTION

A critique of prevention in mental health would focus on (1) feasibility, (2) effectiveness, and (3) ethical and economic considerations. Effectiveness is extremely important and will be described in the next paragraph. Here we focus on what sort of interventions would be appropriate to prevent depression among older adults; how we should organize health care in such a way that this may be feasible; and, given both ethical and economic constraints, whether preventing depression is indeed a core business-type activity of mental health care or whether this goes beyond health care. The third point is discussed last because the answer to this question involves proportionality: The cost and impact of a preventative intervention should be proportional to the health risk avoided by those participating.

Universal Prevention

Universal prevention of late-life depression targets the whole population of older people. Although the risk of depression is considerable at all ages, the vast majority of older people will never be depressed. Therefore, any universal preventative action for late-life depression should be a light intervention: both in terms of cost and in terms of impact. A good example is a public awareness campaign, such as has been launched in many countries in the world. Cuijpers (2003) has described that, even in a disorder like depression, which has quite a high incidence, studies testing the effects of universal prevention in depression are unlikely to be feasible. Among other methodological constraints, such a study would require too many participants and be too costly to be run, given current methods of research. This does not imply that universal prevention may not be useful, but it does suggest that universal prevention is probably best seen as a primer—a way to prepare the public that depression is a disorder that one can do something about. Given the rapid technological advances and the widespread access to electronic media among older people, e-health preventative interventions especially catering for older people are being developed. This may shift preventative action toward universal prevention. With regard to feasibility and effectiveness the conclusion so far is that it is feasible to launch universal preventive programs aiming to prevent depression, but that current methods of research do not allow rigorous testing of their effects.

Selective Prevention

Selective prevention aims to reach older people who are exposed to known risk factors for depression. Their a priori risk to become depressed is elevated, tipping the balance of proportionality more toward intervention. Examples are older people with chronic disease, those who have lost their spouse, and those who have been depressed before. If, through education, the public knows that these are risk factors for depression, and that it is a good idea to invest in prevention, selective prevention may become more mainstream.

Several tested interventions are available. They usually involve (1) a way of identifying and engaging those at risk and (2) the intervention proper. Identification of older people at risk and engaging them effectively depends very much on local factors. In high-resource countries with well-developed health services, the optimal point of contact for selective prevention may be the health service. In the Netherlands there are (as yet) very few financial barriers to health care. All citizens have compulsory health insurance and there is almost universal coverage by general practitioners (GPs). Epidemiological data have shown that the vast majority of older people with known risk factors for depression do contact their GP regularly and that GPs have reliable data about many known risk factors in their files. In the Netherlands, therefore, the optimal point of contact for selective prevention of late-life depression would be the GP practice. This is described here because a similar line of reasoning could lead to a very different optimal point of contact for selective prevention in other places in the world.

Engaging older people who are currently not depressed in an intervention is not easy. This partly involves the same reasons why the majority of those with full-blown affective disorders remain untreated. Known factors include a combination of (1) lack of knowledge about affective disorders; (2) lack of trust in mental health intervention; (3) lack of time, trained personnel, and resources; and (4) the stigma that remains attached to mental illness. Besides these factors, barriers to engage people in depression prevention are consonant with the difficulties in engaging people in any type of prevention. The reality of being human may be that we tend to dislike doing things now to avoid harm later.

The interventions that have been designed are mostly light versions of interventions known to be effective in treating depression. This involves light or self-help versions of cognitive therapy, interpersonal therapy, reminiscence, and problem solving. Often these are modified to cater for people exposed to specific risk factors and circumstances (such as having recently lost a partner or living with a chronic illness). Other ingredients involve engaging in pleasant activities, physical activity, using nutritional supplements such as vitamin D and fish oils, and exposure to bright light.

Indicated Prevention

Indicated prevention engages older people who do have symptoms of depression but who have not (yet) developed a full-blown affective disorder. Given the ongoing discussion as to where exactly the boundary between affective symptoms and disorders should be drawn, drawing a firm line between indicated prevention and treatment is hazardous. However, in a staging model this may not be so problematic. The idea is that any intervention should be proportional and that the aim is to generate health benefit for those involved. Older people with subthreshold or subclinical depressive symptoms are at very high risk to develop full-blown disorders whichever way we define these states (Beekman et al., 2002). Moreover, they do have symptoms and these symptoms interfere with their well-being and daily functioning. These two considerations help to tip proportionality even more toward active intervention. It is therefore no wonder that, when epidemiological data are used to empirically search out which preventative approach may be most fruitful, indicated prevention is a prominent outcome (Schoevers et al., 2006; Smit, Ederveen, Cuijpers, Deeg, & Beekman, 2006). Similarly, these considerations have probably resulted in the fact that the majority of prevention trials conducted so far involve indicated prevention (see earlier discussion).

A drawback of indicated prevention is that participants need to be diagnosed with "symptoms but no disorder." The trials that have been conducted in this area mostly recruited participants through screening. A positive screen on a depression screener implies that some significant symptoms are there. In a next diagnostic step, the outcome may either be that there exists a full-blown affective disorder (in which case the patient is referred for treatment) or that there is no such disorder (in which case the patient is offered the preventative intervention). Considering the staging model (Fig. 25.1), we are now one step further downstream from selective prevention. This means that those eligible for indicated prevention are a subset of those with known risk factors. One may therefore start identifying those with risk factors (preferably through existing records) and then screen out those with ultra high risk (offering them indicated prevention) or fully developed disorders (offering these people treatment).

The interventions that have been tested are similar to those described for selective prevention. Given the lower numbers involved, the higher a priori risk of disease, and the fact that there are symptoms already, more incisive interventions may be acceptable here. A study in the Netherlands tested a program that was organized along the lines of stepped care. In this program all the older participants with "depressive symptoms but no disorder" were offered a choice of educational and self-help interventions first, slowly stepping up the intensity of the intervention if the symptoms remained present (van 't Veer et al., 2009).

Relapse Prevention

Having been depressed before is one of the most consistent risk factors for depression in the future. This is true at all ages and the risk becomes especially strong if recovery was not complete, involving residual symptoms (Reynolds et al., 2011). In terms of the staging model, we now progress to an area beyond treatment. Given the damage a depressive episode can do and the high risk of recurrence, relapse prevention should be part of any treatment plan of affective disorders. This is especially true in older people, as the risk of relapse appears to rise with age (Hardeveld, Spijker, de Graaf, Nolen, & Beekman, 2010).

Besides the interventions mentioned earlier, here the option of maintenance treatment is, of course, important. However, as was discussed in the introduction, this is beyond the scope of this chapter.

EFFECTIVENESS OF PREVENTION IN LATE-LIFE DEPRESSION

Is there an evidence base with regard to thoroughly tested interventions in the area of preventing late-life depression? If there is, does this provide the necessary data to make evidence-based policy decisions as to where limited funds should be directed? During the past decade a number of well-designed randomized clinical trials have been conducted to test the effects of prevention of depression among older people (Beekman et al.,

2010; Cuijpers, van Straten, Smit, Mihalopoulos, & Beekman, 2008).

Universal Prevention

In the area of universal prevention, van de Rest et al. (2008) conducted a three-armed randomized controlled trial testing whether low or higher dose supplementation with n-3 polyunsaturated fatty acids (PUFAs) would help to prevent depression among healthy older people in the community. Over 26 weeks, 302 participants were randomized to consume placebo, 400 mg, or 1,800 mg doses of PUFA. Although the plasma concentrations demonstrated high intake fidelity, there were no effects at either the 13-week or 26-week evaluation.

Selective Prevention

Pitceathly et al. (2009) conducted a randomized controlled trial to test whether a brief psychological intervention may help preventing anxiety or depressive disorders among recently diagnosed cancer patients. Although not primarily aimed at older people, this trial is of interest as it targets cancer patients. The trial was large (465 patients were recruited, of whom 313 completed the study), testing (1) whether the brief intervention would be effective and (2) whether the timing of the start of the intervention may make a difference, while (3) stratifying the participating patients with regard to their a priori risk for depression and anxiety. This trial is one of very few studies in which the effect of the level of a priori risk of depression on the effect could be examined. After 12 months there was no overall difference between those exposed to the intervention and the controls. However, among patients at high risk for depression or anxiety the intervention was effective (OR = 0.54, 95% CI 0.29–1.00), while in the low-risk patients there was no difference. All the patients included were at risk for depression due to their recent cancer diagnosis, which means this trial is an example of selective prevention. However, the results of the stratified analyses suggest that there is a gradient of effect in favor of those with the highest a priori risk.

Robinson et al. (2008) tested the effect of escitalopram and problem solving to prevent depression in patients with stroke. The rationale for this study was that more than half of the patients experiencing a stroke develop depression later on. This is a further example of selective prevention among older people at high risk due to a physical illness. Within 3 months after a stroke, 176 nondepressed patients were randomized to escitalopram, placebo, or problem-solving therapy. Over the 12-month intervention period, the patients receiving placebo were significantly more likely to develop depression than both those receiving escitalopram (HR 4,5; 95% CI 2,4–8,2) and problem-solving therapy (HR 2,2, 95% CI 1,4–3,5).

A further example is the study by Rovner et al. (2007), in which the effect of problem-solving therapy among patients with macular degeneration was tested. The rationale here was that macular degeneration leads to irreversible loss of vision and corresponding disability, which carries a high risk of concomitant depression. In this randomized controlled trial, 206 nondepressed patients with existing macular degeneration in one eye, plus a recent manifestation in the other eye, were randomized to either care as usual or problem-solving therapy (eight weekly sessions). After 8 weeks, the incidence of depressive disorders was lower among those exposed to problem-solving therapy (HR 0,39, 95% CI 0,17–0,92).

Yet another example of selective prevention among older people with chronic disease is a study by de Jonge et al. (2009). They administered a multifaceted nurse-led intervention to prevent major depression in 100 patients with diabetes or rheumatism, who were considered to be medically complex. At 1 year follow-up the incidence of those randomized to the intervention was 36%, as compared to 63% in the usual care group.

Indicated Prevention

Moving on to indicated prevention, van 't Veer et al. (2009) tested the effect of a stepped-care program to prevent depression and anxiety among older GP patients with subthreshold depressive symptoms. In this randomized controlled trial 170 patients with subthreshold symptoms were randomized to either care as usual or a stepped-care prevention program. The steps lasted 3 months each and included (1) watchful waiting, (2) guided self-help, (3) problem solving, and (4) referral to the GP for further evaluation or treatment. Over the year the intervention lasted it was successful in reducing the incidence of *DSM* anxiety or depressive disorders (HR 0,49; 95 CI 0,24–0,98). A year later these effects had persisted.

Walker et al. (2010) tested the effects of (1) mental health literacy, (2) folic acid and vitamin B12 supplementation, and (3) physical activity against placebo conditions among elderly with elevated distress scores in the community. This was a huge trial (909 older adults randomized) in which a factorial design was used, which allowed the authors to test each intervention against placebo, while also testing for interactions between the interventions. As no diagnostic measures were available, some of the participants may have had full-blown disorders and, moreover, it remains unknown what the effect of the interventions may have been on the incidence of full-blown disorders. The results were that, at 24 months follow-up, none of the interventions had any effect on the level of depressive symptoms. During the 24 months follow-up, the only significant effect that was noted was a small effect ($d = 0,12$) of the health literacy intervention at 6 weeks. Although trends remained after that, they were not significant.

Two recent studies (Konnert, Dobson, & Stelmach, 2009; Pot et al., 2010) tested whether psychological interventions (cognitive-behavioral therapy and life review) were effective to reduce depressive symptoms in those with elevated symptoms but no diagnosis. Both found effects, but it remains unsure whether this had an effect on the incidence of affective disorders.

To summarize, the past decade has seen a series of high-quality preventive trials conducted in the area of late-life depression. The trials published have generally shown effects that are both statistically and clinically relevant, and there are indications that the efficacy and the efficiency of interventions are better when elderly with higher a priori risk of depression are included.

CONCLUSION

Providing adequate care to older people is one of the huge challenges facing society all over the world. Depression is a treatable disorder at any age, and it has enormous impact on well-being, functioning, morbidity, and mortality of older people. Despite this, even in the current time and in the richer parts of the world, only a minority of older people with depression are treated adequately. Being able to prevent depression efficiently with interventions that can be feasibly scaled up to be useful at a community level would constitute a way out of the dilemma that treating all older

patients with depression will remain impossible in the future. The present chapter was written with a developmental framework in mind. Depression is a very heterogeneous disorder with an extremely variable course. This is especially true in later life, where the palette of risk and prognostic factors becomes much more varied than among younger adults. A staging and profiling approach to diagnosis is advocated, thereby drawing attention to the early stages of development of affective disorders. The (as yet untested) premises behind this are that, during the early stages of development, relatively light interventions may be effective in averting the development of full-blown disorders, while these interventions lose their effectiveness later on. Examples of the interventions that have been tested to prevent depression were described, as were their effects. It appears that, indeed, relatively cheap, low-intensity interventions may be effective in the early stages of development of depression among older adults. Although much work remains to be done in this area, it seems that the efficiency and also feasibility of intervention program may be better when targeting groups of elderly at higher a priori risk for depressive disorders. As epidemiological data demonstrating which groups of elderly are at high risk are in place, these could be translated into strategies to effectively identify and engage elders at risk. Trials also show that there are personal, practical, ethical, and economic barriers to engaging large numbers of elderly. Increasing the reach of prevention is probably one of the most important issues at this time. Given known risk factors and strategies to engage older people, designing working prevention programs depends very much on fitting the data with local circumstances. Implementing effective prevention programs that make a lasting, demonstrable, and truly significant difference in the incidence of depression has remained elusive as yet. This probably takes more than a combination of good science and good intentions. However, being able to demonstrate that prevention is feasible and that it works is a necessary first step toward that goal, and we should applaud the work that has gone into coming this far.

Disclosures
Dr Beekman has received unrestricted research grants from Eli Lilly, Astra Zeneca, and Jansen and Shire. He has served on the speakers bureaus for Eli Lilly and Lundbeck.
  Dr. Cuipers has nothing to disclose.
  Dr. Smit has nothing to disclose.

REFERENCES

Alexopoulos, G. S., Meyers, B. S., Young, R. C., Campbell, S., Silbersweig, D., & Charlson, M. (1997). "Vascular depression" hypothesis *Archives of General Psychiatry, 54*(10), 915–922.

Beekman, A. T. F. (2004). Psychiatrische epidemiologie: van observatie naar experiment. [Psychiatric epidemiology: From observation to experiment]. Inaugural lecture Vrije Universiteit, September 17, 2003. *Maandblad Geestelijke Volksgezondheid, 59,* 587–599.

Beekman, A. T. F., Geerlings, S. W., Deeg, D. J. H., Smit, J. H., Schoevers, R. S., de Beurs, E., & van Tilburg, W. (2002) The natural history of late-life depression: A 6-year prospective study in the community. *Archives of General Psychiatry, 59,* 605–611.

Beekman, A. T. F., Smit, F., Stek, M. S., Reynolds, C. F., & Cuijpers, P. (2010) Preventing depression in high risk groups. *Current Opinion in Psychiatry, 23,* 8–11.

Cuijpers, P. (2003). Examining the effects of prevention programmes on the incidence of new cases of mental disorders: the lack of statistical power. *American Journal of Psychiatry, 160,* 1385–1391.

Cuijpers, P., van Straten, A., Smit, F., Mihalopoulos, C., & Beekman, A. (2008). Preventing the onset of depressive disorders: A meta-analytic review of psychological interventions. *American Journal of Psychiatry, 165,* 1272–1280.

De Jonge, P., Hadj, F. B., Boffa, D., Zdrojewski, C., Dorogi, Y., So, A.,... Stiefel, F. (2009). Prevention of major depression in complex medical ill patients: Preliminary results from a randomized controlled trial. *Psychosomatics, 50,* 227–233.

Dighe, S., Purkayastha, S., Swift, I., Tekkis, P. P., Darzi, A., A'Hern, R., & Brown, G. (2010). Diagnostic precision of CT in local staging of colon cancers: A meta-analysis. *Clinical Radiology, 65*(9), 708–719.

Fava, G. A., & Kellner, R. (1993). Staging: A neglected dimension in psychiatric classification. *Acta Psychiatrica Scandinavica 87,* 225–230.

Fukui, S., Ogawa, K., Ohtsuka, M., & Fukui, N. (2008). A randomized study assessing the efficacy of communication skill training on patients' psychologic distress and coping: Nurses' communication with patients just after being diagnosed with cancer. *Cancer, 113,* 1462–1470.

Hardeveld, F., Spijker, J., de Graaf, R., Nolen, W., & Beekman, A. T. F. (2010) Prevalence and predictors of recurrence of major depressive disorder in the adult population. *Acta Psychiatrica Scandinavica, 122,* 184–191.

Hariharan, D., Constantinides, V. A., Froeling, F. E., Tekkis, P. P., & Kocher, H. M. (2010). Ppreoperative staging of pancreatico-biliary cancers—A meta-analysis. *European Journal of Surgical Oncology, 36*(10), 941–948.

Hetrick, S. E., Parker, A. G., Hickie, I. B., Purcell, R., Yung, A. R., & McGorry, P. D. (2008). Early identification and intervention in depressive disorders: Towards a clinical stagingmodel. *Psychotherapy and Psychosomatics, 77*(5), 263–270.

Konnert, C., Dobson, K., & Stelmach, L (2009). The prevention of depression in nursing home residents: A randomized clinical trial of cognitive-behavioral therapy. *Aging and Mental Health, 13*(2), 288–299.

Lamers, F., de Jonge, P., Nolen, W. A., Smit, J. H., Zitman, F. G., Beekman, A. T. F., & Penninx, B. W. J. H. (2010). Identifying depressive subtypes is a large cohort study: Results from the Netherlands Study of Depression and Anxiety. *Journal of Clinical Psychiatry, 71,* 1582–1589.

Licht-Strunk, E., van Marwijk, H. W. J., Hoekstra, T., Twisk, J. W. R., de Haan, M., & Beekman, A. T. F. (2009) The prognosis of late life depression in primary care patients. *British Medical Journal, 338,* a3079.

McGorry, P. D. (2007). Issues for DSM-V: Clinical staging: A heuristic pathway to valid nosology and safer, more effective treatment in psychiatry. *American Journal of Psychiatry, 164,* 859–860.

Mrazek, P. J., & Haggerty, R. J. (Eds.). (1994). *Reducing risks for mental disorders.* Washington, DC: National Academic Press.

Paesmans, M., Berghmans, T., Dusart, M., Garcia, C., Hossein-Foucher, C., Lafitte, J. J.,... European Lung Cancer Working Party. (2010). Primary tumor standardized uptake value measured on fluorodeoxyglucose positron emission tomography is of prognostic value for survival in non-small cell lung cancer: Update of a systematic review and meta-analysis by the European Lung Cancer Working Party for the International Association for the Study of Lung Cancer Staging Project. *Journal of Thoracic Oncology, 5*(5), 612–619.

Pitceathly, C., Maguire, P., Fletcher, I., Parle, M., Tomenson, B., & Creed, F. (2009). Can a brief psychological intervention prevent anxiety or depressive disorders in cancer patients? A randomised controlled trial. *Annals of Oncology, 20,* 928–934.

Pot, A. M., Bohlmeijer, E. T., Onrust, S., Melenhorst, A. S., Veerbeek, M., & De Vries, W. (2010). The impact of life review on depression in older adults: a randomized controlled trial. *International Psychogeriatrics, 22*(4), 572–81.

Reynolds, C. F., III, Butters, M. A., Lopez, O., Pollock, B. G., Dew, M. A., Mulsant, B. H.,… DeKosky, S. T. (2011). Maintenance treatment of depression in old age: A randomized, double-blind, placebo-controlled evaluation of the efficacy and safety of donepezil combined with antidepressant pharmacotherapy. *Archives of General Psychiatry*, *68*(1), 51–60.

Riemersma-van der Lek, R. F., Swaab, D. F., Twisk, J., Hol, E. M., Hoogendijk, W. J., & Van Someren, E. J. (2008). Effect of bright light and melatonin on cognitive and noncognitive function in elderly residents of group care facilities: A randomized controlled trial. *Journal of the American Medical Association*, *299*, 2642–2655.

Robinson, R. G., Jorge, R. E., Moser, D. J., Acion, L., Solodkin, A., Small, S. L.,… Arndt, S. (2008). Escitalopram and problem solving therapy for prevention of post stroke depression: A randomised controlled trial. *Journal of the American Medical Association*, *299*, 2391–2400.

Rovner, B. W., Casten, R. J., Hegel, M. T., Leiby, B. E., & Tasman, W. S. (2007). Preventing depression in age-related macular degeneration. *Archives of General Psychiatry*, *64*, 886–892.

Schoevers, R. A., Smit, F., Deeg, D. J. H., Cuijpers, P., Dekker, J., van Tilburg, W., & Beekman, A. T. (2006). Do we know where to start? Prevention of late-life depression in primary care. *American Journal of Psychiatry*, *163*, 1611–1621.

Smit, F., Ederveen, A., Cuijpers, P., Deeg, D., & Beekman, A. (2006). Opportunities for cost-effective prevention of late-life depress ion: An epidemiological approach. *Archives of General Psychiatry*, *63*, 290–296.

Spijker, J., de Graaf, R., Bijl, R. V., Beekman, A. T., Ormel, J., & Nolen, W. A. (2003). Duration of major depressive episodes in the general population. Results from the Netherlands Mental Health Survey and Incidence Study (NEMESIS). *British Journal of Psychiatry*, *181*, 208–213.

Sun, X., Steffens, D. C., Au, R., Folstein, M., Summergrad, P., Yee, J.,… Qiu, W. Q. (2008). Amyloid-associated depression: a prodromal depression of Alzheimer disease? *Archives of General Psychiatry*, *65*(5), 542–550.

van de Rest, O., Geleijnse, J. M., Kok, F. J., van Staveren, W. A., Hoefnagels, W. H.,… de Groot, L. C. (2008). Effect of fish oil supplementation on mental well-being in older subjects: a randomised, double-blind, placebo-controlled trial. *American Journal of Clinical Nutrition*, *88*, 706–713.

van 't Veer, P. J., van Marwijk, H. W. J., Smit, F., van Hout, H. P., van der Horst, H. E., Cuijpers, P.,… Beekman, A. T. (2009). Stepped care prevention of anxiety and depression in late life: A randomised controlled trial. *Archives of General Psychiatry*, *66*, 297–304.

Vogelzangs, N., Beekman, A. T., Boelhouwer, I. G., Bandinelli, S., Milaneschi, Y., Ferrucci, L., & Penninx, B. W. (2011). Metabolic depression: a chronic depressive subtype? Findings from the InCHIANTI study of older persons. *Journal of Clinical Psychiatry*. *72*, 598–604.

Walker, J. G., Mackinnon, A. J., Batterham, P., Jorm, A. F., Hickie, I., McCarthy, A.,… Christensen, H. (2010). Mental health literacy, folic acid and vitamin B12, and physical activity for the prevention of depression in older adults: Randomised controlled trial. *British Journal of Psychiatry*, *197*(1), 45–54.

Xing, Y., Bronstein, Y., Ross, M. I., Askew, R. L., Lee, J. E., Gershenwald, J. E.,… Cormier, J. N. (2011). Contemporary diagnostic imaging modalities for the staging and surveillance of melanoma patients: A meta-analysis. *Journal of the National Cancer Institute*, *103*(2), 129–42.

26

DEPRESSION MEDICATION TREATMENT ADHERENCE IN LATER LIFE

Kara Zivin, Janet Kavanagh, Susan Maixner, Jo Anne Sirey, and Helen C. Kales

MRS. A was referred to the university Geriatric Psychiatry Clinic. She is 70 years old, was born in an Eastern European country, and immigrated in her early 30s. She reports a 3-year history of depressive symptoms, the onset of which was concurrent with psychosocial stressors and medical problems. Her symptoms include low mood (rated as a 4/10), tearfulness, irritability, middle-of-the-night awakening and insomnia, low appetite and weight loss, hopelessness, and the thought that she "doesn't know why she is living." She scores 28/30 on the Mini-mental Status Exam, missing 1 of the short-term memory items and having difficulty with copying a design. Initially, she is prescribed a starting dose of citalopram (10 mg); however, she decides to take half the starting dose (5 mg) and then stops it after 2 days due to "feeling foggy." On return to the clinic several weeks later, she describes anxiety about taking psychiatric medications in general, as well as fears that they may decrease her cognitive function. She is then prescribed escitalopram oral solution at a dose of 2 mg/day with instructions to titrate up by 2 mg every 4 days

with a target dosage of 10 mg/day. Mrs. A is asked to return to the clinic in 4 weeks. When seen for the return visit, she and her daughter state that they were "not able to fill the prescription" but are unclear as to why. Mrs. A's daughter also mentions that she has her own "concerns" about her mother being on medication. A new prescription for sertraline 12.5 mg per day is given with instructions to titrate to 25 mg in 2 weeks and to follow up in 4 weeks. Mrs. A is lost to psychiatric follow-up until 2 years later, when she is on a medical service within the university system and the psychiatry consult-liaison service is called to see her. She reveals that she stopped the sertraline several days after beginning treatment due to "side effects." The consultants diagnose the patient with depression with anxious features, prescribe a new trial of mirtazapine 7.5 mg per day, and schedule her for a follow-up in outpatient Geriatric Psychiatry. The patient and daughter cancel the follow-up in psychiatry. The patient is re-referred to the clinic by her primary care physician, but she does not show for the appointment.

INTRODUCTION

While there is evidence that providers are increasingly diagnosing depression and recommending treatment for older patients (Crystal, Sambamoorthi, Walkup, & Akincigil, 2003; Mamdani, Rapoport, Shulman, Herrmann, & Rochon, 2005) (addressing a "first-generation" problem), a "second-generation" problem has emerged (Datto et al., 2002), that of depression medication treatment nonadherence as demonstrated in the case of Mrs. A. Estimates of such nonadherence, with older patients either never initiating or discontinuing depression medication prematurely, range from 40% (Ivanova et al., 2011) to 75% (Salzman, 1995). Thus, greater effort is needed to ensure that patients actually initiate and continue appropriate care throughout the course of their depressive illness, such that patients may maximize improvement in both emotional and physical quality of life domains (Doraiswamy, Khan, Donahue, & Richard, 2001).

What has been labeled as "treatment-resistant" depression may, in fact, represent undertreatment resulting from poor adherence (Mulsant & Pollock, 1998). Poor depression treatment adherence is an important source of drug exposure variability, but it is often inadequately measured in both research trials and clinical practice. Thus, even with improvements in the screening and diagnosis of late-life depression in health care settings, a large treatment gap remains. Depression treatment nonadherence limits the extent to which older patients with depression realize the benefits of efficacious treatment options. Thus, efforts to improve it can be viewed as the next frontier in the treatment of late-life depression (Zivin & Kales, 2008).

While provider-level (Collins, Westra, Dozois, & Burns, 2004; Cruz & Pincus, 2002; Moride et al., 2002) and system-level factors (Docherty, 1997; Solberg, Korsen, Oxman, Fischer, & Bartels, 1999) can create barriers to depression treatment adherence, this chapter focuses on the key *patient-level* factors associated with depression treatment adherence among older adults. Although other effective modalities exist for treatment of late-life depression, such as electroconvulsive therapy and evidence-based psychotherapy, given the ubiquity of their use in primary care and other treatment settings, our primary focus is adherence to *antidepressant medications*. We then discuss potential investigation and implementation of intervention strategies to improve late-life adherence.

CONCEPTUAL MODEL

Models of health behaviors help us to understand how the beliefs and actions of individuals influence treatment seeking. There are many such models, including the Health Behavior Model (Becker, 1974), The Theory of Reasoned Action (Ajzen, 1996), and the Transtheoretical Model (Prochaska, 1983). Brewer and Rimer (Glanz, Rimer, & Viswanath, 2008) have noted that with regard to a particular construct such as adherence, in the absence of data about which theory is better, researchers should select their model based upon an assessment of its merits and appropriateness to the particular question. We have chosen to apply the Theory of Reasoned Action (Ajzen, 1996) to adherence behaviors because of its emphasis on attitudes and beliefs, as from our research, those appear to be key factors underlying adherence in later life. Furthermore, because many important beliefs and attitudes may be modifiable, they are ideal targets for subsequent interventions (Glanz et al., 2008).

The Theory of Reasoned Action hypothesizes that behavioral intention and eventual treatment seeking are determined by a person's weighing of potential risks and benefits of getting treatment (Cooper, Gonzales, et al., 2003; Van Voorhees et al., 2005). Howland (1997) further adapted the Theory of Reasoned Action to divide factors affecting health behaviors into *external* and *internal*. External factors either are not modifiable (e.g., race) or modifiable only with significant effort or specialized interventions (e.g., depression level, social support; Cooper, Gonzales, et al., 2003). Internal factors are potentially modifiable through education or other experiences and include beliefs (e.g., spirituality), attitudes, and social norms (e.g., family opinions, social stigma). External factors may affect treatment seeking through interaction with a person's internal attitudes and beliefs (e.g., race may be associated with spirituality, which may in turn impact a decision to seek treatment). The net individual balance of favorable and unfavorable factors to treatment seeking determines intentions, which in turn lead to action (Ajzen, 1996). Halgin, Weaver, Edell, and Spencer (1987) suggested that this model can provide a framework for understanding why many patients will not accept a diagnosis of depression. Previous work by Cooper and colleagues using the Theory of Reasoned Action emphasized the importance of patient beliefs about spirituality, stigma, social support, provider relationships, and physical health in determining attitudes toward and acceptance of depression treatment

(Cooper-Patrick et al., 1997; Cooper, Brown, Vu, Ford, & Powe, 2001; Cooper, Gonzales, et al., 2003; Cooper, Hill, & Powe, 2002; Cooper, Roter, et al., 2003; Van Voorhees et al., 2006).

Table 26.1 depicts how we have organized these internal and external factors according to *modifiability*—the potential for influence on patient characteristics or resulting adherence to antidepressants by specialized treatment approaches or interventions. Modifiable factors include attitudes such as perceptions and preferences for treatment, beliefs regarding etiology of depression and effectiveness of depression treatments, spiritual beliefs, and social norms such as impact of caregivers on patient beliefs and stigma. Other factors may be less modifiable per se, but their impact on adherence might be reduced with specialized interventions. These include comorbid anxiety, substance use, cognitive impairment, perception of medication side effects, polypharmacy, social support, and treatment cost. Truly nonmodifiable factors include patient race and gender.

MODIFIABLE FACTORS

Preferences/Attitudes Toward Depression Treatment

As seen in the case of Mrs. A, attitudes toward depression treatment can have a significant impact on adherence in later life. Until recently, they have been little explored (Cooper-Patrick et al., 1997; Kessing, Hansen, Demyttenaere, & Bech, 2005). Mrs. A expressed "worries" about taking antidepressants that may have been a significant barrier to her initiation of and adherence to medications. Personal preferences largely impact treatment acceptability and willingness to engage. Older adults may be both unwilling to take antidepressants or participate in psychotherapy. Arean, Alvidrez, Barrera, Robinson, and Hicks (2002) found that the primary care physician remained the most frequently endorsed choice of provider for psychosocial problems, with only 44% of the sample willing to talk to mental health providers about such problems. Furthermore, many minority elders may be even less willing to engage in specialized mental health treatment than their non-minority counterparts (Gum & Arean, 2004).

Patient preconceptions about depression or antidepressant medications (Givens et al., 2006; Katon et al., 1995; Kessing et al., 2005), treatment acceptability and effectiveness (Aikens & Klinkman, 2012; Aupperle, Lifchus, & Coyne, 1998; Prabhakaran & Butler, 2002), and concern for side effects or potential addiction (Angermeyer & Dietrich, 2006; Cooper, Gonzales, et al., 2003; Fawzi et al., 2012; Givens et al., 2006) may also negatively impact antidepressant adherence and adequate antidepressant titration in older adults. A British study found that

Table 26.1 Factors affecting patient level adherence to depression treatment among older adults

ABILITY TO MODIFY	FACTOR
Modifiable	Preferences / attitudes toward depression treatment
	Spiritual beliefs
	Beliefs about the etiology of depression / effectiveness of depression treatment
	Perceived stigma
	Social norms, family caregiver opinions
	Patient / provider communication
Modifiable with Difficulty / Potentially Modifiable	Social support
	Affordability/costs of treatment
	Cognitive status
	Polypharmacy and medical comorbidity
	Comorbid anxiety
	Substance use
Non-modifiable	Race
	Gender

adherence in older patients with depression was negatively associated with concern about side effects, level of psychological distress, less strong beliefs about the necessity of taking antidepressants, lack of understanding about the nature of depression, and concerns about taking antidepressant medication (Maidment, Livingston, & Katona, 2002). A qualitative study using a purposive sample of older patients who participated in either the PROSPECT or PRISM-E studies of collaborative care noted four main themes characterizing resistance to the use of antidepressants: (1) fear of dependence; (2) resistance to viewing depressive symptoms as a medical illness; (3) concern that antidepressants will prevent natural sadness; and (4) prior negative experiences with depression medications (Givens et al., 2006).

While collaborative care models such as PROSPECT (Bruce & Pearson, 1999) and IMPACT (Unützer et al., 2002) do improve the recognition, treatment, and outcomes of depressive illness in older primary care patients, patient attitudes likely influence how and whether such interventions will succeed in real-world settings (National Advisory Mental Health Council's Workgroup on Aging Research, 2003). Taken together, these findings suggest that patient preferences and attitudes can have a significant and potentially negative effect on depression treatment adherence among older adults.

Spiritual Beliefs

Determinants of help-seeking behavior and treatment preferences for depression care may differ based on a patient's level and intensity of spiritual or religious beliefs. Beliefs about reliance on spiritual aid solely or preferentially in relieving depression symptoms may reduce medical help seeking or increase rates of treatment refusal (Neighbors, Musick, & Williams, 1998). Several mixed-age studies by Cooper et al. (Cooper-Patrick et al., 1997; Cooper et al., 2001; Cooper, Gonzales, et al., 2003) found that spirituality was an important determinant of acceptance of medical depression care for some patients, who endorsed statements such as "prayer can heal depression." Other studies, however, have noted a significant association between religious participation and improved depression outcomes in the elderly (Bosworth, Park, McQuoid, Hays, & Steffens, 2003; Cruz et al., 2009; Koenig, 1998; Koenig et al., 1992; Koenig, George, & Peterson, 1998). In a number of these

studies, religious and spiritual beliefs have been significantly associated with race (e.g., higher spirituality in African American patients). While race is not modifiable, attitudes and beliefs about antidepressants associated with race may be. The extent to which spirituality or other beliefs serve as barriers to effective depression care still is not clear. More research needs to be done to examine the relationship between older age, race, preferences for depression treatment, adherence to depression treatment, and depression treatment outcomes.

Beliefs About the Etiology of Depression/Effectiveness of Depression Treatment

Patients' beliefs about the cause(s) of their depression have been a little studied area. Although Mrs. A felt that her depression was the result of family conflicts as well as medical problems, she received primarily "biological" neurotransmitter-based explanations of her depression from her providers. Perhaps it was difficult for her to connect how an antidepressant would improve her symptoms of interpersonal and physical distress. In a recent study examining the relationship of patient-level factors and depression treatment adherence (Kales et al., 2011) in older adults, only 9% of participants identified biological factors as the cause of their depression. The most frequently cited reasons included personal loss, poor physical health, interpersonal discord, burden of being a caregiver for others, and financial difficulty. A Swedish study in a mixed-age primary care sample seemed to also confirm this hypothesis about patients' beliefs, finding that biological explanations of depression were rare and that common beliefs about etiology centered on life stressors.

Stigma

Depression stigma is based on the belief that most people will devalue and discriminate against individuals who use mental health services and/or have a mental illness. The Surgeon General's report on mental health argues that stigma is the most formidable obstacle to further progress in the arena of mental illness and health (United States Department of Health and Human Services, 1999). There has been limited work examining the role of stigma in adherence to depression care among older adults.

Sirey et al. (2001b) examined the effects of stigma, age, and treatment discontinuation. In this study of younger (n = 63) and older (n = 29) patients with depression, stigma was actually higher in younger patients but affected treatment discontinuation only in older patients (Sirey et al., 2001b). In another study of recently widowed/bereaved older adults, concerns about having a mental health diagnosis substantially decrease the likelihood of mental health service use (Bambauer & Prigerson, 2006). More work is needed to determine how stigma differentially influences treatment initiation, continuation, and adherence among older adults, as well as how patient beliefs and concerns regarding stigmatization may be modified to improve depression outcomes (Sirey, Bruce, & Kales, 2010).

Social Norms

Caregiver agreement with treatment recommendations (Bogardus et al., 2004) can also impact antidepressant adherence and adequate antidepressant titration. As illustrated by the case of Mrs. A, her daughter had her own concerns about Mrs. A being on an antidepressant, and this may have impacted both adherence and the lack of follow-up in the clinic. Caregivers' characterization of the cause of a patient's depression may also influence medication adherence (Sher, McGinn, Sirey, & Meyers, 2005). For example, when caregivers attribute a patient's depression to attitudinal or cognitive factors, a patient may be less likely to be adherent to antidepressants (Sher et al., 2005). Caregivers have also been shown to overestimate levels of patient adherence, reducing the likelihood of recognition of the problem and subsequent intervention (Ownby, Hertzog, Crocco, & Duara, 2006). It is also worth noting that patients with cognitive limitations are also subject to greater influence by caregivers. Given that caregiver beliefs about patient treatment and treatment recommendations can have a substantial impact on patient adherence, including caregivers in treatment plans is an essential component of promoting patient adherence (Bogardus et al., 2004).

Patient/Provider Communication

The relationship between the patient and the health professional is also part of the subjective experience of the patient that can influence adherence. The manner in which the provider introduces and discusses depression and its treatment may affect patients'

willingness to initiate and maintain antidepressant use. Mrs. A appeared to have the longest-standing relationship with her primary care physician. Her primary care physician's attempts to refer her to geriatric psychiatry were less than successful— older patients like Mrs. A often prefer to discuss emotional problems with established primary care providers rather than seek treatment from mental health specialists (Arean et al., 2002). However, primary care providers have limited time to discuss all relevant physical and emotional conditions. Within the context of a brief return visit it may be difficult for the primary care physician to pay sufficient attention to discussing depression and the importance of adherence to treatment. One small mixed-methods study found that older adults who achieved and sustained a remission of their depressive symptoms attributed their improvement to clear psychoeducational support from their depression care providers (Barg et al., 2010). Future research should focus on identifying efficient and effective ways for providers to communicate with older patients about antidepressant adherence, as well as to identify individual barriers that could prevent patients from adhering.

FACTORS WITH POTENTIALLY MODIFIABLE IMPACT ON ADHERENCE

Social Support

Social support, a complex construct, has been shown to be an important factor influencing the presence and levels of depression, and a key contributor associated with an individual's ability to manage stressful situations (Berkman & Syme, 1979; House, Landis, & Umberson, 1988; Mendes de Leon et al., 1999; Seeman, 1996; Thoits, 1995). Older adults may be isolated and lack necessary support. Such isolation may be magnified by circumstances such as caregiving for a loved one or being widowed. Sickness or death in one marital partner can cause substantial stress and loss of social support for the other spouse. In the case of Mrs. A, while she had a large family network, much of her psychosocial conflict centered on a significant rift that had occurred within her extended family, thus reducing opportunity for positive social interaction.

While greater social support has been found to be associated with better antidepressant adherence in older patients with depression (Voils, Steffens,

Flint, & Bosworth, 2005), it should be noted that as in the case of Mrs. A, social networks may not always promote depression medication adherence. Mrs. A's daughter appeared to have ambivalent feelings about her mother's depression treatment, and she had made comments to the provider that she had "concerns" about her mother taking medication. Given that the daughter was her mother's caregiver and provided transportation to the appointments (many of which were missed), her ambivalence may have played a role in her mother's medication nonadherence.

The relationship between depression, social support, and public religious practice is also complex. Some researchers have suggested that public religious practice may be a proxy for social support, while others suggest religious practice and social support independently influence coping with geriatric depression (Bosworth et al., 2003).

Cost of Treatment

Older adults who are more likely to be taking multiple daily medications and living on fixed incomes may not fill certain prescription medications because of cost (Soumerai et al., 2006). Until 2006, Medicare beneficiaries did not have access to a prescription drug benefit. In addition, public insurance does not adequately cover the preventive care services that may increase the likelihood of the detection, diagnosis, and treatment of geriatric depression (Alexopoulos, 2005; Bartels, 2003).

Cost-related nonadherence to medications (CRN) has been estimated to occur in 13% to 25% of elderly populations (Safran et al., 2002, 2005; Soumerai, et al., 2006). A study using nationally representative data demonstrated that 21% of individuals with depression did not fill an initial treatment-related prescription in the last year due to cost, and 14% did not refill an ongoing medication due to cost (Piette, Heisler, & Wagner, 2004). The rates of CRN reported by individuals with depression are significantly higher than among patients with a variety of other medical disorders (Piette et al., 2004). Another study confirmed that depressive symptoms were associated with CRN in elderly Medicare enrollees (Bambauer et al., 2007). Since elderly patients are known to take multiple daily medications, and psychiatric medications are some of the more costly (Bartels, 2003), it is not surprising that late-life depression is associated with CRN. Again, clinical time

limitations may cause providers to infrequently consider affordability when determining which antidepressants to recommend for their elderly patients (Butler, Collins, Katona, & Orrell, 2000). Recently Zivin et al. (Zivin, Madden, Graves, Zhang, & Soumerai, 2009) compared CRN among those with and without depressive symptoms both before and following the implementation of Medicare Part D. They found that despite the fact that Part D aimed to improve adherence among the mentally ill, the prevalence of CRN did not improve. Kennedy, Maciejewski, Liu, and Blodgett (2011) also found that the younger Medicare participants as well as those with depression, in poor health, and with multiple comorbidities were more likely to report CRN following Part D. Given the association between cost and nonadherence, providers should be sensitive to possible financial barriers and explore lower cost medications and therapies.

Cognitive Status

Medication adherence involves taking a prescribed medication at the appropriate time in the correct amount and manner (Insel, Morrow, Brewer, & Figueredo, 2006). Thus, adhering to medications requires intact executive function, working memory, and encoding and storage of information. Because of the impact of memory domains relevant to medication use, cognitive impairment is a uniquely burdensome influence on depression treatment adherence in many older adults.

Patients with cognitive impairment may forget what they have been told about their medications and whether they took them (Murray et al., 2004). They may also have difficulty accurately reporting adherence to treatment. Cooper et al (2005) found that although decreased adherence was associated with cognitive impairment, it was not a linear relationship; adherence was lowest in those with moderate impairment. They hypothesized that those with mild impairment might use memory aids such as pillboxes while those with more severe impairment might have caregivers assisting them. New assistive technologies, such as computerized medication dispensers, can assist patients both with remembering to take medications and preventing excessive medication use (Barat, Andreasen, & Damsgaard, 2001). Some of these devices can communicate to caregivers if patients do not take their medications properly.

Polypharmacy and Medical Comorbidity

Polypharmacy, or taking multiple medications, is the norm among older adults; the average older American uses three prescription and four over-the-counter (OTC) medications daily (Lotrich & Pollock, 2005). Eleven percent of the elderly take 10 or more medications (Kaufman, Kelly, Rosenberg, Anderson, & Mitchell, 2002). Those with depression may take more medications than those without depression (Lotrich & Pollock, 2005). Polypharmacy can have particularly detrimental effects on older adults, including adverse drug events, drug–drug interactions, the influence of aging on pharmacokinetics in older adults through increased sensitivity to toxicity, and contributing to confusion about medication regimen (Gareri et al., 1998; Lotrich & Pollock, 2005; Loya, González-Stuart, & Rivera, 2009; Williams, 2002).

Medication adherence problems increase with the total number of drugs prescribed (Barat et al., 2001). Key risk factors for poor outcomes associated with polypharmacy in the elderly may include lack of a medication administration routine, therapeutic duplication, hoarding, confusion between generic and trade names, multiple prescribers, discontinued medications being refilled or retained, and multiple storage locations (Sorensen, Stokes, Purdie, Woodward, & Roberts, 2005). Patients may also supplement their physician's recommended regimen with OTC drugs or herbal preparations, thus, further increasing regimen complexity (Murray et al., 2004).

Drug interactions and side effects may also impact the ability of the older patient to continue to adhere to depression medications. Patients may decide to limit the total number of medications taken and may view taking their antidepressant for mental health reasons as discretionary, while viewing the medication(s) taken for other medical or physical illnesses as necessary or more important. Mrs. A was taking a number of medications for medical problems, but she seemed to view taking her antidepressant as elective.

Additional difficulty in managing more medications and creation of more complex medication regimens resulting from medical comorbidity may also contribute to decreased depression treatment adherence in the elderly (MacLaughlin et al., 2005; Weintraub, 1990). Among older adults with significant medical burden, depression may also have a compounding adverse effect on medication adherence and health outcomes (DiMatteo, Lepper, & Croghan, 2000; Kilbourne et al., 2005). For example, in a study of depressed older patients with diabetes, they were found to be less able or motivated to obtain medication refills (Kilbourne et al., 2005). The authors of this study noted that worry about side effects may also prevent depressed patients with comorbidity from adhering to medications. Such worry about side effects may be multidimensional: (1) the likelihood of adverse drug reactions increases with increasing numbers of medications and this risk may be exponential (Hohl, Dankoff, Colacone, & Afilalo, 2001) and (2) worry about side effects may also be anticipatory and relate to anxiety and somatization (Lenze, 2003).

Comorbid Anxiety

Clinically significant anxiety is common in older adults with depression, primarily generalized anxiety disorder or subsyndromal anxiety characterized by generalized anxiety or panic symptoms. Such anxiety is found in 30%–60% of older outpatients with depression (Flint & Rifat, 1997; Lenze et al., 2000, 2005; Mulsant, Reynolds, Shear, Sweet, & Miller, 1996; Salzman, 2004). Older depressed patients with anxiety may be less likely to remit than nonanxious depressed patients (Steffens & McQuoid, 2005). In the PROSPECT care management of late-life depression study, the intervention was more effective than usual care in patients with low anxiety, but it added little benefit for patients with higher anxiety severity (Alexopoulos et al., 2005). Thus, those with comorbid anxiety may be at increased risk for poor adherence and negative outcomes in late-life depression. Care management without specific attention to anxiety symptoms may be insufficient treatment for patients with significant anxiety like Mrs. A.

Promisingly, comorbid anxiety is potentially modifiable if appropriately identified. Symptoms of psychic and somatic anxiety may actually show the greatest change during adequate antidepressant treatment of late-life depression (Nelson, Clary, Leon, & Schneider, 2005). Tailored and structured support of older patients with anxious depression appears critical to achieving outcomes similar to those for patients without anxiety (Lenze et al., 2003).

Substance Use

Although many depressed patients have comorbid substance use disorders (Thase, 2003; Zivin et al., 2007), data on addictive behaviors of older adults are scarce (Graham et al., 1996), and studies of comorbid depression, treatment adherence, and comorbid alcoholism or substance use are virtually nonexistent for patients of all ages. Limited existing data suggest a negative relationship between problem drug or alcohol use and adherence to depression treatment. One study of nearly 4,000 older adults in 11 countries (Cooper et al., 2005) found that non-adherence was associated with problem drinking. In a recent study, medication nonadherence at 4 months was found to be lowest among older adults who believed that substance use was the reason they became depressed (Kales et al., 2011). Mixed-age substance abusers have been found to have lower rates of adherence to outpatient follow-up referrals after being discharged from a VA psychiatric emergency room (Dobscha, Delucchi, & Young, 1999). Future research should focus on further elucidating the relationship between addictive disorders and depression treatment adherence in older adults.

NONMODIFIABLE FACTORS

While clearly race and gender are not themselves modifiable, the attitudes, beliefs, and other factors associated with gender and race may be modifiable. To appropriately manage symptoms of late-life depression, strategies to address the unique diagnosis and treatment needs by gender and race need to be considered.

Race

Prior studies have consistently shown that in clinical settings, elderly African Americans have significantly lower rates of depression diagnoses as compared to Caucasians (Fabrega et al., 1994; Kales et al., 1997; Mulsant et al., 1993). These findings echo disparities found in research among younger adults. Few studies have evaluated *why* these differences are found. In clinical settings, it is likely that there is a complex interplay of provider and patient factors such as variation in use of health care services, alternative symptom presentations, and patient preferences.

A previous study examining antidepressant use among community-dwelling elderly found that African Americans were significantly less likely to take antidepressants than Whites (Blazer, Hybels, Simonsick, & Hanlon, 2000). Even after controlling for health coverage and income, it appeared that elderly African Americans were significantly

less likely to be taking selective serotonin reuptake inhibitors than Whites. However, the study's methodology could not determine whether rates of initiation or adherence to antidepressants differed by race. In a subsequent study, data were compared from two follow-up intervals (1986–1987 to 1989–1990 and 1992–1993 to 1996–1997) of the same community-based cohort (Blazer, 2005). While antidepressant use markedly increased overall between the time intervals studied, there was an *increasing* disparity by race. Given that the frequency of depression did not vary by race, the authors concluded that community-dwelling older African Americans may be significantly undertreated. The authors also suggested that older African Americans may view antidepressants as discretionary or less critical to their health care than their need for other medications. Other research has found that appropriate depression treatment was not only less likely in African Americans but also in those 60 years old or over (Ladson Hinton et al., 2012; Young, Klap, Sherbourne, & Wells, 2001).

African American patients with depression may find antidepressant treatment less acceptable than White patients and hence be less likely to initiate such treatment when recommended by physicians. Cooper, Gonzales, et al. (2003) found that while 74% of White patients with depression found antidepressant medication acceptable, only 51% of African American patients with depression did. African American patients with depression were more likely to agree with the statement that "antidepressant medications are addictive" and less likely to agree that "antidepressants are effective."

In terms of the relationship between ethnicity and treatment adherence in older patients, investigators from the PROSPECT trial found that non-White race was the factor most strongly associated with nonadherence to citalopram (Bogner, Lin, & Morales, 2006). In a small study of African American and Latino elderly patients taking antidepressants (Ayalon, Arean, & Alvidrez, 2005), 35% of the African American sample and 29% of the Latino sample were intentionally nonadherent. Intentional nonadherence was associated with concerns about side effects, stigma, and attribution of lesser importance to antidepressants than other medications. Thus, this work, as well as that from mixed-age samples, suggests that modifiable factors discussed earlier, such as spirituality, beliefs, and stigma, may be among the most significant factors that impact treatment seeking and adherence in African American patients (Marwaha & Livingston, 2002).

In a prospective, observational study comparing rates of depression medication adherence for older African American and White primary care patients, we followed 188 subjects aged 60 and over, diagnosed with clinically significant depression with a new recommendation for antidepressant treatment by their primary care physician (Kales et al., 2011; Maixner, Struble, Blazek, & Kales, 2011). Study participants were assessed at study entry and at 4-month follow-up (encompassing the acute treatment phase). Depression medication adherence was based on a well-validated self-report measure. At 4 months follow-up, 61.2% of subjects reported that they were adherent with antidepressant medication. In unadjusted and two of the three adjusted analyses, African American subjects ($n = 82$) had significantly lower rates of 4-month antidepressant adherence than White subjects ($n = 106$). African American females had the lowest adherence rates (44.4%) followed by African American males (56.8%), White males (65.3%), and White females (73.7%). In logistic regression models controlling for demographic, illness, and functional status variables, significant differences persisted between African American women and White women in reported 4-month antidepressant adherence (OR 3.58, 95% CI 1.27–10.07, $p < .02$). Our results demonstrate racial and gender differences in adherence behaviors for depression medication treatment in the elderly.

In another study of Medicare enrollees, African American subjects were more likely than Whites to report running out of medications before refilling them; however, this difference did not persist in adjusted analyses. Race did remain associated with not following physician instructions on how to take medications in adjusted models (Gerber, Cho, Arozullah, & Lee, 2010).

Gender

The relationship between gender, depression, and outcomes such as treatment adherence is undoubtedly complex. The Improving Mood-Promoting Access to Collaborative Treatment (IMPACT) trial of collaborative care in older primary care patients with depression found that older women were significantly more likely to endorse depressive symptoms and to have received prior depression treatment than were older men (Hinton, Zweifach,

Oishi, Tang, & Unützer, 2006). Furthermore, antidepressant use is more prevalent in older women (Mamdani, Herrmann, & Austin, 1999; Pratt, Brody, & Gu, 2011). It is unclear whether these gender differences are due to a higher prevalence of depression in women, greater detection of depression in women, or greater willingness of women to engage in antidepressant treatment as compared to men (Moller-Leimkuhler, 2002; Rutz, von Knorring, Pihlgren, Rihmer, & Walinder, 1995; Steffens et al., 2000). A recent VA study with a sample composed of primarily middle-aged and older men found that antidepressant discontinuation was associated with concerns about side effects and lack of efficacy (Fortney et al., 2010).

OTHER FACTORS POTENTIALLY AFFECTING ADHERENCE

The studies included in this chapter cover a variety of individuals and settings, from clinic based and general population samples, veterans, low-income patients, and those fully covered and treated by managed care health insurance. Therefore, we note that treatment setting may also influence patient adherence. Further included studies were conducted in a variety of countries, which can influence a wide range of factors from insurance coverage and cost to norms and beliefs about antidepressant medication.

Patients in the included studies vary in their level of depressive symptoms with a range in severity from depressive symptoms to mild depression to major depressive disorder. Symptom severity may also influence willingness to initiate and adhere to treatment. Furthermore, some studies may include patients with newly diagnosed depression, while others focus on patients with ongoing or recurrent depression. These factors may influence adherence to antidepressants in older adults and underscore the need for more rigorous studies in this area.

PROMISING INTERVENTIONS TO IMPROVE RATES OF LATE-LIFE DEPRESSION TREATMENT ADHERENCE

In terms of the factors discussed earlier, perhaps the most modifiable and thus most likely targets for interventions are patient attitudes and beliefs. Attitudes and beliefs, especially perceived stigma at the initiation of depression care, predict poor medication adherence and higher rates of mental health treatment discontinuation among the depressed elderly during the acute treatment period (Ayalon et al., 2005; Sirey et al., 2001a, 2001b). Perceptions of stigma are associated with feelings of social exclusion and poorer quality of life for older adults, both of which may be interlinked with depression. Although older adults face tangible barriers (e.g., transportation, medication copayments, and mobility), often it is the attitudes and beliefs that contribute to these barriers becoming insurmountable (Sirey et al., 2010).

Based upon the data linking attitudes and beliefs with adherence in later life, Sirey et al. developed the Treatment Initiation and Participation Program (TIP) (Sirey, Bruce, & Alexopoulos, 2005). TIP is a brief, individualized intervention designed as an adjunct to pharmacotherapy prescribed by a physician for depression treatment. TIP specifically targets modifiable factors such as psychological barriers (e.g., stigma, beliefs about treatment self-efficacy, and resignation about limitations), concerns about treatment, fears of antidepressants, attributions regarding depression etiology, and attribution of depressive symptoms to other causes, which would make treatment unnecessary. TIP is designed to

be tailored to the particular barriers presented by a given older adult, and to empower the older adult to self-manage his or her medication treatment. The potential impact of the TIP intervention on attitudes and beliefs is depicted in Figure 26.1.

As primary care physicians (PCPs) provide the majority of care for late-life depression, the TIP intervention was originally tested in two urban primary care clinics (Sirey et al., 2010). The sample consisted of adults aged 60 years and older with major depression who were recommended antidepressant therapy by their PCPs. All participants were randomly assigned to either the intervention (TIP) or the treatment-as-usual (TAU) group. Study participants were assessed at entry, 6, 12, and 24 weeks later. Adherence was measured based on self-report with chart verification. Participants in TIP were significantly more adherent to their antidepressant pharmacotherapy at all assessment time points and had a significantly greater decrease in depressive symptoms than older adults who received TAU.

Currently, TIP is being tested in a larger randomized controlled study (Sirey and Kales are co-PIs) with inclusion of geographic diversity. Intervention delivery is by social work staff within primary care clinics, demonstrating portability and potential ease of dissemination. If this study reinforces that TIP

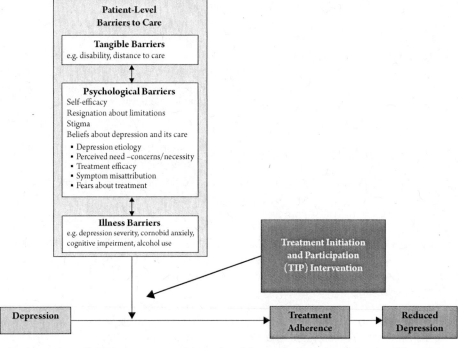

FIGURE 26.1 Impact of TIP Intervention on Patient-Level Barriers to Depression Care in Older Adults.

Table 26.2 Suggested approaches to selected barriers to treatment adherence.

BARRIER	INTERVENTION	TECHNIQUE
Stigma ("If I take depression medication, other people might think I am crazy.")	* Validate concern (stigma is real) * Define disclosure options * Emphasize personal choice	MI-reflective listening and empathy PS-Brainstorming PS-Identify pro's and con's
Concerns about treatment efficacy ("What's medication going to do? Nothing can change.")	* Identify symptoms of depression present in patient * Identify what s/he wishes to change * Link goal with treatment outcome	PE-Education about depression PS-Identify a treatment goal PE-Review antidepressant efficacy and discuss importance of adherence
Misattribution of depression symptoms ("It's my age and other medical problems that cause all of my troubles")	* Validate overlap of medical and psychological symptoms * Describe symptoms of depression * Review myths about depression and misattributions	PE-Depression symptoms and medical overlap PE-Information about depression PE-Discuss myths and aging stereotypes
Fears about treatment ("I am worried this medication will make me more forgetful")	* Validate worries about memory * Discuss potential side effects as well as potential improvement in memory/function with treatment * Reassure regarding close monitoring of side effects in follow-up	MI-reflective listening and empathy PE-Review antidepressant side effects; review impact of depression on attention, memory and function

Technique key: MI = motivational interviewing; PS = problem-solving; PE = psychoeducation.

(NIMH R01-MH-087557–02, Co-PIs Sirey and Kales)

significantly improves patient adherence in primary care, this will represent a significant advance for the second-generation problem of poor adherence to depression medication in older adults like Mrs. A.

In the meantime, how can clinicians in resource-limited settings intervene with their individual patients to improve depression medication adherence? Based upon clinical and research experience, including the TIP program, the first step is a brief discussion to identify any potential barriers to adherence at the time of first depression medication prescription.

For a patient like Mrs. A, the barrier assessment might reveal concerns about stigma, concerns about treatment efficacy, fears about treatment, and misattributed depression etiology and symptoms. Some of these concerns might be related to both cultural factors and family influence. Aspects of psychoeducation, motivational interviewing, problem-solving, and treatment goal-setting would assist Mrs. A in understanding the benefit of depression treatment to her particular set of symptoms. Given the likely influence of Mrs. A's daughter in this case, including her in this discussion would likely be most helpful.

Nonattitudinal barriers such as polypharmacy or comorbid anxiety should also be explored. For polypharmacy, mental health providers should work with primary care providers to consolidate medication regimens as much as possible. Anxious depression can be effectively managed via (1) pretreatment accounting of physical symptoms of anxiety for comparison with later side effects (Stanley, Diefenbach, & Hopko, 2004); (2) altered antidepressant titration schedules ("start low, go slow, aim high, treat long"); (3) psychoeducation (Lenze et al., 2005);

(4) early supportive contact (Lenze, et al., 2005; Lenze, Mulsant, Shear, Houck, & Reynolds, 2002); and (5) cognitive-behavioral treatment strategies modified for anxious-elderly patients (Wetherell, Sorrell, Thorp, & Patterson, 2005).

Finally, for most of the barriers discussed, early supportive contact with the patient after the prescription, even if only a brief phone contact, is key. It appears that with Mrs. A, this did not occur, leading either to no-shows or appearing at the follow-up appointment and disclosing that she had stopped medication altogether. During such contacts, key concepts can be reinforced with the patient as well as objective discussion of any side effect concerns.

CONCLUSIONS: RECOMMENDATIONS/RESEARCH AGENDA

Depression treatment adherence in older adults is complex and is likely associated with multiple factors even for individual patients. While physicians may struggle with how to optimally prescribe antidepressant treatment in a population that often includes patients on complicated medication regimens, they should determine whether the patient is even taking the medication in the first place. Should providers find that the patient is nonadherent to treatment, factors suggested in this chapter may provide possible barriers to assess and discuss with their patients.

In terms of a research agenda, a further understanding of both the characteristics of older depressed patients that lead to optimal treatment adherence, and those that create barriers to adherence will provide the evidence base for crafting novel interventions to improve the effectiveness of antidepressant management. Interventions must target the specific type of nonadherence presented by elderly patients (Ayalon et al., 2005). Strategies to improve patient adherence need to be multidimensional, including consideration of age-related cognitive, comorbidity, environmental, and social factors (Murray, et al., 2004). Such interventions should also include consideration of a patient's disability, functional impairment, and depression characteristics—symptom profile, subtype, severity, age of onset, single episode versus recurrent, presence of family history, presence of suicide ideation, and prior experience with antidepressants.

Research should specifically focus on interventions that can be deployed within primary care practices, where depression in general, and geriatric depression specifically, is often missed or overlooked because clinical time is at a premium, and providers face competing demands for their attention when meeting with patients (Nutting, Rost, Smith, Werner, & Elliot, 2000). Time pressure may prevent the type of interaction that would help identify depression, determine the most acceptable course of treatment, or improve adherence.

On a policy level, disease management programs created and targeted specifically for older adults may also be a promising approach to effectively treating geriatric depression. While important progress has been made in increasing the detection of depression in elderly adults, greater focus now needs to shift toward treatment engagement and continuation to improve quality of life, reduce suffering, and achieve better outcomes.

Disclosures

Dr. Zivin has no conflicts to disclose. She is funded by the following grants: Department of Veterans Affairs (IIR 10–176–3 and CD2 07–206–1), NIH (P01 AG031098–01A1), and NIMH (R01MH087557–01).

Dr. Sirey has no conflicts to disclose. She is supported by individual grants from the National Institute for Mental Health (R01 MH087557 and R01 MH079265) and the Weill Cornell ACISR (P30 MH086943).

REFERENCES

Aikens, J. E., & Klinkman, M. S. (2012). Changes in patients' beliefs about their antidepressant during the acute phase of depression treatment. *General Hospital Psychiatry, 34*(3), 221–226.

Ajzen, I. (1996). The directive influence of attitudes on health behavior. In P. M. Gollwitzer & J. A. Bargh (Eds.), *The psychology of action: Linking cognition and motivation to behavior* (pp. 385–403). New York: Guilford Press.

Alexopoulos, G. S. (2005). Depression in the elderly. *Lancet, 365*(9475), 1961–1970.

Alexopoulos, G. S., Katz, I. R., Bruce, M. L., Heo, M., Ten Have, T., Raue, P., ... Reynolds, C. F., III. (2005). Remission in depressed geriatric primary care patients: A report from the PROSPECT study. *American Journal of Psychiatry, 162*(4), 718–724.

Angermeyer, M. C., & Dietrich, S. (2006). Public beliefs about and attitudes towards people with mental illness: A review of population studies. *Acta Psychiatrica Scandinavica, 113*(3), 163–179.

Arean, P. A., Alvidrez, J., Barrera, A., Robinson, G. S., & Hicks, S. (2002). Would older medical patients use psychological services? *Gerontologist, 42*(3), 392–398.

Aupperle, P. M., Lifchus, R., & Coyne, A. C. (1998). Past utilization of geriatric psychiatry outpatient services by a cohort of patients with major depression. *American Journal of Geriatric Psychiatry, 6*(4), 335–339.

Ayalon, L., Arean, P. A., & Alvidrez, J. (2005). Adherence to antidepressant medications in black and Latino elderly patients. *American Journal of Geriatric Psychiatry, 13*(7), 572–580.

Bambauer, K. Z., & Prigerson, H. G. (2006). The Stigma Receptivity Scale and its association with mental health service use among bereaved older adults. *Journal of Nervous and Mental Disease, 194*(2), 139–141.

Bambauer, K. Z., Safran, D. G., Ross-Degnan, D., Zhang, F., Adams, A. S., Gurwitz, J.,... Soumerai, S. B. (2007). Depression and cost-related medication nonadherence in Medicare beneficiaries. *Archives of General Psychiatry, 64*(5), 602–608.

Barat, I., Andreasen, F., & Damsgaard, E. M. (2001). Drug therapy in the elderly: What doctors believe and patients actually do. *British Journal of Clinical Pharmacology, 51*(6), 615–622.

Barg, F. K., Mavandadi, S., Givens, J. L., Knott, K., Zubritsky, C., & Oslin, D. W. (2010). When late-life depression improves: What do older patients say about their treatment? *American Journal of Geriatric Psychiatric, 18*(7), 596.

Bartels, S. J. (2003). Improving the system of care for older adults with mental illness in the United States. Findings and recommendations for the President's New Freedom Commission on Mental Health. *American Journal of Geriatric Psychiatry, 11*(5), 486–497.

Becker, M. H. (Ed.). (1974). The health belief model and personal health behavior. *Health Education Monographs, 2*.

Berkman, L. F., & Syme, S. L. (1979). Social networks, host resistance, and mortality: A nine-year follow-up study of Alameda County residents. *American Journal of Epidemiology, 109*(2), 186–204.

Blazer, D. G. (2005). The association between successful treatment of depression and physical functioning in older people seeking primary care. *Journal of the American Geriatrics Society, 53*(3), 543–544.

Blazer, D. G., Hybels, C. F., Simonsick, E. M., & Hanlon, J. T. (2000). Marked differences in antidepressant use by race in an elderly community sample: 1986–1996. *American Journal of Psychiatry, 157*(7), 1089–1094.

Bogardus, S. T., Jr., Bradley, E. H., Williams, C. S., Maciejewski, P. K., Gallo, W. T., & Inouye, S. K. (2004). Achieving goals in geriatric assessment: Role of caregiver agreement and adherence to recommendations. *Journal of the American Geriatrics Society, 52*(1), 99–105.

Bogner, H. R., Lin, J. Y., & Morales, K. H. (2006). Patterns of early adherence to the antidepressant citalopram among older primary care patients: The prospect study. *International Journal of Psychiatry in Medicine, 36*(1), 103–119.

Bosworth, H. B., Park, K. S., McQuoid, D. R., Hays, J. C., & Steffens, D. C. (2003). The impact of religious practice and religious coping on geriatric depression. *International Journal of Geriatric Psychiatry, 18*(10), 905–914.

Bruce, M. L., & Pearson, J. L. (1999). Designing an intervention to prevent suicide: PROSPECT (Prevention of Suicide in Primary Care Elderly: Collaborative Trial). *Dialogues in Clinical Neuroscience, 1*(2), 100–112.

Butler, R., Collins, E., Katona, C., & Orrell, M. (2000). How do general practitioners select antidepressants for depressed elderly people? *International Journal of Geriatric Psychiatry, 15*(7), 610–613.

Collins, K. A., Westra, H. A., Dozois, D. J., & Burns, D. D. (2004). Gaps in accessing treatment for anxiety and depression: Challenges for the delivery of care. *Clinical Psychology Review, 24*(5), 583–616.

Cooper, C., Carpenter, I., Katona, C., Schroll, M., Wagner, C., Fialova, D., & Livingston, G. (2005). The AdHOC Study of older adults' adherence to medication in 11 countries. *American Journal of Geriatric Psychiatry, 13*(12), 1067–1076.

Cooper, L. A., Brown, C., Vu, H. T., Ford, D. E., & Powe, N. R. (2001). How important is intrinsic spirituality in depression care? A comparison of white and African-American primary care patients. *Journal of General Internal Medicine, 16*(9), 634–638.

Cooper, L. A., Gonzales, J. J., Gallo, J. J., Rost, K. M., Meredith, L. S., Rubenstein, L. V.,... Ford, D. E. (2003). The acceptability of treatment for depression among African-American, Hispanic, and white primary care patients. *Medical Care, 41*(4), 479–489.

Cooper, L. A., Hill, M. N., & Powe, N. R. (2002). Designing and evaluating interventions to eliminate racial and ethnic disparities in health care. *Journal of General Internal Medicine, 17*(6), 477–486.

Cooper, L. A., Roter, D. L., Johnson, R. L., Ford, D.
E., Steinwachs, D. M., & Powe, N. R. (2003).
Patient-centered communication, ratings of care,
and concordance of patient and physician race.
Annals of Internal Medicine, 139(11), 907–915.

Cooper-Patrick, L., Powe, N. R., Jenckes, M. W.,
Gonzales, J. J., Levine, D. M., & Ford, D. E. (1997).
Identification of patient attitudes and preferences
regarding treatment of depression. *Journal of
General Internal Medicine, 12*(7), 431–438.

Cruz, M., & Pincus, H. A. (2002). Research on the
influence that communication in psychiatric
encounters has on treatment. *Psychiatric Services,
53*(10), 1253–1265.

Cruz, M., Schulz, R., Pincus, H. A., Houck, P. R.,
Bensasi, S., & Reynolds, C. F., III. (2009).
The association of public and private religious
involvement with severity of depression and
hopelessness in older adults treated for major
depression. *American Journal of Geriatric
Psychiatry, 17*(6), 503.

Crystal, S., Sambamoorthi, U., Walkup, J. T., &
Akincigil, A. (2003). Diagnosis and treatment of
depression in the elderly medicare population:
Predictors, disparities, and trends. *Journal of the
American Geriatrics Society, 51*(12), 1718–1728.

Datto, C. J., Oslin, D. W., Streim, J. E., Scheinthal,
S. M., DiFilippo, S., & Katz, I. R. (2002).
Pharmacologic treatment of depression in
nursing home residents: A mental health services
perspective. *Journal of Geriatric Psychiatry and
Neurology, 15*(3), 141–146.

DiMatteo, M. R., Lepper, H. S., & Croghan,
T. W. (2000). Depression is a risk factor for
noncompliance with medical treatment:
Meta-analysis of the effects of anxiety and
depression on patient adherence. *Archives of
Internal Medicine, 160*(14), 2101–2107.

Dobscha, S. K., Delucchi, K., & Young, M. L.
(1999). Adherence with referrals for outpatient
follow-up from a VA psychiatric emergency
room. *Community Mental Health Journal, 35*(5),
451–458.

Docherty, J. P. (1997). Barriers to the diagnosis of
depression in primary care. *Journal of Clinical
Psychiatry, 58*(Suppl 1), 5–10.

Doraiswamy, P. M., Khan, Z. M., Donahue, R. M., &
Richard, N. E. (2001). Quality of life in geriatric
depression: A comparison of remitters, partial
responders, and nonresponders. *American Journal
of Geriatric Psychiatry, 9*(4), 423–428.

Fabrega, H., Jr., Mulsant, B. M., Rifai, A. H., Sweet,
R. A., Pasternak, R., Ulrich, R., & Zubenko, G. S.
(1994). Ethnicity and psychopathology in an
aging hospital-based population. A comparison of
African-American and Anglo-European patients.
Journal of Nervous and Mental Disease, 182(3),
136–144.

Fawzi, W., Mohsen, M. Y. A., Hashem, A. H.,
Moussa, S., Coker, E., & Wilson, K. C. M. (2012).
Beliefs about medications predict adherence
to antidepressants in older adults. *International
Psychogeriatrics, 24*(1), 159–169.

Flint, A. J., & Rifat, S. L. (1997). Effect of
demographic and clinical variables on time to
antidepressant response in geriatric depression.
Depression and Anxiety, 5(2), 103–107.

Fortney, J. C., Pyne, J. M., Edlund, M. J., Stecker, T.,
Mittal, D., Robinson, D. E., & Henderson, K. L.
(2010). Reasons for antidepressant nonadherence
among veterans treated in primary care clinics.
Journal Clinical Psychiatry, 72(6), 827–834.

Gareri, P., Stilo, G., Bevacqua, I., Mattace, R., Ferreri,
G., & De Sarro, G. (1998). Antidepressant drugs in
the elderly. *General Pharmacology, 30*(4), 465–475.

Gerber, B. S., Cho, Y. I., Arozullah, A. M., & Lee, S.
Y. D. (2010). Racial differences in medication
adherence: A cross-sectional study of medicare
enrollees. *American Journal of Geriatric
Pharmacotherapy, 8*(2), 136–145.

Givens, J. L., Datto, C. J., Ruckdeschel, K., Knott, K.,
Zubritsky, C., Oslin, D. W., ... Barg, F. K. (2006).
Older patients' aversion to antidepressants.
A qualitative study. *Journal of General Internal
Medicine, 21*(2), 146–151.

Glanz, K., Rimer, B. K., & Viswanath, K. (2008).
*Health behavior and health education: Theory,
research, and practice.* San Francisco, CA:
Jossey-Bass.

Graham, K., Clarke, D., Bois, C., Carver, V., Dolinki,
L., Smythe, C., ... Brett, P. (1996). Addictive
behavior of older adults. *Addictive Behaviors,
21*(3), 331–348.

Gum, A., & Arean, P. A. (2004). Current status of
psychotherapy for mental disorders in the elderly.
Current Psychiatry Reports, 6(1), 32–38.

Halgin, R. P., Weaver, D. D., Edell, W. S., & Spencer,
P. G. (1987). Relation of depression and
help-seeking history to attitudes toward seeking
professional psychological help. *Journal of
Counseling Psychology, 34*(2), 177–185.

Hinton, L., Apesoa-Varano, E. C., González, H. M.,
Aguilar-Gaxiola, S., Dwight-Johnson, M., Barker,
J. C., ... Unützer, J. (2012). Falling through the
cracks: Gaps in depression treatment among older
Mexican-origin and white men. *International
Journal of Geriatric Psychiatry,* doi: 10.1002/
gps.3779. ePub ahead of print.

Hinton, L., Zweifach, M., Oishi, S., Tang, L., &
Unutzer, J. (2006). Gender disparities in the

treatment of late-life depression: Qualitative and quantitative findings from the IMPACT trial. *American Journal of Geriatric Psychiatry, 14*(10), 884–892.

Hohl, C. M., Dankoff, J., Colacone, A., & Afilalo, M. (2001). Polypharmacy, adverse drug-related events, and potential adverse drug interactions in elderly patients presenting to an emergency department. *Annals of Emergency Medicine, 38*(6), 666–671.

House, J. S., Landis, K. R., & Umberson, D. (1988). Social relationships and health. *Science, 241*(4865), 540–545.

Howland, M. J. (1997). *Examining the decision to seek professional psychological help: A comparison of attribution and attitude theory in predicting help-seeking intention using the theory of reasoned action.* Urbana-Champaign: University of Illinois.

Insel, K., Morrow, D., Brewer, B., & Figueredo, A. (2006). Executive function, working memory, and medication adherence among older adults. *Journals of Gerontology Series B, Psychological Sciences and Social Sciences, 61*(2), P102–107.

Ivanova, J. I., Bienfait-Beuzon, C., Birnbaum, H. G., Connolly, C., Emani, S., & Sheehy, M. (2011). Physicians decisions to prescribe antidepressant therapy in older patients with depression in a US managed care plan. *Drugs and Aging, 28*(1), 51–62.

Kales, H. C., Blow, F. C., Bingham, C. R., Copeland, L. A., & Mellow, A. M. (2000). Race and inpatient psychiatric diagnoses among elderly veterans. *Psychiatric Services, 51*(6), 795–800.

Kales, H. C., Nease, D. E., Jr, Sirey, J. A., Zivin, K., Kim, H. M., Kavanagh, J., Lynn, S., Chiang, C., Neighbors, H. W., Valenstein, M., Blow, F. C. Racial Differences in Adherence to Antidepressant Treatment in Later Life. *Am J Geriatr Psychiatry.* 2012 Oct 10. [Epub ahead of print]

Katon, W., Von Korff, M., Lin, E., Walker, E., Simon, G. E., Bush, T., ... Russo, J. (1995). Collaborative management to achieve treatment guidelines. Impact on depression in primary care. *Journal of the American Medical Association, 273*(13), 1026–1031.

Kaufman, D. W., Kelly, J. P., Rosenberg, L., Anderson, T. E., & Mitchell, A. A. (2002). Recent patterns of medication use in the ambulatory adult population of the United States: The Slone survey. *Journal of the American Medical Association, 287*(3), 337–344.

Kennedy, J. J., Maciejewski, M., Liu, D., & Blodgett, E. (2011). Cost-related nonadherence in the Medicare program: The impact of Part D. *Medical Care, 49*(5), 522.

Kessing, L. V., Hansen, H. V., Demyttenaere, K., & Bech, P. (2005). Depressive and bipolar disorders: Patients' attitudes and beliefs towards depression and antidepressants. *Psychological Medicine, 35*(8), 1205–1213.

Kilbourne, A. M., Reynolds, C. F., III, Good, C. B., Sereika, S. M., Justice, A. C., & Fine, M. J. (2005). How does depression influence diabetes medication adherence in older patients? *American Journal of Geriatric Psychiatry, 13*(3), 202–210.

Koenig, H. G. (1998). Religious attitudes and practices of hospitalized medically ill older adults. *International Journal of Geriatric Psychiatry, 13*(4), 213–224.

Koenig, H. G., Cohen, H. J., Blazer, D. G., Pieper, C., Meador, K. G., Shelp, F., ... DiPasquale, B. (1992). Religious coping and depression among elderly, hospitalized medically ill men. *American Journal of Psychiatry, 149*(12), 1693–1700.

Koenig, H. G., George, L. K., & Peterson, B. L. (1998). Religiosity and remission of depression in medically ill older patients. *American Journal of Psychiatry, 155*(4), 536–542.

Lenze, E. J. (2003). Comorbidity of depression and anxiety in the elderly. *Current Psychiatry Reports, 5*(1), 62–67.

Lenze, E. J., Karp, J. F., Mulsant, B. H., Blank, S., Shear, M. K., Houck, P. R., & Reynolds, C. F. (2005). Somatic symptoms in late-life anxiety: Treatment issues. *Journal of Geriatric Psychiatry and Neurology, 18*(2), 89–96.

Lenze, E. J., Mulsant, B. H., Dew, M. A., Shear, M. K., Houck, P., Pollock, B. G., & Reynolds, C. F., III. (2003). Good treatment outcomes in late-life depression with comorbid anxiety. *Journal of Affective Disorders, 77*(3), 247–254.

Lenze, E. J., Mulsant, B. H., Shear, M. K., Houck, P., & Reynolds, C. F., III. (2002). Anxiety symptoms in elderly patients with depression: What is the best approach to treatment? *Drugs Aging, 19*(10), 753–760.

Lenze, E. J., Mulsant, B. H., Shear, M. K., Schulberg, H. C., Dew, M. A., Begley, A. E., ... Reynolds, C. F., III. (2000). Comorbid anxiety disorders in depressed elderly patients. *American Journal of Psychiatry, 157*(5).

Leo, R. J., Narayan, D. A., Sherry, C., Michalek, C., & Pollock, D. (1997). Geropsychiatric consultation for African-American and Caucasian patients. *General Hospital Psychiatry, 19*(3), 216–222.

Lotrich, F. E., & Pollock, B. G. (2005). Aging and clinical pharmacology: Implications for antidepressants. *Journal of Clinical Pharmacology, 45*(10), 1106–1122.

Loya, A. M., González-Stuart, A., & Rivera, J. O. (2009). Prevalence of polypharmacy, polyherbacy, nutritional supplement use and potential product interactions among older adults living on the United States-Mexico border a descriptive, questionnaire-based study. *Drugs and Aging, 26*(5), 423–436.

MacLaughlin, E. J., Raehl, C. L., Treadway, A. K., Sterling, T. L., Zoller, D. P., & Bond, C. A. (2005). Assessing medication adherence in the elderly: Which tools to use in clinical practice? *Drugs and Aging, 22*(3), 231–255.

Maidment, R., Livingston, G., & Katona, C. (2002). Just keep taking the tablets: Adherence to antidepressant treatment in older people in primary care. *International Journal of Geriatric Psychiatry, 17*(8), 752–757.

Maixner, S. M., Struble, L., Blazek, M., & Kales, H. C. (2011). Later-life depression and heart failure. *Heart Failure Clinics, 7*(1), 47–58.

Mamdani, M., Herrmann, N., & Austin, P. (1999). Prevalence of antidepressant use among older people: Population-based observations. *Journal of the American Geriatrics Society, 47*(11), 1350–1353.

Mamdani, M., Rapoport, M., Shulman, K. I., Herrmann, N., & Rochon, P. A. (2005). Mental health-related drug utilization among older adults: Prevalence, trends, and costs. *American Journal of Geriatric Psychiatry, 13*(10), 892–900.

Marwaha, S., & Livingston, G. (2002). Stigma, racism or choice. Why do depressed ethnic elders avoid psychiatrists? *Journal of Affective Disorders, 72*(3), 257–265.

Mendes de Leon, C. F., Glass, T. A., Beckett, L. A., Seeman, T. E., Evans, D. A., & Berkman, L. F. (1999). Social networks and disability transitions across eight intervals of yearly data in the New Haven EPESE. *Journals of Gerontology Series B, Psychological Sciences and Social Sciences, 54*(3), S162–172.

Moller-Leimkuhler, A. M. (2002). Barriers to help-seeking by men: A review of sociocultural and clinical literature with particular reference to depression. *Journal of Affective Disorders, 71*(1–3), 1–9.

Moride, Y., Du Fort, G. G., Monette, J., Ducruet, T., Boivin, J. F., Champoux, N., & Crott, R. (2002). Suboptimal duration of antidepressant treatments in the older ambulatory population of Quebec: Association with selected physician characteristics. *Journal of the American Geriatrics Society, 50*(8), 1365–1371.

Mulsant, B. H., & Pollock, B. G. (1998). Treatment-resistant depression in late life. *Journal of Geriatric Psychiatry and Neurology, 11*(4), 186–193.

Mulsant, B. H., Reynolds, C. F., III, Shear, M. K., Sweet, R. A., & Miller, M. (1996). Comorbid anxiety disorders in late-life depression. *Anxiety, 2*(5), 242–247.

Mulsant, B. H., Stergiou, A., Keshavan, M. S., Sweet, R. A., Rifai, A. H., Pasternak, R., & Zubenko, G. S. (1993). Schizophrenia in late life: Elderly patients admitted to an acute care psychiatric hospital. *Schizophrenia Bulletin, 19*(4), 709–721.

Murray, M. D., Morrow, D. G., Weiner, M., Clark, D. O., Tu, W., Deer, M. M.,... Weinberger, M. (2004). A conceptual framework to study medication adherence in older adults. *American Journal of Geriatric Pharmacotherapy, 2*(1), 36–43.

National Advisory Mental Health Council's Workgroup on Aging Research. (2003). *Mental health for a lifetime: Research for the mental health needs of older Americans.* Rockville, MD: US Dept of Health and Human Services.

Neighbors, H. W., Musick, M. A., & Williams, D. R. (1998). The African American minister as a source of help for serious personal crises: Bridge or barrier to mental health care? *Health Education Behavior, 25*(6), 759–777.

Nelson, J. C., Clary, C. M., Leon, A. C., & Schneider, L. S. (2005). Symptoms of late-life depression: Frequency and change during treatment. *American Journal of Geriatric Psychiatry, 13*(6), 520–526.

Nutting, P. A., Rost, K., Smith, J., Werner, J. J., & Elliot, C. (2000). Competing demands from physical problems: Effect on initiating and completing depression care over 6 months. *Archives of Family Medicine, 9*(10), 1059–1064.

Ownby, R. L., Hertzog, C., Crocco, E., & Duara, R. (2006). Factors related to medication adherence in memory disorder clinic patients. *Aging and Mental Health, 10*(4), 378–385.

Piette, J. D., Heisler, M., & Wagner, T. H. (2004). Cost-related medication underuse among chronically Ill adults: The treatments people forgo, how often, and who is at risk. *American Journal of Public Health, 94*(10), 1782–1787.

Prabhakaran, P., & Butler, R. (2002). What are older peoples' experiences of taking antidepressants? *Journal of Affective Disorders, 70*(3), 319–322.

Pratt, L. A., Brody, Debra J, & Gu, Q. (2011). *Antidepressant use in persons aged 12 and over: United States, 2005–2008.* NCHS Data Brief 76. Hyattsville, MD: US Department of Health and Human Services.

Prochaska, J. O., & Di Clemente, C. C. (1983). Stages and processes of self-change of smoking: Toward an integrative model of change. *Journal of Consulting and Clinical Psychology, 51*, 390–395.

Rutz, W., von Knorring, L., Pihlgren, H., Rihmer, Z., & Walinder, J. (1995). Prevention of male suicides: Lessons from Gotland study. *Lancet, 345*(8948), 524.

Safran, D. G., Neuman, P., Schoen, C., Kitchman, M. S., Wilson, I. B., Cooper, B., … Rogers, W. H. (2005). Prescription drug coverage and seniors: Findings from a 2003 national survey. *Health Affairs*, W5–152–163.

Safran, D. G., Neuman, P., Schoen, C., Montgomery, J. E., Li, W., Wilson, I. B., … Rogers, W. H. (2002). Prescription drug coverage and seniors: How well are states closing the gap? *Health Affairs, Suppl Web Exclusives*, W253–268.

Salzman, C. (1995). Medication compliance in the elderly. *Journal of Clinical Psychiatry, 56*(Suppl 1), 18–22; discussion 23.

Salzman, C. (2004). Late-life anxiety disorders. *Psychopharmacology Bulletin, 38*(1), 25–30.

Seeman, T. E. (1996). Social ties and health: The benefits of social integration. *Annals of Epidemiology, 6*(5), 442–451.

Sher, I., McGinn, L., Sirey, J. A., & Meyers, B. (2005). Effects of caregivers' perceived stigma and causal beliefs on patients' adherence to antidepressant treatment. *Psychiatric Services, 56*(5), 564–569.

Sirey, J. A., Bruce, M. L., & Alexopoulos, G. S. (2005). The Treatment Initiation Program: An Intervention to Improve Depression Outcomes in Older Adults. *American Journal of Psychiatry, 162*(1), 184–186.

Sirey, J. A., Bruce, M. L., Alexopoulos, G. S., Perlick, D. A., Friedman, S. J., & Meyers, B. S. (2001a). Stigma as a barrier to recovery: Perceived stigma and patient-rated severity of illness as predictors of antidepressant drug adherence. *Psychiatric Services, 52*(12), 1615–1620.

Sirey, J. A., Bruce, M. L., Alexopoulos, G. S., Perlick, D. A., Raue, P., Friedman, S. J., & Meyers, B. S. (2001b). Perceived stigma as a predictor of treatment discontinuation in young and older outpatients with depression. *American Journal of Psychiatry, 158*(3), 479–481.

Sirey, A. J., Bruce, M. L., & Kales, H. C. (2010). Improving antidepressant adherence and depression outcomes in primary care: The Treatment Initiation and Participation (TIP) program. *American Journal of Geriatric Psych, 18*(6), 554–562

Solberg, L. I., Korsen, N., Oxman, T. E., Fischer, L. R., & Bartels, S. (1999). The need for a system in the care of depression. *Journal of Family Practice, 48*(12), 973–979.

Sorensen, L., Stokes, J. A., Purdie, D. M., Woodward, M., & Roberts, M. S. (2005). Medication management at home: Medication-related risk factors associated with poor health outcomes. *Age and Ageing, 34*(6), 626–632.

Soumerai, S. B., Pierre-Jacques, M., Zhang, F., Ross-Degnan, D., Adams, A. S., Gurwitz, J., … Safran, D. G. (2006). Cost-related medication nonadherence among elderly and disabled Medicare beneficiaries: A national survey 1 year before the Medicare drug benefit. *Archives of Internal Medicine, 166*(17), 1829–1835.

Stanley, M. A., Diefenbach, G. J., & Hopko, D. R. (2004). Cognitive behavioral treatment for older adults with generalized anxiety disorder. A therapist manual for primary care settings. *Behavior Modification, 28*(1), 73–117.

Steffens, D. C., & McQuoid, D. R. (2005). Impact of symptoms of generalized anxiety disorder on the course of late-life depression. *American Journal of Geriatric Psychiatry, 13*(1), 40–47.

Steffens, D. C., Skoog, I., Norton, M. C., Hart, A. D., Tschanz, J. T., Plassman, B. L., … Breitner, J. C. S. (2000). Prevalence of depression and its treatment in an elderly population: The Cache County study. *Archives of General Psychiatry, 57*(6), 601–607.

Thase, M. E. (2003). New approaches to managing difficult-to-treat depressions. *Journal of Clinical Psychiatry, 64*(Supp 1), 3–4.

Thoits, P. A. (1995). Stress, coping, and social support processes: Where are we? What next? *Journal of Health and Social Behavior, 35*(extra issue), 53–79.

US Department of Health and Human Services. (1999). *Mental health: A report of the Surgeon General*. Rockville, MD: US Department of Health and Human Services, National Institutes of Health, National Institutes of Mental Health.

Unützer, J., Katon, W., Callahan, C. M., Williams, J. W., Jr., Hunkeler, E., Harpole, L., … Treatment, Impact Investigators. (2002). Collaborative care management of late-life depression in the primary care setting: A randomized controlled trial. *Journal of the American Medical Association, 288*(22), 2836–2845.

Van Voorhees, B. W., Fogel, J., Houston, T. K., Cooper, L. A., Wang, N. Y., & Ford, D. E. (2005). Beliefs and attitudes associated with the intention to not accept the diagnosis of depression among young adults. *Annals of Family Medicine, 3*(1), 38–46.

Van Voorhees, B. W., Fogel, J., Houston, T. K., Cooper, L. A., Wang, N-Y., & Ford, D. E. (2006). Attitudes and illness factors associated with low perceived need for depression treatment among young adults. *Social Psychiatry and Psychiatric Epidemiology, 41*(9), 746–754.

Voils, C. I., Steffens, D. C., Flint, E. P., & Bosworth, H. B. (2005). Social support and locus of control as predictors of adherence to antidepressant medication in an elderly population. *American Journal of Geriatric Psychiatry, 13*(2), 157–165.

Weintraub, M. (1990). Compliance in the elderly. *Clinics in Geriatric Medicine, 6*(2), 445–452.

Wetherell, J. L., Sorrell, J. T., Thorp, S. R., & Patterson, T. L. (2005). Psychological interventions for late-life anxiety: A review and early lessons from the CALM study. *Journal of Geriatric Psychiatry and Neurology, 18*(2), 72–82.

Williams, C. M. (2002). Using medications appropriately in older adults. *American Family Physician, 66*(10), 1917–1924.

Young, A. S., Klap, R., Sherbourne, C. D., & Wells, K. B. (2001). The quality of care for depressive and anxiety disorders in the United States. *Archives of General Psychiatry, 58*(1), 55–61.

Zivin, K., & Kales, H.C. (2008). Adherence to depression treatment in older adults: a narrative review. *Drugs and Aging, 25*(7), 559–571.

Zivin, K., Kim, H. M., McCarthy, J. F., Austin, K. L., Hoggatt, K. J., Walters, H., & Valenstein, M. (2007). Suicide mortality among individuals receiving treatment for depression in the Veterans Affairs health system: Associations with patient and treatment setting characteristics. *American Journal of Public Health, 97*(12), 2193–2198.

Zivin, K., Madden, J., Graves, A., Zhang, F., & Soumerai, S. (2009). Cost-related medication nonadherence among beneficiaries with depression following Medicare Part D. *American Journal of Geriatric Psychiatry, 17*(12), 1068–1076.

SECTION 4

CARE DELIVERY SYSTEMS

27

DEPRESSION IN LONG-TERM CARE

Christina Hui and David L. Sultzer

THE POPULATION of older adults receiving long-term care (LTC) is growing rapidly. In 2009, 9 million Americans over the age of 65 required LTC, defined as "services and supports that meet health or personal needs over an extended period of time." This number is expected to reach 12 million by 2020 (Tumilson & Woods, 2007; US Department of Health and Human Services, 2009). The majority of people who require LTC are over 65 years old (Komisar & Rogers, 2003). LTC can be provided in the community or by a facility, and it includes a wide range of services. Eighty-three percent of people requiring LTC live in the community, and most receive help from informal caregivers, typically relatives. Options for facility-based care include assisted living facilities (ALFs), continuing-care retirement communities, and nursing homes (NHs). NHs provide 24-hour skilled nursing care, and NH care accounts for over 60% of federal LTC spending (Sahyoun, Pratt, Lentzner, Dey, & Robinson, 2001; Tumilson & Woods, 2007).

NHs are a special venue in which to provide psychiatric care. They are a unique psychosocial environment for a distinct patient population that is vulnerable to particular disorders. NHs are continually staffed, are governed by rules, and subject to federal legislation. These characteristics must be factored into any mental health treatment plan for a NH resident. This chapter describes the NH environment and offers recommendations for the psychiatric assessment and treatment of common mood syndromes. The mental health consultant's role and the changing nature of LTC are also discussed.

WHO RESIDES IN NURSING HOMES?

The Centers for Disease Control and Prevention (CDC) estimate that there are 16,000 NHs with 1.5 million residents in the United States (Centers for Disease Control and Prevention, 2008). The number of NH residents is expected to double by 2030 (Sahyoun et al., 2001). The proportion of residents older than 85 has increased, and this age group currently comprises the largest percentage (37.1%) of the NH population (Centers for Medicare & Medicaid Services, 2010). NH residents have also progressively required more assistance with basic activities of daily living, which includes dressing, bathing, toileting, eating, and mobility (Jones, Dwyer, Bercovitz, & Strahan, 2009). Over the past two decades, the mean length of NH stay has declined (Jones et al., 2009; Tumilson & Woods, 2007), although the number of those who reside in NHs for more than 3 years has remained stable (Decker, 2005), comprising 25%–30% of the NH population (Jones et al., 2009).

In the United States and other developed countries, an average of 58% of NH residents have Alzheimer's disease or other dementia syndrome (Centers for Medicare & Medicaid Services, 2010; Seitz, Purandare, & Conn, 2010). NH placement often occurs as a result of severe cognitive impairment, multiple care needs, frequent behavior problems (including psychosis, aggression, and restlessness), and caregiver burden (Etters, Goodall, & Harrison, 2008; Gaugler, Duval, Anderson, & Kane, 2007; Gaugler, Yu, Krichbaum, & Wyman, 2009; Gaugler et al., 2011; Sörensen & Conwell, 2011). Other chronic medical illnesses associated with NH admission are diabetes, hypertension, cancer, and stroke (Gaugler et al., 2007). Because the NH population is advanced in years, with substantial functional disability, cognitive impairment, and medical burden, involvement of mental health providers with subspecialty training in geriatrics can be beneficial.

PSYCHIATRIC DISORDERS IN THE NURSING HOME

Estimated prevalence rates of mental illness in the NH range from 65% to 91% (American Geriatrics Society and American Association for Geriatric Psychiatry, 2003). Dementia is the most common psychiatric disorder, and neuropsychiatric symptoms of dementia (NPS) affect 61%–92% of NH residents worldwide (Seitz et al., 2010). Mood symptoms are also common. Recent estimates indicate that 50% of residents have clinically significant depression, 21% have anxiety, 6% have schizophrenia, and 4% have mania (Centers for Medicare & Medicaid Services, 2010). This chapter focuses on the presentation, assessment, and treatment of depressive symptoms specifically in the NH setting.

FEDERAL LEGISLATION FOR THE NURSING HOME

The federal government has established guidelines to promote optimal detection and treatment of psychiatric disorders in NHs. In the 1980s, the public was concerned about the institutionalization of patients with chronic mental illness in NHs and the subsequent use of restraints or psychotropic medications for controlling undesired behavior (Borson, Loebel, Kitchell, Domoto, & Hyde, 1997; Mintzer, Kennedy et al., 2003). The federal government passed the Omnibus Budget Reconciliation Act in 1987 (OBRA-87), which was implemented by the Health Care Financing Administration, now known as the Centers for Medicare and Medicaid Services (CMS). OBRA-87 created the Preadmission Screening and Resident Review (PASRR) for all CMS-certified NHs, which evaluates whether individuals with "serious mental illness" require 24-hour skilled nursing care and recommends appropriate psychiatric follow-up (Centers for Medicare & Medicaid Services, 2011; Linkins, Lucca, Housman, & Smith, 2006; Snowden, Piacitelli, & Koepsell, 1998). OBRA-87 also created the Minimum Data Set (MDS), a biopsychosocial assessment that describes NH residents' demographics, cognitive deficits, physical needs, and customary routines. The MDS documents all medical information and tracks mood, behavior, and psychosocial well-being. MDS is typically administered by a nurse at admission and updated quarterly (Centers for Medicare & Medicaid Services, 2010; Fullerton, McGuire, Feng, Mor, & Grabowski, 2009; Horgas & Margrett 2001; Reichman & Katz, 2009; Ruckdeschel, Thompson et al., 2004). The most recent version of MDS, 3.0, implemented in October 2010, includes the Patient Health Questionnaire-9 (PHQ-9), a standardized rating scale that has been used to identify major depressive disorder (MDD) in elderly primary care outpatients (Phelan et al., 2010). For MDS 3.0, PHQ-9 is administered as a self-report interview, and the PHQ-9 observer version is used for noncommunicative residents (Saliba & Buchanan, 2008).

PREVALENCE, RISK, AND CONSEQUENCES OF DEPRESSION IN THE NURSING HOME

Depressive symptoms in older adults can present as *Diagnostic Statistical and Manual of Mental Disorders* (*DSM*) defined disorders, such as major depressive disorder (MDD), dysthymia, and depression secondary to a general medical condition (American Psychiatric Association, 2000). Also common is minor depression, which describes symptoms that do not meet the criteria for MDD but results in similar subjective distress and disability (Blazer, 2003). Rates of MDD in NH range from 10% to 25%, and up to 70% of NH residents report depressive symptoms (Jones et al., 2009; Reichman & Katz, 2009). Because dementia is common in NHs, "depression without sadness," characterized by apathy, "vascular depression," manifested by cerebral white matter disease and executive dysfunction, and depression in Alzheimer's disease are also present

(Olin et al., 2002; Reichman & Katz, 2009; Thakur & Blazer, 2008)

Late-life depression is linked to multiple medical comorbidities, cognitive impairment, disability, and physical relocation (Alexopoulos, 2005), and thus LTC populations are vulnerable. Significant risk factors for depression in NH populations include visual impairment, stroke, loneliness, lack of social support, negative life events, and perceived inadequacy of care (Jongenelis et al., 2004). Prior antidepressant treatment showed the strongest association with incident depression after NH admission in one study, followed by prior institutionalization and daily pain (Hoover et al., 2010). For both community- and NH-dwelling elderly, depressive symptoms are associated with increased mortality (Bruce & Leaf, 1989; Cooper, Harris, & McGready, 2002), suggesting that treating depression may decrease mortality risk (Cooper et al., 2002; Kane, Yochim, & Lichtenberg, 2010).

THE EFFECT OF NURSING HOME LIFE ON DEPRESSION

Admission to an LTC setting has been associated with depressive symptoms. Some authors have described an adjustment period to NH residence, which may last as long as 12 months, involve emotional upheaval, and conclude when residents are able to extend support to incoming residents

(Brooke, 1989; Patterson, 1995; Wilson, 1997). Studies have examined the incidence and prevalence of depression from time of NH admission to the end of the first year of residence. In some samples, depression rates decrease over time. Among 201 patients admitted to an LTC facility, approximately 20% had depression at admission, and after 12 months, only 8% of the original group remained depressed. The incidence of depression was 6.4% at 1 year. This decline could be due to detection and treatment of depression (Payne et al., 2002). On the other hand, Hoover et al. noted that one third of newly admitted LTC residents had depression, and by 12 months, 54% were diagnosed with depression (Hoover et al., 2010). Certainly, the NH setting is stressful, as patients potentially face many losses, including independence, privacy, possessions, connection to the outside world, and ability to maintain a personal schedule. Emotional distress can arise when residents interact with severely demented peers or when their peers die (Choi, Ransom, & Wyllie, 2008). Few studies have examined the association between characteristics of the NH facility and depression. Results have suggested that urban settings (Dobalian, Tsao, & Radcliff, 2003) and high staff turnover rates (Doyle, 1995) may contribute to mood symptoms in residents. Understanding risk factors and vulnerable times for depression can guide clinicians to effectively intervene. Subjective patient distress seems greatest early after admission (Patterson, 1995), and residents with a past history of depression, antidepressant treatment, or psychiatric hospitalizations may benefit from closer monitoring.

DETECTION AND ASSESSMENT OF DEPRESSION IN NURSING HOMES

Detecting depression in the NH population can be challenging. Older adults may minimize depressive symptoms (Blazer, 2003). Neurovegetative symptoms of depression, such as weight loss, fatigue, and poor appetite, may be misattributed to medical conditions. Depressive symptoms may be partly masked and manifest as social isolation, uncooperativeness, pain, somatic preoccupations, excessive sedative use, and cognitive complaints (Alexopoulos et al., 2002; Reichman & Katz, 2009). Patients with dementia may be unable to communicate emotional distress. Also, depression tends to be underreported in NHs, despite the continuous presence of care providers.

In a sample of 319 NH residents, 44% had some type of depression, but nursing aides, nurses, and social workers all estimated depressive symptoms in fewer than 32% of these patients (Teresi, Abrams, Holmes, Ramirez, & Eimicke, 2001).

Mental health clinicians in the LTC setting must be aware of the heterogeneity of mood symptoms and confounding etiologies for depression. For NH residents, assessment includes a thorough evaluation of all observed behaviors. Collateral information comes predominantly from the NH staff who care for residents daily, and the consulting psychiatrist should incorporate staff observations to help with diagnosis (Loebel et al., 1991).

The American Geriatric Society (AGS) and American Association for Geriatric Psychiatry (AAGP) created an expert panel to establish guidelines for the optimal assessment and treatment of depression and NPS in the NH setting (American Geriatrics Society and American Association for Geriatric Psychiatry, 2003; Snowden, Sato, & Roy-Byrne, 2003). The panel recommended that depression assessment occur within the first month of NH admission, with serial screenings every 6 months thereafter. Standardized scales, such as the Geriatric Depression Scale (GDS), used for patients with mild cognitive impairment, or the Cornell Scale for Depression in Depression (CSDD), which is appropriate for residents with moderate to severe dementia, can be used to screen for depression (American Geriatrics Society and American Association for Geriatric Psychiatry, 2003). While the MDS includes several mood items, depression rating scales derived from MDS versions prior to 3.0 have demonstrated only poor to fair validity for the diagnosis of depression (Burrows, Morris, Simon, Hirdes, & Phillips, 2000; Reichman & Katz, 2009; Ruckdeschel, Thompson, Datto, Streim, & Katz, 2004) and should not be the sole source of information for diagnosing depression (American Geriatrics Society and American Association for Geriatric Psychiatry, 2003). Although there are no controlled studies of the utility or cost-effectiveness of medical evaluation for depression in NH residents (Snowden et al., 2003), standard diagnostic workup of late-life depression includes a thorough history, a physical exam, and basic laboratory studies to rule out other medical causes of depressive symptoms (Birrer & Vemuri, 2004; Blazer, 2003; Blazer & Steffens, 2009). This standard of care has been incorporated into the AGS/AAGP guidelines and additional international recommendations (American Geriatrics Society and American Association for Geriatric Psychiatry, 2003; Koopmans, Zuidema, Leontjevas, & Gerritsen, 2010). Table 27.1 summarizes the approach to assessing depression in the NH resident.

History should encompass current depressive symptoms, suicidal ideas, comorbid substance abuse disorders, past history of mood syndromes, and treatment response. Psychosocial stressors of the NH milieu involving changes in staff, routines, or environment should be investigated. Medical information should review current medications, pain management, nutritional status, and onset of new physical illnesses (American Geriatrics Society and American Association for Geriatric Psychiatry, 2003). Various classes of drugs, including steroids, cardiovascular, chemotherapeutic, anti-Parkinson's, antipsychotics, anticonvulsants, and hormones have been associated with depressive symptoms. Medical conditions such as dementia, Parkinson's disease, and malignancies can present with depressive symptoms (Birrer & Vemuri, 2004). Laboratory workup recommended for NH residents includes electrolytes, complete blood count, thyroid function, vitamin B12, and relevant serum drug levels (American Geriatrics Society and American Association for Geriatric Psychiatry, 2003). While not addressed specifically in LTC, additional diagnostic studies recommended for some patients with late-life depression include electrocardiogram, brain magnetic resonance imaging to evaluate for vascular dementia, and polysomnography to identify sleep disorders (Blazer, 2003; Blazer & Steffens, 2009). Finally, a mental health professional should be consulted if there is psychosis, suicidal ideation, or poor response to the medication treatment (American Geriatrics Society and American Association for Geriatric Psychiatry, 2003).

PHARMACOLOGICAL TREATMENT OF DEPRESSION IN LONG-TERM CARE

Antidepressants are commonly prescribed in the NH. Recent cross-sectional MDS data indicate that nationwide, 49.5% of NH residents were prescribed an antidepressant daily during the prior week (Centers for Medicare & Medicaid Services, 2010). Selective serotonin reuptake inhibitors (SSRIs) accounted for 68% of antidepressant prescriptions in US NHs in 2004 (Brown, Lapane, & Luisi, 2002; Karkare, Bhattacharjee, Kamble, & Aparasu, 2011).

Table 27.1 Assessment of Depression in Nursing Homes

Screening: At time of nursing home admission, and subsequent 6-month intervals, or when there is concern for depressive symptoms

- Geriatric Depression Scale: self-report, for mild to moderate cognitively impaired
- Cornell Scale for Depression in Dementia: observer rated, for moderate to severe dementia

Diagnostic Interview: Performed when depressive symptoms (new onset or worsening of symptoms) are identified

- Symptom history: symptoms during current depressive episode; suicidal ideation
- Past psychiatric history: past episodes of depression, mania, psychotic features; past treatment response
- Social history: substance abuse disorders
- Changes in nursing home milieu: visitors or staff, changes in physical environment, participation in social activities, possible unmet needs, other psychosocial stressors

Medical Workup: rule out any underlying condition that may be causing/exacerbating symptoms

- History and Physical:
  - Include assessment for pain, nutritional status, cognitive screening
  - Current management of chronic medical conditions
  - Onset of new medical conditions
  - Review medication list for medications that can contribute to mood symptoms
- Labs:
  - Basic metabolic panel
  - Complete blood count
  - Thyroid-stimulating hormone

Mental Health Referral:

- Suicidal ideation
- Presence of psychotic symptoms
- Diagnostic uncertainty or mixed syndromes
- Minimal response after adequate trial (6–12 weeks) of antidepressant medications

Sources: American Geriatrics Society and American Association for Geriatric Psychiatry, 2003; Birrer & Virduma, 2004; Blazer, 2009; Blazer, Steffens, et al., 2009; Koopmans et al., 2010.

Findings From Clinical Trials—Efficacy

Despite the frequent use of antidepressants and the unique LTC population, only 12 controlled trials of antidepressants in the NH setting have been published. Six antidepressants have been studied, in decreasing order of frequency: sertraline, nortriptyline, fluoxetine, paroxetine, mirtazapine, and venlafaxine (Burrows, Salzman, Satlin, Noble, Pollock, & Gersh, 2002; Datto et al., 2002; Katz, Simpson, Curlik, Parmelee, & Muhly, 1990; Magai, Kennedy, Cohen, & Gomberg, 2000; Nelson et al., 2006; Reichman & Katz, 2009; Oslin et al., 2000, 2003; Roose et al., 2003; Rosen, Mulsant et al., 2000; Streim et al., 2000; Trappler &

Cohen, 1996, 1998; Weintraub et al., 2003). Sample sizes in trials ranged from 12 to 115 patients, with most including fewer than 50 subjects. Trial duration ranged from 7 to 12 weeks. Among nine studies reporting Mini-Mental Status Exam (MMSE) score, the weighted average score at baseline (representing 409 patients) was 21.6, and 39 of those patients had either Alzheimer's or vascular dementia. The Hamilton Depression Rating Scale (HAM-D) was consistently used to measure treatment outcome. Overall, the trials included small samples for short treatment periods, and most lacked placebo control. Summary findings of the 12 antidepressant trials are provided in Tables 27.2–27.5. Overall, approximately 50% of patients

Table 27.2 Randomized, Double-Blind, Controlled Trials of Antidepressant Treatment in Nursing Homes

STUDY	DRUG	DURATION	SAMPLE CHARACTERISTICS	OUTCOME MEASURES	COMMENTS
Katz et al., 1990	Nortriptyline Flexible dosing: titrate to plasma level 80–120 Mean dose: 65 mg Mean plasma level: 76 ng/ml	7 weeks	N = 30 Mean age: 84 Depression: MDD[1] (*DSM-III* criteria) Mild to moderate cognitive impairment included 23/30 completed	HAM-D[2] CGI[3] GDS[4]	Improvement from baseline on HAM-D and CGI in both groups Greater improvement in the nortriptyline group 34% dropout secondary to side effects in nortriptyline group
Magai et al., 2000	Sertraline Fixed dosing: 100 mg week	8 weeks	N = 31 Mean age: 89 Depression: MDD, minor depression (CSDD)[5] Alzheimer's Disease required 27/31 completed	CSDD GS[6] CMAI[7] AFBS[8] Facial behaviors, "knit-brow"	Improvement from baseline on CSDD in both groups; no significant difference between groups No significant improvement in target symptoms of agitation or feeding
Burrows et al., 2002	Paroxetine Flexible dosing: 10–30 mg Mean dose: 23 mg	8 weeks	N = 20 Mean age: 88 Depression: minor depression (GDS) Mild to moderate cognitive impairment included, but not required (MMSE[9] range: 16–30)	Nurse-rated CGI HAM-D CSDD GDS	Improvement from baseline on CGI and HAM-D for both groups; no significant difference between groups Two cases of delirium in paroxetine group Mean decrease of 2 points in MMSE for paroxetine group ($p = .03$)

[1]Major Depressive Disorder, [2]Hamilton Depression Rating Scale, [3]Clinical Global Impression, [4]Geriatric Depression Scale, [5]Cornell Scale for Depression in Dementia, [6]Gestalt Scale, [7]Cohen-Mansfield Agitation Inventory, [8]Aversive Feeding Behavior Scale, [9]Mini Mental Status Examination.

Table 27.3 Open-Label Antidepressant Trials in Nursing Homes

STUDY	DRUG	DURATION	SAMPLE CHARACTERISTICS	OUTCOME MEASURES	COMMENTS
Trappler & Cohen, 1996	Fluoxetine Flexible dosing: 10–40 mg Mean dose: 19 mg	12 weeks	N = 29 Mean age: 89 Depression: MDD[1] (*DSM-IV*) Dementia: Alzheimer's disease and vascular dementia included, but not required 26/29 completed	HAM-D[2] Zung depression scale	50% attained a 50% decline in HAM-D scores Nonresponders more likely to have underlying neurological disease Side effects, in decreasing frequency: anorexia, sedation, insomnia, nervousness, sweating
Rosen et al., 2000	Sertraline Flexible dosing: 50–100 mg Mean dose: 58 mg	6 weeks	N = 12 Mean age: 83 Depression: Minor depression (*DSM-IV*) Mild to moderate cognitive impairment included, but not required (MMSE[3] range: 11–29) 12/12 completed	HAM-D GAS[4]	75% attained 50% decline or endpoint <10 score on HAM-D Side effects: constipation, diarrhea, nausea, dizziness, tremor
Nelson et al., 2006 *subgroup from Roose et al. 2003	Mirtazapine Flexible dosing: 15 to 45 mg Mean dose:19 mg	12 weeks	N = 50 Mean age: 89 Depression: Physician-diagnosed Cognitive status: MMSE >10 included; average: 20 36/50 completed	HAM-D CSDD[5] CGI[6]	Mean HAM-D scores declined from 17 to 7 55% response on CGI 10% discontinued because of adverse events Mean increase in weight of 0.6 kg
Roose et al., 2003	Mirtazapine Flexible dosing: 15–45 mg Mean dose: 19 mg	23 weeks	N = 124 Mean age: 83 Depression: physician diagnosed Cognitive status: MMSE >10 included, average: 22 110/124 completed	CGI HAM-D CSDD	47% with ≥ 50% decline in HAM- score ($p < .0001$) 54% "very much" or "much" improved on CGI Adverse events: fall (18%) 10% with ≥ 7% weight gain; 4% with ≥7% weight loss

[1]Major Depressive Disorder, [2]Hamilton Depression Rating Scale, [3]Mini Mental Status Examination, [4]Global Assessment Scale, [5]Cornell Scale of Depression in Dementia, [6]Clinical Global Impression.

Table 27.4 Comparison Trials of Antidepressants in the Nursing Home

STUDY	DRUG	DURATION	SAMPLE CHARACTERISTICS	OUTCOME MEASURES	COMMENTS
Trappler & Choen, 1996	Fluoxetine Flexible dosing: 10–20 mg Mean dose: 18 mg Sertraline Flexible dosing: 50–100 mg Mean dose: 77 mg Paroxetine Flexible dosing: 10–20 mg Mean dose: 19 mg	12 weeks, open label	N= 50 Mean age: 89 Depression: MDD[1] (DSM-IV) Dementia: Alzheimer's disease and vascular dementia included, but not required 50/50 completed	HAM-D[2] Zung depression scale	Overall, 42% with at least 50% improvement on HAM-D No significant difference between groups Side effects: 15%–25% with anorexia; <10%: with somnolence, nausea, diarrhea, headache, anxiety, sweating, insomnia
Oslin et al., 2000	Sertraline Flexible dosing: 50 to 100 mg Mean dose: 83 mg Nortriptyline (see Streim, et al. 2000)	10 weeks, open label	N = 28 Mean age: 81 Depression: MDD, minor depression, or dysthymia (GDS or HAM-D & DSM-III) Cognition: Blessed Information-Memory-Concentration test score ≤18 15/28 completed	HAM-D	Overall, 45% obtained ≥33% improvement on HAM-D 68% of regular dose nortriptyline, 18% low dose nortriptyline, and 33% sertraline responded No difference in tolerability
Oslin, Ten Have, et al., 2003	Venlafaxine Fixed dosing: 150 mg Sertraline Fixed dosing: 100 mg	10 weeks RCT, double-blind, no placebo	N = 52 Mean age: 83 Depression: MDD, minor depression, dysthmia (DSM-IV) Depression in dementia included 33/52 completed	HAM-D CSDD[3] nurse rated CGI[4]	Both groups showed improvement in HAM-D scores (p = .069) Higher rate of dropout due to side effects in the venlafaxine group than in the sertraline group

[1] Major Depressive Disorder, [2] Hamilton Depression Rating Scale, [3] Cornell Scale of Depression in Dementia, [4] Clinical Global Impression.

Table 27.5 Trials Examining Dose and Duration in Nursing Homes

STUDY	DRUG	DURATION	SAMPLE CHARACTERISTICS	OUTCOME MEASURES	COMMENTS
Streim et al., 2000	Nortriptyline Flexible dosing High dose: 60–80 mg, plasma range 80–110 ng/ml Low dose: 10–13 mg, plasma range: 1/6 of high dose	10 weeks Randomized, double-blind no placebo control	N = 69 Mean age: 80 Depression: MDD[1], minor depression, or dysthymia (DSM-IV) Mild to moderate cognitive impairment included but not required (mean MMSE[2]: 21) 47/69 completed	HAM-D[3] GDS[4] CGI[5]	Improvement on HAM-D & GDS in both groups, but no difference between low-dose and high-dose groups Greater improvement on HAM-D and GDS with higher MMSE scores in high-dose group only
Weintraub et al., 2003	Sertraline Fixed dosing: 200 mg *prior treatment sertraline 100 mg	8 weeks	N = 23 Mean age: 82 Depression: HAM-D ≥ 12 and persistence of depressive symptoms Severe cognitive impairment excluded (Blessed Information-Memory-Concentration test score >23) 16/23 completed	HAM-D	52% with >50% response on HAM-D 39% responded during extension phase Rate of discontinuation due to side effects comparable between both doses

[1] Major Depressive Disorder, [2] Mini-mental Status Exam, [3] Hamilton Depression Rating Scale, [4] Geriatric Depression Scale, [5] Clinical Global Impression.

met the criteria for substantial improvement in depressive symptoms, predominantly in open-label and drug comparison trials. Patients with minor depression and those with cognitive disorders did not appear to respond as robustly as cognitively intact patients with major depression.

Nortriptyline, sertraline, and paroxetine were each examined in a randomized, double-blind, placebo-controlled trial (Burrows et al., 2002; Katz et al., 1990; Magai et al., 2000). Significant improvement in depression was noted only in the nortriptyline trial, which included patients with major depression and mild to moderate cognitive impairment. In contrast, the sertraline sample recruited late-stage Alzheimer's disease patients, and the paroxetine study only included patients with minor depression. In the paroxetine study, there was a trend for patients with more severe depressive symptoms to have greater improvement after treatment ($p = .06$) (Burrows et al., 2002). Response rates in the paroxetine trial were 77.7% and 45.5% for the treatment and placebo groups, respectively (Burrows et al., 2002). In the sertraline trial, response rates were approximately 50% for both groups (Magai et al., 2000). These placebo rates are higher than the placebo rate of 34.7% noted in a meta-analysis of 10 antidepressant trials in late-life depression (Nelson, Delucchi, & Schneider, 2008).

In open-label trials, sertraline, mirtazapine, and fluoxetine have been beneficial, although there are no placebo controls for comparison. Based on HAM-D score criteria, approximately 50% of patients responded in each trial, and in one study 81% of patients no longer met criteria for MDD at the end of the trial (Roose et al., 2003; Rosen, Mulsant, & Pollock, 2000; Trappler & Cohen, 1996). To determine whether patient characteristics influence treatment response, investigators re-examined the mirtazapine study data. Advanced age, medical burden, and cognitive impairment did not predict poorer outcome in this study (Nelson et al., 2007), suggesting that antidepressants can be effective in the older, frail NH population. Studies have also examined the effects of medication dose and duration in the NH population. Sixty-nine patients randomized to either a regular (60–80 mg) or low (10–13 mg) daily dose of nortriptyline had comparable significant improvement in HAM-D and GDS scores. Improvement among those with MMSE >18 was greater in the regular dose group, suggesting that routine dosing is effective for older adults who are cognitively intact (Streim et al., 2000). In a group of NH patients with residual depressive symptoms

after 10 weeks of treatment with sertraline 100 mg daily, treatment with an increased dose of sertraline 200 mg daily for an additional 8 weeks led to clinical response in 39% of prior nonresponders (Weintraub et al., 2003). Similar to standard practice in geriatric depression, while initial dosing should be low, final effective antidepressant doses in some NH residents may be comparable to those used in younger adults (Alexopoulos, 2005).

Reminiscent of general truths regarding antidepressants, small open-label studies in NH patients have found no difference in efficacy among SSRIs. For 50 patients randomized to receive paroxetine, sertraline, or fluoxetine, 42% had at least a 50% decline in HAM-D scores, with no significant differences between groups (Trappler & Cohen, 1998). However, there may be a difference in tolerability between SSRIs and selective serotonin-norepinephrine reuptake inhibitors (SNRIs). Sertraline and venlafaxine were similarly effective in treating depressive symptoms in NH residents, but time to discontinuation due to side effects was shorter for venlafaxine (Oslin et al., 2003).

Findings From Clinical Trials—Adverse Effects

The available clinical trials data do not precisely define the side-effect profile of antidepressants in the NH population, due to variable reporting of adverse events across studies, low frequency of events among small sample sizes, and frequent absence of placebo controls. However, while side effects occur, antidepressants appear to be reasonably well tolerated by the "oldest old" of NH residents.

There were two reports of hyponatremia, which is less than the rate of 12.5% of SSRI-induced hyponatremia seen among elderly psychiatric inpatients. (Bouman, Pinner, & Johnson, 1998). There were no reports of serotonin syndrome, which presents with mental status changes, autonomic instability, and neuromuscular rigidity and can be fatal. Particularly relevant to cognitively impaired NH residents, there were six cases of delirium reported, two patients each treated with paroxetine, sertraline, and venlafaxine (Burrows et al., 2002; Oslin et al., 2003; Weintraub et al., 2003). Confusion was also noted in two patients treated with regular dose nortriptyline (Streim et al., 2000). Finally, paroxetine-treated patients had a two-point MMSE score decline, compared to the placebo group (Burrows et al., 2002). Falls are also a problem in the LTC population, and both tricyclic antidepressants (TCAs) and SSRIs appear to increase the risk of falls in NH residents (Thapa, Gideon, Cost, Milam, & Ray, 1998). Across the 12 NH antidepressant trials, there were 27 falls, three with venlafaxine, two with sertraline, and 22 with mirtazapine. There were no placebo groups in the trials that recorded falls as an adverse event (Oslin et al., 2003; Roose et al., 2003).

Typical SSRI side effects, including gastrointestinal distress, sedation, and headache, were tracked in three studies and noted as clinically insignificant (Rosen et al., 2000; Trappler & Cohen, 1996, 1998). Interestingly, Burrows et al. (2002) noted that their placebo group experienced statistically significantly higher rates of restlessness ($p < .01$), insomnia ($p = 0.3$), and drowsiness ($p < .01$).

More severe medical events noted during these trials include pneumonia, cerebrovascular events, worsening congestive heart failure, and urinary tract infections. These events were not assessed in a placebo group, and no detailed analysis was conducted to correlate these events with antidepressant treatment. The lowest effective dose should be prescribed to avoid side effects and potential drug interactions.

Clinical Approach to Medication Treatment

Pharmacological treatment of depression in the LTC setting should take into account each individual's past psychiatric history and treatment response. It may be worthwhile to consider prescribing antidepressants that have been studied in the NH population, such as sertraline and mirtazapine, or those with few drug interactions, such as citalopram. Some patients may respond to lower doses, but others, perhaps those who are more cognitively intact, may benefit from usual adult dosing and treatment beyond 8 weeks. Because older adults treated for depression are at risk for residual symptoms and relapse, monitoring the treatment response over time with input from NH staff is important. For severe treatment-refractory depression or psychotic depression, electroconvulsive therapy (ECT) should be considered (Blazer, 2003). The AGS/AAGP treatment guidelines indicate that antidepressants are first-line treatment for major depression, and SSRIs are the preferred drug class. The panel advises against the use of sedating and anticholinergic TCAs, such as amitriptyline and doxepin, and monoamine oxidase inhibitors. Psychotic depression requires treatment with antipsychotic medications (American Geriatrics Society

and American Association for Geriatric Psychiatry, 2003). Antidepressant prescriptions in NHs have increased over time, which may reflect improved attention to managing depression, perhaps encouraged by practice guidelines and regulatory efforts. However, the ideal NH candidate for antidepressant treatment, specific symptoms that respond best to treatment, time course of treatment response, medication side effects, and strategies to manage residual symptoms are not entirely clear. Additional placebo-controlled trials that include larger patient samples are needed to better understand the optimal use of antidepressants in the NH populations.

Regulatory Considerations

OBRA-87 established guidelines for the use of medications in NHs, published in CMS's State of Operations Manual for LTC facilities, under the F329 amendment, section 483.25(l). F329 focuses on the "necessity" of medications prescribed and restricts the use of antipsychotic medications. Antipsychotic medications must be used to treat a specific diagnosis, and alternative treatments, such as behavioral interventions must be tried. F329 explains that "unnecessary" drugs are those prescribed at "excessive dose, excessive duration, without adequate monitoring, without adequate indications, or in the presence of adverse consequences which indicate the dose should be reduced or discontinued" and lists CMS-accepted indications, contraindications, monitoring, dosing, and side effects for each medication class. F329 also outlines a protocol by which state surveyors can assess compliance with CMS regulations as they review NH patient records. Documentation by the mental health clinician should include, as is consistent with good clinical practice, rationale for medication choice and dosing, progress toward therapeutic goals, adjustments for side effects, and whether trial reductions of medications were attempted (Centers for Medicare & Medicaid Services, 2011). Ultimately, claims for Medicare reimbursement from facilities found noncompliant with guidelines may be denied (Gurvich & Cunningham, 2000). Since OBRA-87 implementation, there has been a steady, linear increase in the number of nursing home patients prescribed antidepressants and a concomitant increase in the diagnosis of depression (Gaboda, Lucas, Siegel, Kalay, & Crystal, 2011). In contrast, prescriptions for antipsychotic medications and sedatives have declined (Borson & Doane, 1997). However, certain patient

Table 27.6 Nonpharmacological Prevention/Treatment of Depression in Long-Term Care

STUDY	INTERVENTION (I) / CONTROL (C)	DURATION	SAMPLE CHARACTERISTICS	OUTCOME MEASURES	COMMENTS
Sumaya, Rienzi, Deegan, & Moss, 2001 Placebo-controlled, crossover	*Alternative treatment with bright light* 5 days: no light 5 days: 300 lux 5 days: 10,000 lux *1 week washout between each phase	6 weeks	N = 11 Mean age: 84 Wheelchair bound Depression: moderate to severe on GDS[1] (mean GDS: 14.7) Cognition: demonstrated capacity to consent to study 10/11 completed	GDS	Significant decrease in GDS scores after 5 days of treatment at 10,000 lux 50% had normal GDS score after 10,000 lux treatment
Konnert, Dobson, & Stelmach, 2009 Randomized control	*Cognitive-Behavioral Therapy (CBT)* I: 13 sessions of group CBT C: treatment as usual	7 weeks	N = 64 Mean age: 81 Depression: clinical diagnosis not required; GDS scores >9 Dementia excluded, MMSE[2] ≥ 21 43/64 completed	GDS CES-D[3]	Significant decline in GDS scores but not CES-D post intervention and at 6 month follow-up
Rosen et al., 1997 Randomized Blinded raters	*Scheduled leisure activities* I: individuals choose activities for structured leisure time C: wait list	8 weeks	N = 31 Mean age: 78 Depression: MDD[4] and minor depression (*DSM-III*)[5] MMSE ≥ 18 22/31 completed	HAM-D[6] GDS	45% responded with signifcant improvement in HAM-D & GDS scores Improved scores not sustained at 2 months

Study / Design	Duration	Intervention	Sample	Outcome measures	Results
Williams & Tappen, 2008 Randomized, blind, three groups	16 weeks	*Physical Exercise* Comprehensive exercise program Supervised walking Social conversation .	N = 54 Mean age: 88 Depression: CSDD[7] > 7 Moderate to severe Alzheimer's dementia only (NINCDS-ADRDA[8] criteria): mean MMSE: 7.3 45/54 completed study	CSDD DMAS9 OAS[10] – positive affect OAS – negative affect AMS[11] – positive mood AMS – negative mood	CSDD scores improved across all groups Some mood outcome scales suggest exercise was more beneficial than social conversation Social conversation may be considered intervention, not control
Chiang et al., 2010 Randomized, control	8 weeks	*Reminiscence Therapy (RT)* I: 90 minute structured group sessions of RT every week C: waiting list	N = 130 Mean age: 77 Mean MMSE: 23 Depression: not required MMSE ≥ 20 92/130 completed	CES-D SCL-90-R[12] RULA-V3[13]	Outcomes well-being, depressive mood, loneliness Experimental group —mean scores on all scales improved & significantly different from control group at 8 weeks Sustained improvement at 3 month follow-up

Sumaya et al study of bright light (no light compared to 300 lux and to 10,000 lux) groups, including non-Hispanic Blacks, those with comorbid dementia, and those with advanced functional disability continue to be less likely to receive antidepressant treatment, even if diagnosed with depression (Gaboda et al., 2011).

NONPHARMACOLOGICAL TREATMENT OF DEPRESSION IN NURSING HOMES

Nonpharmacological treatment (NPT) of depression in the LTC setting encompasses a wide variety of interventions that may be administered by volunteers, nursing staff, recreational therapists, or mental health professionals (American Geriatrics Society and American Association for Geriatric Psychiatry, 2003; Bharucha, Dew, Miller, Borson, & Reynolds, 2006; Snowden et al., 2003; Stinson, 2009). NPT includes psychotherapy, organized activities to increase social support, and alternative treatments, such as bright light and physical exercise (Snowden et al., 2003; Thakur & Blazer, 2008). The variety of interventions, differing inclusion and exclusion criteria, and specific psychological and behavioral symptoms assessed in NPT studies limit the conclusions that can be drawn about treatment efficacy. Nevertheless, evidence from the trials and clinical experience suggest that NPT can offer positive benefits with few side effects (see Table 27.6).

A review commissioned by AGS and AAGP to help guide their consensus statement demonstrates the aforementioned limits to the research. The review included six controlled studies, representative of different types of NPTs. Four were randomized controlled trials. Only one included patients who had been diagnosed with major or minor depression. Trials lasted from 2 to 24 weeks, and sample sizes ranged from 22 to 85 participants (Snowden et al., 2003). Each study described a unique type of intervention: a geriatric nurse-supervised volunteer program in the NH, group cognitive therapy, taking participants outside in a wheelchair attached to a bicycle, and allowing residents to choose leisure time activities (Fitzsimmons, 2001; McCurren, Dowe, Rattle, & Looney, 1999; Rosen et al., 1997; Zerhusen, Boyle, & Wilson, 1991). For each intervention listed, the treated groups showed significant improvement in depressive symptoms. Across the four randomized controlled trials, GDS scores declined by 30–45%, compared to controls, whose GDS scores declined 0–8%, or worsened (Snowden et al., 2003).

Psychotherapy, including CBT and reminiscence therapy (RT), has been used effectively to treat late-life depression (Duffy & Karlin, 2006). Bharucha et al. (2006) reviewed 18 controlled trials of psychotherapy in LTC residents published between 1967 and 2001. There were 1074 participants. The most studied technique was reminiscence therapy (RT), described in seven trials, followed by control-relevant measures, cognitive-behavioral therapy (CBT), and "miscellany" interventions. Control-relevant measures mediate adverse effects of the NH environment by restoring decision making to the resident (Rosen et al., 1997). Sixteen of the studies described group therapy. Trials were short, lasting between 3 and 28 weeks, and only two studies collected 12 and 18 month follow-up data (Haight, 1998; Toseland, 1997). Half of the studies reported improvement in at least one of the psychological variables examined, including depression, helplessness, participation, perceived control, communication skills, or life satisfaction. Within the RT studies, over half reported significant decline in GDS scores after treatment, and among the control-relevant trials all reported significant improvement in the psychological variables measured (Bharucha, 2006). This review suggests that particular therapeutic modalities may be more useful than others in improving depressive symptoms in NH residents. However, little is known about the characteristics of the optimal candidate for NPT, which elements of the therapy contribute to symptoms reduction, or how nuances in the administration of therapy may influence outcome. Manualized treatments may help standardize interventions in controlled trials, and a preliminary depression treatment protocol that combines various NPT techniques has been examined in a small pilot study of five NH residents (Meeks, Looney, Van Haitsma, & Teri, 2008; Meeks & Looney, 2011).

NPTs can be hindered by the NH setting itself (American Geriatrics Society and American Association for Geriatric Psychiatry, 2003; Choi et al., 2008; Cody, Beck, & Svarstad, 2002). Staff may not implement NPT because of personal biases, education level, training, and patient load. The physical layout of the NH may also hamper the ability to enact NPT, and there may be financial constraints (Cody et al., 2002).

In summary, NPT can improve psychological well-being in some NH residents. Psychotherapy, including CBT and RT, can be tailored to each patient, and behavioral interventions can be emphasized if cognitive abilities are limited (Duffy & Karlin, 2006). While larger controlled trials using standardized treatment protocols and outcomes will further elucidate efficacy, techniques, and optimal candidates for NPT in the NH, NPT remains first-line therapy for LTC patients with minor depression, dysthymia, or heterogeneous depressive symptoms. NPT can also be combined with medication treatment, if indicated (American Geriatrics Society and American Association for Geriatric Psychiatry, 2003).

SUICIDE AND LONG-TERM CARE

Known risk factors for suicide, including older age, multiple medicalproblems, and depression are common in NH populations. Moreover, NH placement can trigger suicidal ideation (Malfent, Wondrak, Kapusta, & Sonneck, 2010; Reiss & Tishler, 2008), and residential care has been independently associated with the wish to die (Jorm et al., 1995). Suicide awareness should be routine, but suicide has not been emphasized in the LTC literature, and there is no required reporting of suicide events in NHs. Epidemiologic studies in the early 1990s suggested that completed suicide rates in NHs were lower than among community-dwelling older adults, with a nationwide estimate of 15.8/ 100,000 in the NH, compared to 19.2/100,000 in the community (Abrams, Young, Holt, & Alexopoulos, 1988; Osgood, Brant, & Lipman, 1991). Limited access to lethal weapons and close medical attention in NHs were thought to protect against suicide (Scocco, 2006; Suominen, 2003). More recent studies, however, suggest completed suicide rates in the NH are twice those in the community (Scocco et al., 2006). In New York, the suicide rate between 1990 and 2005 declined in the community but remained constant in local NHs (Mezuk, Prescott, Tardiff, Vlahov, & Galea, 2008). Furthermore, suicidal ideation, an important prerequisite to suicide behaviors, is substantially more common among NH residents with prevalence rates ranging from 31% to 43%, compared to 6.7%–9.2% in the general elderly population (Malfent et al., 2010; O'Connell, Chin, Cunningham, & Lawlor, 2004; Scocco, Fantoni, Rapattoni, de Girolamo, & Pavan, 2009).

Suicidal behaviors in the NH are complex. In addition to "direct" suicidal behaviors that cause immediate harm, 29% to 88% of NH residents regularly engage in "indirect" self-destructive behaviors (Draper et al., 2002; Mahgoub, Klimstra, Kotbi, &

Docherty, 2011; Osgood et al., 1991; Szanto et al., 2002). This typically refers to food or medication refusal (Reiss & Tishler 2008). Indirect behaviors can be "aggressive" (e.g., punching walls), "disorganized" (e.g., ingesting nonfood items), or "risk taking" (e.g., walking without assistance) (Draper et al., 2002; Osgood et al., 1991). These self-harm behaviors are estimated to cause 80/100,000 deaths among the LTC population (Osgood et al., 1991), a rate that is substantially higher than estimated suicide rates. The intention of indirect behaviors is not always obvious. Food refusal may be a manifestation of medical illness, and ignoring medical advice or environmental safeguards may be an effort to reassert control (Draper et al., 2002; Szanto et al., 2002).

Risk factors for suicide in LTC settings include one or more Axis I diagnoses, one or more Axis III diagnoses, depression, and past suicide attempts (Suominen, Henriksson, Rienzi, Deegan, & Moss, 2003). NH residents with a past history of suicidal ideation or behavior require careful monitoring. Tracking patients' recent losses, social support changes, and functional decline may help determine periods when they are at increased risk for suicidal ideation. Mood disorders should be actively treated. Determining the intent of indirect self-harm behaviors is important, and potential medical etiologies should be considered. For example, optimizing dentition, cutting food into manageable sizes, and changing the diet may help mitigate food refusal (Reiss & Tishler, 2008).

DEPRESSION AND DEMENTIA IN LONG-TERM CARE

Depression in the context of dementia is commonly encountered in the LTC setting. Despite its frequent occurrence and contribution to functional disability, comorbid depression in dementia is not well defined and can be difficult to treat. Rates of depressive symptoms among LTC residents with Alzheimer's disease (AD) range from 20% to 29% (Bartels et al., 2003; Rhodes-Kropf, Cheng, Castillo, & Fulton, 2011; Zuidema, Derksen, Verhey, & Koopmans, 2007). Qualitatively, psychomotor retardation, fatigue, and lack of motivation are more prominent in depression with AD (Engedal, Barca, Laks, & Selbaek, 2010; Teng et al., 2008). Provisional diagnostic criteria for depression of AD have been created, which includes social withdrawal and irritability as symptoms (Olin et al., 2002). Irritability occurs in up to two thirds of NH patients (Bergh, Engedal, Røen, & Selbæk, 2011; Youn et al., 2011) and may occur as an independent symptom of dementia, an element of psychosis or aggression, or an aspect of depression. Aggressive physical behavior among community-dwelling elderly with dementia has been associated with moderate to severe depressive symptoms (Lyketsos et al., 1999).

Few studies have assessed the efficacy of antidepressant treatment for depression in patients with dementia, and evidence for efficacy is thin. The one nursing home-based randomized controlled trial of antidepressant use for depression with comorbid dementia was an 8-week, placebo-controlled trial of sertraline that included 31 women with probable or possible AD, and either major or minor depression. There were no between-group outcome differences (Magai et al., 2000). Two recent large, randomized, placebo-controlled treatment trials of depression in AD found no efficacy between those treated with antidepressants versus placebo, with higher adverse effects noted in the treated groups. The first trial studied sertraline (Weintraub et al., 2010), and the second treated participants with either mirtazapine, citalopram, or placebo (Banerjee et al., 2011). These findings suggest that use of antidepressants as a first-line treatment of depression in AD ought to be reconsidered.

Nonpharmacological interventions may benefit patients with dementia and depression, although the evidence base is small. The impact of traditional psychotherapy can be limited by cognitive deficits of dementia. Interventions targeting depressive symptoms in later stage dementia patients in LTC have been behavioral, with focus on physical exercise (Underwood et al., 2011). In a 16-week study, 45 LTC residents with advanced AD and depressive symptoms randomized to a comprehensive exercise program, supervised walking, or social conversation (the control group). There was greater improvement in the active exercise groups than the control group on some depression ratings, although the social contact provided in the control group may have alleviated depressive symptoms (Williams & Tappen, 2008). Additional controlled studies of behavioral interventions to target depressive symptoms in NH residents with AD are needed, particularly in light of the limited efficacy seen in antidepressant medication trials. Overall, the conceptual framework for depression in dementia needs further

development, and more effective treatment awaits additional controlled trials in both community and LTC settings.

DELIVERY OF MENTAL HEALTH SERVICES IN THE NURSING HOME

Optimal delivery of mental health services in LTC can improve care outcomes in the NH. Uncontrolled studies in NHs suggest that certain models of care are preferred over others yet may be difficult to implement secondary to staff availability, reimbursement, and government surveillance. In addition, the mental health clinician needs to consider how to provide care in other types of LTC facilities, with assisted-living facilities (ALFs) being the fastest growing group over the past two decades (Reichman & Katz, 2009).

At least six models of psychiatric care have been described in the NH setting. In practice, the most common is "consultative," where the psychiatrist evaluates specific NH patients when requested and makes recommendations to the primary team. Consultative services can extend to meetings with NH staff to discuss general psychiatric management. Consultants can also consist of a "multidisciplinary mental health team," which expands the scope of psychiatric care by including representatives from different specialties, such as psychiatry, psychiatric nursing, psychology, and social work. A "geropsychiatric nurse" may also serve as the primary consultant who makes routine visits to the NH. Another model of facilitating psychiatric care involves electing a NH staff member—perhaps with advanced formal training in geriatrics, or trained by a consulting geropsychiatric nurse—to coordinate with psychiatric consultants and help train NH staff to manage mental health care. Finally, "telepsychiatry" may improve delivery of mental health services to NHs in remote locations (Bartels et al., 2003; Snowdon, 2010).

Outcomes that have been used to assess the quality of mental health NH interventions include patients' clinical improvement, physician prescribing patterns, use of acute emergency or inpatient psychiatry services, and NH staff performance. Limited evidence suggests that over half of NH residents who receive psychiatric care have symptomatic improvement. Treatment is also associated with lower rates of hospitalizations and emergency services. Staff training and education seem to be associated with improved knowledge and job performance, and lower staff turnover (Bartels et al., 2003). The particular method of psychiatric consultation in the NH that yields the best patient outcomes is not known (Reichman & Katz, 2009). However, when surveyed, NH directors prefer certain models of care. The least preferred model is "consultative," with a one-time patient assessment and limited follow-up (Bartels et al., 2003). In a six-state survey of over 2,600 NH directors conducted in the 1990s, nearly 50% reported that the frequency of psychiatric consultation was inadequate (Reichman et al., 1998). In a more recent survey of NH home medical, nursing, and social work directors, 67% of respondents reported access to psychiatrists as a problem, and the top-rated quality of a psychiatric consultant was "accessibility." Over 80% of respondents felt that psychiatric consultants' diagnostic formulations and medication recommendations were helpful. Staff education in behavioral problems of dementia, depression, suicide, and caregiver stress were frequently requested (Muramatsu & Goebert, 2011). Psychiatric services to provide staff support, nonpharmacological interventions, and negotiating family conflicts are also requested by NH directors (Reichman et al., 1998).

Federal legislation and Medicare reimbursement policy influence both the delivery and type of MH services provided in the NH. A recent Office of Inspector General (OIG) report suggested that off-label use and costs of atypical antipsychotics in NH patients with dementia were excessive (Office of Inspector General, 2011). In a prior OIG report in 2001, high billing rates for individual and group psychotherapy, which can be alternatives to medication management of disruptive NPS behaviors, were found to be "most problematic." Medicare does not reimburse for psychotherapy in patients with dementia, and these services are deemed "medically unnecessary." There are no alternative codes to bill for services that NH directors would like psychiatry to provide, such as nonpharmacological interventions and staff education (Mintzer, Kennedy et al., 2003), which limits their use.

Similar to the NH population, the ALF population is also older, with cognitive impairment rates between 40% and 63%, and rates of mood disorders between 13% and 24% (Reichmann & Katz, 2009). There are 36,451 ALFs in the United States, with over 900,000 total beds (Tumilson & Woods, 2007). Rates of psychotropic use in ALFs range from 34% to 55% and unlike NHs, ALFs are not subject to federal surveillance. The ALF population will also need psychiatric care, and studies are needed to define how best to render mental health services in that setting

THE CHANGING NATURE OF LONG-TERM CARE

The aging population is a growing contingent, whose wishes will continue influence LTC services. Information collected by CMS regarding individual NHs are available to the public online (Castle, 2009); in mainstream media, US News and World Report devoted an entire issue to ranking NHs and ALFs (Comarow, 2011). Catering to potential LTC residents as consumers may be another way by which facilities attend to quality care. Recent trends in LTC emphasize patient autonomy, least restrictive care, home-like environments, and quality of life, which will also likely influence the culture of NHs (Kane, 2001).

The mental health clinician in the LTC setting should remain adaptable and knowledgeable, able to inject his or her expertise into multidisciplinary teams. Efforts should focus on providing quality care for residents, in the context of the evolving landscape of long-term care.

Disclosures

Christina Hui, MD, has no conflicts to disclose. She is partially funded by the Department of Health and Human Services Health Resources and Services Administration, Geriatric Training for Physicians, Dentists, and Behavioral and Mental Health Professionals.

Dr. Sultzer has received research grant support from the National Institutes of Health, the Department of Veterans Affairs, and Eli Lilly. He has been a consultant for Eli Lilly and Otsuka Pharmaceuticals.

REFERENCES

Abrams, R. C., Young, R. C., Holt, J. H., & Alexopoulos, G. S. (1988). Suicide in New York City nursing homes: 1980–1986. American Journal of Psychiatry, 145(11), 1487–1488.

Alexopoulos, G. S. (2005). Depression in the elderly. Lancet, 365(9475), 1961–1970.

Alexopoulos, G. S., Borson, S., Cuthbert, B. N., Devanand, D. P., Mulsant, B. H., Olin, J. T., & Oslin, D. W. (2002). Assessment of late life depression. Biological Psychiatry, 52(3), 164–174.

American Geriatrics Society and American Association for Geriatric Psychiatry. (2003a). The American Geriatrics Society and

American Association for Geriatric Psychiatry recommendations for policies in support of quality mental health care in U.S. nursing homes. *Journal of the American Geriatrics Society, 51*(9), 1299–1304.

American Geriatrics Society and American Association for Geriatric Psychiatry. (2003b). Consensus statement on improving the quality of mental health care in U.S. nursing homes: Management of depression and behavioral symptoms associated with dementia. *Journal of the American Geriatrics Society, 51*(9), 1287–1298.

American Psychiatric Association. (2000). *Diagnostic criteria from DSM-IV-TR.* Washington, DC: American Psychiatric Association.

Banerjee, S., Hellier, J., Dewey, M., Romeo, R., Ballard, C., Baldwin, R.,… Burns, A. (2011). Sertraline or mirtazapine for depression in dementia (HTA-SADD), a randomised, multicentre, double-blind, placebo-controlled trial. *Lancet, 378*(9789), 403–411.

Bartels, S. J., Horn, S. D., Smout, R. J., Dums, A. R., Flaherty, E., Jones, J. K.,… Voss, A. C. (2003). Agitation and depression in frail nursing home elderly patients with dementia: Treatment characteristics and service use. *American Journal of Geriatric Psychiatry, 11*(2), 231–238.

Bergh, S., Engedal, K., Røen, I., & Selbæk, G. (2011). The course of neuropsychiatric symptoms in patients with dementia in Norwegian nursing homes. *International Psychogeriatrics, 23*(8), 1231–1239.

Bharucha, A. J., Dew, M. A., Miller, M. D., Borson, S., & Reynolds, C. F., III. (2006). Psychotherapy in long-term care: A review. *Journal of the American Medical Directors Association, 7*(9), 568–580.

Birrer, R. B., & Vemuri, S. P. (2004). Depression in later life: A diagnostic and therapeutic challenge. *American Family Physician, 69*(10), 2375–2382.

Blazer, D. G. (2003). Depression in late life: Review and commentary. *Journals of Gerontology Series A, Biological Science Medical Science, 58*(3), 249–265.

Blazer, D. G., & Steffens, D. C. (2009). *The American Psychiatric Publishing textbook of geriatric psychiatry.* Washington, DC: American Psychiatric Publishing.

Borson, S., & Doane, K. (1997). The impact of OBRA-87 on psychotropic drug prescribing in skilled nursing facilities. *Psychiatric Services, 48*(10), 1289–1296.

Borson, S., Loebel, J. P., Kitchell, M., Domoto, S., & Hyde, T. (1997). Psychiatric assessments of nursing home residents under OBRA-87: Should PASARR be reformed? Pre-Admission Screening and Annual Review. *Journal of the American Geriatrics Society, 45*(10), 1173–1181.

Bouman, W. P., Pinner, G., & Johnson, H. (1998). Incidence of selective serotonin reuptake inhibitor (SSRI) induced hyponatraemia due to the syndrome of inappropriate antidiuretic hormone (SIADH) secretion in the elderly. *International Journal of Geriatric Psychiatry, 13*(1), 12–15.

Brooke, V. (1989). How elders adjust. *Geriatric Nursing, 10*(2), 66–68.

Brown, M. N., Lapane, K. L., & Luisi, A. F. (2002). The management of depression in older nursing home residents. *Journal of the American Geriatrics Society, 50*(1), 69–76.

Bruce, M. L., & Leaf, P. J. (1989). Psychiatric disorders and 15-month mortality in a community sample of older adults. *American Journal of Public Health, 79*(6), 727–730.

Burrows, A. B., Morris, J. N., Simon, S. E., Hirdes, J. P., & Phillips, C. (2000). Development of a minimum data set-based depression rating scale for use in nursing homes. *Age and Ageing, 29*(2), 165–172.

Burrows, A. B., Salzman, C., Satlin, A., Noble, K., Pollock, B. G., & Gersh, T. (2002). A randomized, placebo-controlled trial of paroxetine in nursing home residents with non-major depression. *Depress and Anxiety, 15*(3), 102–110.

Castle, N. G. (2009). Consumers' use of internet-based nursing home report cards. *Joint Commission Journal on Quality and Patient Safety, 35*(6), 316–323.

Centers for Disease Control and Prevention. (2008, June). National Nursing Home Survey, resident tables. Retrieved June 18, 2011, from http://www.cdc.gov/nchs/nnhs/resident_tables.htm

Centers for Medicare & Medicaid Services. (2010a). MDS Active Resident Information Report-Days received the following medications— antidepressant. Winter Quarter 2010. Retrieved May 18, 2011, from https://www.cms.gov/MDSPubQIandResRep/04_activeresreport.asp?isSubmitted=res3&var=O4c&date=32

Centers for Medicare & Medicaid Services. (2010b). MDS Active Resident Information Report—Age of resident. Winter Quarter 2010. Retrieved May 11, 2011, from https://www.cms.gov/MDSPubQIandResRep/04_activeresreport.asp?isSubmitted=res3&var=RSaGE&date=32

Centers for Medicare & Medicaid Services. (2010c). MDS Active Resident Information Report—Disease -Neurological—Alzheimer's Disease. Winter Quarter 2010. Retrieved May 18, 2011, from https://www.cms.gov/MDSPubQIandResRep/04_activeresreport.asp?isSubmitted=res3&var=I1q&date=32;http

s://www.cms.gov/MDSPubQIandResRep/04_
activeresreport.asp?isSubmitted=res3&var=I1u&
date=32 .

Centers for Medicare & Medicaid Services. (2010d).
MDS Active Resident Information Report
-Diseases Diagnosis—Diseases—Psychiatric/
Mood. Winter Quarter 2010. Retrieved
May 18, 2011, from https://www.cms.gov/
MDSPubQIandResRep/04_activeresreport.asp
?date=32&isSubmitted=res2;https://www.cms.
gov/MDSPubQIandResRep/04_activeresreport.
asp?isSubmitted=res3&var=I1dd&date=32;http
s://www.cms.gov/MDSPubQIandResRep/04_
activeresreport.asp?isSubmitted=res3&va
r=I1ee&date=32;https://www.cms.gov/
MDSPubQIandResRep/04_activeresreport.a
sp?isSubmitted=res3&var=I1ff&date=32;http
s://www.cms.gov/MDSPubQIandResRep/04_
activeresreport.asp?isSubmitted=res3&var=I1gg
&date=32 .

Centers for Medicare & Medicaid Services. (2011a).
Preadmission screening and resident review.
Retrieved 25 June 2011, from https://www.cms.
gov/pasrr/.

Centers for Medicare & Medicaid Services (2011b).
State operations manual .

Chiang K., Chu, H., Chang, H. J., Chung, M.
H., Chen, C. H., Chiou, H. Y., & Chou, K. R.
(2010). The effects of reminiscence therapy
on psychological well-being, depression, and
loneliness among the institutionalized aged.
International Journal of Geriatric Psychiatry, 25(4),
380–388.

Choi, N. G., Ransom, S., & Wyllie, R. J. (2008).
Depression in older nursing home residents:
The influence of nursing home environmental
stressors, coping, and acceptance of group and
individual therapy. *Aging and Mental Health,
12*(5), 536–547.

Cody, M., Beck, C., & Svarstad, B. L. (2002).
Challenges to the use of nonpharmacologic
interventions in nursing homes. *Psychiatric
Services, 53*(11), 1402–1406.

Comarow, A. (2011). Best nursing homes: Behind the
rankings. *US News and World Report*, .

Cooper, J. K., Harris, Y., & McGready, J. (2002).
Sadness predicts death in older people.
Journal of Aging and Health, 14(4),
509–526.

Datto, C. J., Oslin, D. W., Streim, J. E., Scheinthal,
S. M., DiFilippo, S., & Katz, I. R. (2002).
Pharmacologic treatment of depression in
nursing home residents: A mental health services
perspective. *Journal of Geriatric Psychiatry and
Neurology, 15*(3), 141–146.

Decker, F. (2005). Nursing homes, 1977–99: *What
has changed, what has not?* Hyattsville, MD:
National Center for Health Statistics.

Dobalian, A., Tsao, J. C., & Radcliff, T. A. (2003).
Diagnosed mental and physical health conditions
in the United States nursing home population:
Differences between urban and rural facilities.
Journal of Rural Health, 19(4), 477–483.

Doyle, C. J. (1995). Effect of staff turnover and the
social environment on depressive symptoms
in nursing home residents. *International
Psychogeriatrics, 7*(1), 51–61.

Draper, B., Brodaty, H., Low, L. F., Richards, V., Paton,
H., & Lie, D. (2002). Self-destructive behaviors
in nursing home residents. *Journal of the American
Geriatrics Society, 50*(2), 354–358.

Duffy, M., & Karlin, B. (2006). Treating depression
in nursing homes: beond the medical model. In
L. Hyer & R. Intrieri (Eds.), *Geropsychological
interventions in long-term care* (pp. 109–138).
New York: Springer.

Engedal, K., Barca, M. L., Laks, J., & Selbaek, G.
(2010). Depression in Alzheimer's disease:
Specificity of depressive symptoms using three
different clinical criteria. *International Journal of
Geriatric Psychiatry, 26*(9), 944–951.

Etters, L., Goodall, D., & Harrison, B. E. (2008).
Caregiver burden among dementia patient
caregivers: A review of the literature. *Journal of
the American Academy of Nurse Practitioners, 20*,
423–428.

Fitzsimmons, S. (2001). Easy rider wheelchair biking.
A nursing-recreation therapy clinical trial for the
treatment of depression *Journal of Gerontology and
Nursing, 27*(5), 14–23.

Fullerton, C. A., McGuire, T. G., Feng, Z., Mor, V.,
& Grabowski, D. C. (2009). Trends in mental
health admissions to nursing homes, 1999–2005.
Psychiatric Services, 60(7), 965–971.

Gaboda, D., Lucas, J., Siegel, M., Kalay, E., & Crystal,
S. (2011). No longer undertreated? Depression
diagnosis and antidepressant therapy in elderly
long-stay nursing home residents, 1999 to 2007.
Journal of the American Geriatrics Society, 59(4),
673–680.

Gaugler, J. E., Duval, S., Anderson, K. A., &
Kane, R. L. (2007). Predicting nursing home
admission in the US: A meta-analysis. *BMC
Geriatrics, 7*, 13.

Gaugler, J. E., Wall, M. M., Kane, R. L., Menk, J. S.,
Sarsour, K., Johnston, J. A.,… Newcomer, R.
(2011). Does caregiver burden mediate the effects
of behavioral disturbances on nursing home
admission? *American Journal of Geriatric Psychiatry,
19*(6), 497–506.

Gaugler, J. E., Yu, F., Krichbaum, K., & Wyman, J. F. (2009). Predictors of nursing home admission for persons with dementia. *Medical Care, 47*(2), 191–198.

Gurvich, T., & Cunningham, J. A. (2000). Appropriate use of psychotropic drugs in nursing homes. *American Family Physician, 61*(5), 1437–1446.

Hoover, D. R., Siegel, M., Lucas, J., Kalay, E., Gaboda, D., Devanand, D. P., & Crystal, S. (2010). Depression in the first year of stay for elderly long-term nursing home residents in the USA. *International Psychogeriatrics, 22*(7), 1161–1171.

Horgas, A. L., & Margrett, J. A. (2001). Measuring behavioral and mood disruptions in nursing home residents using the Minimum Data Set. *Outcomes Management for Nursing Practice, 5*(1), 28–35.

Jones, A. L., Dwyer, L. L., Bercovitz, A. R., & Strahan, G. W. (2009). The National Nursing Home Survey: 2004 overview. *Vital Health Statistics 13*(167), 1–155.

Jongenelis, K., Pot, A. M., Eisses, A. M., Beekman, A. T., Kluiter, H., & Ribbe, M. W. (2004). Prevalence and risk indicators of depression in elderly nursing home patients: The AGED study. *Journal of Affective Disorders, 83*(2–3), 135–142.

Jorm, A. F., Henderson, A. S., Scott, R., Korten, A. E., Christensen, H., & Mackinnon, A. J. (1995). Factors associated with the wish to die in elderly people. *Age and Ageing, 24*(5), 389–392.

Kane, K. D., Yochim, B. P., & Lichtenberg, P. A. (2010). Depressive symptoms and cognitive impairment predict all-cause mortality in long-term care residents. *Psychology and Aging, 25*(2), 446–452.

Kane, R. A. (2001). Long-term care and a good quality of life: Bringing them closer together. *Gerontologist, 41*(3), 293–304.

Karkare, S. U., Bhattacharjee, S., Kamble, P., & Aparasu, R. (2011). Prevalence and predictors of antidepressant prescribing in nursing home residents in the United States. *American Journal of Geriatric Pharmacotherapy, 9*(2), 109–119.

Katz, I. R., Simpson, G. M., Curlik, S. M., Parmelee, P. A., & Muhly, C. (1990). Pharmacologic treatment of major depression for elderly patients in residential care settings. *Journal of Clinical Psychiatry, 51*(Suppl) 41–47; discussion 48.

Komisar, H., & Rogers, S. (2003). *Who needs long-term care?* G. U. Health Policy Institute. Washington DC: Georgetown University Long-term Care Financing Project.

Konnert, C., Dobson, K., & Stelmach, L. (2009). The prevention of depression in nursing home residents: A randomized clinical trial of cognitive-behavioral therapy. *Aging and Ment Health, 13*(2), 288–299.

Koopmans, R. T., Zuidema, S. U., Leontjevas, R., & Gerritsen, D. L. (2010). Comprehensive assessment of depression and behavioral problems in long-term care. *International Psychogeriatrics, 22*(7), 1054–1062.

Linkins, K. W., Lucca, A. M., Housman, M., & Smith, S. A. (2006). Use of PASRR programs to assess serious mental illness and service access in nursing homes. *Psychiatric Services, 57*(3), 325–332.

Loebel, J. P., Borson, S., Hyde, T., Donaldson, D., Van Tuinen, C., Rabbitt, T. M., & Boyko, E. J. (1991). Relationships between requests for psychiatric consultations and psychiatric diagnoses in long-term-care facilities. *American Journal of Psychiatry, 148*(7), 898–903.

Lyketsos, C. G., Steele, C., Galik, E., Rosenblatt, A., Steinberg, M., Warren, A., & Sheppard, J. M. (1999). Physical aggression in dementia patients and its relationship to depression. *American Journal of Psychiatry, 156*(1), 66–71.

Magai, C., Kennedy, G., Cohen, C. I., & Gomberg, D. (2000). A controlled clinical trial of sertraline in the treatment of depression in nursing home patients with late-stage Alzheimer's disease. *American Journal of Geriatric Psychiatry, 8*(1), 66–74.

Mahgoub, N., Klimstra, S., Kotbi, N., & Docherty, J. P. (2011). Self-injurious behavior in the nursing home setting. *International Journal of Geriatric Psychiatry, 26*(1), 27–30.

Malfent, D., Wondrak, T., Kapusta, N. D., & Sonneck, G. (2010). Suicidal ideation and its correlates among elderly in residential care homes. *International Journal of Geriatric Psychiatry, 25*(8), 843–849.

McCurren, C., Dowe, D., Rattle, D., & Looney, S. (1999). Depression among nursing home elders: Testing an intervention strategy. *Applied Nursing Research, 12*(4), 185–195.

Meeks, S., & Looney, S. W. (2011). Depressed nursing home residents' activity participation and affect as a function of staff engagement. *Behavior Therapy, 42*(1), 22–29.

Meeks, S., Looney, S. W., Van Haitsma, K., & Teri, L. (2008). BE-ACTIV: A staff-assisted behavioral intervention for depression in nursing homes. *Gerontologist, 48*(1), 105–114.

Mezuk, B., Prescott, M. R., Tardiff, K., Vlahov, D., & Galea, S. (2008). Suicide in older adults in long-term care: 1990 to 2005. *Journal of the American Geriatrics Society, 56*(11), 2107–2111.

Mintzer, J., Kennedy, G., (2003). Long-term care forum: care of the psychiatric patient in the nursing home: Challenges and oportunities. A. A. f. G. Psychiatry. 3.

Muramatsu, R. S., & Goebert, D. (2011). Psychiatric services: experience, perceptions, and needs of nursing facility multidisciplinary leaders. *Journal of the American Geriatrics Society*, 59(1), 120–125.

Nelson, J. C., Delucchi, K., & Schneider, L. S. (2008). Efficacy of second generation antidepressants in late-life depression: A meta-analysis of the evidence. *American Journal of Geriatric Psychiatry*, 16(7), 558–567.

Nelson, J. C., Holden, K., Roose, S., Salzman, C., Hollander, S. B., & Betzel, J. V. (2007). Are there predictors of outcome in depressed elderly nursing home residents during treatment with mirtazapine orally disintegrating tablets? *International Journal of Geriatric Psychiatry*, 22(10), 999–1003.

Nelson, J. C., Hollander, S. B., Betzel, J., Smolen, P., & Mirtazapine Nursing Home Study Group. (2006). Mirtazapine orally disintegrating tablets in depressed nursing home residents 85 years of age and older. *International Journal of Geriatric Psychiatry*, 21(9), 898–901.

O'Connell, H., Chin, A. V., Cunningham, C., & Lawlor, B. A. (2004). Recent developments: Suicide in older people. *British Medical Journal*, 329(7471), 895–899.

Office of Inspector General. (2011). *Medicare atypical antipsychotic drug calimes for elderly nursing home residents*. Washington, DC: US Department of Health and Human Services.

Olin, J. T., Schneider, L. S., Katz, I. R., Meyers, B. S., Alexopoulos, G. S., Breitner, J. C., ... Lebowitz, B. D. (2002). Provisional diagnostic criteria for depression of Alzheimer disease. *American Journal of Geriatric Psychiatry* 10(2), 125–128.

Osgood, N. J., Brant, B. A., & Lipman, A. P. (1991). *Suicide among the elderly in long-term care facilities*. New York: Greenwood Press.

Oslin, D. W., Streim, J. E., Katz, I. R., Smith, B. D., DiFilippo, S. D., Ten Have, T. R., & Cooper, T. (2000). Heuristic comparison of sertraline with nortriptyline for the treatment of depression in frail elderly patients. *American Journal of Geriatric Psychiatry*, 8(2), 141–149.

Oslin, D. W., Ten Have, T. R., Streim, J. E., Datto, C. J., Weintraub, D., DiFilippo, S., & Katz, I. R. (2003). Probing the safety of medications in the frail elderly: Evidence from a randomized clinical trial of sertraline and venlafaxine in depressed nursing home residents. *Journal of Clinical Psychiatry*, 64(8), 875–882.

Patterson, B. J. (1995). The process of social support: Adjusting to life in a nursing home. *Journal Advanced Nursing*, 21(4), 682–689.

Payne, J. L., Sheppard, J. M., Steinberg, M., Warren, A., Baker, A., Steele, C., ... Lyketsos, C. G. (2002). Incidence, prevalence, and outcomes of depression in residents of a long-term care facility with dementia. *International Journal of Geriatric Psychiatry*, 17(3), 247–253.

Phelan, E., Williams, B., Meeker, K., Bonn, K., Frederick, J., Logerfo, J., & Snowden, M. (2010). A study of the diagnostic accuracy of the PHQ-9 in primary care elderly. *BMC Family Practice*, 11, 63.

Reichman, W. E., Coyne, A. C., Borson, S., Negrón, A. E., Rovner, B. W., Pelchat, R. J., ... Hamer, R. M. (1998). Psychiatric consultation in the nursing home. A survey of six states. *American Journal of Geriatric Psychiatry*, 6(4), 320–327.

Reichman, W. E., & Katz, P. R. (2009). *Psychiatry in long-term care*. Oxford, England and New York: Oxford University Press.

Reiss, N., & Tishler, C. (2008). Suicidality in nursing home residents: Part 1. prevalence, risk factors, methods, assessment, and management. *Professional Psychology: Research and Practice*, 39(3), 264–270.

Rhodes-Kropf, J., Cheng, H., Castillo, E. H., & Fulton, A. T. (2011). Managing the patient with dementia in long-term care. *Clinical Geriatric Medicine*, 27(2), 135–152.

Roose, S. P., Nelson, J. C., Salzman, C., Hollander, S. B., Rodrigues, H., & Mirtazapine in the Nursing Home Study Group. (2003). Open-label study of mirtazapine orally disintegrating tablets in depressed patients in the nursing home. *Current Medical Research Opinion*, 19(8), 737–746.

Rosen, J., Mulsant, B. H., & Pollock, B. G. (2000). Sertraline in the treatment of minor depression in nursing home residents: A pilot study. *International Journal of Geriatric Psychiatry*, 15(2), 177–180.

Rosen, J., Rogers, J. C., Marin, R. S., Mulsant, B. H., Shahar, A., & Reynolds, C. F., III. (1997). Control-relevant intervention in the treatment of minor and major depression in a long-term care facility. *American Journal of Geriatric Psychiatry*, 5(3), 247–257.

Ruckdeschel, K., Thompson, R., Datto, C. J., Streim, J. E., & Katz, I. R. (2004). Using the minimum data set 2.0 mood disturbance items as a self-report screening instrument for depression in nursing home residents. *American Journal of Geriatric Psychiatry*, 12(1), 43–49.

Sahyoun, N. R., Pratt, L. A., Lentzner, H., Dey, A., & Robinson, K. N. (2001). The changing profile of nursing home residents: 1985–1997. *Aging Trends*, (4), 1–8.

Saliba, D., & Buchanan, J. (2008). Development and validation of a revised nursing home assessment tool: MDS 3.0.

Scocco, P., Fantoni, G., Rapattoni, M., de Girolamo, G., & Pavan, L. (2009). Death ideas, suicidal thoughts, and plans among nursing home residents. *Journal of Geriatric Psychiatry and Neurology, 22*(2), 141–148.

Scocco, P., Rapattoni, M., Fantoni, G., Galuppo, M., De Biasi, F., de Girolamo, G., & Pavan, L. (2006). Suicidal behaviour in nursing homes: A survey in a region of north-east Italy. *International Journal of Geriatric Psychiatry, 21*(4), 307–311.

Seitz, D., Purandare, N., & Conn, D. (2010). Prevalence of psychiatric disorders among older adults in long-term care homes: A systematic review. *International Psychogeriatrics, 22*(7), 1025–1039.

Snowden, M., Piacitelli, J., & Koepsell, T. (1998). Compliance with PASARR recommendations for Medicaid recipients in nursing homes. Preadmission Screening and Annual Resident Review. *Journal of the American Geriatrics Society, 46*(9), 1132–1136.

Snowden, M., Sato, K., & Roy-Byrne, P. (2003). Assessment and treatment of nursing home residents with depression or behavioral symptoms associated with dementia: A review of the literature. *Journal of the American Geriatrics Society, 51*(9), 1305–1317.

Snowdon, J. (2010). Mental health service delivery in long-term care homes. *International Psychogeriatrics, 22*(7), 1063–1071.

Sörensen, S., & Conwell, Y. (2011). Issues in dementia caregiving: Effects on mental and physical health, intervention strategies, and research needs. *American Journal of Geriatric Psychiatry, 19*(6), 491–496.

Sumaya, I. C., Rienzi, B. M., Deegan, J. F., II, & Moss, D. E. (2001). Bright light treatment decreases depression in institutionalized older adults: A placebo-controlled crossover study. *Journals of Gerontology Series A, Biological Science Medical Science, 56*(6), M356–M360.

Stinson, C. K. (2009). Structured group reminiscence: An intervention for older adults. *Journal of Continuing Education in Nursing, 40*(11), 521–528.

Streim, J. E., Oslin, D. W., Katz, I. R., Smith, B. D., DiFilippo, S., Cooper, T. B., & Ten Have, T. (2000). Drug treatment of depression in frail elderly nursing home residents. *American Journal of Geriatric Psychiatry, 8*(2), 150–159.

Suominen, K., Henriksson, M., Isometsä, E., Conwell, Y., Heilä, H., & Lönnqvist, J. (2003). Nursing home suicides-a psychological autopsy study. *International Journal of Geriatric Psychiatry, 18*(12), 1095–1101.

Szanto, K., Gildengers, A., Mulsant, B. H., Brown, G., Alexopoulos, G. S., & Reynolds, C. F., III.. (2002). Identification of suicidal ideation and prevention of suicidal behaviour in the elderly. *Drugs and Aging, 19*(1), 11–24.

Teng, E., Ringman, J. M., Ross, L. K., Mulnard, R. A., Dick, M. B., Bartzokis, G.,... Alzheimer's Disease Research Centers of California-Depression in Alzheimer's Disease Investigators. (2008). Diagnosing depression in Alzheimer disease with the national institute of mental health provisional criteria. *American Journal of Geriatric Psychiatry, 16*(6), 469–477.

Teresi, J., Abrams, R., Holmes, D., Ramirez, M., & Eimicke, J. (2001). Prevalence of depression and depression recognition in nursing homes. *Social Psychiatry and Psychiatric Epidemiology, 36*(12), 613–620.

Thakur, M., & Blazer, D. G. (2008). Depression in long-term care. *Journal of the American Medical Directors Association, 9*(2), 82–87.

Thapa, P. B., Gideon, P., Cost, T. W., Milam, A. B., & Ray, W. A. (1998). Antidepressants and the risk of falls among nursing home residents. *New England Journal of Medicine, 339*(13), 875–882.

Trappler, B., & Cohen, C. (1996). Using fluoxetine in very old depressed nursing home residents. *American Journal of Geriatric Psychiatry, 4*(3), 258–262.

Trappler, B., & Cohen, C. I. (1998). Use of SSRIs in very old depressed nursing home residents. *American Journal of Geriatric Psychiatry, 6*(1), 83–89.

Tumilson, A., & Woods, S. (2007). Long-term care: An introduction. N. C. f. Q. L.-t. Care, Avelere Health LLC .

Underwood, M., Eldridge, S., Lamb, S., Potter, R., Sheehan, B., Slowther, A. M.,... Weich, S. (2011). The OPERA trial: protocol for a randomised trial of an exercise intervention for older people in residential and nursing accommodation. *Trials, 12*, 27.

US Department of Health and Human Services. (2009, 25 March). *What is long-term care?* Retrieved ay 2011, from http://www.medicare.gov/longtermcare/static/home.asp

Weintraub, D., Rosenberg, P. B., Drye, L. T., Martin, B. K., Frangakis, C., Mintzer, J. E.,... DIADS-2 Research Group. (2010). Sertraline for the treatment of depression in Alzheimer disease: Week-24 outcomes. *American Journal of Geriatric Psychiatry, 18*(4), 332–340.

Weintraub, D., Streim, J. E., Datto, C. J., Katz, I. R., DiFilippo, S. D., & Oslin, D. W. (2003). Effect of increasing the dose and duration of sertraline trial in the treatment of depressed nursing home residents. *Journal of Geriatric Psychiatry and Neurology, 16*(2), 109–111.

Williams, C. L., & Tappen, R. M. (2008). Exercise training for depressed older adults with Alzheimer's disease. *Aging and Mental Health, 12*(1), 72–80.

Wilson, S. A. (1997). The transition to nursing home life: A comparison of planned and unplanned admissions. *Journal of Advanced Nursing, 26*(5), 864–871.

Youn, J. C., Lee, D. Y., Jhoo, J. H., Kim, K. W., Choo, I. H., & Woo, J. I. (2011). Prevalence of neuropsychiatric syndromes in Alzheimer's disease (AD). *Archives of Gerontology and Geriatrics, 52*(3), 258–263.

Zerhusen, J. D., Boyle, K., & Wilson, W. (1991). Out of the darkness: Group cognitive therapy for depressed elderly. *Journal of Psychosocial Nursing and Mental Health Services, 29*(9), 16–21.

Zuidema, S. U., Derksen, E., Verhey, F. R., & Koopmans, R. T. (2007). Prevalence of neuropsychiatric symptoms in a large sample of Dutch nursing home patients with dementia. *International Journal of Geriatric Psychiatry, 22*(7), 632–638.

28

LATE-LIFE DEPRESSION IN THE PRIMARY CARE SETTING

TOWARD A PATIENT-CENTERED FUTURE

Marsha Wittink, Paul Duberstein, and Jeffrey M. Lyness

THE PRIMARY care setting is critical for recognizing and addressing a wide range of depression symptoms in late life. However, multiple factors discourage older adults and their primary care physicians from taking a proactive role in addressing depression. In this chapter, we explain the limitations of a biomedical approach to depression care, which emphasizes particular treatments but ignores fundamental behaviors, namely communication and decision making, that are vital to patient-centered treatment outcomes. We introduce an alternative approach to patient-centered mental health care that leverages recent developments in communication and decision making and is consistent with the legitimization of patients as decision makers with expertise in their own circumstances.

THE IMPORTANCE OF THE PRIMARY CARE SETTING AND PHYSICIAN

Most areas of medicine are defined by a particular organ system (e.g., cardiology), period of the life course (e.g., pediatrics), or gender (e.g., obstetrics and gynecology) to the exclusion of others. Primary care medicine is defined by *inclusion* rather than exclusion and is one of the few areas of medicine that attends to the whole patient. At its best, the primary care setting is the place where emphasis is placed on the person more so than disease. Unlike other physicians, primary care physicians are expected to consider all components of health and well-being. In addition, the longitudinal primary care physician–patient relationship affords primary care physicians a perspective that is often not available to specialty mental health providers. Not surprisingly, the primary care setting has been targeted as a critical venue for improving depression outcomes by the pharmaceutical industry, nonprofit foundations, and governmental organizations.

These initiatives are particularly important for older Americans, because primary care is their portal of entry into the health care system (Gallo, Marino, Ford, & Anthony, 1995; Harman, Crystal, Walkup, & Olfson, 2003). Primary care physicians are charged with understanding the "whole patient"

(Fortin, Hudon, Bayliss, Soubhi, & Lapointe, 2007; McGaw, 2008), including the broader psychosocial and cultural contexts in which depression symptoms are experienced. Interventions in the primary care setting can be offered in a more familiar environment with minimal stigma, and in the context of an ongoing relationship that enhances continuity of care, as well as the capacity to monitor the change and impact of symptoms over time.

Symptoms of depression place older adults at increased risk for functional and cognitive decline (Paterniti, Verdier-Taillefer, Duvouil, & Alperovitch, 2002). Whereas older adults are unlikely to utilize specialty mental health services, most do see their primary care physicians regularly (Simning et al., 2010). Primary care physicians are positioned to identify depression as but one element of the full spectrum of human distress ranging from the transient and normative to the intractable and dysfunctional. In contrast to specialty care physicians, who see patients who have already gone through a defining "filter" (Marino, Gallo, Ford, & Anthony, 1995), primary care physicians see many patients who present with a wide spectrum of depression symptoms that have not yet been characterized or "defined."

THE SPECTRUM OF DEPRESSION IN THE PRIMARY CARE SETTING

Estimates of the prevalence of major depression among older primary care patients range between 5% and 10% (Lyness, Caine, King, Cox, & Yoediono, 1999; Steffens, David, Fisher, et al., 2009). An even greater proportion have a history of major depressive episodes but are currently not fully syndromic. The point prevalence of major depression in partial or full remission is approximately 12%. Thus, one fifth of all older persons seen in primary care have a depressive condition that requires ongoing vigilance and careful monitoring if not maintenance therapy.

Estimates of the prevalence of depressive symptoms not meeting criteria for major depression range as high as four times that of major depression (Gallo & Lebowitz, 1999; Shim, Baltrus, Ye, & Rust, 2011). Such symptomatic states have been termed minor, subsyndromal, or subthreshold depression, referred to here as "non-major depression." Although concerns have been raised that diagnostic labels pathologize normal human experience, many patients with non-major depression have significant functional disability and poor quality of life

(Lyness, Chapman, McGriff, Drayer, & Duberstein, 2009; Meeks, Vahia, Lavretsky, Kulkarni, & Jeste, 2011) comparable to or worse than that of adults with chronic medical conditions such as heart and lung disease, arthritis, hypertension, and diabetes (Nierenberg et al., 2010; Wells & Burnam, 1999). Moreover, while community-based rates of major depression decline in older cohorts, rates of depressive symptoms overall may increase with age (Fiske, Gatz, & Pedersen, 2003; Gallo & Lebowitz, 1999). Non-major depression is similarly highly prevalent among older primary care patients and of considerable clinical importance to primary care, with point prevalences greater than major depression (Blazer, 2000; Meeks et al., 2011).

DEPRESSION IN THE CONTEXT OF MEDICAL COMORBIDITIES AND SOCIAL STRAINS

Comorbidity complicates the detection, assessment, and management of late-life depression (Krishnan et al., 2002; Lyness, Niculescu, Tu, Reynolds, & Caine, 2006). Indeed, the reality that faces many older primary care patients, and their primary care physicians, is that most suffer from more than one chronic medical condition (Wolff, Starfield, & Anderson, 2002). The prevalence of multimorbidity (defined as having two or more chronic medical conditions) among older adults in primary care is estimated to be as high as 97%–99% (Fortin, Bravo, Hudon, Vanasse, & Lapointe, 2005; Fortin, Hudon, Haggerty, van den Akker, & Almirall, 2010), having steadily increased over the last two decades as the population is aging and living longer with chronic disease (Mercer, Smith, Wyke, O'Dowd, & Watt, 2009). Patients with multimorbidity have more frequent and longer hospitalizations, higher health expenditures, and use a greater range of health care services (Bodenheimer & Fernandez, 2005; Vogeli et al., 2007).

Psychological distress increases with multimorbidity, with the severity of the multimorbid conditions associated inversely with mental health functioning (Fortin et al., 2006a). Psychological distress can worsen chronic disease progression and contribute to increased pain, functional limitations, and disability (McVeigh, Mostashari, Thorpe, & CDC, 2005; Shih, Hootman, Strine, Chapman, & Brady, 2006; Strine et al., 2004); conversely, pain and disability exacerbate psychological distress.

Competing demands can be a major deterrent to depression treatment for both patients and physicians (Nutting, Rost, Smith, Werner, & Elliot, 2000; Rost et al., 2000). Physicians are under pressure to adhere to guidelines for each chronic disorder, while patients must manage multiple medical appointments and remember to pick up and take their medications. Although physicians are obligated to mind the health of their patients, patients themselves often have other things on their mind—finances, caregiving, children, grandchildren, their living conditions, and more. Indeed, the extensive literature on "nonmedical" factors associated with health (Chapman, Fiscella, Kawachi, & Duberstein, 2010; Meara, Richards, & Cutler, 2008; Phelan, Link, & Tehranifar, 2010; vanRyn & Fu, 2003) raises questions about approaches to the prevention and treatment of depression that ignore the social, economic, and psychological circumstances that confer risk for poor outcomes. These same factors make it difficult for patients to engage in two behaviors that are vital to improving depression outcomes: communicating with health care providers and making decisions. More specifically, it is important for patients to be engaged in the process of making decisions about depression prevention and treatment. They must also communicate with doctors about depression as well as the circumstances that confer risk for depression.

Depression treatment may also be avoided for reasons that have little to do with their social, economic, and psychological circumstances, including concerns about drug–drug interactions (Ereshefsky, 1996; Sloan & Ereshefsky, 2009) and drug–disease interactions (Andersohn, Konzen, Bronder, Klimpel, & Garbe, 2009; Atlantis, Grayson, Browning, Sims, & Kendig, 2011). Consequently, even though the treatment of depression among patients with comorbidities reduces morbidity and mortality in some treatment contexts (Fortin et al., 2006b; Min et al., 2005), many depressed patients receive no intervention. The solutions that have been proposed to improve depression outcomes have not simultaneously considered the implications of multimorbidity, social stressors, and the nature of the care delivery system. The latter issue has been overlooked, but it is critical. *Collaborative care* is a term that has been used to describe a range of structured depression treatment programs that co-localize depression care managers, often nurses or other mental health trained personnel, within primary care. Collaborative care approaches are effective (Gilbody, Bower, Fletcher, Richards, & Sutton, 2006), but they are not pragmatic solutions for most ordinary primary care settings in the United States, outside of large integrated systems such as the VA (the largest public system) or Kaiser Permanente (the largest private system). Few practices hire specialty mental health providers (e.g., psychologists, social workers) or pay nurses to take on extra duties—and they have not been incentivized to do so.

The solutions offered to mitigate or solve problems are inextricably (and too often insidiously) tied to problem definition. We believe there is a need to reconceptualize the problem of depression by taking into consideration broader contextual issues, including the patient's context (medical, social, cultural, etc) and the care-delivery context (e.g., well-resourced vs. poorly resourced). Table 28.1 outlines the major distinction between simple, complicated, and complex problems. When depression is unaccompanied by comorbidities and treated in an integrated care system like the Veterans Administration where collaborative care is readily available, it is a complicated problem. In contrast, when depression is accompanied by multimorbidity and treated in a comparatively small practice, it is complex. Whereas commonly drawn analogies between depression and diabetes or asthma (Andrews, 2001; Klinkman, Schwenk, & Coyne, 1997) reinforce the idea that depression is complicated, depression in late life, when encountered in an ordinary (underresourced) primary care setting, is a complex problem.

Complexity's hallmark is uncertainty (R. M. Epstein & Gramling, 2012; Glouberman & Zimmerman, 2002), which poses significant challenges for decision makers, patients, and physicians alike (Gigerenzer, 2007; Kahneman, 2011). To begin with, there is fundamental uncertainty about whether depression is a genuine condition (Horwitz & Wakefield, 2007; Karp, 1997; Kleinman, 2004), and if so, whether it should be treated by a specialist (Pincus, 2003). Moreover, the diagnosis of depression in the context of chronic physical illness is riddled with uncertainty. No gold-standard diagnostic tool exists, the tools that do exist are largely dependent on patient self-report, and many items on mental health assessment tools are themselves symptoms of chronic disease. Furthermore, no single treatment has been proven superior to others (Pinquart, Duberstein, & Lyness, 2006). Patients and primary care physicians thus have numerous subpar treatment options as opposed to a single effective intervention.

Table 28.1 Simple, Complicated and Complex Problems (Epstein & Gramling, In press; Glouberman & Zimmerman, 2002)

	SIMPLE PROBLEM	COMPLICATED PROBLEM	COMPLEX PROBLEM
Non-clinical example	Following a recipe	Sending a rocket to the moon	Raising a child
Clinical example	Treating uncomplicated urinary tract infection	Choosing prostate cancer screening	Considering third-line chemotherapy
Mental Health example	Simple phobia in mental health setting	Major depression without co-morbidity in integrated care system	Late-life depression associated with co-morbidity in ordinary primary care settings
Cognitive desiderata	Knowledge	Expertise	Attunement to others' priorities
Role of rules and recipes	Recipes are essential	Formulae are critical and necessary	Formulae have a limited application
Results	Good recipes give good results every time	There is a high degree of certainty of outcome	Uncertainty of outcome remains

From the perspective of the primary care physician, the heterogeneity among patients in their attitudes and preferences (Cooper et al., 2003; Gum et al., 2006; Wittink, Cary, Tenhave, Baron, & Gallo, 2010) means that routinely referring patients to a specialty mental health provider, absent a systematic assessment of patient's priorities and values, has a highly uncertain outcome. Patients may or may not show up for appointments. Likewise, primary care physicians differ in their willingness to make specialty mental health referrals, due in part to their uncertainty of locating a reliable and competent specialty mental health provider (Cunningham, 2009). Outcomes of depression treatment are uncertain even when post hoc algorithms are applied (Andreescu et al., 2008).

When uncertainty is present, there are no clear right and wrong answers. Decision-making research suggests that too much choice is often experienced as emotionally burdensome, on account of uncertainty (Botti, Orfali, & Iyengar, 2009; Luce, 2005). The ethical imperative in the context of uncertainty, particularly when equipoise is present, is for primary care physicians to become attuned to patients' expectations, values, beliefs, and priorities by engaging in patient-centered care.

PATIENT EXPECTATIONS, VALUES, BELIEFS, AND PRIORITIES

Patient-centered care has been defined as care that treats the "whole person," supports and empowers patients, and enhances coordination and communication between patients and physicians (Bechtel & Ness, 2010). Arguably, the most important step to implementing patient-centered approaches is to become attuned to patient's values, beliefs, and priorities (Reuben & Tinetti, 2012).

In the primary care setting, patients come to the clinical encounter with particular expectations about health care and the give and take between patient and physician (Wittink, Dahlberg, Biruk, & Barg, 2008). Stigma remains the most commonly cited barrier to the disclosure of depression symptoms (Barney, Griffiths, Jorm, & Christensen, 2006) and subsequent identification of and treatment for depression (*Mental Health: A Report of the Surgeon General*, 1999). However, the factors underlying decisions to discuss depression and its treatment are more nuanced than fear of stigmatization alone. Though certainly patients come to their physicians looking for information and services, they are also looking for reassurance, some times more so than diagnostic action (Backenstrass, Joest, Rosemann, & Szecsenyi, 2007). Because physical symptoms are the lingua franca of the physician visit (Lawrence et al., 2006; Wittink, Barg, & Gallo, 2006), patients may focus exclusively on somatic symptoms. Patients who have had symptoms such as chest pain are keenly aware of the attention and reassurance they receive. They are reinforced for discussing their chest pain. Discussions of depression are rarely rewarded in the same manner.

Older patients may additionally expect their doctor to be able to detect depression if present (Wittink, Barg, & Gallo, 2006), even though physicians themselves rely on patients to disclose their emotional symptoms (O'Connor, Rosewarne, & Bruce, 2001). When patients explicitly request treatment for depression, they are likely to receive it (Kravitz et al., 2005), but most patients, and older adults in particular, are not likely to ask for treatment. Patients often do not know they are "depressed" (Epstein et al., 2010), and those who do acknowledge that something is wrong with their mood will often attribute it to a chronic medical condition or to social causes believed irrelevant to medical care.

For older adults, who grew up in a time when mental health was less openly discussed, psychological terms may be unfamiliar and they may feel particularly uncomfortable describing emotional symptoms to professionals (Murray et al., 2006). Patients tend to want care to be consistent with their illness experiences and causal attributions (Wittink et al., 2008). Older adults often hold nonbiomedical explanations of their depressive symptoms (Barg et al., 2006; Switzer, Wittink, Karsch, & Bargh, 2006), which rarely provide an impetus to seek medical interventions (Wittink et al., 2008; Wittink, Joo, Lewis, & Bargh, 2009). For example, some older adults believe they must take sole responsibility for depression, rather than involve a physician (Switzer et al., 2006). Older African Americans may be more likely to endorse a spiritual explanatory model of depression and describe depression as a "loss of faith" (Wittink et al., 2009a). Yet, among patients who ascribe a spiritual etiology to their depression, there is willingness to see how depression treatment can be helpful (Wittink et al., 2009), the key issue being the adaptability of the treatment to accommodate the patient's perceptions and worldview. Indeed, some patients are comfortable incorporating biomedical and personal knowledge into their explanatory models for depression, in part because they feel supported by their physicians'

willingness to talk about their beliefs (Wittink et al., 2008, 2009; Wittink, Givens, Knott, Coyne, & Barg, 2011). Respect for the patient's model of illness is important in creating a therapeutic alliance. Indeed, a stronger alliance and better communication quality are associated with a range of good outcomes (Bertakis & Azari, 2011; Crits-Christoph, Gibbons, Hamilton, 2011; Zonierek & DiMatteo, 2009). Despite the importance of these issues, patient's priorities, expectations, values, and beliefs are rarely elicited and considered, perhaps because physicians are thinking about other things.

PRIMARY CARE PHYSICIAN PERSPECTIVES

In the primary care setting, short office visits and multiple demands on primary care physicians put immense time pressure on primary care physicians. Physicians are thus likely to experience high cognitive load. Under such conditions they can fall into default patterns, which make it difficult for them to become attuned to the patient's priorities. The common flow of the primary care visit allows the patient to voice the "chief complaint," after which the physician is given the floor to ask focused (and typically close-ended) questions leading to diagnostic and management strategies. When patients have multiple chronic medical conditions, the default option requires the physician to focus on the patient's physical symptoms (M. N. Wittink, Barg, & Gallo, 2006). Physicians are taught to force symptoms into either physical or mental categories; the emphasis on parsing out categories lies in the largely prevailing biomedical worldview that most physicians learn and internalize. When making a depression diagnosis, physicians must consider the number and severity of symptoms, the patient's life circumstances, and the relationship between depression symptoms and physical and social problems over the course of time. Yet the current health care system constrains reimbursement for talking or counseling. In contrast, a complaint of "chest pain" or "shortness of breath" warrants a longer discussion both because of the perceived urgency of such physical matters as well as the reimbursable management steps required to evaluate these symptoms. Even when physicians suspect depression symptoms are present, they may avoid addressing emotional issues due to concerns about labeling patients with a diagnosis (Baik, Bowers, Oakley, & Susman, 2005) or feeling as though they will then need to convince them of a biomedical explanation in order to implement a treatment (Wittink et al., 2011).

In addition, physicians are tasked with eliciting and identifying symptoms in a manner that is amenable to diagnostic categorization and application of specific disease guidelines, yet there is little guidance for how to adapt guidelines to specific needs (e.g., when patients have multiple conditions) and individualized patient preferences. Disentangling depression from other conditions is a difficult and ethically challenging task, as reflected in the ongoing debate about the nature of depression (Dowrick, 2009) and concern about the medicalization of distress or "misery" (Pilgrim & Bental, 1999). In fact, primary care physicians have been criticized for missing depression, especially among older adults, while overtreating normal distress (Parker, 2007). One reason for this apparent discrepancy may be related to the fact that most primary care physicians in the United States are in small practices with limited resources; antidepressants, as opposed to counseling or psychotherapy, remain the most readily available remedy. Even in urban areas where there is more access to specialty mental health services, the existing infrastructure for specialty mental health care in the United States remains separate from the general health care system. The fragmented system and limited and variable mental health care coverage of many insurance plans impose significant barriers to the uptake of specialty mental health care, even as other elements of the reimbursement system disincentivize the exploration of psychosocial and economic considerations.

Briefer office visits, the availability of newer antidepressants and other pharmacological treatments, direct to consumer advertising (Donohue, Berndt, Rosenthal, Epstein, & Frank, 2004; Mintzes et al., 2002), and primary care physicians' dissatisfaction with referrals to mental health specialists (Gallo, Ryan, & Ford, 1999) have all skewed primary care depression treatment toward medication. These trends have implications for how depression is discussed with patients in practice. Physicians now spend more time trying to convince patients of the biomedical etiology of depression rather than exploring patient symptoms and values (Wittink et al., 2011). They use screening tools not as a way to distinguish "true cases" but as way to convince patients of a diagnosis (Baik et al., 2010), which, some have argued, represents a threat to the doctor–patient relationship (Leydon et al., 2011).

Nonetheless, the use of these tools merely reflects the fact that most service-oriented interventions targeted to depression in the primary care setting have taken a decidedly biomedical, disease-oriented approach.

PRIMARY CARE–BASED INTERVENTIONS FOR DEPRESSION

One exemplar of a primary-care based intervention is the collaborative care model. Collaborative care interventions such as IMPACT (Unutzer et al., 2002), PROSPECT (Bruce et al., 2004), PRISM-E (Gallo et al., 2004), and RESPECT-D (Dietrich et al., 2004) involve the integration of mental health care specialists within primary care (Bruce et al., 2004; Dietrich et al., 2004; Unutzer et al., 2002). Collaborative care offers one solution to a fundamental problem with detecting and managing depression in the primary care setting, namely, the separation between mental and general health services. It has been extensively tested in randomized controlled trials and is associated with improved depression outcomes in primary care (Gilbody et al., 2006; Katon, et al., 1999; Rost, Nutting, Smith, Elliott, & Dickinson, 2002). The model provides direct support to primary care providers in managing depression treatment with medications, and it facilitates counseling referral, enhancing uptake. By co-localizing a specialty mental health provider (e.g., nurse, social worker, or psychologist) in primary care settings, the collaborative care model reassures primary care providers that their patients' mental health concerns will be addressed, freeing up primary care provider time and energy to focus on their patients' other concerns.

Under ideal conditions, primary care practices, or the health systems in which they are embedded, would pay for the services provided by psychiatrists, nurses, psychologists, social workers, or others with expertise in mental health care. Indeed, collaborative care has gained traction in comparatively large integrated care systems (e.g., VA, Kaiser Permanente, Group Health). It is thus an appealing option for patients seen in settings where, due to economies of scale and practice-design considerations, specialty mental health services can be paid for without financially burdening primary care practice. Such settings are truly extraordinary, however, and it remains to be seen whether they will become more commonplace with the advent of accountable care organizations.

In the meantime, most depressed patients are seen in smaller practices (Hing & Burt, 2007) outside of integrated care systems (Lee & Mongan, 2009). Furthermore, although most physicians who have experience with collaborative care find it is helpful (Kilbourne, Schulberg, Post, Wittenberg, & Burgers, 2004), some physicians note the increased strain on their workload because more communication with the specialist is required (Belnap et al., 2006). Moreover, the viability of having yet another care-management program that focuses on improvements in one disease at a time (e.g., in addition to chronic diabetes management programs, chronic asthma programs, etc.) has been questioned (Nutting et al., 2008). Finally, collaborative care reinforces the idea that depression is a separate component of health, the treatment of which should be outsourced to or aided by a mental health specialist. Physicians are left with prioritizing depression among competing demands but then relegating it to others to manage. This effectively signals to patients that the primary care physician will selectively focus on their other (physical) health issues (Henke et al., 2008; Nutting et al., 2008; Post, Wittenberg, & Burgers, 2009). While this may help flow and efficiency of care, it may be detrimental to the doctor–patient relationship and undermine patient-centered care. If the management of emotional distress is not viewed as a core component of the primary care physician's role, physicians are deprived of the personal context in which patients experience health and disease. Consequently, patients may feel less understood by their physicians, which raises difficult questions about the implications of collaborative care, as it is currently constituted, for the provision of patient-centered care. Modifications to collaborative care may thus be warranted to mitigate these problems.

Whereas research on collaborative care has focused on improving outcomes among depressed patients, stepped care is a primary care–based intervention that has shown promise in reducing the risk of onset of depression (van't Veer -Tazelaar et al., 2009). The aim of stepped care is to identify primary care patients with subthreshold depression (patients who did not meet the *DSM-IV* criteria for depressive or anxiety disorder according to the MINI) in order to offer them low-intensity treatment options (e.g., watchful waiting, psychoeducation, self-help, counseling, exercise, problem-solving treatment). Patients are monitored closely and if they do not successfully respond to these approaches, or if their symptoms worsen, more intensive treatment options (e.g., antidepressants, psychotherapy, electroconvulsive therapy) are offered. The Netherlands, where stepped care was developed, has devoted national resources to preventing depression and led the way in dissemination of depression prevention strategies, yet only a small proportion of patients with depressive symptoms have taken advantage of the services (Reynolds, 2009). One reason for this may be that the intervention is too narrowly focused on depression treatment goals and therefore does not meet the needs of many patients. Primary care physicians who were part of an implementation study of stepped care felt that labeling and treating the symptoms as a psychiatric disease "could have the negative effect of adopting too narrow of an approach to the patient's problems, offering medical solutions without considering the patient's story and contextual factors"(Franks, Oud, deLange, Wensing, & Grol, 2012). Patient-centered approaches, which explicitly address the context in which depressive symptoms occur, could be particularly helpful for improving depression outcomes.

PATIENT-CENTERED MENTAL HEALTH CARE: BRINGING COMMUNICATION AND DECISION MAKING TO THE FORE

Depression in the context of medical comorbidities and social strains generates uncertainty; this may be particularly true in underresourced primary care settings. With increasing uncertainty, patient–provider communication and decision making become increasingly important, and there is a need for a different model of health care delivery that places these two behaviors front and center. The prevailing "treatment-centered" approach to depression in primary care largely ignores fundamental behaviors, namely communication and decision making, that are vital to patient-centered treatment outcomes. Our conceptualization of patient-centered mental health care teverages recent developments in communication and decision making and is consistent with the legitimization of patients as decision makers with expertise in their own circumstances

This patient-centered approach makes sharply different assumptions (Table 28.2) not only about

Table 28.2 Treatment Centered vs. Patient Centered Care

DOMAIN	TREATMENT CENTERED CARE	PATIENT CENTERED CARE
Intervention Level	Health system organization/ practice infrastructure	Doctor- patient interaction
Resources Required	Co-localized space, psychiatrists, other specialty mental health (MH) providers (S. Gilbody, P. Bower, J. Fletcher, D. Richards, & A. J. Sutton, 2006)	Technology-based tools (e.g. computerized decision-aid)
Burdens that Must be Mitigated	Primary care physicians' competing demands (Rost, et al., 2000)	Patients' experiences of fragmented medical care and MH care that is divorced from psychosocial care (May, Montori, & Mair, 2009)
PCPs' Attitudes About Specialist MH Care	No assumptions made	Ambivalent about specialist involvement in MH care; concerned about autonomy erosion (Gallo, et al., 2002)
Patients' Attitudes About Specialist MH Care	No assumptions made	Ambivalent about specialized MH treatment; want to receive care from PCP (Alexopoulis., 2001)
Patient Expertise	No assumptions made	Have expertise that should be brought to bear in clinical encounters and in research (Coulter, 2011)
Involvement of Mental Health Specialists	Paid to provide a structured, manualized treatment (W. J. Katon, et al., 2010)	No assumptions made
Patient-PCP Communication	No assumptions made	Quality of patient-PCP communication is an important driver of health outcomes (Epstein, et al., 2005; Street, et al., 2009)
Framing of the Problem	PCP and MH specialists frame the problem; requires diagnostic screening tests to determine a case of depression	Patient frames the problem; requires patient expression of health priorities which could be facilitated by computerized decision aid and customized feedback (Wirtz, Cribb, & Barber, 2006)

decision making and communication but also about primary care physicians, patients, and the roles of community stakeholders and resources. Patient-centered care holds that communication and decision making, perhaps more so than the diagnosis and treatment, ought to be targeted in the patient–provider encounter.

To date, most primary care interventions for depression focus explicit communication and decision-making interventions only on treatment discussions and relegate these discussions to a depression care manager (Oxman, 2005; van't Veer-Tazelaar et al., 2009). For example, in the IMPACT trial, a care manager discussed patient preferences for treatment and gave patients the option of either medication or problem-solving therapy. The conversations and decisions thus tend to be framed by mental health providers, not patients (Wirtz, Cribb, & Barber, 2006), a framing problem that patient-centered care seeks to rectify. By default, in most medical encounters, physicians, not patients, frame the options for discussion without explicitly empowering patients to express their health-related priorities. Doctors typically frame the encounter in medical terms, reflecting their training and professional socialization, but not the entirety of their expertise or interests. This "framing problem" (Coulter & Collins, 2011; Wirtz, Cribb, & Barber, 2006) not only impedes patient involvement in decision making but may also undermine patient outcomes.

This problem might best be understood by drawing an analogy to a common experience: the purchase of food. Most health care providers tend to frame the options for patients in much the same way that a restaurant such as Red Lobster, Macaroni Grill, or The Olive Garden, frames the options for its clientele: A menu is provided; some restaurants will permit consumers to order "off the menu" but such orders are merely combinations or modifications of items that are already on the menu or ingredients that are present in those items. In contrast, our patient-centered conceptualization of option-framing is analogous to one's experience in food retail superstores. A recent development in food retailing, food superstores offer a customized approach to shopping. Superstores typically include restaurant-style prepared foods, as well as retail food products, nonfood products, and fresh ingredients from around the world. The food superstore not only provides a much wider array of options, but it does so in a manner that gives the consumer the choice to adopt a more active or less active role in preparing a meal. One can purchase sushi "to go" or the ingredients required to prepare Thai-style prawn tom yam with coconut milk from scratch.

Whereas the options typically available in primary care depression interventions are relatively limited (medication, psychotherapy, medication plus psychotherapy, watchful waiting), there has been incremental progress in the approach to decision making. For example, collaborative care encourages the development of a personalized treatment and an assessment of patient preferences. In advocating for patient-centered care, we encourage further developments of personalized treatment planning that explodes the option set beyond mere combinations, permutations, and types of medication, psychotherapy, and watchful waiting. Other interventions must be considered (modification of health and social behaviors, meditation, self-help, bibliotherapy) in conjunction with social service, community, and other nonprofit agencies. The key issue is to get patients more engaged in the decision-making process. When they do become more engaged, by, for example, expressing their priorities, their outcomes are better. One observational study suggested that the effect of patient decisional participation on outcomes is mediated by treatment adherence (Loh, Leonhart, Wills, Simon, & Harter, 2007). Adherence is only part of the story, however. Another observational study showed that patient involvement in decision making about depression led to better depression outcomes, but the provision of guideline concordant care did not (Clever et al., 2006). The authors speculated that "physicians' willingness to involve patients in decision making might have a direct therapeutic effect because it may signal to patients that their opinions are valuable, thereby improving self-esteem." Just as a strong patient–therapist alliance is associated with better outcomes in specialty mental health care (Crits-Christoph, Gibbons, Hamilton, Ring-Kurtz, & Gallop, 2011, p. 403; Flückiger, Del Re, Wampold, Symonds, & Horvath, 2011), a strengthened alliance and improved communication between patient and primary care physician can lead to better outcomes. That patient-centered communication is associated with fewer specialist referrals, yet better outcomes suggests that the health-promoting effects of physician–patient communication cannot be ascribed to more specialty care (Bertakis & Azari, 2011). Involving the patient in the decision-making process increases patient autonomy and competence, both of which have been shown to drive positive health outcomes (Williams, Lynch, & Glasgow, 2007). This conceptualization of patient-centered care is designed to exploit patients' expertise "in their own circumsances" (Coulter & Collins, 2011) and empower patients to improve doctor–patient communication and doctor–patient decision making. Improvements in the basic processes of communication and decision making are hypothesized to lead to improvements in depression outcomes.

Our field could take advantage of developments in decision making (O'Connor et al., 2009) and technology-based tools (O'Connor, Graham, & Visser, 2005), to experiment with novel health care system redesigns. Drawing from community psychology (Levine, 1998), patient-centered care assumes that interventions often work by changing social norms. For example, the norm of the patient–provider encounter could be modified in a manner that empowers and enables patients to express their health priorities, while supporting the autonomy needs of physicians as well (Street, 2007). Given the central role of behavior (communication and decision making) in patient-centered mental health care, interventions designed to modify patient–provider communication or decision-making norms must be informed by a theory of behavior change, such as self-determination theory (Ryan & Deci, 2000), the theory of planned behavior (Ajzen, 2011), or the transtheoretical model (Prochaska & Velicer, 1997).

We predict that such initiatives will improve patient outcomes in part by enhancing the quality of communication between patients and primary care physicians. Recent research in molecular genetics (Cole et al., 2010) underscores the biological plausibility of a behavioral model of health care that emphasizes supportive patient–provider communication, and epidemiological research on social support (Holt-Lunstad, Smith, & Layton, 2010) highlights its public health significance.

TOWARD A PATIENT-CENTERED FUTURE

Patients may be inherently less likely than health providers to see mental health or psychological symptoms as separated from their physical health (Dahlberg, Barg, Gallo, & Wittink, 2009), but they receive different signals from their physicians and from the structure of the health care system. Considerable effort has been devoted to the development and examination of practice redesign innovations, such as collaborative care, aimed at improving depression outcomes by overcoming poor access to specialty mental health care, stigma, and other barriers. Less costly, point-of-care interventions are needed to facilitate patient-centered communication and help patients and physicians integrate mental health management strategies with overall health care.

Primary care physicians require new tools and skills to help them manage the wider spectrum of depression in a manner that is patient centered, and this is particularly true of physicians working in smaller "mom-and-pop" care settings. There is a need for novel tools designed to help patients and physicians talk about mental health issues, including depression, without forcing them to commit to treatment or diagnostic categorization. Using standard decision-making principles such as trade-offs and prioritization, decision tools (also called decision aids) can be used to empower and enable patients to identify and communicate their informed preferences. While decision tools are typically construed as facilitating the process of informed consent, they might also be used to strengthen relationships between patients and clinicians by helping patients bring up important questions, concerns, and opinions (Epstein, Fiscella, Lesser, & Stange, 2010). Randomized trials show that decision aids lead patients to feel more informed and involved in the decision-making process (Stacey et al., 2011); this idea has gained traction in mental health services research (Adams & Drake, 2006; Raue et al., 2010; Raue & Sirey, 2011). Tools that help patients identify and articulate their health priorities could help patients and physicians determine the best next steps and goals in line with their priorities as well.

Patient-centered care has gained traction, yet most patients and physicians are not ready to reframe the encounter in a manner that is patient centered. Physicians are not well prepared to assess or elicit patients' health priorities, while patients are not prepared to articulate their priorities and have never been systematically empowered to do so. Although the legitimization of patients as decision makers with expertise in their own circumstances (Coulter & Collins, 2011) bodes well for the involvement of patients in their care, it is not wise to take a laissez-faire approach and expect patients to advocate for themselves or doctors to become more patient centered, absent intervention. Decision support tools could be used to empower and enable patients to express their priorities, an idea that has gained traction outside the mental health arena, as reflected in The Patient Protection and Affordable Care Act. Indeed, research on interventions to improve communication and decision making in the primary care setting is needed to shape the development and growth of accountable care organizations and other efforts to centralize service delivery in the United States.

Disclosures

Drs. Wittink, Duberstein, and Lyness have no conflicts to disclose. Drs. Wittink and Duberstein have funding from the NIMH (R34085906-Wittink; R25MH074898-Duberstein). Dr. Lyness has funding from the NIA (R01 AG033202, Y. Li, PI)

ACKNOWLEDGMENTS

Supported by NIMH-funded, patient-oriented career development award K23 MH073658 (Dr. Wittink) and the Hendershot Research Development Fund, Department of Psychiatry, University of Rochester Medical Center.

REFERENCES

Adams, J. R., & Drake, R. E. (2006). Shared decision-making and evidence-based practice. *Community Mental Health Journal, 42*(1), 87–105.

Ajzen, I. (2011). The theory of planned behaviour: reactions and reflections. *Psychology and Health, 26*(9), 1113–1127.

Alexopoulos , G. (2001). Interventions for depressed elderly primary care patients. *International Journal of Geriatric Psychiatry, 16*(1), 553–559

Andersohn, F., Konzen, C., Bronder, E., Klimpel, A., & Garbe, E. (2009). Citalopram-induced bleeding due to severe thrombocytopenia. *Psychosomatics, 50*(3), 297–298.

Andreescu, C., Mulsant, B. H., Houck, P. R., Whyte, E. M., Mazumdar, S., Dombrovski, A. Y., … Reynolds, C. F., III. (2008). Empirically derived decision trees for the treatment of late-life depression. *American Journal of Psychiatry, 165*(7), 855–862.

Andrews, G. (2001). Should depression be managed as a chronic disease? *British Medical Journal (Clinical Research Edition), 322*(7283), 419–421.

Atlantis, E., Grayson, D. A., Browning, C., Sims, J., & Kendig, H. (2011). Cardiovascular disease and death associated with depression and antidepressants in the Melbourne Longitudinal Studies on Healthy Ageing (MELSHA). *International Journal of Geriatric Psychiatry, 26*(4), 341–350.

Backenstrass, M., Joest, K., Rosemann, T., & Szecsenyi, J. (2007). The care of patients with subthreshold depression in primary care: Is it all that bad? A qualitative study on the views of general practitioners and patients. *BMC Health Services Research, 7*, 190.

Baik, S-Y., Bowers, B. J., Oakley, L. D., & Susman, J. L. (2005). The recognition of depression: The primary care clinician's perspective. *Annals of Family Medicine, 3*(1), 31–37.

Baik, S. Y., Gonzales, J. J., Bowers, B. J., Anthony, J. S., Tidjani, B., & Susman, J. L. (2010). Reinvention of depression instruments by primary care clinicians. *Annals of Family Medicine, 8*(3), 224–230.

Barg, F. K., Huss-Ashmore, R., Wittink, M. N., Murray, G. F., Bogner, H. R., & Gallo, J. J. (2006). A mixed-methods approach to understanding loneliness and depression in older adults. *Journals of Gerontology Series B, Psychological Science Social Science, 61*(6), S329–339.

Barney, L. J., Griffiths, K. M., Jorm, A. F., & Christensen, H. (2006). Stigma about depression and its impact on help-seeking intentions. *Australian and New Zealand Journal of Psychiatry, 40*(1), 51–54.

Bechtel, C., & Ness, D. L. (2010). If you build it, will they come? Designing truly patient-centered health care. *Health Affairs (Project Hope), 29*(5), 914–920.

Belnap, B. H., Kuebler, J., Upshur, C., Kerber, K., Mockrin, D. R., Kilbourne, A. M., & Rollman, B. L. (2006). Challenges of implementing depression care management in the primary care setting. *Administration and Policy in Mental Health, 33*(1), 65–75.

Bertakis, K. D., & Azari, R. (2011). Patient-centered care is associated with decreased health care utilization. *Journal of the American Board of Family Medicine, 24*(3), 229–239.

Blazer, D. G. (2000). Psychiatry and the oldest old. *American Journal of Psychiatry, 157*(12), 1915–1924.

Bodenheimer, T., & Fernandez, A. (2005). High and rising health care costs. Part 4: Can costs be controlled while preserving quality? *Annals of Internal Medicine, 143*(1), 26–31.

Botti, S., Orfali, K., & Iyengar, S. S. (2009). Tragic choices: Autonomy and emotional responses to medical decisions. *Journal of Consumer Research, 36*(3), 337–352.

Bruce, M. L., Ten Have, T. R., Reynolds, C., Katz, I. I., Schulberg, H. C., Mulsant, B. H., … Alexopoulos, G. S. (2004) Reducing suicidal ideation and depression symptoms in depressed older primary care patients. *Journal of the American Medical Association, 291*, 1081.

Chapman, B. P., Fiscella, K., Kawachi, I., & Duberstein, P. R. (2010). Personality, socioeconomic status, and all-cause mortality in the United States. *American Journal of Epidemiology, 171*(1), 83–92.

Clever, S. L., Ford, D. E., Rubenstein, L. V., Rost, K. M., Meredith, L. S., Sherbourne, C. D., ... Cooper, L. A. (2006). Primary care patients' involvement in decision-making is associated with improvement in depression. *Medical Care, 44*(5), 398–405.

Cole, S. W., Arevalo, J. M. G., Takahashi, R., Sloan, E. K., Lutgendorf, S. K., Sood, A. K., ... Seeman, T. E. (2010). Computational identification of gene–social environment interaction at the human IL6 locus. *Proceedings of the National Academy of Sciences USA, 107*(12), 5681.

Cooper, L. A., Gonzales, J. J., Gallo, J. J., Rost, K. M., Meredith, L. S., Rubenstein, L. V., ... Ford, D. E. (2003). The acceptability of treatment for depression among African-American, Hispanic, and white primary care patients. *Medical Care, 41*(4), 479–489.

Coulter, A., & Collins, A. (2011). *Making shared decision-making a reality: No decision about me, without me*. London: The King's Fund.

Crits-Christoph, P., Gibbons, M. B. C., Hamilton, J., Ring-Kurtz, S., & Gallop, R. (2011). The dependability of alliance assessments: The alliance–outcome correlation is larger than you might think. *Journal of Consulting and Clinical Psychology, 79*(3), 267.

Cunningham, P. (2009) Beyond parity: Primary care physicians' perspectives on access to mental health care. *Health Affairs, 28*(3), w490–w501.

Dahlberg, B., Barg, F. K., Gallo, J. J., & Wittink, M. N. (2009). Bridging psychiatric and anthropological approaches: The case of "nerves" in the United States. *Ethos, 37*(3), 282–313.

Dietrich, A. J., Oxman, T. E., Williams, J. W., Jr., Schulberg, H. C., Bruce, M. L., Lee, P. W., ... Nutting, P. A. (2004). Re-engineering systems for the primary care treatment of depression: A cluster randomized controlled trial. *British Medical Journal, 329*, 602.

Donohue, J. M., Berndt, E. R., Rosenthal, M., Epstein, A. M., & Frank, R. G. (2004). Effects of pharmaceutical promotion on adherence to the treatment guidelines for depression. *Medical Care, 42*(12), 1176–1185.

Dowrick, C. (2009). Reasons to be cheerful? Reflections on GPs' responses to depression. *British Journal of General Practice, 59*(568), 869–867.

Epstein, R. M., Fiscella, K., Lesser, C. S., & Stange, K. C. (2010). Why the nation needs a policy push on patient-centered health care. *HealthAffairs, 29*(8), 1489–1495.

Epstein, R. M., Duberstein, P. R., Feldman, M. D., Rochlen, A. B., Bell, R. A., Kravitz, R. L., ... Paterniti, D. A. (2010). "I didn't know what was wrong:" How people with undiagnosed depression recognize, name and explain their distress. *Journal of General Internal Medicine, 25*(9), 954–961.

Epstein, R. M., & Gramling, R. E. (2012). What is shared in shared decision-making? Eliciting and constructing patients' preferences when the evidence is unclear. *Medical Care Research and Review*.

Ereshefsky, L. (1996). Drug-drug interactions involving antidepressants: Focus on venlafaxine. *Journal of Clinical Psychopharmacology, 16*(3), S37-S50.

Fiske, A., Gatz, M., & Pedersen, N. L. (2003). Depressive symptoms and aging: the effects of illness and non-health-related events. *Journals of Gerontology Series B, Psychological Sciences and Social Sciences, 58*(6), P320–328.

Flückiger, C., Del Re, A. C., Wampold, B. E., Symonds, D., & Horvath, A. O. (2011). How central is the alliance in psychotherapy? A multilevel longitudinal meta-analysis. *Journal of Counseling Psychology, 59*, 10–17.

Fortin, M., Bravo, G., Hudon, C., Lapointe, L., Almirall, J., Dubois, M. F., & Vanasse, A. (2006a). Relationship between multimorbidity and health-related quality of life of patients in primary care. *Quality of Life Research, 15*(1), 83–91.

Fortin, M., Bravo, G., Hudon, C., Lapointe, L., Dubois, M-F., & Almirall, J. (2006b). Psychological distress and multimorbidity in primary care. *Annals of Family Medicine, 4*(5), 417–422.

Fortin, M., Bravo, G., Hudon, C., Vanasse, A., & Lapointe, L. (2005). Prevalence of multimorbidity among adults seen in family practice. *Annals of Family Medicine, 3*(3), 223–228.

Fortin, M., Hudon, C., Bayliss, E. A., Soubhi, H., & Lapointe, L. (2007). Caring for body and soul: The importance of recognizing and managing psychological distress in persons with multimorbidity. *International Journal of Psychiatry in Medicine, 37*(1), 1–9.

Fortin, M., Hudon, C., Haggerty, J., van den Akker, M., & Almirall, J. (2010). Prevalence estimates of multimorbidity: A comparative study of two sources. *BMC Health Services Research, 10*, 111.

Franks, G., Oud, M., de Lange, J., Wensing, M., & Grol, R. (2012). *Implementation Science, 7*(8).

Gallo, J. J., & Coyne, J. C. (2000). The challenge of depression in late life: Bridging science and service in primary care. *Journal of the American Medical Society*, 284(12), 1570–1572.

Gallo, J. J., & Lebowitz, B. D. (1999a). The epidemiology of common late-life mental disorders in the community: Themes for the new century. *Psychiatric Services*, 50(9), 1158–1166.

Gallo, J. J., Marino, S., Ford, D., & Anthony, J. C. (1995). Filters on the pathway to mental health care, II. Sociodemographic factors. *Psychological Medicine*, 25(6), 1149–1160.

Gallo, J. J., Ryan, S. D., & Ford, D. E. (1999). Attitudes, knowledge, and behavior of family physicians regarding depression in late life. *Archives of Family Medicine*, 8(3), 249–256.

Gallo, J. J., Zubritsky, C. Maxwell, J., Nazar, M., Bogner, H. R., Quijano, L. M., ... PRISM-E Investigators. (2004) Primary care clinicians evaluate intergrated and referral models of behavioral health care of older adults: Results from a multisite effectiveness trial (PRISME-E). *Annals of Family Medicine*, 2(4), 305–309.

Gigerenzer, G. (2007). *Gut feelings: The intelligence of the unconscious.* New York: Penguin.

Gilbody, S., Bower, P., Fletcher, J., Richards, D., & Sutton, A. J. (2006). Collaborative care for depression: A cumulative meta-analysis and review of longer-term outcomes. *Archives of Internal Medicine*, 166(21), 2314.

Glouberman, S., & Zimmerman, B. (2002). Complicated and complex systems: What would successful reform of Medicare look like? *Changing Health Care in Canada: The Romanow Papers*, 2, 21–53.

Gum, A. M., Arean, P. A., Hunkeler, E., Tang, L. Q., Katon, W., Hitchcock, P., ... Unützer, J. (2006). Depression treatment preferences in older primary care patients. *Gerontologist*, 46(1), 14–22.

Harman, J. S., Crystal, S., Walkup, J., & Olfson, M. (2003). Trends in elderly patients' office visits for the treatment of depression according to physician specialty: 1985–1999. *Journal of Behavioral Health Services and Research*, 30(3), 332–341.

Henke, R. M., McGuire, T. G., Zaslavsky, A. M., Ford, D. E., Meredith, L. S., & Arbelaez, J. J. (2008). Clinician- and organization-level factors in the adoption of evidence-based care for depression in primary care. *Health Care Management Review*, 33(4), 289–299.

Hing, E., & Burt, C. W. (2007). Office-based medical practices: Methods and estimates from the national ambulatory medical care survey. *Advance Data*, (383), 1–15.

Holt-Lunstad, J., Smith, T. B., & Layton, J. B. (2010). Social relationships and mortality risk: A meta-analytic review. *PLoS Medicine*, 7(7), e1000316.

Horwitz, A. V., & Wakefield, J. C. (2007). *The loss of sadness: How psychiatry transformed normal sorrow into depressive disorder.* New York: Oxford University Press.

Kahneman, D. (2011). *Thinking, fast and slow.* New York: Farrar, Strauss, and Giroux.

Karp, D. A. (1997). *Speaking of sadness: Depression, disconnection, and the meanings of illness.* New York: Oxford University Press.

Katon, W., Von Korff, M., Lin, E., Simon, G., Walker, E., Unutzer, J., ... Ludman, E. (1999). Stepped collaborative care for primary care patients with persistent symptoms of depression—A randomized trial. *Archives of General Psychiatry*, 56(12), 1109–1115.

Katon, W., Von Korff, M., Lin, E., Walker, E., Simon, G. E., Bush, T., ... Russo, J. (1995). Collaborative management to achieve treatment guidelines. Impact on depression in primary care. *Journal of the American Medical Association*, 273(13), 1026–1031.

Katon, W. J., Lin, E. H. B., Von Korff, M., Ciechanowski, P., Ludman, E. J., Young, B., ... McCulloch, D. (2010). Collaborative care for patients with depression and chronic illnesses. *New England Journal of Medicine*, 363(27), 2611–2620.

Kessler, R. C., Zhao, S., Blazer, D. G., & Swartz, M. (1997). Prevalence, correlates, and course of minor depression and major depression in the National Comorbidity Survey. *Journal of Affective Disorders*, 45(1–2), 19–30.

Kilbourne, A. M., Schulberg, H. C., Post, E. P., Rollman, B. L., Belnap, B. H., & Pincus, H. A. (2004). Translating evidence-based depression management services to community-based primary care practices. *Milbank Quarterly*, 82(4), 631–659.

Kleinman, A. (2004). Culture and depression. *New England Journal of Medicine*, 351(10), 951–953.

Klinkman, M. S., Schwenk, T. L., & Coyne, J. C. (1997). Depression in primary care—More like asthma than appendicitis: The Michigan Depression Project. *Canadian Journal of Psychiatry*, 42(9), 966–973.

Kravitz, R. L., Epstein, R. M., Feldman, M. D., Franz, C. E., Azari, R., Wilkes, M. S., ... Franks, P. (2005). Influence of patients' requests for direct-to-consumer advertised antidepressants—A randomized controlled trial. *Journal of the American Medical Association*, 293(16), 1995–2002.

Krishnan, K. R. R., Delong, M., Kraemer, H., Carney, R., Spiegel, D., Gordon, C., ... Wainscott, C. (2002). Comorbidity of depression with other medical diseases in the elderly. *Biological Psychiatry, 52*(6), 559–588.

Lawrence, V., Murray, J. A., Benerjee, S., Turner, S., Sangha, K., Byng, R., … Macdonald, A. (2006). Concepts and causation of depression: A cross-cultural study of the beliefs of older adults. *Gerontologist, 46*(1), 23–32.

Lee, T. H., & Mongan, J. J. (2009). *Chaos and organization in health care.* Cambridge, MA: MIT Press.

Levine, M.(1998). Prevntion and community. *American Journal of Community Psychology, 26,* 189–206

Leydon, G. M., Dowrick, C. F., McBride, A. S., Burgess, H. J., Howe, A. C., Clarke, P. D., … QOF Depression Study Team. (2011) Questionnaire severity measures for depression: A threat to the doctor-patient relationship? *British Journal of General Practice, 61,* 117–123.

Loh, A., Leonhart, R., Wills, C. E., Simon, D., & Harter, M. (2007). The impact of patient participation on adherence and clinical outcome in primary care of depression. *Patient Education and Counseling, 65*(1), 69–78.

Luce, M. F. (2005). Decision making as coping. *Health Psychology, 24*(4), S23-S28.

Lyness, J. M., Caine, E. D., King, D. A., Cox, C., & Yoediono, Z. (1999). Psychiatric disorders in older primary care patients. *Journal of General Internal Medicine, 14*(4), 249–254.

Lyness, J. M., Chapman, B. P., McGriff, J., Drayer, R., & Duberstein, P. R. (2009). One-year outcomes of minor and subsyndromal depression in older primary care patients. *International Psychogeriatrics, 21*(1), 60–68.

Lyness, J. M., Niculescu, A., Tu, X., Reynolds, C. F., & Caine, E. D. (2006). The relationship of medical comorbidity and depression in older, primary care patients. *Psychosomatics, 47*(5), 435–439.

Marino, S., Gallo, J. J., Ford, D., & Anthony, J. C. (1995). Filters on the pathway to mental health care, I. Incident mental disorders. *Psychological Medicine, 25*(6), 1135–1148.

May, C., Montori, V. M., & Mair, F. S. (2009). We need minimally disruptive medicine. *British Medical Journal, 339.* doi: 10.1136/bmj.b2803.

McGaw, J.L. Whole patient care: reaching beyond traditional healthcare. *Frontiers of Health Service Management. 25*(2), 39–46

McVeigh, K., Mostashari, F., Thorpe, L. E., & CDC. (2005). Serious psychological distress among persons with diabetes—New York City, 2003 (Reprinted from MMWR, 53, 1089–1092, 2004). *Journal of the American Medical Association, 293*(4), 419–420.

Meara, E. R., Richards, S., & Cutler, D. M. (2008). The gap gets bigger: Changes on mortality and life expectancy, by education, 1981–2000. *Health Affairs, 27*(2), 350–360.

Meeks, T. W., Vahia, I. V., Lavretsky, H., Kulkarni, G., & Jeste, D. V. (2011). A tune in "a minor" can "b major": A review of epidemiology, illness course, and public health implications of subthreshold depression in older adults. *Journal of Affective Disorders, 129*(1–3), 126–142.

Mental Health: A Report of the Surgeon General. (1999). U.S. Department of Health and Human Services. Rockville, MD.

Mercer, S. W., Smith, S. M., Wyke, S., O'Dowd, T., & Watt, G. C. M. (2009). Multimorbidity in primary care: Developing the research agenda. *Family Practice, 26*(2), 79–80.

Min, L., Reuben, D., MacLean, C., Shekelle, P., Solomon, D., Higashi, T., … Wenger, N. S. (2005). Predictors of overall quality of care provided to vulnerable older people. *Journal of the American Geriatric Society, 53*(10), 1705–1711.

Mintzes, B., Barer, M. L., Kravitz, R. L., Kazanjian, A., Bassett, K., Lexchin, J., … Marion, S. A. (2002). Influence of direct to consumer pharmaceutical advertising and patients' requests on prescribing decisions: Two site cross sectional survey. *British Medical Journal, 324*(7332), 278–279.

Mrazek, P. J., & Haggerty, R. J. (Eds.), & Committee on Prevention of Mental Disorders, Institute of Medicine. (1994). *Reducing risks for mental disorders: Frontiers for preventive intervention research.* Washington, DC: National Academies Press.

Murray, J., Banerjee, S., Byng, R., Tylee, A., Bhugra, D., & Macdonald, A. (2006). Primary care professionals' perceptions of depression in older people: A qualitative study. *Social Science and Medicine (1982), 63*(5), 1363–1373.

Nierenberg, A. A., Rapaport, M. H., Schettler, P. J., Howland, R. H., Smith, J. A., Edwards, D., … Mischoulon, D. (2010). Deficits in psychological well-being and quality-of-life in minor depression: Implications for DSM-V. *CNS Neuroscience and Therapeutics, 16*(4), 208–216.

Nutting, P. A., Gallagher, K., Riley, K., White, S., Dickinson, W. P., Korsen, N., & Dietrich, A. (2008). Care management for depression in primary care practice: Findings from the RESPECT-Depression trial. *Annals of Family Medicine, 6*(1), 30–37.

Nutting, P. A., Rost, K., Smith, J., Werner, J. J., & Elliot, C. (2000). Competing demands from physical problems—Effect on initiating and completing depression care over 6 months. *Archives of Family Medicine, 9*(10), 1059–1064.

O'Connor, A. M., Bennett, C. L., Stacey, D., Barry, M., Col, N. F., Eden, K. B.,… Rovner, D. (2009). Decision aids for people facing health treatment or screening decisions. *Cochrane Database of Systematic Reviews*, (3), CD001431.

O'Connor, A. M., Graham, I. D., & Visser, A. (2005). Implementing shared decision making in diverse health care systems: The role of patient decision aids. *Patient Education and Counseling, 57*(3), 247–249.

O'Connor, D.W., Rosewarne, R., & Bruce, A. (2001). Depression in primary care. 2: General practitioners' recognition of major depression in elderly patients. *International Psychogeriatrics, 13*(3), 367–74.

Oxman, T. (2005) Evidence-based models of integrated management of depression in primary care. *Psychiatric Clinics of North America, 28*(4), 1061–77.

Parker, G. (2007). Is depression overdiagnosed? Yes. *British Medical Journal, 335*(7615), 328.

Paterniti, S., Verdier-Taillefer, M., Duvouil, C., & Alperovitch, A. (2002) Depresive symptoms and cognitive decline in elderly people. *British Journal of Psychiatry, 181*(5), 406–410.

Phelan, J. C., Link, B. G., & Tehranifar, P. (2010). Social conditions as fundamental causes of health inequalities: Theory, evidence, and policy implications. *Journal of Health and Social Behavior, 51*, S28–S40.

Pilgrim, D., & Bental, R. P. (1999). The medicalisation of misery: A critical realist analysis of the concept of depression. *Journal of Mental Health, 8*(3), 260–274.

Pincus, H. A. (2003). The future of behavioral health and primary care: Drowning in the mainstream or left on the bank? *Psychosomatics, 44*(1), 1–11.

Pinquart, M., Duberstein, P. R., & Lyness, J. M. (2006). Treatments for later-life depressive conditions: A meta-analytic comparison of pharmacotherapy and psychotherapy. *American Journal of Psychiatry, 163*(9), 1493–1501.

Post, P. N., Wittenberg, J., & Burgers, J. S. (2009). Do specialized centers and specialists produce better outcomes for patients with chronic diseases than primary care generalists? A systematic review. *International Journal for Quality in Health Care, 21*(6), 387–396.

Prochaska, J. O., & Velicer, W. F. (1997). The transtheoretical model of health behavior change. *American Journal of Health Promotion, 12*(1), 38–48.

Raue, P. J., Schulberg, H. C., Lewis-Fernandez, R., Boutin-Foster, C., Hoffman, A. S., & Bruce, M. L. (2010). Shared decision-making in the primary care treatment of late-life major depression: A needed new intervention? *International Journal of Geriatric Psychiatry, 25*(11), 1101–1111.

Raue, P. J., & Sirey, J. A. (2011). Designing personlized treatment engagement interventions for depressed older adults. *Psychiatric Clinics of North America, 34*(2), 489–500.

Reuben, D. B., &Tinetti, M. E. (2012) Goal-oriented patient care—an alternative health outcomes paradigm. *New England Journal of Medicine, 366*, 777–770

Reynolds, C. F. (2009). Prevention of depressive disorders: A brave new world. *Depression and Anxiety, 26*(12), 1062–1065.

Rost, K., Nutting, P., Smith, J., Coyne, J. C., Cooper-Patrick, L., & Rubenstein, L. (2000). The role of competing demands in the treatment provided primary care patients with major depression. *Archives of Family Medicine, 9*(2), 150–154.

Rost, K., Nutting, P., Smith, J. L., Elliott, C. E., & Dickinson, M. (2002). Managing depression as a chronic disease: A randomised trial of ongoing treatment in primary care. *British Medical Journal, 325*(7370), 934–937.

Robert Wood Johnson Foundation. (2011). *Health care's blind side: The overlooked connection between social needs and good health.* CITY: Author.

Ryan, R. M., & Deci, E. (2000) Self-determination theory and the facilitation of intrinsic motivation, social development, and well-being. *American Psychologist, 55*(1), 68–78.

Shih, M., Hootman, J. M., Strine, T. W., Chapman, D. P., & Brady, T. J. (2006). Serious psychological distress in US adults with arthritis. *Journal of General Internal Medicine, 21*(11), 1160–1166.

Shim, R. S., Baltrus, P., Ye, J., & Rust, G. (2011). Prevalence, treatment, and control of depressive symptoms in the United States: results from the National Health and Nutrition Examination Survey (NHANES), 2005–2008. *Journal of the American Board of Family Medicine, 24*(1), 33–38.

Simning, A., Richardson, T.M., Friedman, B., Boyle, L. Podgorski, C., & Conwell, Y. (2010). Mental distress and service utilization among help-seeking, community dwelling older adults. *International Psychogeriatrics, 22*(5) 739–49.

Sloan, D. M., & Ereshefsky, L. (2009). Drug-drug interactions with the use of psychotropic medications. *CNS Spectrums, 14*(8), 1–8.

Stacey, D., Bennett, C. L., Barry, M. J., Col, N. F., Eden, K. B., Holmes-Rovner, M.,… Thomson, R. (2011). Decision aids for people facing health treatment or screening decisions. *Cochrane Database of Systematic Reviews*, (10), CD001431.

Street, R. L., Jr. (2007). Aiding medical decision making: A communication perspective. *Medical Decision Making, 27*(5), 550–553.

Steffens, D. C. Fisher, G. G., Langa, K. M., Potter, G. G., & Plassman, B, L. (2009). Prevalence of depression among older Americans: the Aging, Demographics and Memory Study. *International Psychogeriatrics, 21*(5), 879–888.

Street , R. L., Jr., Makoul, G., Arora, N. K., & Epstein, R. M. (2009). How does communication heal? Pathways linking clinician-patient communication to health outcomes. *Patient Education and Counseling, 74*(3), 295–301.

Strine, T. W., Hootman, J. M., Okoro, C. A., Balluz, L., Moriarty, D. G., Owens, M., & Mokdad, A. (2004). Frequent mental distress status among adults with arthritis age 45 years and older, 2001. *Arthritis and Rheumatism, 51*(4), 533–537.

Switzer, J. F., Wittink, M. N., Karsch, B. B., & Barg, F. K. (2006). "Pull yourself up by your bootstraps": A response to depression in older adults. *Qualitative Health Research, 16*(9), 1207–1216.

Unutzer, J., Katon, W., Callahan, C. M., Williams, J. W., Jr., Hunkeler, E., Harpole, L.,… IMPACT Investigators. (2002). Collaborative care management of late-life depression in the primary care setting: A randomized controlled trial. *Journal of the American Medical Association, 288*(22), 2836–2845.

van Ryn, M., & Fu, S. S. (2003). Paved with good intentions: do public health and human service providers contribute to racial/ethnic disparities in health? *American Journal of Public Health, 93*(2), 248–255.

Van't Veer-Tazelaar, P. J., van Marwijk, H. W., van Oppen, P., van Hout, H. P., van der Horst, H. E., Cuijpers, P.,… Beekman, A. T. (2009). Stepped-care prevention of anxiety and depression in late life: A randomized controlled trial. *Archives of General Psychiatry, 66*(3), 297–304.

Vogeli, C., Shields, A. E., Lee, T. A., Gibson, T. B., Marder, W. D., Weiss, K. B., & Blumenthal, D. (2007). Multiple chronic conditions: Prevalence, health consequences, and implications for quality, care management, and costs. *Journal of General Internal Medicine, 22*, 391–395.

Wells, K. B., & Burnam, M. A. (1991). Caring for depression in America—Lessons learned from early findings of the medical outcomes study. *General Hospital Psychiatry, 13*(6), 361–361.

Williams, G. C., Lynch, M., & Glasgow, R. E. (2007). Computer-assisted intervention improves patient-centered diabetes care by increasing autonomy support. *Health Psychology, 26*(6), 728–734.

Wirtz, V., Cribb, A., & Barber, N. (2006). Patient-doctor decision-making about treatment within the consultation—a critical analysis of models. *Social Science and Medicine, 62*(1), 116–124.

Wittink, M. N., Barg, F. K., & Gallo, J. J. (2006). Unwritten rules of talking to doctors about depression: Integrating qualitative and quantitative methods. *Annals of Family Medicine, 4*(4), 302–309.

Wittink, M. N., Cary, M., Tenhave, T., Baron, J., & Gallo, J. J. (2010). Towards patient-centered care for depression: Conjoint methods to tailor treatment based on preferences. *Patient, 3*(3), 145–157.

Wittink, M. N., Dahlberg, B., Biruk, C., & Barg, F. K. (2008). How older adults combine medical and experiential notions of depression. *Qualitative Health Research, 18*(9), 1174–1183.

Wittink, M. N., Givens, J. L., Knott, K. A., Coyne, J. C., & Barg, F. K. (2011). Negotiating depression treatment with older adults: Primary care providers' perspectives. *Journal of Mental Health, 20*(5), 429–437.

Wittink, M. N., Joo, J. H., Lewis, L. M., & Barg, F. K. (2009). Losing faith and using faith: older African Americans discuss spirituality, religious activities, and depression. *Journal of General Internal Medicine, 24*(3), 402–407.

Wolff, J. L., Starfield, B., & Anderson, G. (2002). Prevalence, expenditures, and complications of multiple chronic conditions in the elderly. *Archives of Internal Medicine, 162*(20), 2269–2276.

Zonierek, K. B., & Dimatteo, M. R. (2009). Physician communication and patient adherence to treatment: A meta-analysis. *Medical Care, 47*(8), 826–834.

29

DEPRESSION IN OLDER ADULTS RECEIVING HOSPICE CARE

Abhilash K. Desai, Daphne Lo, and George T. Grossberg

THE WORD *hospice* is derived from the Latin word *hospitium*, meaning "hospitality." Centuries ago, hospice care referred to care provided to weary travelers who were sick or frail. Hospice care as we know it today was founded by the physician Dame Cicely Saunders at St. Christopher's hospice in London, United Kingdom in 1986. Since then, hospice care has grown to become a routine part of medical care in most industrialized countries and is increasingly becoming recognized in developing countries. Along with palliative care, hospice care has become a specialty in medicine. Hospice care as defined by Medicare is provided to patients with terminal illness who have less than 6 months to live if the disease runs its normal course (and this requires physician certification). The philosophy of palliative and hospice care involves improving patients' quality of life (helping patients live their remaining life to the fullest), rather than focusing on increasing the quantity (duration) of life (Desai & Grossberg, 2011). Palliative care is similar to hospice care but does not require a physician to certify that the patient has less than 6 months to live. Patients receiving hospice care are expected to relinquish life-prolonging treatment related to the terminal illness (e.g., chemotherapy for cancer), although palliative treatments (such as radiation treatment to reduce pain from metastatic cancer) may be allowed. Hospice care involves a multidisciplinary team consisting of a physician, registered nurse, psychologist, social worker, and trained volunteers. Often, psychologists, psychiatrists, physical therapists, occupational therapist, and clergy are also involved. The patient and family are the focus of care and services are available on a 24-hr, 7-day-a-week basis at the patient's home, in a long-term care facility, or in an inpatient unit dedicated to hospice care. Bereavement/counseling services to the patient's family members are available even after the death of the patient as part of comprehensive hospice care.

Physicians are often unsure about predicting remaining life expectancy for terminal illnesses (especially for non-cancer-related illness such as terminal-stage dementia). This results in most patients receiving hospice late in the course of their terminal illness (the last 4–8 weeks). This is often inadequate time to help patients and family prepare for death by addressing the physical, emotional, and spiritual needs of the patient and emotional and spiritual needs of their family members. Some patients with terminal illness may not require hospice care as their symptoms are easily controlled, they are psychologically at peace, and have come to terms with their situation. However, for a majority of patients, there is considerable suffering due to undertreated pain, unrecognized depression, and other physical and psychosocial-spiritual problems (Ita, Keorney, & O'Slorain, 2003). Hospice care provides an excellent adjunct to the current medical team and should not be a replacement as many older adults with terminal illness have complex needs that are not solely due to terminal illness. The majority of the patients receiving hospice care are older adults.

Sadness, grieving loss of health, and worrying about pain and discomfort are normal feelings experienced universally during the dying process (Axtell, 2008; Wilson et al., 2007). When these feelings become severe and interfere with the person's daily functioning and capacity to engage with life (henceforth referred to as "depression"), they are in need of clinical attention as they may be abnormal responses to stresses in the final phase of life.

The prevalence of depression in older adults receiving hospice care is not well studied. Eighteen percent of recently admitted hospice residents in a nursing home had depression (Buchanan, Choi, Wang, & Huang, 2002). Many of these residents had daily pain and at least moderate cognitive impairment. In a prospective study of 58 patients (average age was not given) with terminal cancer, 7% had major depressive disorder at study entry and 14% developed major depression almost exclusively at their final visit before death (Rabkin, McElhiney, Moran, Acree, & Folkman, 2009). The approximate prevalence of depression (minor and major depression) in terminally ill adults is around 18% (Block, 2010). The prevalence of depression in adults receiving inpatient hospice care may be higher in men than in women, and it is highest in men who are dependent in activities of daily living (Hayes et al., 2011). In a study involving veterans (n = 88, age 45–93) receiving hospice care at home, 14% were found to have suicidal ideas, 34% were diagnosed with depression, and 19% who were not depressed initially developed depression during the course of hospice care (Goy & Ganzini, 2011). In this study,

the Structured Clinical Interview for *DSM-IV* for depression (past and current) and the Hospital Anxiety Depression Scale (HADS) (Zigmond & Snaith, 1983) were used. A retrospective study of older adults receiving hospice care concluded that depression in older adults (average age 70–78 years) receiving hospice care is underdiagnosed (Irwin et al., 2008). This conclusion was based on findings of lower prevalence of prescription of antidepressants in this population compared to the expected prevalence of depression in such a population. The authors recommended improved assessment of depression in patients enrolled in hospice to reduce the negative impact of depression on patients' quality of life (Irwin et al., 2008).

In this chapter, we discuss the importance of diagnosing depression in older adults receiving hospice care, barriers to diagnosis of depression in this setting, causes and clinical manifestations of depression in older adults receiving hospice care, its assessment and management, and a brief discussion about treating depression in special populations and future directions. We conducted a literature review on this topic by searching PubMed from 1990 to 2011 using the Medical Subject Headings terms *hospice, depression, older adult, elderly, terminal illness,* and *palliative care.*

WHY TREAT DEPRESSION IN OLDER ADULTS RECEIVING HOSPICE CARE?

The impact of untreated depression in older adults receiving hospice care has not been well studied to date. Depression in hospice patients may reduce motivation to complete advance care directives (Resnick et al., 2011). Depression in patients with advanced cancer has been found to reduce quality of life, and this was independent of other factors (e.g., anxiety, pain) that also reduced quality of life (Smith et al., 2003). Depression in hospice patients with cancer is an important predictor of other symptoms (e.g., pain, nausea, vomiting; Lasheen, Walsh, Hauser, Gutgsell, & Karafa, 2009). Depression in hospice cancer patients (43% were above age 60) may cause fatigue or exacerbate fatigue caused by other factors (e.g., medications) (Tsai et al., 2007). In patients with advanced cancer (average age 58, some were up to 72 years of age), preparatory grief, depression, and older age were predictors of hopelessness (Mystakidou et al., 2009). Comorbid depression in cancer patients can exacerbate pain, hasten cancer progression, and result in suicide (Weinberger, Bruce, & Roth, 2011).

A study of 100 patients admitted to hospice (average age 68 years) found that many patients were in pain (even severe pain) but did not mention pain as a cause of their suffering (Terry & Olson, 2004). On the other hand, many of these hospice patients who had pain scores of 0/10 did identify pain as a cause of "suffering." Although this study did not clarify whether the latter group had coexisting depression, they suggest that some of the suffering experienced by older adults receiving hospice care is not related to pain but possibly related to depression. Our clinical experience has indicated that depression often further impairs the ability of older adults with terminal illness to make medical decisions in their own best interest, especially in those who also have significant cognitive impairment. Suicide is one of the most serious complications of depression in any setting (including for older adults receiving hospice care) and its impact can be devastating on family members long after the death of the person. Our clinical experience has shown that depression in adults (including older adults) receiving hospice care may trigger requests for physician-assisted suicide, euthanasia, and requests to family members to end the patient's misery by assisting them in dying or actively causing their death (homicide). Thus, depression in older adults receiving hospice care is a serious health concern.

BARRIERS TO DIAGNOSIS OF DEPRESSION IN OLDER ADULTS RECEIVING HOSPICE CARE

We did not find any studies that examined similarities and differences between the manifestations of depression and grief in older adults receiving hospice care. Much of the information mentioned here is from extrapolation of findings from younger adults with terminal illness. Accurate differentiation between grief and depression is an essential part of routine hospice care, because undertreated depression can be fatal and inappropriate treatment of grief (e.g., antidepressants) may cause more harm (Periyakoil & Hallenbeck, 2002).

Depression is often mistaken for normal grief. Although differentiating between them is challenging, a systematic assessment allows for accurate diagnosis (Noorani & Montagnini, 2007). Depression

needs to be differentiated not only from grief but also from delirium (another prevalent syndrome in older adults receiving hospice care). Many patients have a combination of these syndromes (e.g., depression and delirium, grief and delirium, depression, grief and delirium) (Block, 2000; Breitbart & Strout, 2000; Periyakoil & Hallenbeck, 2002). Diagnosing depression is difficult in terminally ill persons because of the high prevalence of pain, other physical symptoms, delirium, and grief. Many palliative medicine physicians have reported difficulties with distinguishing symptoms of depression from sadness and whether it was appropriate to treat patients for these symptoms when life expectancy was short (Lawrie et al., 2004). Forty-seven percent of these physicians reported difficulties accessing psychiatric input (Lawrie et al., 2004). In addition, many health care providers (HCPs) recognize the importance of diagnosing and treating depression but are inadequately trained in screening, diagnosing, and managing depression in this population. In a study of clinical nurse specialists in the United Kingdom who are involved in assessing and managing depression in patients needing hospice and palliative care for cancer, 79% believed their skills in assessment of depression were poor, and 92% felt they required further training (Lloyd-Williams & Payne, 2002). In a survey of oncologists (n = 895) in Europe and the United States, 42% felt that they were trained inadequately in providing palliative care for patients with advanced and incurable cancer, and 15% of respondents had pervasively negative views about palliative care (Cherny & Catane, 2003). A qualitative study involving individual interviews with physicians and nurses working in two hospices in the United Kingdom found that the majority of staff reported very limited experience and/or training in the field of mental health and expressed a lack of confidence when dealing with mental health–related issues (Hackett & Gaitan, 2007). In our experience, a deeper problem is the pervasive therapeutic nihilism regarding depression treatment that underlies current care practices and poses one of the most formidable barriers to high-quality management of depression in older adults receiving hospice care.

There are no biological markers, characteristic symptoms or signs, or diagnostic tests (e.g., cutoff scores on a depression scale) that can definitively establish the diagnosis of depression and distinguish it from normal grief or sadness in the terminally ill (Lloyd-Williams, 2000). Patients and families often do not recognize or give adequate credence to depressive symptoms in the context of a terminal illness (Block, 2000). Many HCPs, patients, and family members believe that depression is a normal part of terminal illness (thus confusing it with grief) and do not appreciate the sequelae or complications of untreated depression or believe that nothing can be done about it (therapeutic nihilism) (Block, 2001). In our experience it is not uncommon to hear HCPs stating that "the patient is already on so many medications, why give more?" when patients or their family members request antidepressants. Education and training of HCPs in assessment and management of depression in older adults receiving hospice care and routinely screening all hospice patients for depression are two key strategies recommended to improve diagnosis and treatment of depression during end-of-life care (Block, 2000; Rao et al., 2011). Culture and ethnicity have a considerable influence over the meanings attributed to suffering and communication patterns, and this can further complicate recognition of depression (Bosma, Apland, & Kazzanjian, 2010). Thus, diagnosis of depression should be done in the context of a broader understanding of suffering and dying that includes cultural, spiritual, and existential issues.

CLINICAL MANIFESTATIONS OF DEPRESSION IN OLDER ADULTS RECEIVING HOSPICE CARE

We could not find a single study that focused on clinical manifestations of depression in older adults receiving hospice care and compared it to other populations (e.g., younger adults receiving hospice care, older adults not receiving hospice care). Much of the information mentioned here is from extrapolation of findings from adults having terminal illness. A majority of older adults experience at least some psychological distress (anxiety, fear, sadness, anger, agitation) during the last phase of a terminal illness (Sheehan & Schirm, 2003). Terminally ill adult patients experience a host of distressing symptoms along with depression in their last days/weeks/ months of life (Ferris, 2004). Anxiety is thought to occur in more than 70% of terminally ill adult patients and often accompanies depression (Wilson et al., 2007).

Depression is not a normal part of the dying process, though grief (e.g., anticipatory/preparatory grief) is a normal and universal part of the dying process (Block, 2000). In terminally ill older adults,

depression manifests with the same tetrad of physical, affective, behavioral, and cognitive symptoms seen in older patients who are not terminally ill and younger patients who are terminally ill (Block, 2000, 2010). Many, but not all, of these symptoms are seen in any terminally ill person who is experiencing grief related to the impending end of his or her life. Table 29.1 lists the similarities and the differences in these symptoms in grief versus depression (Block, 2000; Chochinov, 1995; Periyakoil, n.d.). As illustrated in Table 29.1, affective symptoms are one of the best ways to differentiate depression from grief. In addition, the greater the number of symptoms (including physical symptoms) and/or greater the impairment of function, the more likely the patient has depression rather than grief. Although physical symptoms may be due to the terminal illness, comorbid illness, or adverse effects of medications, in the presence of cognitive symptoms of depression, we recommend considering them as part of depression syndrome. In general, we recommend a low threshold for diagnosing depression.

Occasional thoughts of suicide or a desire for death are fairly common among older adults living with a terminal illness (Hawton & van Heeringen, 2009). Sadness, loss of interest, and thoughts that one would be better off dead in the last days of life should not be assumed to be due to major depression (Rabkin et al., 2009). On the other hand, preoccupation with a wish to die and/or request for a hastened death are often expressions of fear of suffering (e.g., due to pain, loss of dignity and or control, fear of being a burden) during end of life rather than fear of death and need to be considered psychiatric emergencies (Block, 1994). Terminal illness through its physical manifestations and its psychosocial effects threatens the "intactness" of the person like no other illness and in many patients eventually triggers depression (Cassell, 2004). In addition, facing one's own death in a matter of hours, days, or weeks is not a simple journey of decline in function or awareness but involves complex emotions and a variety of behavioral manifestations and patterns of decline in awareness and function (Lunney, Lynn, Foley, Lipson, & Guralnik, 2003).

Spiritual pain is common in older adults receiving end-of-life (EOL) care and often contributes to depression (Delgado-Guay et al., 2011). A study of 31 inpatients (average age: 60.7 years) who were referred to the palliative care consult service found that negative religious coping (i.e., statements regarding punishment or abandonment by God) was

Table 29.1 Differences in Clinical Manifestations of Grief and Depression

SYMPTOMS	GRIEF	DEPRESSION
Physical		
Loss of appetite	++	+++
Loss of weight	++	+++
Sleep disturbances	++	+++
Loss of libido	++	+++
Fatigue, loss of energy	++	+++
Affective		
Crying spells	Waxes and wanes	Pervasive/persistent
Irritability	Waxes and wanes	Pervasive/persistent
Apathy	–/+	+/++
Hopelessness	–/+	++/+++
Worthlessness	–/+	++/+++
Active desire for an early death	–/+	++/+++
Request for assisted suicide	Absent	Not uncommon
Behavioral		
Agitation	+/++	++/+++
Psychomotor retardation	+/++	++/+++
Aggression	–/+	+/++

Source: Block, 2000; Chochinov, 1995; Periyakoil, 2005.

associated positively with distress and depression (Hills, Paice, Cameron, & Shott, 2005). Women with breast cancer (some in stage IV) who used negative religious coping (e.g., feeling abandoned or anger at God) had worse overall mental health, more depressive symptoms, and lower life satisfaction compared to women with breast cancer who used positive religious coping (i.e., partnering with God or looking to God for strength, support, or guidance) (Hebert, Zdaniuk, Schulz, & Scheier, 2009). It is unclear whether depression causes negative coping or vice versa. Using the Spiritual Well-Being Scale, the existential aspect of spirituality (existential well-being) was found to negatively correlate with anxiety and depression in a study of 85 patients with advanced cancer (average age 68), but religious well-being and strength of belief had no impact on psychological well-being in this study (McCoubrie & Davies, 2006). These data indicate that depression in some older adults receiving hospice care may manifest as spiritual pain or spiritual distress.

Little is known about the natural course of depressive symptoms over time in older adults

receiving hospice care. Over 12 weeks, patients (younger and older adults) attending a palliative care day unit were evaluated for stability of their depression over time (Lloyd-Williams & Riddleston, 2002). The study found that depression scores remained largely unchanged during this period, indicating that depressive symptoms may not resolve spontaneously.

WISH TO HASTEN DEATH

Requests to hasten death are not uncommon in older adults receiving hospice care (Block & Billings, 1994; Chochinov et al., 1995). In our clinical practice, such requests have even come from family members who have witnessed the prolonged suffering of their loved one having terminal illness. In one study of terminally ill cancer patients (n = 256), 14% reported a wish to hasten death (Kelly et al., 2003). In this study, higher levels of depressive symptoms, being admitted to an inpatient hospice setting, a greater perception of being a burden on others, lower family cohesion, lower levels of social support, higher levels of anxiety, and greater impact of physical symptoms were associated with higher wishes to hasten death (Kelly et al., 2003).

Addressing requests to hasten death are emotionally challenging for physicians. Generally, there are multiple issues (e.g., pain, sense of being a burden emotionally and financially, dignity concerns, concerns with dependency, one's desire to be in control of one's life) that are influencing the patient's emotional distress and desire to hasten death (Hudson et al., 2006). Physicians should take time to understand these issues, evaluate for depression as well as for existential suffering, and make care plans that address these issues (Gallagher, 2009).

SCALES TO ASSESS DEPRESSION IN TERMINALLY ILL OLDER ADULTS

Currently, no validated tools exist to screen for depression in older adults with terminal illness (Braun, Kunik, & Pham, 2008; Lloyd-Williams, 2000; Nelson et al., 2009). One reason for the lack of screening tools is that symptoms normally associated with depression in older adults can overlap substantially with symptoms associated with terminal illness. Weight loss, fatigue, and pain are typically caused by terminal illness or therapies (e.g., medications, radiation, chemotherapy) used for palliative care of the terminal illness, but they may also be indicators of depression (Weinberger et al., 2011). Scales used for evaluation of depression in older adults such as the Geriatric Depression Scale (GDS) (Yesavage et al., 1982) have not been rigorously studied in elderly persons receiving hospice care. The Hospital Anxiety and Depression Scale (HADS) (Zigmond & Snaith, 1983) is often used in medically ill patients to assess depression but may not be appropriate for routine screening in terminally ill patients (Lloyd-Williams, 2000). A simple question such as "Are you depressed?" may be a reliable way of screening for depression in patients receiving hospice care (Chochinov, Wilson, Enns, & Lander, 1997). We recommend that caregivers (professional and family) of older terminally ill patients begin their screening by assessing for anhedonia and depressed mood in each individual and basing further screening and treatment on the initial impression. Desire for hastened death may

Table 29.2 Suggested Questions to Assess Desire for Hastened Death

QUESTION	LIKERT SCALE*
I go to sleep hoping that I won't wake up	–
I think of ending my life, but I would not do it	–
I would end my life if I had a chance	–
I wish the doctors would do something to end my life	–

*Likert scale: 0 = never, 1 = some of the time, 2 = a lot of the time, 3 = all the time.

be explored systematically by asking four questions and using a Likert scale (see Table 29.2) (Tiernan et al., 2002). For research purposes, the Terminally Ill Grief or Depression Scale (TIGDS) (Periyakoil et al., 2005) is useful in differentiating between grief and depression, and some questions (see Table 29.3) may be used in clinical practice. A cross-sectional study of 200 hospice inpatients (average age 65 years) found that short assessment scales to evaluate for hopelessness (3-item, 7-item) may be considered in this population (Abbey, Rosenfeld, Pessin, & Breitbart, 2006).

Table 29.3 Selected Items From the Terminally Ill Grief of Depression Scale

Restoration-oriented grief
I hope to die peacefully
I pray for a miracle that will cure me

Loss-oriented grief
I am more concerned for my loved ones than for myself
I have felt numb ever since I was told about my diagnosis

Depression
The world would be a better place without me
I do not know why anyone bothers with me

Source: Adapted from the Terminally Ill Grief or Depression Scale (TIGDS) (Periyakoil, 2005).

MANAGEMENT OF DEPRESSION: GENERAL PRINCIPLES

We did not find any studies that focused on pharmacological strategies. Only four studies focused on non-pharmacological strategies to manage depression in older adults receiving hospice care. Our recommendations are based primarily on studies involving terminally ill adults (the majority being patients with cancer) and adults receiving palliative and or hospice care.

Hospice care has been shown to generate a renewed sense of meaning and purpose for patients. To date, the impact of hospice on depressive symptoms has not yet been well studied (Candy, Holman, Leurent, Davis, & Jones, 2011). Management of depression in older adults receiving hospice care is very challenging because these individuals are often frail, suffer from numerous other comorbidities besides their terminal illness, and are taking multiple medications. We recommend a holistic multidimensional approach to the treatment of depression in older adults receiving hospice care. Treatment includes biological, psychological, social, spiritual, environmental, and cultural dimensions of suffering and healing. These interventions should be used in addition to standard care for hospice patients that include supportive interventions for patients and caregivers (family and professional), spiritual care, and interventions to address financial and other problems (Rousseau, 2000). Optimal control of physical distress (e.g., pain, constipation, dyspnea), financial stressors, and environmental factors (e.g., wish to die at home) are necessary for pharmacological and psychosocial interventions to be successful in relieving depression in this population (Block, 2006).

From the patient's perspective, here-and-now comfort, relief of pain, and small pleasures, including not having to think about his or her terminality, are some of the simple interventions that should be routinely employed to prevent and treat EOL depression. The hospice treatment team needs to convey through words and nonverbal behaviors that every elderly person is worthy of honor and there is meaning in life of all elderly persons, irrespective of their cognitive, physical, and/or emotional condition. These basic tenets of kindness, humanity, and respect are often overlooked in our time-pressured culture and can be reinstated by dignity conserving care (Chochinov, 2007). The final stage of life holds remarkable possibilities for psychological and spiritual growth; for strengthening bonds with one's family and friends; to repair broken relationships; and to create meaning (Byock, 2004; Chochinov, 2003). As the treatment team makes the effort to know the terminally ill person, the person begins to feel that his or her existence matters, and that he or she is valued (Lustbader, 2000).

A desire to die at home in familiar surroundings with family and friends in attendance is common, and depression is often a reaction to not being able to do so. Often the patient's needs are such that adequate care cannot be provided at home by family members and/or the experience of a death at home would be too difficult for family members. Discussions about place of death may help alleviate stress, and availability of hospice may increase the chances of allowing the patient to die at home if this is in keeping with his or her wishes. The choices involving interventions for pain and depression (as well as other EOL care decisions) may be influenced more by ethnicity and culture than the person's age, education, socioeconomic status, or other variables (Baker, 2002). Improved understanding of the patient's ethnic and cultural factors may lead HCPs to change the choice of their interventions. Existential concerns (e.g., loss of dignity, loss of sense of meaning in life remaining) can be addressed by inviting patients to discuss issues that they value and to express their thoughts about what they would most want remembered about themselves as their death draws near (Chochinov et al., 2005). Spiritual beliefs and practices may help relieve depression by improving one's understanding of meaning in one's suffering (Kandasamy, Chaturvedi, & Desai, 2011). Interventions to reduce psychosocial distress of family members may also improve the patient's depression.

Many older adults are depressed because of a sense of helplessness regarding their inability to control circumstances surrounding their death. Palliative sedation and voluntary refusal of nutrition and hydration may be appropriate in some patients (e.g., patient's with intractable severe pain due to metastases) and may relieve their depression by giving them the control they desire (Olsen, Swetz, & Mueller, 2010). Availability and discussion of these interventions will vary based on the physicians' religious characteristics, ethnicity, and experience in caring for dying patients (Curlin, Nwodim, Vance, Chin, & Lantos, 2008).

Psychosocial Interventions Research

We found only four studies that evaluated the impact of psychosocial (non-drug) interventions on depression in older adults receiving hospice care.

Anticipatory grief therapy was found to improve depression (using the Geriatric Depression Scale) over 4 weeks in older adults (n = 26) receiving hospice care as well as long-term care residents with terminal illness (Cheng, Lo, Chan, & Woo, 2010). A review of 20 studies (6 of them were randomized) of home-based music therapy found that the intervention reduced symptoms of depression in elderly receiving hospice and palliative care (Schmid & Ostermann, 2010). Clements-Cortes has reported three cases (ages 71, 72, and 76 years) where terminally ill patients showed improved mood, anxiety, and reduced social isolation with individual music therapy (Clements-Cortes, 2004). Geisler has described improvement in mood (not assessed formally) in two hospice patients (one patient in her 70s and another 60 years old) with the use of pet therapy (Geisler, 2004).

The largest study to date that looked at the impact of non-drug interventions on depression in adults receiving palliative care involved dignity therapy. Dignity therapy is a short-term psychotherapy specifically designed for patients with terminal illness (Chochinov et al., 2005). It involves engaging patients in reviewing current and past events and experiences that were most meaningful to them and to document their legacy. Compared to standard palliative care, dignity therapy was found to improve spiritual well-being and sadness but did not improve scores on a depression scale (HADS) in adults (n = 441) receiving palliative care (Chochinov et al., 2011). Restorative natural environments (such as forests and coastlines) can promote stress reduction, and multisensory computer-generated restorative environments may reduce depression in adult patients receiving hospice care who were unable to access and experience real environments (Depledge, Stone, & Bird, 2011). Aromatherapy massage in adult patients (n = 42) receiving hospice care was found to modestly improve depression using HADS (Soden, Vincent, Craske, Lucas, & Ashley, 2004). A 4-week randomized trial of guided self-help versus waitlist control in adults (n = 38) receiving hospice care found improvement in anxiety but not depression (Galfin, Watkins, & Harlow, 2011).

Psychotherapeutic strategies are effective in treating EOL depression, especially if counselors visit patients several times a week and are present frequently at the time of death (Linn, Linn, & Harris, 1982). Psychotherapy in patients receiving EOL care may involve social support (especially from other patients as seen in group therapy),

emotional expression, cognitive restructuring, and training in coping skills (Spiegel, 1996). Problem-solving therapy may also be considered to treat depression in terminally ill patients (Wood & Mynors-Wallis, 1997). Palliative care nurses who received cognitive-behavioral therapy (CBT) training reported greater confidence and effectiveness in treating anxiety and depression in patients receiving palliative care (Cort et al., 2009). In a small study (n = 11), patients receiving palliative care were provided with CBT after brief training of palliative care professionals (Anderson, Watson, & Davidson, 2008). Anxiety and depression improved in eight patients.

Despite the limited evidence relative to the use of nonpharmacologic therapies for depression in hospice patients, one should not dismiss the benefit of nonpharmacologic therapy in the treatment of depression (Stagg & Lazenby, 2012). While antidepressants take on average up to 8 weeks to be fully effective, nonpharmacologic therapies can provide benefit almost immediately and have few adverse effects.

In a recent study, hospice staff reporting of data from the standardized assessments of depression to interdisciplinary team improved treatment of depression (e.g., prescription of antidepressants, follow-up for response to treatment) in adults (n = 709) receiving hospice care (McMillan, Small, & Haley, 2011). Hospice and hospital staff training programs (Jenkins et al., 2010) improved staff confidence in detection and management of psychological distress. Thus, systematic assessment and staff training are recommended as interventions to improve detection and treatment of depression in older adults receiving hospice care.

An interdisciplinary approach to treatment of depression in older adults receiving hospice care is recommended but has not been studied. One study evaluated the role of psychologists in caring for patients receiving hospice care (Alexander, 2004). The psychologist helped the hospice team manage not only depression but also anxiety, marital / family stresses, problems of alcohol misuse, and dementia-related challenging behaviors. Our clinical experience has found similar benefits with not only involvement of a psychologist but also a social worker. Although high quality empirical studies are lacking, rehabilitation (such as physical and occupational therapy, speech therapy), meditation, massage therapy, music therapy, and aromatherapy may improve mood and prevent depression by improving ability to do daily activities, thus reducing dependence (Javier & Montagnini, 2011; Lafferty, Downey, McCarty, Standish, & Patrick, 2006; Louis & Lowalski 2002; Romo & Gifford, 2007).

HCPs engaged in providing hospice care must also attend to their own sense of grief and loss, proactively engaging in strategies that reduce the likelihood of burnout and enhance their capacity to reap the rewards that helping patients during their last days of life provides (Pantilat & Isaac, 2008).

ROLE OF ANTIDEPRESSANTS AND ELECTROCONVULSIVE THERAPY

We found only one controlled study that looked at effectiveness of antidepressants in older adults receiving hospice care. In this randomized, double-blind, placebo-controlled study ($n = 34$), methylphenidate was found to improve depression and fatigue in patients receiving hospice care (median age: 74.5; age range: 51–90) (Kerr et al., 2012). Hardy (2009) studied 26 hospice inpatients (median age: 63.8; age range: 42–79) with depression and found that methylphenidate improved depression in 46% of these patients, but depression improved only in 7% of those who died within 6 weeks. In a 2-week case series of 18 adults with cancer receiving hospice care, selective serotonin reuptake inhibitors (SSRIs) improved depression (on the Hamilton Depression Rating Scale) and the improvement correlated with presence of "s/s" and "s/I" variants of 5-HTTLPR genetic polymorphism of the serotonin transporter gene (SERT) (Schillani et al., 2011). Approximately 11.5% of adults receiving hospice care were found to be on antidepressants over 18 months (cumulative probability), and SSRIs were the most common class of antidepressants (Shiroma, Geda, Mohan, & Richardson, 2011). In this study, longer stays in hospice were associated with higher likelihood of receiving antidepressants. A single oral dose of the anesthetic agent ketamine was found to improve depression in two older adults (age 64 and 70) receiving hospice care (Irwin & Iglewicz, 2010).

Antidepressants such as SSRIs and mirtazapine may cause hyponatremia and methylphenidate may cause delirium in older adults receiving hospice care (Ladino, Guardiola, & Paniagua, 2006; Macleod, 1998; Miller, Adams, & Miller, 2006). In a study by Lawrie et al., 73% of palliative medicine physicians assessed for depression, 27% used a standardized

scale (HAD scale), and most prescribed antidepressants were SSRIs (80%).

Despite the dearth of controlled studies evaluating efficacy of antidepressants in older adults receiving hospice care, a trial of antidepressants should be considered for the treatment of depression in all older adults receiving hospice care who have depression. A trial of antidepressants is especially recommended if the patient has a past history of good response to antidepressants and or if depression is moderate to severe. Appropriate antidepressant therapy can not only provide relief from depressive symptoms but may also promote reengagement in the remaining days of one's life.

There is no research to support favoring the use of one antidepressant over another in older adults receiving hospice care. Choice of antidepressants depends on matching the patient's physical health problems with adverse effects of antidepressants so that they complement rather than increase the risk of toxicity. For example, in patients with constipation, tricyclic antidepressants (TCAs) should be avoided, and in patients with diarrhea, SSRIs should be avoided. In patients with insomnia and weight loss, mirtazapine may be preferred as it may promote sleep and increase appetite and weight gain. In patients with chronic pain, serotonin norepinephrine reuptake inhibitors (e.g., venlafaxine, duloxetine) may be preferred. All antidepressants take 4–6 weeks or longer before they are optimally effective and in patients with a very short life expectancy, stimulants (methylphenidate) may be preferred as they have a faster onset of action (in days). Concomitant use of stimulants and antidepressants (e.g., SSRIs) may also be considered as stimulants may accelerate response to standard antidepressants (Lavertsky et al., 2006). Stimulants may also help overcome other symptoms that frequently co-occur with depression, such as fatigue, apathy, and daytime sedation due to use of opiates (Hardy, 2009; Kerr et al., 2012).

Electroconvulsive therapy (ECT) is appropriate even in the terminally ill older adult if the patient is having psychotic depression or is actively suicidal or has life-threatening complications of depression (e.g., not eating or drinking due to depression) (Rasmussen & Richardson, 2010). Based on our clinical experience, we would recommend ECT for severe depression in this population, especially if there is a past history of good response to ECTs.

Some antidepressants may interact with analgesics causing toxicity and or loss of efficacy. SSRIs or

TCAs, if used concomitantly with tramadol, may result in serotonin syndrome (e.g., myoclonus, fever, agitation, autonomic instability) and seizures (Pierce & Brahm, 2011). Antidepressants that significantly inhibit the cytochrome P450 2D6 isoenzyme system (e.g., paroxetine, fluoxetine, bupropion) may lessen the analgesic effect of analgesics that need this enzyme system to be converted to active metabolites (e.g., tramadol, codeine) (Pierce & Brahm, 2011). Antidepressants with mild to moderate P450 3A4 inhibiting effects (e.g., fluoxetine, fluvoxamine) may cause opiate toxicity when administered to patients taking opiates metabolized by the 3A4 isoenzyme (e.g., oxycodone, fentanyl) (Pierce & Brahm. 2011). Antidepressants with only mild inhibitory effect on 2D6 isoenzyme system (e.g., citalopram, sertraline, escitalopram, venlafaxine) and mirtazapine (does not seem to inhibit the major CYP isoforms) are preferred in patients taking opiates. Input from a pharmacist is recommended in patients using antidepressants and opioid analgesics, especially if the patient's depression and pain are not improving.

Psychotic depression does not respond to antidepressant monotherapy and generally needs ECT or antipsychotics along with antidepressants. Antidepressants may not be effective for bipolar depression, and treatment options for bipolar depression include quetiapine or a combination of olanzapine and fluoxetine (Sachs, Dupuy, & Wittman, 2011). ECT is also effective for bipolar depression.

DEPRESSION AND ADVANCED DEMENTIA

Older adults receiving hospice care for dementia require special consideration because severe cognitive impairment makes diagnosing and treating depression even more challenging. In the only study we found that studied depression in patients with dementia receiving hospice care, the prevalence of depression was found to be 45% (Kverno et al., 2008). It is important to consider depression as a cause for agitation, anxiety, and aggression in patients with dementia (Prado-Jean et al., 2010). Clinical experience suggests that co-occurrence of psychotic symptoms (e.g., delusions, hallucinations) with depression is not uncommon.

As with older adults with other terminal illnesses, there continues to be no "gold standard" for screening depression in older adults with advanced dementia. The Cornell Scale for Depression in

Dementia (CSDD) (Alexopoulos, Abrams, Young, & Shamoian, 1988) is widely used and validated (Muller-Thomsen et al., 2005). A difficulty with using the CSDD is that it requires input from both the patient and a caregiver, meaning the caregiver must know the patient well enough to evaluate any subtle changes from baseline. This may be difficult when an older adult is receiving institutional care where the staff frequently changes and family members are unable to visit often. Nursing home staff members need education in determining when a patient is appropriate for hospice care as 4% of nursing home residents are designated as being at the end of life and only 2% are shown to be receiving hospice care (Parker-Oliver et al., 2003). Conditions of hospice and nonhospice residents in nursing homes and assisted living facilities are largely similar, indicating that there are limited clinical reasons for low utilization of hospice in nursing home settings (Cartwright, Miller, & Volpin, 2009; Parker-Oliver et al., 2003). We did not find any studies that investigated interventions to treat depression in older adults having dementia who are receiving hospice care. A recent multicenter, randomized, double-blind, placebo-controlled study of patients with mild to moderate dementia of the Alzheimer's type with depression (CSDD score of 8 or more) did not find sertraline (average dose 95 mg) or mirtazapine (average dose 30 mg) to be better than placebo (Banerjee et al., 2011). The active drug group did have more adverse effects than the placebo group. Despite the negative results, a trial of antidepressants may be appropriate in patients with dementia receiving hospice care who have significant depressive symptoms.

The majority of residents in long-term care (LTC) have advanced dementia and their average life expectancy is 2–3 years (Desai & Grossberg, 2010). Similar to cognitively intact older adults, depression in patients with advanced dementia may be in response to physical discomfort such as pain (e.g., due to decubitii), dyspnea, and constipation. Dyspnea rather than pain may be the most prevalent symptoms during the final 48 hours of life because most older adults in long-term care facilities die of non-cancer-related causes (Hall, Schroder, & Weaver, 2002). Relieving dyspnea may reduce anxiety and depression and obviate any need for antidepressants. Meaningful structured activities and sensory stimulation (e.g., hand massage or back rub with an aromatic lotion) for depression may augment antidepressant therapy and may even reduce its use (Volicer, 2001). Geriatric psychiatrists can play a central role in diagnosing depression in patients with dementia and working with the hospice team in instituting appropriate interventions and follow-up (Aupperle, MacPhee, Strozeski, Finn, & Heath, 2004).

FUTURE RESEARCH

The evidence base for prevalence, assessment, and management of depression in older adults receiving hospice care is largely extrapolated from other populations (especially terminally ill cancer patients and patients receiving palliative care, many of whom are younger than 65), and a majority of this research is drawn from small, single-institution studies and case reports. The studies reviewed were primarily descriptive. The findings indicate that little is known about the effectiveness of antidepressants in treating depression in older adults receiving hospice care. There is an urgent need for research to better understand depression in older adults receiving hospice care, including the rigorous development and evaluation of service models and therapeutic interventions (both antidepressants and non-drug interventions). Future research needs to address the generalizability of research findings regarding depression in older adults receiving hospice care from one group of terminal disorders (e.g., metastatic cancer) to other conditions (e.g., advanced heart failure, end-stage renal disease, advanced dementia) and across different settings (e.g., home vs. long-term care facilities; Kurella Tamura, & Cohen, 2010; Lorenz et al., 2008; Selman, Beynon, Higginson, & Harding, 2007). Research will also need to be conducted over an at least 8- to 12-week period of time to fully understand the impact of pharmacotherapy on depression at the EOL. Research is needed to identify valid and clinically practical measures for diagnosing depression in older adults receiving hospice care, especially in those with cognitive impairment. Efforts to understand the constructs of hope, meaning, and dignity, and to correlate them with depression and normal grief, are warranted.

CONCLUSION

Depression is prevalent, underrecognized, and undertreated in older adults receiving hospice care for terminal illnesses such as advanced cancer, heart failure, end-stage renal disease (ESRD), and dementia. The two key reasons are difficulty differentiating depression from normal grief and lack of adequate training of HCPs, including physicians, in diagnosing and treating depression in patients receiving palliative care. Depression can be reliably differentiated from normal grief. There is an urgent need for improved education and training of HCPs to diagnose and manage depression in older adults receiving EOL care. Systematic routine assessment of depression is recommended for all hospice patients, including older adults. Treatment of depression can reduce suffering, improve quality of life, and provide an opportunity to prepare for death. Treatment of depression may lessen desire for early death. Treatment of depression may also reduce emotional distress in family members of the patient. More research is needed before clear guidelines about antidepressant class and dosages for treatment of depression in older adults receiving hospice care can be provided.

Disclosures
Dr. Desai has no conflicts of interest to disclose.
Dr. Lo has no conflicts of interest to disclose.
Dr. Grossberg

REFERENCES

Abbey, J. G., Rosenfeld, B., Pessin, H., & Breitbart, W. (2006). Hopelessness at the end of life: the utility of the hopelessness scale with terminally ill cancer patients. *British Journal of Health Psychology*, 11,173–183.

Alexander, P. (2004). An investigation of inpatient referrals to a clinical psychologist in a hospice. *European Journal of Cancer Care*, 13, 36–44.

Alexopoulos, G. S., Abrams, R. C., Young, R. C., & Shamoian, C. A. (1988). Cornell Scale for Depression in Dementia. *Biological Psychiatry, 23,* 271–284.

Anderson, T., Watson, M., & Davidson, R. (2008). The use of cognitive behavioral therapy techniques for anxiety and depression in hospice patients: A feasibility study. *Palliative Medicine, 22,* 814–821.

Aupperle, P. M., MacPhee, E. R., Strozeski, J. E., Finn, M., & Heath, J. M. (2004). Hospice use for the patient with advanced Alzheimer's disease: The role of the geriatric psychiatrist. *American Journal of Hospital Palliative Care, 21*(6),427–437.

Axtell, A. JPM patient information. Depression in palliative care. *Journal of Palliative Medicine, 11*(3), 529–530.

Baker, M. (2002). Economic, political and ethnic influences on end-of-life decision-making: A decade in review. *Journal of Health and Social Policy, 14*(3), 27–39.

Banerjee, S., Hellier, J., Dewey, M., Romeo, R., Ballard, C., Baldwin, R., ... Burns, A. (2011). Sertraline or mirtazapine for depression in dementia (HTA-SADD): A randomised, multicentre, double-blind, placebo-controlled trial. *Lancet, 378,* 403–411

Block, S. D. (2000). Assessing and managing depression in the terminally ill patient. ACP-ASIM End-of-Life Care Consensus Panel. American College of Physicians—American Society of Internal Medicine. *Annals of Internal Medicine, 132,* 209–218.

Block, S. D. (2001). Perspectives on care at the close of life. Psychological considerations, growth, and transcendence at the end of life: The art of the possible. *Journal of the American Medical Association, 285*(22),2898–2905.

Block, S. D. (2006). Psychological issues in end-of-life care. *Journal of Palliative Medicine, 9*(3), 751–772.

Block, S. D. (2010). Diagnosis and treatment of depression in patients with advanced illness. *Epidemiologia e Psichiatria Sociale, 19,* 103–109.

Block, S. D., & Billings, J. A. (1994). Patient request to hasten death: Evaluation and management in terminal care. *Archives of Internal Medicine, 154,* 2039–2047.

Bosma, H., Apland, L., & Kazzanjian, A. (2010). Cultural conceptualizations of hospice palliative care: More similarities than differences. *Palliative Medicine, 24*(5), 510–522.

Braun, U. K., Kunik, M. E., & Pham, C. (2008). Treating depression in terminally ill patients can optimize their physical comfort at the end of life and provide them the opportunity to confront and prepare for death. *Geriatrics, 63,* 25–27.

Breitbart, W., & Strout, D. (2000). Delirium in the terminally ill. *Clinics in Geriatric Medicine, 16*(2), 357–372.

Buchanan, R. J., Choi, M., Wang, S., & Huang, C. (2002). Analyses of nursing home residents in hospice care using the minimum data set. *Palliative Medicine, 16*(6), 465–480.

Byock, I. (2004). *The four things that matter most: A book about living.* New York: Free Press.

Candy, B., Holman, A., Leurent, B., Davis, S., & Jones, L. (2011). Hospice care delivered at home, in nursing home and in dedicated hospice facilities: A systematic review of quantitative and qualitative evidence. *International Journal of Nursing Studies, 48*(1), 121–133.

Cartwright, J. C., Miller, L., & Volpin, M. (2009). Hospice in assisted living: Promoting good quality care at end of life. *Gerontologist, 49*(4), 508–516.

Cassell, E. J. (2004). *The nature of suffering and the goals of medicine.* New York: Oxford University Press.

Cheng, J. O., Lo, R., Chan, F., & Woo, J. (2010). A pilot study on the effectiveness of anticipatory grief therapy for elderly facing end of life. *Journal of Palliative Care, 26*(4), 261–269.

Cherny, N. I., & Catane, R. (2003). European Society of Medical Oncology Taskforce on Palliative and Supportive Care. Attitudes of medical oncologists toward palliative care for patients with advanced and incurable cancer: Report on a survey by the European Society of Medical Oncology Taskforce on Palliative and Supportive Care. *Cancer, 98*(11), 2502–2510.

Chochinov, H. M. (2003). Thinking outside the box: depression, hope and meaning at the end of life. *Journal of Palliative Medicine, 6,* 973–977.

Chochinov, H. M. (2007). Dignity and the essence of medicine: The A, B, C, and D of dignity conserving care. *British Medical Journal, 335,* 184–187.

Chochinov, H. M., Hack, T., Hassard, T., Kristjanson, L. J., McClement, S., & Harlos, M. (2005). Dignity therapy: A novel psychotherapeutic intervention for patients near the end of life. *Journal of Clinical Oncology, 23*(24), 5520–5525.

Chochinov, H. M., Kristjanson, L. J., Breitbart, W., McClement, S., Hack, T. F., Hassard, T., & Harlos, M. (2011). Effect of dignity therapy on distress and end-of-life experience in terminally ill patients: A randomized controlled trial. *Lancet Oncology, 12*(8), 753–762.

Chochinov, H. M., Wilson, K. G., Enns, M., & Lander, S. (1997). "Are you depressed?" Screening for depression in the terminally ill. *American Journal of Psychiatry, 154*(5), 674–676.

Chochinov, H. M., Wilson, K. G., Enns, M., Mowchun, N., Lander, S., Levitt, M., & Clinch, J. J. (1995). Desire for death in the terminally ill. *American Journal of Psychiatry, 152,* 1185–1191.

Cort, E., Moorey, S., Hotopf, M., Kapari, M., Monroe, B., & Hansford, P. (2009). Palliative care nurses' experience of training in cognitive behavior therapy and taking part in a randomized controlled trial. *International Journal of Palliative Nursing 15*(6), 290–298.

Clements-Cortes, A. (2004). The use of music in facilitating emotional expression in the terminally ill. *American Journal of Hospital Palliative Care, 21*(4), 255–260.

Curlin, F. A., Nwodim, C., Vance, J., Chin, M., & Lantos, J. D. (2008). To die, to sleep: US physicians' religious and other objections to physician-assisted suicide, terminal sedation, and withdrawal of life support. *American Journal of Hospital Palliative Care, 25*(2), 112–120.

Delgado-Guay, M. O., Hui, D., Parsons, H. A., Govan, K., De la Cruz, M., Thorney, S., & Bruera, E. (2011). Spirituality, religiosity, and spiritual pain in advanced cancer patients. *Journal of Pain Symptom Management, 41*(6), 986–994.

Depledge, M. H., Stone, R. J., & Bird, W. J. (2011). Can natural and virtual environments be used to promote improved human health and wellbeing? *Environmental Science Technology, 45*(11), 4660–4665.

Desai AK, Grossberg GT. (2011). Palliative and end-of-life care in psychogeriatric patients. *Aging and Health, 7*(3), 395–408

Desai, A. K., & Grossberg, G. T. (Eds.) (2010). Palliative and end-of-life care. In *Psychiatric consultation in long term care. A guide for healthcare professionals* (pp. 267–295). Baltimore, MD: Johns Hopkins Press.

Ferris, F. D. (2004). Last hours of living. *Clinics in Geriatric Medicine, 20*, 641–667.

Galfin, J. M., Watkins, E. R., & Harlow, T. (2011). A brief guided self-help intervention for psychological distress in palliative care patients: A randomized controlled trial. *Palliative Medicine, 26*(3), 197–205.

Gallagher, R. (2009). Can't we get this over with? An approach to assessing the patient who requests hastened death. *Canadian Family Physician, 55*(3), 260–261.

Geisler, A. M. (2004). Companion animals in palliative care: Stories from the bedside. *American Journal of Hospital Palliative Care, 21*(4), 285–288.

Goy, E. R., & Ganzini, L. (2011). Prevalence and natural history of neuropsychiatric syndromes in veteran hospice patients. *Journal of Pain Symptom Management, 41*(2), 394–401.

Hackett, A., & Gaitan, A. (2007). A qualitative study assessing mental health issues in two hospices in the UK. *International Journal of Palliative Nursing, 13*(6), 273–281.

Hall, P., Schroder, C., & Weaver, L. (2002). The last 48 hours of life in long-term care: A focused chart audit. *Journal of the American Geriatrics Society, 50*(3), 501–506.

Hardy, S. E. (2009). Methylphenidate for treatment of depressive symptom, apathy, and fatigue in medically ill older adults and terminally ill adults. *American Journal of Geriatric Pharmacotherapy, 7*(1), 34–59.

Hawton, K., & van Heeringen, K. (2009). Suicide. *Lancet, 373*(9672), 1372–1381.

Hayes, R. D., Lee, W., Rayner, L., Price, A., Monroe, B., Hansford, P., … Hotopf, M. (2011). Gender differences in prevalence of depression among patients receiving palliative care: The role of dependency. *Palliative Medicine.* 2011 Jul 20 ePub ahead of print.

Hebert, R., Zdaniuk, B., Schulz, R., & Scheier, M. (2009). Positive and negative religious coping and well-being in women with breast cancer. *Journal of Palliative Medicine, 12*(6), 537–545.

Hills, J., Paice, J. A., Cameron, J. R., & Shott, S. Spirituality and distress in palliative care consultation. *Journal of Palliative Medicine, 8*(4), 782–788.

Hudson, P. L., Kristjanson, L. J., Ashby, M., Kelly, B., Schofield, P., Hudson, R., … Street, A. (2006). Desire for hastened death in patients with advanced disease and the evidence base of clinical guidelines: A systematic review. *Palliat Med 20*(7), 693–701.

Irwin, S. A., & Iglewicz, A. (2010). Oral ketamine for the rapid treatment of depression and anxiety in patients receiving hospice care. *Journal of Palliative Medicine, 13*(7), 903–908.

Irwin, S. A., Rao, S., Bower, K., Palica, J., Rao, S. S., Maglione, J. E., … Ferris, F. D. (2008). Psychiatric issues in palliative care: Recognition of depression in patients enrolled in hospice care. *Journal of Palliative Medicine, 11*(2), 158–163.

Ita, D., Keorney, M., & O'Slorain, L. (2003). Psychiatric disorder in a palliative care unit. *Journal of Palliative Medicine, 17*(2), 212–218.

Javier, N. S., & Montagnini, M. L. (2011). Rehabilitation of the hospice and palliative care patient. *Journal of Palliative Medicine, 14*(5), 638–648.

Jenkins, K., Alberry, B., Daniel, J., Dixie, L., North, V., Patterson, L., … North, N. (2010). Beyond communication: The development of a training program for hospital and hospice staff in the detection and management of psychological distress—preliminary results. *Palliative Support Care, 8*(1), 27–33.

Kandasamy, A., Chaturvedi, S. K., & Desai, G. (2011). Spirituality, distress, depression, anxiety, and quality of life in patients with advanced cancer. *Indian Journal of Cancer, 48*(1), 55–59.

Kelly, B., Burnett, P., Pelusi, D., Badger, S., Varghese, F., & Robertson, M. (2003). Factors associated with the wish to hasten death: A study of patients with terminal illness. *Psychology Medicine, 33*(1), 75–81.

Kerr, C. W., Drake, J., Milch, R. A., Brazeau, D. A., Skretny, J. A., Brazeau, G. A., & Donnelly, J. P. (2012). Effects of methylphenidate on fatigue and depression: A randomized, double-blind, placebo-controlled trial. *Journal of Pain Symptom Management*, 43(1), 68–77.

Kurella Tamura, M., & Cohen, L. M. (2010). Should there be an expanded role for palliative care in end-stage renal disease? *Current Opinion in Nephrology and Hypertension*, 19(6), 556–560.

Kverno, K., Black, B., Blass, D., Geiger-Brown, J., & Rabins, P. (2008). Neuropsychiatric symptom patterns in hospice-eligible nursing home residents with advanced dementia. *Journal of the American Medical Directors Association*, 9, 509–515.

Ladino, M., Guardiola, V. D., & Paniagua, M. (2006). Mirtazapine-induced hyponatremia in an elderly hospice patient. *Journal of Palliative Medicine*, 9(2), 258–260.

Lafferty, W. E., Downey, L., McCarty, R. L., Standish, L. J., & Patrick, D. L. (2006). Evaluating CAM treatment at the end of life: A review of clinical trials for massage and meditation. *Complementary Therapies in Medicine*, 14(2), 100–112.

Lasheen, W., Walsh, D., Hauser, K., Gutgsell, T., & Karafa, M. T. (2009). Symptom variability during repeated measurement among hospice patients with advanced cancer. *American Journal of Hospital Palliative Care*, 26(5), 368–375.

Lavertsky, H., Park, S., Siddarth, P., Kumar, A., & Reynolds, C. F., III. (2006). Methylphenidate-enhanced antidepressant response to citalopram in the elderly: A double-blind, placebo-controlled pilot trial. *American Journal of Geriatric Psychiatry*, 14(2), 181–185.

Lawrie, I., Lloyd-Williams, M., & Taylor, F. (2004). How do palliative medicine physicians assess and manage depression. *Palliative Medicine*, 18(3), 234–238.

Linn, M., Linn, B., & Harris, R. (1982). Effects of counseling for late stage cancer patients. *Cancer*, 49, 1048–1055.

Lloyd-Williams, M. (2000). Difficulties in diagnosing and treating depression in the terminally ill cancer patient. *Postgraduate Medicine Journal*, 76, 555–558.

Lloyd-Williams, M., & Payne, S. (2002). Nurse specialist assessment and management of palliative care patients who are depressed—a study of perceptions and attitudes. *Journal of Palliative Care*, 18(4), 270–274.

Lloyd-Williams, M., & Riddleston, H. (2002). The stability of depression scores in patients who are receiving palliative care. *Journal of Pain Symptom Management*, 24(6), 593–597.

Lorenz, K. A., Lynn, J., Dy, S. M., Shugarman, L. R., Wilkinson, A., Mularski, R. A., Shekelle, P. G.

(2008). Evidence for improving palliative care at the end of life: A systematic review. *Annals of Internal Medicine* 148(2), 147–159.

Louis, M., & Lowalski, S. D. (2002). Use of aromatherapy with hospice patients to decrease pain, anxiety, and depression and to promote an increased sense of well-being. *American Journal of Hospital Palliative Care*, 19(6), 381–386.

Lunney, J. R., Lynn, J., Foley, D. J., Lipson, S., & Guralnik, J. M. (2003). Patterns of functional decline at the end of life. *Journal of the American Medical Association*, 289, 2387–2392.

Lustbader, W. (2000). Thoughts on the meaning of frailty. Reasons to grow old: Meaning in later life. *Generations, Winter*, 21–24.

Macleod, A. D. (1998). Methylphenidate in terminal depression. *Journal of Pain Symptom Management*, 16, 193–198.

McCoubrie, R. C., & Davies, A. N. Is there a correlation between spirituality and anxiety and depression in patients with advanced cancer. *Supportive Care in Cancer*, 14(4), 379–385.

McMillan, S. C., Small, B. J., & Haley, W. E. (2011). Improving hospice outcomes through systematic assessment: A clinical trial. *Cancer Nursing*, 34(2), 89–97.

Miller, K. E., Adams, S. M., & Miller, M. M. (2006). Antidepressant medication use in palliative care. *American Journal of Hospital Palliative Care*, 23(2), 127–133.

Muller-Thomsen, T., Arlt, S., Mann, U., Mass, R., & Ganzer, S. (2005). Detecting depression in Alzheimer's disease: Evaluation of four different scales. *Archives of Clinical Neuropsychology*, 20, 271–276.

Mystakidou, K., Tsilika, E., Parpa, E., Athanasouli, P., Galanos, A., Anna, P., & Vlahos, L. (2009). Illness-related hopelessness in advanced cancer: Influence of anxiety, depression and preparatory grief. *Archives of Psychiatric Nursing*, 23(2), 138–147.

Nelson, C. J., Cho, C., Berk, A. R., Holland, J., & Roth, A. J. (2009). Are gold standard depression measures appropraite for use in geriatric cancer patients? A systematic evaluation of self-report depression instruments used with geriatric, cancer, and geriatric cancer samples. *Journal of Clinical Oncology*, 28(2), 348–356.

Noorani, N. H., & Montagnini, M. (2007). Recognizing depression in palliative care patients. *Journal of Palliative Medicine*, 10(2), 458–464.

Olsen, M. L., Swetz, K. M., & Mueller, P. S. (2010). Ethical decision making with end-of-life care: Palliative sedation and withholding or withdrawing life-sustaining treatments. *Mayo Clinic Proceedings*, 85(10), 949–954.

Pantilat, S. Z., & Isaac, M. (2008). End-of-life care for the hospitalized patient. *Medical Clinics of North America, 92*(2), 349–370.

Parker-Oliver, D., Porock, D., Zweig, S., Rantz, M., & Petroski, G. F. (2003). Hospice and nonhospice nursing home residents. *Journal of Palliative Medicine, 6*(1), 69–71.

Periyakoil, V. J. (n. d.). *Fast facts and concepts #43: Is it grief or depression?* 2nd ed. Retrieved October 2012, from the End-of-Life Physician Education Resource Center Web site: http://www.eperc. mcw.edu/EPERC/FastFactsIndex/ff_043.htm

Periyakoil, V. S., & Hallenbeck, J. (2002). Identifying and managing preparatory grief and depression at the end of life. *American Family Physician, 65*(5), 883–890.

Periyakoil, V. S., Kraemer, H. C., Noda, A., Moos, R., Hallenbeck, J., Webster, M., & Yesavage, J. A. (2005). The development and initial validation of the Terminally Ill Grief of Depression Scale (TIGDS). *International Journal of Methods in Psychiatric Research, 14*(4), 202–212.

Pierce, A. M., & Brahm, N. C. (2011). Opiates and psychotropics: Pharmacokinetics for practitioners. *Current Psychiatry, 10*(6), 83–86.

Prado-Jean, A., Couratier, P., Druet-Cabanac, M., Nubukpo, P., Bernard-Bourzeix, L., Thomas, P., ... Clément, J. P. (2010). Specific psychological and behavioral symptoms of depression in patients with dementia. *International Journal of Geriatric Psychiatry, 25*, 1065–1072.

Rabkin, J. G., McElhiney, M., Moran, P., Acree, M., & Folkman, S. Depression, distress and positive mood in late-stage cancer: A longitudinal study. *Psycho-oncology, 18*(1), 79–86.

Rao, S., Ferris, F. D., & Irwin, S. A. (2011). Ease of screening for depression and delirium in patients enrolled in inpatient hospice care. *Journal of Palliative Medicine, 14*(3), 275–279.

Rasmussen, K. G., & Richardson, J. W. (2010). Electroconvulsive therapy in Palliative care. *American Journal of Hospital Palliative Care.* 2010 Nov 17, ePub ahead of print.

Resnick, H. E., Hickman, S., & Foster, G. L. (2011). Documentation of advance directives among home health and hospice patients in United States, 2007. *American Journal of Hospital Palliative Care,* 2011 May 15 ePub ahead of print.

Romo, R., & Gifford, L. (2007). A cost-benefit analysis of music therapy in a home hospice. *Nursing Economics, 25*(6), 353–358.

Rousseau, P. (2000). The losses and suffering of terminal illness. *Mayo Clinic Proceedings, 75*, 197–198.

Sachs, G. S., Dupuy, J. M., & Wittman, C. W. (2011). The pharmacologic treatment of bipolar disorder. *Journal of Clinical Psychiatry, 72*(5), 704–715.

Schillani, G., Capozzo, M. A., Era, D., De Vana, M., Grassi, L., Conte, M. A., & Giraldi, T. (2011). Pharmacogenetics of escitalopram and mental adaptation to cancer in palliative care: Report of 18 cases. *Tumori, 97*(3), 358–361.

Schmid, W., & Ostermann, T. (2010). Home-based music therapy—a systematic overview of settings and conditions for innovative service in healthcare. *BMC Health Services Research, 10*, 291.

Selman, L., Beynon, T., Higginson, I. J., & Harding, R. (2007). Psychological, social and spiritual distress at the end of life in heart failure patients. *Current Opinion in Supportive Palliative Care, 1*(4), 260–266.

Sheehan, D. K., & Schirm, V. (2003). End of life care of older adults: Debunking some common misconceptions about dying in old age. *American Journal of Nursing, 103*(11), 48–58.

Shiroma, P. R., Geda, Y. E., Mohan, A., & Richardson, J. (2011). Antidepressant prescription pattern in a hospice program. *American Journal of Hospital Palliative Care, 28*(3), 193–197.

Smith, E. M., Gomm, S. A., & Dickens, C. M. (2003). Assessing the independent contribution to quality of life from anxiety and depression in patients with advanced cancer. *Palliative Medicine, 17*(6), 509–513.

Soden, K., Vincent, K., Craske, S., Lucas, C., & Ashley, S. (2004). A randomized controlled trial of aromatherapy massage in a hospice setting. *Palliative Medicine, 18*(2), 87–92.

Spiegel, D. (1996). Cancer and depression. *British Journal of Psychiatry, 168*, 109–116.

Stagg, E. K., & Lazenby, M. (2012). Best practices for the nonpharmacological treatment of depression at the end of life. *American Journal of Hospital Palliative Care, 29*, 183–194.

Terry, W., & Olson, L. G. (2004). Unobvious wounds: The suffering of hospice patients. *Internal Medicine Journal, 34*(11), 604–607.

Tiernan, E., Casey, P., O'Boyle, C., Birkbeck, G., Mangan, M., O'Siorain, L., & Kearney, M. (2002). Relations between desire for early death, depressive symptoms and antidepressant prescribing in terminally ill patients with cancer. *Journal of the Royal Society of Medicine, 95*, 386–390.

Tsai, L. Y., Li, I. F., Lai, Y. H., Liu, C. P., Chang, T. Y., & Tu, C. T. Fatigue and its associated factors in hospice cancer patients in Taiwan. *Cancer Nursing, 30*(1), 24–30.

Volicer, L. (2001). Management of severe Alzheimer's Disease and end-of-life issues. *Clinics of Geriatric Medicine, 17*(2), 377–391.

Weinberger, M. I., Bruce, M. L., Roth, A. J., (2011). Depression and barriers to mental health care in older cancer patients. *International Journal of Geriatric Psychiatry, 26,* 21–26.

Wilson, K. G., Chochinov, H. M., Skirko, M. G., Allard, P., Chary, S., Gagnon, P. R., ... Clinch, J. J. (2007). Depression and anxiety disorders in palliative cancer care. *Journal of Pain Symptom Management, 33*(2), 118–129.

Wood, B. C., & Mynors-Wallis, L. M. (1997). Problem-solving therapy in palliative care. *Palliative Medicine, 11*(1), 49–54.

Yesavage, J. A., Brink, T. L., Rose, T. L., Lum, O., Huang, V., Adey, M., & Leirer, V. O. (1982). Development and validation of a geriatric depression screening scale: A preliminary report. *Journal of Psychiatric Res, 83*(17), 37–49.

Zigmond, A. S., & Snaith, R. P. (1983). The hospital anxiety and depression scale. *Acta Psychiatrica Scandinavica, 67,* 361–370.

30

LATE-LIFE MOOD DISORDERS AND HOME-BASED SERVICES AND INTERVENTIONS

Kisha N. Bazelais, Yolonda R. Pickett, and Martha L. Bruce

OF THE almost 40 million people over the age of 65 in the United States, nearly 10% (9.2%) are considered housebound and in need of home-based care (Qiu et al., 2010; US Census Bureau, 2012). Based on epidemiological studies of community-dwelling older adults, the burden of depression and other mood disorders in this population is exceptionally high (Bruce & Hoff, 1994; Bruce & McNamara, 1992; Charlson et al., 2008; Ganguli, Fox, Gilby, & Belle, 1996; Johnson, Sharkey, & Dean, 2011). This high prevalence of major depression and clinically significant depressive symptoms is consistent with the homebound population's significant medical burden, disability, and social isolation, conditions that are both risk factors and outcomes of depression (Alexopoulos, 2005; Bruce, 2001, 2002). Whether a cause or an effect of homebound status, depression left untreated may lead to a number of consequences, including but not limited to an increase in personal suffering, risk of caregiver burden, medical illness, disability, social isolation, adverse falls, hospitalization, institutionalization,

suicide, and nonsuicide mortality (Byers et al., 2008; Cohen-Mansfield, Shmotkin, & Hazan, 2010; Husain et al., 2005; Lyness et al., 2006, 2007; Meredith, Cheng, Hickey, & Dwight-Johnson, 2007; Sheeran, Byers, & Bruce, 2010; Wilson, Mottram, & Hussain, 2007). Regardless of its severity, untreated or undertreated depression among older adults exacerbates medical, functional, and social problems, and leads to higher rates of health care use, premature institutionalization, and mortality (Arean, Hegel, Vannoy, Fan, & Unuzter, 2008; Cuijpers, van Straten, & Warmerdam, 2007; Lyness, Chapman, McGriff, Drayer, & Duberstein, 2009; Malouff, Thorsteinsson, & Schutte, 2007).

Ironically, although community-dwelling older adults who are homebound have a high prevalence of depression, their homebound status is a significant barrier to the detection of mental health problems and mental health services delivery. The multiple and often chronic medical illnesses and disabilities that characterize this population restrict their mobility and their ability to access mental health resources that ambulatory older adults more readily utilize. For many, inadequate financial resources and lack of transportation further restrict access to depression care. Thus, depression in homebound older adults tends to be untreated or inappropriately treated with insufficient monitoring or follow-up care.

To address these challenges and the mental health need of a growing number of homebound seniors, researchers and care providers across the mental health, health, and aging services sectors are testing new strategies to improve the identification, care, and outcomes of depression in homebound older adults. A common goal is to develop interventions that efficiently reach as many depressed homebound older adults as possible. To that end, many build upon existing home-based care in the health or aging services sector and/or take advantage of remote communication technologies.

In this chapter, we review the data on prevalence, the types of treatments, and the service delivery approaches. We use the term "homebound" to encompass the various definitions used by different stakeholders (Qiu et al., 2010). Medicare defines an individual as homebound if leaving the home requires substantial effort or assistance, and if this limitation is due to an illness or injury. Older (age >65) individuals who satisfy this definition leave home briefly and infrequently, or leave only when in need of medical care (Donelson, Murtaugh et al., 2001). The Administration of Aging (AoA) provides meals and other social services to older (age >60) adults who are homebound "due to illness, disability, or geographic isolation." Researchers have operationalized homebound status based on self-reported degrees of confinement (Bruce & McNamara, 1992; Donelson, Murtaugh et al., 2001; Ganguli et al., 1996; Gilbert, Branch, & Orav, 1992; Lindesay & Thompson, 1993; Williams & Butters, 1992). These criteria can vary in terms of the minimum duration of confinement (e.g., 1 week, 1 month), the maximum frequency of departure from the home (e.g., never except in the case of emergencies, or no more than 2 days per week), and even in terms of what type of criteria are included in the definition (e.g., some definitions do not mention a minimum duration of confinement).

NEED AND PREVALENCE OF MOOD DISORDERS

Data on the prevalence of depression in homebound older adults come from community samples and studies of recipients of home-based services.

Community-based epidemiologic studies can both provide prevalence estimates of depression in homebound older adults as well as compare their rates of depression to individuals who are not homebound. Such studies have generally reported that depression is over twice as prevalent in the homebound as in others. Data from the New Haven site of the Epidemiologic Catchment Area (ECA) study (N = 2,553 elderly subjects) found 2.3% of seniors who reported being confined to a bed or chair met criteria for major depression compared to 0.7% of other seniors (Bruce & McNamara, 1992). Among individuals without a reported history of depression, homebound status was also independently associated with an increased risk of incident depression in the following year (Bruce & Hoff, 1994). An epidemiological study conducted in rural Pennsylvania showed that, controlling for potential confounding variables, homebound older adults had a 2.1 higher rate of depressive symptoms than those who were not homebound (Ganguli et al., 1996).

Other studies have estimated the prevalence of depression in older adults who receive in-home health or social services. Rates of depression in these populations are higher than those reported by homebound older adults in community samples as the subset of homebound older adults who need such services are usually experiencing higher levels of other conditions (e.g., medical illnesses and disability) or circumstances (e.g., social isolation, poverty) that contribute to their service needs. Such a high concentration of risk factors is understandably associated with a higher prevalence of depression, and depression itself may contribute to the need for health or social services.

Our study of the home health care (e.g., visiting nurse services) population assessed the prevalence of major depression using the Structured Clinical Interview for *DSM-IV* Axis I Disorders (SCID) (American Psychiatric Association, 1994; Spitzer, Gibbon, & Williams, 1995) in a representative sample of 539 new Medicare patients (age 65–102, mean = 78.4 years). We estimated that approximately 15% were in a current episode of major depression (using *DSM-IV* inclusive criteria) and another 10% met provisional criteria for minor depression (Bruce et al., 2002). The majority (71%) of patients with major depression were in the midst of their first depressive episode. Over one third of the sample reported clinically significant depressives symptoms (>5 on the 15-item Geriatric Depression Scale) (Marc, Raue, & Bruce, 2008; Sheikh & Yesavage,

1986). Fewer than 22% of the patients with major depression were being treated with either antidepressants or psychotherapy and most were not recognized as depressed by chart diagnoses or nurse reports (Brown et al., 2004; Brown, McAvay, Raue, Moses, & Bruce, 2003; Bruce et al., 2002).

Regarding agencies in the AoA service network, most studies (regardless of the instrument and whether the assessment was conducted by a social service provider or researcher) have estimated rates of major depression from approximately 9%–13% and rates of clinically significant depressive symptoms at about 33% (Charlson et al., 2008; Choi, Teeters, Perez, Farar, & Thompson, 2010; Gum et al., 2009; Richardson, He, Podgorski, Tu, & Conwell, 2010; Sirey et al., 2008). For example, in a study conducted in Westchester County, New York, of 403 home-delivered meal recipients (age 60–101, mean 83.3 years), 12.2% of older adults reported clinically significant depression (Patient Health Questionnaire; PHQ-9> 9) (Kroenke, Spitzer, & Williams, 2001) and 13.4% reported suicidal thoughts (Sirey et al., 2008). Almost one third of those endorsing suicide ideation did not report clinically significant depressive symptoms. Only one third of recipients with significant depressive symptoms were currently taking an antidepressant. Similarly, a study of home-delivered meal recipients in Austin, Texas, reported a 9% prevalence of major depression (Choi et al., 2010). In central Florida, 11.9% of 141 older adults receiving home-based aging services received a SCID depression diagnosis (Gum et al., 2009). A higher rate (27%) of major depression was reported in 378 homebound clients of an aging services provider network in upstate New York, although the rate of clinically significant depressive symptoms (31%) was similar to the other studies (Richardson et al., 2010). Among patients with major depression, 61% were being treated with medication and 25% by a mental health provider.

Their high prevalence of depression, coupled with lower rates of depression recognition and treatment, underscores the profound level of unmet need for mental health care in the nation's population of homebound older adults. Meeting those needs requires both an effective treatment and feasible programs to increase access to those treatments.

DEPRESSION TREATMENTS

Experts in the field of geriatric mental health have recommended a number of strategies to treat depression in older adults, most commonly pharmacotherapy, individual psychotherapy, or a combination of medication and psychotherapy (Alexopoulos et al., 2001; Steinman et al., 2007). The use of antidepressants in homebound older adults has risen three-fold over the past decade; in a recently collected national sample of geriatric home health care patients, over one third of patients were taking an antidepressant regardless of whether a depression diagnosis was documented on their home health care chart (Bruce, 2002; Weissman, Meyers, Ghosh, & Bruce, 2011). The majority of homebound seniors who take antidepressants have received their prescriptions from a primary care physician (Choi, Bruce, Sirrianni, Marinucci, & Kunik, 2012; Ciechanowski et al., 2004).

While medication treatment is feasible in homebound older adults, evidence suggests that they have a limited response to antidepressants alone, in part because of poor patient adherence or inadequate monitoring by the treating clinicians. Poor response may also reflect medication treatment's lack of attention to the psychosocial needs of this population, such as having to deal with multiple chronic medical conditions, disability, social isolation, and limited financial resources (Arean & Reynolds, 2005; Cohen et al., 2006; Miranda, Azocar, Organista, Dwyer, & Areane, 2003). Psychotherapies are designed to address these issues. But before advocating their use with depressed homebound seniors, evidence is needed of their effectiveness and feasibility with this population.

Home-Based Psychotherapy

Although at first blush there may be no reason to expect that in-person psychotherapy would be any less effective conducted in a patient's home than in an office, several factors may hinder home-based psychotherapy, such as privacy and confidentiality, distractions, and role ambiguity (e.g., Is the visiting therapist a clinician or guest? Is the depressed older adult a patient or host?). An additional challenge for conducting behavioral therapies with homebound older adults is the more limited span of doable activities for patients with physical disabilities or restricted mobility.

A number of different psychotherapies such as problem-solving therapy (PST), problem adaptation therapy (PATH), and supportive-interpersonal therapy have been adapted for in-home use with homebound seniors. Several randomized control treatment (RCT) studies, described later, have reported significant greater reduction in depression symptoms among older adults in the treatment group compared to usual care or control conditions.

PST, with or without antidepressant medications, has been found effective for treating late-life depression in both ambulatory and homebound older adults (Ciechanowski et al., 2004; Malouff et al., 2007; Nezu, Nezu, & Perri, 1989). Focusing on cognitive and behavioral activation of practical, "here-and-now" problem-solving coping skills, PST can be offered to most individuals without prompting any significant medical or other side effects (Alexopoulos, Raue, & Areán, 2003; D'Zurilla & Nezu, 2007). PST is especially well suited to depressed, financially disadvantaged older adults as they often have coping skill deficits compromising their ability to cope with adversity.

A 40-patient randomized trial of brief PST conducted by social workers of a home health care agency with depressed older patients reported significantly greater reduction in depression scores over time after involvement in the intervention arm (Gellis, McGinty, Horowitz, Bruce, & Misener, 2007). Similarly, a study evaluating the use of PST in home health care for older adults with heart disease found a significant improvement in depressive symptoms in the intervention group in comparison to the elders receiving usual care, which were enhanced by two educational sessions and a brochure on depression (Gellis & Bruce, 2010). Moreover, in this study, intervention group patients reported greater satisfaction with treatment and also showed improvements on subscales assessing mental health and emotional role function, thus providing additional support for the use of psychosocial interventions in home-based settings.

Depressed older adults, especially those with the kinds of mobility restrictions and disabilities that characterize the homebound, often also have cognitive impairments in their executive functioning that further contribute to poor response to pharmacological treatments (Alexopoulos, Kiosses, Murphy, & Heo, 2004; Kalayam & Alexopoulos, 1999; Simpson, Baldwin, Jackson, & Burns, 1998; Sneed et al., 2007). In response, Kiosses and colleagues (2010) developed problem adaptation therapy (PATH), a home-delivered intervention designed to address depression and disability in this subsection of the older adult population (Kiosses, Arean, Teri, & Alexopoulos, 2010). PATH is a 12-week, home-delivered intervention designed specifically to reduce depression and disability in depressed,

cognitively impaired, disabled elders. The PATH model is grounded in Lawton's ecological model of adaptive functioning (Lawton, Windley, & Byerts, 1982), which places an emphasis on the patient's ecosystem (i.e., the patient, caregiver, and home environment) and uses environmental adaptations to help patients gain a sense of competence within their home environment despite the various functional and behavioral limitations that they struggle with. In a 12-week randomized control trial design in which 30 patients were assigned to either the PATH intervention group or home-delivered supportive therapy (ST) group, Kiosses and colleagues found that while both groups were equally satisfied with their respective treatments, the PATH intervention group demonstrated greater decrease in depressive symptoms and disability over the 12-week period compared to the ST group (Kiosses et al., 2010).

Telephone and Telehealth Psychotherapy

While face-to-face psychotherapies, such as PST and PATH, have demonstrated effectiveness in reducing their depressive symptoms, many mental health agencies are not fully capable or equipped to provide ongoing in-person therapy to homebound seniors. A major challenge to in-person psychotherapy is the added financial burden on both homebound seniors and the agencies given the need to transport disabled individuals to outpatient settings, or reimbursing therapists for travel to the home setting. This problem is compounded by the homebound seniors' medical burden that can often compromise their ability to fully participate in sessions when the clinician arrives at their homes, which then multiples the transportation cost for the agencies. A potential cost-effective alternative to in-home visits is conducting psychotherapy using remote communication technologies such as telephone, Internet, or videophone (Bee et al., 2008). Despite the growing evidence that psychotherapies such as cognitive-behavioral therapy can be delivered effectively over the telephone in a broad age range (including older, depressed primary care patients; Simon, Ludman, Tutty, Operskalski, & Von Korff, 2004), few studies have tested this approach with homebound older adults.

Research on the psychotherapy over the telephone (without visual aides) in homebound seniors is needed as this population's high prevalence of sensory impairments, cognitive problems, or socioeconomic circumstances may undermine effectiveness. One study of telephone psychotherapy for patients with depression in Parkinson's disease noted that although patients preferred telephone to making weekly in-person office visits, clinicians often found it difficult to "read emotion in participants'" voices (Veazey, Cook, Stanley, Lai, & Kunik, 2009). Similarly, with depressed, geriatric home-delivered meal clients, Choi and colleagues report that treatment engagement and adherence in telephone sessions were not easy for both patient- and therapist-related factors (Choi, Hegel, Marti, Marinucci, Sirrianni, & Bruce, 2012). Without the visual contact, patients did not feel as connected to their therapists as they did in televideo sessions. Many patients only had cellular phones and were reluctant to use their "minutes" on calls. The therapists could not tell whether the patients were truly engaged in sessions (vs. watching TV at the same time). The therapists also had difficulty understanding some patients without seeing their facial expression and body language, and could not tell whether the patients were actually filling out the worksheets.

An alternative long-distance approach is the use of remote video technology, such as Skype, to deliver psychotherapy to homebound older adults. In her study of televideo PST with depressed home-delivered meal recipients, Choi and colleagues reported preliminary evidence that televideo PST was as effective as in-person PST and that participants equally accepted and enjoyed the two delivery models (Choi et al., 2012). In comparison to telephone PST, televideo technology allowed both parties to be aware of each other's nonverbal behaviors, an essential part of communication and establishing rapport. Also, being able to see the therapist rather than strictly hearing a voice over the phone may have helped strengthen the therapeutic relationship. Although the use of televideo technology was a feasible approach to psychotherapy, technical problems (i.e., poor audio/video quality, slow Internet connections) could be disruptive to therapy sessions. Overall, the cost-effectiveness, feasibility, and the potential for long-term sustainability associated with integrating a telehealth model into home-base mental health care seemed to outweigh some of the potential drawbacks.

DEPRESSION SERVICE DELIVERY MODELS

Evidence of the potential effectiveness of various types of depression treatment with homebound older adults underscores the need for feasible and sustainable models of identifying individuals who need depression care and delivering that care effectively. Although there are some independent psychiatrists or psychotherapists who conduct home visits for geriatric depression, most of depression service delivery models for homebound older adults are embedded within either mental health programs or programs that already provide home-based services. These models generally include a screening or case identification component, access to depression treatment, and strategies for ongoing depression care management (DCM). A small but rapidly growing body of research offers support that home-based mental health services are effective in improving mental health outcomes, such as depression, among homebound seniors (Bruce, Van Citters, & Bartels, 2005; Steinman et al., 2007).

Outreach, Screening, and Referral

Nearly all depression care service delivery models involve some form of depression screening or case identification. Effective screening and case identification strategies require procedures that answer the question, "What do I do when a homebound older adult screens positive to depression?" Both clinicians and nonprofessionals commonly express their unwillingness to screen for depression unless such procedures are in place. Whether these procedures focus on referral and consultation or direct intervention, their success relies upon being well integrated into routine care.

GATEKEEPER MODELS

In the "gatekeeper" model, nonprofessionals (e.g., hairdressers, mail carriers) whose work routinely brings them in contact with high-risk individuals are trained to identify mental health problems. One of the first studies to document the effectiveness of this model with community-dwelling frail older adults was conducted by the Spokane Mental Health Center (Florio et al., 1996). Gatekeepers and other outreach activities may be most successful when embedded in a mental health services infrastructure. The Psychogeriatric Assessment and Treatment in City Housing (PATCH) in Baltimore, Maryland, trained workers within senior housing development sites to recognize and refer older residents in need of psychiatric care. These older adults then received home-based care by a psychiatric nurse. A randomized trial found that elderly residents in the PATCH intervention had a greater reduction in depression compared to the usual care residents (Rabins et al., 2000).

INTEGRATING SCREENING INTO ROUTINE CARE

An alternative to adapting mental health programs to reach homebound older adults is to integrate depression screening into the routine services already provided to homebound seniors. The service sectors that provide in-home care are home health care (providing skilled nursing, social work, physical and occupational therapy, and home health aides) and AoA home-based aging services (providing services such as home-delivered meals, geriatric case management, and home assistance). The past three decades have seen a significant increase in the use of home-based services by older adults. The primary factors contributing to this rise include the longer life expectancy of the elderly population, shorter duration of hospital stays, expansion of Medicare eligibility criteria, and advances in technology that provide health care professionals the ability to deliver comprehensive home-based care (Bruce et al., 2002). While home-based services allow homebound older adults to continue living within their community, often mental health care is not a primary component of the community-based and health care agencies that provide these services to seniors (Zeltzer & Kohn, 2006). The challenge in these service sectors is to develop sustainable programs that provide homebound older adults access to quality mental health care.

Both home health care and aging services routinely required standardized routine assessments of patients and clients. These assessments have typically included a checkbox for depression. Without sufficient clinical guidance or a standardized depression screening instrument, providers often ignore the checkbox or use it inconsistently. Using home health care data, we found that the checkboxes on Medicare's standardized Outcome and Assessment Information Set (OASIS) had poor sensitivity and poor specificity compared to clinical research assessments of depression (Brown et al., 2004).

In home health care, our group addressed these concerns by collaborating with several home health care agencies to identify factors that would facilitate better depression assessment. Through our discussions with the agencies, we opted not to add a standardized scale to routine practice because it would increase the already time consuming and unpopular burden of formal nurse assessments. Instead, the focus of our intervention was to train nurses in the brief, yet clinically meaningful, use of existing required assessments, specifically the depression section of the OASIS. An essential component that made this training effective was that the nurses were trained to assess depression in the context of the OASIS, thus taking advantage of the nurses' clinical skills and reducing any extra steps that may be seen as cumbersome or incongruous with the rest of the routine care. Also important was ensuring that each agency had developed clear policies and procedures for referring depressed patients (e.g., to the patients' physicians or mental health specialists) and including the referral process in the skill training (Brown, Raue et al., 2010).

The first component of Weill Cornell's intervention, TRIAD (Training in the Assessment of Depression), was operationalizing the gateway depression items (depressed mood and anhedonia) in the OASIS to be consistent with *DSM-IV* criteria with appropriate questions and, when indicated, clinical probes (Brown, Raue et al., 2010). The clinical goal was for nurses to identify patients with clinically significant depressive symptoms (i.e., persistent depressed mood or anhedonia) warranting further evaluation for possible diagnosis of depression. The training emphasized factors that commonly complicate depression assessment in home health care patients (e.g., medical illness, disability, pain) in order to increase sensitivity to the presence of depressive symptoms. Nurses were taught to ask follow-up questions about duration and persistence of symptoms as evidence of clinical relevance. Nurses were also encouraged to observe behavioral or nonverbal signs such as flat affect or facial expression, lack of eye contact, and tendency to cry or become teary. Training procedures used techniques with demonstrated effectiveness in continuing education, including didactic instruction, role play, tool kits, and a video developed specifically for this training that demonstrates different scenarios of depression assessment in the context of the OASIS (Robertson, Umble, & Cervero, 2003).

In a nurse-randomized trial conducted in three home health care agencies comparing TRIAD to a minimal intervention consisting of a training video only and to a control condition, we tested the effectiveness of the TRIAD intervention in improving home care nurses' depression assessment and the rates of referral for patients with clinically significant depression (Bruce et al., 2007). The study compared nurses' assessments with assessment conducted by research associates. Based upon review of patients' records, the full TRIAD intervention improved the likelihood that a patient with persistent depressed mood or anhedonia would be successfully referred for a mental health evaluation. Half (50.0%) of depressed TRIAD patients received a referral, versus 18.5% of depressed patients in the minimal and 21.4% of the depressed control patients ($p = .047$). Furthermore, the referral rates for nondepressed patients were not significantly different (4.9%, 2.0%, and 5.8%, respectively), indicating that the intervention did not promote false positives in mental health referrals. Exploratory analyses demonstrated that patients with a depression diagnosis demonstrated that patients who were referred had better clinical outcomes, specifically reduction in depressive symptoms.

In 2010, Medicare required home health care agencies to use a revised version of the OASIS that includes the two-item version of the Patient Health Questionnaire (PHQ-2) (Kroenke, Spitzer, & Williams, 2003). Similarly, many offices of aging (for example, New York City) have begun augmenting their standardized assessments with the PHQ-2 or PHQ-9 (Berman & Furst, 2010; Gum et al., 2009; Richardson et al., 2010; Sirey et al., 2008). These new initiatives should improve the reliability of routine depression screening in homebound older adults.

Our experience, however, suggests that while the use of standardized assessments has increased the reliability of depression screening in these sectors, barriers to screening persist, leading to underidentification of depressed homebound older adults. For that reason, the strategy used by TRIAD of helping providers understand the importance of depression to their patients' care, giving them an opportunity to practice their assessments, and building upon their existing skills, remains relevant to the use of standardized assessments. We have used these strategies in developing training curriculum and resources for the use of the PHQ-2 (and PHQ-9) with older adults (Bruce, Sheeran et al., 2012; Delaney, Fortinsky et al., 2011).

Home-Based Treatment Delivery and Care Management Models

In their review of community-based interventions for depression in older adults, an expert panel consensus recommended strategies that include DCM as most effective in reducing late-life depression symptoms and promoting quality of life (Steinman et al., 2007). The Hartford Foundation-funded IMPACT and the NIMH-funded PROSPECT randomized controlled trials demonstrated the effectiveness of primary care–based multifaceted interventions for late-life depression (Bruce et al., 2004; Unutzer et al., 2002). Both interventions are based on the Collaborative Depression Care model, an evidenced-based approach shown effective in improving quality of care and clinical outcomes (Katon, Unutzer, Wells, & Jones, 2010). The model's cornerstone is managing depression as a chronic—rather than acute—illness. Thus, patients benefit from not only active treatments (e.g., pharmacological and/or psychotherapy) but also ongoing care, for example, monitoring symptoms and adherence, and teaching patients self-management skills. Primary care clinicians are supported both by a "depression care manager" (e.g., nurse or social worker), who provides much of the direct care and by access to mental health specialists for consultation as needed.

HOME HEALTH CARE

While some home health care agencies offer psychiatric nursing care, most do not. And when they do, these resources focus on patients who have been referred with a primary psychiatric diagnosis (representing less than 1% of Medicare home health care patients). Few agencies have the resources to provide specialty services to the far larger number of medically ill/surgical patients who suffer co-occurring depression. A strategy for most agencies, then, is to integrate broader DCM functions into home health care.

Ell and colleagues implemented a randomized intervention, modeled on the IMPACT model from primary care, that included nurse training in depression assessment, designated depression care specialists, and the option of home-based PST (Ell et al., 2007). Their experience confirmed the feasibility and potential effectiveness of conducting depression interventions in home health care. However, as the authors acknowledged, barriers to implementing their model confirmed the need for further adaptation of the primary care model of DCM to fit the needs of home health care patients and the organization and practice of home health care.

There are a number of obstacles to integrating DCM within home health care agencies, including organizational and individual factors. For example, organizational factors that may serve as a barrier include the lack of nursing on-site supervision, infrequent contact between physicians and home care nurses, the limited time constraints, and the lengthy documents that nurses are required to complete. Some individual factors that may also serve to impede changes to traditional home care practice include nurse attitudes/beliefs about mental illness that may make them resistant to asking about depression symptoms in their patients, and the patients' medical problems, which make it difficult to recognize possible mental health symptoms (Alexopoulos, 2005; Bartels et al., 2004). As a way of addressing these challenges, our group adopted an approach to intervention development that has been shown to be effective. This approach was based on the theory that working in partnership with home health care agencies would increase the acceptability, feasibility, and effectiveness of intervention efforts (Wallerstein, 2006; Wells, Miranda, Bruce, Alegria, & Wallerstein, 2004).

The following section describes our group's adaptation of the IMPACT and PROSPECT to home health care. As with TRIAD, the Depression CAREPATH (CARE for PATients at Home) was developed using the evidence-based practice partnership model (Bruce, Sheeran et al., 2011).

In an attempt to fit our interventions into the existing structure of the home health care agencies, the Weill Cornell group collaborated with home health care agencies to adapt the IMPACT and PROSPECT models of DCM from primary care to home health care. The Depression CAREPATH is designed for medical/surgical home health care patients who suffer clinically significant depressive symptoms (Bruce, Raue et al., 2011; Bruce, Sheeran et al., 2011). The underlying premise in developing the Depression CAREPATH is that successful implementation requires an intervention that "fits" how home health care is organized and practiced. We found that the basic model fits naturally with home health care that already uses a team approach to develop and follow a patient's Medicare-mandated "Care Plan" (Hennessey & Suter, 2011). The patient's physician authorizes the Care Plan and is responsible for treatment decisions. The home health care nurse supports the physician by providing in-home patient care and consulting with the physician and experts as clinically indicated both during care and at discharge.

The unique component of the Depression CAREPATH intervention is that all the basic clinical functions of DCM are integrated into the routine care practice of *all* medical/surgical nurses, rather than having only one depression care manager who handles the clinical assessments. The advantage of training all nurses in DCM is related to two factors: (1) *Cost*: Home health care agencies are reimbursed based on a prospective payment system for fee-for-service Medicare patients. Additional home visits by a new provider would likely increase patient costs relative to reimbursement; (2) *Skills*: Nurses commonly manage chronic diseases regardless of the formal reason for home care (e.g., diabetes management with patients receiving wound care). Managing depression is fundamentally comparable to managing other chronic diseases, making nurses clinically prepared to practice DCM and fitting DCM easily into routine care (Hennessey & Suter, 2009; Suter, Hennessey, Florez, & Newton Suter, 2011).

The Depression CAREPATH protocol was developed to be easily implemented and sustained in real-world home health care practice. In addition to training home health care nurses in DCM skills, the intervention also includes guidelines and resources to help home health care agencies develop the infrastructure needed to support the use of the DCM protocol in routine care (Bruce, Sheeran et al., 2011). As part of infrastructure development, home health care agencies are helped to tailor the guidelines to fit their own policies and local resources, including (1) case coordination guidelines that designate whom to contact (e.g., patients' physician, specialist) for referral or consultation; (2) suicide risk protocols that operationalize responses to levels of risk; (3) mental health resources directories for communities that serve their patients; (4) supervision strategies, including consultation, on how to oversee the nurses' use of the protocol; and (5) benchmark reports for use in supervision and quality improvement.

The dissemination and effective implementation of best practices commonly entail face-to-face involvement by the implementation staff (Davies, Walker, & Grimshaw, 2010; McHugh & Barlow, 2010; Thompson, Estabrooks, Scott-Findlay, Moore, & Wallin, 2007). Such intensity, however, may limit their availability, affordability, or acceptability, especially to agencies that are small, geographically dispersed, decentralized, or resource poor. Most of the >10,000 Medicare certified home health care agencies in the United States are freestanding, small, and without resources to support advanced quality improvement. This situation leads to the unequal distribution of evidence-based care.

In response to these concerns, our group has developed a long-distance implementation strategy designed to reach home health care agencies regardless of size, affiliation, or location. It uses a Web-based platform to support the implementation of Weill Cornell's Depression CAREPATH Intervention by home health care agencies. The implementation strategy employs e-learning modules, webinars, e-mail/telephone consultation, toolkits, and social networking technology for long-distance delivery of four implementation activities: (1) infrastructure development, (2) training in the Depression CAREPATH protocol, (3) supervision and performance feedback on nurses' use of the Depression CAREPATH protocol, and (4) social learning among home health care agencies that use the Depression CAREPATH. Future research will evaluate the effectiveness of using such long-distance strategies to support the implementation of evidence-based practices.

AGING SERVICES NETWORK AND MENTAL HEALTH CARE

Two related interventions, described below, have been developed for mild to moderately depressed homebound clients of the aging services sector. Both these interventions refer clients with more serious depression to medical or specialty services, a policy that is consistent with their level of need and the lack of formal linkages between social and health sectors of care. Both interventions, however, are developing strategies to strengthen these linkages with the aim of improving the quality of care for depressed homebound seniors with greatest need. Both have been disseminated widely to communities throughout the United States.

PEARLS is a home-based program for treating minor depression and dysthymia, developed at the University of Washington based in the Wagner Chronic Care Model (Wagner, Austin, & Von Korff, 1996). In a randomized clinical trial of aging services clients, Ciechanowski and colleagues (2004) also found a significant decrease (50%) in depressive symptoms, as well as an increase in quality of life and emotional well-being (Ciechanowski et al., 2004). Three main components include PST psychotherapy, social and physical activation, and pleasant activity scheduling.

Healthy *IDEAS* (Identifying Depression, Empowering Activities for Seniors) is a successful program that integrates depression awareness and management into existing case management services provided to older adults. The model includes screening for symptoms of depression and assessing their severity, educating older adults and caregivers about depression, linking older adults to primary care and mental health providers, and a behavioral activation approach that encourages involvement in meaningful activities (Quijano et al., 2007).

TELEPHONE AND TELEHEALTH CARE MANAGEMENT

Even in the context of agencies that provide home-based care, depression interventions that require in-home visits limit the reach of these services. Several groups are investigating ways to increase both the reach and efficiency of DCM interventions for homebound older adults by using telephones or other remote communication technologies. For example, Sheeran and colleagues embedded DCM components (e.g., assessment of depressive symptoms, antidepressant treatment adherence, and side effects) into remote monitoring devices commonly used by home health care agencies to transmit temperature, blood pressure, and other health-related information to telehealth nurses based at the agency (Sheeran et al., 2011). They reported high levels of feasibility, acceptability by patients and nurses, and preliminary evidence of effectiveness.

Kroenke developed a telecare management intervention that includes nurse telephone care management, automated symptom monitoring, and medication management (Kroenke et al., 2010). In a trial of 309 patients (mean age, 58 years), patients in the intervention group had significantly greater decrease in depressive symptom improvement than those in the usual-care group (over 12 months). Although not designed specifically for homebound older adults, the trial demonstrated the feasibility of providing DCM across multiple geographically dispersed community-based practices in both urban and rural areas by coupling human with technology-augmented patient interactions.

CONCLUSION

The prevalence of major depression and clinically significant depressive symptoms is twice as high in homebound older adults as in other community-dwelling seniors. Hidden from much of the world, depressed homebound older adults are unlikely to have their depressive symptoms recognized or appropriately treated. But while out of sight, their lack of appropriate mental health care affects both the individual and society as a whole given the increased risk of functional and psychosocial impairment, adverse falls, hospitalization, premature institutionalization, suicide, and nonsuicide mortality.

This chapter described the growing number of strategies being developed and tested to improve access to quality of mental health care for homebound older adults. Successful interventions generally involve collaboration across the mental health, health, and aging service sectors. To maximize effectiveness, they build on existing evidence-based depression treatments and care management, taking into account the unique needs and limitations of depressed homebound seniors. To maximize reach, they integrate depression screening into existing standardized assessments, train gatekeepers in depression screening, or take advantage of new communication technologies. To maximize feasibility and sustainability, they build these interventions in partnership with community providers so they will fit seamlessly into routine care.

Innovative approaches such as the ones reviewed in this chapter are essential to addressing what is quickly becoming a major public health concern among older adults. As with any intervention that seeks to have a large-scale impact, there are inherent strengths as well as limitations that need to be addressed in future research in order to increase the likelihood of successful implementation across multiple sectors and with diverse populations.

Disclosures

Dr. Bruce has no conflicts to disclose. She is funded by NIMH only. Grant Support: R01 MH082425, R25 MH068502, and R25 MH01994.

Dr. Pickett has no conflicts to disclose. She is funded by NIMH only. Grant Support: NIMH T32 Geriatric Mental Health Services Fellowship (NIMH T32 MH73553).

Dr. Bazelais has no conflicts to disclose. She is funded by NIMH only. Grant Support: National Institute of Mental Health (T32 MH073553-07).

Partial funding for this work came from P30 MH085943 and T32 MH073553.

REFERENCES

Alexopoulos, G. S. (2005). Depression in the elderly. *Lancet, 365*(9475), 1961–1970.

Alexopoulos, G. S., Katz, I. R., Reynolds, C. F., III, Carpenter, D., Docherty, J. P., & Ross, R. W. (2001). Pharmacotherapy of depression in older patients: A summary of the expert consensus guidelines. *Journal of Psychiatric Practice, 7*(6), 361–376.

Alexopoulos, G. S., Kiosses, D. N., Murphy, C., & Heo, M. (2004). Executive dysfunction, heart disease burden, and remission of geriatric depression. *Neuropsychopharmacology, 29*(12), 2278–2284.

Alexopoulos, G. S., Raue, P., & Areán, P. (2003). Problem-solving therapy versus supportive therapy in geriatric major depression with executive dysfunction. *American Journal of Geriatric Psychiatry, 11*(1), 46–52.

American Psychiatric Association. (1994.). *Diagnostic and statistical manual of mental disorders* (4th ed.). Washington, DC: Author.

Arean, P., Hegel, M., Vannoy, S., Fan, M. Y., & Unuzter, J. (2008). Effectiveness of problem-solving therapy for older, primary care patients with depression: Results from the IMPACT project. *Gerontologist, 48*(3), 311–323.

Arean, P. A., & Reynolds, C. F., III. (2005). The impact of psychosocial factors on late-life depression. *Biological Psychiatry, 58*(4), 277–282.

Bartels, S. J., Coakley, E. H., Zubritsky, C., Ware, J. H., Miles, K. M., Areán, P. A., ... PRISM-E Investigators. (2004). Improving access to geriatric mental health services: A randomized trial comparing treatment engagement with integrated versus enhanced referral care for depression, anxiety, and at-risk alcohol use. *American Journal of Psychiatry, 161*(8), 1455–1462.

Bee, P. E., Bower, P., Lovell, K., Gilbody, S., Richards, D., Gask, L., & Roach, P. (2008). Psychotherapy mediated by remote communication technologies: A meta-analytic review. *BMC Psychiatry, 8*, 60.

Berman, J., & Furst, L. M. (2010). *Depressed older adults: Education and screening*. New York: Springer.

Brown, E. L., Bruce, M. L., McAvay, G. J., Raue, P. J., Lachs, M. S., & Nassisi, P. (2004). Recognition of late-life depression in home care: Accuracy of the outcome and assessment information set. *Journal of the American Geriatrics Society, 52*(6), 995–999.

Brown, E. L., McAvay, G., Raue, P. J., Moses, S., & Bruce, M. L. (2003). Recognition of depression among elderly recipients of home care services. *Psychiatric Services, 54*(2), 208–213.

Brown, E. L., Raue, P. J., Roos, B. A., Sheeran, T., & Bruce, M. L. (2010). Training nursing staff to recognize depression in home healthcare. *Journal of the American Geriatrics Society, 58*(1), 122–128.

Bruce, M. L. (2001). Depression and disability in late life: Directions for future research. *American Journal of Geriatric Psychiatry, 9*(2), 102–112.

Bruce, M. L. (2002). Psychosocial risk factors for depressive disorders in late life. *Biological Psychiatry, 52*(3), 175–184.

Bruce, M. L., Brown, E. L., Raue, P. J., Mlodzianowski, A. E., Meyers, B. S., Leon, A. C.,... Nassisi, P. (2007). A randomized trial of depression assessment intervention in home health care. *Journal of the American Geriatrics Society, 55*(11), 1793–1800.

Bruce, M. L., & Hoff, R. A. (1994). Social and physical health risk factors for first-onset major depressive disorder in a community sample. *Social Psychiatry and Psychiatric Epidemiology, 29*(4), 165–171.

Bruce, M. L., McAvay, G. J., Raue, P. J., Brown, E. L., Meyers, B. S., Keohane, D. J.,... Weber, C. (2002). Major depression in elderly home health care patients. *American Journal of Psychiatry, 159*(8), 1367–1374.

Bruce, M. L., & McNamara, R. (1992). Psychiatric status among the homebound elderly: An epidemiologic perspective. *Journal of the American Geriatrics Society, 40*(6), 561–566.

Bruce, M. L., Raue, P. J., Sheeran, T., Reilly, C., Pomerantz, J. C., Meyers, B. S.,... Zukowski, D. (2011). Depression care for patients at home (Depression CAREPATH), home care depression care management protocol, part 2. *Home Healthcare Nurse, 29*(8), 480–489.

Bruce, M. L., Sheeran, T., Raue, P. J., Reilly, C. F., Greenberg, R. L., Pomerantz, J. C.,... Johnston, C. L. (2011). Depression care for patients at home (Depression CAREPATH), intervention development and implementation, part 1. *Home Healthcare Nurse, 29*(7), 416–426.

Bruce, M. L., Sheeran, T., (March 2012). Patient Health Questionnaire for Depression Screening: Training Module. Retrieved Month, YYYY, from https://www.mentalhealthtrainingnetwork.org/phq/intro/7416.

Bruce, M. L., Ten Have, T. R., Reynolds, C. F., III, Katz, I. I., Schulberg, H. C., Mulsant, B. H.,... Alexopoulos, G. S. (2004). Reducing suicidal ideation and depressive symptoms in depressed older primary care patients: A randomized controlled trial. *Journal of the American Medical Association, 291*(9), 1081–1091.

Bruce, M. L., Van Citters, A. D., & Bartels, S. J. (2005). Evidence-based mental health services for home and community. *Psychiatric Clinics of North America, 28*(4), 1039–1060, x-xi.

Byers, A. L., Sheeran, T., Mlodzianowski, A. E., Meyers, B. S., Nassisi, P., & Bruce, M. L. (2008).

Depression and risk for adverse falls in older home health care patients. *Research in Gerontological Nursing, 1*(4), 245–251.

Charlson, M. E., Peterson, J. C., Syat, B. L., Briggs, W. M., Kline, R., Dodd, M.,... Dionne, W. (2008). Outcomes of community-based social service interventions in homebound elders. *International Journal of Geriatric Psychiatry, 23*(4), 427–432.

Choi, N. G., Bruce, M. L., Sirrianni, L., Marinucci, M. L., & Kunik, M. E. (2012). Self-reported antidepressant use among low-income homebound older adults: Class, type, correlates, and perceived effectiveness. *Brain and Behavior, 2*(2), 178–186.

Choi, N.G., Hegel, M.T., Marti, C.N., Marinucci, M.L., Sirraianni, L., & Bruce, M.L. (2012). "Telehealth problem-solving therapy for depressed low-income homebound older adults." *American Journal of Geriatric Psychiatry*, Epub ahead of print

Choi, N. G., Teeters, M., Perez, L., Farar, B., & Thompson, D. (2010). Severity and correlates of depressive symptoms among recipients of meals on wheels: Age, gender, and racial/ethnic difference. *Aging and Mental Health, 14*(2), 145–154.

Ciechanowski, P., Wagner, E., Schmaling, K., Schwartz, S., Williams, B., Diehr, P.,... LoGerfo, J. (2004). Community-integrated home-based depression treatment in older adults: A randomized controlled trial. *Journal of the American Medical Association, 291*(13), 1569–1577.

Cohen, A., Houck, P. R., Szanto, K., Dew, M. A., Gilman, S. E., & Reynolds, C. F., III. (2006). Social inequalities in response to antidepressant treatment in older adults. *Archives of General Psychiatry, 63*(1), 50–56.

Cohen-Mansfield, J., Shmotkin, D., & Hazan, H. (2010). The effect of homebound status on older persons. *Journal of the American Geriatrics Society, 58*(12), 2358–2362.

Cuijpers, P., van Straten, A., & Warmerdam, L. (2007). Problem solving therapies for depression: A meta-analysis. *European Psychiatry, 22*(1), 9–15.

D'Zurilla, T. J., & Nezu, A. M. (2007). *Problem-solving therapy: A positive approach to clinical intervention.* New York: Springer.

Davies, P., Walker, A. E., & Grimshaw, J. M. (2010). A systematic review of the use of theory in the design of guideline dissemination and implementation strategies and interpretation of the results of rigorous evaluations. *Implementation Science, 5*, 14.

Delaney, C., Fortinsky, R., Doonan, L., Grimes, R. Pearson, T., Rosenberg, S., & Bruce, M. L. (2011). Depression screening and interventions for older home health care patients: Program design and training outcomes for a train-the-trainer model. *Home Health Care Management and Practice*, 23(6), 435–445.

Donelson, S. M., Murtaugh, C. M., Feldman, P. H., Hijjazi, K., Bruno, L., Zeppie, S., ... Clark, A. (2001). *Clarifying the definition of homebound and medical necessity using OASIS data*. Final Report prepared for the Office of the Assistant Secretary for Planning and Evaluation, U.S. Department of Health and Human Services (Contract #HHS-100–99–0020). New York: Center for Home Care Policy and Research, Visiting Nurse Service of NY.

Ell, K., Unutzer, J., Aranda, M., Gibbs, N. E., Lee, P. J., & Xie, B. (2007). Managing depression in home health care: A randomized clinical trial. *Home Health Care Service Quality*, 26(3), 81–104.

Florio, E. R., Rockwood, T. H., Hendryx, M. S., Jensen, J. E., Raschko, R., & Dyck, D. G. (1996). A model gatekeeper program to find the at-risk elderly. *Journal of Case Management*, 5(3), 106–114.

Ganguli, M., Fox, A., Gilby, J., & Belle, S. (1996). Characteristics of rural homebound older adults: A community-based study. *Journal of the American Geriatrics Society*, 44(4), 363–370.

Gellis, Z. D., & Bruce, M. L. (2010). Problem solving therapy for subthreshold depression in home healthcare patients with cardiovascular disease. *American Journal of Geriatric Psychiatry*, 18(6), 464–474.

Gellis, Z. D., McGinty, J., Horowitz, A., Bruce, M. L., & Misener, E. (2007). Problem-solving therapy for late-life depression in home care: A randomized field trial. *American Journal of Geriatric Psychiatry*, 15(11), 968–978.

Gilbert, G. H., Branch, L. G., & Orav, E. J. (1992). An operational definition of the homebound. *Health Services Research*, 26(6), 787–800.

Gum, A. M., Petkus, A., McDougal, S. J., Present, M., King-Kallimanis, B., & Schonfeld, L. (2009). Behavioral health needs and problem recognition by older adults receiving home-based aging services. *International Journal of Geriatric Psychiatry*, 24(4), 400–408.

Hennessey, B., & Suter, P. (2009). The home-based chronic care model. *Caring*, 28(1), 12–16.

Hennessey, B., & Suter, P. (2011). The Community-Based Transitions Model: One agency's experience. *Home Healthcare Nurse*, 29(4), 218–230; quiz 231–212.

Husain, M. M., Rush, A. J., Sackeim, H. A., Wisniewski, S. R., McClintock, S. M., Craven, N., ... Hauger, R. (2005). Age-related characteristics of depression: A preliminary STAR*D report. *American Journal of Geriatric Psychiatry*, 13(10), 852–860.

Johnson, C. M., Sharkey, J. R., & Dean, W. R. (2011). Indicators of material hardship and depressive symptoms among homebound older adults living in North Carolina. *Journal of Nutrition, Gerontology, and Geriatrics*, 30(2), 154–168.

Kalayam, B., & Alexopoulos, G. S. (1999). Prefrontal dysfunction and treatment response in geriatric depression. *Archives of General Psychiatry*, 56(8), 713–718.

Katon, W., Unutzer, J., Wells, K., & Jones, L. (2010). Collaborative depression care: History, evolution and ways to enhance dissemination and sustainability. *General Hospital Psychiatry*, 32(5), 456–464.

Kiosses, D. N., Arean, P. A., Teri, L., & Alexopoulos, G. S. (2010). Home-delivered problem adaptation therapy (PATH) for depressed, cognitively impaired, disabled elders: A preliminary study. *American Journal of Geriatric Psychiatry*, 18(11), 988–998.

Kroenke, K., Spitzer, R. L., & Williams, J. B. (2001). The PHQ-9: Validity of a brief depression severity measure. *Journal of General Internal Medicine*, 16(9), 606–613.

Kroenke, K., Spitzer, R. L., & Williams, J. B. (2003). The Patient Health Questionnaire-2: Validity of a two-item depression screener. *Medical Care*, 41(11), 1284–1292.

Kroenke, K., Theobald, D., Wu, J., Norton, K., Morrison, G., Carpenter, J., & Tu, W. (2010). Effect of telecare management on pain and depression in patients with cancer: A randomized trial. *Journal of the American Medical Association*, 304(2), 163–171.

Lawton, M. P., Windley, P. G., & Byerts, T. O. (1982). *Aging and the environment: Theoretical approaches*. New York: Springer.

Lindesay, D. M., & Thompson, C. (1993). Housebound elderly people: Definition, prevalence and characteristics. *International Journal of Geriatric Psychiatry*, 8(3), 231–237.

Lyness, J. M., Chapman, B. P., McGriff, J., Drayer, R., & Duberstein, P. R. (2009). One-year outcomes of minor and subsyndromal depression in older primary care patients. *International Psychogeriatrics*, 21(1), 60–68.

Lyness, J. M., Heo, M., Datto, C. J., Ten Have, T. R., Katz, I. R., Drayer, R., ... Bruce, M. L. (2006). Outcomes of minor and subsyndromal depression among elderly patients in primary care settings. *Annals of Internal Medicine*, 144(7), 496–504.

Lyness, J. M., Kim, J., Tang, W., Tu, X., Conwell, Y., King, D. A., & Caine, E. D. (2007). The clinical significance of subsyndromal depression in older primary care patients. *American Journal of Geriatric Psychiatry, 15*(3), 214–223.

Malouff, J. M., Thorsteinsson, E. B., & Schutte, N. S. (2007). The efficacy of problem solving therapy in reducing mental and physical health problems: A meta-analysis. *Clinical Psychology Review, 27*(1), 46–57.

Marc, L. G., Raue, P. J., & Bruce, M. L. (2008). Screening performance of the 15-item geriatric depression scale in a diverse elderly home care population. *American Journal of Geriatric Psychiatry 16*(11), 914–921.

McHugh, R. K., & Barlow, D. H. (2010). The dissemination and implementation of evidence-based psychological treatments. A review of current efforts. *American Psychologist, 65*(2), 73–84.

Meredith, L. S., Cheng, W. J., Hickey, S. C., & Dwight-Johnson, M. (2007). Factors associated with primary care clinicians' choice of a watchful waiting approach to managing depression. *Psychiatric Services, 58*(1), 72–78.

Miranda, J., Azocar, F., Organista, K. C., Dwyer, E., & Areane, P. (2003). Treatment of depression among impoverished primary care patients from ethnic minority groups. *Psychiatric Services, 54*(2), 219–225.

Nezu, A. M., Nezu, C. M., & Perri, M. G. (1989). *Problem-solving therapy for depression: Theory, research, and clinical guidelines.* New York: Wiley.

Qiu, W. Q., Dean, M., Liu, T., George, L., Gann, M., Cohen, J., & Bruce, M. L. (2010). Physical and mental health of homebound older adults: An overlooked population. *Journal of the American Geriatrics Society, 58*(12), 2423–2428.

Quijano, L. M., Stanley, M. A., Petersen, N. J., Casado, B. L., Steinberg, E. H., Cully, J. A., & Wilson, N. L. (2007). Healthy IDEAS: A depression intervention delivered by community-based case managers serving older adults. *Journal of Applied Gerontology, 26*, 139–156.

Rabins, P. V., Black, B. S., Roca, R., German, P., McGuire, M., Robbins, B., … Brant, L. (2000). Effectiveness of a nurse-based outreach program for identifying and treating psychiatric illness in the elderly. *Journal of the American Medical Association, 283*(21), 2802–2809.

Richardson, T. M., He, H., Podgorski, C., Tu, X., & Conwell, Y. (2010). Screening depression aging services clients. *American Journal of Geriatric Psychiatry, 18*(12), 1116–1123.

Robertson, M. K., Umble, K. E., & Cervero, R. M. (2003). Impact studies in continuing education for health professions: Update. *Journal of Continuing Education in the Health Professions, 23*(3), 146–156.

Sheeran, T., Byers, A. L., & Bruce, M. L. (2010). Depression and increased short-term hospitalization risk among geriatric patients receiving home health care services. *Psychiatric Services, 61*(1), 78–80.

Sheeran, T., Rabinowitz, T., Lotterman, J., Reilly, C. F., Brown, S., Donehower, P., … Bruce, M. L. (2011). Feasibility and impact of telemonitor-based depression care management for geriatric homecare patients. *Telemedicine Journal and E-Health, 17*(8), 620–626.

Sheikh, J. A., & Yesavage, J. A. (Eds.). (1986). *Geriatric Depression Scale (GDS), Recent findings and development of a shorter version. Clinical gerontology: A guide to assessment and intervention.* New York: Haworth Press.

Simon, G. E., Ludman, E. J., Tutty, S., Operskalski, B., & Von Korff, M. (2004). Telephone psychotherapy and telephone care management for primary care patients starting antidepressant treatment: A randomized controlled trial. *Journal of the American Medical Association, 292*(8), 935–942.

Simpson, S., Baldwin, R. C., Jackson, A., & Burns, A. S. (1998). Is subcortical disease associated with a poor response to antidepressants? Neurological, neuropsychological and neuroradiological findings in late-life depression. *Psychological Medicine, 28*(5), 1015–1026.

Sirey, J. A., Bruce, M. L., Carpenter, M., Booker, D., Reid, M. C., Newell, K. A., & Alexopoulos, G. S. (2008). Depressive symptoms and suicidal ideation among older adults receiving home delivered meals. *International Journal of Geriatric Psychiatry, 23*(12), 1306–1311.

Sneed, J. R., Roose, S. P., Keilp, J. G., Krishnan, K. R., Alexopoulos, G. S., & Sackeim, H. A. (2007). Response inhibition predicts poor antidepressant treatment response in very old depressed patients. *American Journal of Geriatric Psychiatry, 15*(7), 553–563.

Spitzer, R., Gibbon, M., & Williams, J. B. W. (1995). *Structured clinical interview for Axis I DSM-IV disorders (SCID).* Washington, DC: American Psychiatric Association Press.

Steinman, L. E., Frederick, J. T., Prohaska, T., Satariano, W. A., Dornberg-Lee, S., Fisher, R., … Late Life Depression Special Interest Project (SIP) Panelists. (2007). Recommendations for treating depression in community-based older adults. *American Journal of Preventive Medicine, 33*(3), 175–181.

Suter, P., Hennessey, B., Florez, D., & Newton Suter, W. (2011). Review series: Examples of chronic care model: The home-based chronic care model:

Redesigning home health for high quality care delivery. *Chronic Respiratory Disease, 8*(1), 43–52.

Thompson, D. S., Estabrooks, C. A., Scott-Findlay, S., Moore, K., & Wallin, L. (2007). Interventions aimed at increasing research use in nursing: A systematic review. *Implementation Science, 2*, 15.

US Census Bureau. (2012). USA quick facts. Retrieved October 2012, from http://quickfacts.census.gov/qfd/states/00000.html

Unutzer, J., Katon, W., Callahan, C. M., Williams, J. W., Jr., Hunkeler, E., Harpole, L.,... IMPACT Investigators. (2002). Collaborative care management of late-life depression in the primary care setting: A randomized controlled trial. *Journal of the American Medical Association, 288*(22), 2836–2845.

Veazey, C., Cook, K. F., Stanley, M., Lai, E. C., & Kunik, M. E. (2009). Telephone-administered cognitive behavioral therapy: A case study of anxiety and depression in Parkinson's disease. *Journal of Clinical Psychology in Medical Settings, 16*(3), 243–253.

Wagner, E. H., Austin, B. T., & Von Korff, M. (1996). Improving outcomes in chronic illness. *Managed Care Quarterly, 4*(2), 12–25.

Wallerstein, N. (2006). Commentary: Challenges for the field in overcoming disparities through a CBPR approach. *Ethnicity and Disease, 16*(1 Suppl 1), S146–148.

Weissman, J., Meyers, B. S., Ghosh, S., & Bruce, M. L. (2011). Demographic, clinical and functional factors associated with antidepressant use in the home healthcare elderly. *American Journal of Geriatric Psychiatry, 19*(12), 1042–1045.

Wells, K., Miranda, J., Bruce, M. L., Alegria, M., & Wallerstein, N. (2004). Bridging community intervention and mental health services research. *American Journal of Psychiatry, 161*(6), 955–963.

Williams, J. N., & Butters, J. M. (1992). Sociodemographics of homebound people in Kentucky. *Special Care in Dentist, 12*(2), 74–78.

Wilson, K., Mottram, P., & Hussain, M. (2007). Survival in the community of the very old depressed, discharged from medical inpatient care. *International Journal of Geriatric Psychiatry 22*(10), 974–979.

Zeltzer, B. B., & Kohn, R. (2006). Mental health services for homebound elders from home health nursing agencies and home care agencies. *Psychiatric Services, 57*(4), 567–569.

31

NOVEL PLATFORMS FOR CARE DELIVERY

INTERNET-BASED INTERVENTIONS AND TELEPSYCHIATRY

Pim Cuijpers, Heleen Riper, and Aartjan T. F. Beekman

DESPITE THE considerable impact of depressive disorders on the quality of life of patients suffering from these disorders, a considerable number of patients do not seek any professional help, even in high-income countries (Bijl & Ravelli, 2000; Wang et al., 2005). This is true for patients of all age groups, but the number of older adults with depression who seek help is considerably lower than any other adult age group (Conner et al., 2010; Crabb & Hunsley, 2006). It has been estimated that the chance of visiting a mental health professional in older adults is half of the chance in younger adults, despite evidence demonstrating their need for such services (Robb, Haley, Becker, Polivka, & Chwa, 2003).

There are several intrinsic and extrinsic barriers to mental health care among older adults (Pepin, Segal, & Coolidge, 2009). An important intrinsic barrier is that older adults feel more responsible for solving their own problems. Although they recognize the symptoms of mental illness, they are less inclined than younger adults to consider outpatient services as appropriate treatment (Pepin et al.,

2009), although there are also indications that older adults in general have positive attitudes toward treatment of depression (Mackenzie, Scott, Mather, & Sareen, 2008). Furthermore, some older adults consider depression to be a normal part of aging and therefore do not report it to a professional. Stigma associated with mental illness is also an important obstacle to seeking help (Conner et al., 2010), but it is not clear whether this barrier is stronger in older than in younger adults (Pepin et al., 2009).

Extrinsic barriers to help-seeking operate outside of an individual seeking mental health services (Pepin et al., 2009). These include concerns about the payment of these services but also scarcity in clinicians specialized in treating older adults, concerns about transportation to treatment centers, ageist attitudes by general practitioners and other professionals, and the idea that depression is part of a normal aging process and does not require treatment (Robb et al., 2003).

Because of the low rates of receiving adequate treatment among older adults, and the intrinsic and extrinsic barriers to mental health care, it is important to develop evidence-based treatments that are easily accessible for patients and that keep time and costs at a minimum. Telemedicine and Internet-based treatments have been proposed to be such interventions (Andrews, Cuijpers, Craske, McEvoy, & Titov, 2010; Leach & Christensen, 2006; Spek et al., 2007a). In the past decade, dozens of trials have examined the feasibility, acceptability, and effects of such interventions. Although most of them have been conducted with younger and middle-aged adults, the available evidence suggests that these are also useful and effective in older adults.

In this chapter, we will describe what telemedicine and Internet-guided interventions are, the different types that exist, advantages and disadvantages of these treatments, and the evidence for the efficacy and effectiveness. We will also describe future directions for research and practice.

WHAT ARE INTERNET-GUIDED AND TELEMEDICINE INTERVENTIONS

According to the American Telemedicine Association, telemedicine can be defined as "the use of medical information exchanged from one site to another via electronic communications to improve patients' health status" (http://www.americantelemed.org/i4a/pages/index.cfm?pageid=3333; approached at June 21, 2011). Telepsychiatry can be seen as the subfield that applies telemedicine to the field of psychiatry (Monnier, Knapp, & Frueh, 2003). Usually, videoconferencing between a patient and a psychiatrist or therapist is considered to be the most exemplary form of telepsychiatry. Professional consultation, for example, between a psychiatrist and a general practioner, is also considered to be a form of telepsychiatry (Yellowlees et al., 2010). However, telephone-supported psychotherapy also falls within the definition of telepsychiatry, and it is, in fact, the best examined type of telepsychiatry (Leach & Christensen, 2006; Monnier et al., 2003).

Internet-based therapies can be seen as a specific type of guided self-help intervention. A self-help intervention can be defined as a psychological treatment, where the patient or client takes home a standardized psychological treatment and works through it more or less independently (Cuijpers & Schuurmans, 2007; Marrs, 1995). In the standardized psychological treatment, the patient can follow step-by-step instructions on what to do in applying a generally accepted psychological treatment to

himself or herself. The standardized psychological treatment can be written down in book form, but it can also be made available through other media, such as a personal computer, CD-ROM, television, video, or the Internet. Contact with therapists is not a necessity for the completion of the self-help therapy. If contact with a therapist takes place, it should only be of a supportive or facilitative nature. Contact is not aimed at developing a traditional relationship between therapist and patient, and it is only meant to support the carrying out of the standardized psychological treatment. Interaction between patient and therapist can take place through face-to-face contact, by telephone, by e-mail, or any other communication method.

Internet-guided self-help is a specific form of self-help. The contents are often comparable to those of self-help books. The technical possibilities of the Internet are used to improve the contents, for example, by adding video and audio files for illustrative purposes, by easing the use and scoring of self-rating questionnaires, and by providing easy ways to complete homework assignments. The Internet also offers the possibility to facilitate peer support.

DIFFERENT TYPES OF INTERNET-GUIDED AND TELEPSYCHIATRY INTERVENTIONS

Internet-guided and telemedicine interventions can be delivered in many different formats and settings (Cuijpers & Schuurmans, 2007). Without trying to be exhaustive, we will describe the most important types of self-help that have been examined in effect studies:

- *Internet-based self-help without professional support.* There are several examples of unguided Internet-based treatments (Cuijpers et al., 2011). In these interventions, there is no professional or paraprofessional support, and patients can stop the treatment whenever they want.
- *Internet-based self-help as partial replacement of face-to-face therapy.* Internet-based self-help interventions can also be used to support regular treatment. Therapists can give a patient access to an Internet program in order to speed up treatment or to allow the patient to practice with and learn the principles of the therapy in his or her own time. Therapists can also advise the patient to have an Internet-based treatment for a specific problem, such as disturbed sleep or mild alcohol

problems, which might not be the focus of therapy but do interfere with the patient's functioning (Cuijpers & Schuurmans, 2007).

- *Internet-based self-help as an independent intervention.* Internet-based self-help can be delivered as an independent intervention or as part of a stepped-care approach in mood disorders (Scogin, Hanson, & Welsh, 2003). Usually, there is some support from a professional or paraprofessional. Most empirical studies have used these interventions (Andersson & Cuijpers, 2009; Andrews et al., 2010). The patient gets access to an Internet-based therapy and works it through independently, while keeping in contact with a professional by e-mail or chatting, at regular times. These contacts are brief and not aimed at developing a traditional relationship between patient and therapist, but only at answering questions about the method and stimulating the patient to continue with treatment.
- *Telephone-supported psychotherapies and other telepsychiatry interventions.* There are several studies in which psychotherapies are conducted through the telephone, without any face-to-face contact between patient and therapist (Leach & Christensen, 2006). Although most of these studies have been conducted with middle-aged and younger adults, there is no reason to assume that it is not effective in older adults. Telepsychiatry interventions with videoconferencing have been examined in several pilot studies in geriatric populations (Johnston & Jones, 2001; Tang, Chiu, Woo, Hjelm, & Hui, 2001; Yeung et al., 2009).

This list of Internet-based and telepsychiatry interventions is not exhaustive. Several other types are available, such as online support groups, and several others are currently being developed, such as serious gaming interventions and mobile interventions. However, the interventions described in the aforementioned list are the ones that are already available and have been examined in randomized controlled trials, although the number of trials still is limited for most of these interventions.

ADVANTAGES, DISADVANTAGES, AND DANGERS

Internet-guided and telepsychiatry interventions have both advantages and disadvantages. One important advantage is that they may save time. In telepsychiatry interventions there is no travelling time for patients or therapists. In Internet-based guided self-help interventions, even more time can be saved, because most of the therapy is conducted by the patient himself. The therapist only has to check whether the patient has done his or her homework and to have brief contact by e-mail or telephone to give feedback about the homework assignments. In one study it was found that the number of therapy sessions for depression could be reduced with about 50% if patients were given computer-assisted therapy as opposed to regular therapy (Wright et al., 2005). Another important advantage related to this is that self-help interventions can reduce the costs of treatment considerably.

Maybe even more important is that Internet-guided and telepsychiatry interventions extend the reach to populations with mood and anxiety disorders who are not reached with more traditional forms of treatment. As indicated earlier, many patients do not seek professional help for a number of reasons. Internet-guided and telemedicine interventions may be able to solve some of the problems associated with help-seeking. First, possible concerns about transportation to treatment centers are not relevant in Internet-guided and telemedicine interventions because these interventions can be conducted without leaving home. Second, Internet-based treatments are based on the principle that patients solve their problems themselves. The treatments are only meant to support patients in helping themselves. The coaches are not traditional therapists; they only help patients work through the interventions. Because older adults feel more responsible for solving their own problems, these interventions may be more suitable for them than traditional mental health treatments. Third, the stigma associated with mental illness, which is a barrier in all age groups, may be less of a problem in Internet-guided and telemedicine interventions, because receiving these interventions is not visible for anyone else, and Internet-based interventions may be even conducted at the time the patient chooses, even if this is in the middle of the night. Fourth, especially Internet-guided interventions are cheaper for the patient than traditional therapies, because less time per patient is spent by the therapists. Because of these reasons, Internet-guided and telepsychiatry interventions may reach a segment of the population that is not reached by traditional treatment methods.

There are several other advantages. These interventions may reduce waiting lists, allow patients to work at their own pace, and abolish the need to

Table 31.1 Common Components of Internet-Guided and Telepsychiatry Interventions

	COGNITIVE RESTRUCTURING	BEHAVIORAL ACTIVATION	PROBLEM-SOLVING THERAPY
Goal	Learn about dysfunctional thoughts and their relationship with mood, thoughts, and behavior:	Learn about the relationship between mood and activities:	Learn about the relationship between mood and problems experienced:
Components	Identify dysfunctional thoughts	Identify different types of activities	Identify and relate problems, psychological complaints, and important goals in life
	Evaluate the appropriateness of these dysfunctional thoughts	Register pleasant activities	
		Aim and plan for an increase of pleasant activities (calendar)	Learn to distinguish between problems that are solvable, unsolvable, and unimportant problems
	Challenge these dysfunctional thoughts with more appropriate ones	Decrease unpleasant or perceived necessary activities	Learn techniques to cope with the three types of problems
	Modify existing dysfunctional thoughts into more functional ones	Develop reward system for conduct of pleasant activities	Learn to focus on solvable problems and systematic solving strategies
		Conduct and maintain plan	Apply these alternative strategies in daily life
		Train social skills	

schedule appointments with a therapist. Additionally, Internet-based therapies make it easier to treat the hard of hearing because these treatments typically work more with visual than auditory information (Marks, Cavanagh, & Gega, 2007). Even more advantages of Internet-based therapies can be named. For example, it may be programmed to enhance patients' motivation by presenting a wide range of attractive audiovisual information, adaptable to fit a client's preferences in whatever gender, age, accent, language, and game format. Furthermore, it can quickly and automatically report patient progress and self-ratings.

There are, of course, also some disadvantages and dangers worth mentioning. Patients may not be able to finish an Internet-based self-help intervention, which may result in a negative experience that could have a detrimental effect on their condition. Also, a patient's problems may be too severe for an (unguided) self-help intervention, which may prevent the provision of adequate help. Or the patient may suffer from a different disorder than the one aimed at by the intervention at stake.

Internet-based self-help interventions may have other disadvantages. Although the Internet is

available for most people in Western countries, and is expected to grow even further, there is still a large group of older people who do not have Internet access or for whom the intervention is not acceptable. The last group may have access to the Internet, but it will not work with it because of technophobia. Furthermore, the subtle nonverbal and verbal clues to clients' misunderstandings are not detected, and it may stimulate clients to cherry-pick from a range of homework options presented (Marks et al., 2007). Whether telepsychiatry and Internet-interventions may yield negative effects has not been properly examined in empirical research, and it should be the focus of future research.

COMMON COMPONENTS

Most Internet-guided and telepsychiatry interventions are based on cognitive-behavioral techniques, such as cognitive restructuring and behavioral activation. Cognitive-behavioral interventions represent current state-of-the-art treatment for depressive disorders, as they have been shown to be effective in large numbers of well-designed randomized studies and meta-analyses (Churchill et al., 2001; Wampold, Minami, Baskin, & Tierney, 2002). A far more pragmatic reason for choosing cognitive-behavioral techniques is the fact that these techniques tend to be very straightforward and can therefore be readily broken up into relatively easy steps, as opposed to most other common psychological interventions, such as psychodynamic or interpersonal therapies. In Table 31.1, the goals and content of the most common components of Internet-guided and telepsychiatry interventions are presented.

The core of cognitive-behavioral therapy is cognitive restructuring. The intervention is focused on the impact a patient's present dysfunctional thoughts have on current behavior and future functioning. Cognitive restructuring is aimed at evaluating, challenging, and modifying a patient's dysfunctional beliefs. Behavioral activation is aimed at increasing positive interactions between a person and his or her environment. Registration of pleasant activities is an important part of behavioral activation, as well as the development of a plan to increase the number of pleasant activities in daily schedules. Social skills training can be a part of behavioral activation. Apart from cognitive restructuring and behavioral activation, problem-solving techniques are also often included in Internet-guided and telepsychiatry interventions. Systematic problem solving is usually considered to be one of the techniques in cognitive-behavioral therapy. In problem-solving therapy, a patient learns to solve currently existing personal problems. First, the existing problems are defined as well as possible, then a list of possible solutions is generated, the best solution is selected, a plan is made to solve it, and the plan is executed; if the problem is not solved by this, there is a loop back to the first step.

Although most telepsychiatry interventions are also based on cognitive-behavioral therapy, the telephone offers more opportunities to use other psychological techniques. For example, pilot projects have been conducted in which social support has been provided through the telephone (Hunkeler et al., 2000), as well as broader disease management programs (Datto, Thompson, Horowitz, Disbot, & Oslin, 2003).

THE EFFECTS OF INTERNET-GUIDED INTERVENTIONS FOR MOOD DISORDERS

There are a growing number of randomized controlled trials showing that telepsychiatry and Internet-based therapies are effective. However, almost all of this research has been conducted in younger and middle-aged adults (Diamond et al., 2010). There are only few studies specifically aimed at older adults (e.g., Egede et al., 2009). On the other hand, there is no a priori reason to assume that these interventions are less effective in older adults.

Several recent meta-analyses have show that Internet-interventions are effective for mood and anxiety disorders (Andersson & Cuijpers, 2009; Andrews et al., 2010; Cuijpers et al., 2009; Spek et al., 2007a). The effect size found for Internet-based interventions is comparable to those found for face-to-face therapies, ranging from 0.78 (Hedges's g; Andrews et al., 2010) to 0.61 (Cohen's d; Andersson & Cuijpers, 2009) for supported Internet-interventions. This is very comparable to face-to-face therapies, which result in effect sizes in the same ranges (Churchill et al., 2001; Cuijpers et al., 2010).

Most Internet-based therapies can be considered to be guided self-help interventions in which the patient applies the intervention to himself or herself more or less independently. In a recent meta-analysis of studies in which guided self-help intervention was directly compared with face-to-face therapies for depression or anxiety, no significant difference was found between the two types of therapy, despite sufficient statistical power (Cuijpers et al., 2010). Because only a few studies actually used Internet-based interventions (most used self-help books), we have to be cautious with definite conclusions. These results do, however, provide suggestive evidence that Internet-based therapies may be as effective as face-to-face therapies.

Almost all of the studies examining Internet-therapies for depressive disorders have been conducted with middle-aged and younger adults. Until now, only one study has been conducted with older adults (Spek et al., 2007b, 2008a, 2008b), and although the study was aimed at older adults (50 years or older), most of the 301 participants were 60 years or younger (mean age was 55). In this study a cognitive-behavioral Internet-based therapy was compared with the same intervention in group format (the "Coping with Depression" course), and a waiting list control group. No significant difference between the two treatment conditions was found, and both were superior to the waiting list control group (Spek et al., 2007b). At 1-year follow-up, both treatment conditions still showed a significantly better outcome than the control group, and still no significant difference between the active conditions was found.

Despite the positive results of this study, it is the only study on an Internet-based treatment for depression aimed at older adults. Furthermore, the participants in this study are relatively young and should not be compared, for example, with the "older old" of 80 years and older. On the other hand, there is no a priori reason to assume that these interventions are less effective in older adults compared to middle-aged and younger adults. In a recent metaregression analysis, considerable evidence was found that psychological treatments in general are as just as effective in older adults as they are in middle-aged and younger adults (Cuijpers et al., 2009).

Several meta-analyses in this field find that guided Internet-based interventions are more effective than interventions without any type of support by a professional (Andersson & Cuijpers, 2009; Spek et al., 2007a). Internet-based interventions with support by a coach are about as effective as face-to-face therapies, even when this support is given by students (Warmerdam, van Straten, Twisk, & Cuijpers, 2008) or technicians (Titov et al., 2010). Unguided Internet-based interventions, on the other hand, also have significant effects on depression, but these are considerably smaller (effect size, $d = 0.28$, which corresponds to an NNT of 6; Cuijpers et al., 2011). This difference between guided and self-guided Internet-interventions is not a principal one. It is very possible that in the near future self-guided therapies will be developed that are as effective as guided therapies. However, the currently available unguided therapies are not yet as effective as the guided therapies.

The effects of Internet-based therapies for depression have been supported by a growing number of studies in this field. The research in this area is not limited to depression. Since the year 2000 and especially since 2005, the number of studies examining the effects of Internet-based therapies for all kinds of mental health and physical problems is exploding. At this moment dozens of randomized controlled trials have examined the effects of Internet-based therapies for generalized anxiety disorder, panic disorder, social phobia, sleep problems, pain, migraine, eating problems, and problems with smoking and lifestyle (Cuijpers, van Straten, & Andersson, 2008; Marks et al., 2007).

While the effects of Internet-based treatments for depression and other problems are relatively well established, we have to remember that only patients who are motivated to be treated with such interventions participate in these studies. Patients who are not motivated for Internet treatments will not participate in such trials. At the same time very little is known about how many patients are motivated to participate in Internet-based interventions and how many are not. Although it is true for all treatments that studies are limited to patients who are willing to receive the studied intervention, Internet-interventions are new and it is not known whether patients who are now being treated with regular psychotherapy are willing to be treated with Internet therapies. Nor do we know how many patients who are now untreated will be treated when Internet interventions are widely available.

THE EFFECTS OF TELEPSYCHIATRY INTERVENTIONS FOR MOOD DISORDERS

The effects of telepsychiatry interventions with videoconferencing for depression have not yet been examined extensively in randomized controlled trials. In one randomized trial, 119 depressed veterans referred for outpatient treatment were randomly assigned to either telepsychiatry or face-to-face treatment. Both treatments lasted 6 months and consisted of pharmacotherapy, psychoeducation, and brief supportive counseling. No significant differences were found between these two conditions, suggesting that telepsychiatry may be as effective as face-to-face therapies (Ruskin et al., 2004). Although several other randomized controlled trials have been conducted with telepsychiatry with videoconferencing (García-Lizana & Muñoz-Mayorga, 2010; Hailey, Roine, & Ohinmaa, 2008; O'Reilly et al., 2007; Westphal, Dingjana, & Attoe, 2010), no other trials have examined treatments of depression in older nor in middle-aged and younger adults.

Several more randomized controlled trials have examined the effects of telephone-supported psychological treatment. A recent systematic review identified 14 randomized trials examining the effects of telephone-supported psychological treatments (Leach & Christensen, 2006). Six of these trials were focused on depressive disorders, although none of these were aimed at older adults. Although the results of these studies indicate that telephone-supported psychological treatments may be effective as treatments for depression, the sample sizes of these studies were small and the quality was not optimal. Therefore, no definite conclusions can be drawn at this moment. Larger and better randomized trials are needed to establish the effects of telepsychiatry interventions with and without videoconferencing.

DIRECTIONS FOR THE FUTURE

Internet-based interventions and telepsychiatry are promising interventions. They may reduce the costs of treatments for mood and other mental health problems in older adults considerably. They may also reach patients who are now untreated, they may simplify treatments considerably, and stimulate self-management. At this moment however, too few well-designed randomized trials have established the effectiveness of these interventions. In older adults almost no trials have been conducted. Internet-based interventions and, to a lesser extent, telephone-supported interventions have been examined and there are sufficient indications that these are effective. The multiple settings in which telepsychiatry interventions can be used for the elderly, such as at home or nursing homes or homes for the elderly, are not yet studied sufficiently either.

However, modern technologies offer much more possibilities than currently used. Direct contact between therapists and the patient through the television are technically possible, serious gaming is becoming a serious alternative for regular mental health interventions, and the Internet is now moving quickly toward mobile connections to the Web. The bigger screen of tablet handheld technologies accommodates the use of mobile devices especially by the elderly. This offers new technological possibilities for assessing mental health problems and implementing interventions into daily life, and many new pilot studies are currently developed. Clearly, technological developments go much faster in these areas than research in general and randomized controlled efficacy trials specifically. In the next decade we will see how this field develops.

One important issue is to improve the understanding of how Internet interventions stimulate behavior change and symptom improvement. A careful examination and testing of changes in behavior that lead to symptom improvement is essential for the understanding of how Internet interventions, and even treatments in general, work. To realize this, models specific to Internet interventions are needed,

as there are obvious differences in treatment delivery from traditional interventions. We also have to do more research specifically aimed at older adults and develop interventions in such a way they are feasible and acceptable for older patients.

Another important research issue concerns implementation and dissemination of Internet interventions. The research in this area has progressed considerably in the past decade, and it is time to think about dissemination and implementation in routine care, although this may not yet be true for specific interventions for older adults. Most health care systems are not equipped to finance the interventions. Models for the dissemination and implementation of scalable interventions are needed. Making Internet interventions available to the public is an important goal. It is important to examine models of commercialization that help determine how to efficiently disseminate these programs. A range of business models should be made available to develop research prototypes into fully scaled applications.

It is also important to develop an understanding of who will use Internet interventions and how to encourage adherence. By closely examining the characteristics of its users a better understanding should emerge on who will use the interventions and who will not. Furthermore, it will help improve the tailored nature of these programs, and to predict outcomes. Poor adherence and early dropout are issues of major concern for most health interventions, perhaps even more so for Internet interventions. Developing ways to reduce attrition, improve adherence, and maintain compliance are major objectives for research in this area.

CONCLUSION

Mood disorders are highly prevalent in older adults and result in huge losses in quality of life and high levels of service use. Internet-based interventions and telepsychiatry are important new tools to reduce the disease burden of these disorders. They may save considerable amounts of therapist time, reach populations with mood and anxiety disorders who cannot be reached otherwise, reduce waiting lists, simplify the organization of care, save traveling time, and reduce the stigma of going to a therapist. A growing body of research shows that Internet interventions are as effective as the more traditional face-to-face therapies, although more research is needed in older adults.

Not all questions regarding Internet-based interventions and telepsychiatry have been answered. The disadvantages, such as lack of adequate diagnostics, lack of access to the Internet, and technophobia, may result in negative effects for some patients or clients. More research is needed on core areas of these interventions. These include the effective ingredients and behavioral change processes, optimal ways of implementing and disseminating such interventions, the profiles of users for whom this type of intervention is effective, and the improvement of adherence.

There is no doubt, however, that Internet-based interventions and telepsychiatry will change mental health care for older adults considerably, especially with the new developments of mobile technologies and the integration of the Internet in the television.

Disclosures

Dr. Cuijpers has nothing to disclose.

Dr. Riper has nothing to disclose.

Dr. Beekman has received unrestricted research grants from Eli Lilly, Astra Zeneca, and Jansen and Shire. He has served on the speakers bureaus for Eli Lilly and Lundbeck.

REFERENCES

Andersson, G., & Cuijpers, P. (2009). Internet-based and other computerized psychological treatments for adult depression: A meta-analysis. *Cognitive Behaviour Therapy, 38,* 196–205.

Andrews, G., Cuijpers, P., Craske, M. G., McEvoy, P., & Titov, N. (2010). Computer therapy for the anxiety and depressive disorders is effective, acceptable and practical health care: A meta-analysis and pilot implementation. *PLoS One, 5*(10), e13196.

Bijl, R. V., & Ravelli, A. (2000). Psychiatric morbidity, service use, and need for care in the general population: Results of the Netherlands Mental Health Survey and Incidence Study. *American Journal of Public Health, 90,* 602–07.

Churchill, R., Hunot, V., Corney, R., Knapp, M., McGuire, H., Tylee, A., & Wessely, S. (2001). A systematic review of controlled trials of the effectiveness and cost-effectiveness of brief psychological treatments for depression. *Health Technology Assessment, 5,* 35.

Conner, K. O., Copeland, V. C., Grote, N. K., Koeske, G., Rosen, D., Reynolds, C. F., III, & Brown C (2010). Mental health treatment seeking among older adults with depression: The impact of stigma and race. *American Journal of Geriatric Psychiatry, 18*(6), 531–543.

Crabb, R., & Hunsley, J. (2006). Utilization and mental health care services among older adults with depression. *Journal of Clinical Psychology, 62,* 299–312.

Cuijpers, P., Donker, T., Johansson, R., Mohr, D. C., van Straten, A., & Andersson, G. (2011). Self-guided psychological treatment for depressive symptoms: A meta-analysis. *PloS One, 6*(6), e21274.

Cuijpers, P., Donker, T., van Straten, A., Li, J., & Andersson, G. (2010). Is guided self-help as effective as face-to-face psychotherapy for depression and anxiety disorders? A systematic review and meta-analysis of comparative outcome studies. *Psychological Medicine, 40,* 1943–1957.

Cuijpers, P., Marks, I., van Straten, A., Cavanagh, K., Gega, L., & Andersson, G. (2009). Computer-aided psychotherapy for anxiety disorders: A meta-analytic review. *Cognitive Behaviour Therapy, 38,* 66–82.

Cuijpers, .P, & Schuurmans, J. (2007). Self-help interventions for anxiety disorders: An overview. *Current Psychiatry Reports, 9,* 284–290.

Cuijpers, P., van Straten, A., & Andersson, G (2008). Internet-administered cognitive behavior therapy for health problems: A systematic review. *Journal of Behavioral Medicine, 31,* 169–177.

Cuijpers, P., van Straten, A., Smit, F., & Andersson, G (2009). Is psychotherapy for depression equally effective in younger and older adults? A meta-regression analysis. *International Psychogeriatrics, 21,* 16–24

Datto, C. J., Thompson, R., Horowitz, D., Disbot, M., & Oslin, D. W. (2003). The pilot study of a telephone disease management program for depression. *General Hospital Psychiatry, 25,* 169–177.

Diamond, J. M., & Bloch, R. M. (2010). Telepsychiatry assessments of child or adolescent behavior disorders: A review of evidence and issues. *Telemedicine and Journal of E-Health, 16*(6), 712–716.

Egede, L. E., Frueh, C. B., Richardson, L. K., Acierno, R., Mauldin, P. D., Knapp, R. G., & Lejuez, C. (2009). Rationale and design: Telepsychology service delivery for depressed elderly veterans. *Trials, 10,* 22

García-Lizana, F., & Muñoz-Mayorga, I. (2010). Telemedicine for depression: A systematic review. *Perspectives in Psychiatric Care, 46,* 119–126.

Hailey, D., Roine, R., & Ohinmaa, A. (2008). The effectiveness of telemental health applications:

A review. *Canadian Journal of Psychiatry, 53,* 769–778.

Hunkeler, E. M., Meresman, J. F., Hargreaves, W. A., Fireman, B., Berman, W. H., Kirsch, A. J., . . . Salzer M.. (2000). Efficacy of nurse telehealth care and peer support in augmenting treatment of depression in primary care. Archives of Family Medicine, 9, 700–708.

Johnston, D., & Jones, B. N., III. (2001). Telepsychiatry consultations to a rural nursing facility: A 2-year experience. *Journal of Geriatric Psychiatry and Neurology, 14,* 72–75.

Leach, L. S., & Christensen, H. (2006). A systematic review of telephone-based interventions for mental disorders. *Journal of Telemedicine and Telecare, 12,* 122–129.

Mackenzie, C. S., Scott, T., Mather, A., & Sareen, J. (2008). Older adults' help-seeking attitudes and treatment beliefs concerning mental health problems. *American Journal of Geriatric Psychiatry, 16*(12), 1010–1019.

Marks, I. M., Cavanagh, K., & Gega, L. (2007). *Hands-on help: Computer-aided psychotherapy.* Maudsley Monographs No. 45. Hove, England: Psychology Press.

Marrs, R. W. (1995). A meta-analysis of bibliotherapy studies. *American Journal of Community Psychology, 23,* 843–870.

Monnier, J., Knapp, R. G., & Frueh, B. C. (2003). Recent advances in telepsychiatry: An updated review. *Psychiatric Services, 54,* 1604–1609.

O'Reilly, R., Bishop, J., Maddox, K., Hutchinson, L., Fisman, M., & Takhar, J. (2007). Is telepsychiatry equivalent to face-to-face psychiatry? Results from a randomized controlled equivalence trial. *Psychiatric Services, 58,* 836–843.

Pepin, R., Segal, D. L., & Coolidge, F. L. (2009). Intrinsic and extrinsic barriers to mental health care among community-dwelling younger and older adults. *Aging and Mental Health, 13,* 769–777

Robb, C., Haley, W. E., Becker, M. A., Polivka, L. A., & Chwa, J. (2003). Attitudes towards mental health care in younger and older adults: Similarities and differences. *Aging and Mental Health, 7,* 142–152.

Ruskin, P. E., Silver, A. M., Kling, M. A., Reed, S. A., Bradham, D. D., Hebel, J. R., & Hauser, P. (2004). Treatment outcomes in depression: Comparison of remote treatment through telepsychiatry to in-person treatment. *American Journal of Psychiatry, 161,* 1471–1476.

Scogin, F. R., Hanson, A., & Welsh, D. (2003). Self-administered treatment in stepped-care models of depression treatment. *Journal of Clinical Psychology, 59,* 341–349.

Spek, V., Cuijpers, P., Nyklíček, I., Riper, H., Keyzer, J., & Pop, V. (2007a). Internet-based cognitive behavior therapy for mood and anxiety disorders: A meta-analysis. *Psychological Medicine, 37,* 319–328.

Spek, V., Nyklíček, I., Smits, N., Cuijpers, P., Riper, H., Keyzer, J., & Pop, V. (2007b). Internet-based cognitive behavioural therapy for sub-threshold depression in people over 50 years old: A randomized controlled clinical trial. *Psychological Medicine, 37,* 1797–1806.

Spek, V., Nyklíček, I., Smits, N., Cuijpers, P., Riper, H., Keyzer, J., & Pop, V. (2008a). Follow-up results of an internet-based cognitive behavioural therapy for sub-threshold depression in people over 50 years old: A randomized controlled clinical trial. *Psychological Medicine, 38,* 635–639.

Spek, V., Nyklíček, I., Cuijpers, P., & Pop, V. J. (2008b). Predictors of outcome of group and internet-based cognitive behaviour therapy. *Journal of Affective Disorders, 105,* 137–145.

Tang, W. K., Chiu, H., Woo, J., Hjelm, M., & Hui, E. (2001). Telepsychiatry in psychogeriatric service: A pilot study. *International Journal of Geriatric Psychiatry 16,* 88–93.

Wampold, B. E., Minami, T., Baskin, T. W., & Tierney, S. C. (2002). A meta-(re)analysis of the effects of cognitive therapy versus "other therapies" for depression. *Journal of Affective Disorders, 68,* 159–165.

Wang, P. S., Lane, M., Olfson, M., Pincus, H. A., Wells, K. B., & Kessler, R. C. (2005). Twelve-month use of mental health services in the United States; Results from the National Comorbidity Survey Replication. *Archives of General Psychiatry, 62,* 629–640.

Warmerdam, L., van Straten, A., Twisk, J., & Cuijpers, P. (2008). Internet-based treatment for adults with depressive symptoms: a randomized controlled trial. *Journal of Medical Internet Research, 10*(4), e44.

Westphal, A., Dingjana, P., & Attoe, R. (2010). What can low and high technologies do for late-life mental disorders? *Current Opinion in Psychiatry, 23,* 510–515.

Wright, J. H., Wright, A. S., Albano, A. M., Basco, M. R., Goldsmith, L. J., Raffield, T., & Otto, M. W. (2005). Computer-assisted cognitive therapy for depression: Maintaining efficacy while reducing therapist time. *American Journal of Psychiatry, 162,* 1158–1164.

Yellowlees, P. M., Odor, A., Parish, M. B., Iosif, A. M., Haught, K., & Hilty, D. (2010) A feasibility study of the use of asynchronous telepsychiatry for psychiatric consultations. *Psychiatric Services*, 61(8),838–840.

Yeung, A., Johnson, D. P., Trinh, N. H., Weng, W. C. C., Kvedar, J., & Fava, M. (2009). Feasibility and effectiveness of telepsychiatry services for chinese immigrants in a nursing home. *Telemedicine and Jounral of E-Health*, 15, 336–341.

SECTION 5

NEUROBIOLOGY AND BIOMARKERS

32

STRUCTURAL NEUROIMAGING IN LATE-LIFE MOOD DISORDERS

Sean J. Colloby and John T. O'Brien

FOR OVER two decades there has been an increasingly widespread application of structural neuroimaging research in affective disorders. Early observations suggested ventricular enlargement in the brains of older subjects with affective disorders using computed tomography (CT) and were key to paving the way for future research in this area (Jacoby & Levy, 1980; Jacoby, Levy, & Bird, 1981). The development of brain magnetic resonance imaging (MRI) offered a significant improvement over CT in terms of higher resolution, particularly in subcortical regions, and in differentiating gray and white matter, allowing for a more accurate measurement of brain structures than with CT. Affective disorder research has mainly focused on studying many of the structures implicated within neuroanatomical circuits hypothesized to regulate mood. In particular, the limbic-cortical-striatal-pallidal-thalamic circuit, which is extensively interconnected, has been implicated (Sheline, 2003). This chapter concentrates on structural MRI brain changes associated with unipolar major depression and bipolar disorder (BD) of late life, with particular attention to structural imaging, white matter hyperintensities (WMHs), and diffusion tensor imaging (DTI).

STRUCTURAL MAGNETIC RESONANCE STUDIES

Using T1-weighted MRI data, volumetric changes in cortical and subcortical structures have been investigated in late-life affective disorders. The most common of these techniques are region of interest (ROI) and voxelwise procedures. Other more recent methods are surface-based approaches that measure, for example, cortical thickness. Region of interest involves manual or semi-automated tracing of specific brain regions but does not evaluate the entire brain volume and cannot determine whether any changes in volume are due to alterations in gray matter (GM), white matter (WM), or both. Voxelwise methods such as voxel-based morphometry (VBM) allow the separate assessment of GM and WM concentrations in an unbiased manner across the whole brain. Cortical thickness is a relatively new procedure for assessing brain structure and has been reported to represent alterations in cortical surface area and folding (Voets et al., 2008; Winkler et al., 2010), reflecting the underlying deficits in the cortical laminae that may characterize disease-specific neuroanatomical changes.

Cortical Structures

GENERALIZED ATROPHY

Following CT studies suggesting atrophy and ventricular enlargement in older depressed subjects, early MRI studies also found greater structural changes in older subjects with depression compared to healthy aged-matched individuals. Rabins et al. (1991) showed that 21 older depressed subjects had greater cerebral and temporal sulcal atrophy, larger sylvian fissures, and larger lateral and third ventricles relative to 14 similar aged healthy persons. Similarly, Dahabra et al. (1998) found atrophic changes in the lateral and third ventricles in 12 subjects with late-life depression (LLD) versus 11 early-onset depressed and 15 controls. Significantly lower whole-brain volumes and higher cerebrospinal fluid volumes have also been observed in older depressed subjects compared to age-matched controls (Pantel et al., 1998).

In late-life bipolar disorder (LLBD) studies have reported mixed findings. McDonald et al. (1991) showed similar sized ventricles between 12 subjects with late-onset BD and 12 similar aged healthy subjects. In contrast, Young et al. (1999), using visual rating of CT scans, reported larger lateral ventricles and greater cortical sulcal widening in 30 older BD subjects relative to 18 healthy controls. They also observed cortical sulcal widening was positively associated with age at illness onset and age at first manic episode.

FRONTAL LOBE

The frontal lobe comprises nearly 30% of the neocortex and has long been implicated in the regulation of mood. Using ROI methods, numerous studies have reported reduced frontal lobe volume in subjects with late-onset depression relative to similar aged healthy subjects. Kumar et al. (1998) showed significantly smaller prefrontal lobe volumes in their depressed subjects that inversely correlated with illness severity and later found similar results

in a larger cohort (Kumar, Bilker, Jin, & Udupa, 2000). Others observed volumetric reductions to bilateral orbital frontal cortex (Lai, Payne, Byrum, Steffens, & Krishnan, 2000) and right frontal lobe (Almeida, Burton, Ferrier, McKeith, & O'Brien, 2003). Andreescu et al. (2008) identified decreased volumes in orbital, inferior, and medial superior regions of the frontal lobe that negatively correlated with age of onset. Voxel-based analyses have also revealed reduced GM volumes to specific frontal structures, including bilateral middle frontal gyrus (Bell-McGinty et al., 2002), bilateral orbitofrontal cortex that was associated with depression severity (Egger et al., 2008), and right superior frontal cortex (Yuan et al., 2008). However, some did not detect changes in the frontal lobes of late-life depressed subjects compared to older healthy subjects using ROI (Pantel et al., 1998) and voxel morphometry or cortical thickness methods (Colloby, Firbank, et al., 2011b; Koolschijn et al., 2010).

Few studies have focused on exploring frontal lobe deficits in BD, and therefore it is difficult to draw any accurate conclusions regarding the extent that such structural changes have on the neuropathology of LLBD. A recent voxel morphometry study demonstrated a decrease in GM concentration in the right frontal orbital cortex in 19 subjects relative to 47 healthy older subjects (Haller et al., 2011). However, a longitudinal voxel morphometry study showed that over 2 years follow-up, LLBD subjects did not progress cognitively or structurally (frontal GM volume) (Delaloye et al., 2011). Frontal cortical thinning has been observed in younger individuals with BD and was shown to be positively correlated with duration of illness (Lyoo et al., 2006).

TEMPORAL LOBE

Models of neuroanatomical circuitry of mood disorders have implicated the involvement of temporal lobe structures, particularly the hippocampus and amygdala. The overwhelming evidence from ROI and voxel morphometric studies suggests that abnormalities of the temporal lobe are associated with late-life depressive illness. Using ROI, hippocampal atrophy has been shown in subjects relative to healthy older subjects in the right hemisphere (O'Brien, Lloyd, McKeith, Gholkar, & Ferrier, 2004; Steffens et al., 2000) and bilaterally (Andreescu et al., 2008; Hickie et al., 2005; Lloyd et al., 2004; Sheline, Wang, Gado, Csernansky, & Vannier, 1996). Left medial temporal atrophy in LLD compared to age-matched healthy persons has also been reported (Greenwald et al., 1997). Hippocampal atrophy was shown to be related to duration of depressive illness (Lloyd et al., 2004; Sheline et al., 1996), continuing memory deficits (O'Brien et al., 2004), and visual and verbal memory impairment (Hickie et al., 2005). Recently, another study showed that depression in later life was also shown to be associated with smaller amygdala volumes bilaterally, which was independent of age of initial onset of depression (Burke et al., 2011). Findings from voxel morphometric analyses have generally been consistent with ROI methods, with studies demonstrating atrophic changes to the right hippocampus (Bell-McGinty et al., 2002; Egger et al., 2008) and right middle temporal gyrus (Yuan et al., 2008). Using other techniques, cortical pattern matching identified right lateral temporal GM deficits (Ballmaier et al., 2004), while shape analysis revealed smaller left hippocampal volumes (Zhao et al., 2008) in LLD compared to healthy older subjects. Other temporal structures shown to be affected in LLD include the amygdala (Andreescu et al., 2008; Egger et al., 2008; Hickie et al., 2005), entorhinal cortex (Bell-McGinty et al., 2002), and insula (Hwang et al., 2010). However, some investigators did not detect any significant differences in hippocampal volumes between their patient and healthy cohorts (Ashtari et al., 1999; Pantel et al., 1998). Similarly, no temporal GM deficits were found between late-life depressed subjects relative to older healthy individuals (Colloby, Firbank, et al., 2011b; Koolschijn et al., 2010).

Due to limited research, evidence of temporal abnormalities in LLBD is less clear. Delaloye et al. (2009) compared 17 older BD with 17 healthy older individuals and reported no volumetric differences in amygdala, hippocampus, and entorhinal cortex. Fifteen of these BD subjects were then followed up after 2 years showing no deterioration in their cognitive and limbic structures (Delaloye et al., 2011). One previous study has reported structural deficits in LLBD, where reduced GM concentration in the right anterior insula was observed relative to age-matched controls (Haller et al., 2011).

OTHER CORTICAL REGIONS

Using cortical pattern matching, GM deficits in right parietal cortex were observed in late-onset depression compared to healthy older subjects (Ballmaier et al., 2004). Andreescu et al. (2008) showed using

ROI reduced inferior parietal lobe volumes in their depressed group compared to healthy age-matched subjects, which also correlated with age of onset and duration of depression. However, a voxel morphometric analysis revealed significant differences in GM volumes in posterior cingulate (Hwang et al., 2010). In contrast, others reported no significant differences in GM volume in nonfrontotemporal regions in late-life depressed subjects relative to older healthy persons (Colloby, Firbank, et al., 2011b; Koolschijn et al., 2010).

Significant thinning of the corpus callosum in both the genu and splenium regions was found in subjects with late-onset depression, which significantly correlated with memory and attention functioning. Such structural alterations in callosal morphology could distinguish late-onset from early-onset depression (Ballmaier et al., 2008). Other regions that have shown significant cortical thinning include the right cingulate cortex in persons with late-life minor depression compared to similar aged healthy individuals (Kumar, Ajilore, Zhang, Pham, & Elderkin-Thompson, 2012).

Subcortical Structures

Subcortical structures such as the striatum and thalamus form an integral part of neural circuits thought to regulate mood, and therefore they are important in the pathophysiology of affective disorders of late life (Strakowski, Adler, & DelBello, 2002). Most studies investigating subcortical structures in late-onset depression have identified striatal abnormalities. Krishnan et al. (1993) found reduced caudate and putamen volumes relative to older healthy subjects. Greenwald et al. (1997) showed greater caudate atrophy in late-onset subjects compared to early-onset subjects and controls of similar age. Decreased putamen volumes have also been observed and found to be associated with a later age of onset of depression (Andreescu et al., 2008). Bilateral atrophy of the caudate has also been described and found to be correlated with depression severity (Butters et al., 2009). In a large older depressed cohort of 182 subjects, Hannestad et al. (2006) demonstrated a link between reduced caudate volumes and increased white matter lesions (WMLs), thereby suggesting one mechanism by which WMLs may disrupt frontostriatal circuits. In another study, reduced caudate volumes in older subjects with depression were shown to be associated with the short allele of the serotonin transporter promoter polymorphism (5-HTT) gene, which has been linked to increased risk for major depression in early adults (Hickie et al., 2007). Two studies with contradictory results have specifically investigated the thalamus for structural changes in LLD. Andreescu et al. (2008) found reduced thalamic volumes in 71 subjects compared to 32 older healthy subjects, while conversely Krishnan et al. (1993) observed no significant differences between 25 subjects and 20 comparison subjects. Using voxel morphometry analysis, studies reported no evidence of subcortical GM changes between late-life depressed subjects relative to older healthy subjects (Colloby, Firbank, et al., 2011b; Koolschijn et al., 2010).

At present, there is some evidence for subcortical involvement in late-life bipolar disorder, with one recent study reporting reduced GM concentrations in LLBD subjects in head of caudate, nucleus accumbens, and ventral putamen compared to similar aged healthy subjects (Haller et al., 2011). Further research is required to investigate subcortical abnormalities and their role in the pathophysiology of LLBD.

Summary

Structural brain abnormalities are present in subjects with late-life major depression. The evidence points to an atrophic frontal and temporal (hippocampal) pattern. Striatal atrophy also appears to characterize late-life major depression and thus supports the notion of a "fronto-temporo-striatal" dysfunction in older depression. Since other brain structures may be implicated in the pathophysiology of LLD, it would be important for more studies using unbiased methods like voxel morphometric studies that can explore the entire brain volume. Despite the concordance between studies, there is still variability in results. Such discrepancies may be due to differences in populations, depression severity, illness duration, and/or (antidepressant) medications as well as differences in MR acquisition and analysis methods. The cause of such structural changes is not clear, nor is it known if they predate depression, and different hypotheses suggest they may result from developmental problems, prolonged raised cortisol levels as a result of depression, the results of treatments, vascular factors, degenerative changes, or a combination thereof. The evidence for structural abnormalities in LLBD is limited at present,

though studies to date suggest a different pattern from LLD with frontostriatal atrophy but not temporal involvement, which contrasts with findings in younger bipolar subjects. However, further studies are required to investigate the frontostriatal contribution to the pathophysiology of LLBD before firm conclusions can be drawn.

WHITE MATTER HYPERINTENSITIES

Cerebral WMHs are focal areas of increased signal intensity, detectable on either T2-weighted or fluid-attenuated inversion recovery (FLAIR) MRI scans. Such lesions are typically located in periventricular and deep white matter regions as well as in subcortical structures such as the basal ganglia (Pantoni & Garcia, 1997). WMHs are classified into three major groups: periventricular hyperintensities (PVHs), deep white matter hyperintensities (DWMHs), and subcortical gray matter hyperintensities (SCHs). These lesions appear to be associated with aging (de Leeuw et al., 2001; Ylikoski et al., 1995) and may be linked to cognitive decline (Garde, Mortensen, Krabbe, Rostrup, & Larsson, 2000; Marshall, Hendrickson, Kaufer, Ivanco, & Bohnen, 2006). There is also evidence that WMHs in older populations are related to cerebrovascular disease (Fukuda & Kitani, 1995; Pantoni & Garcia, 1997; Thomas et al., 2002; Veldink, Scheltens, Jonker, & Launer, 1998), suggesting ischemic mechanisms may underlie these lesions in old age. In late-life mood disorders, interpretation of images to quantify the extent of WMH burden usually involves either standard visual rating procedures or semiautomated segmentation techniques to calculate WMH lesion volumes. The majority of visual rating studies used the Fazekas/Coffey criteria, while the remaining studies largely adopted their own rating system or Scheltens (Herrmann, Le Masurier, & Ebmeier, 2008).

Periventricular Hyperintensities and Deep White Matter Hyperintensities

WMH findings were an important part of the early work on LLD. Results from visual rating studies have consistently reported increased prevalence of DWMHs in subjects with LLD. Greater occurrences of DWMHs in subjects with LLD compared to early-onset depressed subjects have been reported (Figiel et al., 1991; Tupler et al., 2002), while others showed a greater severity of DWMHs in older depressed subjects relative to healthy older persons (Lesser et al., 1996; O'Brien et al., 1996). Regional changes in DWMHs have also been found to distinguish geriatric depressed from healthy subjects in the left frontal lobe (Greenwald et al., 1998), while a later multicenter study of 626 older subjects revealed depressive symptoms were associated with increase WMH burden in frontal and temporal areas (O'Brien et al., 2006). Utilizing semiautomated segmentation methods, Taylor et al. showed that in depressed subjects a significant association between age and DWMH occurred in bilateral frontal and left parietal regions, whereas in comparison subjects associations appeared only in bilateral parietotemporal areas, not frontal (Taylor, MacFall, et al., 2003); Firbank et al. (2004) demonstrated greater frontal lobe WMH volume in depressed subjects than in healthy comparison subjects; and in a large cohort (n = 253), Taylor et al. (2005) found older depressed subjects exhibited significantly greater total DWMH volumes in both hemispheres than in control subjects. Greater WMHs have also been shown in the following white matter tracts: the superior longitudinal fasciculus, fronto-occipital fasciculus, uncinate fasciculus, extreme capsule, and inferior longitudinal fasciculus (Sheline et al., 2008). Moreover, Dalby et al. (2010) indicated that it was WMH localization rather than WMH burden that discriminates subjects with late-onset major depression from age-matched healthy persons. They showed significantly higher WMH volumes in regions, including the left superior longitudinal fasciculus and right frontal projections of the corpus callosum, in subjects than comparison subjects but not for total number and volume of WMH. Others reported no significant differences in PVH and DWMH volumes in LLD relative to comparison subjects, although an association between orthostatic blood pressure changes and WMH volume was found, suggesting that such changes may be a factor contributing to lesions in LLD (Colloby, Vasudev, et al., 2011).

DWMHs may also relate to poorer outcomes of LLD (O'Brien et al., 1998). Greater severity of DWMH predicted increased mortality in depressed older subjects (Levy et al., 2003), while greater change in DWMH volume was shown to be significantly associated with chronicity or relapse of depression (Taylor, Steffens, et al., 2003). Another study showed late-life depressives with greater WMH burden had significantly higher depression scores, more severe longitudinal courses of depression, and lower

Mini-Mental State Examination (MMSE) scores (Heiden et al., 2005). Similarly, Kohler et al. (2010) demonstrated that WMHs rather than cortisol levels or brain atrophy were associated with continuing cognitive impairments in older depressed persons. There remains debate about whether lesions predate depression or are a consequence of being depressed. Only a few prospective studies address this. A longitudinal multicenter investigation of 639 older persons revealed that baseline severity of WMH volume appeared to independently and significantly predict depressive symptoms at 1 year, controlling for baseline depression (Teodorczuk et al., 2007), and similarly for depressive symptoms at years 2 and 3 (Teodorczuk et al., 2010). A large French study (Godin et al., 2008) also found that WMH at baseline predicted future depression in those with no prior history, strongly arguing that they have an etiological role. This is an important finding, since it may allow the targeting of preventative strategies to those not currently depressed but at high risk.

In contrast to the evidence describing WMHs in late-life major depression, only a small number of studies have investigated the presence of WMHs in LLBD. McDonald et al. (1991) using visual rating observed no significant differences in the frequency of PVHs between older subjects with mania and older healthy individuals. In a later study they reported increased prevalence of PVH and DWMH in 70 older BD subjects than in comparison subjects (McDonald et al., 1999). Significantly greater DWMHs have been identified in bilateral parietal lobes of LLBD subjects relative to controls, while higher right frontal DWMH ratings correlated with a later age of onset of mania (de Asis et al., 2006). Similarly, a greater incidence of parietal DWMH was apparent in late-onset BD subjects than in age-matched early-onset BD group and healthy subjects (Tamashiro et al., 2008). In addition, they reported more severe frontal and parietal DWMH in late-onset BD compared to the other groups and showed that more severe parietal DWMH was related to an older age of onset of illness.

Subcortical Gray Matter Hyperintensities

Rabins et al. showed a particular increase in subcortical WMHs in older subjects with depression, with predominance of lesions in basal ganglia (Rabins, Pearlson, Aylward, Kumar, & Dowell, 1991). Figuel et al. (1991) revealed increased SCH in caudate in subjects with LLD compared to early-onset older depressed subjects. Krishnan et al. (1993) also reported greater frequency of subcortical hyperintensities in older depressed than controls. Putamen hyperintensities have also been shown to feature in LLD, with one study demonstrating greater burden in the left putamen in a geriatric depressed group relative to older healthy subjects (Greenwald et al., 1998), and one reporting more severe subcortical hyperintensity ratings, particularly in putamen, in a late-onset depressed group compared to a similar aged healthy cohort (Tupler et al., 2002). Using semiautomated procedures, some investigations found no WMH volume differences in the basal ganglia between older depressed subjects and older nondepressed subjects (Colloby et al., 2011c; Firbank, Lloyd, Ferrier, & O'Brien, 2004), while in another, depressed subjects exhibited significantly greater total SCH volumes in both hemispheres than control subjects (Taylor et al., 2005). Subcortical WML in older depressed subjects have also been reported to be associated with poor treatment outcome (Chen, McQuoid, Payne, & Steffens, 2006; Steffens et al., 2001; Taylor, Steffens, et al., 2003) and greater risk of subsequent dementia (Steffens et al., 2007). SCHs in LLD have been shown to correlate with psychomotor slowing (Simpson, Jackson, Baldwin, & Burns, 1997) and executive dysfunction (Salloway et al., 1996).

In LLBD, the existence of subcortical WMHs is a consistent finding, although the number of imaging studies remains at present low. A greater number of bilateral SCHs were observed in a small group of subjects with an onset of manic symptoms after the age of 50 years compared to age- and gender-matched healthy subjects (McDonald, Krishnan, Doraiswamy, & Blazer, 1991); then a larger BD cohort reported greater presence of hyperintense

lesions in subcortical structures relative to population-, age-, and gender-matched healthy controls (McDonald et al., 1999). Higher frequency of SCH in caudate, putamen, and globus pallidus differentiated late-onset BD from older early-onset subjects and healthy subjects (Tamashiro et al., 2008). However, others observed that signal hyperintensities in subcortical GM regions did not distinguish older BD subjects from comparison subjects (de Asis et al., 2006).

Summary

Individuals with late-onset depression have generally greater WMH burden than older people with early-onset depressed and healthy nondepressed subjects, and these lesions appear to play a role in their depressive illness. Figure 32.1 illustrates axial FLAIR images depicting subcortical (A), periventricular and deep WMH (B, C) in a subject with LLD. WMH may disrupt neural circuits, or fiber tracts connecting frontal and subcortical regions; such disruptions may alter the function of circuits involved in mood regulation, contributing to the pathogenesis of depression. In addition, although disease severity and lesion burden may be important, a more critical factor in LLD could be in their strategic location. Further studies comparing regional WMH volume measures and their effects on depressive symptoms in LLD are required to investigate this hypothesis. Although studies remain small, LLBD seem to be associated with increased WMH burden; a pattern similar to subjects with LLD and may disrupt several selective neural circuits that describes some of the symptoms of LLBD. However, the apparent WMH burden may to a large degree be mirroring the increased cerebrovascular risk associated with LLD and LLBD.

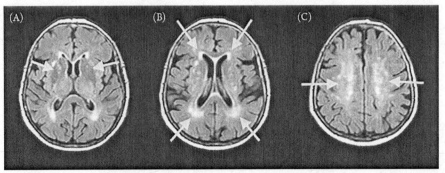

FIGURE 32.1 Axial FLAIR images depicting subcortical (A), periventricular and deep WMH (B, C) in a subject with LLD.

DIFFUSION TENSOR IMAGING

DTI has become the method of choice for detecting white matter changes in the human brain. DTI, which is sensitive to the diffusion of water, captures the microstructural alterations of biological tissue by measuring directional changes in water diffusivity. The directionality of diffusion is typically expressed as fractional anisotropy (FA), which ranges from zero for isotropic diffusion to unity for diffusion exclusively in one direction. Well-organized, strongly myelinated white matter tracts thus have high FA values as water diffuses more freely in the direction of the axonal fiber tracts, while diffusion perpendicular to the fibers is relatively limited. Therefore, as fibers deteriorate, diffusion becomes less directional and the value of FA decreases. Figure 32.2 presents coronal (A) and axial (B) views of a color-coded DTI fractional anisotropy (FA) image map. Notice signal intensity varies according to FA, and the color coding according to the direction of the principal eigenvector, with red being left to right, blue being inferior to superior, and green being anterior to posterior. Another parameter commonly derived is mean diffusivity (MD), which measures the overall displacement of water molecules from multiple directions and

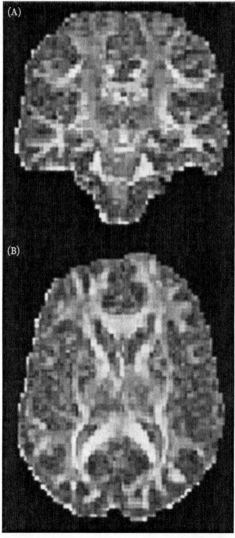

FIGURE 32.2   Coronal (A) and axial (B) views of a color coded DTI fractional anisotropy (FA) image map. Notice signal intensity varies according to FA, and color coding according to the directionality of the principal eigenvector, with red being left-to-right, blue being inferior-to-superior and green anterior-to-posterior (See color insert).

is increased in abnormal fiber tracts. Such measures can be extracted globally using voxel-based analysis or tract-based spatial statistics (TBSS) (Smith et al., 2006), or locally using defined ROI analysis or tractography. ROI usually requires the manual placement of a region of fixed size and shape over a predefined area, which avoids registration errors but is sensitive to user bias. Tractography automatically reconstructs white matter tracts, though user bias remains a consideration if target regions are manually defined. Regarding voxel-based approaches, the technique may be limited by intersubject image registration and the amount of spatial smoothing of data (Smith et al., 2006). TBSS projects all subjects' FA data onto an average FA tract skeleton before applying voxelwise cross subjects statistics. It is more robust and sensitive than voxel-based approaches but is restricted to investigating local changes in white matter integrity (Smith et al., 2006).

Late-Life Depression

The majority of previous studies have adopted the ROI approach to study the microstructural changes in late-life mood disorders relative to comparison subjects. An early investigation showed no significant differences in DTI parameters (FA, MD) in several regions, including frontal, parietal, caudate, and thalamus between older depressed subjects and healthy older subjects (Taylor et al., 2001). In much larger depressed and control cohorts, Bae et al. (2006) using ROI found significantly lower FA in right anterior cingulate, bilateral superior frontal gyri, and left middle frontal gyrus in depressed elders relative to healthy similar aged individuals. In partial agreement, Taylor et al. (2004) observed lower FA in the superior frontal gyrus in LLD than in comparison subjects. Others have also demonstrated that in a group of LLD subjects compared to healthy controls, reduced FA in frontal and temporal lobes was apparent in subjects (Nobuhara et al., 2006). Using tractography methods, the left uncinate fasciculus a region believed to connect frontal and limbic structures was examined revealing lower FA in early-onset depression than in mid and late-onset subjects and nondepressed subjects (Taylor, MacFall, Gerig, & Krishnan, 2007). Two studies using distinct analysis techniques observed WM microstructural abnormalities in frontal and temporal structures (Yang, Huang, Hong, & Yu, 2007; Yuan et al., 2007), with other regions being implicated such as parietal, occipital,

caudate, and putamen (Yuan et al., 2007). Diffuse abnormalities have also been described in LLD, predominantly to prefrontal regions in measures of FA and MD (Shimony et al., 2009). Other procedures using voxelwise TBBS analysis have revealed similar regional reductions in FA in frontal and temporal lobes as well as midbrain in LLD (Colloby, Firbank, et al., 2011a).

Evidence of inferior frontal abnormalities being inversely correlated with severity of depression, possibly implicating the orbitofrontal circuit in symptom severity, has been described (Nobuhara et al., 2006). Poor antidepressant response in geriatric depressed individuals has also been shown to be associated with lower FA in several frontal limbic structures (Alexopoulos et al., 2008). Conversely, others revealed poor treatment response in LLD was associated with higher FA values in frontolimbic regions (Taylor et al., 2008). In addition, stroke risk factors have been found to correlate with impairments in WM integrity in corpus callosum and cortico-spinal tracts in LLD (Allan et al., 2011).

Late-Life Bipolar Disorder

One recent study observed that FA was the most sensitive DTI marker and decreased significantly in the ventral part of the corpus callosum in patients with LLBD, although axial, radial, and mean diffusivity showed no significant group differences (Haller et al., 2011). Currently, there is a lack of studies where previous DTI reports have mainly focused on adult populations.

Summary

It appears that microstructural disturbances to frontal and to lesser extent temporal regions are a consistent finding in LLD. Different parts of the frontal lobes have afferent and efferent connections with other neocortical, limbic, and subcortical regions and participate in the limbic-cortico-striatal-pallidal-thalamic circuits. Thus, disruptions to these neuroanatomical circuits are likely to be important in the pathogenesis of LLD. However, it is not entirely understood whether the observed DTI changes mirror some of the WMH changes in these subjects. Further DTI studies are needed to examine the integrity of non-WMH (i.e., normal appearing) white matter and determine how these microstructural changes contribute to depressive outcomes in LLD.

CONCLUSIONS

Structural brain deficits are associated with LLD and LLBD, with a pattern supporting the notion of "frontostriatal" disturbances in affective disorders of late life. Increased prevalence of WMH is another characteristic of LLD and LLBD, with perhaps location rather than burden being more important to their pathogeneses, but it may also indicate their increased cerebrovascular risk factors. Limited evidence to date suggests that WMH predate development of depression and therefore represent an important risk factor. Whether other structural changes predate depression, or are consequences of illness, remains unclear. Microstructural DTI changes are largely in frontal regions in LLD but in LLBD have not been investigated. Longitudinal studies could clarify whether the volumetric reductions, WMHs, and DTI changes are static or progressive and to what extent factors such as antidepressant medication, illness duration, age of onset, and illness severity have on structural imaging in late-life mood disorders. The variability in studies may represent the heterogeneity of LLD. Future studies with larger clinically representative populations will further aid in elucidating the specific anatomy and etiology of structural MRI changes in late-life mood disorders and investigate their relationship with clinical factors.

Disclosures

Dr. Colloby has no conflicts to disclose.

Professor O'Brien has acted as a consultant for GE and Bayer Healthcare and has received honoraria for lectures from GE Healthcare, Pfizer, Eisai, Lundbeck, Lilly, and Novartis.

ACKNOWLEDGMENTS

This work was supported by the UK NIHR Biomedical Research Centre for Ageing and Age-related disease award to the Newcastle upon Tyne Hospitals NHS Foundation Trust and Northumberland Tyne and Wear NHS Foundation Trust.

REFERENCES

Alexopoulos, G. S., Murphy, C. F., Gunning-Dixon, F. M., Latoussakis, V., Kanellopoulos, D., Klimstra, S., ... Hoptman, M. J. (2008). Microstructural white matter abnormalities and remission of geriatric depression. *American Journal of Psychiatry*, 165(2), 238–244.

Allan, C. L., Sexton, C. E., Kalu, U. G., McDermott, L. M., Kivimaki, M., Singh-Manoux, A., ... Ebmeier, K. P. (2011). Does the Framingham Stroke Risk Profile predict white-matter changes in late-life depression? *International Psychogeriatrics*, 1–8.

Almeida, O. P., Burton, E. J., Ferrier, N., McKeith, I. G., & O'Brien, J. T. (2003). Depression with late onset is associated with right frontal lobe atrophy. *Psychological Medicine*, 33(4), 675–681.

Andreescu, C., Butters, M. A., Begley, A., Rajji, T., Wu, M., Meltzer, C. C., ... Aizenstein, H. (2008). Gray matter changes in late life depression—a structural MRI analysis. *Neuropsychopharmacology*, 33(11), 2566–2572.

Ashtari, M., Greenwald, B. S., Kramer-Ginsberg, E., Hu, J., Wu, H., Patel, M., ... Pollack, S. (1999). Hippocampal/amygdala volumes in geriatric depression. *Psychological Medicine*, 29(3), 629–638.

Bae, J. N., MacFall, J. R., Krishnan, K. R., Payne, M. E., Steffens, D. C., & Taylor, W. D. (2006). Dorsolateral prefrontal cortex and anterior cingulate cortex white matter alterations in late-life depression. *Biological Psychiatry*, 60(12), 1356–1363.

Ballmaier, M., Kumar, A., Elderkin-Thompson, V., Narr, K.L., Luders, E., Thompson, P. M., ... Toga, A. W. (2008). Mapping callosal morphology in early- and late-onset elderly depression: An index of distinct changes in cortical connectivity. *Neuropsychopharmacology*, 33(7), 1528–1536.

Ballmaier, M., Kumar, A., Thompson, P. M., Narr, K. L., Lavretsky, H., Estanol, L., ... Toga, A. W. (2004). Localizing gray matter deficits in late-onset depression using computational cortical pattern matching methods. *American Journal of Psychiatry*, 161(11), 2091–2099.

Bell-McGinty, S., Butters, M. A., Meltzer, C. C., Greer, P. J., Reynolds, C. F., III, & Becker, J. T. (2002). Brain morphometric abnormalities in geriatric depression: Long-term neurobiological effects of illness duration. *American Journal of Psychiatry*, 159(8), 1424–1427.

Burke, J., McQuoid, D. R., Payne, M. E., Steffens, D. C., Krishnan, R. R., & Taylor, W. D. (2011). Amygdala volume in late-life depression: Relationship with age of onset. *American Journal of Geriatric Psychiatry*, 19(9), 771–776.

Butters, M. A., Aizenstein, H. J., Hayashi, K. M., Meltzer, C. C., Seaman, J., Reynolds, C. F., III, ... Becker, J. T. (2009). Three-dimensional surface mapping of the caudate nucleus in late-life depression. *American Journal of Geriatric Psychiatry*, 17(1), 4–12.

Chen, P. S., McQuoid, D. R., Payne, M. E., & Steffens, D. C. (2006). White matter and subcortical gray matter lesion volume changes and late-life depression outcome: A 4-year magnetic resonance imaging study. *International Psychogeriatrics*, *18*(3), 445–456.

Colloby, S. J., Firbank, M. J., Thomas, A. J., Vasudev, A., Parry, S. W., & O'Brien, J. T. (2011a). White matter changes in late-life depression: A diffusion tensor imaging study. *Journal of Affective Disorders*, *135*(1–3), 216–220.

Colloby, S. J., Firbank, M. J., Vasudev, A., Parry, S. W., Thomas, A. J., & O'Brien, J. T. (2011b). Cortical thickness and VBM-DARTEL in late-life depression. *Journal of Affective Disorders*, *133*(1–2), 158–164.

Colloby, S. J., Vasudev, A., O'Brien, J. T., Firbank, M. J., Parry, S. W., & Thomas, A. J. (2011). Relationship of orthostatic blood pressure to white matter hyperintensities and subcortical volumes in late-life depression. *British Journal of Psychiatry*, *199*(5), 404–410.

Dahabra, S., Ashton, C. H., Bahrainian, M., Britton, P. G., Ferrier, I. N., McAllister, V. A., ... Moore, P. B. (1998). Structural and functional abnormalities in elderly patients clinically recovered from early- and late-onset depression. *Biological Psychiatry*, *44*(1), 34–46.

Dalby, R. B., Chakravarty, M. M., Ahdidan, J., Sorensen, L., Frandsen, J., Jonsdottir, K. Y., ... Videbech, P. (2010). Localization of white-matter lesions and effect of vascular risk factors in late-onset major depression. *Psychological Medicine*, *40*(8), 1389–1399.

de Asis, J. M., Greenwald, B. S., Alexopoulos, G. S., Kiosses, D. N., Ashtari, M., Heo, M., & Young, R. C. (2006). Frontal signal hyperintensities in mania in old age. *American Journal of Geriatric Psychiatry*, *14*(7), 598–604.

de Leeuw, F. E., de Groot, J. C., Achten, E., Oudkerk, M., Ramos, L. M., Heijboer, R., ... Breteler, M. M. (2001). Prevalence of cerebral white matter lesions in elderly people: A population based magnetic resonance imaging study. The Rotterdam Scan Study. *Journal of Neurology, Neurosurgery, and Psychiatry*, *70*(1), 9–14.

Delaloye, C., de Bilbao, F., Moy, G., Baudois, S., Weber, K., Campos, L., ... Gold, G. (2009). Neuroanatomical and neuropsychological features of euthymic patients with bipolar disorder. *American Journal of Geriatric Psychiatry*, *17*(12), 1012–1021.

Delaloye, C., Moy, G., de Bilbao, F., Weber, K., Baudois, S., Haller, S., ... Giannakopoulos, P. (2011). Longitudinal analysis of cognitive performances and structural brain changes in late-life bipolar disorder. *International Journal of Geriatric Psychiatry*, *26*(12), 1309–1318.

Egger, K., Schocke, M., Weiss, E., Auffinger, S., Esterhammer, R., Goebel, G., ... Marksteiner, J. (2008). Pattern of brain atrophy in elderly patients with depression revealed by voxel-based morphometry. *Psychiatry Research*, *164*(3), 237–244.

Figiel, G. S., Krishnan, K. R., Doraiswamy, P. M., Rao, V. P., Nemeroff, C. B., & Boyko, O. B. (1991). Subcortical hyperintensities on brain magnetic resonance imaging: A comparison between late age onset and early onset elderly depressed subjects. *Neurobiology of Aging*, *12*(3), 245–247.

Firbank, M. J., Lloyd, A. J., Ferrier, N., & O'Brien, J. T. (2004). A volumetric study of MRI signal hyperintensities in late-life depression. *American Journal of Geriatric Psychiatry*, *12*(6), 606–612.

Fukuda, H., & Kitani, M. (1995). Differences between treated and untreated hypertensive subjects in the extent of periventricular hyperintensities observed on brain MRI. *Stroke*, *26*(9), 1593–1597.

Garde, E., Mortensen, E. L., Krabbe, K., Rostrup, E., & Larsson, H. B. (2000). Relation between age-related decline in intelligence and cerebral white-matter hyperintensities in healthy octogenarians: a longitudinal study. *Lancet*, *356*(9230), 628–634.

Godin, O., Dufouil, C., Maillard, P., Delcroix, N., Mazoyer, B., Crivello, F., ... Tzourio, C. (2008). White matter lesions as a predictor of depression in the elderly: The 3C-Dijon study. *Biological Psychiatry*, *63*(7), 663–669.

Greenwald, B. S., Kramer-Ginsberg, E., Bogerts, B., Ashtari, M., Aupperle, P., Wu, H., ... Patel, M. (1997). Qualitative magnetic resonance imaging findings in geriatric depression. Possible link between later-onset depression and Alzheimer's disease? *Psychological Medicine*, *27*(2), 421–431.

Greenwald, B. S., Kramer-Ginsberg, E., Krishnan, K. R., Ashtari, M., Auerbach, C., & Patel, M. (1998). Neuroanatomic localization of magnetic resonance imaging signal hyperintensities in geriatric depression. *Stroke*, *29*(3), 613–617.

Haller, S., Xekardaki, A., Delaloye, C., Canuto, A., Lovblad, K. O., Gold, G., & Giannakopoulos, P. (2011). Combined analysis of grey matter voxel-based morphometry and white matter tract-based spatial statistics in late-life bipolar disorder. *Journal of Psychiatry and Neuroscience*, *36*(6), 391–401.

Hannestad, J., Taylor, W. D., McQuoid, D. R., Payne, M. E., Krishnan, K. R., Steffens, D. C., & Macfall, J. R. (2006). White matter lesion volumes and caudate volumes in late-life depression. *International Journal of Geriatric Psychiatry, 21*(12), 1193–1198.

Heiden, A., Kettenbach, J., Fischer, P., Schein, B., Ba-Ssalamah, A., Frey, R., ... Kasper, S. (2005). White matter hyperintensities and chronicity of depression. *Journal of Psychiatry Research, 39*(3), 285–293.

Herrmann, L. L., Le Masurier, M., & Ebmeier, K. P. (2008). White matter hyperintensities in late life depression: A systematic review. *Journal of Neurology, Neurosurgery, and Psychiatry, 79*(6), 619–624.

Hickie, I., Naismith, S., Ward, P. B., Turner, K., Scott, E., Mitchell, P., ... Parker, G. (2005). Reduced hippocampal volumes and memory loss in patients with early- and late-onset depression. *British Journal of Psychiatry, 186,* 197–202.

Hickie, I. B., Naismith, S. L., Ward, P. B., Scott, E. M., Mitchell, P. B., Schofield, P. R., ... Parker, G. (2007). Serotonin transporter gene status predicts caudate nucleus but not amygdala or hippocampal volumes in older persons with major depression. *Journal of Affective Disorders, 98*(1–2), 137–142.

Hwang, J. P., Lee, T. W., Tsai, S. J., Chen, T. J., Yang, C. H., Lirng, J. F., & Tsai, C. F. (2010). Cortical and subcortical abnormalities in late-onset depression with history of suicide attempts investigated with MRI and voxel-based morphometry. *Journal of Geriatric Psychiatry and Neurology, 23*(3), 171–184.

Jacoby, R. J., & Levy, R. (1980). Computed tomography in the elderly. 3. Affective disorder. *British Journal of Psychiatry, 136,* 270–275.

Jacoby, R. J., Levy, R., & Bird, J. M. (1981). Computed tomography and the outcome of affective disorder: A follow-up study of elderly patients. *British Journal of Psychiatry, 139,* 288–292.

Kohler, S., Thomas, A. J., Lloyd, A., Barber, R., Almeida, O. P., O'Brien, J. T., ... O'Brien, J. T. (2010). White matter hyperintensities, cortisol levels, brain atrophy and continuing cognitive deficits in late-life depression. *British Journal of Psychiatry, 196*(2), 143–149.

Koolschijn, P. C., van Haren, N. E., Schnack, H. G., Janssen, J., Hulshoff Pol, H. E., & Kahn, R. S. (2010). Cortical thickness and voxel-based morphometry in depressed elderly. *European Neuropsychopharmacology, 20*(6), 398–404.

Krishnan, K. R., McDonald, W. M., Doraiswamy, P. M., Tupler, L. A., Husain, M., Boyko, O. B., ... Ellinwood, E. H., Jr. (1993). Neuroanatomical substrates of depression in the elderly. *European Archives of Psychiatry and Clinical Neuroscience, 243*(1), 41–46.

Kumar, A., Ajilore, O., Zhang, A., Pham, D., & Elderkin-Thompson, V. (2012). Cortical thinning in patients with late-life minor depression. *American Journal of Geriatric Psychiatry.* 2012 Feb 23, ePubh ahead of print.

Kumar, A., Bilker, W., Jin, Z., & Udupa, J. (2000). Atrophy and high intensity lesions: Complementary neurobiological mechanisms in late-life major depression. *Neuropsychopharmacology, 22*(3), 264–274.

Kumar, A., Jin, Z., Bilker, W., Udupa, J., & Gottlieb, G. (1998). Late-onset minor and major depression: Early evidence for common neuroanatomical substrates detected by using MRI. *Proceedings of the National Academy of Sciences USA, 95*(13), 7654–7658.

Lai, T., Payne, M. E., Byrum, C. E., Steffens, D. C., & Krishnan, K. R. (2000). Reduction of orbital frontal cortex volume in geriatric depression. *Biological Psychiatry, 48*(10), 971–975.

Lesser, I. M., Boone, K. B., Mehringer, C. M., Wohl, M. A., Miller, B. L., & Berman, N. G. (1996). Cognition and white matter hyperintensities in older depressed patients. *American Journal of Psychiatry, 153*(10), 1280–1287.

Levy, R. M., Steffens, D. C., McQuoid, D. R., Provenzale, J. M., MacFall, J. R., & Krishnan, K. R. (2003). MRI lesion severity and mortality in geriatric depression. *American Journal of Geriatric Psychiatry, 11*(6), 678–682.

Lloyd, A. J., Ferrier, I. N., Barber, R., Gholkar, A., Young, A. H., & O'Brien, J. T. (2004). Hippocampal volume change in depression: Late- and early-onset illness compared. *British Journal of Psychiatry, 184,* 488–495.

Lyoo, I. K., Sung, Y. H., Dager, S. R., Friedman, S. D., Lee, J. Y., Kim, S. J., ... Renshaw, P. F. (2006). Regional cerebral cortical thinning in bipolar disorder. *Bipolar Disorder, 8*(1), 65–74.

Marshall, G. A., Hendrickson, R., Kaufer, D. I., Ivanco, L. S., & Bohnen, N. I. (2006). Cognitive correlates of brain MRI subcortical signal hyperintensities in non-demented elderly. *International Journal of Geriatric Psychiatry, 21*(1), 32–35.

McDonald, W. M., Krishnan, K. R., Doraiswamy, P. M., & Blazer, D. G. (1991). Occurrence of subcortical hyperintensities in elderly subjects with mania. *Psychiatry Research, 40*(4), 211–220.

McDonald, W. M., Tupler, L. A., Marsteller, F. A., Figiel, G. S., DiSouza, S., Nemeroff, C. B. & Krishnan, K. R. (1999). Hyperintense lesions on magnetic resonance images in bipolar disorder. *Biological Psychiatry, 45*(8), 965–971.

Nobuhara, K., Okugawa, G., Sugimoto, T., Minami, T., Tamagaki, C., Takase, K., ... Kinoshita, T. (2006)

Frontal white matter anisotropy and symptom severity of late-life depression: A magnetic resonance diffusion tensor imaging study. *Journal of Neurology, Neurosurgery, and Psychiatry, 77*(1), 120–122.

O'Brien, J., Ames, D., Chiu, E., Schweitzer, I., Desmond, P., & Tress, B. (1998). Severe deep white matter lesions and outcome in elderly patients with major depressive disorder: Follow up study. *British Medical Journal, 317*(7164), 982–984.

O'Brien, J., Desmond, P., Ames, D., Schweitzer, I., Harrigan, S., & Tress, B. (1996). A magnetic resonance imaging study of white matter lesions in depression and Alzheimer's disease. *British Journal of Psychiatry, 168*(4), 477–485.

O'Brien, J. T., Firbank, M. J., Krishnan, M. S., van Straaten, E. C., van der Flier, W. M., Petrovic, K., … Inzitari, D. (2006). White matter hyperintensities rather than lacunar infarcts are associated with depressive symptoms in older people: The LADIS study. *American Journal of Geriatric Psychiatry, 14*(10), 834–841.

O'Brien, J. T., Lloyd, A., McKeith, I., Gholkar, A., & Ferrier, N. (2004). A longitudinal study of hippocampal volume, cortisol levels, and cognition in older depressed subjects. *American Journal of Psychiatry, 161*(11), 2081–2090.

Pantel, J., Schroder, J., Essig, M., Schad, L. R., Popp, D., Eysenbach, K., … Knopp, M. V. (1998). [Volumetric brain findings in late depression. A study with quantified magnetic resonance tomography]. *The Neurologist, 69*(11), 968–974.

Pantoni, L., & Garcia, J. H. (1997). Pathogenesis of leukoaraiosis: A review. *Stroke, 28*(3), 652–659.

Rabins, P. V., Pearlson, G. D., Aylward, E., Kumar, A. J., & Dowell, K. (1991). Cortical magnetic resonance imaging changes in elderly inpatients with major depression. *American Journal of Psychiatry, 148*(5), 617–620.

Salloway, S., Malloy, P., Kohn, R., Gillard, E., Duffy, J., Rogg, J., … Westlake, R. (1996). MRI and neuropsychological differences in early- and late-life-onset geriatric depression. *Neurology, 46*(6), 1567–1574.

Sheline, Y. I. (2003). Neuroimaging studies of mood disorder effects on the brain. *Biological Psychiatry, 54*(3), 338–352.

Sheline, Y. I., Price, J. L., Vaishnavi, S. N., Mintun, M. A., Barch, D. M., Epstein, A. A., … McKinstry, R. C. (2008). Regional white matter hyperintensity burden in automated segmentation distinguishes late-life depressed subjects from comparison subjects matched for vascular risk factors. *American Journal of Psychiatry, 165*(4), 524–532.

Sheline, Y. I., Wang, P. W., Gado, M. H., Csernansky, J. G., & Vannier, M. W. (1996). Hippocampal atrophy in recurrent major depression. *Proceedings of the National Academy of Sciences USA, 93*(9), 3908–3913.

Shimony, J. S., Sheline, Y. I., D'Angelo, G., Epstein, A. A., Benzinger, T. L., Mintun, M. A., … Snyder, A. Z. (2009). Diffuse microstructural abnormalities of normal-appearing white matter in late life depression: A diffusion tensor imaging study. *Biological Psychiatry, 66*(3), 245–252.

Simpson, S. W., Jackson, A., Baldwin, R. C., & Burns, A. (1997). 1997 IPA/Bayer Research Awards in Psychogeriatrics. Subcortical hyperintensities in late-life depression: Acute response to treatment and neuropsychological impairment. *International Psychogeriatrics, 9*(3), 257–275.

Smith, S. M., Jenkinson, M., Johansen-Berg, H., Rueckert, D., Nichols, T. E., Mackay, C. E., … Behrens, T. E. (2006). Tract-based spatial statistics: Voxelwise analysis of multi-subject diffusion data. *Neuroimage, 31*(4), 1487–1505.

Steffens, D. C., Byrum, C. E., McQuoid, D. R., Greenberg, D. L., Payne, M. E., Blitchington, T. F., … Krishnan, K. R. (2000). Hippocampal volume in geriatric depression. *Biological Psychiatry, 48*(4), 301–309.

Steffens, D. C., Conway, C. R., Dombeck, C. B., Wagner, H. R., Tupler, L. A., & Weiner, R. D. (2001). Severity of subcortical gray matter hyperintensity predicts ECT response in geriatric depression. *Journal of ECT, 17*(1), 45–49.

Steffens, D. C., Potter, G. G., McQuoid, D. R., MacFall, J. R., Payne, M. E., Burke, J. R., … Welsh-Bohmer, K. A. (2007). Longitudinal magnetic resonance imaging vascular changes, apolipoprotein E genotype, and development of dementia in the neurocognitive outcomes of depression in the elderly study. *American Journal of Geriatric Psychiatry, 15*(10), 839–849.

Strakowski, S. M., Adler, C. M., & DelBello, M. P. (2002). Volumetric MRI studies of mood disorders: Do they distinguish unipolar and bipolar disorder? *Bipolar Disorder, 4*(2), 80–88.

Tamashiro, J. H., Zung, S., Zanetti, M. V., de Castro, C. C., Vallada, H., Busatto, G. F., & de Toledo Ferraz Alves, T. C. (2008). Increased rates of white matter hyperintensities in late-onset bipolar disorder. *Bipolar Disorder, 10*(7), 765–775.

Taylor, W. D., Kuchibhatla, M., Payne, M. E., Macfall, J. R., Sheline, Y. I., Krishnan, K. R., & Doraiswamy, P. M. (2008). Frontal white matter anisotropy and antidepressant remission in late-life depression. *PLoS One, 3*(9), e3267.

Taylor, W. D., MacFall, J. R., Gerig, G., & Krishnan, R. R. (2007). Structural integrity of the uncinate fasciculus in geriatric depression: Relationship with age of onset. *Neuropsychiatric Disease and Treatment, 3*(5), 669–674.

Taylor, W. D., MacFall, J. R., Payne, M. E., McQuoid, D. R., Provenzale, J. M., Steffens, D. C., & Krishnan, K. R. (2004). Late-life depression and microstructural abnormalities in dorsolateral prefrontal cortex white matter. *American Journal of Psychiatry, 161*(7), 1293–1296.

Taylor, W. D., MacFall, J. R., Payne, M. E., McQuoid, D. R., Steffens, D. C., Provenzale, J. M., & Krishnan, R. R. (2005). Greater MRI lesion volumes in elderly depressed subjects than in control subjects. *Psychiatry Research, 139*(1), 1–7.

Taylor, W. D., MacFall, J. R., Steffens, D. C., Payne, M. E., Provenzale, J. M., & Krishnan, K. R. (2003). Localization of age-associated white matter hyperintensities in late-life depression. *Progress in Neuropsychopharmacology and Biological Psychiatry, 27*(3), 539–544.

Taylor, W. D., Payne, M. E., Krishnan, K. R., Wagner, H. R., Provenzale, J. M., Steffens, D. C., & MacFall, J. R. (2001). Evidence of white matter tract disruption in MRI hyperintensities. *Biological Psychiatry, 50*(3), 179–183.

Taylor, W. D., Steffens, D. C., MacFall, J. R., McQuoid, D. R., Payne, M. E., Provenzale, J. M., & Krishnan, K. R. (2003). White matter hyperintensity progression and late-life depression outcomes. *Archives of General Psychiatry, 60*(11), 1090–1096.

Teodorczuk, A., Firbank, M. J., Pantoni, L., Poggesi, A., Erkinjuntti, T., Wallin, A., … O'Brien, J. T. (2010). Relationship between baseline white-matter changes and development of late-life depressive symptoms: 3-year results from the LADIS study. *Psychological Medicine, 40*(4), 603–610.

Teodorczuk, A., O'Brien, J. T., Firbank, M. J., Pantoni, L., Poggesi, A., Erkinjuntti, T., … Inzitari, D. (2007). White matter changes and late-life depressive symptoms: longitudinal study. *British Journal of Psychiatry, 191*, 212–217.

Thomas, A. J., O'Brien, J. T., Davis, S., Ballard, C., Barber, R., Kalaria, R. N., & Perry, R. H. (2002). Ischemic basis for deep white matter hyperintensities in major depression: A neuropathological study. *Archives of General Psychiatry, 59*(9), 785–792.

Tupler, L. A., Krishnan, K. R., McDonald, W. M., Dombeck, C. B., D'Souza, S., & Steffens, D. C. (2002). Anatomic location and laterality of MRI signal hyperintensities in late-life depression. *Journal of Psychosomatic Research, 53*(2), 665–676.

Veldink, J. H., Scheltens, P., Jonker, C., & Launer, L. J. (1998). Progression of cerebral white matter hyperintensities on MRI is related to diastolic blood pressure. *Neurology, 51*(1), 319–320.

Voets, N. L., Hough, M. G., Douaud, G., Matthews, P. M., James, A., Winmill, L., … Smith, S. (2008). Evidence for abnormalities of cortical development in adolescent-onset schizophrenia. *Neuroimage, 43*(4), 665–675.

Winkler, A. M., Kochunov, P., Blangero, J., Almasy, L., Zilles, K., Fox, P. T., … Glahn, D. C. (2010). Cortical thickness or grey matter volume? The importance of selecting the phenotype for imaging genetics studies. *Neuroimage, 53*(3), 1135–1146.

Yang, Q., Huang, X., Hong, N., & Yu, X. (2007). White matter microstructural abnormalities in late-life depression. *International Psychogeriatrics, 19*(4), 757–766.

Ylikoski, A., Erkinjuntti, T., Raininko, R., Sarna, S., Sulkava, R., & Tilvis, R. (1995). White matter hyperintensities on MRI in the neurologically nondiseased elderly. Analysis of cohorts of consecutive subjects aged 55 to 85 years living at home. *Stroke, 26*(7), 1171–1177.

Young, R. C., Nambudiri, D. E., Jain, H., de Asis, J. M., & Alexopoulos, G. S. (1999). Brain computed tomography in geriatric manic disorder. *Biological Psychiatry, 45*(8), 1063–1065.

Yuan, Y., Zhang, Z., Bai, F., Yu, H., Shi, Y., Qian, Y., … You, J. (2007). White matter integrity of the whole brain is disrupted in first-episode remitted geriatric depression. *Neuroreport, 18*(17), 1845–1849.

Yuan, Y., Zhu, W., Zhang, Z., Bai, F., Yu, H., Shi, Y., … Liu, Z. (2008). Regional gray matter changes are associated with cognitive deficits in remitted geriatric depression: An optimized voxel-based morphometry study. *Biological Psychiatry, 64*(6), 541–544.

Zhao, Z., Taylor, W. D., Styner, M., Steffens, D. C., Krishnan, K. R., & MacFall, J. R. (2008). Hippocampus shape analysis and late-life depression. *PLoS One, 3*(3), e1837.

33

MOLECULAR IMAGING IN LATE-LIFE DEPRESSION

Anand Kumar, Olusola Ajilore, Brent Forester, Jaime Deseda,
Matthew Woodward, and Emma Rhodes

VARIOUS NEUROIMAGING approaches have been used to characterize the neurobiological underpinnings of late-life major depression. These include approaches associated with magnetic resonance imaging (MRI) and positron emission tomography (PET). While the early approaches focused on global measures such as regional glucose metabolism, lobar brain volumes, and high-intensity lesion volume, the more recent methods have focused on more discrete biological processes. These techniques, which can be collectively called "molecular imaging," study more precise biological mechanisms, including the levels of proteins in the brain, measures of axonal and myelin integrity, and biochemical pathways whose perturbations result in clinical brain disorders.

In this chapter, we describe three specific neuroimaging approaches and their application to late-life major depression. We begin by describing the study of proteins in the brain, both amyloid and tau using PET. This is followed by diffusion tensor imaging studies of the integrity of axons and myelin in specific white matter tracts and is followed by an

emphasis on spectroscopic imaging of the brain in mood disorders. Collectively, they provide a window into the state of the science of human neuroimaging as it relates to depression in the elderly.

POSITRON EMISSION TOMOGRAPHY

Interest in the role of proteins in the pathophysiology of mood disorders is a relatively new area of scientific enquiry. Neuritic plaques (NPs) and neurofibrillary tangles (NTs) provided the sine qua non for the pathological diagnosis of Alzheimer's disease (AD). A history and mental status examination consistent with dementia and the neuropathological correlates of AD, both NP and NT in key brain regions, are required for a diagnosis of definitive AD. Biochemically, the $A\beta$ component of the amyloid precursor molecule (APP) and hyperphosphorylated Tau provide the neural substrates for NP and NT, respectively. Until recently, both

NP and NT were believed to be exclusively involved in the pathophysiology of AD and related cognitive disorders.

Over the last several years, evidence has accumulated about the possible role of both Aβ and NP in the pathophysiology of late-life depression (Kumar et al., in press). Sweet et al. followed a small group of patients who initially presented with symptoms and signs of major depression without clinical evidence of dementia and reported that over time this group developed cognitive impairment with eventual neuropathological evidence of atrophy together with NPs, NTs, and vascular changes. More recently, investigators have used peripheral markers of Aβ (Aβ 42:40 ratios) to identify patients with major depressive disorder (MDD) who present with unique cognitive and neuroimaging findings and who may be "at risk" for developing AD over time (Pomara et al., 2006; Qiu et al., 2007). These findings have led to the amyloidogenic theory of depression in the elderly, which asserts that abnormalities in the biology of amyloid, including deposition of amyloid in critical brain regions, may contribute to mood disorders in the elderly. This thesis suggests that abnormal amyloid biology, together with vascular and degenerative mechanisms, provides a pathway to depression in the elderly.

While the plasma results are intriguing, direct visualization and quantitation of protein in the brain is necessary to directly and more precisely understand the role of amyloid in clinical brain disorders. Positron emission tomography (PET) with specific radioligands has been used to characterize and estimate the in vivo protein load in the brain (Klunk et al., 2004; Shoghi-Jadid et al., 2002; Verhoeff et al., 2004). Two ligands emerged as primary candidates for imaging protein aggregates in the living brain. These are 1,1-dicyano-2-[6-(d imethylamino)-2-naphthalenyl]-propene([18F] FDDNP) and N-methyl-[11C]2-(4'-methylamino phenyl)-6-hydroxybenzothiazole (Pittsburgh compound B or PIB) (Klunk et al., 2004; Shoghi-Jadid et al., 2002).

[18F]FDDNP (2-(1-{6-[(2-[18F]fluoroethyl) (methyl)amino]-2-naphthyl}-ethylidene) malononitrile) is a molecular imaging probe sensitive for detection of amyloid and tau protein deposition in the brain (Shin, Lee, Kim, Kim, & Cho, 2008; Shoghi-Jadid et al., 2002; Small et al., 2006). [18F] FDDNP binding in vivo correlates well with patterns of amyloid and tau distribution known to exist in AD and determined postmortem (Small et al., 2006). [18F]FDDNP has also shown the expected binding progression from myocardial infarction (MCI) to dementia that is supported by neuropathological data in MCI and AD. [18F]FDDNP binding is also increased in patients diagnosed with Down syndrome (Nelson et al., 2011; Small et al., 2006). Interestingly, higher [18F]FDDNP binding in the temporal and frontal lobes has been demonstrated, in preliminary findings, in both MCI and cognitively intact elderly subjects with higher depression and anxiety ratings (Lavretsky et al., 2009).

[11C]PIB (2-(4'-[11C]methylamino)phenyl-6-hydroxybenzothiazole) labels plaques but not tangles. In autoradiographic studies of postmortem brain tissue (Klunk et al., 2004), PIB shows specific and displaceable binding to AD cortical areas containing amyloid deposits, but not to control cortex (Klunk et al., 2004). In vivo binding patterns of PIB retention are consistent with amyloid plaque distribution in postmortem tissue from AD patients and, like [18F]FDDNP, has the ability to discriminate between patients diagnosed with AD and controls (Morris et al., 2009).

Our laboratory recently completed a preliminary study of FDDNP binding in a small sample of patients diagnosed with late-life MDD. Our samples comprised of 20 patients (9 male and 11 female) diagnosed with MDD using established *DSM* criteria and 19 healthy control subjects (8 male and 11 female). All subjects, patients and controls, were recruited from the community in response to advertisements placed in local newspapers, newsletters, and radio advertisement. All subjects received a structured diagnostic interview (SCID) based on the *Diagnostic and Statistical Manual of Mental Disorders* (*DSM*), met criteria for MDD with a Hamilton Depression Score of >15, and were free of antidepressant medication for at least 2 weeks. Patients were free of other brain disorders and did not have a history and mental status consistent with dementia. Several patients did have other stable medical disorders, including diabetes and hypertension. All subjects were screened for dementia based on the clinical evaluation of history, current mental status, and MMSE score <26. MCI was operationally defined as scoring −1.5 standard deviations from the mean on two or more tests of verbal or visual delayed recall. One subject with MDD met criteria for MCI.

QUANTITATIVE POSITRON EMISSION TOMOGRAPHY DATA ANALYSIS

After the injection of the PET tracer (320–410 MBq) as a bolus via the in-dwelling venous catheter the consecutive dynamic PET scans were performed for up to 2 hours. Image data were analyzed and ROIs determined with investigators blind to clinical findings. Quantification of the data on [18F]FDDNP binding was performed with the Logan graphic method, with the cerebellum as the reference region for time points between 30 and 125 minutes (Kepe et al., 2006; Logan et al., 1996). Similar results were obtained when analyses are performed between 30 and 60 min. The slope of the linear portion of the Logan plot is the relative distribution volume (DVR), which is equal to the distribution volume of the tracer in a region of interest (ROI) divided by the distribution volume of the tracer in the reference region. Early frame [18F]FDDNP PET images (sum 0–5 min) were oriented in AC-PC orientation by rigid co-registration with SPM2 software package to the PET template provided in the package. The parameters determined in this step were used to orient the [18F]FDDNP DVR images in the same, co-registered orientation.

A set of regions of interest was drawn bilaterally on frontal, parietal, posterior cingulate, anterior cingulate, medial temporal, and lateral temporal lobe areas as well as cerebellum on each co-registered early frame [18F]FDDNP PET image separately using the ROI set shown in Figure 33.1 as a guide. The resulting ROI sets were imported in their corresponding [18F]FDDNP DVR images, and DVR

values were extracted. Drawing of regions of interest and extraction of DVR values were performed using the AMIDE software package (Kepe et al., 2006). Each regional DVR or binding value was expressed as an average of the left and right regions, and global DVR values were calculated as averages of the values for all these regions. Rules for ROI drawing were based on the identification of gyral and sulcal landmarks with respect to the atlas of Talairach and Tounoux (1988).

The groups, patients with MDD and controls, did not differ on demographic variables. Subjects ranged in age from 60 to 82 years (mean [SD] age = 67.0 [7.2]) and were well educated (mean [SD] education years = 16.3 [2.7]). They showed minimal impairment on cognitive testing (mean [SD] Mini-Mental State Exam scores = 29.0 [1.3]; mean [SD] Verbal IQ scores = 114.6 [10.1]).

The global [18F]FDDNP binding value was significantly higher in our MDD group (N = 20) when compared with controls (N = 19; Fig. 33.1). The groups were also significantly different in their regional [18F]FDDNP binding levels, as revealed by the mixed effects model ($F(1,37) = 9.52$, $p = .004$). Post-hoc t-tests demonstrated that the depressed group had significantly higher binding in the lateral temporal and posterior cingulate regions when compared with controls (Cohen's d effect sizes of 0.92 and 0.67, respectively; Table 33.2 and Fig. 33.2). Group differences in [18F]FDDNP binding levels in the anterior cingulate and mesial temporal regions approached statistical significance. Fig. 33.3 shows scans of a control subject (low levels of [18F]FDDNP binding) and a subject with MDD (areas of high frontal, posterior cingulate, and parietal binding). [18F]FDDNP binding values in the one MDD

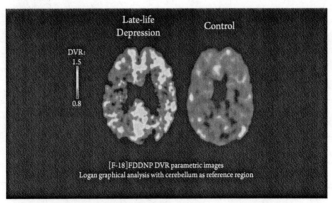

FIGURE 33.1 Visual representation of [18F]FDDNP binding in a healthy control and patient with MDD (See color insert).

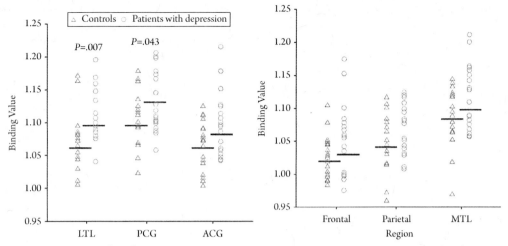

FIGURES 33.2 Plot of [18F]FDDNP binding values in six regions of interest in MDD patients and controls. Abbreviations: LTL= Lateral Temporal; PCG = Posterior Cingulate; ACG= Anterior Cingulate, MTL = Mesial Temporal.

patient who met criteria for MCI were close to the mean for the MDD group in all regions examined. Furthermore, all findings remained the same when we eliminated this subject from the analyses.

The key finding of this exploratory study is that patients with late-life MDD demonstrated significantly higher [18F]FDDNP binding globally in the cortex with regional accentuation in the lateral temporal and posterior cingulate regions when compared with healthy control subjects (Fig. 33.2). Other regions, notably the anterior cingulate and mesial temporal, also showed higher [18F]FDDNP binding

when compared with controls, though the differences did not reach statistical significance. These findings, along with plasma studies of amyloid and [18F] FDDNP binding correlates of anxiety and depression symptoms in patients diagnosed with mild cognitive impairment and cognitively intact elderly subjects (Lavretsky et al., 2009; Pomara et al., 2006; Qiu et al., 2007), indicate that neuronal injury, secondary to amyloid and tau, may represent a pathophysiological pathway that, together with vascular compromise, may predispose to mood and related behavioral syndromes and disorders in the elderly.

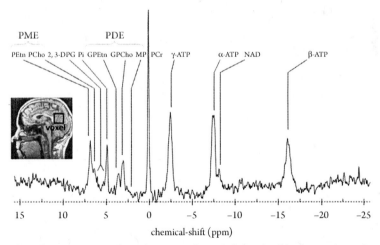

FIGURES 33.3 Phosphorus spectrum from the occipital cortex from a healthy human brain depicting the phosphomonoester (PME) resonances: Phosphoethanolamine (PEtn), Phosphocholine (PCho), the phosphodiester (PDE) resonances: Glycerfophosphoethanolamine (GPEtn), Glycerophosphocholine (GPCho), as well as inorganic phosphate (Pi), diphosphoglyerate (2,3-DPG), Phosphocreatine (PCr), Dinucleotides (NAD) and Adenosine Tri-phosphate (ATP). Reprinted courtesy of Dr. Eric Jensen.

An earlier PET study using [¹¹C]PIB and a small sample of patients with late-life MDD and controls identified higher [¹¹C]PIB brain retention in MDD patients when compared with controls (Butters et al., 2008). In this study, MDD patients with concurrent amnestic MCI had PIB binding patterns that were comparable to patients diagnosed with AD and higher binding in multiple cortical areas (Butters et al., 2008). MDD patients who did not meet the clinical criteria for MCI had [¹¹C]PIB brain retention parameters comparable to those for controls. MDD patients who presented with nonamnestic MCI demonstrated binding that was in between the cognitively intact and amnestic MCI subgroups. In our sample, only one of the 20 MDD patients met criteria for MCI and that patient's [¹⁸F]FDDNP binding parameters and distribution were similar to those of other MDD patients. Our primary findings indicate that in MDD patients who do not meet established criteria for MCI, [¹⁸F]FDDNP cortical binding is higher than that of controls, indicative that brain neuropathological aggregate deposition is present in MDD even in patients without discernible cognitive impairment.

Lavretsky and colleagues reported a correlation between depression and trait anxiety scores and FDDNP binding in the temporal, frontal, and posterior cingulate regions in patients with MCI and cognitively intact subjects (Lavretsky et al., 2009). While these studies are not directly comparable because of differences in the binding characteristics of the ligands and the cognitive status of the subjects, they do point to the previously unidentified role of proteins, both Aβ and Tau in the pathophysiology of depression in the elderly. While this pathway may be relevant to s subgroup of patients with MDD, these findings have broader implications for both the biology and treatment, especially in the area of targeted drug development, for patients with mood disorders.

DIFFUSION TENSOR IMAGING

A hallmark of structural brain change associated with geriatric mood disorders are white matter hyperintensities. An imaging technique that has been useful for the study of white matter integrity and brain microstructural changes is diffusion tensor imaging (DTI). DTI works on the principle that water diffuses randomly in unrestricted environments resulting in isotropic movement (or movement that is equivalent in all directions). This movement is restrained in white matter tracts; thus, water diffusion tends to move along the axis of the axon sheath, leading to anisotropy. DTI can be quantified in several ways, including fractional anisotropy (FA), which represents a measure of directional coherence and in white matter tracts, the degree of structural alignment. Another quantification technique is the apparent diffusion coefficient (ADC) or mean diffusivity (MD), which measures the average diffusion of water in a voxel. Few studies have correlated changes detected using DTI with actual histopathology, but it has been speculated that that lower FA is associated with axonal loss, demyelination, and expansion of extracellular space (Moseley, 2002).

Several studies have utilized DTI to examine microstructural changes in white matter associated with geriatric mood disorders, including subtle white matter damage not detected using more conventional MR imaging techniques. One of the first studies to apply this technique to our understanding of mood disorders found evidence of increased ADC in white matter hyperintensities in patients with major depression and healthy elderly control subjects (Taylor et al., 2001). Lower FA has also been found in normal appearing white matter, in frontal regions such as the right superior frontal gyrus, middle frontal gyrus, and temporal regions such as right parahippocampal gyrus (Taylor et al., 2004; Yang, Huang, Hong, & Yu, 2007).

In addition to detecting lower FA and increased ADC in region of interests, there have been efforts to find evidence of altered white matter microstructure in specific fiber tracts. For example, the uncinate fasciculus, an important fiber tract linking frontal and limbic structures in the temporal lobes, has been shown to have lower FA in the left hemisphere (Taylor, Macfall, Gerig, & Krishnan, 2007). DTI-based parameters also appear to be related to mood changes as evidenced by studies showing that FA is negatively correlated with measures of depressions severity, even in nondepressed older adults (Dalby et al., 2010; Lamar, Charlton, Morris, & Markus, 2010). However, there is also evidence that these changes may represent trait features of major depression. In a study by Yuan et al., lower FA was found in a number of prefrontal regions in remitted geriatric depression subjects (Yuan et al., 2007). There is a dearth of similar studies applied to geriatric bipolar depression. One recent paper found lower FA in the ventral part of the corpus callosum in euthymic bipolar subjects using tract-based spatial statistics (TBSS), which allows for group averaging of DTI parameters (Haller et al., 2011).

In addition to depression severity, clinical research has found decreased FA to be associated with treatment response and resistance as well as cognitive impairment.

The first study to correlate DTI-related changes and clinical variables found that lower FA in left frontal regions was associated with poorer remission rates in late-life depressed patients treated with citalopram (Alexopoulos, Kiosses, Choi, Murphy, & Lim, 2002). This finding was replicated in a larger study demonstrating reduced FA in the medial prefrontal cortex, limbic regions, and the genu of the corpus callosum was associated with poor response to escitalopram (Alexopoulos et al., 2008). In a study by Taylor and colleagues, it was shown that higher FA in the superior frontal gyri and bilateral anterior cingulate were associated with treatment resistance in geriatric depressed patients treated with sertraline (Taylor et al., 2008). In a subsequent longitudinal study, the authors found that geriatric depressed subjects who did not remit after treatment with sertraline showed *less* of a decline in FA in the anterior cingulate over time, and declines in FA were significantly positively correlated with symptom improvement (Taylor et al., 2011). It is interesting to note that while lower FA was associated with poor remission to oral antidepressant treatment, FA has been shown to *increase* in response to ECT treatment. Nobuhara et al. demonstrated that lower frontal white matter FA seen in elderly depressed patients increased within 2 weeks after the cessation of ECT treatment. Although the authors found lower FA in temporal white matter, FA in that region did not change in response to ECT treatment (Nobuhara et al., 2004). With results contrary to previous cross-sectional studies, this highlights the need for more longitudinal studies to better understand the relationship between DTI-based measures and treatment response.

Cognitive performance in late-life depression has also been correlated with DTI measures. For example, processing speed was significantly correlated with prefrontal mean diffusivity in depressed subjects, but not healthy controls (Shimony et al., 2009). Performance on the Stroop task has also been associated with white matter integrity in late-life depression. In a study by Murphy et al., FA in several prefrontal, temporal, and occipital regions was significantly correlated with Stroop Color-Word Interference Score in elderly depressed subjects

(Murphy et al., 2007). When examining specific tracts, FA in the left cingulate bundle was associated with performance on Trail Making Test A in subjects with late-life depression who were even in remission (Yuan et al., 2010).

There have also been genotype associations with DTI-based measures. The s-allele of the serotonin transporter in depressed subjects is associated with lower FA in frontolimibc regions (Alexopoulos et al., 2009). This association has yet to been seen with other polymorphisms associated with major depression. For example, no association between DTI-based measures of the BDNF val66met polymorphism was reported in a recent study by Alexopoulos and colleagues (Alexopoulos et al., 2010).

In conclusion, DTI is a sensitive technique for detecting alterations in white matter microstructure. In late-life depression, DTI-based measures have been associated with disease severity, treatment response/resistance, and cognitive impairment. Future studies will utilize DTI to understand how structural connectivity is impaired in geriatric mood disorders.

MAGNETIC RESONANCE SPECTROSCOPY

Magnetic resonance spectroscopy (MRS), also known as nuclear magnetic resonance spectroscopy, is a noninvasive, in vivo tool for measuring biochemical information in different organs, including the brain (Arnold & Stefano, 1997). MRS data can provide information to assist with diagnostic assessment and therapeutic monitoring. Biochemical alterations in late-life mood disorders may be demonstrated despite virtually normal appearing brain structure (Dager et al., 2004).

The MRS signals arise from atomic nuclei within densely concentrated, low molecular weight molecules that have the ability to move freely in fluid compartments. Molecules found within energy pathways have such characteristics, thus making MRS a prime candidate to measure bioenergetic metabolism (Alger, 2010). ^{31}P (phosphorus) MRS measures high-energy phosphate metabolites such as adenosine triphosphate (ATP), phosphocreatine (PCr), and inorganic phosphorus (Pi), whereas ^1H (proton) MRS is used to quantify nonphosphorus metabolites such as N-acetyl aspartate (NAA), choline (Cho),

Table 33.1 Summary of Metabolites and Their Respective Markers

METABOLITE	MARKER/UTILITY
NAA	Neuronal integrity and mitochondrial function
Cho	Neuronal membrane integrity
mI	Glial function and neurotoxicity
Cr	Often used an internal reference standard; may have bioenergetic relevance
Glu/Gln	Glutamatergic neurotransmission and energy metabolism

creatine (Cr), and myo-inositol (mI). Other MRS techniques utilize various isotopes as probes, including ^{7}Li, ^{13}C, ^{15}N, ^{19}F, and ^{23}Na, that can be employed when measuring pharmaceuticals containing the nonisotope form of these atoms.

The biochemical molecules discussed have been quantified and correlated with specific tissue characteristics and may be used as biomarkers (Table 33.1). NAA is an amino acid that serves as a marker of both the structural integrity of neurons and mitochondrial function (Clark, 1998; Stefano, Matthews, & Arnold, 1995), reflecting the site of NAA synthesis. Choline (Cho) represents neuronal membrane integrity and an increase can be attributed to myelin and membrane breakdown (Klein, 2000). Myoinositol (mI) is related to glial function, and concentration abnormalities may indicate neurotoxicity (Malhi, Valenzuela, Wen, & Sachdev, 2002). Creatine (Cr) is an organic acid synthesized from amino acids that enhances the storage of phosphocreatine increasing the muscle's ability to resynthesize ATP (adenosine triphosphate) from ADP (adenosine diphosphate) to meet increased cellular energy demands (Persky & Brazeau, 2001). Cr has commonly been used as an internal reference standard in which metabolite data are expressed as a ratio to Cr (Mandal, 2011). However, metabolite data may alternatively be represented as absolute values. More recent studies at higher MRI scanner field strength (3T and above) using sophisticated spectral editing techniques have allowed for the individual measurement of the neurotransmitters glutamate and glutamine. Earlier work at 1.5T quantified Glx, an acronym that included the combination of glutamate, glutamine, and γ-aminobutyric acid (GABA). These three metabolites are increasingly a primary outcome in studies of neuropsychiatric disorders to better understand glutamatergic neurotransmission (Yüksel & Öngür, 2010). ^{13}C-MRS may be the most direct method to quantify glutamate and glutamine, but this complex MRS method is not widely available at many academic medical centers.

MRS has the potential to yield insights into many facets of the biochemistry of neuropsychiatric disorders, including neurotransmission, bioenergetic metabolism, and cell membrane integrity. The challenge is to standardize MRS techniques so they can be widely implemented with reliable and valid measurement methods. Such widespread collection of MRS data from neuropsychiatric populations would increase the power of this evolving technology to improve our understanding of the neurobiology of psychiatric illness (Wei, 2009).

GERIATRIC DEPRESSION AND BIPOLAR DISORDER

MRS has been increasingly used to study mood disorders in geriatric populations (Table 33.2). Comparing older adults with depression or bipolar disorder with healthy control subjects may offer insight into the pathophysiology of geriatric depression and predictors of treatment response, and aid the development of more specific therapeutic interventions.

Most of the studies of geriatric depression utilize ^{1}H MRS. In different areas of the brain, changes in mI, Cho, and NAA have been observed in association with major depression. In the prefrontal region, increased mI and decreased NAA have been observed (Fig. 33.3) (Binesh, Kumar, Hwang, Mintz, & Thomas, 2004; Chen et al., 2009; Kumar et al., 2002; Venkatraman, Krishnan, Steffens, Song, & Taylor, 2009). These findings are hypothesized to be associated with changes in myelination and/or neuronal loss. However, there have been inconsistent findings for Cho in the frontal lobe. Venkatraman et al. (2009) found a significant reduction of Cho and Kumar et al. a significant increase

Table 33.2 Summary of Clinical Studies With Their Author, MRS Type Used, and Respective Relevant Findings

AUTHOR	MRS USED	FINDINGS
Geriatric depression studies		
Venkatraman	¹H	NAA decreased in prefrontal cortex
		NAA increased in left medial temporal lobe
		Cho decreased in prefrontal cortex
		Cr decreased in prefrontal cortex
		mI increased in left medial temporal lobe
Kumar	¹H	mI/Cr increased in frontal white matter
		Cho/Cr increased in frontal white matter
Binesh	¹H	mI increased in dorsolateral prefrontal region
		PE increased in dorsolateral prefrontal region
		Glx increased in dorsolateral prefrontal region
Chen	¹H	NAA/Cr ratio decrease in the frontal white matter
		Cho/Cr increase in basal ganglia
		mI/Cr increase in the basal ganglia
Vythilingam	¹H	NAA decreased in caudate
		Cho increased in putamen
Huang	¹H	NAA/Cr levels increased in left hippocampus and bilateral thalamus post antidepressant treatment
		Cho/Cr levels decreased in left hippocampus and bilateral thalamus post antidepressant treatment
Wyckoff	¹H, MT, and MRS	Inverse relationship between MTR and mI/Cr in left dorsolateral white matter
Murata	¹H	Correlation between increased WMH severity and decreased NAA/Cr in frontal white matter
Ajilore	¹H	Significantly decreased Glu and Gln for DM+MDD and DM vs. HC in subcortical nuclei
Haroon	¹H	Increased mI in DM and DM+MDD correlated with visuospatial dysfunction in frontal white matter
Moore	³¹P	Beta NTP decreased in basal ganglia
		Total NTP decreased in basal ganglia
Volz	³¹P	Beta NTP decreased in frontal lobes
		Total NTP decreased in frontal lobes
Renshaw	¹H and ³¹P	Average purine levels were not different between depressed and comparison groups in basal ganglia; however, female responders to fluoxetine treatment had 30% lower purine levels than nonresponders.
		Beta NTP 21% lower in responders to fluoxetine than non-responders, correlated with purine levels

(Continued)

Table 33.2 (Continued)

AUTHOR	MRS USED	FINDINGS
Iosifescu	^{31}P	Mg^{2+} decreased at baseline in frontal and parietal slice superior to corpus callosum of depressed subjects
		Total NTP increased in frontal and parietal slice superior to corpus callosum of T3 responders
		PCr decreased in frontal and parietal slice superior to corpus callosum of T3 responders
Pettegrew	^{31}P	Prefrontal phosphomonoesters levels increased at baseline; decreased with ALCAR treatment, trend between HDRS and phosphomonoester
		ALCAR increased PCr in prefrontal region, PCr levels correlated with HDRS
Forester	^{31}P	Whole-brain total NTP decreased in geriatric depressed vs controls, difference in WM, not GM
		Total NTP decreased with treatment
		Whole-brain beta NTP decreased in MDD
		Whole-brain pH increased in GM for pre-treatment depressed; pH decreased following treatment
Geriatric bipolar disorder studies		
Forester	^{7}Li	Increased brain Li in the superior edge of the corpus callosum associated with increased HDRS scores and frontal lobe dysfunction
FORESTER	^{7}LI	Brain Li levels in the anterior cingulate gyrus associated with increased NAA and mI in BP

ALCAR, acetyl-L-carnitine; BP, bipolar disorder; Cho, choline; Cre, creatine; DM, diabetes mellitus; Gln, glutamine; Glu, glutamate; Glx, glutamate + glutamine; GM, gray matter; H, hydrogen; HDRS, Hamilton Depression Rating Scale; Li, lithium; MDD, major depressive disorder; Mg^{2+}, magnesium ion; mI, myo-inositol; MT, magnetization transfer; MTR, magnetization transfer ratio; NAA, N-acetylaspartate; NAAG, N-acetylaspartylglutamate; NTP, nucleotide triphosphate; P, phosphorus; PCr, phosphocreatine; T3, triiodothyronine.

(2002). Two proposed reasons for these differences include variability in the severity of depression and region of interest. The subjects that participated in the Venkatraman study were depressed older adults who were responsive to treatment and had only residual symptoms, whereas Kumar and colleagues studied acutely depressed older adults. Additionally, Venkatraman et al. focused on the anterior cingulate, while Kumar's findings were based in the dorsolateral prefrontal cortex. An additional novel finding for Venkatraman and colleagues was increased NAA in the left medial temporal lobe, which may reflect increased amygdala activity via diminished frontal lobe inhibition. Furthermore, changes in metabolite concentrations were found in the basal ganglia, where NAA was decreased in the caudate and Cho was increased in the putamen (Vythilingam et al., 2003).

In a study conducted by Huang et al, 1H-MRS was used to measure metabolites in patients with post-stroke depression before and after treatment with an antidepressant. Although the location of the stroke and baseline levels of NAA and Cho varied among the participants, the results suggest that antidepressant treatment may have neurotrophic effects since NAA/Cr levels increased and Cho/Cr levels decreased in the left hippocampus and bilateral thalamus associated with improvement in depression symptoms as measured by the Hamilton Depression Rating Scale (HDRS) (Huang et al., 2010).

A negative correlation was found between magnetization transfer ratio (MTR) and NAA+NAAG/Cr (N-acetylaspartylglutamate) and between mI/Cr and MTR (Wyckoff et al., 2003) in white matter. MTR is associated with structural tissue integrity, and it is hypothesized that changes in mI and NAA pools may result in the observed changes in macromolecular protein pools. Decreases in NAA were also found to be positively correlated with increased severity of white matter hyperintensities (Murata et al., 2001).

Changes in Glu and Gln concentrations have also been observed in mood disorders. In particular, a recent review observed that Glx levels are reduced in major depressive disorder subjects, whereas they are increased in bipolar disorder subjects (Yüksel & Öngür, 2010). In comparing older adults with major depression, diabetes mellitus, and healthy controls, subcortical nuclei Glu and Gln levels were significantly decreased in subjects with diabetes mellitus and depression compared with diabetic subjects and healthy controls. It is hypothesized that reduced Glu and Gln may be a result of glial dysfunction as well as impaired glucose metabolism (Yüksel & Öngür, 2010). Also of note, mI was significantly increased in depressed patients with and without diabetes mellitus versus controls (Ajilore et al., 2006). In another study examining mI levels and visuospatial functioning, it was found that increased frontal white matter mI levels, present in both depressed and nondepressed diabetes mellitus subjects, were correlated with visuospatial dysfunction (Haroon et al., 2009). Patients with diabetes are at an increased risk of suffering from depression, and increased medical burden may be a risk factor for poor response to antidepressant treatment (Iosifescu et al., 2005).

These metabolic changes associated with major depression seem to be clinically relevant as demonstrated by treatment effect studies. For example, an increase in amygdala region NAA was seen in depressed patients who exhibited a positive response to electroconvulsive therapy (Michael et al., 2003). In addition, Glx concentrations in the left dorsal lateral prefrontal cortex were negatively correlated with the severity of depression and increased significantly after electroconvulsive treatment (Michael et al., 2003). In a report examining the effect of antidepressant treatment, it was shown that decreased NAA levels in the anterior cingulate cortex in depressed patients were reversed with venlafaxine treatment (Gonul et al., 2006).

Previous ^{31}P-MRS studies have demonstrated lower levels of beta and total NTP (nucleotide triphosphate) in the basal ganglia (Moore, Christensen, Lafer, Fava, & Renshaw, 1997) and the frontal lobes (Volz et al., 1998) of depressed adults. Bioenergetic changes have also been demonstrated to correlate with response to pharmacological treatment (Fig. 33.4) (Iosifescu et al., 2008; Renshaw et al., 2001). Earlier studies have been inconclusive regarding whether differences in bioenergetic metabolism reflect a trait condition for those individuals at risk for depression or a state condition related to depression severity (Iosifescu et al., 2008).

Studies examining changes in high-energy phosphate metabolites with treatment in geriatric depression are limited. In prefrontal tissue, phosphomonoester concentration was increased in two male older depressed subjects compared with six male controls of similar age. In the depressed group, prefrontal phosphomonoester levels decreased with acetyl-L-carnitine (ALCAR) treatment (Pettegrew et al., 2002). In addition, following ALCAR treatment there was a significant increase in PCr levels. In this study, a trend level correlation was also found between phosphomonoester levels and HDRS scores (Pettegrew et al., 2002). A recent [13]P-MRS study of 13 older depressed adults and 10 healthy older controls at 4T demonstrated that both total NTP and β-NTP (which primarily reflects levels of ATP) were decreased in the geriatric depressed subjects. More specifically, total NTP among depressed subjects was significantly decreased in white matter, but there was no significant difference in gray matter versus controls. Following sertraline treatment, there was a significant decrease (2%) in total NTP. In addition, intracellular pH in gray matter, which was significantly greater in depressed subjects versus controls before treatment, decreased to levels similar to that of healthy controls following treatment (Forester, Harper, et al., 2009). The authors propose that further study of high-energy phosphate alterations in geriatric depression is warranted, and this may lead to bioenergetically based treatment approaches in late-life major depression.

MRS studies in late-life bipolar disorder are more limited, though recent findings using ^{7}Li (lithium) MRS hold promise for a clinical application of this method to help regulate lithium dosing more accurately in older bipolar adults. Examining the superior edge of the corpus callosum in a 4T MRS study of older adults with bipolar disorder treated with Li, increased brain but not serum Li levels were associated with increased depression symptoms (measured by the HDRS) as well as frontal executive dysfunction (measured by the Stroop Interference Tests, Trails B, and Wisconsin Card Sort) (Forester et al., 2008). In addition, brain Li levels were associated with increased mI and NAA levels (Forester, Streeter, et al., 2009). Increased NAA suggests potential neuroprotective and neurotrophic effects of Li treatment, while increased mI levels were thought to reflect increased inositol monophosphatase activity in the setting of chronic Li treatment.

Studies utilizing proton (1H) MRS have identified changes in cerebral concentrations of NAA, Glx, choline-containing compounds, mI, and lactate in adult bipolar subjects compared with normal controls (Stork & Renshaw, 2005). Other studies using ^{31}P MRS have examined additional alterations in levels of PCr, phosphomonoesters, and intracellular pH (pHi) (Stork & Renshaw, 2005). Based on these findings, some have hypothesized that the majority of MRS findings in bipolar disorder can be explained by a cohesive bio energetic and neurochemical model that is focused on central nervous system energy metabolism (Stork & Renshaw, 2005). Treatment studies examining bioenergetics changes in geriatric bipolar depressed individuals utilizing both ^{1}H- and ^{31}P- MRS at 4T are currently underway and may provide further insight into the pathophysiology of late-life bipolar disorder.

Disclosures

Dr. Kumar receives grants from the NIH, an honorarium from the American Association for Geriatric Psychiatry for Associate Editorship of the American Journal Geriatric Psychiatry, and an honorarium for participating in the "Chair's Summit"—a 2-day CME event with several chairs of academic departments of psychiatry.

Dr. Ajilore has nothing to disclose. He receives funding from NIMH grant K23 MH081175.

Dr. Forester has research funding from the National Institutes of Mental Health and the Rogers Family Foundation. He serves as a nonpaid volunteer on the Board of Directors for the American Association for Geriatric Psychiatry and the Board of the Alzheimer's Association for MA and NH. Dr. Forester is also the chair of the Council of Geriatric Psychiatry for the American Psychiatric Association.

Dr. Deseda has no conflicts to disclose.

Mr. Woodward has no conflicts to disclose.

Ms. Rhodes has no conflicts to disclose.

REFERENCES

Ajilore, O., Haroon, E., Kumaran, S., Darwin, C., Binesh, N., Mintz, J., ... Kumar, A. (2006). Measurement of brain metabolites in patients with type 2 diabetes and major depression using proton magnetic resonance spectroscopy. *Neuropsychopharmacology, 32*(6), 1224–1231.

Alexopoulos, G. S., Glatt, C. E., Hoptman, M. J., Kanellopoulos, D., Murphy, C. F., Kelly Jr, R. E., ... Gunning, F. M. (2010). BDNF Val66met polymorphism, white matter abnormalities and remission of geriatric depression. *Journal of Affective Disorders, 125*(1–3), 262–268.

Alexopoulos, G. S., Kiosses, D. N., Choi, S. J., Murphy, C. F., & Lim, K. O. (2002). Frontal white matter microstructure and treatment response of late-life depression: A preliminary study. *American Journal of Psychiatry, 159*(11), 1929–1932.

Alexopoulos, G. S., Murphy, C. F., Gunning-Dixon, F. M., Glatt, C. E., Latoussakis, V., Kelly, R. E., Jr., ... Hoptman, M. J. (2009). Serotonin transporter polymorphisms, microstructural white matter abnormalities and remission of geriatric depression. *Journal of Affective Disorders, 119*(1–3), 132–141.

Alexopoulos, G. S., Murphy, C. F., Gunning-Dixon, F. M., Latoussakis, V., Kanellopoulos, D., Klimstra, S., ... Hoptman, M. J. (2008). Microstructural white matter abnormalities and remission of geriatric depression. *American Journal of Psychiatry, 165*(2), 238–244.

Alger, J. R. (2010). Quantitative proton magnetic resonance spectroscopy and spectroscopic imaging of the brain: A didactic review. *Topics in Magnetic Resonance Imaging, 21*(2), 115–128.

Arnold, D., & Stefano, N. (1997). Magnetic resonance spectroscopy in vivo: Applications in neurological disorders. *Italian Journal of Neurological Sciences, 18*(6), 321–329.

Binesh, N., Kumar, A., Hwang, S., Mintz, J., & Thomas, M. A. (2004). Neurochemistry of late-life major depression: A pilot two-dimensional MR spectroscopic study. *Journal of Magnetic Resonance Imaging, 20*(6), 1039–1045.

Butters, M. A., Klunk, W. E., Mathis, C. A., Price, J. C., Ziolko, S. K., Hoge, J. A., ... Meltzer, C. C. (2008). Imaging Alzheimer pathology in late-life depression with PET and Pittsburgh compound-B. *Alzheimer Disease and Associated Disorders, 22*(3), 261–268.

Chen, C-S., Chiang, I. C., Li, C-W., Lin, W-C., Lu, C-Y., Hsieh, T-J., ... Kuo, Y-T. (2009). Proton magnetic resonance spectroscopy of late-life major depressive disorder. *Psychiatry Research: Neuroimaging, 172*(3), 210–214.

Clark, J. B. (1998). N-acetyl aspartate: A marker for neuronal loss or mitochondrial dysfunction. *Developmental Neuroscience*, 20(4–5), 271–276.

Dager, S. R., Friedman, S. D., Parow, A., Demopulos, C., Stoll, A. L., Lyoo, I. K., ... Renshaw, P. F. (2004). Brain metabolic alterations in medication-free patients with bipolar disorder. *Archives of General Psychiatry*, 61(5), 450–458.

Dalby, R. B., Frandsen, J., Chakravarty, M. M., Ahdidan, J., Sørensen, L., Rosenberg, R., ... Østergaard, L. (2010). Depression severity is correlated to the integrity of white matter fiber tracts in late-onset major depression. *Psychiatry Research: Neuroimaging*, 184(1), 38–48.

Forester, B. P., Finn, C. T., Berlow, Y. A., Wardrop, M., Renshaw, P. F., & Moore, C. M. (2008). Brain lithium, N-acetyl aspartate and myo-inositol levels in older adults with bipolar disorder treated with lithium: A lithium-7 and proton magnetic resonance spectroscopy study. *Bipolar Disorders*, 10(6), 691–700.

Forester, B. P., Harper, D. G., Jensen, J. E., Ravichandran, C., Jordan, B., Renshaw, P. F., & Cohen, B. M. (2009). 31Phosphorus magnetic resonance spectroscopy study of tissue specific changes in high energy phosphates before and after sertraline treatment of geriatric depression. *International Journal of Geriatric Psychiatry*, 24(8), 788–797.

Forester, B. P., Streeter, C. C., Berlow, Y. A., Tian, H., Wardrop, M., Finn, C. T., ... Moore, C. M. (2009). Brain lithium levels and effects on cognition and mood in geriatric bipolar disorder: A lithium-7 magnetic resonance spectroscopy study. *American Journal of Geriatric Psych*, 17(1), 13–23.

Gonul, A. S., Kitis, O., Ozan, E., Akdeniz, F., Eker, C., Eker, O. D., & Vahip, S. (2006). The effect of antidepressant treatment on N-acetyl aspartate levels of medial frontal cortex in drug-free depressed patients. *Progress in Neuro-Psychopharmacology and Biological Psychiatry*, 30(1), 120–125.

Haller, S., Xekardaki, A., Delaloye, C., Canuto, A., Lovblad, K., Gold, G., & Giannakopoulos, P. (2011). Combined analysis of grey matter voxel-based morphometry and white matter tract-based spatial statistics in late-life bipolar disorder. *Journal of Psychiatry and Neuroscience*, 36(1), 100–140.

Haroon, E., Watari, K., Thomas, A., Ajilore, O., Mintz, J., Elderkin-Thompson, V., ... Kumar, A. (2009). Prefrontal myo-inositol concentration and visuospatial functioning among diabetic depressed patients. *Psychiatry Research: Neuroimaging*, 171(1), 10–19.

Huang, Y., Chen, W., Li, Y., Wu, X., Shi, X., & Geng, D. (2010). Effects of antidepressant treatment on N-acetyl aspartate and choline levels in the hippocampus and thalami of post-stroke depression patients: A study using 1H magnetic resonance spectroscopy. *Psychiatry Research: Neuroimaging*, 182(1), 48–52.

Iosifescu, D. V., Bolo, N. R., Nierenberg, A. A., Jensen, J. E., Fava, M., & Renshaw, P. F. (2008). Brain bioenergetics and response to triiodothyronine augmentation in major depressive disorder. *Biological Psychiatry*, 63(12), 1127–1134.

Iosifescu, D. V., Clementi-Craven, N., Fraguas, R., Papakostas, G. I., Petersen, T., Alpert, J. E., ... Fava, M. (2005). Cardiovascular risk factors may moderate pharmacological treatment effects in major depressive disorder. *Psychosomatic Medicine*, 67(5), 703–706.

Kepe, V., Barrio, J. R., Huang, S-C., Ercoli, L., Siddarth, P., Shoghi-Jadid, K., ... Phelps, M. E. (2006). Serotonin 1A receptors in the living brain of Alzheimer's disease patients. *Proceedings of the National Academy of Sciences USA*, 103(3), 702–707.

Klein, J. (2000). Membrane breakdown in acute and chronic neurodegeneration: Focus on choline-containing phospholipids. *Journal of Neural Transmission*, 107(8), 1027–1063–1063.

Klunk, W. E., Engler, H., Nordberg, A., Wang, Y., Blomqvist, G., Holt, D. P., ... Långström, B. (2004). Imaging brain amyloid in Alzheimer's disease with Pittsburgh Compound-B. *Annals of Neurology*, 55(3), 306–319.

Kumar, A., Kepe, V., Barrio, J., Siddarth, P., Manoukian, V., Elderkin-Thompson, V., & Small, G. (in press). Protein binding in patients with late-life depression detected using [18F]FDDNP positron emission tomography. *Archives of General Psychiatry*.

Kumar, A., Thomas, A., Lavretsky, H., Yue, K., Huda, A., Curran, J., ... Toga, A. (2002). Frontal white matter biochemical abnormalities in late-life major depression detected with proton magnetic resonance spectroscopy. *American Journal of Psychiatry*, 159(4), 630–636.

Lamar, M., Charlton, R., Morris, R., & Markus, H. (2010). The impact of subcortical white matter disease on mood in euthymic older adults: A diffusion tensor imaging study. *American Journal of Geriatric Psychiatry*, 18, 634–642.

Lavretsky, H., Siddarth, P., Kepe, V., Ercoli, L. M., Miller, K. J., Burggren, A. C., ... Small, G. W. (2009). Depression and anxiety symptoms are associated with cerebral FDDNP-PET binding in middle-aged and older nondemented adults.

American Journal of Geriatric Psych, 17(6), 493–502.

Logan, J., Fowler, J. S., Volkow, N. D., Wang, G-J., Ding, Y-S., & Alexoff, D. L. (1996). Distribution volume ratios without blood sampling from graphical analysis of PET data. *Journal of Cerebral Blood Flow and Metabolism*, 16(5), 834–840.

Malhi, G. S., Valenzuela, M., Wen, W., & Sachdev, P. (2002). Magnetic resonance spectroscopy and its applications in psychiatry. *Australian and New Zealand Journal of Psychiatry*, 36(1), 31–43.

Mandal, P. K. (2011). In vivo proton magnetic resonance spectroscopic signal processing for the absolute quantitation of brain metabolites. *European Journal of Radiology*. ePub ahead of print, doi: 10.1016/j.ejrad.2011.03.076

Michael, N., Erfurth, A., Ohrmann, P., Arolt, V., Heindel, W., & Pfleiderer, B. (2003). Metabolic changes within the left dorsolateral prefrontal cortex occurring with electroconvulsive therapy in patients with treatment resistant unipolar depression. *Psychological Medicine*, 33(07), 1277–1284

Michael, N., Erfurth, A., Ohrmann, P., Arolt, V., Heindel, W., & Pfleiderer, B. (2003). Neurotrophic effects of electroconvulsive therapy: A proton magnetic resonance study of the left amygdalar region in patients with treatment-resistant depression. *Neuropsychopharmacology*, 28(4), 720–725.

Moore, C. M., Christensen, J. D., Lafer, B., Fava, M., & Renshaw, P. F. (1997). Lower levels of nucleoside triphosphate in the basal ganglia of depressed subjects: A phosphorous-31 magnetic resonance spectroscopy study. *American Journal of Psychiatry*, 154(1), 116–118.

Morris, J. C., Roe, C. M., Grant, E. A., Head, D., Storandt, M., Goate, A. M.,... Mintun, M. A. (2009). Pittsburgh compound B imaging and prediction of progression from cognitive normality to symptomatic Alzheimer disease. *Archives of Neurology*, 66(12), 1469–1475.

Moseley, M. (2002). Diffusion tensor imaging and aging—a review. *NMR in Biomedicine*, 15, 553–560.

Murata, T., Kimura, H., Omori, M., Kado, H., Kosaka, H., Iidaka, T.,... Wada, Y. (2001). MRI white matter hyperintensities, 1H-MR spectroscopy and cognitive function in geriatric depression: A comparison of early- and late-onset cases. *International Journal of Geriatric Psychiatry*, 16(12), 1129–1135.

Murphy, C., Gunning-Dixon, F., Hoptman, M., Lim, K., Ardekani, B., Shields, J.,... Alexopoulos, G. (2007). White-matter integrity predicts stroop performance in patients with geriatric depression. *Biological Psychiatry*, 61, 1007–1010.

Nelson, N. D., Siddarth, P., Kepe, V., Scheibel, K. E., Huang, S-C., Ringman, J. M.,... Small, G. (2011). PET of brain amyloid and tau in adults with Down Syndrome. *Archives of Neurology*, 68(6), 768–774.

Nobuhara, K., Okugawa, G., Minami, T., Takase, K., Yoshida, T., Yagyu, T.,... Kinoshita, T. (2004). Effects of electroconvulsive therapy on frontal white matter in late-life depression: a diffusion tensor imaging study. *Neuropsychobiology*, 50, 48–53.

Persky, A. M., & Brazeau, G. A. (2001). Clinical pharmacology of the dietary supplement creatine monohydrate. *Pharmacological Reviews*, 53(2), 161–176.

Pettegrew, J. W., Levine, J., Gershon, S., Stanley, J. A., Servan-Schreiber, D., Panchalingam, K., & McClure, R. J. (2002). 31P-MRS study of acetyl-L-carnitine treatment in geriatric depression: Preliminary results. *Bipolar Disorders*, 4(1), 61–66.

Pomara, N., Doraiswamy, P., Willoughby, L., Roth, A., Mulsant, B., Sidtis, J.,... Pollock, B. (2006). Elevation in plasma abeta42 in geriatric depression: A pilot study. *Neurochemical Research*, 31(3), 341–349.

Qiu, W. Q., Sun, X., Selkoe, D. J., Mwamburi, D. M., Huang, T., Bhadela, R.,... Folstein, M. (2007). Depression is associated with low plasma Aβ42 independently of cardiovascular disease in the homebound elderly. *International Journal of Geriatric Psychiatry*, 22(6), 536–542.

Renshaw, P. F., Parow, A. M., Hirashima, F., Ke, Y., Moore, C. M., Frederick, B. D.,... Cohen, B. M. (2001). Multinuclear magnetic resonance spectroscopy studies of brain purines in major depression. *American Journal of Psychiatry*, 158(12), 2048–2055.

Shimony, J., Sheline, Y., D'Angelo, G., Epstein, A., Benzinger, T., Mintun, M.,... Snyder, A. (2009). Diffuse microstructural abnormalities of normal-appearing white matter in late life depression: A diffusion tensor imaging study. *Biological Psychiatry*, 66, 245–252.

Shin, J., Lee, S-Y., Kim, S. H., Kim, Y. B., & Cho, S. B. (2008). Multitracer PET imaging of amyloid plaques and neurofibrillary tangles in Alzheimer's disease. [Research Support, Non-US Government]. *Neuroimage.*, 43(2), 236–244.

Shoghi-Jadid, K., Small, G. W., Agdeppa, E. D., Kepe, V., Ercoli, L. M., Siddarth, P.,... Barrio, J. R. (2002). Localization of neurofibrillary tangles and beta-amyloid plaques in the brains of living patients with Alzheimer disease. *American Journal of Geriatric Psych, 10*(1), 24–35.

Small, G. W., Kepe, V., Ercoli, L. M., Siddarth, P., Bookheimer, S. Y., Miller, K. J.,... Barrio, J. R. (2006). PET of brain amyloid and tau in mild cognitive impairment. *New England Journal of Medicine, 355*(25), 2652–2663.

Stefano, N. D., Matthews, P. M., & Arnold, D. L. (1995). Reversible decreases in N-acetylaspartate after acute brain injury. *Magnetic Resonance in Medicine, 34*(5), 721–727.

Stork, C., & Renshaw, P. F. (2005). Mitochondrial dysfunction in bipolar disorder: evidence from magnetic resonance spectroscopy research. *Molecular Psychiatry, 10*(10), 900–919.

Talairach, J., & Tournoux, P. (1988). *Co-planar stereotaxic atlas of the human brain. 3-Dimensional proportional system: An approach to cerebral imaging.* New York: Thieme Medical.

Taylor, W., Kuchibhatla, M., Payne, M., Macfall, J., Sheline, Y., Krishnan, K., & Doraiswamy, P. (2008). Frontal white matter anisotropy and antidepressant remission in late-life depression. *PLoS One, 3*(9), e3267.

Taylor, W., Macfall, J., Boyd, B., Payne, M., Sheline, Y., Krishnan, R., & Murali, D. (2011). One-year change in anterior cingulate cortex white matter microstructure: Relationship with late-life depression outcomes. *American Journal of Geriatric Psychiatry, 19,* 43–52.

Taylor, W., Macfall, J., Gerig, G., & Krishnan, R. (2007). Structural integrity of the uncinate fasciculus in geriatric depression: Relationship with age of onset. *Neuropsychiatric Disorders and Treatment, 3,* 669–674.

Taylor, W., Macfall, J., Payne, M., McQuoid, D., Provenzale, J., Steffens, D., & Krishnan, K. (2004). Late-life depression and microstructural abnormalities in dorsolateral prefrontal cortex white matter. *American Journal of Psychiatry, 161,* 1293–1296.

Taylor, W., Payne, M., Krishnan, K., Wagner, H., Provenzale, J., Steffens, D., & Macfall, J. (2001). Evidence of white matter tract disruption in MRI hyperintensities. *Biological Psychiatry, 50,* 179–183.

Venkatraman, T. N., Krishnan, R. R., Steffens, D. C., Song, A. W., & Taylor, W. D. (2009). Biochemical abnormalities of the medial temporal lobe and medial prefrontal cortex in late-life depression. *Psychiatry Research: Neuroimaging, 172*(1), 49–54.

Verhoeff, N. P. L. G., Wilson, A. A., Takeshita, S., Trop, L., Hussey, D., Singh, K.,... Houle, S. (2004). In-vivo imaging of Alzheimer disease [beta]-amyloid with [11C]SB-13 PET. *American Journal of Geriatric Psych, 12*(6), 584–595.

Volz, H. P., Rzanny, R., Riehemann, S., May, S., Hegewald, H., Preussler, B.,... Sauer, H. (1998). 31P magnetic resonance spectroscopy in the frontal lobe of major depressed patients. *European Archives of Psychiatry and Clinical Neuroscience, 248*(6), 289–295.

Vythilingam, M., Charles, H. C., Tupler, L. A., Blitchington, T., Kelly, L., & Krishnan, K. R. R. (2003). Focal and lateralized subcortical abnormalities in unipolar major depressive disorder: An automated multivoxel proton magnetic resonance spectroscopy study. *Biological Psychiatry, 54*(7), 744–750.

Wei, C. (2009, September 3–6). *Brain imaging developments based on in vivo MRS.* Paper presented at the Annual International Conference of the IEEE, Engineering in Medicine and Biology Society, Minneapolis, Minnesota.

Wyckoff, N., Kumar, A., Gupta, R. C., Alger, J., Hwang, S., & Thomas, M. A. (2003). Magnetization transfer imaging and magnetic resonance spectroscopy of normal-appearing white matter in late-life major depression. *Journal of Magnetic Resonance Imaging, 18*(5), 537–543.

Yang, Q., Huang, X., Hong, N., & Yu, X. (2007). White matter microstructural abnormalities in late-life depression. *International Psychogeriatrics, 19,* 757–766.

Yuan, Y., Hou, Z., Zhang, Z., Bai, F., Yu, H., You, J.,... Jiang, T. (2010). Abnormal integrity of long association fiber tracts is associated with cognitive deficits in patients with remitted geriatric depression: A cross-sectional, case-control study. *Journal of Clinical Psychiatry, 71,* 1386–1390.

Yuan, Y., Zhang, Z., Bai, F., Yu, H., Shi, Y., Qian, Y.,... You, J. (2007). White matter integrity of the whole brain is disrupted in first-episode remitted geriatric depression. *Neuroreport, 18,* 1845–1849.

Yüksel, C., & Öngür, D. (2010). Magnetic resonance spectroscopy studies of glutamate-related abnormalities in mood disorders. *Biological Psychiatry, 68*(9), 785–794.

34

FUNCTIONAL NEUROIMAGING IN LATE-LIFE MOOD DISORDERS

Meenal J. Patel, Howard J. Aizenstein, and Gwenn S. Smith

A WIDE range of neuroimaging techniques allow researchers to investigate the changes in neural circuitries experienced by patients with mood disorders. Two of the most widely used imaging modalities include functional magnetic resonance imaging (fMRI) and positron emission tomography (PET). In this chapter, fMRI and PET biomarkers found to be associated with late-life mood disorders by current and past research studies will be reviewed.

HISTORY OF FUNCTIONAL MAGNETIC RESONANCE IMAGING

Magnetic resonance imaging (MRI) has helped make many advances in studying anatomical changes associated with late-life mood disorders using structural imaging (e.g., T1-weighted, T2-weighted, FLAIR, DTI, etc.). By the early 1990s, methods for tracking dynamic changes in blood oxygenation levels throughout the brain and thus performing functional MRI were also discovered (Ogawa, Lee, Nayak, & Glynn, 1990). This new discovery has

opened many doors for studies, allowing them to investigate neural pathways underlying cognitive and emotional processes (especially in late-life mood disorders) more in depth via an approach denoted as "human brain mapping." In 1992, functional MRI capabilities were further extended to help measure regional cerebral blood flow with the introduction of perfusion MRI and a technique called arterial spin labeling (Detre, Leigh, Williams, &Koretsky, 1992). However, for this chapter, we will focus on BOLD functional MRI studies.

FUNDAMENTALS OF MAGNETIC RESONANCE IMAGING

BOLD Functional Magnetic Resonance Imaging

BOLD functional MRI is used to indirectly measure neuronal activity. The process of measuring neuronal activity starts with performance of a task, followed by corresponding change in regional neural activity, and ends with a change in BOLD MR signal. If the performed task increases the regional neural activity, the BOLD MR signal is also increased in that region in the following order of events: (1) increase in neuronal activity, (2) decrease of deoxyhemoglobin (note that deoxyhemoglobin alters spins of nearby hydrogen nuclei due to presence of magnetic field), and (3) increase in the received BOLD MR signal due to a greater alignment of the spins with the applied magnetic field. Thus, the change in regional neural activity due to a performed task is directly proportional to the change in BOLD MR signal. Consequently, by evaluating changes in the blood oxygenation level dependent (BOLD) signal, studies are able to map brain activity during experimental tasks (e.g., cognitive and affective tasks) and resting state.

COGNITIVE TASKS

Cognitive tasks comprise both executive and memory tasks. However, the focus of this chapter will be on cognitive executive tasks. Executive tasks involve executive control, such as integrating other cognitive activities. Prefrontal brain regions play a prominent role in the performance of executive tasks (see Table 34.1). As a result, executive tasks help analyze reflecting conscious, strategic, and goal-directed cognitive activity (Bryan & Luszcz, 1999). Examples of executive tasks used in functional MR studies include the Stroop task, which is known to test response inhibition, interference resolution, and behavioral conflict resolution (Adleman et al., 2001), and task-switching tests, which help test cognitive efficiency, processing speed, performance, as well as controlling and coordinating execution of goal-directed behavior (DiGirolamo et al.., 2001; Dove, Pollmann, Schubert, Wiggins, & von Cramon, 2000; Sylvester, Wager, & Lacey, 2003), and so on. Figure 34.1 shows an example of results obtained from an fMRI study performed using an executive task.

AFFECTIVE TASKS

Affective tasks are used to evaluate neural systems associated with mood and emotion. Commonly associated regions with affective processes include

Table 34.1 The Roles of Task-Specific Regions in Functional Processes

REGION	ROLE IN EXECUTIVE COGNITIVE PROCESSES (BRYAN & LUSZCZ, 1999)
Prefrontal cortex	Planning and implementing strategies for performance, monitoring performance, adjusting future responses using feedback, vigilance, and inhibiting information irrelevant to a given task

REGION	ROLE IN AFFECTIVE PROCESSES (DAVIDSON ET AL., 2002)
Amygdala	Threat signaling cue perception; producing aversive responding related behavior and autonomic responses
Anterior cingulate cortex	Monitoring conflict (specifically conflict between response options)
Prefrontal cortex	Left hemisphere: approach-based appetitive goal Right hemisphere: maintaining goals involving behavioral inhibition

REGION	ROLE IN DEFAULT MODE NETWORK (BUCKNER ET AL., 2008)
Midtemporal cortex	Provides memories of past experiences as well as associations used for mental simulation
Prefrontal cortex	Facilitates information from temporal cortex to construct self-relevant mental simulations
Cingulate cortex	Helps integrate the two systems: mid-temporal lobe subsystem and prefrontal subsystem

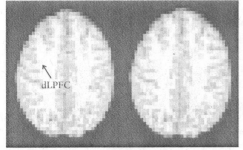

Non-Depressed   Depressed

FIGURE 34.1 Hypoactivation (p < 0.01, K = 8) of the dorsolateral prefrontal cortex (dLPFC) in observed in depressed patients during a Preparing to Overcome Prepotency (POP) task—an executive task derived from the switching Stroop task (Aizenstein et al., 2009) (See color insert).

limbic regions, such as the amygdala and anterior cingulate cortex. Also, because of its role in regulating affect, the prefrontal cortex (especially ventral prefrontal cortex) is also often studied with affective tasks. In addition to studying these regions separately, several studies also focus on the functional connectivity between these regions. Table 34.1 summarizes the involvement of each region in affective processes. Functional affective tasks used to study these regions involve arousal and/or control of emotion and mood (e.g., emotional faces task; Davidson, Pizzagalli, Nitschke, & Putnam, 2002). An example of results obtained from an fMRI study performed using an affective task is shown in Figure 34.2.

RESTING STATE AND THE DEFAULT MODE NETWORK

An important circuitry often focused on by fMRI studies is the default mode network. The default mode network mainly consists of the prefrontal, cingulate, and midtemporal cortices. These regions and their roles are summarized in Table 34.1. In fMRI studies, the BOLD signal is significantly greater in the regions of the network during the resting state, or when no task is being performed, than during cognitive and affective tasks. In other words, regions of the default mode network deactivate during performance of goal-directed tasks. The involvement of this network in functional processes is still up for debate; however, there are two possibilities: (1) it plays a role in forming dynamic internal mental images of perspectives and scenarios not related to the present while the mind is detached from the external world (e.g., planning future actions based on past experiences), or (2) it plays a role in monitoring the external environment in an exploratory manner whenever focused external attention and sensory processes are relaxed (Buckner, Andrews-Hanna, & Schacter, 2008). An example of results obtained from a resting state fMRI study exploring the default mode network is shown in Figure 34.3.

FUNCTIONAL MAGNETIC RESONANCE IMAGING AND BIOMARKERS

Late-Life Depression

FRONTOSTRIATAL AND FRONTOLIMBIC CIRCUITRY

Past functional MRI (fMRI) studies have shown a relationship between geriatric depression (i.e., late-life depression [LLD]) and functional changes in regions associated with the frontostriatal and frontolimbic circuitry. In studying the integrity of this circuitry, these studies have shown geriatric

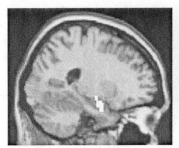
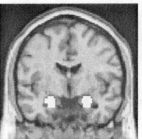
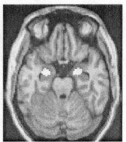

FIGURE 34.2 Significant activation (t > 2.6618, df = 59, p < 0.005) in the amygdala is observed in elderly subjects (depressed + non depressed combined) during an emotional faces affective task. Regions of significant activation are in red (brighter = greater significance) and the amygdala is highlighted in yellow (Aizenstein et al., 2011) (See color insert).

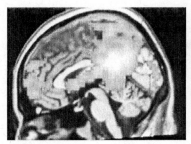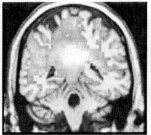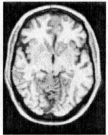

FIGURE 34.3 Resting state functional connectivity maps showing significant activation (corrected p < 0.001) in the default mode network observed in non-depressed elderly subjects. Regions with greatest to least significant activation are scaled from yellow to dark orange respectively (Wu et al., 2011) (See color insert).

depression to be associated with deficits in cognition (via executive cognitive tasks) and emotion (via affective tasks), respectively.

In an fMRI study by Aizenstein et al. (2005), implicit and explicit sequence learning tasks were used to analyze the frontostriatal circuitry. Significant results were only found in the explicit condition. The results showed hypoactivation in the dorsolateral prefrontal cortex bilaterally, and hyperactivation in the right caudate and putamen in elderly depressed patients, thus supporting the frontostriatal dysfunction hypothesis. The decreased activation of the dorsolateral prefrontal cortex (dLPFC) is consistent with hypofrontality associated with executive function deficits, while the increased activation of the striatum (i.e., caudate and putamen) indicates a greater response to negative rewards and altered emotional processes in the patients.

A later fMRI study by Aizenstein et al. (2009) used an executive task to examine the frontostriatal circuit and study executive and cognitive control in LLD. The task was a derivation of the switching Stroop task called Preparing to Overcome Prepotency (POP) task. The findings of this study suggest hypoactivity in the dLPFC as well as a decreased functional connectivity between the dLPFC and the dorsal anterior cingulate cortex (dACC) in LLD patients—once again confirming the frontostriatal dysfunction hypothesis. Taking it a step further, this study also evaluated the posttreatment (treated with the antidepressant paroxetine) effects on activation in the patients. The results indicated the presence of both episodic and persistent neurobiological components of LLD. After treatment, the decreased functional connectivity continued to persist and is thought to be due to vascular damage in frontal white matter and to play a role in recurrences of depressive episodes after treatment.

However, activity in the right dLPFC was found to have increased in comparison to pre-treatment and is thought to be due to response to treatment. An extension of this study was also performed by Andreescu et al. (2009) to examine comorbid anxiety in depressive disorders. The same POP task was used to compare LLD and late-life anxious depression (LLAD) patients. Based on this study, LLAD patients showed greater and more sustained activation in dACC, prefrontal cortex (e.g., supplementary motor area), and posterior cingulate during the task. These results are suggestive of the following in LLAD: increased and more sustained efforts by the ACC to carry out cognitive control tasks, increased anticipatory preparation for initiating movement by the supplementary motor area, and impaired attention and short-term episodic memory due to altered activation in the posterior cingulate.

Extending the analysis to limbic regions, Bobb et al. (2011) studied the frontostriatal-limbic brain circuitry in LLD using another executive task: the stop signal task (SST). The SST is used to study motor response inhibition. According to this study, LLD patients exhibited significantly greater activation bilaterally in the superior frontal gyri, and unilaterally in the frontal gyri, orbitofrontal gyri, insular cortex, cingulate cortex, caudate, and putamen compared to the healthy individuals. In addition, the SST performance of LLD patients was comparable to that of healthy individuals. These results suggest that the increased activity in regions of the frontostriatal-limbic circuitry is a way of compensation in LLD patients to perform similarly to healthy individuals on the SST. More specifically, the increased activity compensates for the deficits in executive functional processing and excessive depression-driven limbic activity due to frontostriatal-limbic dysfunction found in LLD.

Another fMRI study by Wang et al. (2008) studied both affective and executive processes in geriatric depression. This study used an emotional oddball task to analyze both emotional and executive processes. In addition to comparing depressed patients to healthy comparison subjects, this study also included subjects who were fully remitted from major depression. The major findings in this study include the following: (1) depressed patients experienced decreased activation during target detection in the right middle frontal gyrus (associated with the dorsolateral prefrontal cortex); (2) remitted patients showed attenuated activation similar to depressed patients during target detection in the cingulate and inferior parietal areas; (3) greater deactivation was found in the posterior portion of the posterior cingulate than the anterior portion by depressed patients compared to the remitted patients; and (4) remitted patients demonstrated diminished deactivation during target detection in the default mode network. These results (1) verify dysfunction of the frontostriatal circuitry; (2) suggest executive dysfunction (e.g., tested during target detection) is associated with pathological changes (e.g., cerebrovascular disease or white matter lesions) in geriatric depression; (3) indicate the anterior (perhaps important in attention and cognition due to interconnection with the dorsal anterior cingulate cortex and dorsolateral prefrontal cortex) and posterior (perhaps important in self-consciousness and memory retrieval due to connections with the retrosplenial cortex and the hippocampal complex) portions of the posterior cingulate play different roles in geriatric depression—where the anterior portion may be more closely related to the pathology; and (4) normalization of activation in the default mode network after remission, respectively. All significant findings indicate that the fMRI signal during performance of executive tasks is a prominent marker of geriatric depression.

In an fMRI study by Brassen et al. (2008), the emotional processing involved in geriatric depression was further studied. The task involved presentation of neutral, positive, and negative adjectives (i.e., affective or emotional evaluation of emotional words). The goal of the study was to evaluate activation of the ventromedial prefrontal cortex (vmPFC) during emotional processing. Based on the acquired results, patients demonstrated attenuated neural response to positive and negative words in the vmPFC. The same patients, after remission, showed improvement and the neural response normalized in the vmPFC. These results suggest the importance of vmPFC dysfunction as a potential biomarker for geriatric depression, especially since this region is related to evaluating and regulating emotional occurrences and contextual reward processing.

Other more limbic regions (e.g., cingulate, amygdala, and insula) known to play an important role in emotional processing were studied by Aizenstein et al. (2011). This study used an emotional faces paradigm as the affective task for its known potential to activate limbic regions. In addition to functional activity, this study also evaluated the affect of structural changes (i.e., amount of white matter hyperintensity [WMH] burden) on functional activity. The results of the study showed greater limbic activity (significant in the rostral cingulate) in late-life depression patients compared to nondepression subjects. This pattern of activation was found to be proportional to the amount of WMH burden. In other words, patients with greater WMH burden showed greater activation. One possible explanation for this association is that white matter changes in patients alter functional connectivity, leading to disruptions in the ability of the prefrontal cortex to modulate hyperactivity in limbic structures. Regardless, these results are consistent with the vascular depression hypothesis, which supports the associations of ischemic white matter changes with the pathogenesis of late-life depression, thus making WMHs another potential biomarker of LLD.

DEFAULT MODE NETWORK IN LATE-LIFE DEPRESSION

Resting-state fMRI studies are often performed to study brain activity when no activity is being performed. As mentioned earlier, a network that is most studied at rest is the default mode network.

Further examining anxiety in LLD, Andreescu et al. (2011) studied the affects of default mode network connectivity on levels of anxiety. Using a low cognitive load event-related finger-tapping task, the resting-state data for this study were acquired from the fixation periods. The default mode network connectivity was determined via a whole-brain, voxel-wise correlation with the average time series in the posterior cingulate cortex. In this study, functional connectivity was found to be significantly higher in posterior regions (e.g., precuneus) and lower in the anterior regions (e.g., rostral anterior cingulate cortex, medial prefrontal cortex, and orbital frontal cortex) of the network in LLD patients with high anxiety. Based on the hypothesized roles of the default mode network, this study suggests the following: (1) the increased connectivity in the posterior regions indicates that higher anxiety patients scan both the environment and themselves (using occipital and parietal areas, respectively) excessively maintaining a high alert to detect sources of threat; and (2) the decreased connectivity in the frontal regions indicates that higher anxiety patients self-regulate using fewer prefrontal related strategies like reappraisal and reorganization of retrieved and perceived objects. Both observations may be respectively related to (1) the common increase in bias to threat found in anxious subjects, and (2) the perceived poorer response to top-down psychotherapeutic interventions in comorbid anxious depression patients.

Using the same methodology as Andreescu et al. (2011), Wu et al. (2011) investigated the possibility of WMHs as a biomarker of LLD further by studying the association of WMH burden with default mode network connectivity in LLD. The results of the analysis indicate improved, but persistent significant hypoconnectivity between the subgenual anterior and posterior cingulate cortices in depressed patients post treatment (treated with the antidepressant paroxetine and weekly interpersonal psychotherapy). In addition, the abnormal functional connectivity was found to be significantly correlated with greater WMH burden in support of the vascular depression hypothesis. Thus, the study suggests that the hypoconnectivity between the subgenual anterior and posterior cingulate cortices may be a feature of LLD related to structural brain changes.

The relation between brain structure and function in LLD was also studied by Steffens et al. (2011). In this study, diffusion tensor imaging (DTI) was used to examine the structural integrity of the white matter at a more microscopic level as a potential marker for understanding resting-state function connectivity in LLD. Specifically, the association between the integrity of the uncinate fasciculus (UF) white matter tract and functional connectivity among regions connected by the UF was analyzed. The UF tract was chosen because it connects regions thought to be associated with depression. The results of this study show that left UF integrity was (1) significantly positively correlated with resting-state functional connectivity between left ventrolateral PFC (vlPFC) and left amygdala as well as between left vlPFC and left hippocampus; and (2) significantly negatively correlated with left vmPFC and left caudate. These correlations may suggest the following:

(1) reappraisal failure, an essential feature of cognitive bias in depression associated with the vlPFC and amygdala connectivity, may be anatomically explained by UF integrity; and (2) top-down control may be exerted via corticostriatal fiber connections between vmPFC and caudate in a compensatory manner due to poor UF integrity. Overall, these studies show the importance of analyzing functional connectivity and especially its relationship with structural integrity more in depth to better understand LLD and discover new biomarkers of LLD.

Bipolar Disorder

There have not been many fMRI studies specific to late-life bipolar disorder. Nevertheless, there have been several fMRI studies regarding bipolar disorder, which have included subjects of a wide age range. This section summarizes such studies that have included bipolar patients at least 50 years old.

PREFRONTAL CORTEX AND LIMBIC REGIONS

Past studies have shown that patients with bipolar disorder experience both state-related and trait-related functional abnormalities. In a study by Blumberg et al. (2003), neuroimaging was used to examine these abnormalities. Patients of all three states (elevated, depressed, and euthymic mood states) were studied using a color-naming Stroop task. This task was utilized to study the functional activation of the prefrontal cortex and the anterior cingulate cortex, which are involved in focusing attention, inhibiting automatic impulses, and responding appropriately: cognitive and behavior processes associated with abnormalities in bipolar disorder. The results of this study indicated an increased signal in the patients in both the regions of interest. In fact, both state- and trait-related abnormalities in activation were found to differ in location as well as direction of signal change in the ventral prefrontal cortex (VPFC). Specifically, blunted activation in the right caudal VPFC was associated with elevated mood states, and increased left caudal VPFC activation was found to be associated with the depression state. Additionally, the bipolar disorder group compared to the control group showed significantly greater activation in the left rostral VPFC. This region was distinctively in a more dorsal and anterior location than that related to the state-related abnormalities. However, it did not differ significantly between the three different bipolar state groups, thus suggesting an association with trait-related abnormalities. Overall, the presence of abnormalities in the VPFC may be associated with disturbances in stimulus-reward relations, which may explain the emotional, cognitive, and behavioral abnormalities (e.g., emotional liability, thought disorder, and exploration of hedonic activities) of bipolar disorder. In contrast to this study, Roth et al. (2006) showed hypoactivation in bipolar patients compared to healthy controls in the right inferior and medial frontal gyri (also regions of the prefrontal cortex) using the counting Stroop task to study executive control. These results are indicative of disturbances in the cognitive-motor response inhibition circuitry in bipolar disorder. Even though the direction of dysfunction varies, both studies agree upon one common conclusion: Bipolar patients experience dysfunction of the neural circuitry involving the prefrontal cortex, thus making it an essential biomarker for studying bipolar disorder.

In another study, Yurgelun-Todd et al. (2000) examined the control of affective and cognitive processes in the dorsolateral prefrontal cortex and amygdala. In this study, fearful and happy affect recognition tasks were used to test for abnormalities in these processes in bipolar patients. The results showed reduced activation in the right dorsolateral prefrontal cortex (dLPFC) and increased activation in the left amygdalar region in bipolar patients. Past studies have indicated the dLPFC to be involved in mediating mood and attention, as well as higher order functions. Therefore, the decreased activation in dLPFC during the fearful facial affect task in patients agrees with previous hypotheses that suggest bipolar patients experience disruptions in modulating behavior and affect. The results are also suggestive of alterations in the frontolimbic circuitry involved with higher order processes in bipolar patients during fearful affect recognition.

Functional abnormalities during emotional regulation in bipolar disorder have also been studied by Almeida et al. (2009). In this study, a similar task—an emotional judgment task in which participants are led to think about, instead of feel, the presented emotion—was used to examine two neural systems: ventromedial (consisting of right parahippocampal gyrus [PHG] and right subgenual cingulate gyrus [sgCG]) and dorsal/lateral (consisting of dorsolateral prefrontal cortex [dLPFC]) systems. The ventromedial neural system plays a role in the early appraisal and encoding of emotional

significance while regulating the automatic control of behavioral responses to emotional stimuli. The dorsal/lateral neural system, on the other hand, is responsible for the voluntary control and can be simultaneously active for emotional stimuli instigated behavioral responses generated in subcortical limbic regions (e.g., amygdala, ventral striatum, and thalamus). Significant increases in effective connectivity were found in the ventromedial system in bipolar patients, but no difference was found in the effective connectivity in the dorsal/lateral system. In addition to the significant increases in effective connectivity of right PHG-sgCG, this study also found reduced right PHG activity in comparison to healthy controls. These abnormalities are thought to be a result of decreased early appraisal, increased encoding of emotional significance, and greater acknowledgment of emotionally salient stimuli: functional alterations that may explain the pathophysiology for regulating mood in bipolar disorder.

Dysfunctionality of the prefrontal cortex has also been studied in resting state in bipolar disorder since it is also an essential part of the default mode network. Chepenik et al. (2010) used low-frequency, resting-state fMRI to study the ventral prefrontal cortex (vPFC) and amygdala functional connectivity in bipolar patients. Resting state was studied to better examine the natural mental state of the patients rather than a limited state based on an activation task. The study showed that a negative correlation between the left vPFC and amygdala activity in healthy controls, and a decreased significance of the correlation in bipolar patients. The decrease in correlation is suggestive of reduced functional connectivity in bipolar disorder. In agreement with other fMRI studies, this study also indicates bipolar patients experience disruptions in affective regulation represented by the vPFC-amygdala connectivity.

SUMMARY AND FUTURE DIRECTIONS OF FUNCTIONAL MAGNETIC RESONANCE IMAGING FINDINGS ON MOOD DISORDERS

According to past studies, late-life depression patients show signs of altered cognitive, emotional, and resting state processes suggested to be due to dysfunction of the frontostriatal circuit, frontolimbic circuit, and default mode network, respectively. Structural alterations (e.g., WMH burden and WM structural integrity) have also been found to be associated with the functional alterations. Additionally, remittance after treatment has been shown to partially improve these alterations, indicating late-life depression patients experience both episodic and persistent dysfunctionalities. Similarly, bipolar patients also experience alterations in cognitive, emotional, and resting state processes due to dysfunction in the prefrontal cortex and limbic regions. The important brain regions and their observed fMRI activity represented by BOLD signal change—related to the altered functional activity and connectivity—associated with each mood disorder are summarized in Table 34.2.

The aforementioned findings are not conclusive due to limitations involved in all studies. Thus, future studies are required to confirm previous results. Other future directions include testing the association between structural and functional changes related to the mood disorders. Additionally, studies specific to late-life bipolar disorder are necessary to determine how brain activity and connectivity differ in late life. These studies can help determine the functional differences between mood disorders.

HISTORY OF POSITRON EMISSION TOMOGRAPHY

PET is an in vivo molecular imaging technical for the quantitative measurement of physiological processes. A PET scan involves the intravenous administration of a radiotracer and the detection of gamma radioactivity from the position emitting isotope that is labeled to a pharmacologic agent at a tracer (subphysiological dose). The details of the methodology of have been reviewed extensively (Bailey, Townsend, Valk, & Maisey, 2005; Phelps, 2006; Phelps, Mazziota, & Schelbert, 1986; Scott & Hockley, 2011). One of the initial major advances in the field of radiotracer chemistry in the late 1970s was the development of radiotracers to measure the cerebral metabolic rate of glucose and cerebral blood flow. The use of these radiotracers resulted in the initial observations of the functional neuroanatomy of basic brain functions in normal individuals, as well as the deficits observed in a range of neuropsychiatric diseases (e.g., schizophrenia, Alzheimer's disease, depression, obsessive-compulsive disorder). The next major advance was the development of a radiotracer to measure neurotransmitter receptors, with an initial focus on the dopamine (D2) receptor (Arnett et al., 1986; Wagner et al., 1983). These

initial reports had a profound influence on researchers interested in studying the neurochemical basis of psychiatric disorders in the living brain. Over the past two decades, radiotracer development has made possible the visualization of enzymes, synthesis/metabolic processes, transporters, and receptor sites for a variety of neurotransmitter and neuromodulatory systems (as reviewed by Smith et al., 2003; Sacher & Smith, 2010). In the past decade, major advances have been made in the ability to investigate neuropathological mechanisms that have been associated with neurodegenerative diseases. Such mechanisms include inflammation, as measured by radiotracers for the peripheral benzodiazepine receptor, and beta-amyloid deposition, measured by the Pittsburgh B compound (Chauveau, Boutin, Van Camp, Dollé, & Tavitian, 2008; Mathis et al., 2003). Advances in instrumentation that occurred during this same time interval have resulted in substantial improvements in PET spatial resolution. The highest resolution PET scanner is the high-resolution research tomograph (HRRT), a dedicated human brain PET scanner with a resolution of 2.3- and 3.4-mm (Wienhard et al., 2002). Another major innovation in instrumentation has been the development of dual modality imaging, PET/CT, and more recently PET/MR (Townsend, 2008; Wehrl et al., 2010). The promise of simultaneous PET/MR imaging will have important implications for understanding the relationship of neurocircuitry and neurochemistry associated with behavior.

THE FUNCTIONAL NEUROANATOMY OF LATE-LIFE DEPRESSION AND TREATMENT RESPONSE USING POSITRON EMISSION TOMOGRAPHY

The Neural Circuitry of Depression

PET neuroimaging studies in affective disorders have focused on the characterization of regional cerebral blood flow and glucose metabolic alterations in midlife patients with primary, unipolar depression, secondary depression in stroke or movement disorders (Huntington's and Parkinson's disease), as well as the effects of antidepressant interventions. These results have been reviewed extensively (Fitzgerald, Laird, Maller, & Daskalakis, 2008; Mayberg, 2003; Sacher & Smith, 2010). Fewer studies comparing late-life depressed patients to controls or evaluating treatment

Table 34.2 Summary of Brain Regions and Observed Corresponding Alterations in Functional Magnetic Resonance Imaging (fMRI) Activity and Connectivity Represented by BOLD Signal Change in Patients Compared to Controls

LATE-LIFE DEPRESSION	ALTERATIONS IN FMRI BOLD SIGNAL CHANGE

Executive functional activity	Frontostriatal Circuitry:
	    Hypoactivation in dorsolateral prefrontal cortex (dlPFC)
	    Hyperactivation in striatum (caudate + putamen)

Affective functional activity	Frontolimbic Circuitry:
	    Attenuated activation in ventromedial prefrontal cortex (vmPFC)
	    Increased limbic activity (especially rostral cingulate)

Resting-state functional connectivity	Default Mode Network:
	    Greater anxiety results in function connectivity increases between posterior cingulate cortex and posterior brain regions; and decreases between posterior cingulate cortex and frontal brain regions.
	    Improved, yet persistant hypoconnectivity between subgenual anterior and posterior cingulate cortices after treatment may be related to greater structural brain changes (e.g., white matter hyperintensity burden)
	    Left uncinate fasciculus structural integrity is positivity correlated with left ventrolateral prefrontal cortex (vlPFC)-amygdala and left vlPFC-hippocampus connectivity; and negatively correlated with left vmPFC-caudate connectivity.

BIPOLAR DISORDER	ALTERATIONS IN FMRI BOLD SIGNAL CHANGE

Executive functional activity	Trait Specific:
	    Increased signal in prefrontal cortex (specifically left rostral ventral prefrontal cortex [vPFC])
	    Increased signal in anterior cingulate cortex
	    Decreased activation in right dlPFC
	State Specific:
	    Attenuated activation in the right caudal vPFC associated with elevated mood states of bipolar disorder
	    Increased left caudal vPFC activation was found to be associated with the depression state of bipolar disorder

Affective functional activity	Trait Specific:
	    Increased activation in the left amygdalar region
	    Decreased activation in right parahippocampal gyrus
	    Increased connectivity of ventromedial system (i.e., connectivity of right parahippocampal gyrus and right subgenual cingulate gyrus)

Resting-state functional connectivity	Trait Specific: Decreased significance of negative correlation between left vPFC and amygdala activity (i.e., disruptions in vPFC and amygdala connectivity)

effects have been performed (Kumar et al., 1993; Nobler et al., 2000; Smith et al., 1999, 2002, 2008).

A functional neuroanatomic model of depression and of antidepressant effects has been developed based on the data from midlife depressed patients (Mayberg et al., 2009). Many of the brain regions that comprise this model have been implicated in a recent meta-analysis of neuroimaging studies in major depression (Fitzgerald et al., 2008). The regions that are hypoactive at rest, show a lack of activation during negative mood states, and increase with selective serotonin reuptake inhibitor (SSRI) treatment include the dorsal pregenual cingulate gyrus, middle and dorsolateral prefrontal cortex, insula, and superior temporal gyrus. A second network identified was a cortical-limbic network, including the medial and inferior frontal cortex and basal ganglia, structures that were overactive at rest and during induction of negative mood states and reduced in activity with antidepressant treatment. The amygdala and thalamus were also implicated in the network in some studies. Other regions highlighted in the meta-analysis included the cerebellum (which showed increased activity at rest), posterior cingulate, and medial temporal lobe (including the parahippocampal gyrus), all of which show abnormal activation in mood-induction paradigms. The applicability of this model to late-life patients can be tested, given that such data have become available recently (Diaconsecu, Kramer, Hermann, 2011; Smith et al., 2009a, 2009b).

The Functional Neuroanatomy of Late-Life Depression: Comparison With Midlife Depression: Resting State and Antidepressant Effects

Differences between the functional neuroanatomy of older depressed patients compared to younger patients have been observed (Smith et al., 2009a). Relative to younger patients who demonstrate increased glucose metabolism in ventralfrontal cortical regions, late-life depressed patients demonstrate increased glucose metabolism in a more extensive network of both anterior cortical regions, as well as posterior cortical regions (Smith et al., 2009a). Relative to comparison subjects, cerebral glucose metabolism was increased in late-life depressed patients in anterior (right and left superior frontal gyrus) and posterior (precuneus, inferior parietal lobule) cortical regions. The metabolic increases were correlated with greater depression and anxiety symptoms and were observed in regions that demonstrated cerebral atrophy. In contrast to decreased metabolism observed in normal aging and neurodegenerative conditions such as Alzheimer's disease, cortical glucose metabolism was increased in late-life depressed patients relative to controls, particularly in brain regions in which cerebral atrophy was observed, which may represent a compensatory response.

In younger depressed patients, antidepressant treatment increased anterior cortical metabolism and decreased limbic metabolism (as reviewed by Mayberg, 2003; Fitzgerald et al., 2008). Within the cingulate gyrus, effects are observed in rostral areas (BA 24, 25) in midlife depressed patients (Mayberg, 2003). In contrast, studies in older depressed patients (Diaconsecu et al., 2010; Smith et al., 2002a, 2002b, 2009b) observe decreased anterior cortical and limbic metabolism and increases in posterior cortical regions and cerebellum with antidepressant treatment (including SSRIs and total sleep deprivation). Specifically, after chronic citalopram treatment (8–10 weeks), decreases in cerebral glucose metabolism were observed in frontal cortical regions, including the bilateral superior (BA 6) and medial frontal gyrus (BA 10); temporal cortical regions, including left superior and right middle temporal gyrus (BA 22/21); and parietal regions, including the left precuneus (BA 7). Decreased metabolism was observed in limbic regions, including the right anterior cingulate gyrus (BA 24), bilateral posterior cingulate cortex (BA 31), bilateral parahippocampal gyrus (BA 36), left insula (BA 13), and bilateral amygdale. Increased metabolism was observed in the right thalamus (pulvinar and medial dorsal nuclei), dorsal striatum (bilateral putamen), the right cuneus (BA 19), left inferior parietal lobule (BA 40), and bilateral cerebellum (Diaconescu et al., 2011).

With respect to the cingulate gyrus, effects are observed in caudal subregions of the cingulate gyrus (BA 32) with acute treatment and in rostral subregions (BA24) with chronic treatment in late-life depression. Importantly, the cerebral metabolic response to a single dose of an antidepressant (citalopram) is associated with clinical improvement after a 12-week trial (Smith et al., 2011b). The regional differences in metabolic response to antidepressant medications between younger and older depressed patients may be attributable to differences in depression phenomenology, as well as differential compensatory processes in the aging brain.

Mood and Cognitive Networks of Treatment Response in Late-Life Depression

While changes in neural circuitry with antidepressant treatment have been observed in midlife and late-life depression, the relationship to improvement in domains of symptoms is not well understood. Functional connectivity methods have identified neural networks associated with improvement of affective and cognitive symptoms in late-life depressed patients who underwent PET glucose metabolism studies prior to and during a course of treatment with the antidepressant citalopram (Diaconescu et al., 2011). The partial least squares method identified a subcortical-limbic-frontal network was associated with improvement in affect (mood and anxiety), while a medial temporal-parietal-frontal network was associated with improvement in cognition (immediate verbal learning/memory and verbal fluency). The network of regions that correlated with the left anterior cingulate (ACC; BA 24) seed and with improved affect was comprised of the left amygdala, frontal regions (right orbitofrontal cortex [BA 11], bilateral medial frontal gyrus [BA 10], bilateral middle frontal gyrus [BA 46], bilateral superior frontal gyrus [BA 6], and right inferior frontal gyrus [BA 45]), right ACC (BA 24), the bilateral insula (BA13), and left midbrain. The network of regions that correlated with the right PHG seed and with improved scores in the California Verbal Learning Test (CVLT; sum of the first five trials) and Controlled Oral Word Association Test (COWAT) included the left hippocampus, frontal (bilateral middle frontal gyrus [BA 46], bilateral orbitofrontal cortex [BA 11], and left inferior frontal gyrus [BA 47]), temporal regions (left inferior temporal gyrus [BA 20], bilateral middle temporal gyrus [BA 21], and right superior temporal gyrus [BA 22]), parietal regions (left inferior parietal lobule [BA 40] and right postcentral gyrus [BA 2]), and the bilateral cerebellum. In contrast, the bilateral insula and occipital areas (bilateral lateral occipital gyrus [BA 19], right superior occipital gyrus [BA 39], and right fusiform gyrus [BA 37]) showed increased metabolism and also correlated with improvements in the two cognitive measures. The underlying mechanisms of the midbrain-limbic-frontal affective network may involve interactions between monoaminergic and glutamatergic systems. The regions involved in the medial temporal- parietal-frontal cognitive network

overlap with the regions affected in Alzheimer's dementia and may reflect neuronal vulnerability to a neurodegenerative processes (such as beta-amyloid deposition; Buckner et al., 2005). Thus, an understanding of the cerebral metabolic networks associated with the affective and cognitive responses to antidepressant treatment is critical to the design of future mechanistic studies.

In summary, as shown in Table 34.3, PET cerebral glucose metabolism measures have provided a fundamental understanding of the functional neuroanatomic pathways underlying depressive symptomatology and treatment response. This information is critical to inform the design of studies to evaluate specific neurochemical substrates with molecular imaging methods. As cerebral glucose metabolism in the final common pathway of neurochemical activity, these studies identify the neural circuitry of pathophysiology and treatment response to inform the design of mechanistic studies within the pathways identified.

Molecular Imaging in Depression

The initial application of neurochemical imaging methods to affective disorders was to test the hypothesis of decreased monoaminergic function (norepinephrine, dopamine, and in particular, serotonin; Lapin & Oxenkrug, 1969; Schildkraut, 1965) in depression. The majority of the studies have been performed in midlife depressed patients thus far. Advances in radiotracer chemistry over the last decade have made possible the ability to image neuropathological processes that may be relevant to understanding neurodegenerative and cerebrovascular mechanisms involved in late-life depression. The monoamine imaging data in depression will be reviewed briefly in this section with a focus on the serotonin and dopamine systems. The amyloid imaging data will be reviewed next, followed by a discussion of future directions that is based on new developments in radiotracer chemistry.

THE SEROTONIN SYSTEM

The majority of evidence supports serotonin hypofunction in major depression, based on changes in symptoms with acute pharmacologic interventions of the serotonin system, neuroendocrine challenge studies, and measurements of serotonin metabolites in cerebrospinal fluid and plasma (e.g., Mann, 1999; Owens & Nemeroff, 1998). These studies supported

Table 34.3 Summary of Brain Regions and Observed Corresponding Alterations in Positron Emission Tomography Cerebral Glucose Metabolism Measures in Late-Life Depressed Patients Compared to Controls

LATE-LIFE DEPRESSION	ALTERATIONS IN CEREBRAL GLUCOSE METABOLISM
Resting-state cerebral metabolism	Increased cerebral glucose metabolism in right superior and middle frontal gyrus, left superior (BA 9) and inferior frontal gyrus (BA 45), left precentral gyrus, right middle temporal gyrus (BA 22), right precuneus, left precuneus (BA 7), and inferior parietal lobule (BA 40), left cuneus, and right cerebellum
Cerebral metabolic effects of antidepressant treatment	Decreased cerebral glucose metabolism in bilateral superior (BA 6), medial frontal gyrus (BA 10), left superior and right middle temporal gyrus (BA 22/21), left precuneus (BA 7), right anterior cingulate gyrus (BA 24), bilateral posterior cingulate cortex (BA 31), bilateral parahippocampal gyrus (BA 36), left insula (BA 13), and bilateral amygdale
	Increased cerebral glucose metabolism was observed in the right thalamus (pulvinar and medial dorsal nuclei), dorsal striatum (bilateral putamen), left inferior parietal lobule (BA 40), right cuneus (BA 19), and bilateral cerebellum
Affective network associated with antidepressant response	Decreased cerebral glucose metabolism in a subcortical-limbic-frontal network
Cognitive network associated with antidepressant response	Decreased cerebral glucose metabolism in a medial temporal-parietal-frontal network

PET neuroimaging studies to test this hypothesis directly in depressed patients. Neurochemical imaging studies have evaluated serotonin synthesis, serotonin transporter (5-HTT) binding, the initial target site of action of the SSRIs, as well as 5-HT1A and 5-HT2A binding.

Reduced serotonin synthesis in depression has been observed in several studies. Agren et al. (1991) reported lower uptake of [11C]-5-hydroxytryptophan, a radiolabeled precursor for serotonin synthesis, in depressed patients. Serotonin synthesis as measured by trapping of the radiotracer alpha-[11C] methyl-L-tryptophan was shown to be reduced in anterior cingulate gurus (bilaterally in females, left hemisphere in males) and left medial temporal cortex in unmedicated depressed patients (Rosa-Neto et al., 2004).

Studies have evaluated 5-HTT, 5-HT1A, and 5-HT2A binding in midlife unipolar and bipolar depressed patients. Increased 5-HTT (Cannon et al., 2006, 2007), decreased 5-HTT (Oquendo et al., 2007; Parsey et al., 2006; Reimold et al., 2008),

or no difference in 5-HTT has been reported in unmedicated, recovered, or currently depressed patients (Bhagwagar et al., 2007; Meyer et al., 2004). While the direction of the results across studies is different, the regions implicated are remarkably consistent (e.g., cingulate gyrus, frontal cortex, insula, thalamus, and striatum). The factors that may contribute to differences across studies include differences in sample characteristics or the radiotracers used ([11C]-DASB versus [11C]-McN5652). Preliminary studies in two samples of late-life depressed patients show decreased 5-HTT relative to controls in the anterior cingulate (BA 24), middle temporal gyrus, parahippocampal gyrus, amygdala, caudate, and thalamus (Smith et al., unpublished data). Two studies have reported that higher baseline 5-HTT binding predicted remission to acute fluoxetine treatment, as well as remission at 1 year (Kuyagaya et al., 2004; Miller, Oquendo, Ogden, Mann, & Parsey, 2008).

5-HTT occupancy by SSRIs has been evaluated in midlife and late-life depressed patients. Studies in midlife depressed patients treated for 4 weeks with either paroxetine or citalopram have reported significant 5-HTT occupancy in caudate, putamen, thalamus, in addition to prefrontal and anterior cingulate cortices. The magnitude occupancy for both compounds was similar (ranging from 65% to 87% across regions; Meyer et al., 2001). The magnitude of occupancy and the relationship between brain occupancy and plasma concentrations is consistent with that observed in elderly depressed patients treated with the citalopram at steady-state doses (Smith et al., 2011a). Significant overlap between regions of 5-HTT occupancy that were correlated with improvement in depressive symptoms and regions of cerebral metabolic alterations by citalopram was observed (e.g., anterior cingulate gyrus, middle frontal gyrus, precuneus, inferior parietal lobule, cuneus; Diaconescu et al., 2011; Smith et al., 2008). Importantly, positive correlations were observed between the improvement in depressive symptoms and 5-HTT occupancy in the anterior cingulate gyrus (bilaterally), left middle and inferior frontal gyrus, right superior and middle temporal gyrus, right precuneus, left inferior parietal lobule, parahippocampal gyrus (bilaterally), and left cuneus. The findings suggest that cortical and limbic SERT occupancy may be an underlying mechanism for the regional cerebral metabolic effects of citalopram in late-life depression. Furthermore, 5-HTT occupancy in cortical and limbic regions is associated with treatment response, a finding that has not yet been reported in mid-life depressed patients.

Studies of the 5-HT1A receptor have either shown decreased (Drevets et al., 1999; Hirvonen et al., 2007; Sargent et al., 2000) or increased (Parsey et al., 2006a) binding. A correlation between higher baseline 5-HT1A binding and poorer treatment response has been reported (Moses-Kolko et al., 2007; Parsey et al., 2006b). The one study of late-life depressed patients observed decreased 5-HT1A binding in the dorsal raphe, as well as in the middle temporal cortex and hippocampus (Meltzer et al., 2004). Alterations in 5-HT1A binding following SSRI treatment have not been observed in human neuroimaging studies (Moses-Kolko et al., 2007; Sargent et al., 2000), a finding that is not expected based on animal studies showing 5-HT1A desensitization induced by SSRI treatment (Blier et al., 1986). One of the explanations for the lack of an observed effect is that the 5-HT1A antagonist radiotracers bind to low-affinity sites, whereas the change with treatment may be observed in high-affinity sites.

To test this hypothesis, a promising 5-HT1A agonist radiotracer has been developed (Milak et al., 2008). 5-HT2A receptor binding has reported to be unchanged in both midlife and late-life depressed patients (Meltzer et al., 1999; Meyer et al., 2001), decreased in orbitofrontal cortex in one report (Biver et al., 1997), or increased (Bhagwagar et al., 2006; Meyer et al., 1999b). Treatment studies have shown either a decrease (Meyer et al., 2001b; Yatham et al., 1999) or increase in 5-HT2A binding (Massou et al., 1997; Moresco et al., 2000). The discrepancy between studies may be due to differences in antidepressant drugs or radiotracers used. At the present time, there are no published studies on the effects of antidepressant treatment on the 5-HT1A or 5-HT2A receptors in late-life depression.

THE DOPAMINE SYSTEM

Several lines of evidence support dopamine hypofunction in midlife depression (Brown & Gershon, 1993; Nestler & Carlezon, 2006). The data include improvement in depressive symptoms with dopamine agonists, the induction of a depressive relapse by pharmacologic depletion of dopamine, and low cerebrospinal fluid homovanillic acid levels in depressed patients compared to controls. The available imaging data suggest modest decreases or no change in dopamine metabolism, dopamine transporter, and D1 and D2 receptor binding (Agren & Reibring, 1994; Meyer et al., 2001a; Suhara et al., 1992). Dopamine transporter binding was reduced in depressed patients relative to controls (Meyer et al., 2001). Several studies of striatal and extrastriatal D2 receptor availability have not shown differences between patients and controls, including studies in medication naive patients (Hirvonen et al., 2008; Klimke et al., 1999; Montgomery et al., 2007; Parsey et al., 2001). Greater psychomotor slowing has been associated with increased striatal D2 receptor binding, indicating that perhaps differences may be observed in subgroups of depressed patients (Meyer et al., 2006). With respect to the D1 receptor, decreased binding was observed in the left middle caudate in one report (Cannon et al., 2008). In addition, no differences in amphetamine-induced striatal dopamine release have been observed in either euthymic bipolar patients or patients with unipolar depression (Anand et al., 2000; Parsey et al., 2001). Several lines of evidence suggest that dopamine dysfunction may play a more prominent role in late-life depression. A substantial age-related decline in dopamine transporters and receptors is observed (Volkow et al., 1998a, 1998b). Furthermore, the evidence for the augmentation of the antidepressant response by psychostimulants (such as methylphenidate; Lavretsky & Kumar, 2001; Volkow et al., 1998a, 1998b) supports the further investigation of the dopamine system in late-life depression. A better understanding of the nature of the dopaminergic deficits in late-life depression would lead to targeted treatments that would potentially be more effective.

Beta-Amyloid Imaging

The development of radiotracers to image beta-amyloid deposition, one of the pathological hallmarks of AD (in addition to hyperphosphorylated tau), represents a significant advance in neuroimaging studies of neurodegenerative disease. Several PET radiotracers for beta amyloid have been evaluated in human subjects and show good diagnostic sensitivity between normals, MCI, and AD ([18F]-FDDNP, [11C]-SB13, [11C]-PIB; Forsberg et al., 2008; Klunk et al., 2004; Pike et al., 2008; Rowe et al., 2007; Shoghi-Jadid et al., 2002; Small et al., 2006; Verhoeff et al., 2004). [11C]-PIB is the best characterized and most commonly used radiotracer [11C]-PIB has a high binding affinity and specificity to amyloid in AD brain (Ikonomovic et al., 2008; Klunk et al., 2003; Mathis et al., 2003). It is important to note that the radiotracer [18F]-FDDNP binds to other aspects of AD pathology in addition to beta-amyloid, including tau (Shoghi-Jadid et al., 2002). Several lines of evidence suggest that beta-amyloid imaging measures are sensitive to subtle cognitive impairment and may predict subsequent cognitive decline. Higher cortical beta-amyloid concentrations is associated with cognitive impairment in healthy controls, as well as cognitive impairment and cognitive decline in subjects with mild cognitive impairment (Forsberg et al., 2008; Kemppainen et al., 2007; Pike et al., 2007; Villemagne, 2008).

The initial study of beta-amyloid deposition in late-life depression was recently published (Butters et al., 2008). Late-life depressed patients who met criteria for amnestic MCI demonstrated greater binding than those with nonamnestic MCI and subjects who were cognitively normal. These results are consistent with that of nondepressed subjects with cognitive impairment. In a study of late-life depressed patients who do not meet criteria for MCI,

greater beta-amyloid deposition relative to controls was observed in the anterior cingulate gyrus, superior and middle frontal gyrus, left orbitofrontal gyrus, precuneus bilateral insula, and left parahippocampal gyrus (Marano et al., 2010). Interestingly, in patients with MCI and cognitively normal controls, greater depression and anxiety symptoms were associated with higher [18F]-FDDNP binding (Lavretsky et al., 2009). These studies suggest that depressive symptoms in normal control subjects and depressed patients without cognitive impairment may be associated with AD neuropathology. Furthermore, beta-amyloid deposition may underlie the cognitive impairment that persists after mood symptom remission in late-life depression.

SUMMARY AND FUTURE DIRECTIONS OF POSITRON EMISSION TOMOGRAPHY FINDINGS ON MOOD DISORDERS

PET studies in late-life depression have focused on elucidating the functional neuroanatomy and neural circuitry associated with treatment response. The studies using radiotracers for specific neurotransmitters or neuropathological processes are limited. The serotonin and dopamine systems have been the major focus of neurochemical imaging studies in depression; the majority of studies have been performed in younger patients. Recent studies have focused on imaging beta-amyloid deposition in late-life depression as a mechanism underlying cognitive impairment that might be related to the increased risk of Alzheimer's disease in depressed patients. There are several other potentially relevant molecular targets for which radiotracers are in development and/or promising new radiotracers are available. With respect to other monoaminergic targets, radiotracers for other serotonin receptor sites are being evaluated that may elucidate the role of serotonin in affective and cognitive symptoms, including 5-HT1b (Pierson et al., 2008), 5-HT4 (Comley, 2006), and 5-HT6 (Parker, 2008) receptors. The development of radiotracers for the noradrenergic system has been challenging due to the lack of pharmacologically selective agent and the low signal to noise levels of binding in the brain. Recently developed radiotracers for the norepinephrine transporter have been developed and look promising (Ding, 2010). The reports of rapid antidepressant effects of ketamine and scopolamine have renewed interested in the glutamatergic and muscarinic systems (Furey & Drevets, 2006; Mathew, Manji, & Charney, 2008). These systems may be especially relevant to cognitive impairment in late-life depression and may represent a pathophysiological link to Alzheimer's disease (Ondrejcak et al., 2010). Finally, inflammation may be a common underlying mechanism for depression and neurodegeneration, and it may be more relevant to late-life depression given the increasing medical comorbidity in late life (as reviewed by Miller et al., 2009; Smith, Gunning-Dixon, Lotrich, Taylorm, & Evans, 2007). A recent focus in radiotracer chemistry is the development of is peripheral benzodiazepine radiotracers that bind with high affinity to translocator protein. Translocator protein is upregulated in activated microglia and represents a marker of neuroinflammation. A number of radiotracers have been developed and evaluated and applied to neurodegenerative diseases, including Alzheimer's disease (as reviewed by Chauveau et al., 2008). Thus, future studies can test hypotheses using these recently developed radiotracers and mechanisms identified to understand the neurobiology of treatment resistance and of cognitive impairment in both unipolar and bipolar depression. The use of molecular imaging to understand the mechanisms underlying the increased risk of dementia associated with depression is critical to developing strategies for prevention and intervention.

Disclosures

Neither Aizenstein nor Patel have any disclosures to note.

REFERENCES

Adleman , N. E., Menon, V., Blasey, C. M., White, C. D., Warsofsky, I. S., Glover, G. H., & Reiss, A. L. (2002). A developmental fMRI study of the Stroop color-word task. *NeuroImage*, *16*, 61–75.

Agren, H., & Reibring, L. (1994). PET studies of presynaptic monoamine metabolism in depressed patients and healthy volunteers. *Pharmacopsychiatry*, *27*, 2–6.

Agren H., Reibring L., Hartvig P., Tedroff, J., Bjurling, P., Hörnfeldt, K., ... Långström, B. (1991). Low brain uptake of L-[11C]5-hydroxytryptophan in major depression: A positron emission tomography study on patients and healthy volunteers. *Acta Psychiatrica Scandinavica*, *83*, 449–455.

Aizenstein, H. J., Butters, M. A., Figurski, J. L., Stenger, V. A., Reynolds, C. F., III, & Carter, C. S. (2005). Prefrontal and striatal activation during sequence learning in geriatric depression. *Biological Psychiatry*, *58*, 290–296.

Aizenstein, H. J., Butters, M. A., Wu, M., Mazurkewicz, L. M., Stenger, V. A., Gianaros, P. J., ... Carter, C. S. (2009). Altered functioning of the executive control circuit in late-life depression: Episodic and persistent phenomena. *American Journal of Geriatric Psychiatry*, *17*(1), 30–42.

Almeida, J. R., Mechelli, A., Hassel, S., Versace, A., Kupfer, D. J., & Phillips, M. L. (2009). Abnormally increased effective connectivity between parahippocampal gyrus and ventromedial prefrontal regions during emotion labeling in bipolar disorder. *Psychiatry Research: Neuroimaging*, *174*, 195–201.

Anand, A., Verhoeff, P., Seneca, N., Zoghbi, S. S., Seibyl, J. P., Charney, D. S., & Innis, R. B. (2000). Brain SPECT imaging of amphetamine-induced dopamine release in euthymic bipolar disorder patients. *American Journal of Psychiatry*, *157*, 1108–1114.

Andreescu, C., Butters, M., Lenze, E. J., Venkatraman, V. K., Nable, M., Reynolds, C. F., III, & Aizenstein, H. J. (2009). fMRI activation in late-life anxious depression: a potential biomarker. *International Journal of Geriatric Psychiatry*, *24*, 820–828.

Andreescu, C., Wu, M., Figurski, J., Figurski, J., Reynolds, C. F., III, & Aizenstein, H. J. (2011). The default mode network in late-life anxious depression. *American Journal of Geriatric Psychiatry*, *19*(11), 980–983.

Arnett, C. D., Wolf, A. P., Shiue, C. Y., Fowler, J. S., MacGregor, R. R., Christman, D. R., & Smith, M. R. (1986). Improved delineation of human dopamine receptors using [18F]-N-methylspiroperidol and PET. *Journal of Nuclear Medicine*, *27*(12), 1878–1882

Bailey, D., Townsend, D., Valk, P., & Maisey, M. (Eds.). (2005). *Positron emission tomography: Basic sciences*. New York: Springer.

Bhagwagar Z., Hinz R., Taylor M., Fancy, S., Cowen, P., & Grasby, P. (2006). Increased 5-HT(2A) receptor binding in euthymic, medication-free patients recovered from depression: A positron emission study with [(11)C]MDL 100,907. *American Journal of Psychiatry*, *163*, 1580–1587.

Bhagwagar Z., Murthy N., Selvaraj S., Hinz, R., Taylor, M., Fancy, S., ... Cowen, P. (2007). 5-HTT binding in recovered depressed patients and healthy volunteers: A positron emission tomography study with [11C]DASB. *American Journal of Psychiatry*, *164*, 1858–1865.

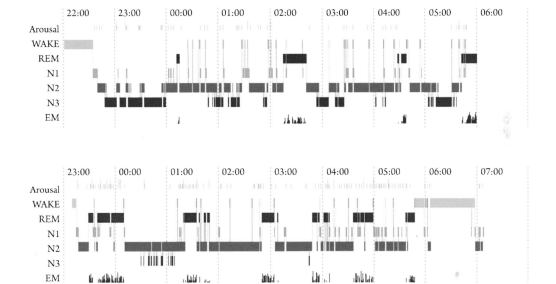

FIGURE 20.1. Comparison of the polysomnographic sleep profile of a healthy good sleeper (upper panel) and a severely depressed patient (lower panel). REM: rapid eye movements sleep; N1: NREM sleep, stage 1; N2: NREM sleep, stage 2; N3: NREM sleep, deep sleep; EM: eye movements.

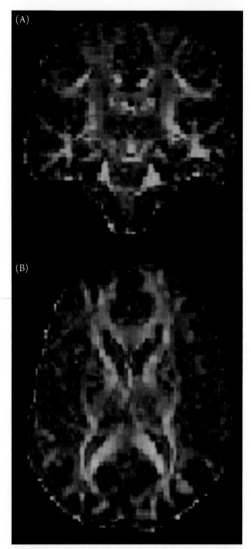

FIGURE 32.2 Coronal (A) and axial (B) views of a color coded DTI fractional anisotropy (FA) image map. Notice signal intensity varies according to FA, and color coding according to the directionality of the principal eigenvector, with red being left-to-right, blue being inferior-to-superior and green anterior-to-posterior.

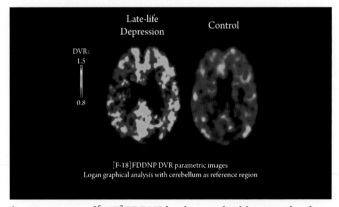

FIGURE 33.1 Visual representation of [18F]FDDNP binding in a healthy control and patient with MDD.

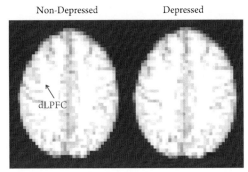

Non-Depressed   Depressed

FIGURE 34.1 Hypoactivation (p < 0.01, K = 8) of the dorsolateral prefrontal cortex (dLPFC) in observed in depressed patients during a Preparing to Overcome Prepotency (POP) task—an executive task derived from the switching Stroop task (Aizenstein et al., 2009).

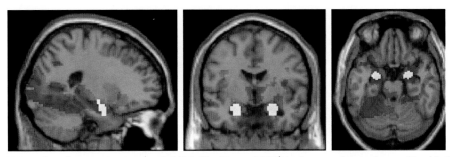

FIGURE 34.2 Significant activation (t > 2.6618, df = 59, p < 0.005) in the amygdala is observed in elderly subjects (depressed + non depressed combined) during an emotional faces affective task. Regions of significant activation are in red (brighter = greater significance) and the amygdala is highlighted in yellow (Aizenstein et al., 2011).

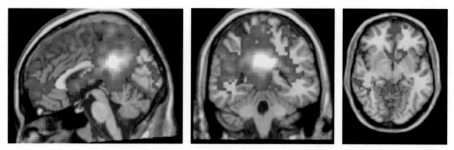

FIGURE 34.3 Resting state functional connectivity maps showing significant activation (corrected p < 0.001) in the default mode network observed in non-depressed elderly subjects. Regions with greatest to least significant activation are scaled from yellow to dark orange respectively (Wu et al., 2011).

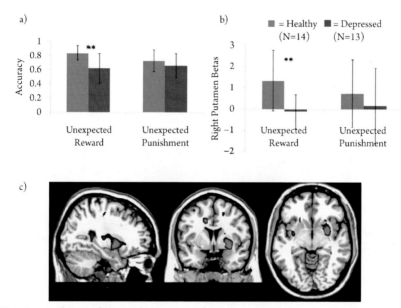

FIGURE 35.1 Impaired Reward Reversal Learning and Attenuated Right Putamen Response to Unexpected Reward in Depressed Individuals Relative to Healthy Comparison Subjects.
As shown in panel A, accuracy is lower on reward ($F = 11.7$, df = 1, 25, $p = 0.002$) but not punishment reversals in depressed individuals relative to healthy individuals. Panel B shows attenuated right (anatomically defined) putamen response during reward reversal trials in depressed individuals relative to healthy individuals ($F = 10.5$, df = 1, 25, $p = 0.003$) but equivalent response during punishment reversal. Error bars indicate standard deviations. In panel C, whole brain analysis confirms that the peak neural response difference between depressed and healthy individuals on reward reversal trials was the right anteroventral putamen (peak voxel $x = 30$, $y = 3$, $z = -8$; image shows SPM t scores ranging from 2.1 to 4.1) (taken by permission from Robinson, Cools, et al., 2012).

Biver F., Wikler D., Lotstra F., Damhaut, P., Goldman, S., & Mendlewicz, J. (1997). Serotonin 5-HT2 receptor imaging in major depression: Focal changes in orbito-insular cortex. *British Journal of Psychiatry, 171*, 444–448.

Blier, P., De Montigny, C., & Azzaro, A. J. (1986). Modification of serotonergic and noradrenergic neurotransmissions by repeated administration of monoamine oxidase inhibitors: Electrophysiological studies in the rat central nervous system. *Journal of Pharmacology and Experimental Therapies, 237*, 987–994.

Blumberg, H. P., Leung, H., Skudlarski, P., Lacadie, C. M., Fredericks, C. A., Harris, B. C.,… Peterson BS. (2003). A functional magnetic resonance imaging study of bipolar disorder. *Archives of General Psychiatry, 60*, 601–609.

Bobb, D. S., Jr., Adinoff, B., Laken S. J., McClintock, S. M., Rubia, K., Huang, H. W.,… Kozel, F. A. (2011). Neural correlates of successful response inhibition in unmedicated patients with late-life depression. *American Journal of Geriatric Psychiatry*, 2011 Oct 12, ePub ahead of print.

Brassen, S., Kalisch, R., Weber-Fahr, W., Braus, D. F., & Büchel, C. (2008). Ventromedial prefrontal cortex processing during emotional evaluation in late-life depression: A longitudinal functional magnetic resonance imaging study. *Biological Psychiatry, 64*, 349–355.

Brown, A. S., & Gershon, S. (1993). Dopamine and depression. *Journal of Neural Transmission, 91*, 75–109.

Bryan, J., Luszcz, M. A., & Pointer, S. (1999). Executive function and processing resources as predictors of adult age differences in the implementation of encoding strategies. *Aging, Neuropsychology, and Cognition, 6*(4), 273–287.

Buckner, R. L., Andrews-Hanna, J. R., & Schacter, D. L. (2008). The brain's default network: Anatomy, function, and relevance to disease. *Annals of the New York Academy of Sciences, 1124*, 1–38.

Buckner, R. L., Snyder, A. Z., Shannon, B. J., LaRossa, G., Sachs, R., Fotenos, A. F.,… Mintun, M. A. (2005). Molecular, structural, and functional characterization of Alzheimer's disease: Evidence for a relationship between default activity, amyloid, and memory. *Journal of Neuroscience, 25*, 7709–7717.

Butters, M. A., Klunk, W. E., Mathis, C. A., Price, J. C., Ziolko, S. K., Hoge, J. A.,… Meltzer, C. C. (2008). Imaging Alzheimer pathology in late-life depression with PET and Pittsburgh compound-B. *Alzheimer's Disease and Associated Disorders, 22*, 261–268.

Cannon, D. M., Ichise, M., Fromm, S. J., Nugent, A. C., Rollis, D., Gandhi, S. K.,… Drevets, W. C. (2006). Serotonin transporter binding in bipolar disorder assessed using [11C]DASB and positron emission tomography. *Biological Psychiatry, 60*, 207–217.

Cannon, D. M., Ichise, M., Rollis, D., Klaver, J. M., Gandhi, S. K., Charney, D. S.,… Drevets, W. C. (2007). Elevated serotonin transporter binding in major depressive disorder assessed using positron emission tomography and [11C]DASB; comparison with bipolar disorder. *Biological Psychiatry, 62*, 870–877.

Cannon, D. M., Klaver, J. M., Peck, S. A., Rallis-Voak, D., Erickson, K., & Drevets, W. C. (2009). Dopamine type-1 receptor binding in major depressive disorder assessed using positron emission tomography and [11C]NNC-112. *Neuropsychopharmacology, 34*, 1277–1287.

Chauveau F., Boutin H., Van Camp N., Dollé, F., & Tavitian, B. (2008). Nuclear imaging of neuroinflammation: A comprehensive review of [(11)C]PK11195 challengers. *European Journal of Nuclear Medicine and Molecular Imaging, 35*, 2304–2319.

Comley, R., Parker, C., Wishart, M ., (2006). In vivo evaluation and quantification of the 5-HT4 receptor PET ligand [11C]SB-207145. *Neuroimage, 31*, T23.

Chepenik, L. G., Raffo, M., Hampson, M., Lacadie, C., Wang, F., Jones, M. M.,… Blumberg, H. P. (2010). Functional connectivity between ventral prefrontal cortex and amygdala at low frequency in the resting state in bipolar disorder. *Psychiatry Research: Neuroimaging, 182*, 207–210.

Davidson, R. J., Pizzagalli, D., Nitschke, J. B., & Putnam, K. (2002). DEPRESSION: Perspectives from affective neuroscience. *Annual Review of Psychology, 53*, 545–574.

Detre, J. A., Leigh, J. S., Williams, D. S., &Koretsky, A. P. (1992). Perfusion imaging. *Magnetic Resonance in Medicine, 23*, 37–45.

Diaconescu, A. O., Kramer, E., Hermann, C., (2011). Distinct functional networks associated with improvement of affective symptoms and cognitive function during citalopram treatment in geriatric depression. *Human Brain Mapping, 32*(10), 1677–1691.

DiGirolamo, G. J., Kramer, A. F., Barad, V., Cepeda, N. J., Weissman, D. H., Milham, M. P.,… McAuley, E. (2001). General and task-speci°c frontal lobe recruitment in older adults during executive processes: A fMRI investigation of task-switching. *NeuroReport, 12*, 2065–2071.

Ding, Y. S., Singhal, T., Planeta-Wilson, B., Gallezot, J. D., Nabulsi, N., Labaree, D.,… Malison, R. T. (2010). PET imaging of the effects of age and cocaine on the norepinephrine transporter in the human brain using (S,S)-[(11)C] O-methylreboxetine and HRRT. *Synapse, 64*(1), 30–38.

Dove, A., Pollmann, S., Schubert, T., Wiggins, C. J., & von Cramon, D. Y. (2000). Prefrontal cortex activation in task switching: An event-related fMRI Study. *Cognitive Brain Research, 9,* 103–109.

Drevets, W.C., Frank, E., Price, J.C., Kupfer, D. J., Holt, D., Greer, P. J.,… Mathis, C. (1999). PET imaging of serotonin 1A receptor binding in depression. *Biological Psychiatry, 46,* 1375–1387.

Endres, C. J., Pomper, M. G., James, M., Uzuner, O., Hammoud, D. A., Watkins, C. C.,… Kassiou, M. (2009). Initial evaluation of 11C-DPA-713, a novel TSPO PET ligand, in humans. *Journal of Nuclear Medicine, 50,* 1276–1282.

Fitzgerald, P. B., Laird, A. R., Maller, J., & Daskalakis, Z. J. (2008). A meta-analytic study of changes in brain activation in depression. *Human Brain Mapping, 29,* 683–695.

Forsberg, A., Engler, H., Almkvist, O., Blomquist, G., Hagman, G., Wall, A.,… Nordberg, A. (2008). PET imaging of amyloid deposition in patients with mild cognitive impairment. *Neurobiology of Aging, 29,* 1456–1465.

Furey, M. L., & Drevets, W. C. (2006). Antidepressant efficacy of the antimuscarinic drug scopolamine: A randomized, placebo-controlled clinical trial. *Archives of General Psychiatry, 63,* 1121–1129.

Hirvonen, J., Karlsson, H., Kajander, J., Markkula, J., Rasi-Hakala, H., Någren, K.,… Hietala, J. (2008). Striatal dopamine D2 receptors in medication-naïve patients with major depressive disorder as assessed with [11C]raclopride PET. *Psychopharmacology (Berlin), 197,* 581–590.

Ikonomovic, M. D., Klunk, W. E., Abrahamson, E. E., Mathis, C. A., Price, J. C., Tsopelas, N. D.,… DeKosky, S. T. (2008). Post-mortem correlates of in vivo PIB-PET amyloid imaging in a typical case of Alzheimer's disease. *Brain, 131,* 1630–1645.

Kemppainen, N. M., Aalto, S., Wilson, I. A., Någren, K., Helin, S., Brück, A.,… Rinne, J. O. (2007). PET amyloid ligand [11C]PIB uptake is increased in mild cognitive impairment. *Neurology, 68,* 1603–1606.

Klimke A., Larisch R., Janz A., Vosberg, H., Müller-Gärtner, H. W., & Gaebel, W. (1999). Dopamine D2 receptor binding before and after treatment of major depression measured by [123I] IBZM SPECT. *Psychiatry Research, 90,* 91–101.

Klunk, W. E., Engler, H., Nordberg, A., Wang, Y., Blomqvist, G., Holt, D. P.,… Långström, B. (2004). Imaging brain amyloid in Alzheimer's

disease with Pittsburgh compound-B. *Annals of Neurology, 55,* 306–319.

Kugaya , A., Sanacora, G., Staley, J. K., Malison, R. T., Bozkurt, A., Khan, S.,… Innis, R. B. (2004). Brain serotonin transporter availability predicts treatment response to selective serotonin reuptake inhibitors. *Biological Psychiatry, 56,* 497–502.

Kumar, A., Newberg, A., Alavi, A., Berlin, J., Smith, R., & Reivich, M. (1993). Regional cerebral glucose metabolism in late-life depression and Alzheimer disease: A preliminary positron emission tomography study. *Proceedings of the National Academy of Sciences USA, 90,* 7019–7023.

Lapin, I. P., & Oxenkrug, G. F. (1969). Intensification of the central serotonergic processes as a possible determinant of the thymoleptic effect. *Lancet, 1,* 132–136.

Lavretsky, H., & Kumar, A. (2001). Methylphenidate augmentation of citalopram in elderly depressed patients. *American Journal of Geriatric Psychiatry, 9,* 298–303.

Lavretsky, H., Siddarth, P., Kepe, V., Ercoli, L. M., Miller, K. J., Burggren, A. C.,… Small, G. W. (2009). Depression and anxiety symptoms are associated with cerebral FDDNP-PET binding in middle-aged and older nondemented adults. *American Journal of Geriatric Psychiatry, 17,* 493–502.

Mann, J. J. (1999). Role of the serotonergic system in the pathogenesis of major depression and suicidal behavior. *Neuropsychopharmacology, 21*(Suppl 2), 99S–105S.

Marano, C., Workman, C., Zhou, Y., (2010, MONTH) *Cortical beta-amyloid deposition in late-life depression.* Paper presented at the American College of Neuropsychopharmacology 49th Annual Meeting, Miami, FL.

Mathew, S. J., Manji, H. K., & Charney, D. S. (2008). Novel drugs and therapeutic targets for severe mood disorders. *Neuropsychopharmacology, 33,* 2080–2092.

Mathis, C. A., Wang, Y., Holt, D. P., Huang, G. F., Debnath, M. L., & Klunk, W. E. (2003). Synthesis and evaluation of 11C-labeled 6-substituted 2-arylbenzothiazoles as amyloid imaging agents. *Journal of Medical Chemistry, 46,* 2740–2754.

Massou, J. M., Trichard, C., Attar-Levy, D., Feline, A., Corruble, E., Beaufils, B., & Martinot, J. L. (1997). Frontal 5-HT2A receptors studied in depressive patients during chronic treatment by selective serotonin reuptake inhibitors. *Psychopharmacology, 133,* 99–101.

Meltzer, C. C., Price, J. C., Mathis, C. A., Greer, P. J., Cantwell, M. N., Houck, P. R.,… Reynolds, C. F., III. (1999). PET imaging of serotonin type 2A receptors in late-life neuropsychiatric disorders. *American Journal of Psychiatry, 156,* 1871–1878.

Meltzer, C. C., Price, J. C., Mathis, C. A., Butters, M. A., Ziolko, S. K., Moses-Kolko, E.,... Reynolds, C. F. (2004). Serotonin 1A receptor binding and treatment response in late-life depression. *Neuropsychopharmacology, 29,* 2258–2265.

Mayberg, H. S. (2003). Modulating dysfunctional limbic-cortical circuits in depression: Towards development of brain-based algorithms for diagnosis and optimised treatment. *British Medical Bulletin, 65,* 193–207.

Mayberg, H. S. (2009). Targeted electrode-based modulation of neural circuits for depression. *Journal of Clinical Investigations, 119*(4), 717–725.

Meyer, J. H., Houle, S., Sagrati, S., Carella, A., Hussey, D. F., Ginovart, N.,... Wilson, A. A. (2004). Brain serotonin transporter binding potential measured with carbon 11-labeled DASB positron emission tomography: Effects of major depressive episodes and severity of dysfunctional attitudes. *Archives of General Psychiatry, 61,* 1271–1279.

Meyer , J. H., Kapur, S., Houle, S., DaSilva, J., Owczarek, B., Brown, G. M.,... Kennedy, S. H. (1999). Prefrontal cortex 5-HT2 receptors in depression: An [18F] setoperone PET imaging study. *American Journal of Psychiatry, 156,* 1029–1034.

Meyer, J. H., Kapur, S., Eisfeld, B., Brown, G. M., Houle, S., DaSilva, J.,... Kennedy, S. H. (2001). The effect of paroxetine on 5-HT2A receptors in depression: An [18F] setoperone PET imaging study. *American Journal of Psychiatry, 158,* 78–85.

Meyer, J. H., Krüeger, S., Wilson, A. A., Christensen, B. K., Goulding, V. S., Schaffer, A.,... Kennedy, S. H. (2001). Lower dopamine transporters binding potential in striatum during depression. *Neuroreport, 12,* 4121–4125.

Meyer, J. H., McNeely, H. E., Sagrati, S., Boovariwala, A., Martin, K., Verhoeff, N. P.,... Houle, S. (2006). Elevated putamen D(2) receptor binding potential in major depression with motor retardation: An [11C]raclopride positron emission tomography study. *American Journal of Psychiatry, 163,* 1594–1602.

Meyer, J. H., Wilson, A. A., Ginovart, N., Goulding, V., Hussey, D., Hood, K., & Houle, S. (2001). Occupancy of SERTs by paroxetine and citalopram during treatment of depression: A [(11)C]DASB PET imaging study. *American Journal of Psychiatry, 158* (11), 1843–1849.

Milak, M. S., Severance, A. J., Ogden, R. T., Prabhakaran, J., Kumar, J. S., Majo, V. J.,... Parsey, R. V. (2008). Modeling considerations for 11C-CUMI-101, an agonist radiotracer for

imaging serotonin 1A receptor in vivo with PET. *Journal of Nuclear Medicine, 49,* 587–596.

Miller, J. M., Oquendo, M. A., Ogden, R. T., Mann, J. J., & Parsey, R. V. (2008). Serotonin transporter binding as a possible predictor of one-year remission in major depressive disorder. *Journal of Psychiatric Research, 42,* 1137–1144.

Moresco, R. M., Colombo, C., Fazio, F., Bonfanti, A., Lucignani, G., Messa, C.,... Smeraldi, E. (2000). Effects of fluvoxamine treatment on the in vivo binding of [F-18]FESP in drug naive depressed patients: A PET study. *Neuroimage, 12,* 452–465.

Moses-Kolko, E. L., Price, J. C., Thase, M. E., Meltzer, C. C., Kupfer, D. J., Mathis, C. A.,... Drevets, W. C. (2007). Measurement of 5-HT1A receptor binding in depressed adults before and after antidepressant drug treatment using positron emission tomography and [11C]WAY-100635. *Synapse, 61,* 523–530.

Nestler, E. J., & Carlezon, W. A., Jr. (2006). The mesolimbic dopamine reward circuit in depression. *Biological Psychiatry, 59,* 1151–1159.

Nobler, M. S., Mann, J. J., & Sackeim, H. A. (1999). Serotonin, cerebral blood flow, and cerebral metabolic rate in geriatric major depression and normal aging. *Brain Research, 30,* 250–263.

Nobler, M. S., Roose, S. P., Prohovnik, I., Moeller, J. R., Louie, J., Van Heertum, R. L., & Sackeim, H. A. (2000). Regional cerebral blood flow in mood disorders, V: Effects of antidepressant medication in late-life depression. *American Journal of Geriatric Psychiatry, 8,* 289–296.

Ondrejcak, T., Klyubin, I., Hu, N. W., Barry, A. E., Cullen, W. K., & Rowan, M. J. (2010). Alzheimer's disease amyloid beta-protein and synaptic function. *Neuromolecular Medicine, 12*(1), 13–26.

Oquendo, M. A., Hastings, R. S., Huang, Y. Y., Simpson, N., Ogden, R. T., Hu, X. Z.,... Parsey, R. V. (2007). Brain serotonin transporter binding in depressed patients with bipolar disorder using positron emission tomography. *Archives of General Psychiatry, 64,* 201–208.

Ogawa, S., Lee, T-M., Nayak, A. S., & Glynn, P. (1990). Oxygenation-sensitive contrast in magnetic resonance image of rodent brain at high magnetic fields. *Magnetic Resonance Medicine, 14,* 68–78.

Parker, C. A., Cunningham, V. J., Martarello, L., (2008). Evaluation of the novel 5-HT6 receptor radioligand, [11C] GSK-215083 in human. *Neuroimage, 41,* T20.

Parsey, R. V., Hastings, R. S., Oquendo, M. A., Huang, Y. Y., Simpson, N., Arcement, J.,... Mann, J. J. (2006). Lower serotonin transporter binding potential in the human brain during major depressive episodes. *American Journal of Psychiatry,* *163,* 52–58.

Parsey, R. V., Olvet, D. M., Oquendo, M. A., Huang, Y. Y., Ogden, R. T., & Mann, J. J. (2006). Higher 5-HT1A receptor binding potential during a major depressive episode predicts poor treatment response: Preliminary data from a naturalistic study. *Neuropsychopharmacology, 31,* 1745–1749.

Parsey, R. V., Oquendo, M. A., Zea-Ponce, Y., Rodenhiser, J., Kegeles, L. S., Pratap, M., . . . Laruelle, M. (2001). Dopamine D(2) receptor availability and amphetamine-induced dopamine release in unipolar depression. *Biological Psychiatry, 50,* 313–322.

Pierson, M. E., Andersson, J., Nyberg, S., McCarthy, D. J., Finnema, S. J., Varnäs, K., . . . Halldin, C. (2008). [11C]AZ10419369: a selective 5-HT1B receptor radioligand suitable for positron emission tomography (PET): Characterization in the primate brain. *Neuroimage, 41,* 1075–1085.

Phelps, M. (Ed.). (2006). *PET: Physics, instrumentation, and scanners.* New York: Springer.

Phelps, M., Mazziota, J., & Schelbert, H. (Eds.). (1986). *Positron emission tomography and autoradiography: Principles and applications for the brain and heart.* San Diego, CA: Raven Press.

Pike, K. E., Savage, G., Villemagne, V. L., Ng, S., Moss, S. A., Maruff, P., . . . Rowe, C. C. (2007). Beta-amyloid imaging and memory in non-demented individuals: Evidence for preclinical Alzheimer's disease. *Brain, 130,* 2837–2844.

Reimold, M., Batra, A., Knobel, A., Smolka, M. N., Zimmer, A., Mann, K., . . . Heinz, A. (2008). Anxiety is associated with reduced central serotonin transporter availability in unmedicated patients with unipolar major depression: A [11C] DASB PET study. *Molecular Psychiatry, 13,* 606–613.

Rosa-Neto, P., Diksic, M., Okazawa, H., Leyton, M., Ghadirian, N., Mzengeza, S., . . . Benkelfat, C. (2004). Measurement of brain regional alpha-[11C]methyl-L-tryptophan trapping as a measure of serotonin synthesis in medication-free patients with major depression. *Archives of General Psychiatry, 61,* 556–563.

Roth, R. M., Koven, N. S., Randolph, J. J., Flashman, L. A., Pixley, H. S., Ricketts, S. M., . . . Saykin, A. J. (2006). Functional magnetic resonance imaging of executive control in bipolar disorder. *NeuroReport, 17,* 1085–1089.

Rowe, C.C., Ng, S., Ackermann, U., Gong, S. J., Pike, K., Savage, G., . . . Villemagne, V. L. (2007). Imaging beta-amyloid burden in aging and dementia. *Neurology, 68,* 1718–1725.

Sacher , J., & Smith,G. (2011). Molecular imaging of depression. In B. Turetsky & M. Shenton (Eds.), *Imaging neuropsychiatric disorders* (pp. 170–196). New York: Cambridge University Press.

Sargent, P. A., Kjaer, K. H., Bench, C. J., Rabiner, E. A., Messa, C., Meyer, J., . . . Cowen, P. J. (2000). Brain serotonin 1A receptor binding measured by positron emission tomography with [11C]WAY-100635: Effects of depression and antidepressant treatment. *Archives of General Psychiatry, 57,* 174–180.

Schildkraut, J. J. (1965). The catecholamine hypothesis of affective disorders: A review of supporting evidence. *American Journal of Psychiatry, 122,* 509–522.

Scott, P., & Hockley, B. (2011). *Radiochemical syntheses, radiopharmaceuticals for positron emission tomography.* (Wiley Series on Radiochemical Syntheses, Vol. 1) New York: Wiley.

Shoghi-Jadid, K., Small, G. W., Agdeppa, E. D., Kepe, V., Ercoli, L. M., Siddarth, P., . . . Barrio, J. R. (2002). Localization of neurofibrillary tangles and beta-amyloid plaques in the brains of living patients with Alzheimer disease. *American Journal of Geriatric Psychiatry, 10,* 24–35.

Small, G. W., Kepe, V., Ercoli, L. M., Siddarth, P., Bookheimer, S. Y., Miller, K. J., . . . Barrio JR. (2006). PET of brain amyloid and tau in mild cognitive impairment. *New England Journal of Medicine, 355,* 2652–2663.

Smith, G., Gunning-Dixon, F., Lotrich, F., Taylorm, W. D., & Evans, J. D. (2007). Translational research in late-life mood disorders: Implications for future intervention and prevention research. *Neuropsychopharmacology, 32,* 1857–1875.

Smith, G. S., Kahn, A., Sacher, J., Rusjan, P., van Eimeren, T., Flint, A., & Wilson, A. A. (2011). Serotonin transporter occupancy and the functional neuroanatomic effects of citalopram in geriatric depression. *American Journal of Geriatric Psychiatry.* 2011 Aug 11, ePub ahead of print.

Smith, G., Kramer, E., Hermann, C., Kingsley, P., Dhawan, V., Chaly, T., & Eidelberg, D. (2009). The functional neuroanatomy of geriatric depression. *International Journal of Geriatric Psychiatry, 24,* 798–808.

Smith, G., Kramer, E., Hermann, C., Ma, Y., Dhawan, V., Chaly, T., & Eidelberg, D. (2009). Serotonin modulation of cerebral glucose metabolism in depressed older adults. *Biological Psychiatry, 66,* 259–266.

Smith, G., Kramer, E., Hermann, C ., (2002). Serotonin modulation of cerebral glucose metabolism in geriatric depression. *American Journal of Geriatric Psychiatry, 45,* 105–112.

Smith, G., Reynolds, C. F., III, Pollock, B., Derbyshire, S., Nofzinger, E., Dew, M. A.,... Kupfer, D. J. (1999). Acceleration of the cerebral glucose metabolic response to antidepressant treatment by total sleep deprivation in geriatric depression. *American Journal of Psychiatry, 156,* 683–689.

Smith, G., Reynolds, C., Houck, P., Dew, M. A., Ma, Y., Mulsant, B. H., & Pollock, B. G. (2002). The glucose metabolic response to total sleep deprivation, recovery sleep and acute antidepressant treatment as functional neuroanatomic correlates of treatment outcome in geriatric depression. *American Journal of Geriatric Psychiatry, 10,* 561–567.

Steffens, D. C., Taylor, W. D., Denny, K. L., Bergman, S. R., & Wang, L. (2011). Structural integrity of the uncinate fasciculus and resting state functional connectivity of the ventral prefrontal cortex in late life depression. *PLoS One, 6*(7), e22697.

Suhara, T., Nakayama, K., Inoue, O., Fukuda, H., Shimizu, M., Mori, A., & Tateno, Y. (1992). D1 dopamine receptor binding in mood disorders measured by positron emission tomography. *Psychopharmacology, 106,* 14–18.

Sylvester, C. C., Wager, T. D., & Lacey, S. C. (2003). Switching attention and resolving interference: fMRI measures of executive functions. *Neuropsychologia, 41,* 357–370.

Townsend, D. W. (2008). Combined positron emission tomography-computed tomography: The historical perspective. *Seminars in Ultrasound, CT, and MRI, 29*(4), 232–235

Verhoeff, N. P., Wilson, A. A., Takeshita, S., Trop, L., Hussey, D., Singh, K.,... Houle, S. (2004). In-vivo imaging of Alzheimer disease beta-amyloid with [11C]SB-13 PET. *American Journal of Geriatric Psychiatry, 12,* 584–595.

Villemagne , V. L., Pike, K. E., Darby, D., Maruff, P., Savage, G., Ng, S.,... Rowe, C. C. (2008). A beta deposits in older non-demented individuals with cognitive decline are indicative of preclinical Alzheimer's disease. *Neuropsychologia, 46,* 1688–1697.

Volkow, N. D ., Wang, G. J., Fowler, J. S., (1998). Parallel loss of presynaptic and postsynaptic dopamine markers in normal aging. *Annals of Neurology, 44,* 143–147.

Wagner, H. N., Jr., Burns, H. D., Dannals, R. F., Wong, D. F., Langstrom, B., Duelfer, T.,... Kuhar, M. J. (1983). Imaging dopamine receptors in the human brain by positron tomography. *Science, 221*(4617), 1264–1266.

Wang, L., Krishnan, K. R., Steffens, D. C., Potter, G. G., Dolcos, F., & McCarthy, G. (2008). Depressive state- and disease-related alterations in neural responses to affective and executive challenges in geriatric depression. *American Journal of Geriatric Psychiatry, 165,* 863–871.

Wienhard, K., Schmand, M., Casey, M. E ., (2002). The ECAT HRRT: Performance and first clinical application of the new high resolution research tomograph. *IEEE Transactions on Nuclear Science, 49,* 104–110.

Wu, M., Andreescu, C., Butters, M. A., Tamburo, R., Reynolds, C. F., III, & Aizenstein, H. (2011). Default-mode network connectivity and white matter burden in late-life depression. *Psychiatry Research: Neuroimaging, 194,* 39–46.

Yatham, L. N., Liddle, P. F., Dennie, J., Shiah, I. S., Adam, M. J., Lane, C. J.,... Ruth, T. J. (1999). Decrease in brain serotonin 2 receptor binding in patients with major depression following desipramine treatment: A positron emission tomography study with fluorine-18-labeled setoperone. *Archives of General Psychiatry, 56,* 705–711.

Yurgelun-Todd, D. A., Gruber, S. A., Kanayama, G., Killgore, W. D., Baird, A. A., & Young, A. D. (2000). fMRI during affect discrimination in bipolar affective disorder. *Bipolar Disorders, 2,* 237–248.

35

COGNITIVE BIOMARKERS IN DEPRESSION

Oliver J. Robinson and Barbara J. Sahakian

MAJOR DEPRESSIVE disorder (MDD) is extremely common (Kessler et al., 2005) and is associated with enormous economic and emotional costs (Greenberg et al., 2003). Depression that occurs in late life is, unfortunately, often neglected in the face of multiple comorbidities (Lebowitz et al., 1997) despite the profound negative impact it has upon late-life well-being and mental capital (Beddington et al., 2008). Reducing the prevalence of late-life depression is therefore of pressing concern.

This chapter discusses how using neurocognitive testing to clarify the effects of depression on cognitive function can help achieve this aim. Specifically, this chapter will discuss how neurocognitive assessment—assessment of both cognitive performance and underlying neural architecture—can reveal cognitive biomarkers that may, in turn, improve the diagnosis, treatment, and prevention of late-life depression.

Cognitive Biomarkers

Cognition is a broad and imprecise term, but in the present context it is perhaps best thought of as

"information processing" (it comes from the Latin *cognoscere*, which means "to conceptualize," "to know," or "to recognize"). The purpose of processing information from the outside world is clear; it increases survival and reproductive chances and improves adaptive strength. From this perspective, it is possible to divide information processing into broad categories. One such category includes information that has direct survival implications and should be acted upon immediately. Such information usually elicits an "emotional" response that drives either approach or withdrawal behavior. This includes, for example, fight or flight responses (in response to immediate threats), withdrawal (in response to uncontrollable threats), or consummatory behavior. This type of cognition is sometimes referred to as "hot" cognition in reference to its immediate, affectively valenced, and arousing value. A broad distinction can be made between this type of information processing and processing that may not be immediately pressing or have immediate affective value. This latter type of cognition might include planning for future responses, changing performance strategies, or storing memories of nonemotional stimuli. This is often referred to as "cold" cognition in reference to its nonaffective and nonimmediate nature. These two broad categories may be subserved by different neural substrates. Hot cognition may recruit the limbic-cortical circuits formed by connections between the orbital and medial prefrontal cortex, amygdala, hippocampus, striatum, and thalamus, whereas cold cognition may utilize neuroanatomical loops involving the dorsolateral prefrontal cortex (Robinson & Sahakian, 2009b; Roiser, Rubinsztein, & Sahakian, 2009; Sahakian & Morein-Zamir, 2011). However, it is worth noting that these broad hot and cold categories are almost certainly an oversimplification and likely demonstrate significant overlap. But since they provide a simple framework within which to think about cognitive processing, this chapter uses them as a starting point to sort the cognitive alterations seen in depression.

A *biomarker* in this context is simply a marker that may prove useful in identifying or treating depression. Biomarkers may help to more precisely define disorders by grounding them in observable biological mechanisms, such as genes or physiological responses, rather than subjective reports of symptoms (for example, see the Research Domain Criteria of the National Institute of Mental Health; Insel & Cuthbert, 2009) or the MRC Review of Mental Health Research Report of the Strategic Review Group, 2010 (Sahakian, Malloch, & Kennard, 2010). Here, however, the focus is on *cognitive biomarkers*. That is, biomarkers that can be revealed using computerized neurocognitive tasks. Such tasks have enormous advantages over self-report or pencil-and-paper testing in that they standardize administration and analysis of results (Clark, Chamberlain, & Sahakian, 2009) and are less likely to suffer from demand characteristics (Orne, 1969). This chapter discusses how individuals with late-life depression show alterations to both hot and cold cognitive function (Elliott, Zahn, Deakin, & Anderson, 2011; Roiser, Rubinsztein, & Sahakian, 2003; Sahakian & Morein-Zamir, 2011) and how this can be revealed via altered accuracy and reaction time (RT) on such computerized neurocognitive tasks.

ALTERED COGNITION IN DEPRESSION

Although not as immediately obvious as the mood changes, depression is associated with altered cognitive function. Indeed, the *Diagnostic and Statistical Manual of Mental Disorders,* fourth edition (*DSM-IV*), criteria list diminished ability to think or concentrate and indecisiveness every day as a key symptom of depression. This impairment may be especially pronounced in late life (Köhler, Thomas, Barnett, & O'Brien, 2010) and is critical because it may reduce the effectiveness of psychological treatments (Murphy et al., 2000) and may impair performance of enjoyable or necessary pursuits (Austin et al., 2001; Taylor Tavares et al., 2007), which further impairs recovery. From a diagnostic perspective, however, this impairment may provide a way to uniquely identify depression. It may, that is to say, provide a "biomarker" for depression. This chapter will discuss depression-linked alterations in both cold and hot cognition, but it will first highlight a potential distinction between state and trait cognitive biomarkers (Maalouf et al., 2011).

State Biomarkers

Some symptoms of depression, mood being the most obvious, are "state" markers that fluctuate with the extent of the depression (Maalouf et al., 2011). For example, during a depressive episode patients experience a negative mood. However, this depressed mood remits with successful treatment. Some neurocognitive biomarkers may track these state changes. For instance, in both middle-aged and elderly patients, some mnemonic and executive functional impairments occur during depression but return to normal upon remission (Abas, Sahakian, & Levy, 1990; Beats, Sahakian, & Levy, 1996; Pizzagalli et al., 2001; Trichard et al., 1995). Such neurocognitive impairments as assessed using computerized tasks may therefore have value as nonsubjective diagnostic markers of depression and represent "efficacy markers" for treatment during drug development or primary care (Clark et al., 2009; Harmer, Cowen, & Goodwin, 2010). Such state biomarkers are therefore valuable from a diagnostic and treatment perspective.

Trait Biomarkers

Trait biomarkers may, by contrast, have predictive value for depression. Genetic predisposition accounts for up to 50% of the risk for depression, so close relatives of patients (especially females; Nolen-Hoeksema, Larson, & Grayson, 1999) may particularly be "at risk" for subsequent illness (Elliott et al., 2011). Some cognitive biomarkers that are present in depression are also present in at risk groups prior to the onset of the disorder and may then persist into remission (i.e., once state biomarkers have normalized). Such patterns of cognitive performance may therefore represent neurodevelopmental predispositions to depression. For instance, some negative affective biases are present before, during, and after mid- or late-life depression, and even in adolescents undergoing a first episode of depression (Elliott et al., 2011; Kyte, Euml, Goodyer, & Sahakian, 2005; LeMoult, Joormann, Sherdell, Wright, & Gotlib, 2009; Neumeister et al., 2006; Rogers et al., 2004). Such markers may represent altered function in underlying neural mechanisms that lead to trait vulnerabilities. The presence of such vulnerabilities in early life and midlife may thus predict late-life depression.

It should be noted that this distinction between state and trait biomarkers has not been fully explored and warrants considerable future research. However, it provides a helpful framework with which to interpret cognitive performance in vulnerable populations and remitted patients as well as in currently depressed patients.

This chapter will now focus upon cognitive biomarkers in late-life depression before broadening the focus to depression "in general," This latter section encompasses a larger number of studies, thereby increasing the breadth of understanding while remaining directly relevant to an understanding of late-life depression. Indeed, as shall be seen, the most severe and diverse depression-linked cognitive impairment is seen in late-life depression (Salloway et al., 1996; Sweeney, Kmiec, & Kupfer, 2000), so these broad findings may be *especially* relevant to late-life depression.

SPECIFIC EFFECTS IN LATE-LIFE DEPRESSION

It should be emphasized that there are at least two types of depression which can occur in elderly individuals. One group of patients develops depression for the first time in their old age, while another group of patients develops chronic relapsing depression earlier in life and it persists into old age (Panza et al., 2010). There may be a number of key differences between these two types of late-life depression.

Late-Onset Depression

Late-onset depression is often precipitated by cerebrovascular disease, which both predisposes and perpetuates depressive symptoms (Alexopoulos et al., 1997; Butters et al., 2008). Such comorbid depression and cerebrovascular disease in late life are associated with greater executive planning, and mnemonic and language impairment (all "cold" impairments) than both depression (Alexopoulos, Meyers, Young, Mattis, & Kakuma, 1993) and cardiovascular disease alone (Kramer-Ginsberg et al., 1999; Potter et al., 2007). As such, late-onset depression may be associated with a uniquely high level of cold cognitive impairment, which may be independent of the neurodegeneration (Aizenstein et al., 2008). Nevertheless it is extremely difficult to separate out neurocognitive impairment caused by the depression (Lebowitz et al., 1997) from that caused by the comorbid vascular dementia (Aizenstein et al., 2011), Alzheimer's, or other old age–associated neurodegenerative disorder. Age in and of itself is associated with cognitive decline (Austin, Mitchell, & Goodwin, 2001; Kennedy, Rodrigue, Head, Gunning-Dixon, & Raz, 2009; Raskin, 1986; Smith, Hillman, & Duley, 2005), and depression may simply facilitate this decline (King, Caine, & Cox, 1993; see Butters et al., 2008 for a summary of possible pathways). It is becoming increasingly recognized, for instance, that there may be a relationship between mild cognitive impairment (MCI) and late-life depression, with each potentially predisposing the other (Steffens et al., 2006).

Chronic Relapsing Depression Extending Into Late Life

A second group of elderly depressed individuals develops chronic relapsing depression when young or middle aged, and it persists into late life. Comparable levels of cognitive impairment during this type of depression seem to be associated with less neurological deterioration than late-onset depressed individuals (Lloyd et al., 2004). However, this type of depression in the elderly is often associated with greater cognitive impairment than same pathology in younger individuals simply by virtue of the fact that depression symptoms get worse with each successive episode (Robinson & Sahakian, 2008; Takami, Okamoto, Yamashita, Okada, & Yamawaki, 2007). This episode-linked decline may be driven, at least in part, by the deleterious effect of prolonged stress on the HPA axis, which leads to a snowballing increase in a wide range of pathologies from sleep impairment to neuronal atrophy (Millan, 2008). The elderly brain is vulnerable and may be particularly susceptible to such prolonged stress. As such, older individuals with recurrent depression may have greater cognitive impairment (Coryell et al., 1995), worse treatment outcomes (Mitchell & Subramaniam, 2005), and increased treatment-related side effects (Cooper et al., 2011), possibly due to aging and a great number of episodes.

Comparative Research

In general, there is a need for more research comparing depression in (a) early versus late life (Blazer, 2003) and (b) across subtypes of late-life depression (Smith, Gunning-Dixon, Lotrich, Taylor, & Evans, 2007). Regarding the early- versus late-life comparison, there is evidence from nondepressed samples that older individuals recruit distinct neural substrates when completing the same cognitive tasks as younger individuals, and there is limited evidence that this extends to depressed individuals (Smith et al., 2007). Specifically, there is an indication that older depressed individuals are more likely than younger patients to demonstrate mnemonic impairment (Goodwin, 1997) and residual impairment following recovery (Austin et al., 2001), alongside increased neuronal structural abnormalities (Beats, Levy, & Förstl, 1991; Rabins, Pearlson, Aylward, Kumar, & Dowell, 1991) and reduced frontal cortical activity. Indeed cognitive impairment comprises a key age-related risk factor for major depression (Goodwin, 1997) and, as highlighted earlier, the severest state cognitive deficits may be specific to comorbid late-onset depression (Feehan, Knight, & Partridge, 1991; Jorm, 1986; Köhler et al., 2010; Sweeney et al., 2000). It is possible, in fact, that younger patients do not show the whole range of cognitive impairments associated with depression that we shall review next (Sweeney et al., 2000). For instance, intact learning and memory, but impaired cognitive flexibility and planning function, have been shown in younger depressed individuals (Purcell, Maruff, Kyrios, & Pantelis, 1997), whereas greater mnemonic impairment is seen in late- compared to early-life depression (Köhler et al., 2010; Salloway et al., 1996). This greater impairment may represent the additive contribution of the cardiovascular disease in late-onset depression (Salloway et al., 1996) or the cumulative effects of stress and HPA axis

"overdrive" in recurrent depression (Millan, 2008). Nevertheless, the differential impact of early- and late-life depression on neurocognitive biomarkers is far from understood (Blazer, 2003).

Regarding the subtypes of late-life depression, there is evidence that cognitive impairment is greater in some elderly subgroups than others (e.g., suicidal elderly; Dombrovski et al., 2008), and that some treatments (e.g., interpersonal psychotherapy; Carreira et al., 2008) are more effective in elderly individuals with worse cognitive impairment, but there is a dearth of evidence examining cognitive performance across putative subtypes of late-life depression (Smith et al., 2007). It is even unclear whether there are in fact multiple subgroups of late-life depression. It is plausible that those who experience depression associated with cardiovascular disease are simply individuals who had enough cognitive reserve and resilience (putatively driven by top-down control of emotional processing) to fend off depression earlier in life, and who only become vulnerable to depression following age-related neural deterioration (e.g., enlarged ventricles or white matter lesions; Butters et al., 2008). Similarly, late-life depression may be seen alongside early symptoms of late-life dementing disorders, like MCI, the prodromal stage of Alzheimer's disease, and other forms of dementia (Panza et al., 2010), although the extent to which this relationship is causal is unclear (Köhler et al., 2010). The longitudinal assessment of cognitive biomarkers from young to late life may thus help resolve this, and other, open questions regarding cognition in late-life depression.

However, as emphasized already, the numbers of studies that directly compare late- and early-life depression are somewhat limited (Cooper et al., 2011), and most neurocognitive impairments are seen in depression across the life course. This chapter therefore moves on to consider cognitive biomarkers for depression irrespective of when they occur. As highlighted earlier, the general pattern is that many of these cognitive biomarkers are potentially *more* relevant to late-life depression when cognitive impairment is at its greatest (Salloway et al., 1996).

"COLD" COGNITION IN DEPRESSION

As highlighted in the introduction, the *DSM-IV* includes "diminished ability to think or concentrate" as a key symptom of depression but cognitive tasks allow us to be more specific than this (Chamberlain & Sahakian, 2004, 2005; Murphy et al., 2000; Taylor Tavares, Drevets, & Sahakian, 2003). Although there are some inconsistencies (see Clark et al., 2009; Rogers et al., 2004, for a review), impairments in "cold" cognitive function can be broadly divided into (1) impairments in learning and memory and (2) impairments in executive function. It has been suggested that some of these impairments increase with increasingly severe depression (Austin et al., 2001) and hence may be especially valuable as state biomarkers.

Learning and Memory

Impairments in learning and memory are often introspectively fairly obvious to depressed individuals, who frequently complain of increased "forgetfulness" and "difficulty remembering things" (Abas et al., 1990; Dalgleish et al., 2007; Elliott et al., 1996; Fossati et al., 2004). Major depression predicts, for instance, significant impairment on Wechsler Memory Scale–Revised (Gorwood, Corruble, Falissard, & Goodwin, 2008). Moreover, using automated neuropsychological testing, elderly (Abas et al., 1990; Beats et al., 1996) and young (Sweeney et al., 2000) depressed individuals show impaired ability to recall abstract patterns and spatial locations that they were shown just moments before. This impairment also scales up to more naturalistic spatial memory situations such as navigation of a "virtual reality" town (Gould et al., 2007) and may vary across major and bipolar depression (Taylor Tavares et al., 2007). Explicit (but not implicit) verbal memory also seems to be impaired in depression (Austin et al., 2001).

Executive Function

Executive function is a more loosely defined group of cognitive functions. It encompasses, frequently but not exclusively, processes that are not automatic, processes that are conscious, and processes that require integration of information from multiple processing domains. Specifically, depressed individuals demonstrate deficits in planning, cognitive flexibility, and attention (Rogers et al., 2004):

1. *Planning* ability can be tested using the Tower of London (TOL) planning task in which individuals must "work out in their minds" the number of moves required to make one group of movable pieces look like another. Both young (Elliott et al., 1996; Fitzgerald et al., 2008; Watts, MacLeod, & Morris, 1988) and elderly (Beats et al., 1996) depressed patients spend considerably longer "working out" problems on this task compared with healthy individuals. It has been argued, in fact, that measures of performance speed (RT) on tasks such as this are those most frequently impaired in depression (Austin et al., 1992; Goodwin, 1997). Depressed patients also, nevertheless, make far more errors (even after taking longer to decide) on this task, especially following a previous error. This increase in errors following errors has been argued to represent a "catastrophic response to failure" in which, after being told that they are wrong, the performance of depressed individuals falls apart and they fail to successfully complete the rest of the task (Beats et al., 1996; Elliott et al., 1996; Elliot, Baker, et al., 1997). This may actually be due to increased impact of punishment on cognitive performance and will be discussed in the section on "Hot Cognition in Depression."

2. *Cognitive flexibility* can be tested by seeing how quickly it takes individuals to learn new rules. Depressed individuals demonstrate impaired rule switching on tasks like the Wisconsin Card Sorting Task (WCST) and the Intradimensional/ Extradimensional Shift Task (IDED) (Clark, Sarna, & Goodwin, 2005; Lockwood, Alexopoulos, & van Gorp, 2002; Martin, Oren, & Boone, 1991; Merriam, Thase, Haas, Keshavan, & Sweeney, 1999; Taylor Tavares et al., 2007), although the impairment on the WCST may be worse in bipolar than major depression (Borkowska & Rybakowski, 2001) and the impairments on the IDED may be greater in major than bipolar depression (Taylor Tavares et al., 2007). Depressed individuals also show reduced ability to flexibly switch and produce lists of words on fluency tasks (Dalgleish et al., 2007; Fossati, Bastard Guillaume, Ergis, & Allilaire, 2003; Okada, Okamoto, Morinobu, Yamawaki, & Yokota, 2003; Videbech et al., 2003) and demonstrate less "conflict adaptation"—that is, decreased ability to recover from distracting (conflicting) stimuli—than healthy individuals (Rogers et al., 2004).

3. *Attention and response inhibition* can be tested using Stroop and go/no-go (GNG) tasks, where subjects are asked to respond to target stimuli and avoid responding to irrelevant stimuli. The degree of attentional focus or inhibitory control can be assessed by the extent to which subjects respond

to targets or are distracted by irrelevant stimuli. Depressed patients are usually impaired on Stroop tasks (Rogers et al., 2004), and this may be worse in bipolar rather than major depression (Borkowska & Rybakowski, 2001).

At-Risk Populations

As highlighted earlier, for a cognitive marker to be valuable as a trait biomarker, it also should be present in individuals at risk of the disorder. First-degree relatives of bipolar depressed individuals demonstrate impairment on the shift stage of the IDED cognitive flexibility task (Clark et al., 2005), and recovered depressed elderly individuals demonstrate planning impairment on the TOL task (Beats et al., 1996). These impairments may be related to the "underlying vulnerability rather than the actual disease phenotype" and hence represent trait biomarkers.

In general, therefore, depressed individuals show impairments in cold cognitive functions. These problems may be especially prominent in late-life depression (Goodwin, 1997; Salloway et al., 1996; Sweeney et al., 2000) in which they may be linked to comorbid vascular disease and/or MCI (Butters et al., 2008; Köhler et al., 2010).

"HOT" COGNITION IN DEPRESSION

In contrast to cold cognition, hot cognition encompasses processing involving emotionally valenced stimuli. Depressed individuals demonstrate "negative affective biases" in favor of negative stimuli. These affective biases are seen in emotional responses, which are specific short-term responses to emotional stimuli and may contribute to (although are not the same as) the negative mood state, which is a long duration and more diffuse state (Mitchell & Phillips, 2007; Robinson & Sahakian, 2009b). Hot cognitive tasks are tasks that recruit such emotional processing and can be divided into two broad processes: (1) reward or appetitive processing and (2) punishment or aversive processing (see Eshel & Roiser, 2010, for a review).

1. *Response to punishment.* Individuals with depression often view life events with greater negativity than do healthy individuals. This can be studied more precisely using cognitive tasks to assess responses to negative, punishing stimuli. For instance, the impairment in planning on the TOL

task highlighted earlier may actually be caused by a "catastrophic response to perceived failure" following the negative feedback received after an error. Specifically, the enhanced impact of punishment in depressed individuals may cause a collapse in subsequent performance. This effect is also been seen on the Simultaneous and Delayed Matching-to-Sample task (SDMTS) and an adapted TOL called the "one-touch tower task" (OTT) in both elderly (Beats et al., 1996; Steffens, Wagner, Levy, Horn, & Krishnan, 2001) and middle-aged (Elliott et al., 1996; Elliott, Sahakian, Herrod, Robbins, & Paykel, 1997) patients. It is also seen on probabilistic reversal-learning tasks in which depressed subjects prematurely reverse following misleading negative feedback (Dombrovski et al., 2010; Murphy, Michael, Robbins, & Sahakian, 2003; Remijnse et al., 2009; Taylor Tavares et al., 2008). Moreover, this enhanced impact of negative feedback correlates with depression severity (Elliott et al., 1996) and might therefore represent a state biomarker for depression. Similarly, depressed individuals demonstrate increased RT following losses on gambling tasks (Steele, Kumar, & Ebmeier, 2007), which correlates with anhedonia and may represent a state biomarker (Taylor Tavares et al., 2007). Indeed, negative biases are pervasive in depression and are also seen on go no-go tasks (GNG) (depressed individuals demonstrate a bias toward sad, relative to happy, words) (Erickson et al., 2005; Murphy et al., 2000), face recognition tasks (depressed interpret neutral faces as sad) (Gur et al., 1992; Hale Iii, 1998; Surguladze et al., 2004), and memory tasks (Bradley, Mogg, & Williams, 1995; Brittlebank, Scott, Williams, & Ferrier, 1993; Lim & Kim, 2005; Nunn, Mathews, & Trower, 1997; Rinck & Becker, 2005). Thus, there is clear evidence that depression is associated with enhanced responses to punishment. Moreover, punishment processing (i.e., the processing of negatively valenced faces) is also altered in daughters of mothers with depression (Joormann, Gilbert, & Gotlib, 2010), indicating that it may underlie vulnerability for depression and thus represent a trait biomarker for depression.

2. *Response to reward.* Depressed individuals also experience anhedonia, or impaired ability to appreciate positive life events. This may be the subjective result of reduced reward processing. In fact, a meta-analysis of behavioral and self-report response to positive and negative stimuli found more evidence for reduced response to positive stimuli than increased response to negative stimuli in depression

(Bylsma, Morris, & Rottenberg, 2008). Depressed individuals make more errors and are slower to respond to reward-related words than punishment-related words on the affective GNG task (Erickson et al., 2005) and show a bias toward recalling less positive self-referent words (Harmer et al., 2009). Moreover, on gambling or rewarded memory tasks, depressed individuals do not adapt behavior in anticipation of reward (Clark et al., 2011; Henriques & Davidson, 2000; Pizzagalli et al., 2009; Steele et al., 2007) and show corresponding reduced happiness in anticipation of monetary reward (McFarland & Klein, 2009). They also show reduced behavioral sensitivity to happy (relative to neutral or sad) faces (Gur et al., 1992; Harmer et al., 2009; Joormann & Gotlib, 2006; Rubinow & Post, 1992; Surguladze et al., 2004). Furthermore, on reversal-learning tasks in which reward and punishment reversals are separated, impairment is seen in reward-, but not punishment-, based reversal learning in depression (Robinson, Cools, Carlisi, Sahakian, & Drevets, 2012). This varies across but not within patient groups, indicating that it might actually represent a stable trait cognitive biomarker. Computed learning rates on probabilistic selection tasks, on the other hand, vary with anhedonia (Chase et al., 2009) and may therefore represent a more state-like impairment.

Depression is therefore associated with enhanced punishment and reduced reward processing. An open question, however, is whether this varies with age. While there is clear evidence for an increase in cold cognitive symptoms in late-life depression, there is little to suggest that these "hot" cognitive symptoms are greater in late-life depression. As such, it is plausible that these "hot" symptoms are common to episodes of depression irrespective of when they occur. Indeed, the presence of a mood-congruent bias may allow for the differential diagnosis of late-life depression and late-life MCI or dementia (Steffens et al., 2006), but this requires further research.

UNDERLYING CAUSES OF ALTERED COGNITION

The core features of cognitive biomarkers in depression are therefore impaired planning, attention, and cognitive flexibility alongside mood-congruent hypersensitivity to punishment and hyposensitivity to reward. This next section outlines the potential underlying neural and pharmacological causes of this altered cognitive performance.

FUNCTIONAL IMAGING

Functional imaging, such as functional magnetic resonance imaging (fMRI) and positron emission tomography (PET), can help localize neural regions involved in the cognitive alterations in depression (see, for example, Drevets et al., 1997, and see Chapter 34 of this book).

Cold Cognition

Cognitive biomarkers in cold cognition tend to be driven by changes in higher cortical regions and may therefore reflect impairments in "top-down" cognitive control (Robinson & Sahakian, 2009c). For instance, when there is an impairment in cold cognition, such as an impairment in learning and memory (Barch, Sheline, Csernansky, & Snyder, 2003; Bremner, Vythilingam, Vermetten, Vaccarino, & Charney, 2004), planning (Elliott, Baker, et al., 1997), or cognitive flexibility (Aizenstein et al., 2009; Okada et al., 2003; Siegle, Thompson, Carter, Steinhauer, & Thase, 2007), *reduced* activity is seen in the prefrontal cortex (PFC) (including the dorsolateral prefrontal cortex [DLPFC] and anterior cingulate cortex [ACC]) (Diener et al., 2012; Rogers et al., 2004), and connected subcortical regions such as the hippocampus, amygdala, and thalamus, which are critical for the same processing in healthy individuals. This may therefore represent a more cortically oriented impairment that underlies the behavioral alteration. Moreover, in the *absence* of behavioral impairment, *increased* activity is seen in the cortical and subcortical regions critical to memory (Harvey et al., 2005), planning (Fitzgerald et al., 2008), attention (Langenecker et al., 2007; Matthews et al., 2009; Wagner et al., 2006), and arithmetic (Hugdahl et al., 2004) tasks. It has been suggested that this increased activity (relative to healthy individuals) may represent compensatory activity required to overcome neural abnormalities and achieve comparable levels of cognitive processing in depression (when there is no behavioral difference across diagnosis) (Clark et al., 2009; George et al., 1997; Thomas & Elliott, 2009). Indeed, this compensatory pattern may serve to distinguish normal aging from late-life depression. Decreased striatal response is seen during sequence learning in normal aging (Aizenstein et al., 2006), while increased striatal response is seen during sequence learning in late-life depression (Aizenstein et al., 2005). There are, moreover, differences between subtypes of late-life depression with greater ACC activity during Stroop tasks in individuals with comorbid anxiety and late-life depression compared to individuals with late-life depression alone (Andreescu et al., 2009)

Hot Cognition

Hot cognition, in contrast to cold cognition, tends to recruit more "limbic" subcortical emotional regions, such as the amygdala and striatum (Elliott et al., 2011; Sahakian & Morein-Zamir, 2011). As such, it may represent a more "bottom-up" pattern of altered processing (Robinson & Sahakian, 2009c). For instance, depression is associated with increased activity in the amygdala during negative words (Siegle, Steinhauer, Thase, Stenger, &

Carter, 2002; Siegle et al., 2007), negative facial expressions (Fales et al., 2008; Sheline et al., 2001; Surguladze et al., 2005), negative feedback (Taylor Tavares et al., 2008), and encoding of subsequently recalled negative pictures (Hamilton & Gotlib, 2008; Roberson-Nay et al., 2006). By contrast, activity in the striatum, which is thought to play a key role in reward and punishment processing in healthy individuals (Robinson, Frank, Sahakian, & Cools, 2010), is attenuated in depressed individuals during wins on gambling tasks (Smoski et al., 2009; Steele et al., 2007), positive pictures (Kumari et al., 2003), reward anticipation (Pizzagalli et al., 2009), and feedback on planning tasks (Elliott, Sahakian, Michael, Paykel, & Dolan, 1998). Reward-based reversal learning impairments in depression, for instance, are associated with attenuated response in the striatum during reward but not punishment reversal (Fig. 35.1) (Robinson, Cools, et al., 2012)

Hot cognition in depression is nevertheless also associated with altered cortical responses, especially

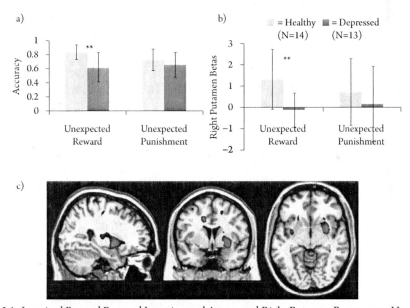

FIGURE 35.1 Impaired Reward Reversal Learning and Attenuated Right Putamen Response to Unexpected Reward in Depressed Individuals Relative to Healthy Comparison Subjects.
As shown in panel A, accuracy is lower on reward ($F = 11.7$, df = 1, 25, $p = 0.002$) but not punishment reversals in depressed individuals relative to healthy individuals. Panel B shows attenuated right (anatomically defined) putamen response during reward reversal trials in depressed individuals relative to healthy individuals ($F = 10.5$, df = 1, 25, $p = 0.003$) but equivalent response during punishment reversal. Error bars indicate standard deviations. In panel C, whole brain analysis confirms that the peak neural response difference between depressed and healthy individuals on reward reversal trials was the right anteroventral putamen (peak voxel $x = 30$, $y = 3$, $z = -8$; image shows SPM t scores ranging from 2.1 to 4.1) (taken by permission from Robinson, Cools, et al., 2012) (See color insert).

regions strongly connected to subcortical limbic regions. Increased activity is seen in the anterior cingulate cortex (ACC) during losses on gambling tasks (Steele et al., 2007; Steele, Kumar, & Ebmeier, 2004), during anticipation of increasing gains (Smoski et al., 2009), and during viewing of evocative pictures (Kumari et al., 2003). This latter study also revealed reduced activity in the subgenual cingulate cortex during viewing of evocative pictures (Kumari et al., 2003), which is consistent with reduced resting blood flow and metabolism in this region in depressed individuals (Drevets et al., 1997). However, in contrast, in a task requiring attention and response to target sad words, increased subgenual cingulate activity was seen in depressed individuals (Elliott, Rubinsztein, Sahakian, & Dolan, 2002). Indeed, in late-life depression increased subgenual activity to fearful faces is associated with greater cerebrovascular white matter change (Aizenstein et al., 2011), linking these cognitive changes to cerebrovascular disease. Reduced responses are seen in the PFC and orbitofrontal cortex (OFC) during negative feedback (Elliott et al., 1998; Kyte et al., 2005), and more recent work has begun to examine the interaction between these higher cortical regions and lower subcortical regions in depression. There is emerging evidence, for instance, that reduced top-down ventromedial PFC / subgenual ACC control of the amygdala in depressed individuals (Clark et al., 2009; Diener et al., 2012; Johnstone, van Reekum, Urry, Kalin, & Davidson, 2007; Taylor Tavares et al., 2008) may underlie a reduced ability to regulate emotional responses. In fact, there may be a distinction between the functions of dorsal and ventral regions of the PFC and ACC, with dorsal regions exciting the amygdala and ventral regions inhibiting the amygdala (Robinson, Charney, Overstreet, Vytal, & Grillon, 2012), potentially as human functional homologues of the rodent prelimbic/infralimbic regions (Sierra-Mercado, Padilla-Coreano, & Quirk, 2011). Indeed, both hot and cold cognition likely recruit neural *circuits*, and the overall pattern of neurocognitive performance likely requires a complex interaction between bottom-up and top-down neural responses.

At-Risk Individuals

Individuals at risk of developing depression also show some of the same patterns of hot neurocognitive processing. There is a lack of ACC activation to positive and negative words during the emotional Stroop task in individuals with a family history of depression (Mannie et al., 2008), and individuals with high neuroticism show greater activity in the amygdala during fearful versus happy faces (Chan, Norbury, Goodwin, & Harmer, 2009). Recovered depressed individuals also show blunted neural response to pleasant stimuli in the ventral striatum, despite no behavioral effect (McCabe, Cowen, & Harmer, 2009). These neural traces may therefore represent trait biomarkers for depression.

MODELING IN HEALTHY INDIVIDUALS

This next section of this review briefly examines the effects of manipulating monoamines and mood state on neurocognitive performance as another way to illuminate the underlying symptomatic causes of the neurocognitive biomarkers.

Monoamine Manipulation

Depression is associated with reduced serotonin (Owens & Nemeroff, 1994) and dopamine function (Eshel & Roiser, 2010; Martin-Soelch, 2009; Price & Drevets, 2009). Putative reduction of serotonin via acute tryptophan depletion (ATD; a technique in which subjects are deprived of the amino acid precursor to serotonin) in healthy individuals can induce memory impairment (Park et al., 1994; Riedel, Klaassen, Deutz, van Someren, & van Praag, 1999; Sambeth et al., 2007; Schmitt et al., 2000), impaired cognitive flexibility (Gallagher, Massey, Young, & McAllister-Williams, 2003; Hughes et al., 2003), and negative biases in hot cognition (Evers, van der Veen, Jolles, Deutz, & Schmitt, 2006; Robinson, Cools, Crockett, & Sahakian, 2009; Robinson, Cools, & Sahakian, 2011; Robinson & Sahakian, 2009c; Roiser et al., 2007; Rubinsztein et al., 2001) comparable to those seen in depression. By comparing manipulations it is also possible to gain insight into the relative contributions of different neurotransmitters. The depressed impairment in probabilistic reversal learning (Murphy et al., 2003) is seen in individuals undergoing dopamine depletion (Hasler, Mondillo, Drevets, & Blair, 2009) but not ATD (Evers et al., 2005; Murphy, Smith, Cowen, Robbins, & Sahakian, 2002), and on the adapted reversal task highlighted earlier (Fig. 35.1), individuals undergoing both ATD and dopaminergic manipulation demonstrate distinct patterns of altered punishment processing (Cools, Roberts, & Robbins, 2008). As such, alterations to both serotonin and dopamine function may underlie some of the neurocognitive impairments seen in depression.

As an aside, it should be noted that recent research has shown that ATD can induce negative mood, but only in certain groups (Robinson & Sahakian, 2009b; Ruhe, Mason, & Schene, 2007). Specifically, ATD seems to reliably induce negative mood in individuals who have suffered from depression and those who are at risk of depression (Booij et al., 2002). As such, a mood response to ATD might actually constitute a trait biomarker for depression. Recent work argues that this may be due to associations that are either prepotent or formed during depressive episodes (Robinson & Sahakian, 2008, 2009a) and which constitute a risk factor for recurrence.

Mood Manipulation

Depression is also, of course, associated with negative mood. Mood can be manipulated in healthy individuals via a variety of mood induction procedures, including emotionally charged music or recall of emotional situations (Mitchell & Phillips, 2007; Robinson et al., 2009; Robinson & Sahakian, 2009c). Individuals undergoing negative mood induction procedures demonstrate impaired memory (Gray, 2001; Gray, Braver, & Raichle, 2002; Spies, Hesse, & Hummitzsch, 1996), impaired cognitive flexibility (Robinson et al., 2007), reduced verbal fluency (Baker, Frith, & Dolan, 1997; Bartolic, Basso, Schefft, Glauser, & Titanic-Schefft, 1999; Vosburg, 1998), and some negative affective biases (Gilboa-Schechtman, Revelle, & Gotlib, 2000; Richards, French, Johnson, Naparstek, & Williams, 1992), including impaired response to negative feedback on the TOL task (Oaksford, Grainger, Morris, & Williams, 1996; Phillips, Smith, & Gilhooly, 2002; Robinson & Sahakian, 2009c; Watts et al., 1988). As such, mood state likely contributes to the overall profile of cognitive performance in depression.

GENETICS

Depression has been linked to a number of different candidate genes (Levinson, 2006) such as brain-derived neurotropic factor (BDNF), the serotonin transporter gene-linked polymorphic region (5-HTTLPR), and catechol-o-methyltransferase (COMT). A number of studies have shown neurocognitive patterns comparable to those seen in depression in healthy individuals possessing certain polymorphisms (Canli & Lesch, 2007; Hariri & Holmes, 2006; Savitz, Solms, & Ramesar, 2006). The 5-HTTLPR, for instance, modulates risky decision making (Roiser, Rogers, Cook, & Sahakian, 2006) and response to aversive stimuli in healthy individuals (Hariri et al., 2005) likely through modulation of the amygdala (Hariri et al., 2005; Roiser, de Martino, et al., 2009); COMT modulates performance on the WCST in healthy individuals (Malhotra et al., 2002); and both BDNF and COMT polymorphisms modulate working memory performance (Strauss et al., 2004). This association between genotype and cognition is controversial (Munafò, Durrant, Lewis, & Flint, 2009), but correspondence with genotype lends particular credence to the idea that some neurocognitive effects represent trait biomarkers.

TREATMENT IMPACT ON MARKERS

The standard treatments for depression are selective serotonin reuptake inhibitors (SSRIs), serotonin–norepinephrine reuptake inhibitors, and psychological therapies (such as cognitive-behavioral therapy). However, newer treatments are emerging such as deep-brain stimulation for intractable depression (Mayberg et al., 2005), ketamine (Berman et al., 2000), and scopolamine (Drevets & Furey, 2010), which is especially important for late-life depression, where failure to respond to a single treatment is common (Cooper et al., 2011). One potential value of state biomarkers in depression is improved assessment of the efficacy of treatment response (Clark et al., 2009; Harmer et al., 2010), but cognitive effects that are impervious to treatment-based mood improvement may reveal trait biomarkers.

State Biomarkers

In general, greater neurocognitive impairment prior to treatment, such as that seen in late-life depression in particular, leads to worse outcomes (Fu et al., 2008; Hale Iii, 1998; Hugdahl et al., 2007; Jaeger, Berns, Uzelac, & Davis-Conway, 2006; Langenecker et al., 2007; Siegle, Carter, & Thase, 2006) and a higher chance of relapse (Bouhuys, Geerts, & Gordijn, 1999). However, successful treatment can improve mnemonic and executive function and normalize the associated neural function in the

ACC, basal ganglia, and PFC and subgenual cingulate (Abas et al., 1990; Aizenstein et al., 2009; Beats et al., 1996; Goldapple et al., 2004; Goodwin, 1997; Goodwin et al., 1993; Kennedy et al., 2007; Linden, 2006; Pizzagalli et al., 2001; Trichard et al., 1995). To take but one example, SSRIs can remove amygdala hyperactivity to aversive stimuli in depressed individuals (Fu et al., 2004; Sheline et al., 2001). For some tasks, treatment-linked improvement of performance also leads to *increased* activity in the neural substrates associated with the neurocognitive impairment in patients, which may reflect compensatory activity (Hugdahl et al., 2007; Matsuo et al., 2006; Walsh et al., 2007).

Trait Markers

There are two types of potential trait markers. The first are neurocognitive impairments that seem impervious to recovery. For instance, despite mood recovery some remitted depressed individuals still require greater emotional intensity to identify happy facial expressions (LeMoult et al., 2009), show amygdala mediated biases in self referential memory (Ramel et al., 2007), and show increased amygdala response to masked sad faces (Neumeister et al., 2006). Stroop impairments, in particular, are thought to be especially promising trait markers (Rogers et al., 2004). A second group of trait markers, however, show a persistent neural trace despite recovery of the associated behavior. For instance, treatment removes a behavioral bias away from positive pictures, but the attenuated striatal response to positive pictures remains (McCabe et al., 2009). This effect may be especially pronounced in individuals treated with SSRIs (Kumar et al., 2008) and may represent a residual trace of the depression, or "kindling," which increases the likelihood of subsequent recurrence (Robinson & Sahakian, 2008).

CONCLUSION AND PERSPECTIVES

This chapter has provided a broad, but by no means exhaustive, overview of the patterns of altered "hot" and "cold" cognition that can be measured in depression, especially late-life depression, using computerized neurocognitive tasks. Specifically, this review began by highlighting some key differences between cognitive biomarkers in late and early life, emphasizing that older patients often demonstrate greater impairments in cold cognitive function.

Widening the focus, the review then highlighted the specific alterations to both cold cognitive functions such as learning, memory, and cognitive flexibility, and hot cognitive functions involving affectively valenced stimuli that are seen in depression irrespective of when it occurs. It was then shown that these alterations are associated with specific patterns of neural activity, and evidence was provided that they may be driven by changes in neurotransmitters, mood state, and linked genetic polymorphisms.

The review also made a distinction between state cognitive biomarkers that can be normalized with treatment and trait markers that are present prior, during, and in remission from depression. Some state markers suggest that neurocognitive impairments may be worse in late-life depression, and these markers may also be of use in determining improvement in treatment efficacy. It was also argued that trait markers, on the other hand, may allow for the detection of vulnerability to late-life depression earlier in life. There is, nevertheless, a clear need for more comparative studies explicitly assessing the extent of the differences between state and trait -biomarkers and between early- and late-life depression (and associated subtypes). A possibility highlighted in this review is that late-life depression is associated with worse cold-cognitive impairment, but that hot cognitive impairment may be specific to depression irrespective of when it occurs, but this requires further research.

Before finishing, however, it is worth highlighting that there is also a need to put the growing body of research on cognitive biomarkers to more practical use. Specifically, cognitive biomarkers could be used for the following:

1. *Better identification.* State and trait cognitive biomarkers could be used to identify abnormal underlying mechanisms (Insel & Cuthbert, 2009). For instance, RT to fearful relative to happy faces could be used to measure the extent of amygdala-mediated negative affective biases in both patients and at-risk individuals and, alongside a battery of other measures, be used to diagnose depression subtypes more accurately. Moreover, more comparative studies across putative subtypes will allow us to determine whether these subtypes are, in fact, distinct. Is there, for instance, a true distinction between late-onset and chronic relapsing late-life depression highlighted earlier? A developing line of research indicates a

strong, potentially reciprocal, link between MCI and late-life depression (Köhler et al., 2010; Panza et al., 2010), and neurocognitive biomarkers may help illuminate this relationship (Steffens et al., 2006). Are certain cold biomarkers common to both MCI and depression, but hot biomarkers restricted to depression?

2. *Improved treatment outcomes.* Neurocognitive biomarkers can be used to more precisely identify, and hence target, impairments to underlying mechanisms (Sahakian et al., 2010). Do the different subtypes of late-life depression (Panza et al., 2010) require, for instance, distinct treatments? Moreover, neurocognitive biomarkers can be used as efficacy markers to assess the treatment outcomes in the development of new treatments (Clark et al., 2009; Harmer et al., 2010).

3. *Promoting resilience.* From a public health perspective, however, the most efficient use of cognitive biomarkers would be to catch vulnerability and protect individuals from succumbing to disorders in the first place (Robinson, 2011; Robinson, Cools, & Sahakian, 2011; Sahakian et al., 2010). In other words, it might be possible to promote resilience to affective disorders (Beddington et al., 2008; Elliott, Sahakian, & Charney, 2008). Work has already begun to outline, for instance, positive affective biases in healthy individuals which may serve to protect against affective disorders (Cools, Robinson, & Sahakian, 2008; Elliott et al., 2008; Erickson et al., 2005; McCabe & Gotlib, 1995; Murphy et al., 2000; Robinson, Letkiewicz, Overstreet, Ernst, & Grillon, 2011). It may therefore be possible to preemptively use, for example, psychological or pharmacological interventions to boost these positive biases in young, healthy individuals at risk of developing late-life depression. The latter pharmacological approach, of course, raises multiple ethical issues in terms of the risks and benefits involved in the treatment of "at-risk" individuals prior to illness onset (see, e.g., Sahakian & Morein-Zamir, 2010), but given the enormous financial and emotional cost of depression, it should not be overlooked. Specifically, if it is possible to promote resilience in younger people they could be prevented from developing late-life depression in the first place. This would greatly enhance well-being and mental capital throughout the life course (Beddington et al., 2008), but especially in the prevalent, yet the often overlooked, instance of late-life depression (Lebowitz et al., 1997).

Disclosures

BJS acknowledges funding by a Wellcome Trust Programme Grant 076274/Z/04/Z awarded to T.W. Robbins, B. J. Everitt, A. C. Roberts, and B. J. Sahakian. OJR is a visiting fellow in the intramural research program of the National Institutes of Mental Health. BJS consults for Cambridge Cognition and a number of pharmaceutical companies. OJR declares that, except for income received from the primary employer, no financial support or compensation has been received from any individual or corporate entity over the past 3 years for research or professional service, and there are no personal financial holdings that could be perceived as constituting a potential conflict of interest

REFERENCES

Abas, M. A., Sahakian, B. J., & Levy, R. (1990). Neuropsychological deficits and CT scan changes in elderly depressives. *Psychological Medicine, 20,* 507–520.

Aizenstein, H. J., Andreescu, C., Edelman, K. L., Cochran, J. L., Price, J., Butters, M. A., ... Reynolds, C. F., III. (2011). fMRI correlates of white matter hyperintensities in late-life depression. *American Journal of Psychiatry, 168,* 1075–1082.

Aizenstein, H. J., Butters, M. A., Clark, K. A., Figurski, J. L., Andrew Stenger, V., Nebes, R. D., ... Carter, C. S. (2006). Prefrontal and striatal activation in elderly subjects during concurrent implicit and explicit sequence learning. *Neurobiology of Aging, 27,* 741–751

Aizenstein, H. J., Butters, M. A., Figurski, J. L., Stenger, V. A., Reynolds, C. F., III, & Carter, C. S. (2005). Prefrontal and striatal activation during sequence learning in geriatric depression. *Biological Psychiatry, 58,* 290–296

Aizenstein, H. J., Butters, M. A., Wu, M., Mazurkewicz, L. M., Stenger, V. A., Gianaros, P. J., ... Carter, C. S. (2009). Altered functioning of the executive control circuit in late-life depression: Episodic and persistent phenomena. *American Journal of Geriatric Psychiatry, 17,* 30–42.

Aizenstein, H. J., Nebes, R. D., Saxton, J. A., Price, J. C., Mathis, C. A., Tsopelas, N. D., ... Klunk, W. E. (2008). Frequent amyloid deposition without significant cognitive impairment among the elderly. *Archives of Neurology, 65,* 1509–1517.

Alexopoulos, G., Meyers, B., Young, R., Mattis, S., & Kakuma, T. (1993). The course of geriatric depression with "reversible dementia": A controlled study. *American Journal of Psychiatry, 150,* 1693–1699

Alexopoulos, G. S., Meyers, B. S., Young, R. C., Campbell, S., Silbersweig, D., & Charlson, M. (1997). "Vascular depression" hypothesis. *Archives of General Psychiatry, 54*, 915–922.

Andreescu, C., Butters, M., Lenze, E. J., Venkatraman, V. K., Nable, M., Reynolds, C. F., & Aizenstein, H. J. (2009). fMRI activation in late-life anxious depression: A potential biomarker. *International Journal of Geriatric Psychiatry, 24*, 820–828

Austin, M-P., Mitchell, P., & Goodwin, G. M. (2001). Cognitive deficits in depression: Possible implications for functional neuropathology. *British Journal of Psychiatry, 178*, 200–206.

Austin, M. P., Ross, M., Murray, C., O'Carroll, R. E., Ebmeier, K. P., & Goodwin, G. M. (1992). Cognitive function in major depression. *Journal of Affective Disorders, 25*, 21–29.

Baker, S. C., Frith, C. D., & Dolan, R. J. (1997). The interaction between mood and cognitive function studied with PET. *Psychological Medicine, 27*, 565.

Barch, D. M., Sheline, Y. I., Csernansky, J. G., & Snyder, A. Z. (2003). Working memory and prefrontal cortex dysfunction: Specificity to schizophrenia compared with major depression. *Biological Psychiatry, 53*, 376–384.

Bartolic, E. I., Basso, M. R., Schefft, B. K., Glauser, T., & Titanic-Schefft, M. (1999). Effects of experimentally-induced emotional states on frontal lobe cognitive task performance. *Neuropsychologia, 37*, 677–683

Beats, B., Levy, R., & Förstl, H. (1991). Ventricular enlargement and caudate hyperdensity in elderly depressives. *Biological Psychiatry, 30*, 452–458.

Beats, B. C., Sahakian, B. J., & Levy, R. (1996). Cognitive performance in tests sensitive to frontal lobe dysfunction in the elderly depressed. *Psychological Medicine, 26*, 591.

Beddington, J., Cooper, C. L., Field, J., Goswami, U., Huppert, F. A., Jenkins, R., ... Thomas, S. M. (2008). The mental wealth of nations. *Nature, 455*, 1057–1060

Berman, R. M., Cappiello, A., Anand, A., Oren, D. A., Heninger, G. R., Charney, D. S., & Krystal, J. H. (2000). Antidepressant effects of ketamine in depressed patients. *Biological Psychiatry, 47*, 351–354.

Blazer, D. G. (2003). Depression in late life: Review and commentary. *Journals of Gerontology Series A, Biological Sciences Medical Sciences, 58*, M249–M265.

Booij, L., Van der Does, W., Benkelfat, C., Bremner, D., Cowen, P. J., Fava, M., ... Van der Kloot, W. A. (2002). Predictors of mood response to acute tryptophan depletion: A reanalysis. *Neuropsychopharmacology, 27*, 852–861.

Borkowska, A., & Rybakowski, J. K. (2001). Neuropsychological frontal lobe tests indicate that bipolar depressed patients are more impaired than unipolar. *Bipolar Disorders, 3*, 88–94.

Bouhuys, A. L., Geerts, E., & Gordijn, M. C. (1999). Depressed patients' perceptions of facial emotions in depressed and remitted states are associated with relapse: A longitudinal study. *Journal of Nervous and Mental Disease, 187*, 595–602.

Bradley, B. P., Mogg, K., & Williams, R. (1995). Implicit and explicit memory for emotion-congruent information in clinical depression and anxiety. *Behaviour Research and Therapy, 33*, 755–770.

Bremner, J. D., Vythilingam, M., Vermetten, E., Vaccarino, V., & Charney, D. S. (2004). Deficits in hippocampal and anterior cingulate functioning during verbal declarative memory encoding in midlife major depression. *American Journal of Psychiatry, 161*, 637–645.

Brittlebank, A. D., Scott, J., Williams, J. M., & Ferrier, I. N. (1993). Autobiographical memory in depression: state or trait marker? *British Journal of Psychiatry, 162*, 118–121.

Butters, M. A., Young, J. B., Lopez, O., Aizenstein, H. J., Mulsant, B. H., Reynolds, C. F., III, ... Becker, J. T. (2008). Pathways linking late-life depression to persistent cognitive impairment and dementia. *Dialogues in Clinical Neuroscience, 10*, 345.

Bylsma, L. M., Morris, B. H., & Rottenberg, J. (2008). A meta-analysis of emotional reactivity in major depressive disorder. *Clinical Psychology Review, 28*, 676–691.

Canli, T., & Lesch, K-P. (2007). Long story short: The serotonin transporter in emotion regulation and social cognition. *Nature Neuroscience, 10*, 1103–1109.

Carreira, K., Miller, M. D., Frank, E., Houck, P. R., Morse, J. Q., Dew, M. A., ... Reynolds, C. F. (2008). A controlled evaluation of monthly maintenance interpersonal psychotherapy In late-life depression with varying levels of cognitive function. *International Journal of Geriatric Psychiatry, 23*, 1110–1113.

Chamberlain, S., & Sahakian, B. (2004). Cognition in mania and depression: Psychological models and clinical implications. *Current Psychiatry Reports, 6*, 451–458.

Chamberlain, S., & Sahakian, B. (2005). Neuropsychological assessment of mood disorders. *Clinical Neuropsychiatry, 2*, 137–148.

Chan, S. W. Y., Norbury, R., Goodwin, G. M., & Harmer, C. J. (2009). Risk for depression and neural responses to fearful facial expressions of emotion. *British Journal of Psychiatry, 194,* 139–145.

Chase, H. W., Frank, M. J., Michael, A., Bullmore, E. T., Sahakian, B. J., & Robbins, T. W. (2009). Approach and avoidance learning in patients with major depression and healthy controls: Relation to anhedonia. *Psychological Medicine, 40,* 433–440.

Clark, L., Chamberlain, S. R., & Sahakian, B. J. (2009). Neurocognitive mechanisms in depression: Implications for treatment. *Annual Review of Neuroscience, 32,* 57–74.

Clark, L., Dombrovski, A. Y., Siegle, G. J., Butters, M. A., Shollenberger, C. L., Sahakian, B. J., & Szanto, K. (2011). Impairment in risk-sensitive decision-making in older suicide attempters with depression. *Psychology and Aging, 26*(2), 321–330.

Clark, L., Sarna, A., & Goodwin, G. M. (2005) Impairment of executive function but not memory in first-degree relatives of patients with bipolar I disorder and in euthymic patients with unipolar depression. *American Journal of Psychiatry, 162,* 1980–1982.

Cools, R., Roberts, A. C., & Robbins, T. W. (2008). Serotoninergic regulation of emotional and behavioural control processes. *Trends in Cognitive Sciences, 12,* 31–40.

Cools, R., Robinson, O. J., & Sahakian, B. (2008) Acute tryptophan depletion in healthy volunteers enhances punishment prediction but does not affect reward prediction. *Neuropsychopharmacology, 33,* 2291–2299.

Cooper, C., Katona, C., Lyketsos, K., Blazer, D., Brodaty, H., Rabins, P.,... Livingston, G. (2011). A systematic review of treatments for refractory depression in older people. *American Journal of Psychiatry, 168*(7), 681–688.

Coryell, W., Endicott, J., Winokur, G., Akiskal, H., Solomon, D., Leon, A.,... Shea, T. (1995). Characteristics and significance of untreated major depressive disorder. *American Journal of Psychiatry, 152,* 1124–1129.

Dalgleish, T., Golden, A. M. J., Barrett, L. F., Yeung, C. A., Murphy, V., Tchanturia, K.,... Elward, R. (2007). Reduced specificity of autobiographical memory and depression: The role of executive control. *Journal of Experimental Psychology, General, 136,* 23.

Diener, C., Kuehner, C., Brusniak, W., Ubl, B., Wessa, M., & Flor, H. (2012). A meta-analysis of neurofunctional imaging studies of emotion and cognition in major depression. *Neuroimage, 61,* 677–685.

Dombrovski, A. Y., Butters, M. A., Reynolds, C. F., III, Houck, P. R., Clark, L., Mazumdar, S., & Szanto,

K. (2008). Cognitive performance in suicidal depressed elderly: Preliminary report. *American Journal of Geriatric Psychiatry, 16,* 109.

Dombrovski, A. Y., Clark, L., Siegle, G. J., Butters, M. A., Ichikawa, N., Sahakian, B. J., & Szanto, K. (2010). Reward/punishment reversal learning in older suicide attempters. *American Journal of Psychiatry, 167,* 699–707.

Drevets, W. C., & Furey, M. L. (2010). Replication of Scopolamine's antidepressant efficacy in major depressive disorder: A randomized, placebo-controlled clinical trial. *Biological Psychiatry, 67,* 432–438.

Drevets, W. C., Price, J. L., Simpson, J. R., Todd, R. D., Reich, T., Vannier, M., & Raichle, M. E. (1997). Subgenual prefrontal cortex abnormalities in mood disorders. *Nature, 386,* 824–827.

Elliott, R., Baker, S. C., Rogers, R. D., O'Leary, D. A., Paykel, E. S., Frith, C. D.,... Sahakian, B. J. (1997). Prefrontal dysfunction in depressed patients performing a complex planning task: A study using positron emission tomography. *Psychological Medicine, 27,* 931–942.

Elliott, R., Rubinsztein, J. S., Sahakian, B. J., & Dolan, R. J. (2002). The neural basis of mood-congruent processing biases in depression. *Archives of General Psychiatry, 59,* 597–604.

Elliott, R., Sahakian, B. J., & Charney, D. S. (2008). *State-of-science review: E7 the neural basis of resilience.* UK Government;s Foresight Project, Mental Capital and Wellbeing, http://www.bis. gov.uk/assets/foresight/docs/mental-capital/ sr-e7_mcw.pdf.

Elliott, R., Sahakian, B. J., Herrod, J. J., Robbins, T. W., & Paykel, E. S. (1997). Abnormal response to negative feedback in unipolar depression: Evidence for a diagnosis specific impairment. *Journal of Neurology, Neurosurgery, and Psychiatry, 63,* 74–82.

Elliott, R., Sahakian, B. J., McKay, A. P., Herrod, J. J., Robbins, T. W., & Paykel, E. S. (1996). Neuropsychological impairments in unipolar depression: The influence of perceived failure on subsequent performance. *Psychological Medicine, 26,* 975–989.

Elliott, R., Sahakian, B. J., Michael, A., Paykel, E. S., & Dolan, R. J. (1998). Abnormal neural response to feedback on planning and guessing tasks in patients with unipolar depression. *Psychological Medicine, 28,* 559–571.

Elliott, R., Zahn, R., Deakin, J. F. W., & Anderson, I. M. (2011). Affective cognition and its disruption in mood disorders. *Neuropsychopharmacology, 36,* 153–182.

Erickson, K., Drevets, W. C., Clark, L., Cannon, D. M., Bain, E. E., Zarate, C. A.,... Sahakian, B. J. (2005).

Mood-congruent bias in affective Go/No-Go performance of unmedicated patients with major depressive disorder. *American Journal of Psychiatry, 162*, 2171-U1.

Eshel, N., & Roiser, J. P. (2010). Reward and punishment processing in depression. *Biological Psychiatry, 68*, 118–124.

Evers, E. A. T., Cools, R., Clark, L., van der Veen, F. M., Jolles, J., Sahakian, B. J., & Robbins, T. W. (2005). Serotonergic modulation of prefrontal cortex during negative feedback in probabilistic reversal learning. *Neuropsychopharmacology, 30*, 1138–1147.

Evers, E. A. T., van der Veen, F. M., Jolles, J., Deutz, N. E. P., & Schmitt, J. A. J. (2006). Acute tryptophan depletion improves performance and modulates the BOLD response during a Stroop task in healthy females. *NeuroImage, 32*, 248–255.

Fales, C. L., Barch, D. M., Rundle, M. M., Mintun, M. A., Snyder, A. Z., Cohen, J. D.,... Sheline, Y. I. (2008). Altered emotional interference processing in affective and cognitive-control brain circuitry in major depression. *Biological Psychiatry, 63*, 377–384.

Feehan, M., Knight, R. G., & Partridge, F. M. (1991). Cognitive complaint and test performance in elderly patients suffering depression or dementia. *International Journal of Geriatric Psychiatry, 6*, 287–293.

Fitzgerald, P. B., Srithiran, A., Benitez, J., Daskalakis, Z. Z., Oxley, T. J., Kulkarni, J., & Egan, G. F. (2008). An fMRI study of prefrontal brain activation during multiple tasks in patients with major depressive disorder. *Human Brain Mapping, 29*, 490–501.

Fossati, P., Bastard Guillaume, L., Ergis, A-M., & Allilaire, J-F. (2003). Qualitative analysis of verbal fluency in depression. *Psychiatry Research, 117*, 17–24.

Fossati, P., Harvey, P-O., Le Bastard, G., Ergis, A-M., Jouvent, R., & Allilaire, J-F. (2004). Verbal memory performance of patients with a first depressive episode and patients with unipolar and bipolar recurrent depression. *Journal of Psychiatric Research, 38*, 137–144.

Fu, C. H. Y., Williams, S. C. R., Cleare, A. J., Brammer, M. J., Walsh, N. D., Kim, J.,... Bullmore, E. T. (2004). Attenuation of the neural response to sad faces in major depression by antidepressant treatment: A prospective, event-related functional magnetic resonance imaging study. *Archives of General Psychiatry, 61*, 877–889.

Fu, C. H. Y., Williams, S. C. R., Cleare, A. J., Scott, J., Mitterschiffthaler, M. T., Walsh, N. D.,... Murray, R. M. (2008). Neural responses to sad facial expressions in major depression following cognitive behavioral therapy. *Biological Psychiatry, 64*, 505–512.

Gallagher, P., Massey, A. E., Young, A. H., & McAllister-Williams, R. H. (2003). Effects of acute tryptophan depletion on executive function in healthy male volunteers. *BMC Psychiatry, 3*, 1–9.

George, M. S., Ketter, T. A., Parekh, P. I., Rosinsky, N., Ring, H. A., Pazzaglia, P. J.,... Post, R. M. (1997). Blunted left cingulate activation in mood disorder subjects during a response interference task (the Stroop). *Journal of Neuropsychiatry and Clinical Neurosciences, 9*, 55–63.

Gilboa-Schechtman, E., Revelle, W., & Gotlib, I. H. (2000). Stroop interference following mood induction: Emotionality, mood congruence, and concern relevance. *Cognitive Therapy and Research, 24*, 491–502.

Goldapple, K., Segal, Z., Garson, C., Lau, M., Bieling, P., Kennedy, S., & Mayberg, H. (2004). Modulation of cortical-limbic pathways in major depression: Treatment-specific effects of cognitive behavior therapy. *Archives of General Psychiatry, 61*, 34–41.

Goodwin, G. M. (1997). Neuropsychological and neuroimaging evidence for the involvement of the frontal lobes in depression. *Journal of Psychopharmacology, 11*, 115–122.

Goodwin, G. M., Austin, M. P., Dougall, N., Ross, M., Murray, C., O'Caroll, R. E.,... Ebmeier, K. P. (1993). State changes in brain activity shown by the uptake of 99mTc-exametazime with single photon emission tomography in major depression before and after treatment. *Journal of Affective Disorders, 29*, 243–253.

Gorwood, P., Corruble, E., Falissard, B., & Goodwin, G. M. (2008). Toxic effects of depression on brain function: Impairment of delayed recall and the cumulative length of depressive disorder in a large sample of depressed outpatients. *American Journal of Psychiatry, 165*, 731–739.

Gould, N. F., Holmes, M. K., Fantie, B. D., Luckenbaugh, D. A., Pine, D. S., Gould, T. D.,... Zarate, C. A., Jr. (2007). Performance on a virtual reality spatial memory navigation task in depressed patients. *American Journal of Psychiatry, 164*, 516–519.

Gray, J. R. (2001). Emotional modulation of cognitive control: Approach-withdrawal states double-dissociate spatial from verbal two-back task performance. *Journal of Experimental Psychology, General, 130*, 436–452.

Gray, J. R., Braver, T. S., & Raichle, M. E. (2002). Integration of emotion and cognition in the lateral prefrontal cortex. *Proceedings of the National Academy of Sciences of the USA, 99*, 4115–4120.

Greenberg, P. E., Kessler, R. C., Birnbaum, H. G., Leong, S. A., Lowe, S. W., Berglund, P. A., & Corey-Lisle, P. K. (2003). The economic burden of depression in the United States: How did it change between 1990 and 2000? *Jounal of Clinical Psychiatry, 64,* 1465–1475.

Gur, R. C., Erwin, R. J., Gur, R. E., Zwil, A. S., Heimberg, C., & Kraemer, H. C. (1992). Facial emotion discrimination: II. Behavioral findings in depression. *Psychiatry Research, 42,* 241–251.

Hale, W. W., III. (1998) Judgment of facial expressions and depression persistence. *Psychiatry Research, 80,* 265–274.

Hamilton, J. P., & Gotlib, I. H. (2008). Neural substrates of increased memory sensitivity for negative stimuli in major depression. *Biological Psychiatry, 63,* 1155–1162.

Hariri, A. R., Drabant, E. M., Munoz, K. E., Kolachana, B. S., Mattay, V. S., Egan, M. F., & Weinberger, D. R. (2005). A susceptibility gene for affective disorders and the response of the human amygdala. *Archives of General Psychiatry, 62,* 146–152.

Hariri, A. R., & Holmes, A. (2006). Genetics of emotional regulation: The role of the serotonin transporter in neural function. *Trends in Cognitive Sciences, 10,* 182–191.

Harmer, C. J., Cowen, P. J., & Goodwin, G. M. (2010). Efficacy markers in depression. *Journal of Psychopharmacology, 25*(9), 1148–1158.

Harmer, C. J., O'Sullivan, U., Favaron, E., Massey-Chase, R., Ayres, R., Reinecke, A., ... Cowen, P. J. (2009). Effect of acute antidepressant administration on negative affective bias in depressed patients. *American Journal of Psychiatry, 166,* 1178–1184.

Harvey, P-O., Fossati, P., Pochon, J-B., Levy, R., LeBastard, G., Lehéricy, S., ... Dubois, B. (2005). Cognitive control and brain resources in major depression: An fMRI study using the n-back task. *NeuroImage, 26,* 860–869.

Hasler, G., Mondillo, K., Drevets, W. C., & Blair, J. R. (2009). Impairments of probabilistic response reversal and passive avoidance following catecholamine depletion. *Neuropsychopharmacology, 34,* 2691–2698.

Henriques, J. B., & Davidson, R. J. (2000). Decreased responsiveness to reward in depression. *Cognition and Emotion, 14,* 711–724.

Hugdahl, K., Rund, B. R., Lund, A., Asbjornsen, A., Egeland, J., Ersland, L., ... Thomsen, T. (2004). Brain activation measured with fMRI during a mental arithmetic task in schizophrenia and major depression. *American Journal of Psychiatry, 161,* 286–293.

Hugdahl, K., Specht, K., Biringer, E., Weis, S., Elliott, R., Hammar, Å., ... Lund, A. (2007). Increased parietal and frontal activation after remission from recurrent major depression: A repeated fMRI study. *Cognitive Therapy and Research, 31,* 147–160.

Hughes, J. H., Gallagher, P., Stewart, M. E., Matthews, D., Kelly, T. P., & Young, A. H. (2003). The effects of acute tryptophan depletion on neuropsychological function. *Journal of Psychopharmacology, 17,* 300–309.

Insel, T. R., & Cuthbert, B. N. (2009). Endophenotypes: Bridging genomic complexity and disorder heterogeneity. *Biological Psychiatry, 66,* 988–989.

Jaeger, J., Berns, S., Uzelac, S., & Davis-Conway, S. (2006). Neurocognitive deficits and disability in major depressive disorder. *Psychiatry Research, 145,* 39–48.

Johnstone, T., van Reekum, C. M., Urry, H. L., Kalin, N. H., & Davidson, R. J. (2007). Failure to regulate: Counterproductive recruitment of top-down prefrontal-subcortical circuitry in major depression. *Journal of Neuroscience, 27,* 8877–8884.

Joormann, J., Gilbert, K., & Gotlib, I. H. (2010). Emotion identification in girls at high risk for depression. *Journal of Child Psychology and Psychiatry, 51,* 575–582.

Joormann, J., & Gotlib, I. H. (2006). Is this happiness I see? Biases in the identification of emotional facial expressions in depression and social phobia. *Journal of Abnormal Psychology, 115,* 705–714.

Jorm, A. F. (1986). Cognitive deficit in the depressed elderly: A review of some basic unresolved issues. *Australian and New Zealand Journal of Psychiatry, 20,* 11–22.

Kennedy, K. M., Rodrigue, K. M., Head, D., Gunning-Dixon, F., & Raz, N. (2009). Neuroanatomical and cognitive mediators of age-related differences in perceptual priming and learning. *Neuropsychology, 23,* 475–491.

Kennedy, S. H., Konarski, J. Z., Segal, Z. V., Lau, M. A., Bieling, P. J., McIntyre, R. S., & Mayberg, H. S. (2007). Differences in brain glucose Metabolism between responders to CBT and Venlafaxine in a 16-week randomized controlled trial. *American Journal of Psychiatry, 164,* 778–788.

Kessler, R. C., Berglund, P., Demler, O., Jin, R., Merikangas, K. R., & Walters, E. E. (2005). Lifetime prevalence and age-of-onset distributions of DSM-IV disorders in the national comorbidity survey replication. *Archives of General Psychiatry, 62,* 593–602.

King, D. A., Caine, E. D., & Cox, C. (1993). Influence of depression and age on selected cognitive functions. *Clinical Neuropsychologist, 7,* 443–453.

Köhler, S., Thomas, A. J., Barnett, N. A., & O'Brien, J. T. (2010). The pattern and course of cognitive impairment in late-life depression. *Psychological Medicine, 40,* 591–602.

Kramer-Ginsberg, E., Greenwald, B. S., Krishnan, K. R. R., Christiansen, B., Hu, J., Ashtari, M.,... Pollack, S. (1999). Neuropsychological functioning and MRI signal hyperintensities in geriatric depression. *American Journal of Psychiatry, 156,* 438–444.

Kumar, P., Waiter, G., Ahearn, T., Milders, M., Reid, I., & Steele, J. D. (2008). Abnormal temporal difference reward-learning signals in major depression. *Brain, 131,* 2084–2093.

Kumari, V., Mitterschiffthaler, M. T., Teasdale, J. D., Malhi, G. S., Brown, R. G., Giampietro, V.,... Sharma, T. (2003). Neural abnormalities during cognitive generation of affect in Treatment-Resistant depression. *Biological Psychiatry, 54,* 777–791.

Kyte, Z., Euml, A., Goodyer, I. M., & Sahakian, B. J. (2005). Selected executive skills in adolescents with recent first episode major depression. *Journal of Child Psychology and Psychiatry and Allied Disciplines, 46,* 995–1005.

Langenecker, S. A., Kennedy, S. E., Guidotti, L. M., Briceno, E. M., Own, L. S., Hooven, T.,... Zubieta, J-K. (2007). Frontal and limbic activation during inhibitory control predicts treatment response in major depressive disorder. *Biological Psychiatry, 62,* 1272–1280.

Lebowitz, B. D., Pearson, J. L., Schneider, L. S., Reynolds, C. F., Alexopoulos, G. S., Bruce, M. L.,... Parmelee, P. (1997). Diagnosis and treatment of depression in late life. *Journal of the American Medical Association, 278,* 1186–1190.

LeMoult, J., Joormann, J., Sherdell, L., Wright, Y., & Gotlib, I. H. (2009). Identification of emotional facial expressions following recovery from depression. *Journal of Abnormal Psychology, 118,* 828–833.

Levinson, D. F. (2006). The genetics of depression: A review. *Biological Psychiatry, 60,* 84–92.

Lim, S-L., & Kim, J-H. (2005). Cognitive processing of emotional information in depression, panic, and somatoform disorder. *Journal of Abnormal Psychology, 114,* 50–61.

Linden, D. E. J. (2006). How psychotherapy changes the brain—the contribution of functional neuroimaging. *Molecular Psychiatry, 11,* 528–538.

Lloyd, A. J., Ferrier, I. N., Barber, R., Gholkar, A., Young, A. H., & O'Brien, J. T. (2004). Hippocampal volume change in depression: Late- and early-onset illness compared. *British Journal of Psychiatry, 184,* 488–495.

Lockwood, K. A., Alexopoulos, G. S., & van Gorp, W. G. (2002). Executive dysfunction in geriatric depression. *American Journal of Psychiatry, 159,* 1119–1126.

Maalouf, F. T., Brent, D., Clark, L., Tavitian, L., McHugh, R. M., Sahakian, B. J., & Phillips, M. L. (2011). Neurocognitive impairment in adolescent major depressive disorder: State vs. trait illness markers. *Journal of Affective Disorders, 133*(3), 625–632.

Malhotra, A. K., Kestler, L. J., Mazzanti, C., Bates, J. A., Goldberg, T., & Goldman, D. (2002). A functional polymorphism in the COMT gene and performance on a test of prefrontal cognition. *American Journal of Psychiatry, 159,* 652–654.

Mannie, Z. N., Norbury, R., Murphy, S. E., Inkster, B., Harmer, C. J., & Cowen, P. J. (2008). Affective modulation of anterior cingulate cortex in young people at increased familial risk of depression. *British Journal of Psychiatry, 192,* 356–361.

Martin-Soelch, C. (2009). Is depression associated with dysfunction of the central reward system? *Biochemical Society Transactions, 37,* 313–317.

Martin, D. J., Oren, Z., & Boone, K. (1991). Major depressives' and dysthymics' performance on the Wisconsin card sorting test. *Journal of Clinical Psychology, 47,* 684–690.

Matsuo, K., Glahn, D. C., Peluso, M. A. M., Hatch, J. P., Monkul, E. S., Najt, P.,... Soares, J. C. (2006). Prefrontal hyperactivation during working memory task in untreated individuals with major depressive disorder. *Molecular Psychiatry, 12,* 158–166.

Matthews, S., Simmons, A., Strigo, I., Gianaros, P., Yang, T., & Paulus, M. (2009). Inhibition-related activity in subgenual cingulate is associated with symptom severity in major depression. *Psychiatry Research: Neuroimaging, 172,* 1–6.

Mayberg, H. S., Lozano, A. M., Voon, V., McNeely, H. E., Seminowicz, D., Hamani, C.,... Kennedy, S. H. (2005). Deep brain stimulation for treatment-resistant depression. *Neuron, 45,* 651–660.

McCabe, C., Cowen, P., & Harmer, C. (2009). Neural representation of reward in recovered depressed patients. *Psychopharmacology, 205,* 667–677.

McCabe, S. B., & Gotlib, I. H. (1995) Selective attention and clinical depression: Performance on a deployment-of-attention task. *Journal of Abnormal Psychology, 104,* 241–245.

McFarland, B. R., & Klein, D. N. (2009). Emotional reactivity in depression: Diminished responsiveness to anticipated reward but not to anticipated punishment or to nonreward or avoidance. *Depression and Anxiety, 26,* 117–122.

Merriam, E. P., Thase, M. E., Haas, G. L., Keshavan, M. S., & Sweeney, J. A. (1999). Prefrontal cortical dysfunction in depression determined by Wisconsin Card Sorting Test performance. *American Journal of Psychiatry, 156,* 780–782.

Millan, M. J. (2008). *State-of-science review: SR-E16 stress-related mood disorder: Novel concepts for treatment and prevention.* UK Government's Foresight Project, Mental Capital and Wellbeing, http://www.bis.gov.uk/assets/foresight/docs/mental-capital/sr-e7_mcw.pdf.

Mitchell, A. J., & Subramaniam, H. (2005). Prognosis of depression in old age compared to middle age: A systematic review of comparative studies. *American Journal of Psychiatry, 162,* 1588–1601.

Mitchell, R. L. C., & Phillips, L. H. (2007). The psychological, neurochemical and functional neuroanatomical mediators of the effects of positive and negative mood on executive functions. *Neuropsychologia, 45,* 617–629.

Munafò, M. R., Durrant, C., Lewis, G., & Flint, J. (2009). Gene × environment interactions at the serotonin transporter locus. *Biological Psychiatry, 65*(3), 211–219.

Murphy, F. C., Michael, A., Robbins, T. W., & Sahakian, B. J. (2003). Neuropsychological impairment in patients with major depressive disorder: The effects of feedback on task performance. *Psychological Medicine, 33,* 455–467.

Murphy, F. C., Sahakian, B. J., Rubinsztein, J. S., Michael, A., Rogers, R. D., Robbins, T. W., & Paykel, E. S. (2000). Emotional bias and inhibitory control processes in mania and depression. *Psychological Medicine, 29,* 1307–1321.

Murphy, F. C., Smith, K. A., Cowen, P. J., Robbins, T. W., & Sahakian, B. J. (2002). The effects of tryptophan depletion on cognitive and affective processing in healthy volunteers. *Psychopharmacology, 163,* 42–53.

Neumeister, A., Drevets, W. C., Belfer, I., Luckenbaugh, D. A., Henry, S., Bonne, O., ... Charney, D. S. (2006). Effects of a [alpha]2C-adrenoreceptor gene polymorphism on neural responses to facial expressions in depression. *Neuropsychopharmacology, 31,* 1750–1756.

Nolen-Hoeksema, S., Larson, J., & Grayson, C. (1999). Explaining the gender difference in depressive symptoms. *Journal of Personal and Social Psychology, 77,* 1061–1072.

Nunn, J. D., Mathews, A., & Trower, P. (1997). Selective processing of concern-related information in depression. *British Journal of Clinical Psychology, 36,* 489–503.

Oaksford, M., Grainger, B., Morris, F., & Williams, J. M. G. (1996). Mood, reasoning, and central executive processes. *Journal of Experimental Psychology: Learning, Memory, and Cognition, 22,* 476–492.

Okada, G., Okamoto, Y., Morinobu, S., Yamawaki, S., & Yokota, N. (2003). Attenuated left prefrontal activation during a verbal fluency task in patients with depression. *Neuropsychobiology, 47,* 21–26.

Orne, M. T. (1969). Demand characteristics and the concept of quasi-controls. In R. Rosenthal & R. L. Rosnow (Eds.), *Artifact in behavioral research* (pp. 143–179). San Diego, CA: Academic Press.

Owens, M., & Nemeroff, C. (1994). Role of serotonin in the pathophysiology of depression: Focus on the serotonin transporter. *Clinical Chemistry, 40,* 288–295.

Panza, F., Frisardi, V., Capurso, C., D'Introno, A., Colacicco, A. M., Imbimbo, B. P., ... Solfrizzi, V. (2010). Late-life depression, mild cognitive impairment, and dementia: Possible continuum? *American Journal of Geriatric Psychiatry, 18,* 98–116.

Park, S. B., Coull, J. T., McShane, R. H., Young, A. H., Sahakian, B. J., Robbins, T. W., & Cowen, P. J. (1994). Tryptophan depletion in normal volunteers produces selective impairments in learning and memory. *Neuropharmacology, 33,* 575–588.

Phillips, L. H., Smith, L., & Gilhooly, K. J. (2002). The effects of adult aging and induced positive and negative mood on planning. *Emotion, 2,* 263–72.

Pizzagalli, D., Pascual-Marqui, R. D., Nitschke, J. B., Oakes, T. R., Larson, C. L., Abercrombie, H. C., ... Davidson, R. J. (2001). Anterior cingulate activity as a predictor of degree of treatment response in major depression: Evidence from brain electrical tomography analysis. *American Journal of Psychiatry, 158,* 405–415.

Pizzagalli, D. A., Holmes, A. J., Dillon, D. G., Goetz, E. L., Birk, J. L., Bogdan, R., ... Fava, M. (2009). Reduced caudate and nucleus accumbens response to rewards in unmedicated individuals with major depressive disorder. *American Journal of Psychiatry, 166,* 702–710.

Potter, G. G., Blackwell, A. D., McQuoid, D. R., Payne, M. E., Steffens, D. C., Sahakian, B. J., ... Krishnan, K. R. R. (2007). Prefrontal white matter lesions and prefrontal task impersistence in depressed and nondepressed elders. *Neuropsychopharmacology, 32,* 2135–2142.

Price, J. L., & Drevets, W. C. (2009). Neurocircuitry of mood disorders. *Neuropsychopharmacology, 35,* 192–216.

Purcell, R., Maruff, P., Kyrios, M., & Pantelis, C. (1997). Neuropsychological function in young patients with unipolar major depression. *Psychological Medicine, 27,* 1277–1285.

Rabins, P., Pearlson, G., Aylward, E., Kumar, A., & Dowell, K. (1991). Cortical magnetic resonance imaging changes in elderly inpatients with major depression. *American Journal of Psychiatry, 148,* 617–620.

Ramel, W., Goldin, P. R., Eyler, L. T., Brown, G. G., Gotlib, I. H., & McQuaid, J. R. (2007). Amygdala reactivity and mood-congruent memory in Individuals at risk for depressive relapse. *Biological Psychiatry, 61,* 231–239.

Raskin, A. (1986). *Partialing out the effects of depression and age on cognitive functions: Experimental data and methodologic issues. Handbook for clinical memory assessment of older adults.* Washington, DC: American Psychological Association.

Remijnse, P. L., Nielen, M. M. A., van Balkom, A. J. L. M., Hendriks, G. J., Hoogendijk, W. J., … Veltman, D. J. (2009). Differential frontal-striatal and paralimbic activity during reversal learning in major depressive disorder and obsessive-compulsive disorder. *Psychological Medicine, 39,* 1503–1518.

Richards, A., French, C. C., Johnson, W., Naparstek, J., & Williams, J. (1992). Effects of mood manipulation and anxiety on performance of an emotional Stroop task. *British Journal of Psychology, 83,* 479–491.

Riedel, W. J., Klaassen, T., Deutz, N. E. P., van Someren, A., & van Praag, H. M. (1999). Tryptophan depletion in normal volunteers produces selective impairment in memory consolidation. *Psychopharmacology, 141,* 362–369.

Rinck, M., & Becker, E. S. (2005). A comparison of attentional biases and memory biases in women with social phobia and major depression. *Journal of Abnormal Psychology, 114,* 62–74.

Roberson-Nay, R., McClure, E. B., Monk, C. S., Nelson, E. E., Guyer, A. E., Fromm, S. J., … Pine, D. S. (2006) Increased amygdala activity during successful memory encoding in adolescent major depressive disorder: An fMRI study. *Biological Psychiatry, 60,* 966–973.

Robinson, O., Letkiewicz, A., Overstreet, C., Ernst, M., & Grillon, C. (2011) The effect of induced anxiety on cognition: Threat of shock enhances aversive processing in healthy individuals. *Cognitive, Affective, and Behavioral Neuroscience, 11*(2), 217–227.

Robinson, O., & Sahakian, B. (2009a) Acute tryptophan depletion evokes negative mood in healthy females who have previously experienced concurrent negative mood and tryptophan depletion. *Psychopharmacology, 205,* 227–235.

Robinson, O., & Sahakian, B. (2009b) A double dissociation in the roles of serotonin and mood in healthy subjects. *Biological Psychiatry, 65,* 89–92.

Robinson, O. J. (2011). Brain burdens: Boost resilience to tackle mental illness. *Nature, 478,* 459–459.

Robinson, O. J., Charney, D. R., Overstreet, C., Vytal, K., & Grillon, C. (2012) The adaptive threat bias in anxiety: Amygdala–dorsomedial prefrontal cortex coupling and aversive amplification. *Neuroimage, 60,* 523–529.

Robinson, O. J., Cools, R., Carlisi, C. O., Sahakian, B. J., & Drevets, W. C. (2012) Ventral striatum response during reward and punishment reversal learning in unmedicated major depressive disorder. *American Journal of Psychiatry, 169,* 152–159.

Robinson, O. J., Cools, R., Crockett, M. J., & Sahakian, B. J. (2009). Mood state moderates the role of serotonin in cognitive biases. *Journal of Psychopharmacology, 24*(4), 573–583.

Robinson, O. J., Cools, R., & Sahakian, B. J. (2011). Tryptophan depletion disinhibits punishment but not reward prediction: Implications for resilience. *Psychopharmacology, 219*(2), 599–605.

Robinson, O. J., Frank, M. J., Sahakian, B. J., & Cools, R. (2010) Dissociable responses to punishment in distinct striatal regions during reversal learning. *NeuroImage, 51,* 1459–1467.

Robinson, O. J., & Sahakian, B. J. (2008) Recurrence in major depressive disorder: A neurocognitive perspective. *Psychological Medicine, 38,* 315–318.

Robinson, O. J., & Sahakian, B. J. (2009c). A double dissociation in the roles of serotonin and mood in healthy subjects. *Biological Psychiatry, 65,* 89–92.

Robinson, R. G., Paradiso, S., Mizrahi, R., Fiedorowicz, J. G., Kouzoukas, D. E., & Moser, D. J. (2007). Neuropsychological correlates of normal variation in emotional response to visual stimuli. *Journal of Nervous and Mental Disease, 195,* 112.

Rogers, M. A., Kasai, K., Koji, M., Fukuda, R., Iwanami, A., Nakagome, K., … Kato, N. (2004). Executive and prefrontal dysfunction in unipolar depression: A review of neuropsychological and imaging evidence. *Neuroscience Research, 50,* 1–11.

Roiser, J., Rogers, R., Cook, L., & Sahakian, B. (2006). The effect of polymorphism at the serotonin transporter gene on decision-making, memory and executive function in ecstasy users and controls. *Psychopharmacology, 188,* 213–227.

Roiser, J. P., de Martino, B., Tan, G. C. Y., Kumaran, D., Seymour, B., Wood, N. W., & Dolan, R. J. (2009). A genetically mediated bias in decision making driven by failure of amygdala control. *Journal of Neuroscience, 29,* 5985–5991.

Roiser, J. P., Levy, J., Fromm, S. J., Wang, H., Hasler, G., Sahakian, B. J., & Drevets, W. C. (2007). The effect of acute tryptophan depletion on the neural correlates of emotional processing in healthy volunteers. *Neuropsychopharmacology, 33*(8), 1992–2006.

Roiser, J. P., Rubinsztein, J. S., & Sahakian, B. J. (2003). Cognition in depression. *Psychiatry, 2,* 43–47.

Roiser, J. P., Rubinsztein, J. S., & Sahakian, B. J. (2009). Neuropsychology of affective disorders. *Psychiatry, 8,* 91–96.

Rubinow, D. R., & Post, R. M. (1992). Impaired recognition of affect in facial expression in depressed patients. *Biological Psychiatry, 31,* 947–953.

Rubinsztein, J. S., Rogers, R. D., Riedel, W. J., Mehta, M. A., Robbins, T. W., & Sahakian, B. J. (2001). Acute dietary tryptophan depletion impairs maintenance of "affective set" and delayed visual recognition in healthy volunteers. *Psychopharmacology, 154,* 319–326.

Ruhe, H. G., Mason, N. S., & Schene, A. H. (2007). Mood is indirectly related to serotonin, norepinephrine and dopamine levels in humans: A meta-analysis of monoamine depletion studies. *Molecular Psychiatry, 12,* 331–359.

Sahakian, B., & Morein-Zamir, S. (2011). Depression and resilience: Insights from cognitive, neuroimaging and psychopharmacological studies. In M. Delgado, E. Phelps, & T. Robbins (Eds.), *Decision making, affect and learning. Attention and Performance XXIII* (pp. 505–532). Oxford, England: Oxford University Press.

Sahakian, B. J., Malloch, G., & Kennard, C. (2010). A UK strategy for mental health and wellbeing. *Lancet, 375,* 1854–1855.

Sahakian, B. J., & Morein-Zamir, S. (2010). Neuroethical issues in cognitive enhancement. *Journal of Psychopharmacology.* 2010 Mar 8, ePub ahead of print.

Salloway, S., Malloy, P., Kohn, R., Gillard, E., Duffy, J., Rogg, J.,… Westlake, R. (1996). MRI and neuropsychological differences in early- and late-life-onset geriatric depression. *Neurology, 46,* 1567–1574.

Sambeth, A., Blokland, A., Harmer, C. J., Kilkens, T. O. C., Nathan, P. J., Porter, R. J.,… Riedel, W. J. (2007). Sex differences in the effect of acute tryptophan depletion on declarative episodic memory: A pooled analysis of nine studies. *Neuroscience and Biobehavioral Reviews, 31,* 516–529.

Savitz, J., Solms, M., & Ramesar, R. (2006). The molecular genetics of cognition: Dopamine, COMT and BDNF. *Genes, Brain and Behavior, 5,* 311–328.

Schmitt, J. A. J., Jorissen, B. L., Sobczak, S., van Boxtel, M. P. J., Hogervorst, E., Deutz, N. E. P., & Riedel, W. J. (2000). Tryptophan depletion impairs memory consolidation but improves focussed attention in healthy young volunteers. *Journal of Psychopharmacology, 14,* 21–29.

Sheline, Y. I., Barch, D. M., Donnelly, J. M., Ollinger, J. M., Snyder, A. Z., & Mintun, M. A. (2001). Increased amygdala response to masked emotional faces in depressed subjects resolves with antidepressant treatment: An fMRI study. *Biological Psychiatry, 50,* 651–658.

Siegle, G. J., Carter, C. S., & Thase, M. E. (2006). Use of fMRI to predict recovery from unipolar depression with cognitive behavior therapy. *American Journal of Psychiatry, 163,* 735–738.

Siegle, G. J., Steinhauer, S. R., Thase, M. E., Stenger, V. A., & Carter, C. S. (2002). Can't shake that feeling: Event-related fMRI assessment of sustained amygdala activity in response to emotional information in depressed individuals. *Biological Psychiatry, 51,* 693–707.

Siegle, G. J., Thompson, W., Carter, C. S., Steinhauer, S. R., & Thase, M. E. (2007). Increased amygdala and decreased dorsolateral prefrontal BOLD responses in unipolar depression: Related and independent features. *Biological Psychiatry, 61,* 198–209.

Sierra-Mercado, D., Padilla-Coreano, N., & Quirk, G. J. (2011). Dissociable roles of prelimbic and infralimbic cortices, ventral hippocampus, and basolateral amygdala in the expression and extinction of conditioned fear. *Neuropsychopharmacology, 36,* 529–538.

Smith, D. P., Hillman, C. H., & Duley, A. R. (2005). Influences of age on emotional reactivity during picture processing. *Journals of Gerontology Series B, Psychological Sciences Social Sciences, 60,* P49-P56.

Smith, G. S., Gunning-Dixon, F. M., Lotrich, F. E., Taylor, W. D., & Evans, J. D. (2007). Translational research in late-life mood disorders: Implications for future intervention and prevention research. *Neuropsychopharmacology, 32,* 1857–1875.

Smoski, M. J., Felder, J., Bizzell, J., Green, S. R., Ernst, M., Lynch, T. R., & Dichter, G. S. (2009). fMRI of alterations in reward selection, anticipation, and feedback in major depressive disorder. *Journal of Affective Disorders, 118,* 69–78.

Spies, K., Hesse, F. W., & Hummitzsch, C. (1996). Mood and capacity in Baddeley's model of human memory. *Zeitschrift Fur Psychologie, 204,* 367–381.

Steele, J. D., Kumar, P., & Ebmeier, K. P. (2007). Blunted response to feedback information in depressive illness. *Brain, 130*, 2367–2374.

Steele, J. D., Meyer, M., & Ebmeier, K. P. (2004). Neural predictive error signal correlates with depressive illness severity in a game paradigm. *NeuroImage, 23*, 269–280.

Steffens, D. C., Otey, E., Alexopoulos, G. S., Butters, M. A., Cuthbert, B., Ganguli, M., ... Yesavage, J. (2006). Perspectives on depression, mild cognitive impairment, and cognitive decline. *Archives of General Psychiatry, 63*, 130–138.

Steffens, D. C., Wagner, H. R., Levy, R. M., Horn, K. A., & Krishnan, K. R. R. (2001). Performance feedback deficit in geriatric depression. *Biological Psychiatry, 50*, 358–363.

Strauss, J., Barr, C., George, C., Ryan, C., King, N., Shaikh, S., ... Kennedy, J. (2004). BDNF and COMT polymorphisms. *NeuroMolecular Medicine, 5*, 181–192.

Surguladze, S., Brammer, M. J., Keedwell, P., Giampietro, V., Young, A. W., Travis, M. J., ... Phillips, M. L. (2005). A differential pattern of neural response toward sad versus happy facial expressions in major depressive disorder. *Biological Psychiatry, 57*, 201–209.

Surguladze, S. A., Young, A. W., Senior, C., Brébion, G., Travis, M. J., & Phillips, M. L. (2004). Recognition accuracy and response bias to happy and sad facial expressions in patients with major depression. *Neuropsychology, 18*, 212–218.

Sweeney, J. A., Kmiec, J. A., & Kupfer, D. J. (2000). Neuropsychologic impairments in bipolar and unipolar mood disorders on the CANTAB neurocognitive battery. *Biological Psychiatry, 48*, 674–684.

Takami, H., Okamoto, Y., Yamashita, H., Okada, G., & Yamawaki, S. (2007). Attenuated anterior cingulate activation during a verbal fluency task in elderly patients with a history of multiple-episode depression. *American Journal of Geriatric Psychiatry, 15*, 594–603.

Taylor Tavares, J. V., Clark, L., Cannon, D. M., Erickson, K., Drevets, W. C., & Sahakian, B. J. (2007). Distinct profiles of neurocognitive function in unmedicated unipolar depression and bipolar II depression. *Biological Psychiatry, 62*, 917–924.

Taylor Tavares, J. V., Clark, L., Furey, M. L., Williams, G. B., Sahakian, B. J., & Drevets, W. C. (2008). Neural basis of abnormal response to negative feedback in unmedicated mood disorders. *NeuroImage, 42*, 1118–1126.

Taylor Tavares, J. V., Drevets, W. C., & Sahakian, B. J. (2003). Cognition in mania and depression. *Psychological Medicine, 33*, 959–967.

Thomas, E. J., & Elliott, R. (2009). Brain imaging correlates of cognitive impairment in depression. *Frontiers in Human Neuroscience, 3*, 30.

Trichard, C., Martinot, J. L., Alagille, M., Masure, M. C., Hardy, P., Ginestet, D., & Féline, A. (1995). Time course of prefrontal lobe dysfunction in severely depressed in-patients: A longitudinal neuropsychological study. *Psychological Medicine, 25*, 79–85.

Videbech, P., Ravnkilde, B., Kristensen, S., Egander, A., Clemmensen, K., Rasmussen, N. A., ... Rosenberg, R. (2003). The Danish PET/depression project: Poor verbal fluency performance despite normal prefrontal activation in patients with major depression. *Psychiatry Research: Neuroimaging, 123*, 49–63.

Vosburg, S. K. (1998). The effects of positive and negative mood on divergent-thinking performance. *Creativity Research Journal, 11*, 165–172.

Wagner, G., Sinsel, E., Sobanski, T., Köhler, S., Marinou, V., Mentzel, H-J., ... Schlösser, R. G. M. (2006). Cortical inefficiency in patients with unipolar depression: An event-related fMRI study with the Stroop task. *Biological Psychiatry, 59*, 958–965.

Walsh, N. D., Williams, S. C. R., Brammer, M. J., Bullmore, E. T., Kim, J., Suckling, J., ... Fu C. H. Y. (2007). A longitudinal functional magnetic resonance imaging study of verbal working memory in depression after antidepressant therapy. *Biological Psychiatry, 62*, 1236–1243.

Watts, F. N., MacLeod, A. K., & Morris, L. (1988). Associations between phenomenal and objective aspects of concentration problems in depressed patients. *British Journal of Psychology, 79*, 241–250.

36

NEUROPATHOLOGICAL MARKERS IN LATE-LIFE DEPRESSION

José Javier Miguel-Hidalgo and Grazyna Rajkowska

MAJOR DEPRESSION is a highly prevalent psychiatric disorder with devastating personal, social, and economic consequences. This high prevalence is underscored by its significant presence at all ages along the life span from adolescence to late life (Beekman, Copeland, & Prince, 1999; Luijendijk et al., 2008). That is, unlike schizophrenia and other psychiatric disorders, the incidence of major depressive disorder (MDD) is still high among the elderly. The persistence of affective disorders in late life suggests a particular insidiousness of the pathophysiological mechanisms of depression and the possibility that age-related alterations in cellular metabolism, neurotransmission, or brain blood supply contribute to late-life onset or to the continued surfacing of depressive symptoms in the elderly. As explained in detail in other chapters of this book, neuroimaging studies have shown that specific alterations in gray and white matter are detectable in cortical and subcortical regions in late-life depression. These alterations suggest that age-dependent, functional and structural changes at the cellular level

occur in specific brain areas and contribute to the pathophysiology of late-life depression. Increased risk for depression is also associated with the manifestation of Alzheimer's disease, stroke, and vascular disorders, which are also age dependent themselves. However, some research suggests that depression in late life is not necessarily a consequence of neuropathology of the Alzheimer's type or of vascular dementia (Hoogendijk et al., 1999; Tsopelas et al., 2011). Psychiatric disorders in late life do not appear to increase the risk for Alzheimer's neuropathology (Damadzic, Shuangshoti, Giblen, & Herman, 2002), or they are associated with this pathology when late-life depression is concurrent with dementia (Sweet et al. 2004), which suggests the existence of age-specific neuropathological alterations in late-life depression (Table 36.1). Most of the studies and evidence reviewed herein concerns depressive symptoms or MDD. Bipolar disorder also occurs late in life, and in a proportion of patients it has a late onset. However, bipolar disorder accounts only for 8%–10% of late-life admissions, and many late-onset cases appear

Table 36.1 Summary of brain postmortem studies with relevant neuropathological findings in late-life major depressive disorder

DISEASE(NO. OF SUBJECTS); AGE IN YEARS	BRAIN REGION OR CORTICAL AREA; HEMISPHERE	METHODS	NEURONS	GLIA	REFERENCES
MDD (12); Age 52.8/CTRL (12); Age 43.3	dlPFC (BA 9); left	Nissl, optical disector	↓Density of large neurons (20% LV, 60% L II, III, VI) ↑Density of small neurons ↓Size (5% L III, 7% LVI)	↓Density (20% – 30% L III, V) ↑Size (6% L IIIa)	Rajkowska et al. 1999
MDD (15); Age 47±9.3/ BPD (15) / CTRL (15);48±10.7	dlPFC (BA 9); left+right	Nissl, Optical disector	↓Size (20% L VI) in MDD ↓Size (14% L V, 18% L VI) in BPD	↓Density (30% L V) in MDD ↔Size in MDD, BPD	Cotter et al. 2002b
MDD (14); Age 52.8/ CTRL (15); 44.6	dlPFC (BA 9); left	GFAP IHC	Not examined	↓Area fraction and density (L III – V) in subgroup of young MDD subjects, ↔Density in older MDD subgroup ↔Area and density in young and old subjects combined	Miguel-Hidalgo et al. 2000
MDD (15); Age 55±17.6/ CTRL (15); Age 54±18.3	dlPFC (BA 9); left	Western blotting		↓Levels of GFAP in younger MDD subjects but not in older Positive correlation of GFAP levels with age in MDD subjects.	Si et al. 2004

Sample	Region	Method	Findings		References
MDD (14); Age 54±16.8/ CTRL (11); Age 47±16.6	dlPFC (BA9), OFC (BA47) left	IHC for calbindin (CB) and parvalbumin (PV); optical disector, nucleator	↓Density CB neurons (50%) dlPFC; ↓size CB neurons (18%) dlPFC. =density size CB neurons in ORB / ↔Density, size of PV neurons in dlPFC and ORB / Density CB neurons negatively correlated with age		Rajkowska et al., 2007
MDD (17); Age 76±7.05/ CTRL (10); Age 77±7.69	dlPFC (BA 9/46); right	Nissl, optical disector, nucleator	↓Volume of pyramidal neurons (17%, L III – V); =non-pyramidal neurons / ↔Density pyramidal, non-pyramidal	↔Density	Khundakar et al., 2009
MDD (36)/CTRL (117); Age >60 years, old	dlPFC (BA 8/9), BA21, BA17/18, BA7, hippocampus;	H&E, Golgi, Four-point subjective scale	↓Hippocampus, ↓Substantia nigra, ↓Raphe nucleus,, No AD neuropathology in neocortex		Tsopelas et. al., 2011
MDD (8)/CTRL (10) Age >60 years old	dlPFC (BA 9); left	Autoradiography of 5-HT transporter binding	↔Density of binding		Thomas et al., 2006
MDD (15); Age 46.5±9.3/ CTRL (15); Age 48.1±10.7	Anterior cingulate cortex (BA 24b); left + right	Nissl, optical disector	↔Density	↓Density (22% L VI)	Cotter et al.,2001
MDD (12); Age 52.8/ CTRL (12); Age 43.3	OFC (BA 10, 47); left	Nissl, optical disector	↓Density of large neurons (20% – 60% L II – IV) / ↑Density of small neurons (L III) / ↓Size (9% L II, III) / ↓Density (L IIIa, Va)	↓Density (15% – 18% L IIIc – VI)	Rajkowska et al., 1999

(Continued)

Table 36.1 Continued

DISEASE(NO. OF SUBJECTS); AGE IN YEARS	BRAIN REGION OR CORTICAL AREA; HEMISPHERE	METHODS	NEURONS	GLIA	REFERENCES
MDD (15); Age 75±9/ CTRL (11); Age 72±8	OFC (BA 47); left	Nissl, optical dissector, nucleator	↓Size (6% L II) ↓Density pyramidal neurons (overall 30%; L III-V) ↔Density non-pyramidal neurons	↔Density	Rajkowska et al., 2005
MDD (13); Age 49±19.9/ CTRL (13); Age 51±14.4	OFC (BA47); left	IHC, Western Blotting of glutamate transporters, glutamine synthetase		↓Levels of glutamate transporters, glutamine synthetase, but positive correlation of EAAT1 levels with age in MDD	Miguel-Hidalgo et al., 2010
MDD (13)/CTRL (9); Age >60 years old	Caudate nucleus (dorsolateral and ventromedial); right	Nissl, optical disector, nucleator	↓Density; ↔volume	↔Density	Khundakar et al., 2011
MDD (14); Age 71.0±8.6/ CTRL (10); Age 77.5±6.7	Dorsal raphe nuclei	IHC for tryptophan hydroxylase, 2-D image analysis	↔Density; ↔dendritic pathology		Hendricksen et al., 2004

MDD (9)/CTRL (18); Age >65 years old	Dorsal raphe; locus coeruleus	IHC tyrosine hydroxilase, IHC phenylalanine hydroxylase, Nissl; 2-D image analysis	↔Density; ↑cell body size	Syed et al., 2005
MDD (10); Age 80.6±8.6/ Dementia alone (56); Age 81.2±6.8	middle and superior frontal gyri, Ant cingulate gyrus, caudate head, hippocampus, substantia nigra, inferior parietal cortex, superior temporal gyrus, BA17, amygdala, transentorhinal cortex	H&E, Bielschowsky, IHC.	Predominant Alzheimer's neuropathology in MDD comorbid with dementia.	Sweet et al, 2004

Notes: Ant = anterior; BA = Brodmann's area; BPD = bipolar disorder; CB = calbindin; CR = calretinin; CTRL = control; dlPFC = dorsolateral prefrontal cortex; EAAT1 = excitatory amino acid transporter 1; f = familial; GFAP = glial fibrillary acidic protein; IHC = immunohistochemistry; L= layer; MDD = major depressive disorder; OFC = orbitofrontal cortex; PV = paravalbumin; ↓, ↑< = significantly different from control; ↔ < = not significantly different from control.

to be related to neurological factors (Depp & Jeste, 2004). Unlike MDD, and despite some structural neuroimaging data suggesting reduced gray matter volume in the orbitofrontal cortex (OFC) in elderly subjects with bipolar disorder (Beyer et al., 2009), there is much less information on brain cell pathological changes in late-life bipolar disorder. Accordingly, most of the discussion and citations herein are related to late-life major depression.

The prefrontal cortex (PFC) has been a major focus of attention in neuropathological studies of late-life affective disorders. As detailed in the sections that follow, several cortical areas within the PFC have been examined for changes in neurons, glia, and blood vessels. Thus, most of the research that we discuss is concerned with the PFC, although we also present less abundant data on relevant subcortical structures. Within the PFC, the OFC has been often targeted because it is a region showing major functional and structural alterations in affective disorders (Drevets, 2007; Lacerda et al., 2004; Lai, Payne, Byrum, Steffens, & Krishnan, 2000; Rajkowska, Miguel-Hidalgo, Dubey, Stockmeier, & Krishnan, 2005; Van Otterloo et al., 2009). In addition, as compared to other prefrontal regions, the OFC undergoes significant regressive changes during late life even in nonpsychiatric healthy subjects (Raz et al., 1997; Resnick, Lamar, & Driscoll, 2007), although other prefrontal regions also suffer significant changes as compared to the rest of the cortex (Fjell et al., 2009; Pieperhoff et al., 2008). Age-related changes in the OFC include a progressive reduction of cortical thickness and volume of the gray matter. Thus, an interaction between age-related vulnerability and the neuropathological and functional disturbances characteristic of affective disorders set the stage for a significant involvement of the OFC, and possibly other prefrontal regions, in the neuropathology and neurophysiology of late-life disorders.

NEURONAL PATHOLOGY

Most of our knowledge on the pathology of late-life-depression is based on clinical investigations or the use of neuroimaging techniques, which provide mostly evidence of macroscopic changes in the brain of elderly subjects. Functional neuroimaging studies of glucose metabolism, neurotransmitter levels, and hemodynamic parameters indicate that in elderly subjects with depression there is a specific enhancement of pathological changes that are observed in various cortical and subcortical brain regions of younger subjects with depression (Drevets, 2001). However, some structural changes in late-onset late-life depression appear to involve cerebrovascular alterations and nonspecific signs of atrophy not observed with as much frequency in age-matched control subjects or MDD subjects with early onset (Drevets, Price, & Furey, 2008). The consequences or involvement of pathological changes at the level of individual neurons or groups of neurons in late-life depression have not been investigated as much as changes observed with neuroimaging techniques. However, in the last decade there have been a few postmortem studies that have focused their attention on late-life depression. These postmortem investigations have targeted changes at the cellular and molecular levels in blood vessels, neurons, and glial cells that should eventually build the foundation to explain functional, structural, and behavioral changes observed by neuroimaging and neuropsychological studies in late-life depression. Some of the studies have specifically focused on neuronal changes in late-life depression (Khundakar, Morris, Oakley, McMeekin, & Thomas, 2009; Rajkowska et al., 2005; Tsopelas et al., 2011). Some of them used a subjective, semiquantitative four-point scale to characterize neuronal pathology specifically in elderly subjects and found that late-life depression is associated with apparent neuronal loss in the hippocampus (Thomas et al., 2001; Tsopelas et al., 2011). However, this research did not find differences in Alzheimer's disease–like neuronal pathology in a region encompassing areas 8/9 of the dorsolateral prefrontal cortex (dlPFC). Using more sensitive three-dimensional morphometric techniques, a quantitative study of the density and size of neurons in the dlPFC (area 9) of late-life depression reported a reduced average volume of the cell bodies of pyramidal neurons in dlPFC areas 9 and 46, but no differences in the density of pyramidal or nonpyramidal neurons, although no data were presented separately for each of the cortical areas 9 and 46 (Khundakar et al., 2009; Van Otterloo et al., 2009). Increased risk for damage or degeneration of pyramidal neurons in late life-depression is also supported by a report of reduced density of pyramidal glutamatergic cells in the OFC of elderly MDD subjects as compared to age-matched healthy comparison subjects (Rajkowska et al., 2005). These reductions in pyramidal cells affect mainly layers IIIc and V (Rajkowska et al., 2005). Research in nonhuman primates has shown that pyramidal neurons in these layers originate efferent connections terminating in the striatum, other association and limbic cortical areas, and the amygdala (Carmichael & Price, 1995a, 1995b; Haber, Kunishio, Mizobuchi, & Lynd-Balta, 1995; Porrino, Crane, & Goldman-Rakic, 1981; Rempel-Clower & Barbas, 2000). Thus, assuming that similar connection pathways occur in the human brain, a reduction of pyramidal cells in layers III and V in late-life depression may result in a disturbed flow of information between the PFC and several key brain regions involved in emotional regulation (Rajkowska et al., 2005).

The research on neuronal pathology mentioned earlier is based on the use of nonspecific histological staining of neurons, with limited ability to determine the neurochemical/physiological phenotype of the neurons under study. However, there is still the possibility that some specific neuronal subpopulations are differentially affected in depression. In line with this possibility, a study targeting subpopulations of putatively GABAergic nonpyramidal neurons with antibodies to different calcium-binding proteins found that the density of calbindin-28k immunoreactive neurons was decreased in area 9 in depression as compared to nonpsychiatric controls (Rajkowska, O'Dwyer, Teleki, Stockmeier, & Miguel-Hidalgo, 2007). Interestingly, the density of these cells was negatively correlated with age, suggesting that depression in late life might involve increased damage to GABAergic, calbindin-28K immunoreactive cells. There was no difference, however, in the density of another subpopulation of GABAergic neurons characterized by parvalbumin immunoreactivity (Rajkowska, O'Dwyer, Teleki, Stockmeier, & Miguel-Hidalgo, 2007). In another prefrontal area, the OFC, there was a nonsignificant tendency for lower numbers of GABAergic, calbindin-28K-immunoreactive neurons (but not of parvalbumin-immunoreactive neurons) (Rajkowska, O'Dwyer, Teleki, Stockmeier, & Miguel-Hidalgo, 2007), which is consistent with changes found in the dlPFC. These differences between subpopulations of GABAergic cells suggest that specific circuits within the PFC might be responsible for the alterations in GABA-related metabolites in the PFC (Hasler et al., 2007; Sanacora et al., 1999), and that these alterations involve a prominent loss of GABAergic cells in late-life MDD.

GLIAL CELL PATHOLOGY

The available evidence suggests that changes in glial cells in depression are also age dependent. At a relatively young age (less than 60 years) most studies on the PFC describe a reduction (more or less restricted to particular layers or affecting most cortical layers) in the density or number of the general population of glial cells in the OFC (Rajkowska et al., 1999), dlPFC (Cotter et al., 2002; Rajkowska et al., 1999), and anterior cingulate cortex (Cotter, Mackay, Landau, Kerwin, & Everall, 2001; Öngür, Drevets, & Price, 1998). Later in life, however, no differences in glial cell densities between nonpsychiatric controls and MDD subjects have been detected (Khundakar et al., 2009; Khundakar & Thomas, 2009; Rajkowska et al., 2005). Since there is no reduction of glial cell numbers during life in nonpsychiatric subjects, it seems that a secondary increase in glial cell numbers or their markers might be occurring in the PFC of MDD subjects in late life. These glial increases might be related to a decrease in neuronal density or to an enhancement of damage to neurons of the OFC and other cortical areas.

The data regarding the general population of glial cells reported earlier does not distinguish among the three major classes of glial cells, that is, astrocytes, oligodendrocytes, or microglial cells, but some studies have addressed involvement of specific glial cell types. One of the studies targeted the population of astrocytes containing the cytoskeletal protein glial fibrillary acidic protein (GFAP) (Miguel-Hidalgo et al., 2000), a specific marker for astrocytes. This study showed that the area fraction and packing density of GFAP astrocytes are lower in younger MDD subjects than in healthy comparison subjects, but that older MDD subjects do not differ significantly from age-matched psychiatrically healthy subjects. A later study focusing on individual cortical layers showed that there is actually an increase in GFAP immunostaining in layer I of elderly MDD subjects as compared to nonpsychiatric controls (Davis et al., 2002). Studies of GFAP levels in the dlPFC also uncovered a steep increase of GFAP protein in elderly subjects with MDD (Si, Miguel-Hidalgo, O'Dwyer, Stockmeier, & Rajkowska, 2004) as compared to younger MDD and healthy control subjects. A possible explanation for the age-related increase of GFAP in late-life MDD would be that the increase in numbers or in glial markers in late-life MDD is a secondary response to an increase in neuronal loss or atrophy. It is well known that astrocytes and microglial cells are sensitive to signals derived from damaged or dying neurons and that the activation is not restricted only to the area directly suffering neurotrauma, ischemia, or manifest neurodegeneration (Giaume, Kirchhoff, Matute, Reichenbach, & Verkhratsky, 2007; McGraw, Hiebert, & Steeves, 2001; Sofroniew, 2009). More subtle degenerative changes in neurons or their connections that do not involve cell death or catastrophic synaptic changes can also trigger the activation of GFAP-immunoreactive glial cells. For example, in some animal models of synaptic damage caused by exposure to toxicants, astrocyte activation occurs without formation of a glial scar at locations distant from the main focus of trauma (Brock & O'Callaghan, 1987; Fernandez et al., 2011; Malhotra & Shnitka, 2002). Likewise, neuronal changes observed in MDD studies may not be related to catastrophic trauma or neurodegeneration, since subjects with patent brain damage or neurodegeneration were excluded in most studies of late-life MDD mentioned earlier. Even in the absence of major neuropathological changes, the available studies on neuropathology of MDD still reported increased degenerative features in specific populations of neurons in late-life MDD, as described earlier. For instance, in the dlPFC, volumes of pyramidal cell bodies were smaller in the dlPFC and their packing density reduced in the ORB, while the density of calbindin-immunoreactive GABAergic neurons was reduced in the dlPFC in older subjects with MDD. Thus, in response to age-related regressive changes, distress signals from neurons in the PFC may trigger the activation of specific glial cell functions that would account for the increased density of glial cells or their markers. However, this hypothesis does not rule out that, since neuronal function might be abnormal, physiological features of glial cells that depend on a healthy neuronal physiology might still be diminished or pathological. Further studies should determine what aspects of the glia–neuron interaction are most important in the pathophysiology of late-life depression.

The studies presented earlier suggest that some areas in the PFC might be preferential sites for age-related neuropathology in late-life depression. However, recent research by Khundakar et al. (2011) has also revealed modest but significantly low neuronal packing density in the caudate nucleus in late-life depression as compared to nonpsychiatric comparison subjects (Khundakar, Morris, Oakley, & Thomas, 2011). Like in the aging PFC, the packing density of glial cells was not changed in the caudate nucleus, suggesting that similar glial responses to neuronal vulnerability might be at work in the caudate nucleus and PFC in late-life depression. In

other brain regions with assumed high relevance to depression pathophysiology or treatment, there is no neuropathological evidence for neuronal changes in late-life depression. For instance, the number of serotonergic neurons and the morphology of their neurites in the dorsal raphe nucleus are not changed in elderly MDD subjects as compared to age-matched controls (Hendricksen, Thomas, Ferrier, Ince, & O'Brien, 2004; Syed et al., 2005). In line with this absence of depression-related changes is the finding that in subjects with Alzheimer's disease, there is loss and marked pathology of neurons in the raphe, but there is no difference between Alzheimer's subjects diagnosed with comorbid depression and those without depression (Hendricksen et al., 2004). Even the levels of serotonin transporters in the PFC, which are carried to the PFC by axons of raphe neurons, appear not to differ in elderly subjects with MDD (Thomas et al., 2006) as compared to nonpsychiatric controls or be correlated with aging (Austin, Whitehead, Edgar, Janosky, & Lewis, 2002). Only in the locus coeruleus (LC) immunoreactivity for corticotropin-releasing hormone has been found positively correlated with age of onset in MDD subjects (Austin, Janosky, & Murphy, 2003). However, as in the raphe, loss of neurons in the LC in Alzheimer's disease is not associated with depression (Hoogendijk et al., 1999). The importance of the PFC as a main site for late-life neuropathology in depression, in comparison to other brain regions, is also supported by the tendency of depression in Alzheimer's disease patients to be associated with disturbed executive functions (Thomas et al., 2009), which depend heavily on the integrity of the PFC (Alexopoulos, 2003).

Astrocytes are major players in the supply of metabolic energy to neurons and in the termination of glutamatergic neurotransmission (Anderson & Swanson, 2000; Araque, Carmignoto, & Haydon, 2001; Harder, Zhang, & Gebremedhin, 2002). The possibility of a role for astrocytes in the pathophysiology of depression is underscored by the proposed pathophysiological role of glutamate changes and reduced brain metabolism in prefrontal areas of subjects with MDD (Auer et al., 2000; Choudary et al., 2005; Hasler et al., 2007; Paul & Skolnick, 2003). In the neocortex, astrocytes are the principal mediators of the reuptake of released glutamate through glutamate transporters EAAT1 and EAAT2 located in their processes. In accordance with reduced numbers or diminished tissue coverage by GFAP-immunoreactive astrocytes in MDD subjects, a recent study has shown that the levels of EAAT2 and EAAT1 in the ORB are lower in MDD subjects as compared to healthy, nonpsychiatric control subjects (Miguel-Hidalgo et al., 2010). Interestingly, the levels of EAAT1 increase significantly with age in MDD subjects, supporting the hypothesis that activity of some astrocytes might be enhanced in late-life depression (Miguel-Hidalgo et al., 2010). Whether initial low levels of EAAT1 and increased EAAT1 levels in late life in subjects with early-onset depression are related to increased concentrations of glutamate in the PFC as revealed by magnetic resonance spectroscopy, and whether the increase might be observed in subjects with late onset of depression, remains to be ascertained.

Unlike astrocytes, the numbers of oligodendrocytes (the glial cells that form myelin in the central nervous system) do not appear to increase late in life in the cortex of MDD subjects. In fact, recent studies indicate that in cortical layer VI and white matter of the PFC (Byne, Tatusov, Yiannoulos, Vong, & Marcus, 2008; Vostrikov & Uranova, 2011) and possibly in some thalamic nuclei (Byne et al., 2008) of MDD, bipolar disorder, and schizophrenia subjects, there is not an aging-related increase of oligodendrocytes. However, in nonpsychiatric healthy subjects there is a significant age-dependent increase in the numbers of oligodendrocytes extending well into late life (Byne et al., 2008; Vostrikov & Uranova, 2011). Both in gray and white matter of the PFC, this interaction with age in psychiatric subjects is highly significant as compared to nonpsychiatric healthy control subjects. It remains to be ascertained whether a deficit in the normal increase of oligodendrocytes in the PFC during aging might be related to the persistence or appearance of late-life depression. Despite reduced numbers of oligodendrocytes in MDD, there could be an activation of myelin-forming mechanisms in the remaining oligodendrocytes. A recent preliminary investigation on the white matter of the ventromedial PFC (adjacent to the gray mater of the OFC) found reduced level of CNPase, an enzyme contained in oligodendrocytes and directly involved in myelin production, and lower density of oligodendrocytes in MDD subjects, as compared to matched controls (Rajkowska, Maciag, Iyo, Austin, & Stockmeier, 2011). However, while in young MDD subjects the levels of CNPase were significantly lower than in their age-matched normal controls, this difference was absent between controls and MDD subjects over 60 years, suggesting the presence of compensatory CNPase expression

in late-life MDD in a similar fashion to the increased GFAP in elderly MDD subjects described earlier. The reported data from Rajkowska et al. (2011) also suggest an increased size of the oligodendrocyte cell bodies in the white matter of MDD subjects. It remains to be determined whether protein level changes in deep white matter are correlated with changes (or absence of changes) in the numbers and size of oligodendrocytes in different brain regions and how the observed changes and correlations relate to the manifestation of late-life depression. Thus, it seems that different types of glial cells would respond or contribute to the prefrontal neuropathology of late-life depression according to the specific roles they play in neuronal function. Sorting out what are the relative contributions of the various types of glial cells will require further studies of each glial cell type and their interaction with the neurons they support.

MARKERS OF CELL DEATH AND CELL PROLIFERATION IN LATE-LIFE DEPRESSION

Enhanced neuronal and glial cell damage in depression, even if progressive and noncatastrophic, would suggest that there is activation of cellular pathways that increases the pathological vulnerability of prefrontal cortical cells. In bipolar disorder, recent research has shown that some proteins involved in the progression of apoptosis are increased in the dlPFC, although the relationship of those increases to aging is still unknown (Kim, Rapoport, & Rao, 2010). In MDD, cross-sectional studies using the TUNEL technique (which labels DNA fragmentation in the nucleus of cells dying by apoptosis) have found only scarce labeling of apoptotic cells in the hippocampus and entorhinal cortex, suggesting that even if vulnerability to apoptosis might be increased, cell death might be occurring at a very low rate in the hippocampal formation (Lucassen et al., 2001). Information on other brain areas is not available, so it is not possible to determine the regional specificity of those changes. It is also unknown whether bursts of cell death or damage might occur that would be difficult to detect in the necessarily cross-sectional postmortem studies. At the protein level, there is some evidence that in major depression or stress (as a factor facilitating the onset of or being associated with depression) proteins involved in the control of apoptosis might be altered in the direction of favoring apoptosis (McKernan, Dinan, & Cryan, 2009). These alterations include reduction of pro-survival factors, such as bcl-2, ERK1, or CREB, although it is still unknown whether age may modify the relationship of depression to changes in cells survival or integrity. Some glial cells, mainly astrocytes, also appear to be activated in the PFC in late-life MDD. This activation would point to mechanisms that affect the proliferation of glial cells or glial cell precursors, which, unlike neocortical neurons, still retain during adulthood the ability to divide. In a first approach to determine whether proteins related to cell death, DNA damage, and proliferation are altered in depression and comorbid conditions across the life span, we have started to determine the levels and distribution of some of those proteins in depression, alcoholism, and comorbid depression and alcoholism. Recently, we have observed that activated caspase 8, a protease that is a major switch in the cascade of cell death by apoptosis (it is an initiator caspase that activates other caspases) is significantly higher in depression, alcoholism, and comorbid depression and alcoholism. However, while there is a small but significant progressive increase in the levels of activated caspase 8 with age in nonpsychiatric subjects, the levels of this protein were consistently high at all ages in all groups of diseased subjects (Miguel-Hidalgo, Whittom, et al., 2011). The increased activation might indicate increased vulnerability to cell death, although not necessarily a high degree of completed cell death, because frequent cell death is not observed in brains from MDD subjects (Lucassen et al., 2001). In the same groups of subjects we determined levels of proliferating cell nuclear antigen (PCNA), which is involved and required in DNA replication and is upregulated in dividing cells. PCNA in some cell types is also a crucial factor involved in DNA repair. PCNA was found in individual cells and its levels were determined in the OFC. Interestingly, the levels of this protein were not changed in controls subjects across the life span, but their levels were positively correlated with age in subjects with depression or alcoholism. At first sight this would indicate increased proliferative activity in cells of the PFC. However, the increased neuronal and/or glial cell damage in the OFC in late life and the absence of neuronal proliferation would not rule out an increase in DNA damage events that would trigger an increase in the PCNA involved in DNA repair.

NEUROVASCULAR AND NEUROIMMUNE CHANGES

Neuroimaging and neuropsychological studies have linked the occurrence of MDD in the elderly to the presence of vascular lesions that are detected as hyperintensities in the prefrontal white matter (Alexopoulos et al., 1997; Krishnan, Hays, & Blazer, 1997; Taylor et al., 2003; Thomas et al., 2002). These lesions are more frequent in elderly MDD subjects than in younger subjects or in matched nonpsychiatric comparison subjects and appear in the deep white matter underneath prefrontal cortical areas directly relevant to depression. The lesions appear to be ischemic in nature (Thomas et al., 2002), supporting the hypothesis that vascular pathology might significantly contribute to depression in the elderly. The presence of increased cerebrovascular pathology in the white matter of the elderly with MDD might suggest that vascular pathology might occur also in vessels of the cortical gray matter. However, histomorphological assessment of pathological changes in small vessels (capillaries, arterioles) either by semiquantitative subjective grading of vascular histopathology or by more quantitative automated morphometric methods (Miguel-Hidalgo et al., 2012) does not support pathology of these vessels in MDD subjects as compared to controls. For instance, Kandahar et al. (2009) used a four-point semiquantitative scale to determine the degree of small-vessel morphological disturbances in the PFC of MDD subjects and did not detect differences as compared to small vessels in nonpsychiatric comparison subjects, in agreement with previous studies using a similar four-point subjective scoring system (Thomas et al., 2001). Likewise, computerized analysis of small vessels in the OFC in elderly subjects with MDD revealed an absence of changes in the density or size of small vessel profiles encompassing capillaries and small arterioles, while suggesting that only in larger vessels a difference between elderly MDD subjects and controls could be detected (Miguel-Hidalgo & Rajkowska et al., 2012). It seems that localized vascular accidents in relevant brain areas increase the risk for depression in the elderly, but that depression in the elderly is not necessarily associated with disease of capillaries and arterioles in the gray matter.

Neuronal and glial pathology arising during normal aging or associated with affective disorders in late life could be related to alterations in the peripheral immune system or to the activation of immuno-competent microglial cells and astrocytes within the brain (Jurgens & Johnson, 2010). Peripheral immune activation can directly affect neuronal physiology and survival (Matsumoto, Watanabe, Suh, & Yamamoto, 2002; Talley et al., 1995), but it also triggers the activation of glial cells within the central nervous system (Henry, Huang, Wynne, & Godbout, 2009) probably involving the extravasation of blood-borne immune cells across the vascular endothelium into the brain parenchyma and the action of inflammatory cytokines released by these cells or glial cells themselves. It is of particular relevance that the priming of glial cells by peripheral immune activation may be exacerbated by age (Deng, Bertini, Xu, Yan, & Bentivoglio, 2006; Henry et al., 2009; Wynne, Henry, & Godbout, 2009). There is also evidence supporting that neuroimmune alterations can be major factors in the pathophysiology of depression regardless of age (Dantzer, O'Connor, Freund, Johnson, & Kelley, 2008). Thus, there is the possibility of an interaction between disorder-specific and age-related immune changes that may result in disruption of particular brain circuits in late-life depression. Most of the effects of neuroimmune alterations on function and structure of neurons and glial cells are mediated by cytokines and related growth factors (Hayley, Poulter, Merali, & Anisman, 2005). These molecules are produced not only in lymphocytes and other peripheral immunocompetent cells but also by activated microglia and astrocytes. Microglia and astrocytes can act as immunocompetent cells in response to neuronal damage, including degeneration of neurites and synapses (Brock & O'Callaghan, 1987; O'Callaghan, Miller, & Reinhard, 1990). Conversely, untimely or excessive activation of neuroimmune properties of microglia and astrocytes may cause neuronal or synaptic damage (Chao, Hu, Molitor, Shaskan, & Peterson, 1992; Deshpande et al., 2005; Markiewicz & Lukomska, 2006). Thus, a positive feedback between neuronal damage and glial activation in late life may lead to substantial damage of neuronal structure and function, and it might explain disturbances found in some regions of the aging brain in depression. Facilitation of late-life depression by inflammatory activation involving blood vessels has been suggested by the finding of increased proportions of blood vessels positive for intercellular adhesion molecule 1 (ICAM-1) in the PFC of subjects with late-life depression (Thomas et al., 2000). ICAM-1 is a main inflammatory mediator of leukocyte extravasation across the vascular endothelium wall. Accordingly, Thomas et al. (2000) have proposed that an increase in the proportion of ICAM-1-positive vessels supports the involvement of prefrontal vascular pathology and inflammation in late-life depression. However, ICAM-1 is not only localized to blood vessels but is also expressed in an inducible manner by astrocytes (Lee & Benveniste, 1999; Satoh, Kim, Kastrukoff, & Takei, 1991; Shrikant, Chung, Ballestas, & Benveniste, 1994). Recent research in our laboratories using a morphometric technique different from that of Thomas et al. (2000) has shown that ICAM-1 in blood vessels of the OFC is detectable at all ages and increases only slightly toward late life. In addition, we also found that the content of extravascular ICAM-1 immunoreactivity in astrocytes is very low in early and middle-age life but dramatically increases after 60 years of age in many nonpsychiatric normal control subjects (Miguel-Hidalgo, Nithuairisg, Stockmeier, & Rajkowska, 2007). The age-dependent small increase of ICAM-1 in vessels and the dramatic increase of ICAM-1 in astrocytes (Miguel-Hidalgo, Nithuairisg, Stockmeier, & Rajkowska, 2007) may be associated with increased extravasation of lymphocytes, dendritic cells, and/or mast cells, which has been shown to be more prominent in late life (Silverman, Sutherland, Wilhelm, & Silver, 2000; Stichel & Luebbert, 2007), although that association remains to be established. Interestingly, we have shown that the dramatic age-dependent increase of extravascular, astrocyte-associated ICAM-1 immunoreactivity is significantly attenuated in the brain of elderly subjects with MDD, particularly in those that died by suicide, suggesting that a change in the immune status of astrocytes may be related to behavioral and emotional alterations in late-life depression (Miguel-Hidalgo, Overholser, et al., 2011). It remains to be ascertained whether the increase of astrocyte-associated ICAM-1 observed in nonpsychiatric, healthy subjects has a protective role against age-related inflammatory activation and whether this role is diminished in late-life depression.

CONCLUSIONS

In summary, there are pathological changes in the neurons, glial cells, and white matter structure in late-life depression, affecting brains areas that are directly relevant to the emotional and behavioral manifestations of depression. In the PFC the size or the packing density of specific populations of pyramidal (glutamatergic) and nonpyramidal (GABAergic) neurons is reduced as compared to age-matched nonpsychiatric control subjects. Interestingly, there is a rebound in the density of glial cells or expression of their markers in late-life depression, which contrasts with the reductions in glial densities observed in younger subjects with depression as compared to nonpsychiatric controls. Damage, possibly of an ischemic nature, to the deep white matter underlying the gray matter of the PFC may explain the association of vascular disturbances to depression in the elderly, although there is no evidence for vascular pathology in capillaries and small arterioles in the gray matter. Neuroimmune and inflammatory changes that are observed during aging and in depression may be involved in neuronal and glial pathology in the elderly, although there is much to be learned about this possible relationship. Likewise, there is a pressing need for a better understanding of how glial changes are mechanistically linked to neuronal pathology in late-life depression and how they may be linked to vascular alterations.

Disclosures

Dr. Rajkowska has no conflicts to disclose.
Dr. Miguel-Hidalgo has no conflicts to disclose.

REFERENCES

Alexopoulos, G. S. (2003). Role of executive function in late-life depression. *Journal of Clinical Psychiatry, 64*(Suppl 14), 18–23.

Alexopoulos, G. S., Meyers, B., Young, R., Campbell, S., Silbersweig, D., & Charlson, M. (1997). "Vascular depression" hypothesis. *Archives of General Psychiatry, 54*, 915–922.

Anderson, C. M., & Swanson, R. A. (2000). Astrocyte glutamate transport: Review of properties, regulation, and physiological functions. *Glia, 32*, 1–14.

Araque, A., Carmignoto, G., & Haydon, P. G. (2001). Dynamic signaling between astrocytes and neurons. *Annual Review of Physiology, 63*, 795–813.

Auer, D. P., Putz, B., Kraft, E., Lipinski, B., Schill, J., & Holsboer, F. (2000). Reduced glutamate in the anterior cingulate cortex in depression: An in vivo proton magnetic resonance spectroscopy study. *Biological Psychiatry, 47*, 305–313.

Austin, M. C., Janosky, J. E., & Murphy, H. A. (2003). Increased corticotropin-releasing hormone immunoreactivity in monoamine-containing pontine nuclei of depressed suicide men. *Molecular Psychiatry, 8*, 324–332.

Austin, M. C., Whitehead, R. E., Edgar, C. L., Janosky, J. E., & Lewis, D. A. (2002). Localized decrease in serotonin transporter-immunoreactive axons in the prefrontal cortex of depressed subjects committing suicide. *Neuroscience, 114*, 807–815.

Beekman, A. T., Copeland, J. R., & Prince, M. J. (1999). Review of community prevalence of depression in later life. *British Journal of Psychiatry, 174*, 307–311.

Beyer, J. L., Kuchibhatla, M., Payne, M. E., Macfall, J., Cassidy, F., & Krishnan, K. R. (2009). Gray and white matter brain volumes in older adults with bipolar disorder. *International Journal of Geriatric Psychiatry, 24*, 1445–1452.

Brock, T. O., & O'Callaghan, J. P. (1987). Quantitative changes in the synaptic vesicle proteins synapsin I and p38 and the astrocyte-specific protein glial fibrillary acidic protein are associated with chemical-induced injury to the rat central nervous system. *Journal of Neuroscience, 7*, 931–942.

Byne, W., Tatusov, A., Yiannoulos, G., Vong, G. S., & Marcus, S. (2008). Effects of mental illness and aging in two thalamic nuclei. *Schizophrenia Research, 106*, 172–181.

Carmichael, S. T., & Price, J. L. (1995a). Limbic connections of the orbital and medial prefrontal cortex in macaque monkeys. *Journal of Comparative Neurology, 363*, 615–641.

Carmichael, S. T., & Price, J. L. (1995b). Sensory and premotor connections of the orbital and medial prefrontal cortex of macaque monkeys. *Journal of Comparative Neurology, 363*, 642–664.

Chao, C., Hu, S., Molitor, T., Shaskan, E., & Peterson, P. (1992). Activated microglia mediate neuronal cell injury via a nitric oxide mechanism. *Journal of Immunology, 149*, 2736–2741.

Choudary, P. V., Molnar, M., Evans, S. J., Tomita, H., Li, J. Z., Vawter, M. P., … Jones, E. G. (2005). Altered cortical glutamatergic and GABAergic signal transmission with glial involvement in depression. *Proceedings of the National Academy of Sciences USA, 102*, 15653–15658.

Cotter, D., Mackay, D., Chana, G., Beasley, C., Landau, S., & Everall, I. P. (2002). Reduced neuronal size and glial cell density in area 9 of the dorsolateral prefrontal cortex in subjects with major depressive disorder. *Cerebral Cortex, 12*, 386–394.

Cotter, D., Mackay, D., Landau, S., Kerwin, R., & Everall, I. (2001). Reduced glial cell density and neuronal size in the anterior cingulate cortex in major depressive disorder. *Archives of General Psychiatry, 58*, 545–553.

Damadzic, R., Shuangshoti, S., Giblen, G., & Herman, M. M. (2002). Neuritic pathology is lacking in the entorhinal cortex, subiculum and hippocampus in middle-aged adults with schizophrenia, bipolar disorder or unipolar depression. *Acta Neuropathologica (Berl), 103*, 488–494.

Dantzer, R., O'Connor, J. C., Freund, G. G., Johnson, R. W., & Kelley, K. W. (2008). From inflammation to sickness and depression: When the immune system subjugates the brain. *Nature Reviews Neuroscience, 9*, 46–56.

Davis, S., Thomas, A., Perry, R., Oakley, A., Kalaria, R. N., & O'Brien, J. T. (2002). Glial fibrillary acidic protein in late life major depressive disorder: an immunocytochemical study. *Journal of Neurology, Neurosurgery, and Psychiatry, 73*, 556–560.

Deng, X. H., Bertini, G., Xu, Y. Z., Yan, Z., & Bentivoglio, M. (2006). Cytokine-induced activation of glial cells in the mouse brain is enhanced at an advanced age. *Neuroscience, 141*, 645–661.

Depp, C. A., & Jeste, D. V. (2004). Bipolar disorder in older adults: A critical review. *Bipolar Disorders, 6*, 343–367.

Deshpande, M., Zheng, J., Borgmann, K., Persidsky, R., Wu, L., Schellpeper, C., & Ghorpade, A. (2005). Role of activated astrocytes in neuronal damage: Potential links to HIV-1-associated dementia. *Neurotoxin Research, 7*, 183–192.

Drevets, W. C. (2001). Neuroimaging and neuropathological studies of depression: Implications for the cognitive-emotional features of mood disorders. *Current Opinion in Neurobiology, 11*, 240–249.

Drevets, W. C. (2007). Orbitofrontal cortex function and structure in depression. *Annals of the New York Academy of Sciences, 1121*, 499–527.

Drevets, W. C., Price, J. L., & Furey, M. L. (2008). Brain structural and functional abnormalities in mood disorders: Implications for neurocircuitry models of depression. *Brain Structure and Function, 213*, 93–118.

Fernandez, L. L., de Lima, M. N., Scalco, F., Vedana, G., Miwa, C., Hilbig, A., ... Schroder, N. (2011). Early post-natal iron administration induces astroglial response in the brain of adult and aged rats. *Neurotoxin Research, 20*, 193–199.

Fjell, A. M., Westlye, L. T., Amlien, I., Espeseth, T., Reinvang, I., Raz, N., ... Walhovd, K. B. (2009). High consistency of regional cortical thinning in aging across multiple samples. *Cerebral Cortex, 19*, 2001–2012.

Giaume, C., Kirchhoff, F., Matute, C., Reichenbach, A., & Verkhratsky, A. (2007). Glia: The fulcrum of brain diseases. *Cell Death and Differentiation, 14*, 1324–1335.

Haber, S. N., Kunishio, K., Mizobuchi, M., & Lynd-Balta, E. (1995). The orbital and medial prefrontal circuit through the primate basal ganglia. *Journal of Neuroscience, 15*, 4851–4867.

Harder, D. R., Zhang, C., & Gebremedhin, D. (2002). Astrocytes function in matching blood flow to metabolic activity. *News in Physiological Sciences, 17*, 27–31.

Hasler, G., van der Veen, J. W., Tumonis, T., Meyers, N., Shen, J., & Drevets, W. C. (2007). Reduced prefrontal glutamate/glutamine and gamma-aminobutyric acid levels in major depression determined using proton magnetic resonance spectroscopy. *Archives of General Psychiatry, 64*, 193–200.

Hayley, S., Poulter, M. O., Merali, Z., & Anisman, H. (2005). The pathogenesis of clinical depression: Stressor- and cytokine-induced alterations of neuroplasticity. *Neuroscience, 135*, 659–678.

Hendricksen, M., Thomas, A. J., Ferrier, I. N., Ince, P., & O'Brien, J. T. (2004). Neuropathological study of the dorsal raphe nuclei in late-life depression and Alzheimer's disease with and without depression. *American Journal of Psychiatry, 161*, 1096–1102.

Henry, C. J., Huang, Y., Wynne, A. M., & Godbout, J. P. (2009). Peripheral lipopolysaccharide (LPS) challenge promotes microglial hyperactivity in aged mice that is associated with exaggerated induction of both pro-inflammatory IL-1beta and anti-inflammatory IL-10 cytokines. *Brain Behavior and Immunity, 23*, 309–317.

Hoogendijk, W. J., Sommer, I. E., Pool, C. W., Kamphorst, W., Hofman, M. A., Eikelenboom, P., & Swaab, D. F. (1999). Lack of association between depression and loss of neurons in the locus coeruleus in Alzheimer disease. *Archives of General Psychiatry, 56*, 45–51.

Jurgens, H. A., & Johnson, R. W. (2010). Dysregulated neuronal-microglial cross-talk during aging, stress and inflammation. *Experimental Neurology, 233*(1), 40–48.

Khundakar, A., Morris, C., Oakley, A., McMeekin, W., & Thomas, A. J. (2009). Morphometric analysis of neuronal and glial cell pathology in the dorsolateral prefrontal cortex in late-life depression. *British Journal of Psychiatry, 195*, 163–169.

Khundakar, A., Morris, C., Oakley, A., & Thomas, A. J. (2011). Morphometric analysis of neuronal and glial cell pathology in the caudate nucleus in late-life depression. *American Journal of Geriatric Psychiatry, 19*, 132–141.

Khundakar, A. A., & Thomas, A. J. (2009). Morphometric changes in early- and late-life major depressive disorder: Evidence from postmortem studies. *International Psychogeriatrics, 21*, 844–854.

Kim, H. W., Rapoport, S. I., & Rao, J. S. (2010). Altered expression of apoptotic factors and synaptic markers in postmortem brain from bipolar disorder patients. *Neurobiological Disorders, 37*, 596–603.

Krishnan, K., Hays, J., & Blazer, D. (1997). MRI-defined vascular depression. *American Journal of Psychiatry, 154*, 497–501.

Lacerda, A. L., Keshavan, M. S., Hardan, A. Y., Yorbik, O., Brambilla, P., Sassi, R. B., … Soares, J. C. (2004). Anatomic evaluation of the orbitofrontal cortex in major depressive disorder. *Biological Psychiatry, 55*, 353–358.

Lai, T., Payne, M. E., Byrum, C. E., Steffens, D. C., & Krishnan, K. R. (2000). Reduction of orbital frontal cortex volume in geriatric depression. *Biological Psychiatry, 48*, 971–975.

Lee, S. J., & Benveniste, E. N. (1999). Adhesion molecule expression and regulation on cells of the central nervous system. *Journal of Neuroimmunology, 98*, 77–88.

Lucassen, P. J., Muller, M. B., Holsboer, F., Bauer, J., Holtrop, A., Wouda, J., … Swaab, D. F. (2001). Hippocampal apoptosis in major depression is a minor event and absent from subareas at risk for glucocorticoid overexposure. *American Journal of Pathology, 158*, 453–468.

Luijendijk, H. J., van den Berg, J. F., Dekker, M. J., van Tuijl, H. R., Otte, W., Smit, F., … Tiemeier, H. (2008). Incidence and recurrence of late-life depression. *Archives of General Psychiatry, 65*, 1394–1401.

Malhotra, S. K., & Shnitka, T. K. (2002). Diversity in reactive astrocytes. In J. de Vellis (Ed.), *Neuroglia in the aging brain* (pp. 17–33). Totowa, NJ: Humana Press.

Markiewicz, I., & Lukomska, B. (2006). The role of astrocytes in the physiology and pathology of the central nervous system. *Acta Neurobiologia Experimentalis (Wars), 66*, 343–358.

Matsumoto, Y., Watanabe, S., Suh, Y-H., & Yamamoto, T. (2002). Effects of intrahippocampal CT105, a carboxyl terminal fragment of β-amyloid precursor protein, alone/with inflammatory cytokines on working memory in rats. *Journal of Neurochemistry, 82*, 234–239.

McGraw, J., Hiebert, G. W., & Steeves, J. D. (2001). Modulating astrogliosis after neurotrauma. *Journal of Neuroscience Research, 63*, 109–115.

McKernan, D. P., Dinan, T. G., & Cryan, J. F. (2009). "Killing the blues": A role for cellular suicide (apoptosis) in depression and the antidepressant response? *Progress in Neurobiology, 88*, 246–263.

Miguel-Hidalgo, J. J., Baucom, C., Dilley, G., Overholser, J. C., Meltzer, H. Y., Stockmeier, C. A., & Rajkowska, G. (2000). Glial fibrillary acidic protein immunoreactivity in the prefrontal cortex distinguishes younger from older adults in major depressive disorder. *Biological Psychiatry, 48*, 861–873.

Miguel-Hidalgo, J. J., Nithuairisg, S., Stockmeier, C., & Rajkowska, G. (2007). Distribution of ICAM-1 immunoreactivity during aging in the human orbitofrontal cortex. *Brain Behavior and Immunity, 21*, 100–111.

Miguel-Hidalgo, J. J., Overholser, J. C., Jurjus, G. J., Meltzer, H. Y., Dieter, L., Konick, L., … Rajkowska, G. (2011). Vascular and extravascular immunoreactivity for intercellular adhesion molecule 1 in the orbitofrontal cortex of subjects with major depression: Age-dependent changes. *Journal of Affective Disorders, 132*(3), 422–431.

Miguel-Hidalgo, J. J., Waltzer, R., Whittom, A. A., Austin, M. C., Rajkowska, G., & Stockmeier, C. A. (2010). Glial and glutamatergic markers in depression, alcoholism, and their comorbidity. *Journal of Affective Disorders, 127*, 230–240.

Miguel-Hidalgo, J. J., Whittom, A. A., Soni, M., Rajkowska, G., Meshram, A., & Stockmeier, C. (2011). Increased ratio of apoptosis marker caspase 8 to a proliferation marker in the orbitofrontal cortex in alcoholism, major depression, and comorbid depression and alcoholism. *Neuropsychopharmacology, 35*, S131.

Miguel-Hidalgo, J. J., Jiang, W., Konick, L., Overholser, J. C., Jurjus, G. J., Stockmeier, C. A., Steffens, D.C., Krishnan, K. R., Rajkowska, G. (2012). Morphometric analysis of vascular pathology in the orbitofrontal cortex of older subjects with major depression. *International Journal of Geriatric Psychiatry*. 2012 Dec 3. doi: 10.1002/gps.3911. [Epub ahead of print].

O'Callaghan, J. P., Miller, D. B., & Reinhard, J. J. F. (1990). Characterization of the origins of astrocyte response to injury using the dopaminergic neurotoxicant, 1-methyl-4-phenyl-1,2,3,6-tetrahydropyridine. *Brain Research, 521*, 73–80.

Öngür, D., Drevets, W. C., & Price, J. L. (1998). Glial reduction in the subgenual prefrontal cortex in mood disorders. *Proceedings of the National Academy of Sciences USA, 95*, 13290–13295.

Paul, I. A., & Skolnick, P. (2003). Glutamate and depression: Clinical and preclinical studies. *Annals of the New York Academy of Sciences, 1003*, 250–272.

Pieperhoff, P., Homke, L., Schneider, F., Habel, U., Shah, N. J., Zilles, K., & Amunts, K. (2008). Deformation field morphometry reveals age-related structural differences between the brains of adults up to 51 years. *Journal of Neuroscience, 28,* 828–842.

Porrino, L. J., Crane, A. M., & Goldman-Rakic, P. S. (1981). Direct and indirect pathways from the amygdala to the frontal lobe in rhesus monkeys. *Journal of Comparitive Neurology, 198,* 121–136.

Rajkowska, G., Maciag, D., Iyo, A., Austin, A., & Stockmeier, C. (2011). Oligodendrocyte gene and protein expression is altered in the medio-ventral prefrontal white matter bundle in major depression. *Neuropsychopharmachology, 35,* S309.

Rajkowska, G., Miguel-Hidalgo, J. J., Dubey, P., Stockmeier, C. A., & Krishnan, K. R. R. (2005). Prominent reduction in pyramidal neurons density in the orbitofrontal cortex of elderly depressed patients. *Biological Psychiatry, 58,* 297–306.

Rajkowska, G., Miguel-Hidalgo, J. J., Wei, J. R., Dilley, G., Pittman, S. D., Meltzer, H. Y.,... Stockmeier, C. A. (1999). Morphometric evidence for neuronal and glial prefrontal cell pathology in major depression. *Biological Psychiatry, 45,* 1085–1098.

Rajkowska, G., O'Dwyer, G., Teleki, Z., Stockmeier, C. A., & Miguel-Hidalgo, J. J. (2007). GABAergic neurons immunoreactive for calcium binding proteins are reduced in the prefrontal cortex in major depression. *Neuropsychopharmacology, 32,* 471–482.

Raz, N., Gunning, F. M., Head, D., Dupuis, J. H., McQuain, J., Briggs, S. D.,... Acker, J. D. (1997). Selective aging of the human cerebral cortex observed in vivo: Differential vulnerability of the prefrontal gray matter. *Cerebral Cortex, 7,* 268–282.

Rempel-Clower, N. L., & Barbas, H. (2000). The laminar pattern of connections between prefrontal and anterior temporal cortices in the Rhesus monkey is related to cortical structure and function. *Cerebral Cortex, 10,* 851–865.

Resnick, S. M., Lamar, M., & Driscoll, I. (2007). Vulnerability of the orbitofrontal cortex to age-associated structural and functional brain changes. *Annals of the New York Academy of Sciences, 1121,* 562–575.

Sanacora, G., Mason, G. F., Rothman, D. L., Behar, K. L., Hyder, F., Petroff, O. A.,... Krystal, J. H. (1999). Reduced cortical gamma-aminobutyric acid levels in depressed patients determined by proton magnetic resonance spectroscopy. *Archives of General Psychiatry, 56,* 1043–1047.

Satoh, J., Kim, S. U., Kastrukoff, L. F., & Takei, F. (1991). Expression and induction of intercellular adhesion molecules (ICAMs) and major histocompatibility complex (MHC) antigens on cultured murine oligodendrocytes and astrocytes. *Journal of Neuroscience Research, 29,* 1–12.

Shrikant, P., Chung, I. Y., Ballestas, M. E., & Benveniste, E. N. (1994). Regulation of intercellular adhesion molecule-1 gene expression by tumor necrosis factor-alpha, interleukin-1 beta, and interferon-gamma in astrocytes. *Journal of Neuroimmunology, 51,* 209–220.

Si, X. H., Miguel-Hidalgo, J. J., O'Dwyer, G., Stockmeier, C. A., & Rajkowska, G. (2004). Age-dependent reductions in the level of glial fibrillary acidic protein in the prefrontal cortex in major depression. *Neuropsychopharmacology, 29,* 2088–2096.

Silverman, A. J., Sutherland, A. K., Wilhelm, M., & Silver, R. (2000). Mast cells migrate from blood to brain. *Journal of Neuroscience, 20,* 401–408.

Sofroniew, M. V. (2009). Molecular dissection of reactive astrogliosis and glial scar formation. *Trends in Neuroscience, 32,* 638–647.

Stichel, C. C., & Luebbert, H. (2007). Inflammatory processes in the aging mouse brain: Participation of dendritic cells and T-cells. *Neurobiology of Aging, 28,* 1507–1521.

Sweet, R. A., Hamilton, R. L., Butters, M. A., Mulsant, B. H., Pollock, B. G., Lewis, D. A.,... Reynolds, C. F., III. (2004). Neuropathologic correlates of late-onset major depression. *Neuropsychopharmacology, 29*(12), 2242–2250.

Syed, A., Chatfield, M., Matthews, F., Harrison, P., Brayne, C., & Esiri, M. M. (2005). Depression in the elderly: Pathological study of raphe and locus ceruleus. *Neuropathology and Applied Neurobiology, 31,* 405–413.

Talley, A. K., Dewhurst, S., Perry, S. W., Dollard, S. C., Gummuluru, S., Fine, S. M.,... Gelbard, H. A. (1995). Tumor necrosis factor alpha-induced apoptosis in human neuronal cells: Protection by the antioxidant N-acetylcysteine and the genes bcl-2 and crmA. *Molecular and Cellular Biology, 15,* 2359–2366.

Taylor, W. D., MacFall, J. R., Steffens, D. C., Payne, M. E., Provenzale, J. M., & Krishnan, K. R. (2003). Localization of age-associated white matter hyperintensities in late-life depression. *Progress in Neuropsychopharmacology and Biological Psychiatry, 27,* 539–544.

Thomas, A. J., Ferrier, I. N., Kalaria, R. N., Perry, R. H., Brown, A., & O'Brien, J. T. (2001). A neuropathological study of vascular factors in late-life depression. *Journal of Neurology, Neurosurgery, and Psychiatry, 70,* 83–87.

Thomas, A. J., Ferrier, I. N., Kalaria, R. N., Woodward, S. A., Ballard, C., Oakley, A.,... O'Brien, J. T. (2000). Elevation in late-life depression of intercellular adhesion molecule-1 expression in the dorsolateral prefrontal cortex. *American Journal of Psychiatry, 157*, 1682–1684.

Thomas, A. J., Hendriksen, M., Piggott, M., Ferrier, I. N., Perry, E., Ince, P., & O'Brien, J. T. (2006). A study of the serotonin transporter in the prefrontal cortex in late-life depression and Alzheimer's disease with and without depression. *Neuropathology and Applied Neurobiology, 32*, 296–303.

Thomas, A. J., O'Brien, J. T., Davis, S., Ballard, C., Barber, R., Kalaria, R. N., & Perry, R. H. (2002). Ischemic basis for deep white matter hyperintensities in major depression: A neuropathological study. *Archives of General Psychiatry, 59*, 785–792.

Thomas, P., Hazif Thomas, C., Billon, R., Peix, R., Faugeron, P., & Clement, J. P. (2009). [Depression and frontal dysfunction: Risks for the elderly?]. *Encephale, 35*, 361–369.

Tsopelas, C., Stewart, R., Savva, G. M., Brayne, C., Ince, P., Thomas, A., & Matthews, F. E. (2011). Neuropathological correlates of late-life depression in older people. *British Journal of Psychiatry, 198*, 109–114.

Van Otterloo, E., O'Dwyer, G., Stockmeier, C. A., Steffens, D. C., Krishnan, R. R., & Rajkowska, G. (2009). Reductions in neuronal density in elderly depressed are region specific. *International Journal of Geriatric Psychiatry, 24*, 856–864.

Vostrikov, V., & Uranova, N. (2011). Age-related increase in the number of oligodendrocytes Ii dysregulated in schizophrenia and mood disorders. *Schizoprenia Research and Treatment*. 2011 Jul 3, ePub ahead of print.

Wynne, A., Henry, C. J., & Godbout, J. P. (2009). Immune and behavioral consequences of microglial reactivity in the aged brain. *Integrated and Comparitive Biology, 49*, 254–266.

37

PHARMACOGENETICS OF LATE-LIFE DEPRESSION

Greer M. Murphy, Jr.

THE GOAL of pharmacogenetics is to identify DNA markers that predict medication response. This chapter will discuss the evidence that DNA can be used to understand why some geriatric patients respond to antidepressant treatments, whereas others do not. We will also review data suggesting that certain DNA markers predict whether patients treated with antidepressants will develop intolerable side effects. Although many pharmacogenetic studies include some geriatric patients in addition to younger ones, this review will focus on studies involving exclusively geriatric patients.

Many DNA polymorphisms have been proposed as pharmacogenetic markers for antidepressant treatment. These have recently been reviewed by Porcelli et al. (2011). The proposed pharmacogenetic markers can generally be grouped into two categories: those with pharmacokinetic effects and those with pharmacodynamic effects (Murphy, Kremer, Rodrigues, & Schatzberg, 2003a).

Pharmacokinetic markers are those that affect the concentration of antidepressant medications in the blood or in the brain. A classic example would be polymorphisms in the genes encoding liver cytochrome enzymes, which affect the concentrations of drugs in the blood by metabolizing them to active or inactive compounds. Pharmacodynamic markers are those that affect the interaction of medications with neurons or other cells. An example would be polymorphisms in genes encoding neurotransmitter receptors that might affect the binding of a drug to the receptor.

Another way to classify pharmacogenetic effects is to consider those that affect medication efficacy versus those that affect medication tolerability. Markers that affect efficacy result in increased or decreased responsiveness to the therapeutic effects of antidepressant medications. Tolerability markers predispose patients to be more or less likely to experience medication side effects than patients without the marker.

PHARMACOKINETIC MARKERS

CYP2D6

Most antidepressant medications are metabolized by liver cytochrome enzymes (Bertilsson, 2007). The concentrations of medications in the blood as well as the concentrations of medication metabolites are affected by the activity of these enzymes. Because the activity of these enzymes varies between individuals, concentrations of drugs and their metabolites may also vary between individuals, which may affect antidepressant efficacy and tolerability. Among the liver cytochrome enzymes, debrisoquine hydroxylase, encoded by the CYP2D6 gene, is the best studied. Of note, the CYP2D6 gene is highly polymorphic, with over 80 allelic variants identified thus far (http://www.cypalleles.ki.se/). Because CYP2D6 is involved in the metabolism of many antidepressants, interest has focused on whether the CYP2D6 genotype, which in part determines enzyme activity, might be a marker for treatment efficacy or adverse events.

The numerous CYP2D6 alleles encode a variety of debrisoquine hydroxylase isoforms that differ in their metabolic activity. CYP2D6 alleles are generally classified as resulting in poor metabolism (no enzyme activity), intermediate metabolism (enzyme activity is present but impaired), extensive metabolism ("wild-type" or normal enzyme activity), and ultra-metabolism (increased enzyme activity, generally due to duplication of the CYP2D6 gene). The frequency of these alleles varies markedly according to ethnic background. In European Caucasians, about 7%–10% of patients are poor metabolizers, 3%–5% are ultrametabolizers, 10%–15% are intermediate metabolizers, and the rest are extensive metabolizers, which is considered the most prevalent phenotype (Bernard, Neville, Nguyen, & Flockhart, 2006; Raimundo et al., 2000). Among Asians, there are few poor metabolizers but many intermediate metabolizers. Mexican Americans generally have more extensive metabolizers than do Caucasians (Luo, Gaedigk, Aloumanis, & Wan, 2005). One study reported that African Americans have a somewhat lower frequency of alleles encoding poor metabolic phenotypes and a higher frequency of alleles encoding ultrametabolic phenotypes in comparison with Caucasians (Cai et al., 2006). Another investigation, however, found overall debrisoquine hydroxylase metabolic activity, determined by phenotyping, was lower in African

Americans than in Caucasians (Gaedigk, Bradford, Marcucci, & Leeder, 2002). Additional studies are needed of CYP2D6 genotype-phenotype correlations in African Americans.

In a pioneering study, Dahl et al. (1996) examined the CYP2D6 genotype as a predictor of nortriptyline levels in younger patients. Genotyping was performed using laborious PCR-RFLP and gel electrophoresis methods to detect three alleles that give rise to impaired metabolism. Although they had only one subject who was a homozygous poor metabolizer (carrying two copies of an allele encoding poor metabolism), subjects who were heterozygous for a poor metabolic allele showed evidence of impaired metabolism of nortriptyline.

Our laboratory expanded on this finding by studying geriatric patients treated with nortriptyline, and by using microarray technology to perform CYP2D6 genotyping (Murphy et al., 2001). Thirty-six patients with a mean age of 73 years and a diagnosis of major depression were treated with nortriptyline. Nortriptyline dosage was adjusted by clinicians who were unaware of genotype so as to achieve a steady-state concentration of between 50 and 150 ng/ml. Oligonucleotide microarrays were used to test for 16 CYP2D6 alleles. In addition, a long-range PCR assay was used to detect CYP2D6 gene deletions. Results showed that patients carrying one or more CYP2D6 alleles that impaired debrisoquine hydroxylase activity had steady-state nortriptyline levels over twice those of patients with two extensive metabolic alleles.

It is important to keep in mind that CYP2D6 genotype may not predict actual debrisoquine hydroxylase metabolic activity. This is because debrisoquine hydroxylase is readily inhibited by a variety of medications. Hence, a patient with an intermediate metabolic genotype may be converted to poor metabolizer status by taking a strong CYP2D6 inhibitor, such as quinidine. This could increase the blood levels of drugs metabolized debrisoquine hydroxylase, like nortriptyline. It is interesting in that in our study the elderly subjects were taking a mean of 8.6 other medications in addition to nortriptyline. Despite the potential for interaction of these medications with debrisoquine hydroxylase to inhibit enzyme activity and alter phenotype, genotyping nevertheless proved to be an adequate predictor of nortriptyline concentrations. Furthermore, the advanced age of these patients did not prevent genotype from providing useful information about drug metabolism.

Although CYP2D6 genotyping can predict nortriptyline levels in geriatric patients, the clinical utility of this finding remains uncertain. Orthostatic hypotension is a frequent side effect of tricyclic treatment in the elderly. However, in our study, there was no significant difference in change in systolic blood pressure on standing between those with genotypes predicting impaired debrisoquine hydroxylase activity and other patients (unpublished results). The most likely explanation for this finding is that the prescribing physicians, who were unaware of genotype, adjusted dosing so as to achieve nortriptyline levels in the recommended therapeutic range, which minimized side effects. Were out-of-range concentrations permitted in the study, there might have been a stronger relationship between CYP2D6 genotype and orthostasis. However, allowing patients to have out-of-range values would not be within the current standard of practice for most prescribers of nortriptyline, and hence would be rare in actual clinical settings.

To test the clinical consequences of CYP2D6 genotype in treating geriatric patients with modern antidepressants, we studied 246 patients over 65 with major depression treated for 8 weeks with paroxetine and mirtazapine. Paroxetine is metabolized primarily by CYP2D6 (Sindrup et al., 1992b), and CYP2D6 plays an important role in the metabolism of mirtazapine (Lind et al., 2009). All subjects were genotyped for 16 CYP2D6 alleles using a microarray platform, as well as for CYP2D6 gene duplications and deletions. We found no evidence that CYP2D6 genotype affected either medication efficacy or side effects in geriatric patients treated with paroxetine or mirtazapine. After 4 weeks of treatment, a significant effect of CYP2D6 genotype on paroxetine serum levels was apparent, with those carrying one or more poor metabolic alleles showing higher levels. However, this difference did not translate into a clinical effect.

It is important to note that there were no differences during the early weeks of treatment between the genotype groups for paroxetine. At high doses, paroxetine saturates debrisoquine hydroxylase, so that differences in enzyme activity might have had no effect on paroxetine concentrations when the patients received higher doses. However, during treatment at low doses, no saturation occurs (Sindrup, Brosen, & Gram, 1992a). It was during initial treatment, when the paroxetine dosage was low, that we expected to see differences among the genotype groups. In fact, paroxetine did cause

significantly more side effects than mirtazapine overall in this elderly cohort (Schatzberg, Kremer, Rodrigues, & Murphy, 2002), but at no time point did CYP2D6 genotype predict side effects for either drug treatment group, or for the combined cohort.

Paroxetine is both an inhibitor and a substrate for debrisoquine hydroxylase. Patients who are genetically intermediate metabolizers would be expected to be readily converted to a poor metabolizer phenotype due to inhibition of debrisoquine hydroxylase when starting paroxetine (Solai et al., 2002). In elderly intermediate metabolic patients also taking a debrisoquine hydroxylase substrate such as an antihypertensive, this might result in increased side effects such as orthostatic dizziness. Or patients who were intermediate metabolizers and already taking a CYP2D6 inhibitor might be expected to experience increased side effects due to paroxetine, because paroxetine metabolism was already inhibited. We tested these hypotheses by examining all concurrent medications taken by our subjects during paroxetine and mirtazapine treatment. All debrisoquine hydroxylase inhibitors and substrates were identified. Overall, 66 patients were taking a concurrent medication classified as a debrisoquine hydroxylase inhibitor or substrate. There was no interaction between CYP2D6 genotype and concurrent treatment with a CYP2D6 substrate or inhibitor on the severity of side effects or number of discontinuations due to adverse events for either medication. Thus, in our cohort, it appears that concurrent treatment with debrisoquine hydroxylase inhibitors or substrates did not interact with CYP2D6 genotype to affect outcomes in paroxetine-treated patients.

Mirtazapine is also metabolized in part by CYP2D6. Although total mirtazapine levels may not be significantly altered by CYP2D6 genotype, ratios of mirtazapine enantiomers may be affected (Lind et al., 2009). In our study, we did not find a significant difference between patients with genotypes encoding impaired debrisoquine hydroxylase activity and those with extensive metabolism in steady-state mirtazapine levels. Even if differences did exist, mirtazapine levels are unlikely to predict clinical outcomes, because we found no differences among the CYP2D6 genotype groups in mirtazapine efficacy or side effects.

In summary, our results do not support the position that CYP2D6 genotype is critical in determining side effects during treatment of elderly patients with paroxetine or mirtazapine. At first glance this result seems surprising. However, it is important to recall that plasma concentrations of these two medications have never been shown to have a strong relationship with either efficacy or adverse events (Gram, 1990; Kaye et al., 1989; Tasker, Kaye, Zussman, & Link, 1989). In fact, the therapeutic windows for serum concentrations of paroxetine and mirtazapine appear to be remarkably wide. It may be that genetic factors affecting the pharmacokinetics of these medications are less important than genetic factors affecting their pharmacodynamic interactions with receptors and transporters in the brain (Murphy et al., 2003a; Murphy, Hollander, Rodrigues, Kremer, & Schatzberg, 2004). Others have reached a similar conclusion (Peters et al., 2008; Serretti et al., 2009).

Whyte et al. (2006) performed a study of the effects of CYP2D6 genotype on clinical outcomes in elderly patients treated with venlafaxine. They collected more detailed pharmacokinetic data than we did in our paroxetine-mirtazapine study. Significant differences among genotype groups were detected for venlafaxine as well as the active metabolite O-desmethylvenlafaxine (which is currently marketed as the antidepressant Pristiq). Patients with impaired debrisoquine hydroxylase activity had higher levels of venlafaxine and lower levels of O-desmethylvenlafaxine. CYP2D6 genotype did not affect blood pressure, orthostatic hypotension, or QTc interval, and it did not affect a measure of overall antidepressant side effects (UKU scale). The authors noted that power to detect a CYP2D6 effect on medication adverse events was limited due to the relatively small number of patients with impaired metabolism. However, these results indicate that if there is a clinical effect of CYP2D6 variation on venlafaxine outcomes, it is probably small.

Although not directly involving patients with geriatric depression, Wessels et al. (2010) studied the metabolism of risperidone in elders with Alzheimer's disease. Risperidone is also frequently used in geriatric patients with psychotic depression, and it is metabolized by CYP2D6 and CYP3A4 to 9-hydroxy-risperidone (currently marketed as the antipsychotic Invega). Wessels et al. found that 9-hydroxy-risperidone concentrations were predictive of medication switching and discontinuations. Because CYP2D6 ultrametabolizers treated with risperidone have higher levels of 9-hydroxy-risperidone, these subjects may be at increased risk for side effects. This hypothesis should be tested in a cohort of depressed geriatric patients genotyped for CYP2D6 and treated with risperidone.

The acetylcholinesterase inhibitor donepezil is approved for the treatment of Alzheimer's disease and is metabolized largely by debrisoquine hydroxylase, although CYP3A4 is also involved (Jann, Shirley, & Small, 2002). Donepezil has been proposed as an augmenting agent for antidepressants in elderly patients (Pelton et al., 2008), although recent evidence indicates that it may lack efficacy in depression (Reynolds et al., 2011). In any case, CYP2D6 genotype affects whether CYP2D6 genotype affects clinical outcomes in geriatric patients treated with antidepressants and donepezil. However, data are conflicting as to whether CYP2D6 genotype affects treatment outcomes in Alzheimer's disease (Chianella et al., 2011; Seripa et al., 2011). Even if donepezil were proven to be an efficacious augmenting agent in geriatric depression, it remains to be seen whether CYP2D6 genotype would be of any value in prescribing the medication.

P-Glycoprotein (ABCB1, MDR1)

Debrisoquine hydroxylase and other liver cytochromes affect the serum concentrations of many medications. However, there are other means by which drug concentrations are regulated in the brain and in the periphery. P-glycoprotein is a membrane-bound transporter that affects the movement of drug molecules from the gut to the bloodstream, excretion of drugs and their metabolites into bile, elimination of drugs from the blood by the kidney, and transport of drugs across the blood–brain barrier (Zhou, 2008). In fact, P-glycoprotein can actively transport drugs out of the brain. P-glycoprotein is encoded by the ABCB1 (MDR1) gene. We examined the effects of 15 single-nucleotide polymorphisms (SNPs) in the ABCB1 gene on response to paroxetine or mirtazapine in 246 geriatric patients with major depression (Sarginson et al., 2010a). Paroxetine is a substrate for P-glycoprotein, whereas mirtazapine is not (Uhr, Grauer, & Holsboer, 2003). Hence, we hypothesized that ABCB1 genetic variation would affect clinical outcomes in paroxetine-treated patients by modifying brain antidepressant concentrations, whereas in mirtazapine-treated patients, we would not see this effect. Interestingly, two ABCB1 SNPs had small but significant effects on time to remission among paroxetine-treated patients, but not among mirtazapine-treated subjects. These results appeared to replicate those reported by Uhr and colleagues in younger depressed patients (Uhr et al., 2008). However, the magnitude of the genetic effect in our cohort was small (approximately 4 points on the 21-item Hamilton Depression Rating Scale), and the clinical application is unclear. Additional studies of the role of p-glycoprotein in antidepressant treatment should be performed.

PHARMACODYNAMIC MARKERS

5HT2A

Neuronal serotonin receptors are thought to be essential in the actions of many antidepressant medications. The serotonin 2A receptor (5HT2A) may mediate SSRI side effects such as insomnia, agitation, gastrointestinal distress, and sexual dysfunction. We studied 246 patients 65 years of age and older treated with either paroxetine or mirtazapine in a double-blind, randomized, 8-week clinical trial (Murphy et al., 2003a). We investigated the 5HT2A locus, because mirtazapine blocks this receptor, whereas paroxetine does not. It has been hypothesized that this difference in 5HT2A binding accounts for differences in side effects between the two drugs. All subjects were genotyped for the 102 T/C polymorphism at the 5HT2A locus, which is in complete linkage disequilibrium (highly linked) with a functional variant (-1438 A/G; rs6311) in the promoter region of the gene, which may affect receptor expression (Serretti, Drago, & De Ronchi, 2007). Although the 102 T/C SNP had no effect on the antidepressant efficacy of either mirtazapine or paroxetine, it had a large effect on adverse events due to paroxetine. We hypothesized that in paroxetine-treated patients, the 102 T/C variant alters the sensitivity of the 5HT2A receptor to synaptic serotonin, resulting in more side effects. Among mirtazapine-treated patients, this effect would not occur, as the 5HT2A receptor is effectively blocked by the drug.

Lenze et al. (2012) recently tested the 5HT2A -1438 A/G variant for effects on escitalopram-induced cognitive changes in 133 patients age 60 and older. They found that the -1438 A allele was associated with deficits in the digit span test in escitalopram-treated patients. Interestingly, the -1438 A allele is linked to the 5HT2A 102 T allele, which was associated with fewer discontinuations due to adverse events in the Murphy et al. (2003a) study. Lenze et al. did not report on adverse events other than cognitive changes, whereas Murphy et al. did not report on cognitive side effects. Hence,

additional work will be required to resolve this apparent discrepancy.

5HTTLPR

The serotonin reuptake transporter (5HTT) affects the concentration of serotonin in the synapse by regulating reuptake into the presynaptic neuron. There is a variable repeat polymorphism in the promoter region of the 5HTT gene that is commonly designated as the 5HTTLPR variant. The "short" or S allele at the 5HTTLPR results in reduced transcription of the 5HTT gene (Lesch & Gutknecht, 2005). This polymorphism has been investigated extensively as a marker for antidepressant response in the nongeriatric population (Serretti, Benedetti, Zanardi, & Smeraldi, 2005). In the older population, Pollock et al. (2000) found that among geriatric patients treated with paroxetine, those carrying the "short" allele of the 5HTTLPR showed a slower antidepressant response than those carrying one or more "long" alleles. This effect was not seen among patients treated with nortriptyline. The 5HTTLPR effect on SSRI response detected by Pollock et al. in elderly depressed patients replicates the original finding in younger patients (Smeraldi et al., 1998).

We tested the effects of the 5HTTLPR on geriatric patients treated with paroxetine or mirtazapine in an 8-week clinical trial (Murphy et al., 2004). We replicated the findings of Pollock et al. (2000), in that among paroxetine-treated patients, carriers of the "short" allele showed a small but significant decrease in antidepressant efficacy compared to noncarriers. However, we also found that among paroxetine-treated patients, carriers of the S allele showed a large increase in the frequency of discontinuations due to adverse events in comparison with noncarriers. For mirtazapine-treated subjects, the 5HTTLPR had no effect on antidepressant efficacy. However, a significant effect was seen on mirtazapine-induced adverse events, with carriers of the S allele showing fewer discontinuations due to adverse events. Thus, the S allele had an opposite effect on adverse events in mirtazapine-treated patients than among paroxetine-treated patients. The differing mechanisms of action in paroxetine and mirtazapine likely account for the difference in 5HTTLPR genetic effects.

Alexopolous et al. (2009) examined remission in depressed geriatric patients treated with escitalopram. Similar to Pollock et al. (2000) and Murphy et al. (2004), they found an impaired antidepressant response among carriers of the 5HTTLPR S allele. S carriers also showed evidence of white matter abnormalities on structural brain imaging. Lavretsky et al. (2008) did not find an effect of the 5HTTLPR on citalopram response in a small sample of geriatric depressed patients.

Kim et al. (2006) examined the effects of the 5HTTLPR in elderly depressed patients of Korean descent treated with fluoxetine or sertraline in a naturalistic setting. In contrast to results in Caucasians, they found that the S allele was associated with a better response to SSRI antidepressants. Kim et al. suggested that the differing effect of the 5HTTLPR in Koreans could be due to differences from Caucasians at other closely linked loci.

Additional Pharmacodynamic Markers

In younger patients, some data suggest that polymorphisms in the norepinephrine reuptake transporter (NET) and the dopamine reuptake transporter (DAT) may affect medication response (Purper-Ouakil et al., 2008; Yoshida et al., 2004). There are few data to address this issue in geriatric patients. Lavretsky et al. (2008) found that in elderly patients treated with citalopram plus methylphenidate, carriers of the DAT VNTR 10/10 variant showed enhanced response. Among Korean elderly depressed patients, Kim et al. (2006) reported that the NET G127A polymorphism was strongly associated with nortriptyline response, but not with SSRI response.

Neurotrophins are thought to be important in the actions of antidepressants. In particular, brain-derived neurotrophic factor (BDNF) is increased in the brain by antidepressants (Nibuya, Morinobu, & Duman, 1995; Russo-Neustadt, Beard, & Cotman, 1999). Delivering BDNF into the brain (Shirayama, Chen, Nakagawa, Russell, & Duman, 2002; Siuciak, Lewis, Wiegand, & Lindsay, 1997) or even to the periphery (Schmidt & Duman, 2010) may result in antidepressant-like effects in animal models of depression. There is a well-studied polymorphism in the BDNF gene that results in a substitution of a methionine for a valine at amino acid 66 in the BDNF protein (Val66Met). This variant results in decreased secretion of BDNF by neurons (Tsai, Hong, Chen, & Yu, 2010). Taylor et al. (2010) studied 229 depressed elderly subjects treated using a prescribing algorithm for at least 4 weeks with an SSRI, venlafaxine, or bupropion. They found that at 6-month follow-up, carriers of the Met allele at the BDNF Val66Met polymorphism were more likely to be in remission. Interestingly, at 3-month follow-up there was no pharmacogenetic effect of BDNF Val66Met. Alexopoulos et al. (2010) treated subjects 60 years and older with escitalopram for 12 weeks. Like Taylor et al., they observed that carriers of the BDNF Met allele showed an increased remission rate, but unlike the Taylor et al. study, Alexopolous and colleagues observed this effect after approximately 3 months of treatment.

There is evidence that the hypothalamic-pituitary-adrenal axis may be activated in depression and may adversely affect mood and possibly antidepressant response (Anacker, Zunszain, Carvalho, & Pariante, 2011; Binder et al., 2009). Mirtazapine can suppress HPA axis activity (Schule et al., 2003), so we hypothesized that genes involved in the regulation of the HPA axis might affect mirtazapine treatment outcomes, but not paroxetine outcomes. One such gene is FK506 binding protein 5 (FKBP5) that encodes a glucocorticoid receptor-regulating co-chaperone of Hsp90 (Zhang, Clark, & Yorio, 2008). FKBP5 polymorphisms were previously shown to affect antidepressant treatment outcomes in a mixed-age cohort of depressed patients (Binder et al., 2004). We tested the effects of two FKBP5 SNPs on paroxetine and mirtazapine clinical outcomes in geriatric depression (Sarginson, Lazzeroni, Ryan, Schatzberg, Murphy, 2010b). These two SNPs had shown large effects on antidepressant outcomes in the mixed-age cohort of Binder et al. (2004). Surprisingly, we found no effects of FKBP5 genetic variation on paroxetine or mirtazapine treatment outcomes in older depressed patients. This difference from the results of Binder et al. (2004) could be due to age-related changes in the effects of FKBP5, or it could indicate that results of Binder et al. were spurious, as other investigators have also failed to replicate their findings (Tsai et al., 2007).

OTHER MARKERS

The APOE ε4 allele is an important risk factor for Alzheimer's disease. Furthermore, nondemented elders who carry the ε4 allele may be at risk for cognitive decline (Lavretsky et al., 2003; Small et al., 2000). We hypothesized that depressed, nondemented ε4 carries might have subtle cognitive deficits that could impair their response to antidepressants.

In our sample of 246 elderly depressed patients treated with paroxetine or mirtazapine, we found that ε4 carriers treated with paroxetine were slow to respond, but that ε4 carriers treated with mirtazapine responded faster than noncarriers (Murphy, Kremer, Rodrigues, & Schatzberg, 2003b). These results suggest that the APOE E4 protein interacts with paroxetine and mirtazapine to affect treatment outcomes in geriatric depression.

Kondo et al. (2007) studied the A1166C polymorphism in the angiotensin II receptor, vascular type 1 (AGTR1), which has been associated with a variety of cardiovascular disorders. Kondo et al. hypothesized that this variant might also predispose to white matter lesions in the brain that could contribute to late-life depression. They reported on 236 geriatric depressed subjects treated using an algorithm that allowed for a variety of antidepressant medications. They found that the 17 subjects with the CC genotype had a much lower remission rate than those with the AC and AA genotypes.

Mood stabilizers are frequently co-prescribed with antidepressants in geriatric depression, particularly if the patient has a history of bipolar disorder. The anticonvulsant carbamazepine has mood-stabilizing properties, but it has been associated with Stevens-Johnson syndrome (SJS) and toxic epidermal necrolysis (TEN), particularly in Asian populations. Chung et al. (2004) identified a common polymorphism (*1502) at the HLA-B locus that dramatically increases the risk of carbamazepine-induced SJS/TEN in certain Asian populations. In the Chung et al. study, the *1502 variant was present in 100% of Chinese patients who developed SJS after carbamazepine treatment, but it was present in only 3% who did not develop SJS after carbamazepine. This result has proven to be extremely robust and has been replicated in many other studies. Furthermore, genotyping for the HLA-B *1502 marker was recently shown to decrease the incidence of SJS/TEN among patients treated with carbamazepine in Taiwan (Chen et al., 2011). In fact, because of the very strong association between the HLA-B *1502 marker and SJS/TEN in Asians, the Food and Drug Administration (FDA) has added a warning to the package insert for carbamazepine instructing physicians to genotype Asian patients before starting carbamazepine (Ferrell & McLeod, 2008). None of the other potential pharmacogenetic markers discussed in this review carry this level of regulatory agency

intervention, and clinicians should not ignore these instructions without good justification.

It is interesting that even though the FDA recommends testing of all Asians for the HLA-B *1502 allele before starting carbamazepine, the strong association with SJS/TEN is present only in certain Asian subgroups. For example, there does not seem to be an association between the *1502 allele and carbamazepine-induced SJS/NEN in Japanese (Kaniwa et al., 2008). Furthermore, although individuals with ancestors from the Indian subcontinent are usually not considered Asian, some subgroups there show a strong effect of the *1502 variant (Mehta et al., 2009). At present, data do not indicate increased risk for carbamazepine-treated European Caucasians carrying the *1502 allele, and indeed this variant is less frequent among Europeans than among Asians. Of note, a recent study indicates that the HLA-A *3101 allele may be a risk factor for hypersensitivity reactions to carbamazepine in those of European ancestry (McCormack et al., 2011). This is an actively evolving field, and all clinicians who prescribe anticonvulsants for mood disorders should review the literature frequently.

ISSUES IN PHARMACOGENETICS OF GERIATRIC DEPRESSION

It is uncertain whether pharmacogenetic results obtained with younger patients apply to the geriatric population. In psychiatric pharmacogenetics overall, there have been many findings that have not been replicated (Drago, De Ronchi, & Serretti, 2009). Some studies with older patients have been unable to replicate results from younger cohorts (Sarginson et al., 2010b), but negative results are difficult to interpret. Negative results could be due to age-related differences in genetic effects or due to methodological issues, such as lack of statistical power or differences in treatment protocols, or they could be due to the original result in younger patients being spurious.

Unfortunately, there is little incentive for investigators to perform well-powered, well-designed replication studies in psychiatric pharmacogenetics. Funding agencies tend to avoid replication studies and favor proposals viewed as innovative. Few psychiatric pharmacogenetic studies are initially designed to test genetic hypotheses. Most are "piggybacked" onto clinical trials designed to answer other questions. The famous "STAR-D" medication algorithm trial produced virtually nothing of certain pharmacogenetic value, despite a large investment in collecting DNA samples and in performing sophisticated genetic analyses (Garriock & Hamilton, 2009). This is no reflection on the many fine scientists involved in the STAR*D clinical trial and in the genetic work, but rather an indication of the difficulties in trying to extract pharmacogenetic "added value" from a nonpharmacogenetic clinical study. Industry-sponsored trials offer opportunities for pharmacogenetic studies in the elderly, but academic investigators may find their results subject to restrictions imposed by pharmaceutical company sponsors. Furthermore, industry sponsors or cash-strapped universities may pressure investigators to seek early patent protection, or even licensing and marketing of pharmacogenetic findings before they are replicated in the scientific forum. Indeed, a dark side to the pharmacogenetic field is that there is money to be made selling pharmacogenetic tests lacking demonstrated clinical utility to unsuspecting patients, as there is little regulatory oversight of this business (Katsanis, Javitt, & Hudson, 2008).

Most psychiatric pharmacogenetic studies have involved one or a handful of SNPs, but the trend is to include larger numbers of SNPs for each candidate gene. It is important that investigators state the method for SNP selection and the degree to which the selected SNPs are representative of all of the known variation in the gene of interest. Investigators should state the percentage of total SNP variation in the gene that is captured through linkage disequilibrium by the selected SNPs that were genotyped. Although genome-wide pharmacogenetic studies of antidepressant effects are technically feasible, the relatively small sample sizes available at present along with the need to control for Type I statistical error make this approach of limited value. Another issue usually not adequately addressed is mode of inheritance of pharmacogenetic effects (Jorgensen & Williamson, 2008). In particular, there is great variation among psychiatric pharmacogenetic studies as to whether heterozygotes are grouped with homozygotes for the dominant allele, homozygotes for the minor allele, or analyzed independently. Different models for mode of inheritance can give very different results. Medication compliance is also critical in any pharmacogenetic study. Ideally, serum drug concentrations should be checked, but if this is not possible, medication usage should be carefully monitored and quantified. Clearly, if patients are not taking the study drug, pharmacogenetic effects will not be valid.

In summary, the small numbers of studies on the pharmacogenetics of late-life depression have resulted in some interesting findings. However, so far there is nothing of demonstrated clinical value to aid in the prescribing of antidepressant medications to the elderly. The field faces of number of barriers to clinical application common to all pharmacogenetic investigations at present. Future studies should focus on replication of existing findings, larger sample sizes, and more comprehensive and better documented approaches to SNP selection.

ACKNOWLEDGMENTS

Supported by an award from the National Institute of Mental Health.

Disclosures

In the past five years, Dr. Murphy received royalty income from a pharmacogenetic test licensed by Stanford University, but currently he receives no income from this source. Currently Dr. Murphy is listed as an inventor on a patent application filed by Stanford University regarding CRHR2 and NR3C1 polymorphisms and the risk for depression. Dr. Murphy is a consultant for Brain Resource, Ltd.

REFERENCES

Alexopoulos, G. S., Glatt, C. E., Hoptman, M. J., Kanellopoulos, D., Murphy, C. F., Kelly, R. E., Jr., ... Gunning, F. M. (2010). BDNF val66met polymorphism, white matter abnormalities and remission of geriatric depression. *Journal of Affective Disorders, 125*, 262–268.

Alexopoulos, G. S., Murphy, C. F., Gunning-Dixon, F. M., Glatt, C. E., Latoussakis, V., Kelly, R. E., Jr., ... Hoptman, M. J. (2009). Serotonin transporter polymorphisms, microstructural white matter abnormalities and remission of geriatric depression. *Journal of Affective Disorders, 119*, 132–141.

Anacker, C., Zunszain, P. A., Carvalho, L. A., & Pariante, C. M. (2011). The glucocorticoid receptor: Pivot of depression and of antidepressant treatment? *Psychoneuroendocrinology, 36*, 415–425.

Bernard, S., Neville, K. A., Nguyen, A. T., & Flockhart, D. A. (2006). Interethnic differences in genetic polymorphisms of CYP2D6 in the U.S. population: Clinical implications. *Oncologist, 11*, 126–135.

Bertilsson, L. (2007). Metabolism of antidepressant and neuroleptic drugs by cytochrome p450s: Clinical and interethnic aspects. *Clinical Pharmacology and Therapeutics, 82*, 606–609.

Binder, E. B., Kunzel, H. E., Nickel, T., Kern, N., Pfennig, A., Majer, M., ... Holsboer, F. (2009). HPA-axis regulation at in-patient admission is associated with antidepressant therapy outcome in male but not in female depressed patients. *Psychoneuroendocrinology, 34*, 99–109.

Binder, E. B., Salyakina, D., Lichtner, P., Wochnik, G. M., Ising, M., Putz, B., ... Muller-Myhsok, B. (2004). Polymorphisms in FKBP5 are associated with increased recurrence of depressive episodes and rapid response to antidepressant treatment. *Nature Genetics, 36*, 1319–1325.

Cai, W. M., Nikoloff, D. M., Pan, R. M., de Leon, J., Fanti, P., Fairchild, M., ... Wedlund, P. J. (2006). CYP2D6 genetic variation in healthy adults and psychiatric African-American subjects: Implications for clinical practice and genetic testing. *Pharmacogenomics Journal, 6*, 343–350.

Chen, P., Lin, J. J., Lu, C. S., Ong, C. T., Hsieh, P. F., Yang, C. C., ... Shen, C. Y. (2011). Carbamazepine-induced toxic effects and HLA-B*1502 screening in Taiwan. *New England Journal of Medicine, 364*, 1126–1133.

Chianella, C., Gragnaniello, D., Delser, P. M., Visentini, M. F., Sette, E., Tola, M. R., ... Fuselli, S. (2011). BCHE and CYP2D6 genetic variation in Alzheimer's disease patients treated with cholinesterase inhibitors. *European Journal of Clinical Pharmacology, 67*, 1147–1157.

Chung, W. H., Hung, S. I., Hong, H. S., Hsih, M. S., Yang, L. C., Ho, H. C., ... Chen, Y. T. (2004). Medical genetics: A marker for Stevens-Johnson syndrome. *Nature, 428*, 486.

Dahl, M. L., Bertilsson, L., & Nordin, C. (1996). Steady-state plasma levels of nortriptyline and its 10-hydroxy metabolite: Relationship to the CYP2D6 genotype. *Psychopharmacology (Berl), 123*, 315–319.

Drago, A., De Ronchi, D., & Serretti, A. (2009). Pharmacogenetics of antidepressant response: An update. *Human Genomics, 3*, 257–274.

Ferrell, P. B., Jr., & McLeod, H. L. (2008). Carbamazepine, HLA-B*1502 and risk of Stevens-Johnson syndrome and toxic epidermal necrolysis: US FDA recommendations. *Pharmacogenomics, 9*, 1543–1546.

Gaedigk, A., Bradford, L. D., Marcucci, K. A., & Leeder, J. S. (2002). Unique CYP2D6 activity distribution and genotype-phenotype discordance in black Americans. *Clinical Pharmacology and Therapeutics, 72*, 76–89.

Garriock, H. A., & Hamilton, S. P. (2009). Genetic studies of drug response and side effects in the STAR*D study, part 2. *Journal of Clinical Psychiatry, 70*, 1323–1325.

Gram, L. F. (1990). Paroxetine: A selective serotonin reuptake inhibitor showing better tolerance, but weaker antidepressant effect than clomipramine in a controlled multicenter study. Danish University Antidepressant Group. *Journal of Affective Disorders, 18*, 289–299.

Jann, M. W., Shirley, K. L., & Small, G. W. (2002). Clinical pharmacokinetics and pharmacodynamics of cholinesterase inhibitors. *Clinical pharmacokinetics, 41*, 719–739.

Jorgensen, A. L., & Williamson, P. R. (2008). Methodological quality of pharmacogenetic studies: Issues of concern. *Statistics in Medicine, 27*, 6547–6569.

Kaniwa, N., Saito, Y., Aihara, M., Matsunaga, K., Tohkin, M., Kurose, K., ... Hasegawa, R. (2008). HLA-B locus in Japanese patients with anti-epileptics and allopurinol-related Stevens-Johnson syndrome and toxic epidermal necrolysis. *Pharmacogenomics, 9*, 1617–1622.

Katsanis, S. H., Javitt, G., & Hudson, K. (2008). Public health. A case study of personalized medicine. *Science, 320*, 53–54.

Kaye, C. M., Haddock, R. E., Langley, P. F., Mellows, G., Tasker, T. C., Zussman, B. D., & Greb, W. H. (1989). A review of the metabolism and pharmacokinetics of paroxetine in man. *Acta Psychiatrica Scandinavica Supplement, 350*, 60–75.

Kim, H., Lim, S. W., Kim, S., Kim, J. W., Chang, Y. H., Carroll, B. J., & Kim, D. K. (2006). Monoamine transporter gene polymorphisms and antidepressant response in Koreans with late-life depression. *Journal of the American Medical Association, 296*, 1609–1618.

Kondo, D. G., Speer, M. C., Krishnan, K. R., McQuoid, D. R., Slifer, S. H., Pieper, C. F., ... Steffens, D. C. (2007). Association of AGTR1 with 18-month treatment outcome in late-life depression. *American Journal of Geriatric Psychiatry, 15*, 564–572.

Lavretsky, H., Ercoli, L., Siddarth, P., Bookheimer, S., Miller, K., & Small, G. (2003). Apolipoprotein epsilon4 allele status, depressive symptoms, and cognitive decline in middle-aged and elderly persons without dementia. *American Journal of Geriatric Psychiatry, 11*, 667–673.

Lavretsky, H., Siddarth, P., Kumar, A., & Reynolds, C. F., III. (2008). The effects of the dopamine and serotonin transporter polymorphisms on clinical features and treatment response in geriatric depression: A pilot study. *International Journal of Geriatric Psychiatry, 23,* 55–59.

Lenze, E. J., Dixon, D., Nowotny, P., Lotrich, F. E., Dore, P. M., Pollock, B. G.,…Butters, M. A. (2012). Escitalopram reduces attentional performance in anxious older adults with high-expression genetic variants at serotonin 2A and 1B receptors. *International Journal of Neuropsychopharmacology,* 1–10.

Lesch, K. P., & Gutknecht, L. (2005). Pharmacogenetics of the serotonin transporter. *Progress in Neuropsychopharmacology and Biological Psychiatry, 29,* 1062–1073.

Lind, A. B., Reis, M., Bengtsson, F., Jonzier-Perey, M., Powell Golay, K., Ahlner, J.,…Dahl, M. L. (2009). Steady-state concentrations of mirtazapine, N-desmethylmirtazapine, 8-hydroxymirtazapine and their enantiomers in relation to cytochrome P450 2D6 genotype, age and smoking behaviour. *Clinical Pharmacokinetics, 48,* 63–70.

Luo, H. R., Gaedigk, A., Aloumanis, V., & Wan, Y. J. (2005). Identification of CYP2D6 impaired functional alleles in Mexican Americans. *European Journal of Clinical Pharmacology, 61,* 797–802.

McCormack, M., Alfirevic, A., Bourgeois, S., Farrell, J. J., Kasperaviciute, D., Carrington, M.,…Pirmohamed, M. (2011). HLA-A*3101 and carbamazepine-induced hypersensitivity reactions in Europeans. *New England Journal of Medicine, 364,* 1134–1143.

Mehta, T. Y., Prajapati, L. M., Mittal, B., Joshi, C. G., Sheth, J. J., Patel, D. B.,…Goyal, R. K. (2009). Association of HLA-B*1502 allele and carbamazepine-induced Stevens-Johnson syndrome among Indians. *Indian Journal of Dermatology, Venereology and Leprology, 75,* 579–582.

Murphy, G. M., Jr., Hollander, S. B., Rodrigues, H. E., Kremer, C., & Schatzberg, A. F. (2004). Effects of the serotonin transporter gene promoter polymorphism on mirtazapine and paroxetine efficacy and adverse events in geriatric major depression. *Archives of General Psychiatry, 61,* 1163–1169.

Murphy, G. M., Kremer, C., Rodrigues, H., & Schatzberg, A. F. (2003b). The apolipoprotein E epsilon4 allele and antidepressant efficacy in cognitively intact elderly depressed patients. *Biological Psychiatry, 54,* 665–673.

Murphy, G. M., Jr., Kremer, C., Rodrigues, H. E., & Schatzberg, A. F. (2003a). Pharmacogenetics of antidepressant medication intolerance. *American Journal of Psychiatry, 160,* 1830–1835.

Murphy, G. M., Jr., Pollock, B. G., Kirshner, M. A., Pascoe, N., Cheuk, W., Mulsant, B. H., &

Reynolds, C. F., III. (2001). CYP2D6 genotyping with oligonucleotide microarrays and nortriptyline concentrations in geriatric depression. *Neuropsychopharmacology, 25,* 737–743.

Nibuya, M., Morinobu, S., & Duman, R. S. (1995). Regulation of BDNF and trkB mRNA in rat brain by chronic electroconvulsive seizure and antidepressant drug treatments. *Journal of Neuroscience, 15,* 7539–7547.

Pelton, G. H., Harper, O. L., Tabert, M. H., Sackeim, H. A., Scarmeas, N., Roose, S. P., & Devanand, D. P. (2008). Randomized double-blind placebo-controlled donepezil augmentation in antidepressant-treated elderly patients with depression and cognitive impairment: A pilot study. *International Journal of Geriatric Psychiatry, 23,* 670–676.

Peters, E. J., Slager, S. L., Kraft, J. B., Jenkins, G. D., Reinalda, M. S., McGrath, P. J., & Hamilton, S. P. (2008). Pharmacokinetic genes do not influence response or tolerance to citalopram in the STAR*D sample. *PloS One, 3,* e1872.

Pollock, B. G., Ferrell, R. E., Mulsant, B. H., Mazumdar, S., Miller, M., Sweet, R. A.,…Kupfer, D. J. (2000). Allelic variation in the serotonin transporter promoter affects onset of paroxetine treatment response in late-life depression. *Neuropsychopharmacology, 23,* 587–590.

Porcelli, S., Drago, A., Fabbri, C., Gibiino, S., Calati, R., & Serretti, A. (2011). Pharmacogenetics of antidepressant response. *Journal of Psychiatry and Neuroscience, 36,* 87–113.

Purper-Ouakil, D., Wohl, M., Orejarena, S., Cortese, S., Boni, C., Asch, M.,…Gorwood, P. (2008). Pharmacogenetics of methylphenidate response in attention deficit/hyperactivity disorder: Association with the dopamine transporter gene (SLC6A3). *American Journal of Medical Genetics B, Neuropsychiatric Genetics, 147B,* 1425–1430.

Raimundo, S., Fischer, J., Eichelbaum, M., Griese, E. U., Schwab, M., & Zanger, U. M. (2000). Elucidation of the genetic basis of the common 'intermediate metabolizer' phenotype for drug oxidation by CYP2D6. *Pharmacogenetics, 10,* 577–581.

Reynolds, C. F., III, Butters, M. A., Lopez, O., Pollock, B. G., Dew, M. A., Mulsant, B. H.,…DeKosky, S. T. (2011). Maintenance treatment of depression in old age: A randomized, double-blind, placebo-controlled evaluation of the efficacy and safety of donepezil combined with antidepressant pharmacotherapy. *Archives of General Psychiatry, 68,* 51–60.

Russo-Neustadt, A., Beard, R. C., & Cotman, C. W. (1999). Exercise, antidepressant medications, and enhanced brain derived neurotrophic factor expression. *Neuropsychopharmacology, 21,* 679–682.

Sarginson, J. E., Lazzeroni, L. C., Ryan, H. S., Ershoff, B. D., Schatzberg, A. F., & Murphy, G. M., Jr. (2010a). ABCB1 (MDR1) polymorphisms and antidepressant response in geriatric depression. *Pharmacogenetics and Genomics, 20,* 467–475.

Sarginson, J. E., Lazzeroni, L. C., Ryan, H. S., Schatzberg, A. F., Murphy, G. M., Jr. (2010b). FKBP5 polymorphisms and antidepressant response in geriatric depression. *American Journal of Medical Genetics B, Neuropsychiatric Genetics, 153B,* 554–560.

Schatzberg, A. F., Kremer, C., Rodrigues, H. E., & Murphy, G. M., Jr. (2002). Double-blind, randomized comparison of mirtazapine and paroxetine in elderly depressed patients. *American Journal of Geriatric Psychiatry, 10,* 541–550.

Schmidt, H. D., & Duman, R. S. (2010). Peripheral BDNF produces antidepressant-like effects in cellular and behavioral models. *Neuropsychopharmacology, 35,* 2378–2391.

Schule, C., Baghai, T., Zwanzger, P., Ella, R., Eser, D., Padberg, F.,...Rupprecht, R. (2003). Attenuation of hypothalamic-pituitary-adrenocortical hyperactivity in depressed patients by mirtazapine. *Psychopharmacology (Berl), 166,* 271–275.

Seripa, D., Bizzarro, A., Pilotto, A., D'Onofrio, G., Vecchione, G., Gallo, A. P.,...Pilotto, A. (2011). Role of cytochrome P4502D6 functional polymorphisms in the efficacy of donepezil in patients with Alzheimer's disease. *Pharmacogenetics and Genomics, 21,* 225–230.

Serretti, A., Benedetti, F., Zanardi, R., & Smeraldi, E. (2005). The influence of serotonin transporter promoter polymorphism (SERTPR) and other polymorphisms of the serotonin pathway on the efficacy of antidepressant treatments. *Progress in Neuropsychopharmacology and Biological Psychiatry, 29,* 1074–1084.

Serretti, A., Calati, R., Massat, I., Linotte, S., Kasper, S., Lecrubier, Y.,...Souery, D. (2009). Cytochrome P450 CYP1A2, CYP2C9, CYP2C19 and CYP2D6 genes are not associated with response and remission in a sample of depressive patients. *International Clinical Psychopharmacology, 24,* 250–256.

Serretti, A., Drago, A., & De Ronchi, D. (2007). HTR2A gene variants and psychiatric disorders: A review of current literature and selection of SNPs for future studies. *Current Medical Chemistry, 14,* 2053–2069.

Shirayama, Y., Chen, A. C., Nakagawa, S., Russell, D. S., & Duman, R. S. (2002). Brain-derived neurotrophic factor produces antidepressant

effects in behavioral models of depression. *Journal of Neuroscience, 22,* 3251–3261.

Sindrup, S. H., Brosen, K., & Gram, L. F. (1992a). Pharmacokinetics of the selective serotonin reuptake inhibitor paroxetine: Nonlinearity and relation to the sparteine oxidation polymorphism. *Clinical Pharmacology and Therapeutics, 51,* 288–295.

Sindrup, S. H., Brosen, K., Gram, L. F., Hallas, J., Skjelbo, E., Allen, A.,...Tasker, T. C., et al. (1992b). The relationship between paroxetine and the sparteine oxidation polymorphism. *Clinical Pharmacology and Therapeutics, 51,* 278–287.

Siuciak, J. A., Lewis, D. R., Wiegand, S. J., & Lindsay, R. M. (1997). Antidepressant-like effect of brain-derived neurotrophic factor (BDNF). *Pharmacology, Biochemistry, and Behavior, 56,* 131–137.

Small, G. W., Ercoli, L. M., Silverman, D. H., Huang, S. C., Komo, S., Bookheimer, S. Y.,...Phelps, M. E. (2000). Cerebral metabolic and cognitive decline in persons at genetic risk for Alzheimer's disease. *Proceedings of the National Academy of Sciences USA, 97,* 6037 6042.

Smeraldi, E., Zanardi, R., Benedetti, F., Di Bella, D., Perez, J., & Catalano, M. (1998). Polymorphism within the promoter of the serotonin transporter gene and antidepressant efficacy of fluvoxamine. *Molecular Psychiatry, 3,* 508–511.

Solai, L. K., Pollock, B. G., Mulsant, B. H., Frye, R. F., Miller, M. D., Sweet, R. A.,...Reynolds, C. F., III. (2002). Effect of nortriptyline and paroxetine on CYP2D6 activity in depressed elderly patients. *Journal of Clinical Psychopharmacology, 22,* 481–486.

Tasker, T. C., Kaye, C. M., Zussman, B. D., & Link, C. G. (1989). Paroxetine plasma levels: Lack of correlation with efficacy or adverse events. *Acta Psychiatrica Scandinavica Supplement, 350,* 152–155.

Taylor, W. D., McQuoid, D. R., Ashley-Koch, A., Macfall, J. R., Bridgers, J., Krishnan, R. R., & Steffens, D. C. (2010). BDNF Val66Met genotype and 6-month remission rates in late-life depression. *Pharmacogenomics Journal, 11*(2), 146–154.

Tsai, S. J., Hong, C. J., Chen, T. J., & Yu, Y. W. (2007). Lack of supporting evidence for a genetic association of the FKBP5 polymorphism and response to antidepressant treatment. *American Journal of Medical Genetics B, Neuropsychiatric Genetics, 144B,* 1097–1098.

Tsai, S. J., Hong, C. J., & Liou, Y. J. (2010). Effects of BDNF polymorphisms on antidepressant action. *Psychiatry Investigation, 7,* 236–242.

Uhr, M., Grauer, M. T., & Holsboer, F. (2003). Differential enhancement of antidepressant penetration into the brain in mice with abcb1ab (mdr1ab) P-glycoprotein gene disruption. *Biological Psychiatry*, 54, 840–846.

Uhr, M., Tontsch, A., Namendorf, C., Ripke, S., Lucae, S., Ising, M., ... Holsboer, F. (2008). Polymorphisms in the drug transporter gene ABCB1 predict antidepressant treatment response in depression. *Neuron*, 57, 203–209.

Wessels, A. M., Pollock, B. G., Anyama, N. G., Schneider, L. S., Lieberman, J. A., Marder, S. R., & Bies, R. R. (2010). Association of 9-hydroxy risperidone concentrations with risk of switching or discontinuation in the clinical antipsychotic trial of intervention effectiveness-Alzheimer's disease trial. *Journal of Clinical Psychopharmacology*, 30, 683–687.

Whyte, E. M., Romkes, M., Mulsant, B. H., Kirshne, M. A., Begley, A. E., Reynolds, C. F., III, &

Pollock, B. G. (2006). CYP2D6 genotype and venlafaxine-XR concentrations in depressed elderly. *International Journal of Geriatric Psychiatry*, 21, 542–549.

Yoshida, K., Takahashi, H., Higuchi, H., Kamata, M., Ito, K., Sato, K., ... Nemeroff, C. B. (2004). Prediction of antidepressant response to milnacipran by norepinephrine transporter gene polymorphisms. *American Journal of Psychiatry*, 161, 1575–1580.

Zhang, X., Clark, A. F., & Yorio, T. (2008). FK506-binding protein 51 regulates nuclear transport of the glucocorticoid receptor beta and glucocorticoid responsiveness. *Investigations in Ophthalmology and Vision Science*, 49, 1037–1047.

Zhou, S. F. (2008). Structure, function and regulation of P-glycoprotein and its clinical relevance in drug disposition. *Xenobiotica*, 38, 802–832.

38

PHARMACOKINETICS AND PHARMACODYNAMICS IN LATE LIFE

Kristin L. Bigos, Robert R. Bies, and Bruce G. Pollock

OLDER PATIENTS are the major recipients of drugs, taking an average of five or more drugs each day (Mulsant et al., 2003); however, most research during drug development is conducted in healthy younger adults. Adverse drug events are common in older adults, but they are often preventable (Gurwitz et al., 2003). Psychotropic medications and anticoagulants are the most common medications associated with preventable adverse drug events in nursing homes (Gurtwitz et al., 2000). In homebound older adults, a group that is at even higher risk of adverse drug events, there is a high prevalence of psychotropic medication use (Golden et al., 1999). Antipsychotics now carry a black-box warning about the increased mortality in elderly patients with dementia-related psychosis after epidemiological studies found an increased risk of death in this cohort (Gill et al., 2007; Schneeweiss, Setoguchi, Brookhart, Dormuth, & Wang, 2007). Geriatric patients are a heterogeneous population, which is evident in the highly variable drug concentrations and differences in dose–concentration–response

relationships; therefore, safe and effective drug therapy requires an understanding of both drug disposition and response in older individuals (Bigos, Chew, & Bies, 2008).

The first requirement for rational therapeutics in an older population is to control for the immense variability in drug concentration (Pollock, 2005). Pharmacokinetics provides a means of describing and predicting drug concentrations in plasma and various tissues over time. Failure to address pharmacokinetic issues resulted in notable difficulties with the introduction of bupropion and clozapine (which produce seizures at high doses) and, for older patients, the introduction of fluoxetine and risperidone (which produce agitation, akathisia, and extrapyramidal syndromes) (Pollock, 2005). There are many physiological changes during aging that can contribute to changes in the pharmacokinetics of a drug, including changes in liver volume and hepatic blood flow (Schmucker, 2001). Declining renal. clearance is the major factor in renally excreted drugs such as lithium, and it can result in the accumulation of active drug metabolites such as 9-OH risperidone.

In addition to age-related physiological changes governing the processes of drug metabolism and elimination, there are also substantial changes in the brain that result in differences in the pharmacodynamics of drugs. The greatest changes in mRNA expression in the brain occur during fetal development and then late life (Colantuoni et al., 2011). These gene expression changes may result in changes from receptor densities to the brain circuitries themselves. The result is that older adults experience a difference in sensitivity to some drugs like alprazolam, even after accounting for differences in drug exposure (Bertz et al., 1997). Moreover, older adults tend to be on multiple medications that compound these differences and increase the potential for drug–drug interactions. This chapter focuses on the age-related differences in the pharmacokinetics and pharmacodynamics of drugs used in the treatment of late-life mood disorders.

AGE-ASSOCIATED PHYSIOLOGICAL CHANGES

There is evidence of physiological changes that result in differences in the pharmacokinetics of a drug across the life span (Pollock, 2004). Age-related physiological changes that affect drug absorption, distribution, metabolism, and excretion are reviewed in this section.

Absorption

While the absorption of nutrients that require active transport, such as iron, thiamine, and calcium, is often impaired in older adults, the rate and extent of passive drug absorption do not appear to be affected by normal aging (Pollock, 2004). Coadministration of antacids, high-fiber supplements, and the cholesterol-binding resin cholestyramine may significantly diminish the absorption of some medications. Additionally, food may have a modest and variable effect on the absorption of some antidepressants (Wright, Aikman, Werts, Seabolt, & Haeusler, 2009).

Distribution

The loss of lean body mass with aging leads to increases in the volume of distribution of lipid-soluble drugs, like most psychotropics. Because the half-life of a drug is directly proportional to its apparent volume of distribution, the result is a longer half-life and accumulation of drug in the tissue. Conversely, for water-soluble drugs such as lithium, the volume of distribution is decreased in older patients, reducing the margin of safety after acute increases in plasma drug concentration (Pollock, 2004). Changes in protein binding can also affect the distribution of a drug. Reductions in serum albumin with age and potential increases in alpha-1-acid glycoprotein with illness can affect the amount of drug bound to plasma proteins. However, as reviewed by Benet and Hoener (2002), changes in plasma protein binding are only clinically significant when therapeutic drug monitoring is used to adjust dosing, since total drug concentrations (free drug plus protein bound drug) are usually reported. Free drug levels in older patients have been found to be useful for lidocaine, theophylline, phenytoin, and digoxin, but most psychotropics are not monitored by free drug levels. Therapeutic plasma levels may benefit older adults treated with valproic acid, due to its increased use in dementia and its increased age-associated potential to produce thrombocytopenia and hepatotoxicity (Conley et al., 2001).

Metabolism

There is no evidence of an age-associated decline in the amount of CYP450 enzymes in the liver, though the efficiency of these enzymes may decrease with aging (Schmucker, 2001). However, there are known reductions in hepatic mass and liver blood flow with aging, which may place a greater emphasis on inter-individual differences in drug metabolizing capacity (Pollock, 2004). CYP2D6 is the primary metabolizing enzyme for tricyclic antidepressants and venlafaxine, as well as some older antipsychotics and risperidone. Studies conducted in older unmedicated subjects have not found an age-associated decline in CYP2D6 activity (Pollock et al., 1992). Patients who carry a CYP2D6 genotype that results in a poor metabolizer phenotype have greater nortriptyline concentrations and lower nortriptyline doses than patients who are not poor metabolizers (Murphy et al., 2001). Older patients who are CYP2D6 poor metabolizers also have greater side effects after treatment with perphenazine than patients without the genotype (Pollock et al., 1995). There is evidence of cardiovascular toxicity after treatment with venlafaxine in CYP2D6 poor metabolizers (Lessard et al., 1999), and concomitant diphenhydramine (a CYP2D6 inhibitor) can alter venlafaxine metabolism (Lessard et al., 2001). CYP2D6 has also been shown to exhibit stereoselectivity toward metabolizing chiral drugs such as venlafaxine. In CYP2D6 extensive metabolizers but not poor metabolizers, oral clearance of the (R)-enantiomer of venlafaxine is two-fold greater than clearance S(-)-venlafaxine (Eap et al., 2003). This stereoselectivity may be clinically relevant since S(-)-venlafaxine inhibits noradrenaline and serotonin presynaptic reuptake, while R(+)-venlafaxine primarily inhibits serotonin reuptake (Holliday & Benfield, 1995).

The CYP450 3A family of enzymes, including CYP3A4, CYP3A5, CYP3A7, and CYP3A43, are responsible for metabolizing the largest number of medications. While it is normally a high-capacity enzyme, serious toxicity can occur when CYP3A-mediated clearance is inhibited for drugs like the benzodiazepines midazolam and triazolam, and it is responsible for drugs like terfenadine, astemizole, and cerivastatin being pulled from the market. Because hepatic metabolism of CYP3A4 drugs is typically very rapid, many of these drugs can be perfusion limited, meaning that the rate of metabolism is dependent on hepatic blood flow, which is known to decline by about 40% from age 25 to 65 years. This may be the mechanism behind the decline in metabolism of drugs primarily metabolized by CYP3A4, such as alprazolam and triazolam, which are cleared 20% to 50% slower in older adults. CYP3A4 activity may be potently inhibited by the antidepressants nefazodone and fluvoxamine and, to a lesser extent, fluoxetine through its demethylated metabolite. The very long half-life of norfluoxetine may result in interactions many weeks after initiation of therapy. Other CYP3A4 inhibitors include grapefruit juice, protease inhibitors, *mycin* antibiotics, and *azole* antifungals. Similarly, the inhibition of the CYP3A4-mediated clearance of *statins*, resulting in muscle weakness, may be misattributed in depressed patients (Pollock, 2004). Other concomitant medications can induce CYP3A4 and thereby decrease drug concentrations of CYP3A4 substrates, including carbamazepine, phenytoin, topiramate, modafinil, barbiturates, steroids, and St. John's wort, which may result in lack of clinical response. This becomes a concern if a patient discontinues the inducing medication, reversing the induction effect, and potentially resulting in supratherapeutic drug levels and adverse events.

CYP1A2 is the primary metabolizing enzyme for olanzapine, clozapine, and fluvoxamine, and contributes to the demethylation of some tertiary tricyclic antidepressants. This isoenzyme undergoes induction by the polyaromatic hydrocarbons in cigarette smoke and charbroiled meats, as well as by some medications, including omeprazole and phenobarbital. The result is an increase in drug metabolism, as shown for olanzapine clearance in smokers (Bigos, Pollock, et al., 2008). Conversely, estrogen replacement therapy in postmenopausal women has been found to inhibit CYP1A2 metabolism (Pollock et al., 1999). Other CYP450 isoenzymes metabolize psychotropics as well; for example, CYP2B6 metabolizes bupropion, CYP2C9 metabolizes fluoxetine, and CYP2C19 metabolizes citalopram (Flockhart, 2012). Additionally the selective serotonin reuptake inhibitors (SSRIs) fluoxetine, paroxetine, and sertraline are CYP2B6 inhibitors in vitro, which could cause a drug interaction with bupropion (Hesse et al., 2000).

Excretion

The well-established age-associated decline in renal clearance (Lindeman, Tobin, & Shock, 1985; Rowe, Andres, Tobin, Norris, & Shock, 1976) may affect excretion of psychotropic drug metabolites and lithium in older patients. The degree of renal decline varies significantly and can be exacerbated by other illnesses such as diabetes and hypertension, as well as medications like nonsteroidal anti-inflammatory medications. There are higher concentrations of bupropion, risperidone, and venlafaxine metabolites in older patients and in patients with renal impairment, though the clinical consequences are unknown (Feng et al., 2008; Sweet et al., 1995).

PHARMACOKINETICS

Controlling for the wide variability in drug concentration is the first step toward optimizing drug therapy. Unfortunately, there is a paucity of data regarding pharmacokinetics of psychotropics in older adults. Most studies in older adults have been designed using classical pharmacokinetic modeling, which requires intensive sampling of a small number of subjects, often after only a single dose. The pharmacokinetic parameters are determined in a two-stage approach, first for each individual separately and then the pharmacokinetic parameters are calculated as the mean of the individual parameters. Most classical pharmacokinetic studies also use a homogenous population and leave out groups of people like women, children, and older adults, which would add to the variability. The results are therefore difficult to generalize to larger populations, including older adults with illnesses and concurrent medications typical of this age group (Devane & Pollock, 1999).

A better approach is population pharmacokinetic modeling, which uses nonlinear mixed-effects modeling. Population pharmacokinetic modeling in geriatric psychiatry has been reviewed by Bigos et al. (2006). The benefit of this approach is the ability to sparsely sample a large number of heterogeneous individuals. This allows for determination of both individual and population pharmacokinetic parameters. Population pharmacokinetic analyses can be included in routine assessments of patients in clinical trials as was done for the CATIE trials (Bigos et al., 2010), which is discussed later in this chapter. This allows us to identify sources of variability in drug exposure, and then covary for differences in drug exposure in the pharmacodynamic analyses. Additionally, the measurement of drug concentrations may have a role in evaluating treatment adherence, especially for drugs like antidepressants that have a delayed onset and variable therapeutic responses.

Antidepressants

While there is a paucity of data regarding the age-related changes in the pharmacokinetics of antidepressants, there is increasing data that clearance of some of these drugs decreases with aging and therefore older patients may experience greater concentrations than younger patients at the same dose (Table 38.1). Many of these are classical pharmacokinetic studies of a single dose and/or in a small number of subjects. However, there are a few studies that use a large number of sparsely sampled subjects in a population pharmacokinetic analysis (Bies et al., 2004; Feng et al., 2006; Jin et al., 2010) or in therapeutic drug monitoring (Gex-Fabry, Balant-Gorgia, Balant, & Garrone, 1990; Reis, Lundmark, & Bengtsson, 2003; Reis, Aamo, Spigset, & Ahlner, 2009).

Pharmacokinetic differences have been described in product label information for each SSRI, although fluoxetine is the only drug to be specifically tested for both disposition and efficacy in an older adult population. There were no differences in fluoxetine disposition found between older and younger adults in single-dose studies; however,

given the long half-life and the nonlinear disposition of the drug, a single-dose study is not adequate to rule out the possibility of altered pharmacokinetics in older adults (Prozac, Eli Lilly and Company: Indianapolis, IN, 2011). A multiple-dose study (20 mg/day for 6 weeks) also did not show pharmacokinetic differences. Despite the lack of evidence of pharmacokinetic differences, the label recommends a lower or less frequent dose be considered for older adults (Prozac, Eli Lilly and Company: Indianapolis, IN, 2011). Pharmacokinetic data in the package inserts from the other SSRIs report a decreased clearance and/or higher concentrations in older adults (Table 38.1). Citalopram clearance is 20% to 30% slower, escitalopram half-life is 50% longer, fluvoxamine clearance is reduced by 50%, minimum paroxetine concentration is 70% to 80% greater, and sertraline plasma clearance is 40% slower in older adults. The label recommendations for these SSRIs are to reduce the initial dose and to titrate doses more slowly in older adults. Despite these pharmacokinetic differences, they report no difference in safety or efficacy measures, or rate of adverse effects in older adults, although admittedly their studies may not have a sufficient number of older subjects to detect a difference.

Antipsychotics

Antipsychotics are often also prescribed as treatment for mood disorders and have quite variable pharmacokinetics. A population pharmacokinetic study was conducted as part of the Clinical Antipsychotic Trials of Intervention Effectiveness (CATIE) to identify the magnitude and sources of variability in antipsychotic clearance. During CATIE, patients with schizophrenia and Alzheimer's disease were treated with antipsychotics and followed for 18 months or until medication discontinuation. Plasma samples were collected during the study visits for determination of drug concentrations, and time and amount of last dose and time of sample were recorded. Population pharmacokinetic models were built for each drug and covariates, including age, were tested as potential sources of variability of antipsychotic clearance. There was no effect of age on the clearance of olanzapine (Bigos, Pollock, et al., 2008), quetiapine (Bigos et al., 2010), ziprasidone (Wessels et al., 2011), perphenazine (Jin et al., 2010), or risperidone (Feng et al., 2008). However, there was an effect of age on the clearance of the active metabolite 9-OH risperidone (Feng et al.,

Table 38.1 Age-Related Pharmacokinetic Differences in Antidepressants

DRUG	STUDY POPULATION AND DESIGN	FINDINGS
Amitriptyline	Therapeutic drug monitoring data; most common daily dose 100 mg; $n = 17 \geq 65$ y and $n = 66 <65$ y	No effect of age on clearance (Reis et al., 2009)
	$n = 7$ (21 to 23y), $n = 5$ (62 to 81y)	Longer half-life in older men compared to young (21.7 vs. 16.2 h) due to larger V_d; no difference in clearance (Schulz, Turner-Tamiyasu, Smith, Giacomini, & Blaschke, 1983)
	$n = 6$ (72 to 83 y); single dose of 125 mg	Clearance was lower than reported for younger subjects (0.18 to 0.45 L/h/kg) (Henry et al., 1981)
Bupropion	$n = 6$ (63 to 76 y), single dose of 100 mg; chronic dosing 100 mg t.i.d.	20% reduction in clearance, longer half-life (mean 32 h); increased metabolite concentrations (Sweet et al., 1995)
Citalopram	24 older adults (69 ± 3.7 y) vs. 8 younger adults (28 ± 4 y)	Plasma concentration to dose ratio of 3.5 is higher (Foglia et al., 1997) than the ratio of 1.96 reported in younger adults (Fredricson Overø, 1982)
	$n = 10$ (77 ± 8 y); 20 mg for 14 d	30% longer half-life in older adults (Gutierrez & Abramowitz, 2000)
	Therapeutic drug monitoring data; $n = 749$	Patients aged >65 y had greater dose-corrected concentrations of citalopram and desmethylcitalopram and lower clearance than younger patients (Margareta Reis et al., 2003)
	Therapeutic drug monitoring data; most common daily dose 20 mg; $n = 590 \geq 65$ y and $n = 1,740 <65$ y	84% increase in median concentration (Margareta Reis et al., 2009)
	$n = 106$ (22 to 93 y); 20 to 45 mg/d	Clearance decreased 0.23 L/h for every year of age (Bies et al., 2004)
	Two normal volunteer studies: single-dose and multiple-dose studies	In a single-dose study, citalopram AUC and half-life were increased in the older subjects (≥ 60 years) by 30% and 50%, respectively, whereas in a multiple-dose study they were increased by 23% and 30%, respectively (Celexa, St. Louis, MO: Forest Pharmaceuticals, Inc., 2011).
Clomipramine	Therapeutic drug monitoring data; $n = 150$	Clearance is 40 to 50% lower for patients ≥ 75 y than for those ≤ 40 y (Gex-Fabry et al., 1990)
	Therapeutic drug monitoring data; most common daily dose 150 mg; $n = 12 \geq 65$ y and $n = 103 <65$ y	71% increase in median concentration (Margareta Reis et al., 2009)

(Continued)

Table 38.1 *(Continued)*

DRUG	STUDY POPULATION AND DESIGN	FINDINGS
Escitalopram	$n = 45$ (<30 y), $n = 84$ (30 to 50 y), $n = 43$ (>50 y); 5 to 20 mg/d	Patients < 30 y cleared escitalopram 20.7% and 42.7% faster than patients 30 to 50 y, and > 50 y respectively; across the population CL decreased with increasing age (Jin et al., 2010)
	Single- and multiple-dose studies (≥65 y)	Half-life increased by approximately 50% in older subjects but no change in C_{max} (Lexapro, St. Louis, MO: Forest Pharmaceuticals, Inc., 2011)
	Therapeutic drug monitoring data; most common daily dose 10 mg; $n = 258$ ≥65 y and $n = 1,212$ <65 y	91% increase in median concentration (Margareta Reis et al., 2009)
Fluoxetine	$n = 11$ (65 to 77 y); single 40 mg dose	Minimal differences (Bergstrom, Lemberger, Farid, & Wolen, 1988)
	Single-dose studies in healthy older adults (≥65 y) and multiple-dose study of 20 mg fluoxetine for 6 weeks in 260 depressed but otherwise healthy patients (≥60 y)	No difference is disposition after single dose compared to younger subjects. In multiple-dose study, combined fluoxetine plus norfluoxetine plasma concentrations were 209.3 ± 85.7 ng/mL at the end of 6 weeks (Prozac, Eli Lilly and Company: Indianapolis, IN, 2011)
	Therapeutic drug monitoring data; most common daily dose 20 mg; $n = 40$ ≥65 y and $n = 293$ <65 y	61% increase in median concentration in older group (Margareta Reis et al., 2009)
Fluvoxamine	$n = 13$ (63 to 77 y); 50 mg b.i.d. for 28 d	No differences in AUC or half-life compared to young (De Vries, Van Harten, Van Bemmel, & Raghoebar, 1993)
	Studies of 50 and 100 mg fluvoxamine maleate tablets in older subjects (66 to 73 y) and young subjects (19 to 35 y)	40% higher mean C_{max} in older adults and multiple dose elimination half-life was 17.4 and 25.9 hours in the older compared to 13.6 and 15.6 hours in the young subjects at steady state for 50 and 100 mg doses, respectively; 50% reduction in clearance in older patients (Luvox, Baudette, MN: ANI Pharmaceuticals, Inc., 2011)
	$n = 30$ (10 young, 10 older adults, 10 older adults with chronic heart failure); single dose 50 mg	Two times higher C_{max} and three times greater AUC in older adults; 63% longer half-life; 50% decrease in clearance; inverse correlation ($r = -.67$) between age and oral clearance (Orlando, De Martin, Andrighetto, Floreani, & Palatini, 2010)
Mianserin	$n = 8$ (60 to 83 y); single 60 mg dose	No difference in clearance or half-life compared to younger subjects but longer absorption and AUC (Maguire, McIntyre, Norman, & Burrows, 1983)

(Continued)

Table 38.1 (*Continued*)

DRUG	STUDY POPULATION AND DESIGN	FINDINGS
Mirtazapine	Therapeutic drug monitoring data; most common daily dose 30 mg; $n = 101 \geq 65$ y and $n = 215 < 65$ y	62% increase in median concentration in older adults (Margareta Reis et al., 2009)
	$n = 16$ (68 ± 3 y); single and multiple 20 mg dose(s)	Half-life lowest in young men (22 h); similar half-life in young and older women and older men (35 h) (Timmer, Paanakker, & Van Hal, 1996)
	$n = 49$; mean age 49.6 ± 13.5 y	No effect of age on clearance (Grasmäder et al., 2004)
Moclobemide	Therapeutic drug monitoring data; most common daily dose 30 mg; $n = 151 \geq 65$ y and $n = 509 < 65$ y	44% increase in median concentration in older adults (Margareta Reis et al., 2009)
	$n = 14$ older adults (65 to 77 y), $n = 6$ young adults (22 to 33 y); single 100 mg dose and multiple 100 mg t.i.d.	No differences in PK parameters of parent or metabolite; no differences in steady-state concentrations (Stoeckel et al., 1990)
Nefazodone	Therapeutic drug monitoring data; most common daily dose 600 mg; $n = 9 \geq 65$ y and $n = 67 < 65$ y	No effect of age on clearance (Margareta Reis et al., 2009)
	$n = 24$ (>65 y) and $n = 24$ (18 to 40 y); single 300 mg dose, and 300 mg b.i.d. for 8 d	After single dose, mean plasma C_{max} and AUC for nefazodone and active metabolite hydroxynefazodone were two-fold higher in older vs. young subjects. At steady state, AUC for nefazodone and hydroxynefazodone was 50% higher in older women compared to other three groups (Barbhaiya, Buch, & Greene, 1996)
Nortriptyline	$n = 20$ older adults, $n = 17$ young adults; single 75 mg dose	Plasma nortriptyline half-life was longer and clearance slower in older adults (Dawling, Crome, & Braithwaite, 1980)
	$n = 25$ (57 to 83 y); 25 to 125 mg/d	No differences in nortriptyline concentrations but age correlates with metabolite concentrations (E-10-hydroxynortriptyline); replicated in a separate sample of 9 subjects (≥ 59 y) (Schneider et al., 1990)
Paroxetine	Therapeutic drug monitoring data; most common daily dose 100 mg; $n = 20 \geq 65$ y and $n = 30 < 65$ y	72% increase in median concentration in older adults (Margareta Reis et al., 2009)
	$n = 21$ (median 72 y); single and multiple dose of 20 or 30 mg	Increased steady-state variability; 20% higher in older adults; half-life increased (30 vs. 21 h) at 20 mg (38 h at 30 mg) (Hebenstreit, Fellerer, Zöchling, Zentz, & Dunbar, 1989; Lundmark et al., 1989)

(*Continued*)

Table 38.1 (*Continued*)

DRUG	STUDY POPULATION AND DESIGN	FINDINGS
	Multiple-dose study in older adults; daily doses of 20, 30, and 40 mg	C_{min} concentrations were about 70% to 80% greater in older adults. Recommended reduced initial dose in older adults (Paxil, Research Triangle Park, NC: GlaxoSmithKline, 2011)
	$n = 171$ (69 to 95 y); 10 to 40 mg/d	No effect of age on clearance as a continuous covariate in subjects with mean age of 77 y, though V_{max} in those ≥ 80 y was lower than those <80 y (275 µg/h vs. 419 µg/h) (Feng et al., 2006)
	Therapeutic drug monitoring data; most common daily dose 20 mg; $n = 159 \geq 65$ y and $n = 545 <65$ y	74% increase in median concentration in older adults (Margareta Reis et al., 2009)
Sertraline	$n = 22$ >65 y; 50 mg increasing to 200 mg/d for 21 d	Concentration higher in older men and women compared with young men but similar to young women (Ronfeld, Tremaine, & Wilner, 1997)
	16 (8 male, 8 female) elderly patients treated for 14 days at a dose of 100 mg/day	40% lower clearance compared to group of younger adults (25 to 32 y), also decreased clearance of desmethylsertraline in older males, but not in older females (Zoloft, New York, NY, 2011)
	Therapeutic drug monitoring data; most common daily dose 100 mg; $n = 166 \geq 65$ y and $n = 905 <65$ y	35% increase in median concentration in older adults (Margareta Reis et al., 2009)
Trimipramine	Therapeutic drug monitoring data; most common daily dose 150 mg; $n = 7 \geq 65$ y and $n = 25 <65$ y	No effect of age on clearance (Margareta Reis et al., 2009)
Venlafaxine	$n = 18$ (60 to 80 y); single 50 mg dose, chronic dosing 50 mg t.i.d.	24% increase in steady-state half-life in older adults; 14% increase in steady-state half-life of metabolite (Klamerus, Parker, Rudolph, Derivan, & Chiang, 1996)
	$n = 35$; 300 mg/d	No effect of age on ratio of O-desmethylvenlafaxine to venlafaxine concentrations (Gex-Fabry et al., 2002)
	Therapeutic drug monitoring data; most common daily dose 150 mg; $n = 102 \geq 65$ y and $n = 614 <65$ y	38% increase in median concentration in older adults (Margareta Reis et al., 2009)

AUC, area under the concentration-time curve; C_{min}, minimum concentration; C_{max}, maximum concentration; d, days; PK, pharmacokinetic; V_d, volume of distribution; V_{max} maximal elimination rate; y, years.
Source: Adapted from Pollock (2005).

2008). Differences in the clearance of 9-OH risperidone, now marketed as the drug paliperidone, result in an average 70-year-old patient having a 20% lower clearance than an average 45-year-old patient, which is likely due to decline in kidney function as measured by creatinine clearance (Feng et al., 2008). According to the drug label, no dosage adjustment is recommended based on age alone; however, age-related decreases in renal clearance affect paliperidone pharmacokinetics (Invega, Mountain View, CA: Alza Corp., 2007).

In a similar population approach, 391 patients with schizophrenia spectrum disorders (age 11 to 79 years) were treated with clozapine at the Centre for Addiction and Mental Health, Toronto, and drug concentrations were analyzed using population pharmacokinetic modeling (Ismail et al., 2012). Age had a significant effect on the clearance of clozapine and the active metabolite norclozapine (Ismail et al., 2012). Clearance of both parent and metabolite decreased exponentially after age 39 years, resulting in increased drug concentrations in plasma (Ismail et al., 2012). These data along with the CATIE data suggest that dosing adjustments may be necessary for risperidone and clozapine for older adults considering their decreased clearance with aging.

There are little data on the age-related pharmacokinetic differences of the newest approved antipsychotic aripiprazole. In formal single-dose pharmacokinetic studies of aripiprazole (15 mg), clearance was 20% lower in older subjects (≥65 years) compared to younger adult subjects (18 to 64 years). However, the pharmacokinetics of aripiprazole after multiple doses in older patients appeared similar to that observed in young, healthy subjects (Abilify Discmelt, Tokyo, Japan: Otsuka Pharmaceutical Co., Ltd., 2006). Aripiprazole has also recently been developed as an intramuscular injectable for acute mania and psychosis, as well as an orally disintegrating tablet (Abilify, Tokyo, Japan: Otsuka Pharmaceutical Co., Ltd., 2006).

Mood Stabilizers

There are few data about the pharmacokinetics of mood stabilizers in older adults. Most studies have not found an effect of age on the clearance of valproic acid (Birnbaum et al., 2004; Blanco-Serrano et al., 1999; Fattore et al., 2006; Stephen, 2003). One study of 208 patients (14 to 95 years) found no relationship between age and valproic acid clearance (Blanco-Serrano et al., 1999), and another study

of 51 older patients (65 to 89 years) and younger matched control subjects (age 21 to 50 years) found no difference between the groups (Fattore et al., 2006). Two small studies have found no difference in total plasma valproic acid concentrations, but significantly higher unbound valproic acid concentrations and decreased clearance of free drug in older adults (Bauer, Davis, Wilensky, Raisys, & Levy, 1985; Perucca et al., 1984), which appear to be a result of a decrease in plasma protein binding. A study of 146 nursing home residents (>65 years) found no association between age and valproic acid clearance, but they found an increased clearance in the patients taking the syrup formulation that is likely due to a decreased bioavailability rather than an increased clearance (Birnbaum et al., 2007), which may be an important consideration when dosing older adults.

Lithium is not biotransformed; therefore, any changes in hepatic metabolism with aging should not alter lithium clearance. However, due to decline in renal function with aging, there are changes in the excretion of lithium. Several studies have shown that older adults need lower doses of lithium and have higher dose-corrected plasma and serum concentrations (Coppen & Abou-Saleh, 1988; Greil, Stoltzenburg, Mairhofer, & Haag, 1985; Hewick, Newbury, Hopwood, Naylor, & Moody, 1977; Slater, Milanes, Talcott, & Okafor, 1984; Sproule, Hardy, & Shulman, 2000; Vestergaard & Schou, 1984). The largest of these studies ($n = 222$) showed that patients aged 65 years needed an average of 34% less lithium to maintain the same serum lithium concentrations as patients aged 25 years (Vestergaard & Schou, 1984). As reviewed by Sproule et al. (2000) and Eastham, Jeste, and Young (1998), a lithium dosage reduction of 25% to 50% is recommended in older adults.

Most of the studies on carbamazepine and lamotrigine in older adults are in patients treated for epilepsy, not mood disorders, but the pharmacokinetics of these drugs should be similar in both patient populations. Several studies have reported a decrease in carbamazepine clearance in older adults (Battino et al., 2003; Cloyd, Lackner, & Leppik, 1994; Graves et al., 1998; Jiao, Zhong, Shi, Hu, & Zhang, 2003; Svinarov & Pippenger, 1996). One study of 157 older adults (65 to 90 years) and 157 younger adults (20 to 50 years) matched for gender, body weight, and comedications, found a 23% decrease in carbamazepine clearance between the older adults and younger adults (Battino et al., 2003). When the groups were combined, there was a significant inverse correlation between carbamazepine clearance and age ($r = 0.32$) (Battino et al., 2003). A population pharmacokinetic study of 585 patients found a similar correlation with age and carbamazepine clearance, and patients 65 years and older had a 15% decrease in clearance compared to other adults (Jiao et al., 2003). One study found no effect of age on carbamazepine clearance though the sample included less than 10% older adults (36 ± 16 years) (Vucicevic et al., 2007). A large study of lamotrigine pharmacokinetics evaluated 247 young adults (16 to 36 years) compared to 155 older adults (55 to 92 years) and found that median lamotrigine clearance was 22% lower in the older adults compared to the younger adults (Arif, Svoronos, Resor, Buchsbaum, & Hirsch, 2011). Other studies have not found an association between age and lamotrigine clearance (Chan, Morris, Ilett, & Tett, 2001; Hussein & Posner, 1997; Rivas et al., 2008), although these studies had a small percentage of patients over 65 years. This highlights the opportunity for population approaches in attempting to understand age-related changes in disposition in a population beset by limited access and opportunity for sampling.

Benzodiazepines

While there are limited data on age differences in the pharmacokinetics of benzodiazepines, most studies of the longer acting benzodiazepines (e.g., alprazolam, diazepam) found few age-related changes, while the shorter acting triazolam has some important age-related changes. Additionally, a recent study found no change in protein binding of the benzodiazepines, lorazepam, oxazepam, and temazepam, with age in healthy subjects (19 to 87 years) (Chin, Jensen, Larsen, & Begg, 2011). One study found that older adults had a slower clearance and longer half-life after acute IV administration of alprazolam but had a similar AUC and C_{max} (Bertz et al., 1997). Another single oral dose study found modest increases in alprazolam plasma concentrations in older adults compared to younger adults shortly after drug administration, but there was no difference in apparent elimination half-life, time of maximum concentration, maximum concentration, volume of distribution, and apparent clearance (Kaplan et al., 1998). There is a reported increase in the mean half-life of orally disintegrating tablets of alprazolam in healthy older subjects compared to healthy younger adult subjects (16.3 vs. 11.0 hours;

Niravam, Milwaukee, WI: Schwarz Pharma, 2005). One study of diazepam found that the half-life and volume of distribution of acute administration were approximately two-fold greater in the older adults compared to younger subjects (Herman & Wilkinson, 1996). However, there were no age differences in diazepam clearance and no age-related differences in the levels of accumulated diazepam and its active metabolites; thus, changes that occur in diazepam disposition after acute administration do not appear to be important during chronic dosing (Herman & Wilkinson, 1996). Another long-acting benzodiazepine, nitrazepam, has also been shown to have similar clearance across the life span (van Gerven et al., 1998).

Unlike the longer acting benzodiazepines, triazolam has some significant age-related differences in its pharmacokinetics. One study found that older subjects had higher plasma concentrations of triazolam, and slower clearance, which resulted in a greater degree of sedation than younger subjects after the same dose (Greenblatt et al., 1991). Another study by this group found an age-by-sex interaction effect on triazolam pharmacokinetics (Greenblatt, Harmatz, von Moltke, Wright, & Shader, 2004). Among the women in their study, age did not have a significant effect on triazolam AUC or clearance. However, among the men, AUC increased and clearance decreased with increasing age (Greenblatt et al., 2004). Based on these data, it may be necessary to decrease the dosage of triazolam for older adults, especially older men (Greenblatt et al., 1991, 2004).

New Drug Formulations

A number of psychoactive drugs have had additional formulations recently approved (Bigos, Chew, & Bies, 2008). The most common of these is an orally disintegrating tablet developed for benzodiazepines (alprazolam), SSRIs (citalopram), and antipsychotics (aripiprazole). Orally disintegrating tablets have made taking medication easier, especially for older adults, who often have difficulties swallowing more conventional dosage forms such as tablets and capsules. An oral suspension has been developed for ziprasidone for similar reasons. However, a disadvantage of an oral suspension is that because it contains undissolved particles of drug, it requires thorough shaking to distribute the drug particles throughout the vehicle. If not mixed properly, the uneven distribution can cause inefficacy or toxicity, as reported in the past with phenytoin.

Extended-release formulations have been made for several drugs. Quetiapine is now available as an extended-release oral tablet, which allows for a reduction in dosing frequency as compared to a conventional immediate-release dosage form. According to the label, there is no indication of any different tolerability of the extended-release formulation of quetiapine (Seroquel XR) in older adults compared to younger adults; however, the mean plasma clearance of quetiapine was reduced by 30% to 50% in older patients when compared to younger patients. Older patients should be started on a lower dose of the immediate-release formulation (25 mg/day) and the dose can be increased depending on the response and tolerance of the individual patient. When an effective dose has been reached, the patient may be switched to the extended-release formulation at an equivalent total daily dose (Seroquel XR, Wilmington, DE: AstraZeneca, 2007).

PHARMACODYNAMICS

Interindividual differences in pharmacodynamics become evident when patients with similar plasma drug concentrations experience different responses, or even after controlling for differences in drug concentrations there are marked differences in the response to a medication. As in younger adults, SSRIs are the first-line therapy for treatment of mood disorders in late life. In general, older patients require similar concentrations to initiate a therapeutic response but are more sensitive than younger patients to adverse effects of antidepressants at lower concentrations (Pollock et al., 1999).

None of the SSRIs are specifically indicated for treatment in the elderly, but many have been tested in older adults. Fluoxetine has been sufficiently tested to determine that there are no differences in response in older adults. Two 6-week randomized placebo-controlled studies (N = 671) showed fluoxetine (20 mg daily) to be effective in the treatment of older patients (≥60 years of age) with major depressive disorder (Prozac, Eli Lilly and Company: Indianapolis, IN, 2011). Studies reported in the label information of paroxetine are not sufficient to determine the differences in response in older adults; however, approximately 700 patients in the preclinical studies were 65 years of age or older, and no overall differences in the adverse event profile or effectiveness were detected between older and younger patients (Paxil, Research Triangle Park, NC: GlaxoSmithKline, 2011). Similarly, there were

947 subjects in placebo-controlled geriatric clinical studies of sertraline in major depressive disorder, and there were no overall differences in the pattern of efficacy between older and younger adults (Zoloft, New York, NY, 2011). Citalopram, escitalopram, and fluvoxamine were not specifically studied, but again no overall differences were found between older and younger adults (Celexa, St. Louis, MO: Forest Pharmaceuticals, Inc., 2011) (Lexapro, St. Louis, MO: Forest Pharmaceuticals, Inc., 2011) (Luvox, Baudette, MN: ANI Pharmaceuticals, Inc., 2011).

Unfortunately, even with treatment with SSRIs, older adults with major depression are at high risk for relapse, as well as disability and even death. Maintenance therapy with paroxetine has shown to be effective in adults over 70 years, but more than one third of patients relapse (Reynolds et al., 2006). Major depression recurred within 2 years more often in patients receiving placebo (68% with and 58% without psychotherapy) than in patients receiving paroxetine (35% with and 37% without psychotherapy) (Reynolds et al., 2006). Another study in the very old (mean age 79.6 years) involved an 8-week trial of citalopram for the treatment of depression (Roose et al., 2004). There was a considerable range in response, and while there was no difference in response to citalopram or placebo overall, there was a significant benefit to treatment with citalopram in the patients with severe depression (HAM-D ≥24), which is consistent with other antidepressant treatment trials (Roose et al., 2004).

SSRIs are also used to treat late-life anxiety disorders. Citalopram has been shown to be effective in 60% of older adults (≥60 years) with anxiety disorders and have improved quality of life and sleep quality (Blank et al., 2006). A similar study of escitalopram in 177 older patients (≥60 years) with generalized anxiety disorder had a mean cumulative response rate of 69%, and patients had improvement in anxiety symptoms and role functioning (Lenze et al., 2009). Benzodiazepines are also used to treat late-life anxiety, and some studies have shown increased sensitivity in older adults. One study designed an infusion of alprazolam to maintain a plateau concentration that did not differ between young and older subjects to eliminate pharmacokinetic differences. The median half-life of offset of drug effect, as measured by digit symbol substitution, was longer for the older adults compared to the young adults (4.9 vs. 2.8 hours), which suggests that aging increases sensitivity to the effects of alprazolam through a mechanism other than pharmacokinetics (Bertz et al., 1997). Another study found modest increases in alprazolam plasma concentrations in older compared to younger adults shortly after drug administration, but no evidence of increased sensitivity to the pharmacodynamic effects of alprazolam in the older adults (Kaplan et al., 1998). A study of the short-acting benzodiazepine, triazolam, found a combination of higher plasma levels and increased intrinsic sensitivity led to greater pharmacodynamic effects of triazolam in older adults (Greenblatt et al., 2004). However, another study from this group found that the relationship between plasma triazolam concentration and the degree of impairment was similar for younger and older subjects (Greenblatt et al., 1991), suggesting that the difference from the previous study may be only a result of differences in triazolam pharmacokinetics.

Adjunctive treatment with antipsychotics has been shown to be effective in some older patients with depression who only have a partial response to SSRIs. In a 12-week open-label study of adjunctive aripiprazole, 50% of previous partial responders achieved remission, and none relapsed during a continuation treatment period (median: 27.6 weeks) (Sheffrin et al., 2009). While very few studies of antipsychotics have focused on comparing older and younger adults, there is evidence that older adults have increased sensitivity to antipsychotics (Uchida, Mamo, Mulsant, Pollock, & Kapur, 2009). Older psychiatric patients have a higher risk of extrapyramidal side effects with typical neuroleptic treatment. In one study of typical neuroleptics (haloperidol, thioridazine, perphenazine) and risperidone, approximately one third of patients developed neuroleptic-induced parkinsonism (Caligiuri, Lacro, & Jeste, 1999). In the subset of patients treated with risperidone, there was no association with extrapyramidal side effects (Caligiuri et al., 1999), which suggests atypical antipsychotics may be a better choice for older adults.

Atypical antipsychotics are also often used for the treatment of late-life bipolar disorder, as well as lithium and other mood stabilizers (Aziz, Lorberg, & Tampi, 2006). There has been very little research on differences in the pharmacodynamics of mood stabilizers, and the available data are in studies of patients with epilepsy. One study found higher rates of lamotrigine intolerability in older (34.8%) versus younger adults (24.2%) (Arif et al., 2011). Older patients had higher rates of intolerability due to imbalance (16% vs. 4%), drowsiness (13% vs. 7%),

and tremor (5% vs. 2%) compared with younger patients; however, rates of 6-month seizure-free were comparable (Arif et al., 2011). These higher rates of intolerability may be due to the decreased clearance of lamotrigine in older adults, which is likely the case with differences found in lithium response as well.

There is increasing evidence that SSRIs may have potential cognitive enhancing effects in patients with Alzheimer's disease, either as a direct effect on cognition or as a secondary effect of mood stabilization (Chow, Pollock, & Milgram, 2007). Paroxetine, due to its chemical structure and not its activity on the serotonin transporter, may also reduce amyloid plaque formations (Chow et al., 2007). Cognitive impairment also sometimes accompanies late-life depression and requires treatment. SSRIs in conjuction with cholinesterase inhibitors may be effective in treating the associated cognitive impairment. A placebo-controlled study of donepezil in conjunction with maintenance antidepressant treatment showed a marginal benefit of the addition of the cholinesterase inhibitor in global cognition and cognitive instrumental activities of daily living (Reynolds et al., 2011).

Side Effects in Older Adults

With aging, a decline in the body's ability to maintain homeostasis, including control of water balance, posture, orthostatic circulatory responses, and thermoregulation, may also interfere with the ability to adapt physiologically to medication. For example, all psychotropics, including SSRIs, increase the risk of falls and hip fracture (Liu et al., 1998). The syndrome of inappropriate antidiuretic hormone secretion (SIADH) is an age-associated adverse effect of all SSRIs and venlafaxine (Kirby & Ames, 2001). SIADH is more prevalent in older adults, and 12% experience some degree of hyponatremia after treatment with paroxetine (Fabian et al., 2004). Hyponatremia through SIADH then contributes to the increased risk of falls and fractures. The use of benzodiazepines in older adults is also associated with an increased risk of falls and fractures due to their sedating effects (Sgadari et al., 2000).

While SSRIs are thought to have a wide therapeutic dosing window, very low or high concentrations result in lack of efficacy or unnecessary side effects, respectively. The most serious side effect is the potential risk of abnormal heart rhythms with higher doses of citalopram or escitalopram in older patients over 60 years of age, patients who are CYP2C19 poor metabolizers, or patients taking concomitant CYP2C19 inhibitors (e.g., cimetidine, omeprazole), because these factors lead to increased blood levels of citalopram or escitalopram (Health Canada, 2012; US Food and Drug Administration, 2011).

High plasma paroxetine and sertraline concentrations have been associated with adverse cognitive and psychomotor effects in healthy older subjects (Furlan et al., 2001). Reductions in dopamine or acetylcholine function with age may increase sensitivity to SSRIs, which indirectly reduce dopamine output. SSRI-induced parkinsonism requires monitoring in older adults, and even low serum anticholinergic levels may be associated with cognitive impairment in depressed and psychiatrically healthy older adults (Fox, Livinston, 2011; Fox, Richardson, et al., 2011; Mulsant et al., 2003; Nebes et al., 1997).

Serious side effects have also been associated with antipsychotic use in older adults. All antipsychotics now carry a black-box warning about the increased mortality in elderly patients with dementia-related psychosis. The increased risk of death while small (adjusted hazard ratio 1.31 to 1.55) was significant in two large epidemiological studies and should be taken into consideration when prescribing antipsychotics in older adults (Gill et al., 2007; Schneeweiss et al., 2007).

Pharmacodynamic Drug Interactions

Because older adults require more medications, the prevalence of pharmacodynamic drug interactions increases, as previously reviewed (Lotrich & Pollock, 2005). A few examples include tricyclic antidepressants and paroxetine that can potentiate the effects of other anticholinergic medications, the combination of SSRIs and antipsychotics increases the likelihood of dyskinesias, and the combination of lithium and SSRIs increases risk of tremors, fever, and leukocytosis. There are also pharmacodynamic interactions between antidepressants and nonpsychotropic medications such as the combination of SSRIs and anticoagulants (including NSAIDs) and the risk of bleeding, or the combination of mirtazapine and clonidine and increased hypertension. The resulting drug interactions can then interplay with the decreased compensatory homeostatic mechanisms in older adults. For example, the anticholinergic effects of some drugs may result in slight

sedation in a younger adult but cause a degree of sedation in an older adult that increases the risk of falls and delirium. Unfortunately, anticholinergic drugs continue to be widely prescribed in older adults (Roe, Anderson, & Spivack, 2002).

The interactions between anticoagulants and antidepressants may be both pharmacokinetic and pharmacodynamic in nature. Among antidepressants, fluvoxamine poses the greatest risk of a pharmacokinetic interaction through inhibition of CYP2C9, reducing the clearance of warfarin's active S-enantiomer (Pollock, 2004). In addition, inhibition of CYP1A2 and CYP3A4 by fluvoxamine causes R-warfarin to accumulate, which also contributes to reduced S-warfarin clearance. However, increased bleeding times with SSRIs alone, or in combination with anticoagulants, may also be possible due to serotonin-depleting platelets and attenuating their aggregation (Pollock, Laghrissi-Thode, & Wagner, 2000). Epidemiological studies of SSRIs have reported concerns of increased risk of gastrointestinal bleeding (van Walraven, Mamdani, Wells, & Williams, 2001), as well as the potential protective effects against myocardial infarction in smokers (Sauer, Berlin, & Kimmel, 2001). Predicting and preventing the potential types of cumulative interactions from the addition of concomitant medications will become increasingly more important in geriatric psychiatry as more medications to treat these disorders become available.

CONCLUSIONS

Effective treatment of late-life mood disorders requires a more thorough understanding of the clinical pharmacology of the available medications, as well as a greater understanding of the pharmacokinetic and pharmacodynamic differences associated with aging and age-related illness, which may be a significant source of variability in clinical response to antidepressant therapy (Lotrich & Pollock, 2005). For example, it is well established that hepatic and or renal function changes contribute to differences in both drug disposition and response in older adults (Turnheim, 2003, 2004). Age-related physiological changes in the liver and kidney could then lead to pronounced interindividual differences related to CYP450 genotype, which can be compounded by the concomitant administration of drugs that are inhibitors or inducers of CYP450 enzymes. Age-associated pharmacokinetic changes that result in higher and more variable drug concentrations may contribute to the wide variability in response found in older adults (Pollock, 2005).

Although pharmacodynamic changes appear to make older adults more sensitive to the side effects of antidepressants, pharmacodynamic differences are not interpretable in the absence of drug concentrations (Pollock, 2004). It is also important to note that classical pharmacokinetic studies are often not sufficient to detect differences due to aging, or illness, or to identify drug interactions, due to the small number of subjects and often single-dose designs. Population pharmacokinetic studies are optimal for the very young and the very old because of the use of sparse sampling strategies. Another advantage is the ability to identify factors that contribute to the variability in pharmacokinetics, including age, weight, sex, race, and concomitant medications. Population pharmacokinetics can also be used to measure patient adherence and evaluate its effect on clinical outcome.

Accounting for differences in drug concentrations can increase the power to detect genetic influences or other factors that modulate drug response. In a study of antidepressant efficacy in late-life depression, patients with the S allele of the serotonin transporter polymorphism (5-HTTLPR) responded less quickly to paroxetine (Pollock, Ferrell, et al., 2000). In contrast to other SSRIs, this polymorphism does not however influence the overall antidepressant response at 12 weeks (Lotrich, Pollock, & Ferrell, 2001; Lotrich, Pollock, Kirshner, Ferrell, & Reynolds, 2008). A subsequent analysis discovered a relationship between paroxetine concentration and response, but only for the S-allele carriers; there was no relationship found in the L/L carriers (Lotrich, Bies, Smith, & Pollock, 2006).

A better understanding of pharmacokinetic and pharmacodynamic differences in older adults will hopefully decrease the prevalence and severity of adverse effects as well as optimize therapy for this fragile group of individuals. Carefully designing population pharmacokinetic studies and accounting for differences in drug concentrations in clinical trials are the first steps in the ultimate goal of safe and effective treatment of late-life mood disorders.

ACKNOWLEDGMENTS

Dr. Bigos is supported by the Lieber Institute for Brain Development, Johns Hopkins University, Baltimore, MD. Dr. Bies is supported by the Indiana Clinical Translational Sciences Institute through a gift from Eli Lilly and Company, as well as NICHD. Dr. Pollock's research is currently supported by the National Institute of Aging (AG031348), the American Psychiatric Association, and the Foundation of the Centre for Addiction and Mental Health.

Disclosures
Dr. Bigos has no conflicts of interest to declare.

Dr. Bies is funded by the Indiana Clinical and Translational Sciences Institute through a gift of Eli Lilly and Company. In addition, he has received funding through NICHD, the FDA ORISE, and Merck (for cardiovascular disease modeling). He serves on the scientific advisory board of Metrum Institute (unpaid).

Dr. Pollock receives research support from the National Institutes of Health, Canadian Institutes of Health Research, American Psychiatric Association, and the Foundation of the Centre for Addiction and Mental Health.

REFERENCES

Arif, H., Svoronos, A., Resor, S. R., Jr., Buchsbaum, R., & Hirsch, L. J. (2011). The effect of age and comedication on lamotrigine clearance, tolerability, and efficacy. Epilepsia, 52(10), 1905–1913.

Aziz, R., Lorberg, B., & Tampi, R. R. (2006). Treatments for late-life bipolar disorder. American Journal of Geriatric Pharmacotherapy, 4(4), 347–364.

Barbhaiya, R. H., Buch, A. B., & Greene, D. S. (1996), A study of the effect of age and gender on the pharmacokinetics of nefazodone after single and multiple doses, Journal of Clinical Psychopharmacology, 16(1), 19–25.

Battino, D., Croci, D., Rossini, A., Messina, S., Mamoli, D., & Perucca, E. (2003), Serum carbamazepine concentrations in elderly patients: A case-matched pharmacokinetic evaluation based on therapeutic drug monitoring data. Epilepsia, 44(7), 923–929.

Bauer, L. A., Davis, R., Wilensky, A., Raisys, V., & Levy, R. H. (1985). Valproic acid clearance: unbound fraction and diurnal variation in young and elderly adults. Clinical Pharmacology and Therapeutics, 37(6), 697–700.

Benet, L. Z., & Hoener, B. A. (2002), Changes in plasma protein binding have little clinical relevance, Clinical Pharmacology and Therapeutics, 71(3), 115–121.

Bergstrom, R. F., Lemberger, L., Farid, N. A., & Wolen, R. L. (1988). Clinical pharmacology and pharmacokinetics of fluoxetine: a review. *British Journal of Psychiatry Supplement, 3*, 47–50.

Bertz, R. J., Kroboth, P. D., Kroboth, F. J., Reynolds, I. J., Salek, F., Wright, C. E., & Smith, R. B. (1997), Alprazolam in young and elderly men: Sensitivity and tolerance to psychomotor, sedative and memory effects, *Journal of Pharmacology and Experimental Therapeutics, 281*(3), 1317–1329.

Bies, R. R., Feng, Y., Lotrich, F. E., Kirshner, M. A., Roose, S., Kupfer, D. J., & Pollock, B. G. (2004), Utility of sparse concentration sampling for citalopram in elderly clinical trial subjects. *Journal of Clinical Pharmacology, 44*, 1352–1359.

Bigos, K. L., Chew, M. L., & Bies, R. R. (2008). Pharmacokinetics in geriatric psychiatry, *Current Psychiatry Reports, 10*(1), 30–36.

Bigos, K. L., Bies, R. R., Marder, S. R., & Pollock, B. G. (2010), Population pharmacokinetics of antipsychotics. In T. S. Stroup & J. A. Lieberman (Eds.), *Antipsychotic trials in schizophrenia: The CATIE project* (pp. 267–280). Cambridge University Press, Cambridge, UK.

Bigos, K. L., Bies, R. R., & Pollock, B. G. (2006), Population pharmacokinetics in geriatric psychiatry. *American Journal of Geriatric Psychiatry, 14*(12), 993–1003.

Bigos, K. L., Pollock, B. G., Coley, K. C., Miller, D. D., Marder, S. R., Aravagiri, M.,... Bies, R. R. (2008), Sex, race, and smoking impact olanzapine exposure, *Journal of Clinical Pharmacology, 48*(2), 157–165.

Birnbaum, A. K., Ahn, J. E., Brundage, R. C., Hardie, N. A., Conway, J. M., & Leppik, I. E. (2007), Population pharmacokinetics of valproic acid concentrations in elderly nursing home residents. *Therapeutic Drug Monitoring, 29*(5), 571–575.

Birnbaum, A. K., Hardie, N. A., Conway, J. M., Bowers, S. E., Lackner, T. E.,... Leppik, I. E. (2004), Valproic acid doses, concentrations, and clearances in elderly nursing home residents. *Epilepsy Research, 62*(2–3), 157–162.

Blanco-Serrano, B., Otero, M. J., Santos-Buelga, D., García-Sánchez, M. J., Serrano, J., & Domínguez-Gil, A. (1999). Population estimation of valproic acid clearance in adult patients using routine clinical pharmacokinetic data. *Biopharmaceutics and Drug Disposition, 20*(5), 233–240.

Blank, S., Lenze, E. J., Mulsant, B. H., Dew, M. A., Karp, J. F., Shear, M. K.,... Reynolds, C. F. (2006), Outcomes of late-life anxiety disorders during 32 weeks of citalopram treatment. *Journal of Clinical Psychiatry, 67*(3), 468–472.

Caligiuri, M. P., Lacro, J. P., & Jeste, D. V. (1999). Incidence and predictors of drug-induced parkinsonism in older psychiatric patients treated with very low doses of neuroleptics. *Journal of Clinical Psychopharmacology, 19*(4), 322–328.

Chan, V., Morris, R. G., Ilett, K. F., & Tett, S. E. (2001), Population pharmacokinetics of lamotrigine. *Therapeutic Drug Monitoring, 23*(6), 630–635.

Chin, P. K., Jensen, B. P., Larsen, H. S., & Begg, E. J. (2011), Adult age and ex vivo protein binding of lorazepam, oxazepam and temazepam in healthy subjects. *British Journal of Clinical Pharmacology, 72*(6), 985–989.

Chow, T. W., Pollock, B. G., & Milgram, N. W. (2007). Potential cognitive enhancing and disease modification effects of SSRIs for Alzheimers disease. *Neuropsychiatric Disease and Treatment, 3*(5), 627–636.

Cloyd, J. C., Lackner, T. E., & Leppik, I. E. (1994). Antiepileptics in the elderly: Pharmacoepidemiology and pharmacokinetics. *Archives of Family Medicine, 3*(7), 589–598.

Colantuoni, C., Lipska, B. K., Ye, T., Hyde, T. M., Tao, R., Leek, J. T., Kleinman, J. E. (2011). Temporal dynamics and genetic control of transcription in the human prefrontal cortex. *Nature, 478*(7370), 519–523.

Conley, E. L., Coley, K. C., Pollock, B. G., Dapos, S. V., Maxwell, R., & Branch, R. A. (2001). Prevalence and risk of thrombocytopenia with valproic acid: Experience at a psychiatric teaching hospital. *Pharmacotherapy, 21*(11), 1325–1330.

Coppen, A., & Abou-Saleh, M. T. (1988). Lithium therapy: From clinical trials to practical management. *Acta Psychiatrica Scandinavica, 78*(6), 754–762.

Dawling, S., Crome, P., & Braithwaite, R. (1980). Pharmacokinetics of single oral doses of nortriptyline in depressed elderly hospital patients and young healthy volunteers. *Clinical Pharmacokinetics, 5*(4), 394–401.

De Vries, M. H., Van Harten, J., Van Bemmel, P., & Raghoebar, M. (1993), Pharmacokinetics of fluvoxamine maleate after increasing single oral doses in healthy subjects. *Biopharmaceutics and Drug Disposition, 14*(4), 291–296.

Devane, C. L., & Pollock, B. G. (1999). Pharmacokinetic considerations of antidepressant use in the elderly. *Journal of Clinical Psychiatry, 60*(Suppl 20), 38–44.

Eap, C. B., Lessard, E., Baumann, P., Brawand-Amey, M., Yessine, M. A., O'Hara, G., & Turgeon, J.

(2003). Role of CYP2D6 in the stereoselective disposition of venlafaxine in humans. *Pharmacogenetics and Genomics, 13*(1), 39–47.

Eastham, J. H., Jeste, D. V., & Young, R. C. (1998). Assessment and treatment of bipolar disorder in the elderly. *Drugs and Aging, 12*(3), 205–224.

Fabian, T. J., Amico, J. A., Kroboth, P. D., Mulsant, B. H., Corey, S. E., Begley, A. E.,... Pollock, B. G. (2004), Paroxetine-induced hyponatremia in older adults—a 12-week prospective study. *Archives of Internal Medicine, 164,* 327–332.

Fattore, C., Messina, S., Battino, D., Croci, D., Mamoli, D., & Perucca, E. (2006). The influence of old age and enzyme inducing comedication on the pharmacokinetics of valproic acid at steady-state: A case-matched evaluation based on therapeutic drug monitoring data. *Epilepsy Research, 70*(2–3), 153–160.

Feng, Y., Feng, Y., Pollock, B. G., Coley, K., Marder, S., Miller, D.,... Bies, R. R. (2008). Population pharmacokinetic analysis for risperidone using highly sparse sampling measurements from the CATIE study. *British Journal of Clinical Pharmacology, 66*(5), 629–639.

Feng, Y., Pollock, B. G., Ferrell, R. E., Kimak, M. A., Reynolds, C. F., III, & Bies, R. R. (2006), Paroxetine: Population pharmacokinetic analysis in late-life depression using sparse concentration sampling, *British Journal of Clinical Pharmacology, 61*(5), 558–569.

Flockhart, D. A. *Drug interactions: Cytochrome P450 drug interaction table*. Retrieved October 15, 2012, from http://medicine.iupui.edu/clinpharm/ddis/clinicalTable.aspx

Foglia, J. P., Pollock, B. G., Kirshner, M. A., Rosen, J., Sweet, R., & Mulsant, B. (1997). Plasma levels of citalopram enantiomers and metabolites in elderly patients. *Psychopharmacology Bulletin, 33*(1), 109–112.

Fox, C., Livingston, G., Maidment, I. D., Coulton, S., Smithard, D. G., Boustani, M., & Katona, C. (2011). The impact of anticholinergic burden in Alzheimers dementia-the Laser-AD study. *Age and Ageing, 40*(6), 730–735.

Fox, C., Richardson, K., Maidment, I. D., Savva, G. M., Matthews, F. E,. Smithard, D.,... Brayne, C. (2011). Anticholinergic medication use and cognitive impairment in the older population: The medical research council cognitive function and ageing study. *Journal of the American Geriatrics Society, 59*(8), 1477–1483.

Fredricson Overø, K. (1982). Kinetics of citalopram in man; plasma levels in patients. *Progress in Neuropsychopharmacology and Biological Psychiatry, 6*(3), 311–318.

Furlan, P. M., Kallan, M. J., Ten Have, T., Pollock, B. G., Katz, I., & Lucki, I. (2001), Cognitive and psychomotor effects of paroxetine and sertraline on healthy elderly volunteers. *American Journal of Geriatric Psychiatry, 9*(4), 429–438.

Gex-Fabry, M., Balant-Gorgia, A. E., Balant, L. P., & Garrone, G. (1990). Clomipramine metabolism: Model-based analysis of variability factors from drug monitoring data. *Clinical Pharmacokinetics, 19*(3), 241–255.

Gex-Fabry, M., Rudaz, S., Balant-Gorgia, A. E., Brachet, A., Veuthey, J. L., Balant, L. P., & Bertschy, G. (2002). Steady-state concentration of venlafaxine enantiomers: Model-based analysis of between-patient variability. *European Journal of Clinical Pharmacology, 58*(5), 323–331.

Gill, S. S., Bronskill, S. E., Normand, S. L., Anderson, G. M., Sykora, K., Lam, K.,... Rochon, P. A. (2007). Antipsychotic drug use and mortality in older adults with dementia. *Annals of Internal Medicine, 146*(11), 775–786.

Golden, A. G., Preston, R. A., Barnett, S. D., Llorente, M., Hamdan, K., & Silverman, M. A. (1999). Inappropriate medication prescribing in homebound older adults. *Journal of the American Geriatrics Society, 47*(8), 948–953.

Grasmäder, K., Verwohlt, P. L., Kühn, K. U., Dragicevic, A., von Widdern, O., Zobel, A.,... Rao, M. L. (2004). Population pharmacokinetic analysis of mirtazapine. *European Journal of Clinical Pharmacology, 60*(7), 473–480.

Graves, N. M., Brundage, R. C., Wen, Y., Cascino, G., So, E., Ahman, P.,... Leppik, I. E. (1998). Population pharmacokinetics of carbamazepine in adults with epilepsy. *Pharmacotherapy, 18*(2), 273–281.

Greenblatt, D. J., Harmatz, J. S., von Moltke, L. L., Wright, C. E., & Shader, R. I. (2004). Age and gender effects on the pharmacokinetics and pharmacodynamics of triazolam, a cytochrome P450 3A substrate[ast], *Clinical Pharmacology and Therapeutics, 76*(5), 467–479.

Greenblatt, D. J., Harmatz, J. S., Shapiro, L., Engelhardt, N., Gouthro, T. A., & Shader, R. I. (1991). Sensitivity to triazolam in the elderly. *New England Journal of Medicine, 324*(24), 1691–1698.

Greil, W., Stoltzenburg, M. C., Mairhofer, M. L., & Haag, M. (1985). Lithium dosage in the elderly: A study with matched age groups. *Journal of Affective Disorders, 9*(1), 1–4.

Gurwitz, J. H., Field, T. S., Harrold, L. R., Rothschild, J., Debellis, K., Seger, A. C.,... Bates, D. W. (2003), Incidence and preventability of adverse drug events among older persons in the ambulatory setting. *Journal of the American Medical Association, 289*(9), 1107–1116.

Gurwitz, J. H., Field, T. S., Avorn, J., McCormick, D., Jain, S., Eckler, M.,… Bates, D. W. (2000). Incidence and preventability of adverse drug events in nursing homes. *American Journal of Medicine, 109*(2), 87–94.

Gutierrez, M., & Abramowitz, W. (2000). Steady-state pharmacokinetics of citalopram in young and elderly subjects. *Pharmacotherapy, 20*(12), 1441–1447.

Health Canada. (2012). *Health antidepressant cipralex (escitalopram): Updated information regarding dose-related heart risk.* Retrieved June 1, 2012, from http://www.hc-sc.gc.ca/ahc-asc/media/advisories-avis/_2012/2012_63-eng.php

Hebenstreit, G. F., Fellerer, K., Zöchling, R., Zentz, A., & Dunbar, G. C. (1989). A pharmacokinetic dose titration study in adult and elderly depressed patients. *Acta Psychiatrica Scandinavica Supplement, 350*, 81–84.

Henry, J. F., Altamura,, C., Gomeni, R., Hervy, M. P., Forette, F., & Morselli, P. L. (1981). Pharmacokinetics of amitriptyline in the elderly. *International Journal of Clinical Pharmacology, Therapy, and Toxicology, 19*(1), 1–5.

Herman, R. J., & Wilkinson, G. R. (1996), Disposition of diazepam in young and elderly subjects after acute and chronic dosing. *British Journal of Clinical Pharmacology, 42*(2), 147–155.

Hesse, L. M., Venkatakrishnan, K., Court, M. H., von Moltke, L. L., Duan, S. X., Shader, R. I., & Greenblatt, D. J. (2000). CYP2B6 mediates the in vitro hydroxylation of bupropion: Potential drug interactions with other antidepressants. *Drug Metabolism and Disposition, 28*(10), 1176–1183.

Hewick, D. S., Newbury, P., Hopwood, S., Naylor, G., & Moody, J. (1977). Age as a factor affecting lithium therapy. *British Journal of Clinical Pharmacology, 4*(2), 201–205.

Holliday, S. M., & Benfield, P. (1995). Venlafaxine: A review of its pharmacology and therapeutic potential in depression. *Drugs, 49*(2), 280–294.

Hussein, Z., & Posner, J. (1997). Population pharmacokinetics of lamotrigine monotherapy in patients with epilepsy: Retrospective analysis of routine monitoring data. *British Journal of Clinical Pharmacology, 43*(5), 457–465.

Ismail, Z., Wessels, A. M., Uchida, H., Ng, W., Mamo, D. C., Rajji, T. K.,… Bies, R. R. (2012). Age and sex impact clozapine plasma concentrations in inpatients and outpatients with schizophrenia. *American Journal of Geriatric Psychiatry, 20*(1), 53–60.

Jiao, Z., Zhong, M. K., Shi, X. J., Hu, M., & Zhang, J. H. (2003). Population pharmacokinetics of carbamazepine in Chinese epilepsy patients. *Therapeutic Drug Monitoring, 25*(3), 279–286.

Jin, Y., Pollock, B. G., Frank, E., Cassano, G. B., Rucci, P., Müller, D. J.,… Bies, R. R. (2010). Effect of age, weight, and CYP2C19 genotype on escitalopram exposure. *Journal of Clinical Pharmacology, 50*, 62–72.

Kaplan, G. B., Greenblatt, D. J., Ehrenberg, B. L., Goddard, J. E., Harmatz, J. S., & Shader, R. I. (1998). Single-dose pharmacokinetics and pharmacodynamics of alprazolam in elderly and young subjects. *Journal of Clinical Pharmacology, 38*(1), 14–21.

Kirby, D., & Ames, D. (2001). Hyponatraemia and selective serotonin re-uptake inhibitors in elderly patients. *International Journal of Geriatric Psychiatry, 16*(5), 484–493.

Klamerus, K. J., Parker, V. D., Rudolph, R. L., Derivan, A. T., & Chiang, S. T. (1996). Effects of age and gender on venlafaxine and O-desmethylvenlafaxine pharmacokinetics. *Pharmacotherapy, 16*(5), 915–923.

Lenze, E. J., Rollman, B. L., Shear, M. K., Dew, M. A., Pollock, B. G., Ciliberti, C., Reynolds, C. F., III. (2009), Escitalopram for older adults with generalized anxiety disorder, *Journal of the American Medical Association, 301*(3), 295–303.

Lessard, É., Yessine, M. A., Hamelin, B. A., O'Hara, G., LeBlanc, J., & Turgeon, J. (1999). Influence of CYP2D6 activity on the disposition and cardiovascular toxicity of the antidepressant agent venlafaxine in humans. *Pharmacogenetics, 9*(4), 435–443.

Lessard, É., Yessine, M. A., Hamelin, B. A., Gauvin, C., Labbé, L., O'Hara, G.,… Turgeon, J. (2001). Diphenhydramine alters the disposition of venlafaxine through inhibition of CYP2D6 activity in humans. *Journal of Clinical Psychopharmacology, 21*(2), 175–184.

Lindeman, R. D., Tobin, J., & Shock, N. W. (1985). Longitudinal studies on the rate of decline in renal function with age. *Journal of the American Geriatrics Society, 33*(4), 278–285.

Liu, B., Anderson, G., Mittmann, N., To, T., Axcell, T., & Shear, N. (1998). Use of selective serotonin-reuptake inhibitors of tricyclic antidepressants and risk of hip fractures in elderly people. *Lancet, 351*(9112), 1303–1307.

Lotrich, F. E., & Pollock, B. G. (2005). Aging and clinical pharmacology: Implications for antidepressants. *Journal of Clinical Pharmacology, 45*, 1106–1122.

Lotrich, F. E., Pollock, B. G., & Ferrell, R. E. (2001). Polymorphism of the serotonin transporter: Implications for the use of selective serotonin reuptake inhibitors. *American Journal of PharmacoGenomics, 1*(3), 153–1164.

Lotrich, F. E., Bies, R. R., Smith, G. S., & Pollock, B. G. (2006). Relevance of assessing drug concentration exposure in pharmacogenetic and imaging studies. *Journal of Psychopharmacology, 20*, 33–40.

Lotrich, F. E., Pollock, B. G., Kirshner, M., Ferrell, R. F., & Reynolds, C. F., III. (2008). Serotonin transporter genotype interacts with paroxetine plasma levels to influence depression treatment response in geriatric patients. *Journal of Psychiatry and Neuroscience, 33*(2), 123–130.

Lundmark, J., Scheel Thomsen, I., Fjord-Larsen, T., Manniche, P. M., Mengel, H., Møller-Nielsen, E. M.,... Wålinder, J. (1989). Paroxetine: Pharmacokinetic and antidepressant effect in the elderly. *Acta Psychiatrica Scandinavica Supplement, 350*, 76–80.

Maguire, K., McIntyre, I., Norman, T., & Burrows, G. D. (1983). The pharmacokinetics of mianserin in elderly depressed patients, *Psychiatry Research, 8*(4), 281–287.

Mulsant, B. H., Pollock, B. G., Kirshner, M., Shen, C., Dodge, H., & Ganguli, M. (2003). Serum anticholinergic activity in a community-based sample of older adults: Relationship with cognitive performance. *Archives of General Psychiatry, 60*, 198–203.

Murphy, G. M., Jr., Pollock, B. G., Kirshner, M. A., Pascoe, N., Cheuk, W., Mulsant, B. H., & Reynolds, C. F., III. (2001). CYP2D6 genotyping with oligonucleotide microarrays and nortriptyline concentrations in geriatric depression, *Neuropsychopharmacology, 25*(5), 737–743.

Nebes, R. D., Pollock, B. G., Mulsant, B. H., Kirshner, M. A., Halligan, E., Zmuda, M., & Reynolds, C. F., III. (1997). Low-level serum anticholinergicity as a source of baseline cognitive heterogeneity in geriatric depressed patients. *Psychopharmacology Bulletin, 33*(4), 715–720.

Orlando, R., De Martin, S., Andrighetto, L., Floreani, M., & Palatini, P. (2010). Fluvoxamine pharmacokinetics in healthy elderly subjects and elderly patients with chronic heart failure. *British Journal of Clinical Pharmacology, 69*(3), 279–286.

Perucca, E., Grimaldi, R., Gatti, G., Pirracchio, S., Crema, F., & Frigo, G. M. (1984). Pharmacokinetics of valproic acid in the elderly. *British Journal of Clinical Pharmacology, 17*(6), 665–669.

Pollock, B. G. (2004). Pharmacokinetics and pharmacodynamics in late life. In S. P. Roose & H. A. Sackeim (Eds.), *Late-life depression* (pp. 185–191). Oxford, UK: Oxford University Press.

Pollock, B. G. (2005). The pharmacokinetic imperative in late-life depression. *Journal of Clinical Psychopharmacology, 25*(1), S19-S23.

Pollock, B. G., Laghrissi-Thode, F., & Wagner, W. R. (2000). Evaluation of platelet activation in depressed patients with ischemic heart disease after paroxetine or nortriptyline treatment, *Journal of Clinical Psychopharmacology, 20*(2), 137–140.

Pollock, B. G., Mulsant, B. H., Sweet, R. A., Rosen, J., Altieri, L. P., & Perel, J. M. (1995). Prospective cytochrome P450 phenotyping for neuroleptic treatment in dementia. *Psychopharmacol Bulletin, 31*(2), 327–331.

Pollock, B. G., Perel, J. M., Altieri, L. P., Kirshner, M., Fasiczka, A. L., Houck, P. R., & Reynolds, C. F., III. (1992). Debrisoquine hydroxylation phenotyping in geriatric psychopharmacology. *Psychopharmacol Bulletin, 28*(2), 163–168.

Pollock, B. G., Wylie, M., Stack, J. A., Sorisio, D. A., Thompson, D. S., Kirshner, M. A., Condifer, K. A. (1999). Inhibition of caffeine metabolism by estrogen replacement therapy in postmenopausal women. *Journal of Clinical Pharmacology, 39*(9), 936–940.

Pollock, B. G., Ferrell, R. E., Mulsant, B. H., Mazumdar, S., Miller, M., Sweet, R. A.,... Kupfer, D. J. (2000). Allelic variation in the serotonin transporter promoter affects onset of paroxetine treatment response in late-life depression. *Neuropsychopharmacology, 23*(5), 587–590.

Reis, M., Lundmark, J., & Bengtsson, F. (2003). Therapeutic drug monitoring of racemic citalopram: A 5-year experience in Sweden, 1992–1997. *Therapeutic Drug Monitoring, 25*(2), 183–191.

Reis, M., Aamo, T., Spigset, O., & Ahlner, J. (2009). Serum concentrations of antidepressant drugs in a naturalistic setting: Compilation based on a large therapeutic drug monitoring database. *Therapeutic Drug Monitoring, 31*(1), 42–56.

Reynolds, C. F., III, Dew, M. A., Pollock, B. G., Mulsant, B. H., Frank, E., Miller, M. D.,... Kupfer, D. J. (2006). Maintenance treatment of major depression in old age. *New England Journal of Medicine, 354*, 1130–1138.

Reynolds, C. F., III, Butters, M. A., Lopez, O., Pollock, B. G., Dew, M. A., Mulsant, B. H.,... DeKosky, S. T. (2011). Maintenance treatment of depression in old age: A randomized, double-blind, placebo-controlled evaluation of the efficacy and safety of donepezil combined with antidepressant pharmacotherapy. *Archives of General Psychiatry, 68*(1), 51–60.

Rivas, N., Buelga, D. S., Elger, C. E., Santos-Borbujo, J., Otero, M. J., Domínguez-Gil, A., & García, M. J. (2008). Population pharmacokinetics of lamotrigine with data from therapeutic drug monitoring in German and Spanish patients with epilepsy. *Therapeutic Drug Monitoring, 30*(4), 483–489.

Roe, C. M., Anderson, M. J., & Spivack, B. (2002). Use of anticholinergic medications by older adults with dementia. *Journal of the American Geriatrics Society, 50*(5), 836–842.

Ronfeld, R. A., Tremaine, L. M., & Wilner, K. D. (1997). Pharmacokinetics of sertraline and its N-demethyl metabolite in elderly and young male and female volunteers. *Clinical Pharmacokinetics, 32*(Suppl 1), 22–30.

Roose, S. P., Sackeim, H. A., Krishnan, K. R., Pollock, B. G., Alexopoulos, G., Lavretsky, H.,... Old-Old Depression Study Group. (2004). Antidepressant pharmacotherapy in the treatment of depression in the very old: A randomize, placebo-controlled trial. *American Journal of Psychiatry, 161,* 2050–2059.

Rowe, J. W., Andres, R., Tobin, J. D., Norris, A. H., & Shock, N. W. (1976). The effect of age on creatinine clearance in men: A cross-sectional and longitudinal study. *Journal of Gerontology, 31*(2), 155–163.

Sauer, W. H., Berlin, J. A., & Kimmel, S. E. (2001). Selective serotonin reuptake inhibitors and myocardial infarction. *Circulation, 104*(16), 1894–1898.

Schmucker, D. L. (2001). Liver function and phase I drug metabolism in the elderly: A paradox. *Drugs and Aging, 18* (11), 837–851.

Schneeweiss, S., Setoguchi, S., Brookhart, A., Dormuth, C., & Wang, P. S. (2007). Risk of death associated with the use of conventional versus atypical antipsychotic drugs among elderly patients. *Canadian Medical Association Journal, 176*(5), 627–632.

Schneider, L. S., Cooper, T. B., Suckow, R. F., Lyness, S. A., Haugen, C., Palmer, R., & Sloane, R. B. (1990), Relationship of hydroxynortriptyline to nortriptyline: Concentration and creatinine clearance in depressed: Elderly outpatients. *Journal of Clinical Psychopharmacology, 10*(5), 333–337.

Schulz, P., Turner-Tamiyasu, K., Smith, G., Giacomini, K. M., & Blaschke, T. F. (1983). Amitriptyline disposition in young and elderly normal men. *Clinical Pharmacology and Therapeutics, 33*(3), 360–366.

Sgadari, A., Lapane, K. L., Mor, V., Landi, F., Bernabei, R., & Gambassi, G. (2000). Oxidative and nonoxidative benzodiazepines and the risk of femur fracture. *Journal of Clinical Psychopharmacology, 20*(2), 234–239.

Sheffrin, M., Driscoll, H. C., Lenze, E. J., Mulsant, B. H., Pollock, B. G., Miller, M. D., Reynolds, C. F., III. (2009). Pilot study of augmentation with

aripiprazole for incomplete response in late-life depression: Getting to remission. *Journal of Clinical Psychiatry, 70*(2), 208–213.

Slater, V., Milanes, F., Talcott, V., & Okafor, K. C. (1984). Influence of age on lithium therapy. *Southern Medical Journal, 77*(2), 153–154.

Sproule, B. A., Hardy, B. G., & Shulman, K. I. (2000). Differential pharmacokinetics of lithium in elderly patients. *Drugs and Aging, 16*(3), 165–177.

Stephen, L. J. (2003). Drug treatment of epilepsy in elderly people: Focus on valproic acid. *Drugs and Aging, 20*(2), 141–152.

Stoeckel, K., Pfefen, J. P., Mayersohn, M., Schoerlin, M. P., Andressen, C., Ohnhaus, E. E.,... Guentert, T. W. (1990). Absorption and disposition of moclobemide in patients with advanced age or reduced liver or kidney function. *Acta Psychiatrica Scandinavica Supplement, 360,* 94–97.

Svinarov, D. A., & Pippenger, C. E. (1996). Relationships between carbamazepine-diol, carbamazepine-epoxide, and carbamazepine total and free steady-state concentrations in epileptic patients: The influence of age, sex, and comedication. *Therapeutic Drug Monitoring, 18*(6), 660–665.

Sweet, R. A., Pollock, B. G., Kirshner, M., Wright, B., Altieri, L. P., & DeVane, C. L. (1995). Pharmacokinetics of single- and multiple-dose bupropion in elderly patients with depression. *Journal of Clinical Pharmacology, 35*(9), 876–884.

Timmer, C. J., Paanakker, J. E., & Van Hal, H. J. M. (1996). Pharmacokinetics of mirtazapine from orally administered tablets: Influence of gender, age and treatment regimen, *Human Psychopharmacology: Clinical and Experimental, 11*(6), 497–509.

Turnheim, K. (2003). When drug therapy gets old: pharmacokinetics and pharmacodynamics in the elderly. *Experimental Gerontology, 38,* 843–853.

Turnheim, K. (2004). Drug therapy in the elderly. *Experimental Gerontology, 39,* 1731–1738.

Uchida, H., Mamo, D. C., Mulsant, B. H., Pollock, B. G., & Kapur, S. (2009). Increased antipsychotic sensitivity in elderly patients: Evidence and mechanisms. *Journal of Clinical Psychiatry, 70*(3), 397–405.

US Food and Drug Administration. (2011). *FDA drug safety communication: Revised recommendations for Celexa (citalopram hydrobromide) related to a potential risk of abnormal heart rhythms with high doses.* Retrieved May 23, 2012, from http://www. fda.gov/Drugs/DrugSafety/ucm297391

van Gerven, J. M., Uchida, E., Uchida, N., Pieters, M. S., Meinders, A. J., Schoemaker, R. C.,... Cohen, A. F. (1998). Pharmacodynamics and pharmacokinetics of a single oral dose of nitrazepam in healthy volunteers: An interethnic comparative study between Japanese and European volunteers. *Journal of Clinical Pharmacology, 38*(12), 1129–1136.

van Walraven, C., Mamdani, M. M., Wells, P. S., & Williams, J. I. (2001). Inhibition of serotonin reuptake by antidepressants and upper gastrointestinal bleeding in elderly patients: Retrospective cohort study. *British Medical Journal, 323*(7314), 655.

Vestergaard, P., & Schou, M. (1984). The effect of age on lithium dosage requirements. *Pharmacopsychiatry, 17*(06), 199–201.

Vucicevic, K., Miljković, B., Velickovć, R., Pokrajac, M., Mrhar, A., & Grabnar, I. (2007). Population pharmacokinetic model of carbamazepine derived from routine therapeutic drug monitoring data. *Therapeutic Drug Monitoring, 29*(6), 781–788.

Wessels, A. M., Bies, R. R., Pollock, B. G., Schneider, L. S., Lieberman, J. A., Stroup, S., ... Marder, S. R. (2011). Population pharmacokinetic modeling of ziprasidone in patients with schizophrenia from the CATIE study. *Journal of Clinical Pharmacology, 51*(11), 1587–1591.

Wright, C. W., Aikman, M. S., Werts, E., Seabolt, J., & Haeusler, J. M. (2009). Bioequivalence of single and multiple doses of venlafaxine extended-release tablets and capsules in the fasted and fed states: Four open-label, randomized crossover trials in healthy volunteers. *Clinical Therapeutics, 31*(11), 2722–2734.

39

PSYCHONEUROIMMUNOLOGY OF DEPRESSIVE DISORDERS

IMPLICATIONS FOR OLDER ADULTS AND LATE-LIFE DEPRESSION

Michael R. Irwin

DEPRESSION IN the elderly is a major public health concern (Alexopoulos, 2005). Given that 1 in 5 women and 1 in 8 men experience a depressive episode across their lifetime (Kessler, Zhao, Blazer, & Swartz, 1997), the disease burden of depression in older adults is enormous (Greenberg et al., 2003). Indeed, as the population ages in high-income countries, depression is projected to increase by 2030 to a position of the second greatest contributor to illness burden (Mathers & Loncar, 2006). Moreover, because elderly persons with depression often do not receive diagnosis and treatment (Alexopoulos, 2005), and only about 30%–35% of older adults achieve remission using current treatment approaches (Roose & Schatzberg, 2005), over two thirds of the disease burden remains intact (Andrews, Issakidis, Sanderson, Corry, & Lapsley, 2004; Chisholm, Sanderson, Ayuso-Mateos, & Saxena, 2004), leading to staggering costs in the health care sector (Vos et al., 2004). Moreover, substantial epidemiologic data indicate that depressive disorders

are associated with marked increases of medical morbidity and mortality.

Clinically relevant alterations in immune responses are found in major depression, which are implicated as a mechanism that might contribute to disease risk (Evans et al., 2002; Irwin, 2002; Irwin & Miller, 2007; Zautra, Yocum, Hong, Chen, & Tsai, 2004). Indeed, depressed persons show reductions of cell-mediated and antiviral immune responses that are associated with infectious disease susceptibility (Cohen, Doyle, Alper, Janicki-Deverts, & Turner, 2009; Leserman, 2003). Additionally, the risk of inflammation-associated cardiovascular, autoimmune, neurodegenerative, and neoplastic diseases is also increased in depression, presumably owing to excessive expression of immune response genes, and activation of innate immune responses (Irwin, 2002; Irwin & Miller, 2007). In turn, the immune system has reciprocal effects on the central nervous system (CNS) with effects on behavior (Irwin & Miller, 2007). Several molecular signaling pathways have been identified to convey peripheral pro-inflammatory and antiviral signals into the brain, and changes in these neurotransmitters activate physiological and behavioral responses that contribute to depressive symptoms and depression (Irwin & Cole, 2011; Irwin & Miller, 2007).

In this chapter, we map the immune alterations found in depression, discuss the implications for disease risk by highlighting the reciprocal regulation of the CNS by inflammatory signaling pathways. We discuss the unique implications of these data for risk of late-life depression given the associations between age, medical morbidity, and inflammation.

IMMUNOLOGICAL ALTERATIONS IN DEPRESSION

As described in a comprehensive meta-analysis of over 180 studies (Zorrilla et al., 2001), multiple enumerative and functional immune response measures have been characterized in patients with major depressive disorder. For example, studies using enumerative measures of white blood cells report increases in total numbers and in the numbers and percentages of neutrophils and lymphocytes in depressed persons (Herbert & Cohen, 1993; Kronfol, Turner, Nasrallah, & Winokur, 1984; Zorrilla et al., 2001). However, analyses of phenotype-specific cell surface markers have yielded mixed results, raising questions about whether depression is associated with alterations in the number and percentage of subpopulations of lymphocytes (B cells, T cells, T helper cells, and T suppressor/cytotoxic cells) (Herbert & Cohen, 1993), as well as cells that express the natural killer cell phenotype (Schleifer, Keller, Bond, Cohen, & Stein, 1989; Zorrilla et al., 2001).

Nonspecific Functional Measures

Substantial evidence indicates that the function of the immune system is altered in depressed patients, as first identified by assay of nonspecific mitogen-induced lymphocyte proliferation and natural killer cell activity. These early data showed reliable evidence of an association between depression and lower proliferative responses to the three nonspecific mitogens, including phytohemaglutinin (PHA), concanavalin-A (Con A), and pokeweed (PWM) (Herbert & Cohen, 1993; Zorrilla et al., 2001), along with decreases of natural killer cell activity (Herbert & Cohen, 1993; Zorrilla et al., 2001). In addition, sex differences in these effects

have been suggested; depressed women are more likely to show changes in natural killer activity as compared to depressed men (Evans et al., 1992). Furthermore, depression-associated decreases of natural killer activity are suggested to have clinical implications, as declines of killer lymphocytes in depressed women infected with human immunodeficiency virus (HIV) correlate with HIV disease progression (Evans et al., 2002).

Whereas it is well recognized that older age is associated with declines in the cell-mediated immune response, less is known about the moderating effects of age on the declines of functional immune measures in depression. Indeed, few studies have systematically examined the role of age on depression-associated changes in functional measures of immunity, but rather have controlled for the effects of age as well as other demographic characteristics (e.g., sex) by the selection of nondepressed controls who are comparable to the depressed patients on such characteristics. Nevertheless, one study has suggested that age, for example, may interact with depression status in altering immune variables, and it found that the presence of comorbid depression may further exacerbate age-related immune alterations (Schleifer et al., 1989).

Stimulated Cytokine Production

The function of various types of immune cells can also be estimated by assay of the ex vivo production of cytokines by various populations of mononuclear cells. For example, the stimulation of mononuclear cells by lipopolysaccharide or other Toll-like receptor ligands induces the production of proinflammatory cytokines such as interleukin-1 (IL-1), IL-6, and tumor necrosis factor-α (TNF). However, findings of differences in such ex vivo expression of proinflammatory cytokines between depressed patients and nondepressed controls are mixed. For example, one study found that peripheral blood mononuclear cells of nonmelancholic depressed patients showed a greater stimulated capacity to produce interleukin-1β and interleukin-1 receptor antagonist as compared to responses from controls and melancholic depressed patients (Kaestner et al., 2005), although earlier work by this group of investigators did not identify increases in IL-1 production (Rothermundt et al., 2001). Variable results in other studies might partly be explained by differences in sample characteristics, which relate to the regulation of stimulated inflammatory responses in depression. For example, depression subtype and/or severity of depressive symptoms are associated with activation of the hypothalamic pituitary adrenal (HPA) axis. In turn, such differential activation of HPA activity influences inflammatory responses. Indeed, melancholic, but not nonmelancholic, depressed patients showed evidence of HPA axis overactivity that is thought to inhibit immune activation and the expression of inflammatory markers, and which might account for the reported differences of inflammatory cytokine production between these two groups of diagnostic depression (Kaestner et al., 2005). Moreover, Miller et al. has found that a laboratory stress protocol reveals differences in the sensitivity of mononuclear cells to glucocorticoid signaling; depressed patients have similar levels of stimulated cytokine production at rest as compared to controls, but they are more resistant to glucocorticoids that typically terminate the inflammatory cascade following stress (Miller, Rohleder, Stetler, & Kirschbaum, 2005). Among depressed women, severity of depressive symptoms correlates with decreases in production of IL-1, IL-6, and TNF independent of health-related variables such as age, body mass index, or physically activity (Cyranowski, 2007). However, when assay methodologies are more refined (i.e., dual-color flow cytometry) to focus solely on the production of these proinflammatory cytokines by monocytes, as opposed to mixed mononuclear populations, a different pattern of results emerges; severity of depressive symptoms correlates with *increases*, rather than decreases, in the expression of IL-1, TNF, and IL-8 (Suarez, Krishnan, & Lewis, 2003). Indeed, the latter findings are consistent with broad evidence of systemic inflammation in depressed patients as will be discussed later in this chapter.

In addition to the stimulated production of proinflammatory cytokines, other studies have examined expression of T-cell cytokines and the relative balance of T helper 1 versus T helper 2 cytokine production. Whereas increases in the capacity of lymphocytes to produce interferon in depression (Seidel et al., 1995) have been found, no difference in the stimulated production of IL-2 is identified (Irwin, Clark, Kennedy, Christian Gillin, & Ziegler, 2003; Seidel et al., 1995).

Inflammation and Circulating Levels of Inflammatory Markers

Meta-analyses now firmly indicate that depression is associated with increases in circulating levels of proinflammatory markers, which suggest that systemic inflammation is present in some depressed patients (Howren, Lamkin, & Suls, 2009; Zorrilla et al., 2001). As compared to controls, elevated levels of IL-6 have been found in adults with major depression (Frommberger et al., 1997; Motivala, Sarfatti, Olmos, & Irwin, 2005; Pike, Hauger et al., 2003), as well in depressed elderly populations (Penninx et al., 2003). Indeed, a high plasma level of IL-6, but not CRP, is associated with an increased prevalence of major depression, both recurrent and new episodes, in older adults, independent of age, chronic diseases, cognitive functioning, and antidepressants (Bremmer et al., 2008). These cross-sectional data provide evidence of an association between depression and IL-6 but do not inform whether IL-6 elevations are capable of predicting depression or depression-associated mortality risk, which will be discussed later.

Similar elevations of inflammatory markers (e.g., IL-6) are found in patients with chronic medical disorders such as rheumatoid arthritis (Zautra et al., 2004), cancer (Musselman et al., 2001), and cardiovascular disease (Empana et al., 2005). It is hypothesized that increases in circulating levels of proinflammatory cytokine are due to activation of monocyte populations, and increases in circulating levels of other proinflammatory cytokines such as tumor necrosis factor-α (TNFα) and interleukin-1β (IL-1β) have been reported in depressed patients (Anisman, Ravindran, Griffiths, & Merali, 1999; Maes, Bosmans, Meltzer, Scharpé, & Suy, 1993), including late-life depressive disorder (Milaneschi et al., 2009; Thomas et al., 2005), although the numbers of studies that have examined these additional cytokines are too few to make firm conclusions, especially in older adults. One study also reported increases of plasma levels of IL-12 in a large cohort of depressed patients (Kim et al., 2002); IL-12 is a heterodimeric cytokine that is produced primarily by monocytes and macrophages and plays a central role in the early phases of inflammation. In addition to circulating levels, levels of IL-6 have also found to be elevated in the cerebrospinal fluid of depressed patients who attempt suicide, in which severity of depressive symptoms correlates with increases of IL-6 (Lindqvist et al., 2009).

Markers of systemic inflammation such as C-reactive protein (CRP) also show consistent elevations in depressed adults who are otherwise healthy (Miller, Stetler, Carney, Freedland, & Banks, 2002), as well as in depressed patients with acute coronary syndrome (Frasure-Smith 2009; Lesperance,

Frasure-Smith, Théroux, & Irwin, 2004; Miller, Freedland, Duntley, & Carney, 2005), although neither Bremmer et al. (2008) nor Whooley et al. (2007) found that depression was associated with increases of CRP in depressed older adults or in those with established coronary heart disease in contrast to increases of IL-6. Nevertheless, if systemic immune activation occurs in depression, it is thought to lead to endothelial activation and drive the increases in the expression of soluble intercellular adhesion molecule (sICAM) that is found in depressed patients (Lesperance et al., 2004; Motivala et al., 2005). Elevated levels of c-reactive protein and sICAM are associated with cardiovascular disease and are prospectively linked to myocardial infarction risk (Ridker, 2001).

Dissociation Between Declines of Innate Immunity and Inflammatory Markers

As reviewed earlier, a number of studies have evaluated cellular immune responses or markers of inflammation in depression, yet little attention has been given to understanding whether these patterns of immune alterations are related (Raison & Miller, 2003; Segerstrom & Miller, 2004). Rather, immune differences have been generated in separate samples of depressed patients with some studies examining levels of cellular immunity, for example, and other studies examining markers of inflammation. One study, however, has evaluated both natural killer activity and markers of inflammation in the same study population of depressed patients and controls and suggested that depression has independent, and nonoverlapping effects in these separate immune indices. For example, major depressive disorder was associated with lower natural killer activity and higher circulating levels of IL-6, yet levels of natural killer activity were not correlated with IL-6 or with other markers of immune activation, including acute phase proteins or IL-2R (Pike & Irwin, 2006). This pattern of independent effects provides insight for the effects of major depressive disorder on risk of infectious disease (Evans et al., 2002), as well as inflammatory disorders (Zautra et al., 2004).

The mechanisms for these divergent effects are not known. HPA activation, which is found in depression, is associated with suppression of both antiviral- and innate response gene profiles (Irwin & Cole, 2011). This paradox that HPA axis activation

fails to dampen inflammatory responses in depression may be due to the down-regulation of glucocorticoid receptor expression in depression similar to that found in chronic stress (Irwin & Cole, 2011; Miller et al., 2008). Alternatively, sympathetic nervous system (SNS) activation also occurs in depression (Irwin et al., 1991). Such adrenergic signaling induces a suppression of antiviral immune responses, with increases of innate immune response genes (Irwin & Cole, 2011). Moreover, SNS activation can induce IL6 gene expression via β-adrenergic activation of the transcription factor, GATA1, and polymorphisms of the gene promoter region of IL-6 (i.e., rs1800795 G/C transversion) moderates the impact of SNS/GATA1 signaling in ways that ultimately protect C allele carriers from the heightened inflammation-related disease risk associated with adverse socioenvironmental conditions, including depressive symptoms (Cole, Hawkley, Arevalo, & Cacioppo, 2011). Together, these findings point to the role of functional polymorphisms of IL-6 expression in predicting gene by socioenvironmental interactions on mortality risk in humans.

Viral Specific Immune Measures

Extension of these nonspecific measures of immunity to viral-specific immune response has begun to yield promising findings relevant to the increased risk of infectious disease in depression and psychological stress. For example, in middle-aged adults major depression is associated with a functional decline in memory T cells that respond to varicella zoster virus (Irwin et al., 1998), and this immune response is a surrogate marker for herpes zoster risk (Levin et al., 2008; Oxman et al., 2005; Weinberg et al., 2009). Furthermore, decreased memory T cell responses to varicella zoster virus have also been found in older adults. In addition to the robust declines of varicella zoster virus immunity in older adults as compared to middle-aged persons, the presence of depression in late life leads to a further decline of varicella zoster–specific immunity, which might further increase the risk of herpes zoster (Irwin, 2011). Such findings are consistent with a broader literature which has demonstrated that psychological stress is associated with decline in specific immune responses to immunization against viral infections (Miller et al., 2004; Vedhara et al., 1999), although extension of this work to major depression has not yet been conducted.

Assays of In Vivo Responses

Basic observations in animals have raised the possibility that depression can alter in vivo immune responses as administration of chronic stress in animals suppresses the delayed type hypersensitivity (DTH) response (Dhabhar, 2000). Indeed, in depressed patients, suppression of the DTH response to a panel of antigenic challenges has been found (Hickie, Hickie, Lloyd, Silove, & Wakefield, 1993). In contrast, Shinkawa et al. (2002) found that older depressed patients were more likely to show positive tuberculin responses than nondepressed patients. To our knowledge, no study has investigated whether depression alters immunological response to vaccination, although several studies have revealed that psychological stress is associated with declines of hepatitis B antibody responses as well as antibody response to influenza immunization (Glaser et al., 1992; Miller et al., 2004; Vedhara et al., 1999).

CLINICAL MODERATING FACTORS OF IMMUNE ALTERATIONS IN DEPRESSION

Depression Treatment: Effects of Antidepressant Medications

Cross-sectional observational studies suggest that treatment with the presence of antidepressant medications such as selective serotonin reuptake inhibitors (SSRIs) is associated with a partial or full normalization of the immune alterations (e.g., varicella zoster virus immunity) found in depression (Irwin et al., 2011), which suggests that alterations in the activity of central serotoninergic pathways may play a role in the modulation of immunity in depression. These observations are consistent with those of Evans et al. (2008), who found that treatment with the SSRI citalopram enhanced natural killer cell activity in HIV-infected subjects, independent of effects on depressive symptom. Other data suggest that SSRI treatment is associated with a normalization of inflammatory cytokine levels (e.g., IL-1β) in patients with posttraumatic stress disorder (Tucker et al., 2004).

Only a limited number of studies have investigated the clinical course of depression and changes of cellular immunity in relation to antidepressant medication treatment and symptom resolution. In one longitudinal case-control study, Irwin and coworkers (Irwin, Lacher, & Caldwell, 1992) found that depressed patients showed an increase in natural killer activity during a 6-month course of tricyclic antidepressant medication treatment and symptom resolution, although the improvements of natural killer activity were correlated with declines of symptoms severity and not treatment status at the time of follow-up. In another longitudinal follow-up study (Schleifer, Keller, & Bartlett, 1999) of young adults with unipolar depression involving 6 weeks of treatment with nortriptyline and alprazolam, clinical improvements in the severity of depressive symptoms was associated with decreased numbers of circulating lymphocytes and decreased responses to PHA and Con A but not PWM. In addition, decreases in T cells, CD4+, and CD29 were found, although there were no changes in B cell numbers or CD8+ cells. None of these changes were related to nortriptyline blood levels (Schleifer et al., 1999). In addition, Frank et al. (1999) found that in vivo and in vitro treatment with fluoxetine, an SSRI, resulted in enhanced natural killer activity along with changes in depressive symptoms, consistent with the finding of Ravidran et al. in which a number of different antidepressants were used, including nafazodone, paroxetine, sertraline, and venlafaxine (Ravindran, Griffiths, Merali, & Anisman, 1995). Finally, in studies of depression-associated inflammation, increased levels of IL-6 during acute depression were normalized after 8 weeks of fluoxetine treatment (Sluzewska et al., 1995). Similarly, production of IL-6 and TNF was decreased in depressed patients treated with amitriptyline, although this decrease was confined to the responders, suggesting that symptom resolution is a relatively more important predictor of the cytokine changes (Sluzewska et al., 1995). In contrast, 4-week treatment with clomipramine was found to be associated with increases in the mononuclear cell production of IL-1 in depressed patients (Weizman et al., 1994).

A few studies have also examined the effects of antidepressant treatment on Th1 versus Th2 cytokine production in depression. Treatments in vivo and in vitro with imipramine, venlafaxine, or fluoxetine increased stimulated cellular production of IL-10, with a decrease in the ratio of interferon (IFN) to IL-10 (Kubera et al., 1996). In hospitalized psychiatric patients (with either schizophrenia, depression, or bipolar disorder), one study found that treatment with psychotropic medications reduced IL-12 expression as compared to controls (Kim et al., 2002), consistent with the view held by Kenis and Maes (2002) that antidepressants decrease proinflammatory cytokine expression and induce a shift toward Th2 cytokine expression.

Smoking: Prevalence and Immune Effects

Cigarette smoking has long been considered a health risk, with effects on immunity via direct actions or possibly endocrine mediated mechanisms (Sopori & Kozak, 1998). Several studies of depressed patients have begun to evaluate the contribution of cigarette smoking to depression-related declines of natural killer activity and increases of IL-6 and other inflammatory markers (Andreoli et al., 1993; Irwin et al., 1990; Lesperance et al., 2004; Miller et al., 2002; Motivala et al., 2005), although none of this work has focused on depression in older adults. In a large study of 245 depressed and comparison controls stratified by smoking status, Jung and Irwin (1999) reported that depression and smoking status interact to produce greater declines of natural killer activity than those found in depressed or smoking groups alone. In addition, smoking status was associated with increases of IL-6 and sICAM in depression (Lesperance et al., 2004; Miller et al., 2002; Motivala et al., 2005), although evidence of immune activation occurs in depression independent of smoking status (Lesperance et al., 2004; Miller et al., 2002; Motivala et al., 2005; Pike & Irwin, 2006). Nevertheless, epidemiologic evidence suggests that depression interacts with cigarette smoking to impact health, rather than the presence of a unitary link between depression and cancer. In a 12-year follow-up of 2,264 adult men and women, depressed mood and cigarette smoking were associated with a marked increase in the relative risk of cancer (Linkins & Comstock, 1990) as compared to the risk associated with smoking or depression status alone.

Alcohol Dependence: Immune Effects in Depression

Alcohol/substance dependence has a number of effects on cellular and innate immune responses. However, little is known about the interaction of such alcohol/substance abuse with affective disorders, and whether there might be a combined effect that results in significantly more immune impairment than either condition alone. In a study by Irwin et al. (1990), individuals with a dual diagnosis of alcoholism and depression have further decreases of natural killer activity compared to individuals diagnosed with only alcoholism or depression. Furthermore, depressed subjects with histories of alcoholism had lower natural killer activity compared with depressed subjects without such histories. Alcoholics with secondary depression showed a further decrease in cytotoxicity compared with alcoholics who are not clinically depressed (Irwin et al., 1990). Strikingly, this result reflects the effects of past consumption of alcohol. Depressed and alcoholic subjects were free of alcohol for a minimum of 2 weeks, and thus the decline of natural killer activity was not due to a direct pharmacological effect of alcohol. More systematic assessment of current alcohol use along with dependence histories is needed.

Activity and Exercise: Immune Consequences in Depression

Activity, or a lack thereof, can have negative consequences on the immune system, and some data suggest that older adults with depression may be especially vulnerable to the harmful effects of sedentary lifestyles. Conversely, exercise has been shown to have potent salutary effects on immune measures and has even been found to promote a remission of depressive symptoms in older adults. In the meta-analysis from Herbert and Cohen (1993), melancholic depression correlated with greater impairments of cellular immunity, which may be due, at least in part, to an increased predominance of neurovegetative symptoms. Cover and Irwin (1994) found that severity of psychomotor retardation uniquely predicted declines of natural killer activity, similar to the effects of insomnia.

Behavioral interventions that include a component of physical activity have been found to boost antibody response to a novel antigen (Smith, Kennedy, & Fleshner, 2004), antibody production in response in to influenza vaccination (Kohut et al., 2005), and viral-specific T cell memory response to the varicella zoster virus (Irwin, Cole et al., 2003), with the latter effects found in older adults who show substantial age-related declines level at rest and following vaccine doses (Irwin, Olmstead, & Oxman, 2007). Similarly, a behavioral intervention that incorporates physical activity and meditative focus, Tai Chi, has been found to reduce circulating levels of IL-6 among older adults with elevated levels (Irwin & Olmstead, 2012). Furthermore, among elderly with late-life depression, the coadministration of Tai Chi and an antidepressant medication, citalopram, led to greater improvements of depressive symptoms along declines of CRP as compared to depressed elderly who received only citalopram (Lavretsky et al., 2011). These data extend other observations that the administration of aerobic exercise has been found to decrease depressive symptoms and to decrease the risk of relapse in major depressive disorder (Babyak et al., 2000; Blumenthal et al., 2005), although no study has examined whether similar benefits can be achieved in older adults with depression.

Disordered Sleep and Immunity: Relevance to Depression

Insomnia is one of the most common complaints of depressed subjects, but its role in moderating and/or mediating immune alterations in depression has been relatively unexplored. Nevertheless, in depressed patients, severity of subjective insomnia, but not with other depressive symptoms, correlates with lower levels of natural killer activity. Similarly, disturbance of electroencephalogram sleep in depressed patients correlated with alterations of natural and cellular immune function (Cover & Irwin, 1994; Irwin, Smith, & Gillin, 1992), with similar findings in bereaved subjects in which disordered sleep mediates the relationship between severe life stress and a decline of natural killer responses (Hall et al., 1998). These findings are consistent with a broader literature that has examined the effects of primary insomnia and sleep deprivation on cellular and innate immune responses and shown, similar to depression, suppression of cellular immunity and increases in markers of inflammation in association with sleep disturbance (Irwin, 2002; Irwin & Cole, 2011).

INFLAMMATORY REGULATION OF DEPRESSIVE SYMPTOMS

The peripheral inflammatory signals that are found in depression have reciprocal effects on the CNS, which are increasingly viewed as contributing to depression. For example, in clinical populations who have underlying inflammation, there is a nearly four-fold increased risk of depression (Miller, Ancoli-Israel, Bower, Capuron, & Irwin, 2008; Miller, Maletic, & Raison, 2009). Within the brain,

proinflammatory cytokines decrease the activity of key behavior-modulating neurotransmitter systems, including norepinephrine, dopamine, and serotonin (Miller et al., 2009), and they activate physiological and behavioral responses such as fever and social withdrawal (Dantzer, O'Connor, Freund, Johnson, & Kelley, 2008; Hart, 1988), inducing a constellation of sickness behaviors. Indeed, the chronic low-grade inflammation of aging is associated with alterations in the enzymatic pathways involved in monoamine metabolism, which correlate with the neurovegetative symptoms of depression such as sleep disturbance and fatigue (Capuron et al., 2011). In turn, dysregulated activation of cytokine-mediated sickness behavior is hypothesized to contribute to some cases of medically unexplained fatigue and sleep impairment (Miller et al., 2009).

Proinflammatory cytokines are also associated with the onset of depressive symptoms. Indeed, large-scale epidemiologic studies in adults show that elevations of IL-6, as well as TNFα, predict the occurrence of major depressive disorders at a later time (Gimeno et al., 2009). Likewise, in older adults, elevations of the inflammatory marker IL-1 receptor antagonist are higher in depressed subjects as compared to nondepressed persons, and those with the highest levels show a nearly three-fold increase in the risk of developing depressed mood during a 6-year follow-up (Milaneschi et al., 2009). Furthermore, elevated levels of CRP associated with over four-fold elevation in the probability of a recurrent depression in men, but not women (Liukkonen et al., 2006). However, other data in women show that elevated levels of CRP longitudinally predict severity of depressive symptoms (Matthews et al., 2007).

Among the inflammatory cytokines most studied in regard to depressive symptoms, IFN-α acts as a potent inducer of inflammatory activity to lead to hallmark symptoms of depression such as anhedonia and feelings of sadness, along with a range of other neurobehavioral changes, including disturbed sleep, fatigue, and loss of appetite (Capuron, Ravaud, & Dantzer, 2000; Capuron et al., 2002). Because these symptoms fully remit after cessation of IFN-α therapy, it is thought that such pharmacologic doses of an inflammatory mediator drive the onset of these symptoms (Anisman & Merali, 2002). Furthermore, other challenges (e.g., typhoid vaccination; endotoxin doses) that provoke the physiologic activation of inflammatory responses also lead to increases in feelings of fatigue and depressed mood, even though such elevations in IL-6 and TNFα are relatively less robust and shorter in duration as compared to treatment with IFNα (Eisenberger et al., 2010; Eisenberger, Inagaki, Mashal, & Irwin, 2010; Eisenberger, Inagaki, Rameson, Mashal, & Irwin, 2009; Harrison et al., 2009a,b). Importantly, such inflammation-driven changes in mood and symptoms of anhedonia, including social withdrawal, appear to be associated with neural changes such as reduced functional connectivity between the subgenual anterior cingulate cortex, amygdala, and medial prefrontal cortex (Harrison et al., 2009a), as well as reduced ventral striatum activity in response to reward cues (Eisenberger et al., 2010). Conversely, biologic therapies such as the TNFα antagonist, etanercept, which is not believed to appreciably enter the brain, was shown to be effective in reducing depressive symptoms in patients with the peripheral immune disorder, psoriasis (Tyring et al., 2006). There is also preliminary evidence for beneficial effects of nonsteroidal anti-inflammatory drugs, omega-3 fatty acids, and minocycline (an antibiotic that has some anti-inflammatory activity) on mood disorder symptoms (Lotrich, 2011).

Genetic factors may also influence the development and onset of depressive symptoms, and functional polymorphisms in the IL-6 gene and serotonin transporter gene may be especially relevant. Indeed, inflammatory biomarkers may identify depressed patients who are less likely to respond to antidepressant treatments. For example, among depressed patients, elevated levels of inflammatory markers prior to treatment prospectively predict poor clinical response to antidepressants medications (Jun et al., 2003; Wong, Dong, Maestre-Mesa, & Licinio, 2008; Yu, Chen, Hong, Chen, & Tsai, 2003). Furthermore, functional allelic variants of the IL-1 and TNFα genes are also found to be associated with an increased risk of depression, as well as reduced responses to antidepressant medications (Benedetti, Lucca, Brambilla, Colombo, & Smeraldi, 2002; Lanquillon, Krieg, Bening-Abu-Shach, & Vedder, 2000).

Given the "main effects" of inflammation-related gene polymorphisms on depression (i.e., mediated via genetic effects on inflammatory cytokine levels), it is also conceivable that inflammatory signaling may interact with brain neurotransmitter systems to affect the risk or severity of depression. Under such a model, polymorphisms in neurotransmitter-related genes (e.g., the serotonin transporter promoter polymorphism *5HTTLPR*, coding polymorphisms in *BDNF* and *COMT* genes; Uher & McGuffin, 2008) might affect CNS vulnerability/resilience to the depression-promoting effects of inflammatory cytokines. With this hypothesis, inflammation could be viewed as a moderator of brain-related genetic risk factors for depression, serving as a physiologic "stress" to actualize a genetic "diathesis," as previously observed in studies of interaction between psychosocial stress and the *5HTTLPR* polymorphism (Caspi et al., 2003). Consistent with this notion, antidepressant medications (e.g., serotonin- and norepinephrine reuptake inhibitors) interact with brain neurotransmitter gene polymorphisms (serotonin transporter gene) to affect monoamine metabolism, which in turn have been shown to influence the development of cytokine-induced depressive symptoms in humans (Bull et al., 2009). Alternatively, variants neurotransmitter genes such as the serotonin transporter gene might influence inflammatory profile and risk for depression. Indeed, it is thought that variants in the serotonin transporter gene (i.e., 5-HTTLPR polymorphisms) influence susceptibility to depression in which those carrying two short alleles of the 5-HTTLPR gene have an increased risk of depression. Recent evidence demonstrated that SS individuals exhibit a proinflammatory bias under resting conditions and/or during laboratory stress (Fredericks et al., 2010). Moreover, among individuals who have the serotonin transporter gene variant, the SLC6A4 gene, increases in both depressive symptoms and IL-6 plasma levels have been identified (Su et al., 2009). Recently, Lotrich et al. found that variants in the serotonin reuptake transporter promoter (5-HTTLPR) interact with the inflammatory system and influence depression risk in nondepressed hepatitis C patients about to receive INF-alpha. In these patients, the L(A) allele was associated with a decreased rate of developing major depressive disorder, with the L(A)/L(A) genotype being the most resilient. In addition, this genotype was also associated with better sleep quality, suggesting that sleep disturbance mediates a possible interaction between inflammatory cytokine (INF-alpha) exposure and 5-HTTLPR variability in risk for depression (Lotrich, Ferrell, Rabinovitz, & Pollock, 2009). Together, these data suggest that inflammatory markers and/or cytokine gene polymorphisms have the potential to be used as biological markers of risk for the onset and perpetuation of depressive symptoms.

CONCLUSION

In conclusion, there is strong evidence that depression involves alterations in multiple aspects of immunity that may not only contribute to the development or exacerbation of a number of medical disorders but also may contribute to the pathophysiology of the disease itself. Accordingly, aggressive management of depressive disorders in older adults may improve age-related disease outcomes. On the other hand, inflammatory processes prominent in older adults may interact with neural pathways known to contribute to depression, suggesting the need for novel approaches to the treatment of depression inclusive of both pharmacologic and behavioral strategies that impact inflammatory biology dynamics. Taken together, psychoneuroimmunology has provided an innovative frame of reference for understanding the impact of depression on health, and for the potential development of targeted interventions for the treatment and possibly prevention of late-life depression.

ACKNOWLEDGMENTS

This work was supported in part by grants HL 079955, AG 026364, CA 10014152, MH 19925, MH55253, M01 RR00827, General Clinical Research Centers Program, and the Cousins Center for Psychoneuroimmunology.

Disclosures

The author has no financial gain related to the outcome of this research, and there are no potential conflicts of interest.

REFERENCES

Surgeon General Report on Mental Health in older adults. 2004;http://www.surgeongeneral.gov/library/mentalhealth/toc.html.

Report of the 2005 White House Conference on Aging: The Booming Dynamics of Aging: From Awareness to Action. 2004; http://www.whcoa.gov.

Alexopoulos, G. S. (2005). Depression in the elderly. *Lancet, 365*(9475), 1961–1970.

Andreoli, A. V., Keller, S. E., Rabaeus, M., Marin, P., Bartlett, J. A., & Taban, C. (1993). Depression and immunity: Age, severity, and clinical course. *Brain Behavior and Immunity, 7*, 279–292.

Andrews, G., Issakidis, C., Sanderson, K., Corry, J., & Lapsley, H. (2004). Utilising survey data to inform public policy: Comparison of the cost-effectiveness of treatment of ten mental disorders. *British Journal of Psychiatry, 184,* 526–533.

Anisman, H., & Merali, Z. (2002). Cytokines, stress, and depressive illness. *Brain Behavior and Immunity, 16*(5), 513–524.

Anisman, H., Ravindran, A. V., Griffiths, J., & Merali, Z. (1999). Endocrine and cytokine correlates of major depression and dysthymia with typical or atypical features. *Molecular Psychiatry, 4*, 182–188.

Babyak, M. A., Blumenthal, J. A., Herman, S., Khatri, P., Doraiswamy, M., Moore, K., ... Krishnan, K. R. (2000). Exercise treatment for major depression: Maintenance of therapeutic benefit at 10 months. *Psychosomatic Medicine, 62*, 633–638.

Benedetti, F., Lucca, A., Brambilla, F., Colombo, C., & Smeraldi, E. (2002). Interleukin-6 serum levels correlate with response to antidepressant sleep deprivation and sleep phase advance. *Progress in Neuropsychopharmacology and Biological Psychiatry, 26*(6), 1167–1170.

Blumenthal, J. A., Sherwood, A., Babyak, M. A., Watkins, L. L., Waugh, R., Georgiades, A., ... Hinderliter, A. (2005). Effects of exercise and stress management training on markers of cardiovascular risk in patients with ischemic heart disease: A randomized controlled trial. *Journal of the American Medical Association 293*(13), 1626–1634.

Bremmer, M. A., Beekman, A. T., Deeg, D. J., Penninx, B. W., Dik, M. G., Hack, C. E., & Hoogendijk, W. J. (2008). Inflammatory markers in late-life depression: Results from a population-based study. *Journal of Affective Disorders, 106*(3), 249–255.

Bull, S. J., Huezo-Diaz, P., Binder, E. B., Cubells, J. F., Ranjith, G., Maddock, C., ... Pariante, C. M. (2009). Functional polymorphisms in the interleukin-6 and serotonin transporter genes, and depression and fatigue induced by interferon-alpha and ribavirin treatment. *Molecular Psychiatry, 14*(12), 1095–1104.

Capuron, L., Gumnick, J. F., Musselman, D. L., Lawson, D. H., Reemsnyder, A., Nemeroff, C. B., & Miller, A. H. (2002). Neurobehavioral effects of interferon-alpha in cancer patients: Phenomenology and paroxetine responsiveness of symptom dimensions. *Neuropsychopharmacology, 26*(5), 643–652.

Capuron, L., Ravaud, A., & Dantzer, R. (2000). Early depressive symptoms in cancer patients receiving interleukin 2 and/or interferon alfa-2b therapy. *Journal of Clinical Oncology, 18*(10), 2143–2151.

Capuron, L., Schroecksnadel, S., Féart, C., Aubert, A., Higueret, D., Barberger-Gateau, P., ... Fuchs, D. (2011). Chronic low-grade inflammation in elderly persons is associated with altered tryptophan and tyrosine metabolism: Role in neuropsychiatric symptoms. *Biological Psychiatry, 70*(2), 175–182.

Caspi, A., Sugden, K., Moffitt, T. E., Taylor, A., Craig, I. W., Harrington, H., ... Poulton, R. (2003). Influence of life stress on depression: Moderation by a polymorphism in the 5-HTT gene. *Science, 301*(5631), 386–389.

Chisholm, D., Sanderson, K., Ayuso-Mateos, J. L., & Saxena, S. (2004). Reducing the global burden of depression: Population-level analysis of intervention cost-effectiveness in 14 world regions. *British Journal of Psychiatry, 184*, 393–403.

Cohen, S., Doyle, W. J., Alper, C. M., Janicki-Deverts, D., & Turner, R. B. (2009). Sleep habits and susceptibility to the common cold. *Archives of Internal Medicine, 169*(1), 62–67.

Cole, S. W., Hawkley, L. C., Arevalo, J. M., & Cacioppo, J. T. (2011). Transcript origin analysis identifies antigen-presenting cells as primary targets of socially regulated gene expression in leukocytes. *Proceedings of the National Academy of Sciences USA, 108*(7), 3080–3085.

Cover, H., & Irwin, M. (1994). Immunity and depress ion:insomnia,retardation, and reduction of natural killer cell activity. *Journal of Behavioral Medicine, 17*(2), 217–223.

Cyranowski JM, Marsland AL, Bromberger JT, Whiteside TL, Chang Y, Matthews KA (2007). Depressive symptoms and production of proinflammatory cytokines by peripheral blood mononuclear cells stimulated in vitro. *Brain Behaviour and Immunity;*21(2):229–237.

Dantzer, R., O'Connor, J. C., Freund, G. G., Johnson, R. W., & Kelley, K. W. (2008). From inflammation to sickness and depression: When the immune system subjugates the brain. *Nature Reviews Neuroscience, 9*(1), 46–56.

Dhabhar, F. S. (2000). Acute stress enhances while chronic stress suppresses skin immunity. The role of stress hormones and leukocyte trafficking. *Annals of the New York Academy of Sciences, 917*, 876–893.

Eisenberger, N. I., Berkman, E. T., Inagaki, T. K., Rameson, L. T., Mashal, N. M., & Irwin, M. R. (2010). Inflammation-induced anhedonia: endotoxin reduces ventral striatum responses to reward. *Biological Psychiatry, 68*(8), 748–754.

Eisenberger, N. I., Inagaki, T. K., Mashal, N. M., & Irwin, M. R. (2010). Inflammation and social experience: An inflammatory challenge induces feelings of social disconnection in addition to depressed mood. *Brain Behavior and Immunity, 24*(4), 558–563.

Eisenberger, N. I., Inagaki, T. K., Rameson, L. T., Mashal, N. M., & Irwin, M. R. (2009). An fMRI study of cytokine-induced depressed mood and social pain: The role of sex differences. *Neuroimage, 47*(3), 881–890.

Empana, J. P., Sykes, D. H., Luc, G., Juhan-Vague, I., Arveiler, D., Ferrieres, J., ... PRIME Study Group. (2005). Contributions of depressive mood and circulating inflammatory markers to coronary heart disease in healthy European men: The Prospective Epidemiological Study of Myocardial Infarction (PRIME). *Circulation, 111*(18), 2299–2305.

Evans, D. L., Folds, J. D., Petitto, J. M., Golden, R. N., Pedersen, C. A., Corrigan, M., ... Ozer, H. (1992). Circulating natural killer cell phenotypes in men and women with major depression. *Archives of General Psychiatry, 49*, 388–395.

Evans, D. L., Lynch, K. G., Benton, T., Dubé, B., Gettes, D. R., Tustin, N. B., ... Douglas, S. D. (2008). Selective serotonin reuptake inhibitor and substance P antagonist enhancement of natural killer cell innate immunity in human immunodeficiency virus/acquired immunodeficiency syndrome. *Biological Psychiatry, 63*(9), 899–905.

Evans, D. L., Ten Have, T. R., Douglas, S. D., Gettes, D. R., Morrison, M., Chiappini, M. S., ... Petitto, J. M. (2002). Association of depression with viral load, CD8 T lymphocytes, and natural killer cells in women with HIV infection. *American Journal of Psychiatry, 159*(10), 1752–1759.

Frank, M. G., Hendricks, S. E., Johnson, D. R., Wieseler, J. L., & Burke, W. J. (1999). Antidepressants augment natural killer cell activity: In vivo and in vitro. *Neuropsychobiology, 39*, 18–24.

Frasure-Smith N, Lesperance F, Irwin MR, Talajic M, Pollock BG. (2009) The relationships among heart rate variability, inflammatory markers and depression in coronary heart disease patients. *Brain Behavior and Immunity.;*23(8):1140–1147.

Fredericks, C. A., Drabant, E. M., Edge, M. D., Tillie, J. M., Hallmayer, J., Ramel, W., ... Dhabhar, F. S. (2010). Healthy young women with serotonin transporter SS polymorphism show a pro-inflammatory bias under resting and stress conditions. *Brain Behavior and Immunity, 24*(3), 350–357.

Frommberger, U. H., Bauer, J., Haselbauer, P., Fräulin, A., Riemann, D., & Berger, M. (1997). Interleukin-6-(IL-6) plasma levels in depression and schizophrenia: Comparison between the acute state and after remission. *European Archives of Psychiatry and Clinical Neuroscience, 247*(4), 228–233.

Gimeno, D., Kivimaki, M., Brunner, E. J., Elovainio, M., De Vogli, R., Steptoe, A.,...Ferrie, J. E. (2009). Associations of C-reactive protein and interleukin-6 with cognitive symptoms of depression: 12-year follow-up of the Whitehall II study. *Psychological Medicine, 39*(3), 413–423.

Glaser, R., Kiecolt-Glaser, J. K., Bonneau, R. H., Malarkey, W., Kennedy, S., & Hughes, J. (1992). Stress-induced modulation of the immune response to recombinant hepatitis B vaccine. *Psychosomatic Medicine, 54*, 22–29.

Greenberg, P. E., Kessler, R. C., Birnbaum, H. G., Leong, S. A., Lowe, S. W., Berglund, P. A., & Corey-Lisle, P. K. (2003). The economic burden of depression in the United States: How did it change between 1990 and 2000? *Journal of Clinical Psychiatry, 64*(12), 1465–1475.

Hall, M., Baum, A., Buysse, D. J., Prigerson, H. G., Kupfer, D. J., & Reynolds, C. F., III. (1998). Sleep as a mediator of the stress-immune relationship. *Psychosomatic Medicine, 60*, 48–51.

Harrison, N. A., Brydon, L., Walker, C., Gray, M. A., Steptoe, A., & Critchley, H. D. (2009a). Inflammation causes mood changes through alterations in subgenual cingulate activity and mesolimbic connectivity. *Biological Psychiatry, 66*(5), 407–414.

Harrison, N. A., Brydon, L., Walker, C., Gray, M. A., Steptoe, A., Dolan, R. J., & Critchley, H. D. (2009b). Neural origins of human sickness in interoceptive responses to inflammation. *Biological Psychiatry, 66*(5), 415–422.

Hart, B. L. (1988). Biological basis of the behavior of sick animals. *Neuroscience and Biobehavioral Reviews, 12*(2), 123–137.

Herbert, T. B., & Cohen, S. (1993). Depression and immunity—A meta-analytic review. *Psychological Bulletin, 113*(3), 472–486.

Hickie, I., Hickie, C., Lloyd, A., Silove, D., & Wakefield, D. (1993). Impaired in vivo immune responses in patients with melancholia. *British Journal of Psychiatry, 162*, 651–657.

Howren, M. B., Lamkin, D. M., & Suls, J. (2009). Associations of depression with C-reactive protein, IL-1, and IL-6: A meta-analysis. *Psychosomatic Medicine, 71*(2), 171–186.

Irwin, M. (2002). Psychoneuroimmunology of depression: Clinical implications (Presidential Address). *Brain Behavior and Immunity, 16*, 1–16.

Irwin, M., Brown, M., Patterson, T., Hauger, R., Mascovich, A., & Grant, I. (1991). Neuropeptide Y and natural killer cell activity: Findings in

depression and Alzheimer caregiver stress. *FASEB Journal, 5*(15), 3100–3107.

Irwin, M., Caldwell, C., Smith, T. L., Brown, S., Schuckit, M. A., & Gillin, J. C. (1990). Major depressive disorder, alcoholism, and reduced natural killer cell cytotoxicity: Role of severity of depressive symptoms and alcohol consumption. *Archives of General Psychiatry, 47*: 713–719.

Irwin, M., Clark, C., Kennedy, B., Christian Gillin, J., & Ziegler, M. (2003). Nocturnal catecholamines and immune function in insomniacs, depressed patients, and control subjects. *Brain Behavior and Immunity, 17*, 365–372.

Irwin, M., Costlow, C., Williams, H., Artin, K. H., Chan, C. Y., Stinson, D. L.,...Oxman, M. N. (1998). Cellular immunity to varicella-zoster virus in patients with major depression. *Journal of Infectious Diseases, 178*(Suppl 1), S104–108.

Irwin, M., Lacher, U., & Caldwell, C. (1992). Depression and reduced natural killer cytotoxicity: A longitudinal study of depressed patients and control subjects. *Psychological Medicine, 22*, 1045–1050.

Irwin, M., Smith, T. L., & Gillin, J. C. (1992). Electroencephalographic sleep and natural killer activity in depressed patients and control subjects. *Psychosomatic Medicine, 54*, 107–126.

Irwin, M. R., & Cole, S. W. (2011). Reciprocal regulation of the neural and innate immune systems. *Nature Reviews Immunology, 11*(9), 625–632.

Irwin, M. R., Levin, M. J., Carrillo, C., Olmstead, R., Lucko, A., Lang, N.,...Oxman MN. (2011). Major depressive disorder and immunity to varicella-zoster virus in the elderly. *Brain Behavior and Immunity, 25*(4), 759–766.

Irwin, M. R., & Miller, A. H. (2007). Depressive disorders and immunity: 20 years of progress and discovery. *Brain Behavior and Immunity, 21*(4), 374–383.

Irwin, M. R., & Olmstead, R. (2011). Mitigating cellular inflammation in older adults. *American Journal of Geriatric Psychiatry, 20*(9), 764–772.

Irwin, M. R., Olmstead, R., & Oxman, M. N. (2007). Augmenting immune responses to varicella zoster virus in older adults: A randomized, controlled trial of Tai Chi. *Journal of the American Geriatrics Society, 55*(4), 511–517.

Irwin MR, Pike JL, Cole JC, Oxman MN (2003). Effects of a behavioral intervention, Tai Chi Chih, on varicella-zoster virus specific immunity and health functioning in older adults. *Psychosom Med* 65(5):824–830

Jun, T. Y., Pae, C. U., Hoon-Han, Chae, J. H., Bahk, W. M., Kim, K. S., & Serretti, A. (2003). Possible association between -G308A tumour necrosis

factor-alpha gene polymorphism and major
depressive disorder in the Korean population.
Psychiatric Genetics, 13(3), 179–181.

Jung, W., & Irwin, M. (1999). Reduction of natural
killer cytotoxic activity in major depression:
Interaction between depression and cigarette
smoking. *Psychosomatic Medicine, 61*, 263–270.

Kaestner, F., Hettich, M., Peters, M., Sibrowski,
W., Hetzel, G., Ponath, G., ... Rothermundt,
M. (2005). Different activation patterns of
proinflammatory cytokines in melancholic and
non-melancholic major depression are associated
with HPA axis activity. *Journal of Affective
Disorders, 87*(2–3), 305–311.

Kenis, G., & Maes, M. (2002). Effects of
antidepressants on the production of cytokines.
*International Journal of Neuropsychopharamacology,
5*, 401–412.

Kessler, R. C., Zhao, S., Blazer, D. G., & Swartz, M.
(1997). Prevalence, correlates, and course of
minor depression and major depression in the
National Comorbidity Survey. *Journal of Affective
Disorders, 45*(1–2), 19–30.

Kim, Y., Suh, I. B., Kim, H., Han, C. S., Lim, C. S.,
Choi, S. H., & Licinio, J. (2002). The plasma
levels of interleukin-12 in schizophrenia,
major depression, and bipolar mania: Effects
of psychotropic drugs. *Molecular Psychiatry, 7*,
1107–1114.

Kohut, M. L., Lee, W., Martin, A., Arnston, B., Russell,
D. W., Ekkekakis, P., ... Cunnick, J. E. (2005).
The exercise-induced enhancement of influenza
immunity is mediated in part by improvements in
psychosocial factors in older adults. *Brain Behavior
and Immunity, 19*(4), 357–366.

Kronfol, Z., Turner, R., Nasrallah, H., & Winokur, G.
(1984). Leukocyte regulation in depression and
schizophrenia. *Psychiatry Research, 13*, 13–18.

Kubera, M., Symbirtsev, A., Basta-Kaim, A., Borycz,
J., Roman, A., Papp, M., & Claesson, M. (1996).
Effect of chronic treatment with imipramine on
interleukin-1 and interleukin-2 production by
splenocytes obtained from rats subjected to a
chronic mild stress model of depression. *Polish
Journal of Pharmacology and Pharmacy, 48*,
503–506.

Lanquillon, S., Krieg, J. C., Bening-Abu-Shach, U.,
& Vedder, H. (2000). Cytokine production and
treatment response in major depressive disorder.
Neuropsychopharmacology, 22(4), 370–379.

Lavretsky, H., Alstein, L. L., Olmstead, R. E., Ercoli,
L. M., Riparetti-Brown, M., Cyr, N. S., & Irwin,
M. R. (2011). Complementary use of Tai Chi
Chih augments escitalopram treatment of geriatric
depression: A randomized controlled trial.

American Journal of Geriatric Psychiatry, 19(10),
839–850.

Leserman, J. (2003). HIV disease progression:
Depression, stress, and possible mechanisms.
Biological Psychiatry, 54(3), 295–306.

Lesperance, F., Frasure-Smith, N., Théroux, P., &
Irwin, M. (2004). The association between major
depression and levels of soluble intercellular
adhesion molecule 1, interleukin-6, and C-reactive
protein in patients with recent acute coronary
syndromes. *American Journal of Psychiatry, 161*(2),
271–277.

Levin, M. J., Oxman, M. N., Zhang, J. H., Johnson, G.
R., Stanley, H., Hayward, A. R., ... Veterans Affairs
Cooperative Studies Program Shingles Prevention
Study Investigators. (2008). Varicella-zoster
virus-specific immune responses in elderly
recipients of a herpes zoster vaccine. *Journal of
Infectious Diseases, 197*(6), 825–835.

Lindqvist, D., Janelidze, S., Hagell, P., Erhardt,
S., Samuelsson, M., Minthon, L., ... Brundin,
L. (2009). Interleukin-6 is elevated in the
cerebrospinal fluid of suicide attempters and
related to symptom severity. *Biological Psychiatry,
66*(3), 287–292.

Linkins, R. W., & Comstock, G. W. (1990). Depressed
mood and development of cancer. *American
Journal of Epidemiology, 132*(5), 962–972.

Liukkonen, T., Silvennoinen-Kassinen, S., Jokelainen,
J., Räsänen, P., Leinonen, M., Meyer-Rochow, V. B.,
& Timonen, M. (2006). The association between
C-reactive protein levels and depression: Results
from the northern Finland 1966 birth cohort study.
Biological Psychiatry, 60(8), 825–830.

Lotrich, F. (2011). Depression symptoms, low-grade
inflammatory activity, and new targets for clinical
intervention. *Biological Psychiatry, 70*(2), 111–112.

Lotrich, F. E., Ferrell, R. E., Rabinovitz, M., &
Pollock, B. G.. (2009). Risk for depression during
interferon-alpha treatment is affected by the
serotonin transporter polymorphism. *Biological
Psychiatry, 65*(4), 344–348.

Maes, M., Bosmans, E., Meltzer, H. Y., Scharpé, S.,
& Suy, E. (1993). Interleukin-1 beta: A putative
meidator of HPA axis hyperactivity in major
depression. *American Journal of Psychiatry, 150*,
1189–1193.

Mathers, C. D., & Loncar, D. (2006). Projections of
global mortality and burden of disease from 2002
to 2030. *PLoS Medicine, 3*(11), e442.

Matthews, K. A., Schott, L. L., Bromberger, J.,
Cyranowski, J., Everson-Rose, S. A., & Sowers,
M. F. (2007). Associations between depressive
symptoms and inflammatory/hemostatic
markers in women during the menopausal

transition. *Psychosomatic Medicine*, 69(2), 124–130.

Milaneschi, Y., Corsi, A. M., Penninx, B. W., Bandinelli, S., Guralnik, J. M., & Ferrucci, L. (2009). Interleukin-1 receptor antagonist and incident depressive symptoms over 6 years in older persons: The InCHIANTI study. *Biological Psychiatry*, 65(11), 973–978.

Miller, A. H., Ancoli-Israel, S., Bower, J. E., Capuron, L., & Irwin, M. R. (2008). Neuroendocrine-immune mechanisms of behavioral comorbidities in patients with cancer. *Journal of Clinical Oncology*, 26(6), 971–982.

Miller, A. H., Maletic, V., & Raison, C. L. (2009). Inflammation and its discontents: The role of cytokines in the pathophysiology of major depression. *Biological Psychiatry*, 65(9), 732–741.

Miller, G. E., Chen, E., Sze, J., Marin, T., Arevalo, J. M., Doll, R., … Cole, S. W. (2008). A functional genomic fingerprint of chronic stress in humans: Blunted glucocorticoid and increased NF-kappaB signaling. *Biological Psychiatry*, 64(4), 266–272.

Miller, G. E., Cohen, S., Pressman, S., Barkin, A., Rabin, B. S., & Treanor, J. J. (2004). Psychological stress and antibody response to influenza vaccination: When is the critical period for stress, and how does it get inside the body? *Psychosomatic Medicine*, 66(2), 215–223.

Miller, G. E., Freedland, K. E., Duntley, S., & Carney, R. M. (2005). Relation of depressive symptoms to C-reactive protein and pathogen burden (cytomegalovirus, herpes simplex virus, Epstein-Barr virus) in patients with earlier acute coronary syndromes. *American Journal of Cardiology*, 95(3), 317–321.

Miller, G. E., Rohleder, N., Stetler, C., & Kirschbaum, C. (2005). Clinical depression and regulation of the inflammatory response during acute stress. *Psychosomatic Medicine*, 67(5), 679–687.

Miller, G. E., Stetler, C. A., Carney, R. M., Freedland, K. E., & Banks, W. A. (2002). Clinical depression and inflammatory risk markers for coronary heart disease. *American Journal of Cardiology*, 90(12), 1279–1283.

Motivala, S. J., Sarfatti, A., Olmos, L., & Irwin, M. R. (2005). Inflammatory markers and sleep disturbance in major depression. *Psychosomatic Medicine*, 67(2), 187–194.

Musselman, D. L., Miller, A. H., Porter, M. R., Manatunga, A., Gao, F., Penna, S., … Nemeroff, C. B. (2001). Higher than normal plasma interleukin-6 concentrations in cancer patients with depression: Preliminary findings. *American Journal of Psychiatry*, 158, 1252–1257.

Oxman, M. N., Levin, M. J., Johnson, G. R., Schmader, K. E., Straus, S. E., Gelb, L. D., … Shingles Prevention Study Group. (2005). A vaccine to prevent herpes zoster and postherpetic neuralgia in older adults. *New England Journal of Medicine*, 352(22), 2271–2284.

Penninx, B. W., Kritchevsky, S. B., Yaffe, K., Newman, A. B., Simonsick, E. M., Rubin, S., … Pahor, M. (2003). Inflammatory markers and depressed mood in older persons: Results from the Health, Aging and Body Composition study. *Biological Psychiatry*, 54(5), 566–572.

Pike, J. L., & Irwin, M. R. (2006). Dissociation of inflammatory markers and natural killer cell activity in major depressive disorder. *Brain Behavior and Immunity*, 20(2), 169–174.

Raison, C., & Miller, A. H. (2003). When not enough is too much: The role of insufficient glucocorticoid signaling in the pathophysiology of stress-related disorders. *American Journal of Psychiatry*, 160, 1554–1565.

Ravindran, A. V., Griffiths, J., Merali, Z., & Anisman, H. (1995). Lymphocyte subsets associated with major depression and dysthymia: Modification by antidepressant treatment. *Psychosomatic Medicine*, 57, 555–563.

Ridker, P. M. (2001). Role of inflammatory biomarkers in prediction of coronary heart disease. [Comment On: Lancet. 2001 Sep 22;358(9286),971–6 UI: 21468341]. *Lancet*, 358(9286), 946–948.

Roose, S. P., & Schatzberg, A. F. (2005). The efficacy of antidepressants in the treatment of late-life depression. *Journal of Clinical Psychopharmacology*, 25(4 Suppl 1), S1–7.

Rothermundt, M., Arolt, V., Peters, M., Gutbrodt, H., Fenker, J., Kersting, A., & Kirchner, H. (2001). Inflammatory markers in major depression and melancholia. *Journal of Affective Disorders*, 63(1–3), 93–102.

Schleifer, S. J., Keller, S. E., & Bartlett, J. A. (1999). Depression and immunity: Clinical factors and therapeutic course. *Psychiatry Research*, 85(1), 63–69.

Schleifer, S. J., Keller, S. E., Bond, R. N., Cohen, J., & Stein, M. (1989). Major depressive disorder and immunity: Role of age, sex, severity, and hospitalization. *Archives of General Psychiatry*, 46, 81–87.

Segerstrom, S. C., & Miller, G. E. (2004). Psychological stress and the human immune system: A meta-analytic study of 30 years of inquiry. *Psychological Bulletin*, 130(4), 601–630.

Seidel, A., Arolt, V., Hunstiger, M., Rink, L., Behnisch, A., & Kirchner, H. (1995). Cytokine production and serum proteins in depression. *Scandanavian Journal of Immunology*, 41, 534–538.

Shinkawa, M., Nakayama, K., Hirai, H., Monma, M., & Sasaki, H. (2002). Depression and immunoreactivity in disabled older patients. *Journal of the American Geriatrics Society, 50,* 198–199.

Sluzewska, A., Rybakowski, J. K., Laciak, M., Mackiewicz, A., Sobieska, M., & Wiktorowicz, K. (1995). Interleukin-6 serum levels in depressed patients before and after treatment with fluoxetine. *Annals of the New York Academy of Sciences, 762,* 474–476.

Smith, T. P., Kennedy, S. L., & Fleshner, M. (2004). Influence of age and physical activity on the primary in vivo antibody and T cell-mediated responses in men. *Journal of Applied Physiology, 97,* 491–498.

Sopori, M. L., & Kozak, W. (1998). Immunomodulatory effects of cigarette smoke. *Journal of Neuroimmunology, 83,* 148–156.

Su, S., Zhao, J., Bremner, J. D., Miller, A. H., Tang, W., Bouzyk, M., ... Vaccarino, V. (2009). Serotonin transporter gene, depressive symptoms, and interleukin-6. *Circulation and Cardiovascular Genetics, 2*(6), 614–620.

Suarez, E. C., Krishnan, R. R., & Lewis, J. G. (2003). The relation of severity of depressive symptoms to monocyte-associated proinflammatory cytokines and chemokines in apparently healthy men. *Psychosomatic Medicine, 65*(3), 362–368.

Thomas, A. J., Davis, S., Morris, C., Jackson, E., Harrison, R., & O'Brien, J. T. (2005). Increase in interleukin-1beta in late-life depression. *American Journal of Psychiatry, 162*(1), 175–177.

Tucker, P., Ruwe, W. D., Masters, B., Parker, D. E., Hossain, A., Trautman, R. P., & Wyatt, D. B. (2004). Neuroimmune and cortisol changes in selective serotonin reuptake inhibitor and placebo treatment of chronic posttraumatic stress disorder. *Biological Psychiatry, 56*(2), 121–128.

Tyring, S., Gottlieb, A., Papp, K., Gordon, K., Leonardi, C., Wang, A., ... Krishnan, R. (2006). Etanercept and clinical outcomes, fatigue, and depression in psoriasis: Double-blind placebo-controlled randomised phase III trial. *Lancet, 367*(9504), 29–35.

Uher, R., & McGuffin, P. (2008). The moderation by the serotonin transporter gene of environmental adversity in the aetiology of mental illness: Review and methodological analysis. *Molecular Psychiatry, 13*(2), 131–146.

Vedhara, K., Cox, N. K., Wilcock, G. K., Perks, P., Hunt, M., Anderson, S., ... Shanks, N. M. (1999). Chronic stress in elderly carers of dementia patients and antibody response to influenza vaccination. *Lancet, 353*(9153), 627–631.

Vos, T., Haby, M. M., Barendregt, J. J., Kruijshaar, M., Corry, J., & Andrews, G. (2004). The burden of major depression avoidable by longer-term treatment strategies. *Archives of General Psychiatry, 61*(11), 1097–1103.

Weinberg, A., Zhang, J. H., Oxman, M. N., Johnson, G. R., Hayward, A. R., Caulfield, M. J., ... US Department of Veterans Affairs (VA) Cooperative Studies Program Shingles Prevention Study Investigators. (2009). Varicella-zoster virus-specific immune responses to herpes zoster in elderly participants in a trial of a clinically effective zoster vaccine. *Journal of Infectious Diseases, 200*(7), 1068–1077.

Weizman, R., Laor, N., Podliszewski, E., Notti, I., Djaldetti, M., & Bessler, H. (1994). Cytokine production in major depressed patients before and after clomipramine treatment. *Biological Psychiatry, 35,* 42–47.

Whooley, M. A., Caška, C. M., Hendrickson, B. E., Rourke, M. A., Ho, J., & Ali, S. (2007). Depression and inflammation in patients with coronary heart disease: Findings from the Heart and Soul Study. *Biological Psychiatry, 62*(4), 314–320.

Wong, M. L., Dong, C., Maestre-Mesa, J., & Licinio, J. (2008). Polymorphisms in inflammation-related genes are associated with susceptibility to major depression and antidepressant response. *Molecular Psychiatry, 13*(8), 800–812.

Yu, Y. W., Chen, T. J., Hong, C. J., Chen, H. M., & Tsai, S. J. (2003). Association study of the interleukin-1 beta (C-511T) genetic polymorphism with major depressive disorder, associated symptomatology, and antidepressant response. *Neuropsychopharmacology, 28*(6), 1182–1185.

Zautra, A. J., Yocum, D. C., Villanueva, I., Smith, B., Davis, M. C., Attrep, J., & Irwin, M. (2004). Immune activation and depression in women with rheumatoid arthritis. *Journal of Rheumatology, 31*(3), 457–463.

Zorrilla, E. P., Luborsky, L., McKay, J. R., Rosenthal, R., Houldin, A., Tax, A., ... Schmidt, K. (2001). The relationship of depression and stressors to immunological assays: A meta-analytic review. *Brain Behavior and Immunity, 15*(3), 199–226.

40

THE HPA AXIS AND LATE-LIFE DEPRESSION

Keith Sudheimer, John Flournoy, Anda Gershon, Bevin Demuth,
Alan Schatzberg, and Ruth O'Hara

AS POINTED out recently by Miller et al. (2011), dysregulation of the hypothalamic-pituitary-adrenal (HPA) axis during depression has been called one of the most reliable findings in all of biological psychiatry. HPA dysregulation may be an important mechanism underlying the pathophysiology of depression itself, and it may also partly explain associated symptoms such as cognitive dysfunction. However, there are multiple sources of HPA dysregulation that may implicate it in affective disorders, including chronic and acute environmental stressors; psychological, physiological, and genetic predispositions; and comorbid medical conditions. HPA disturbances may be a contributing factor, a correlate, or a consequence of depressive symptomatology. Furthermore, despite the bourgeoning basic and animal research investigating the relationships among HPA, stress, and depression, it is relatively unknown when and where perturbations of the HPA axis relate to the progression or etiology of depression. These issues are all the more complex when one considers depression in late life may be due to (1) age-associated changes in

HPA function; (2) the significant number of medical comorbidities experienced by older adults; and (3) increased variability with age in terms of exposure and response to environmental stressors.

Here we provide a review of the current knowledge regarding the relationship of HPA function to late-life depression. This chapter is organized into three parts. We first describe the HPA axis and the effects of aging on this system. Next, we address associations between HPA functioning, depression, and aging. Finally, we discuss potential mediators and moderators that could underlie interactions between HPA axis function, aging, and depression, including genetic markers, stress, and medical comorbidities.

DESCRIPTION OF HPA

Overview

The HPA axis is a term used to describe a series of physiological effects involving interactions among the hypothalamus, the pituitary gland, and adrenal gland

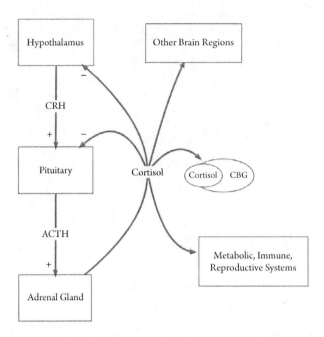

FIGURE 40.1 The relationship of the HPA system to other physiological and brain systems.

(see Fig. 40.1). The hypothalamus, located just underneath the much larger thalamus, has many subnuclei, and it functions both as a neural and as an endocrine structure. It is involved in the regulation of emotion, feeding, reproductive, and homeostatic processes. In managing these systems, the hypothalamus secretes a wide array of different hormones essential to the regulation of multiple physiological systems, including corticotropin-releasing hormone (CRH; also known as corticotropin-releasing factor [CRF]).

The pituitary gland is the most important of several sites of action of CRH signaling. CRH has two main receptors, CRHR1 and CRHR2, which are distributed in the brain and peripheral nervous system. The CRHR1 is expressed in significant concentrations in the amygdala, thalamus, and hippocampus (Hiroi et al., 2001). CRHR2 is also expressed in the brain but at lower levels than CRHR1. The pituitary gland is prompted by CRH to release a second hormone known as adrenocorticotropic hormone (ACTH, also known as corticotropin). The principal target tissue of ACTH is a cortical layer of the adrenal gland known as the zona fasciculata, which secretes glucocorticoid hormones.

The adrenal cortex is the element of the HPA axis that secretes the primary bioactive corticosteroid hormone. Cortisol, the principal corticosteroid in humans, is secreted into the general circulation

and has wide-ranging physiological effects on target tissue in the central nervous system and in the periphery. The mechanisms of cortisol signaling and feedback include at least two main intracellular cytosolic receptors, the mineralcorticoid receptor (MR) and the glucocorticoid receptor (GR). The MR has a higher affinity for cortisol than the GR. MR and GR are distributed throughout the body, including several brain regions: the hippocampus, amygdala, frontal lobe, and temporal lobe (Sarrieau et al., 1986; Watzka, Beyenburg, et al., 2000; Watzka, Bidlingmaier, et al., 2000). Endogenous glucocorticoids cross the blood–brain barrier with high efficiency (Pariante, Thomas, Lovestone, Makoff, & Kerwin, 2004) and affect neural tissue via a variety of mechanisms. These mechanisms include the cytosolic MR and GR signaling by initiating genomic processes mediated by glucocorticoid response elements as well as a variety of other less well-characterized rapid functioning membrane-bound receptors and protein interactions (Evanson, Herman, Sakai, & Krause, 2010). Cortisol is known to have effects on human memory and emotion and the underlying neural systems (Abercrombie et al., 2011; Buchanan & Lovallo, 2001; Reuter, 2002; Wirth, Scherer, Hoks, & Abercrombie, 2011), including the medial temporal lobe (O'Hara et al., 2007), amygdala (Lovallo, Robinson, Glahn, & Fox, 2010), hippocampus (Abercrombie et al., 2011), and prefrontal cortex (Henckens et al., 2011). Animal work also demonstrates that corticosterone affects the morphology and/or physiology of the hippocampus, amygdala, ventral tegmentum, and prefrontal cortex (De Kloet, Vreugdenhil, Oitzl, & Joels, 1998; Karst et al., 2002; Mitra & Sapolsky, 2008; Sapolsky, 2000; Woolley, Gould, & McEwen, 1990).

ACTH and cortisol function as potent feedback inhibitors of the HPA axis. ACTH or cortisol present in the general circulation will act to inhibit the further release of CRH. However, the feedback inhibition process involves additional target tissues as well, such as the hippocampus (Sapolsky & McEwen, 1984). The feedback regulation of the HPA is tightly regulated. Too much or too little HPA activity can have significant detrimental physiological effects as is seen in Cushing's and Addison's diseases. More subtle variability in regulation mediated by genetic and/or physiological influences on receptor efficiency or distribution may also impact cognitive and emotional systems relevant to mood disorders (McEwen, 2007).

Several tests of the efficiency of HPA feedback regulation exist. The dexamethasone (DEX) suppression test (DST) and the combined DEX/CRH suppression test are designed to test for HPA regulation problems. Dexamethasone is given in the evening to simulate the HPA-inhibiting effects of cortisol. Cortisol and ACTH activity are then measured the following morning. If HPA regulation is functioning properly, then low (suppressed) levels of ACTH and cortisol activity should be seen. However, significantly elevated ACTH and cortisol responses indicate reduced efficiency of feedback regulation.

HPA and Aging

Although a limited number of studies have directly examined changes in HPA function with age, some evidence suggests that HPA abnormalities may worsen in the elderly. One large study (N = 177) demonstrated that several parameters of the cortisol circadian rhythm change progressively with age, including the total amount of cortisol being secreted over 24 hours, the magnitude of cortisol released at both the high and low points in the cycle, and the timing of onset of the morning rise in cortisol (Van Cauter et al., 1996). Other studies show that sensitivity to dexamethasone feedback is decreased in the elderly (Hatzinger, Brand,

Herzig, & Holsboer-Trachsler, 2011; Rosenbaum et al., 1984). Studies of aging in animals also show similar patterns of decreased sensitivity to dexamethasone feedback, increasing glucocorticoid secretion over the circadian rhythm, and breakdown of the feedback inhibition mechanism the HPA axis uses to auto-regulate (Hatzinger, Reulf, Landgraf, Holsboer, & Neumann, 1996; Sapolsky & Altmann, 1991). The aspects of this feedback system that involve the hippocampus seem to be particularly susceptible to age-related breakdown (Sapolsky, 1986). Progressive alteration of hippocampal physiology, including volume loss, reduced functional activation, and connectivity in humans, is commonly observed as a function of aging (Ta et al., 2011; Tsukiura et al., 2011) and is associated with declining cognitive abilities. Dysregulation of the HPA system in older adults has been implicated in neuroimpairment in the medial temporal lobes and hippocampus (O'Hara et al., 2007). As normal degenerative changes occur in the hippocampus and medial temporal lobes with age, sensitivity to the glucocorticoid negative feedback circuit may decrease, which in turn may be responsible for a certain degree of dysregulation of the HPA axis.

HPA, DEPRESSION, AND AGING

Several different types of HPA axis abnormalities have been reported in patients with depression, including elevated secretion over the 24-hour cycle (Carroll, Curtis, Davies, Mendels, & Sugerman, 1976), adrenal gland enlargement (Rubin, Phillips, Sadow, & McCracken, 1995), altered patterns in the circadian cycle (Halbreich, Asnis, Shindledecker, Zumoff, & Nathan, 1985a, 1985b), elevated nocturnal secretion (Yehuda, Teicher, Trestman, Levengood, & Siever, 1996), a larger cortisol response to awakening, and reduced sensitivity to inhibitory feedback (Carroll, 1980). Some, but not all, studies have shown that these HPA axis abnormalities are associated with symptoms and resolve with successful treatment.

It is worth noting that not all depressed patients have HPA axis abnormalities and not all patients with HPA axis abnormalities have depression. The "endogenous" and "melancholic" depression subtypes are most closely associated with HPA axis abnormalities. Formal investigations into the sensitivity and specificity of using the DST or other HPA measures as a laboratory test for depression or other psychiatric disorders have yielded mixed results (Carroll, 1982; Heuser, Yassouridis, & Holsboer, 1994; Paslakis et al., 2011). These tests seem to perform best for detecting the endogenous and melancholic subtypes of depression (Stetler & Miller, 2011).

A recent meta-analysis of 414 independent studies of the relationships between a diverse array of HPA axis measures in depression reports that relative to non-depressed controls, depressed persons tend to exhibit increased cortisol levels (Stetler & Miller, 2011). The size of this effect was medium ($d = 0.60$; 95% confidence interval [CI], 0.54–0.66). This meta-analysis also reports that several additional factors are likely to impact the magnitude of the effect size observed in these types of studies. These factors included the time of day cortisol is sampled, the fluid it is sampled in (blood, saliva, urine, CSF), whether it is sampled as part of a challenge test (DST, DEX/CRH), age, gender, and depression subtypes. Within the same meta-analysis the authors also investigated the effect sizes for comparing depressed patients to healthy controls using ACTH and CRH. Positive overall effect sizes ($d = 0.30$) were observed for ATCH measures but not for CRH ($d = 0.02$). The authors suggest that the lack of positive effect sizes of CRH measures, as observed by Binneman et al. (2008), may reflect that both blood and cerebral spinal fluid measures suffer from the inability to distinguish hypothalamic CRH from CRH produced in a wide variety of other tissues in the brain and periphery.

Patients with depression also exhibit reduced hippocampal volume associated with elevated cortisol levels, but these findings are not entirely consistent. Some studies report hippocampal volume loss (Bremner et al., 2000; MacQueen et al., 2003; Steffens et al., 2000), while others found no correlation between decreased hippocampal volume and depression, even though elevated cortisol levels were present (Axelson et al., 1993; O'Brien, Lloyd, McKeith, Gholkar, & Ferrier, 2004; Vakili et al., 2000). Larger hippocampal volume is also associated with faster normalization of HPA hyperactivity when combined with treatment and observed a subsequent decrease in cortisol levels under pharmacotherapy (Colla et al., 2007). Most recently, Abercrombie et al. (2011) demonstrated that cortisol altered hippocampal functional response in depressed but not healthy individuals, suggesting disrupted neural signaling of cortisol in depression.

HPA and Depression in Older Adults

HPA axis dysregulation in the form of higher circadian cortisol secretion and a higher rate of dexamethasone nonsuppression have been observed in studies of aging in healthy subjects and in studies comparing depressed patients to healthy controls. Being of advanced age and having HPA axis dysregulation may independently and interactively contribute to depression. Early studies suggest that dexamethasone nonsuppression rates among depressed patients increase over the life span and are significantly elevated in patients 55 years of age and older, compared to younger patients (Davis et al., 1984). Other studies of young and old healthy controls report nonsuppression rates are marginally higher in the elderly (Rosenbaum et al., 1984). Davis et al. reported a greater than 60% incidence of dexamethasone nonsuppression in depressed patients 55 and older, which is much higher than is ever observed in groups of healthy controls. Two recent studies have directly addressed the interactions between depression, age, and nocturnal circadian secretion of cortisol. One study demonstrated higher nocturnal urinary free cortisol was associated with age, depressive symptoms, and the interaction between age and depressive symptoms (Hartaigh et al., 2011). Another recent study reports higher nocturnal salivary cortisol in older depressed participants compared to either younger or older healthy controls (Balardin, Vedana, Luz, & Bromberg, 2011). Another previous study demonstrated that dexamethasone non-suppression significantly correlates with age in healthy subjects and in subjects with depression (Keitner et al., 1992). In their meta-analysis, Stetler and Miller (2011) found age to be a significant linear predictor of cortisol effect size. When studies of only older participants were examined separately ($n = 11$ studies, ages 65 and over), the average effect size was large ($d = 0.71$, 95% CI, 0.28–1.14).

The cause-and-effect relationships between HPA dysregulation, aging, and depression are not well understood. One theory suggests age-related stressors may result in a viscous cycle of increasing cortisol. Human imaging studies have demonstrated that as cortisol levels rise across the life span, hippocampal volumes decline in parallel (Lupien et al., 1998). Animal studies have demonstrated that repeated stress or sustained exposures to corticosteroids cause decreases in glucocorticoid receptor in the hippocampus and amygdala (Sapolsky,

Krey, & McEwen, 1984) and reshape the structure and physiology of neurons in these regions (Karst et al., 2002; Mitra & Sapolsky, 2008; Woolley et al., 1990). The loss of glucocorticoid sensitivity in the hippocampus can also result in excessive cortisol secretion by interfering with the ability of these neurons to terminate HPA axis activity (Sapolsky, Krey, & McEwen, 1986), forming a feed-forward loop of increasing cortisol effects on the brain. While this theory may explain components of age-related changes in hippocampus and HPA dysregulation, it is incomplete. In addition, not all depressed subjects show signs of HPA dysregulation. A few studies have even demonstrated that subjects exhibiting among the lowest levels of cortisol secretion can present with significant depressive symptoms (Bremmer et al., 2007; Penninx et al., 2007). In an investigation of a large community-dwelling sample of older adults who have recovered from depression, Beluche et al. (2009) found an abnormal HPA response persisted even after recovery from depression, suggesting that cortisol abnormalities may be trait markers for vulnerability to depression.

Pharmacotherapy, Depression, and HPA in Older Adults

It is possible that the therapeutic effects of drug treatments for depression and anxiety are partly due to effects of these drugs on the HPA axis. Additionally, markers of HPA axis regulation markers may useful for predicting response and tailoring treatment.

Antidepressant drugs may work in part by restoring dysfunctional HPA reactivity to normal patterns (Nikisch, 2009). Tricyclic antidepressants (TCAs) such as amitriptyline and desipramine appear to increase GR expression, while selective serotonin reuptake inhibitors (SSRIs) appear to have minimal effect on GR expression and likely alter HPA axis outcomes through MR (Budziszewska, 2002; Pariante, Pearce, Pisell, Su, & Miller, 2001; Pariante et al., 2004). Evidence from studies of TCAs indicates that this class of drugs reduces basal cortisol levels, though whether this correlates with treatment response is as yet unclear. Data on the tetracyclic antidepressant mirtazapine (structurally related to tricyclic antidepressants) indicate that it also reduces cortisol saliva concentrations, but there was no difference between remitters and nonremitters, which indicates that this effect may not related to antidepressant qualities (Horstmann et al., 2009; Scharnholz et al., 2010).

In older adults TCA treatment also reduces cortisol levels, though in contrast to younger populations, treatment response is predicted by absolute cortisol levels. Heuser et al. (1996) found that amitriptyline reduced basal cortisol levels over a 6-week treatment period. Responders differed from nonresponders by total cortisol, though both groups reduced these levels by the same relative amount (responders, –43%; nonresponders, –44%). This is markedly different from research in a younger population in which nonresponders saw no reduction in cortisol (Deuschle et al., 2003). In addition, the older population also saw reductions in an initially elevated response to the DEX/CRH test in basal plasma measures of both ACTH and cortisol. Consistent with findings from younger adults, this evidence is suggestive of TCA reduction of cortisol, though the relationship of age to treatment response merits further elaboration.

Chronic SSRI treatment effects on HPA axis function have been more difficult to specify. Basal cortisol in response to chronic SSRI treatment has been found to be increased (Manthey et al., 2011), decreased (Vythilingam et al., 2004), and unchanged (Deuschle et al., 2003; Scharnholz et al., 2010). Another study suggests that SSRIs may reduce the response magnitude of ACTH and cortisol responses to the DEX/CRH test, and it shows that these reductions are a significant predictor of symptom improvement (Nikisch et al., 2005).

Age-dependent effects of antidepressant drugs on HPA axis function in the animal literature indicate a role for pharmacotherapy in the maintenance of cognition throughout the life span. In a comparison of cognitively impaired aged rats, unimpaired aged rats, and young rats, desipramine, a TCA, brought the elevated levels of blood plasma corticosterone and ACTH in the impaired aged group in line with the levels in unimpaired aged rats and young rats (Rowe et al., 1997). Additionally, cognitive impairment as measured by spatial learning tasks is preserved in aging rats if antidepressant treatment is started in midlife (i.e., at 16 months) and may be in part due to reductions in corticosterone levels (Yau et al., 2002). However, cognition did not improve when treatment was started in late life (Yau, Olsson, Morris, Meaney, & Seckl, 1995). Promisingly, human participants with a diagnosis of depression show cognitive improvement after successful treatment with SSRIs for a mean duration of 7 months (Vythilingam et al., 2004), though neuroprotective effects related to cortisol reductions effected by antidepressants over longer periods of time remain to be evaluated.

Depression, HPA, and Cognitive Function in Older Adults

Cognitive deficits are a key feature of late-life depression. Between 20% and 50% of patients with late-life depression are estimated to have cognitive impairment greater than that observed in age and education-matched controls (Butters et al., 2004; O'Hara et al., 2006). Cognitive deficits associated with late-life depression have significant clinical consequences and have been associated with increased rates of relapse, disability and poorer response to antidepressant treatment (Alexopoulos et al., 2000, 2003; Mehta et al., 2003). The most consistently documented impairments in late-life depression exist in executive functioning, memory, visuospatial ability, and psychomotor speed (O'Hara et al., 2006). Many have proposed interactive and reciprocal effects of glucocorticoid function, brain aging, and cognition in late-life depression (Byers et al., 2011).

In one of the few investigations to examine this issue longitudinally, Hinkelmann et al. (2012) investigated the impact on cortisol and cognition in 52 patients with major depressive disorder before and after 3 weeks of standardized SSRIs and an add-on treatment modulating the mineralocorticoid receptor. SSRI treatment reduced salivary cortisol in patients, and reduction of cortisol significantly correlated with improvement in depressive symptoms, speed of information processing, and cognitive set shifting.

However, although the number of studies investigating this issue is limited, not all studies have observed interactive effects of cortisol and depression on cognitive functioning in late-life depression. Köhler et al. (2010) found that white matter hyperintensities rather than cortisol levels or brain atrophy were associated with continuing cognitive impairments in older adults with depression. Similarly, in an investigation of whether cognitive impairments and structural brain changes in older depressed subjects are related to hypercortisolemia, O'Brien et al. found that hippocampal volume reduction was not associated with increased cortisol levels but was significantly correlated with continuing memory deficits at a 6-month follow-up in over 60 patients with late-life depression (O'Brien, Lloyd, McKeith, Gholkar, & Ferrier,

2004). Mild cognitive impairment at a 6-month follow-up was associated with reduced hippocampal volume but not severity of depression, cortisol levels, or APOE genotype. In our own investigation of 156 older, community-dwelling adults without depression (O'Hara et al., 2007), we found the serotonin polymorphism transporter short allele was associated with significantly higher levels of waking cortisol, poorer memory function, and reduced hippocampal volume. Interactive effects of the serotonin polymorphism transporter, cortisol, and cognition in late-life depression remains to be examined, but this line of work suggests that genetic moderators of these relationships may be of significance in examining stress and cortisol-related affective and cognitive profiles of late-life depression patients.

MEDIATORS AND MODERATORS OF THE RELATIONSHIP OF HPA FUNCTION AND LATE-LIFE DEPRESSION

Over the years there has been increasing interest in identifying potential mediating mechanisms underlying the relationship between HPA dysregulation and late-life depression. Stressful experiences have been proposed as one such key mechanism. Furthermore, moderating variables such as genetic markers, and the medical comorbidities so strongly associated with aging, have been proposed as yet additional sources of the mixed findings in our understanding of the role of HPA in depression in the elderly.

Stress

Severely stressful life events and chronic stress play an important role in precipitating depressive onset throughout the life course. However, physical health–related issues are of particular concern in older populations.

Chronic and acute life stressors have a significant role in the etiology and course of mood disorders (Hammen, Henry, & Daley, 2000) and may be particularly important in late life (Brilman & Ormel, 2001). A meta-analysis of 25 studies examining life stress and depression in people aged 65 and older found that almost all of the categories of stressful events that were measured, including events involving difficulties with health, finances, close others, as well as exposure to abuse or neglect, showed modest but significant relationships with levels of depression (Kraaij, Arensman, & Spinhoven, 2002). In one of the few studies to prospectively examine life stress in relation to depression onset in older adults (55 years or older), the role of life stress in late-life depression was found to be as large as indicated in younger age groups (Brilman & Ormel, 2001). Echoing findings with younger samples, severe life events showed the largest relative risk (22-fold) for association with late-life affective disorders, whereas chronic stress accounted for most depressive episodes.

Acute and chronic physiological and psychological stress activates the HPA axis on top of the circadian rhythm activity. A psychological or physiological stress-induced mobilization of the HPA axis causes the release of CRH, ACTH, and cortisol. As discussed previously, CRH and cortisol have significant effects on brain structure and function related to aging and mood disorders. Thus, stress-related dysregulation of HPA has been proposed as a key mechanism underlying depression in older adults. The majority of life events and chronic stressors in older subjects linked to developing depression are categorized as health related (Wolkowitz, Reus, & Mellon, 2011).

Medical Comorbidities

The HPA axis reactions to stressful life events and interactions with depression pathophysiology can result in substantial comorbidities, including cognitive decline, insomnia, metabolic syndrome, and adverse cardiovascular conditions (Brown, Varghese, & McEwen, 2004). Substantial evidence suggests that the HPA axis abnormalities are present in a number of age-related medical disorders (Wirtz et al., 2007). Abnormally elevated cortisol levels due to persistent stress of the HPA axis constitute a significant risk for serious and age-related medical illnesses (Knoops, van der Graaf, Mali, & Geerlings, 2010). Those living with a chronic disease are two times more likely to report depression (Beekman et al., 1997).

HPA axis hyperactivity in individuals with depression can increase the risk for physiological disease and premature mortality (Evans et al., 2005; Frasure-Smith & Lesperance, 2005). In 2009, Jokinen and Nordström reported elevated cortisol was associated with increased risk of death in individuals with depression and cardiovascular disease.

Stetler and Miller (2011) found individuals who reported specific symptoms such as hypersomnia, hyperphagia, fatigue, and emotional reactivity were less vulnerable to experience hypercortisolemia, and those who reported decreased appetite, insomnia, anhedonia, diurnal mood variability, hallucinations, or delusions were at increased risk for diseases associated with HPA axis hyperactivity (e.g., type 2 diabetes). Here we focus on three of the primary medical disorders proposed as mediators of the relationship of HPA dysregulation to depression in older adults.

METABOLIC SYNDROME

There is mounting evidence individuals with abnormal HPA axis regulation and depression often display elements of metabolic syndrome. Metabolic syndrome is a group of medical disorders that include three or more of the following criteria: central obesity, hypertriglyeridemia, low HDL cholesterol, high blood pressure, and high fasting plasma glucose. Metabolic syndrome increases the risk of cardiovascular disease, stroke, and diabetes. The prevalence of metabolic syndrome increases with age (Hildrum, Mykletun, Hole, Midthjell, & Dahl, 2007) and affects 44% of people over the age of 60 in the United States (Ganne, Arora, Karam, & McFarlane, 2007). HPA axis hyperactivity has been shown to mediate the relationship between central obesity and in metabolic syndrome by influencing cortisol metabolism in adipose tissue (Bose, Oliván, & Laferrère, 2009). Age-related changes in HPA axis function are thought to induce the onset of metabolic syndrome. HPA axis hyperactivity, increased cortisol levels, and depression have been described in several studies and strongly predict metabolic syndrome (McCaffery, Niaura, Todaro, Swan, & Carmelli, 2003; Raikkonen, Matthews, & Kuller, 2002; Vogelzangs & Penninx, 2007).

CARDIOVASCULAR DISEASES

Long-term HPA dysregulation is also suggested as a mediating factor between depression and cardiovascular mortality. Increased cortisol and glucocorticoids levels sustained over time are potential mediators of cardiovascular disease risk factors, including visceral obesity, hypercholesterolemia, hypertriglyceridemia, hypertension, increased heart rate, insulin resistance, and type 2 diabetes (Everson-Rose & Lewis, 2005; Rosmond

& Bjorntorp, 2000). Dysregulation of the HPA is suggested to be a biomarker for meditating depression and cardiovascular disease vulnerability, and depression is indicated as a robust predictor for cardiovascular disease (Barth, Schumacher, & Herrmann-Lingen, 2004; Jokinen & Nordström, 2009). It has been proposed that abnormalities in coagulation and endothelial cell function as a result of HPA axis dysregulation foster the development of artherogenesis in the depressed population (Nemeroff & Musselman, 2000; O'Connor, Gurbel, & Serebruany, 2000). Older men displayed a greater HPA response and cortisol secretion when presented with psychological stress prompting an elevated risk for cardiovascular disease (Traustadottir, Bosch, & Matt, 2003).

SLEEP DISORDERS

The sleep/wake cycle is fundamental for the physiologic process and restorative functions essential for survival. When sleep is continually disrupted, the immune system and metabolism are impacted (Lange, Dimitrov, & Born, 2010), cognitive functions are impaired (Vance, Heaton, Eaves, & Fazeli, 2011), the HPA axis is activated (Spath-Schwalbe, Gofferje, Kern, Born, & Fehm, 1991), and there is an increased risk for the onset of psychiatric disorders, most commonly depression (Maglione et al., 2012). Sleep disturbances affect the HPA axis, and the HPA axis in turn affects sleep patterns. In studies that manipulate sleep quality by introducing sleep disruptions, increases in HPA activity are observed (Spath-Schwalbe et al., 1991). Since sleep problems, disorders, and disruption are a hallmark of late life, continuously disrupted sleep in the elderly may represent a significant form of physical and psychological "stress" (Beaudreau & O'Hara, 2009) that exacerbates HPA axis hyperactivity, creating a "vicious cycle" (Buckley & Schatzberg, 2005). Abnormal functioning of the HPA axis and elevated cortisol levels may induce depression and result in sleep-related problems such as insomnia and other sleep disturbances (Antonijevic, 2008; Steiger & Kimura, 2010), including disrupted sleep, decreased sleep time, short REMS latency, and sleep efficacy (Vgontzas et al., 2001). Since there are many effective treatments for all aspects of sleep disorders, future treatment trials should examine the impact of sleep improvements on the HPA axis and subsequent effects on depression in late life.

Genetic Polymorphisms

Genetic factors may play a role in accounting for some of the individual variation in susceptibility to stress (McEwen, 1998) via individual differences in activation and regulation of the response. An increasing number of studies suggest that genetic differences in Apolipoprotein E (APOE), the serotonin transporter polymorphism, and genes that regulate the corticosteroid receptors may influence the relationships between HPA axis abnormalities, stress, and depression.

Several studies have suggested there may be interplay between the APOE genotype and HPA activity (Gordon et al., 1996). However, findings of APOE, stress, and HPA function have been inconsistent, with Beluche et al. (2010) observing a negative impact of elevated cortisol on cognitive function and decline in nondepressed older adults, independent of APOE status. Similarly, O'Brien et al. (2004) found no association between APOE genotype and HPA function in older, depressed patients.

The serotonergic system in general is implicated in hippocampal regulation of HPA axis activity (Lowry, 2002) and regulation of hippocampal glucocorticoid receptors. Genetic variations in the serotonin promoter polymorphism region (5HTTLPR) have been associated with changes in depressive symptomatology and anxiety (Lenze et al., 2011). The S allele is associated with lower levels of serotonin uptake and transcriptional efficiency of the serotonin transporter. Several studies support the hypothesis of an interaction between stressful life events, 5-HTT genotype, and psychiatric outcomes such as depression and anxiety. Recent evidence suggests the 5HTT short allele may increase vulnerability to stress, with subsequent depression onset (Caspi et al., 2003). Individuals homozygous for the S allele have been shown to be more sensitive to the depressogenic effects of stressful life events compared to carriers of an L allele (Kendler, Kuhn, Vittum, Prescott, & Riley, 2005). The presence of the S allele may also moderate the relationship between HPA dysregulation and depression (Gotlib, Joormann, Minor, & Hallmayer, 2008). In older adults, we found the S allele to be associated with higher waking cortisol and to interact with higher cortisol, resulting in poorer memory and lower hippocampal volume (O'Hara et al., 2007). The 5HTT S allele may thus impact the normal aging process by increasing vulnerability to neuropsychiatric outcomes. Some studies also suggest that the effects of chronic illness-related stress may result in neurodegeneration, and that this neurodegeneration is mediated by glucocorticoid modulation via the serotonin system (Smith et al., 2004).

Glucocorticoid receptor polymorphisms such as Bcl1 (Fleury et al., 2003) have been shown to play a role in the HPA axis response and risk for depression. The G allele has been associated with lower baseline cortisol levels, diminished cortisol responses (van Rossum et al., 2003), and diminished ACTH responses (Wüst et al., 2004). Individuals homozygous for the G allele may also be at greater risk for developing depression (van Rossum et al., 2003). Variations in the FKBP5 gene region have also been observed to affect glucocorticoid sensitivity to stress (Ising et al., 2008). In one study variation, FKBP5, which codes for a glucocorticoid receptor–regulating protein, has been shown to predict antidepressant treatment responses (Binder et al., 2004). However, this result was not reproduced in a recent study (Sarginson, Lazzeroni, Ryan, Schatzberg, & Murphy, 2010). Inconsistency in these results may be due to differing age cohorts or to differences in symptom severity, but they represent an important avenue for future inquiry since prevalence of genetic variants that impact glucocorticoid response may account for the mixed findings regarding the relationship of HPA function and depression in elderly adults.

CONCLUSIONS

Hyperactivity of the HPA axis is one of many changes that occur in response to the psychological experience, and physiological milieu, of individuals in late life. As such, the cumulative evidence suggests that HPA dysfunction is a key pathophysiological system implicated in late-life depression. The HPA axis dysregulation that develops later in life may not only impact mood, but it may also contribute to the decreased cognitive abilities, disrupted sleep, increased risk of cardiovascular disease, and metabolic syndrome so often evident in patients with late-life depression. However, inferences regarding the reciprocal nature and directionality of the relationship among HPA, mood, cognition, sleep, and comorbid medial disorders in late-life depression are limited by a dearth of studies addressing the temporal development of symptomatology. Few studies have addressed whether HPA axis abnormalities are a source or a consequence of depression in late life.

Similarly it is largely unknown whether HPA dysregulation contributes significantly to the development of a variety of medical comorbidities that occur with depression or if HPA axis dysregulation is simply a biomarker of those comorbidities. Utilization of bioinformatic technologies and efficient longitudinal designs such as the accelerated longitudinal design (Thompson, Hallmayer, O'Hara, & Alzheimer's Disease Neuroimaging Initiative, 2011) should be considered to begin to unravel the direction of causality and thus inform treatment and intervention approaches.

Disclosures

Dr. Schatzberg discloses the following financial/intellectual and consulting relationships: Amlyn, Amnestix, Bay City Capital, BrainCells, CeNeRx, Cervel, Corcept, Delpor, Eli Lillt, Forest, Merck, Neurocrine, Neuronetics, NovaDel, Pfizer, PharmaNeuroBoost, Velocity Pharmaceutical Development, Xhale. None of the other coauthor report any disclosures.

REFERENCES

Abercrombie, H. C., Jahn, A. L., Davidson, R. J., Kern, S., Kirschbaum, C., & Halverson, J. (2011). Cortisol's effects on hippocampal activation in depressed patients are related to alterations in memory formation. *Journal of Psychiatric Research*, 45(1), 15–23.

Alexopoulos, G. S. (2003). Role of executive function in late-life depression. *Journal of Clinical Psychiatry*, 64(14), 18–23.

Alexopoulos, G. S., Meyers, B. S., Young, R. C., Kalayam, B., Kakuma, T., Gabrielle, M.,…Hull, J. (2000). Executive dysfunction and long-term outcomes of geriatric depression. *Archives of General Psychiatry*, 57, 285–90.

Antonijevic, I. (2008). HPA axis and sleep: Identifying subtypes of major depression. *Stress*, 11(1), 15–27.

Axelson, D. A., Doraiswamy, P. M., McDonald, W. M., Boyko, O. B., Tupler, L. A., Patterson, L. J., Krishnan, K. R. (1993). Hypercortisolemia and hippocampal changes in depression. *Psychiatry Research*, 47(2), 163–173.

Balardin, J. B., Vedana, G., Luz, C., & Bromberg, E. (2011). Subjective mild depressive symptoms are associated with abnormal diurnal cycle of salivary cortisol in older adults. *Journal of Geriatric Psychiatry and Neurology*, 24(1), 19–22.

Barth, J., Schumacher, M., & Herrmann-Lingen, C. (2004). Depression as a risk factor for mortality in patients with coronary heart disease: A meta-analysis. *Psychosomatic Medicine, 66*(6), 802–813.

Beaudreau, S. A., & O'Hara, R. (2009). The association of anxiety and depressive symptoms with cognitive performance in community-dwelling older adults. *Psychology and Aging, 24*(2), 507–512.

Beekman, A. T., Penninx, B. W., Deeg, D. J., Ormel, J., Braam, A. W., & van Tilburg, W. (1997). Depression and physical health in later life: Results from the Longitudinal Aging Study Amsterdam (LASA). *Journal of Affective Disorders, 46*(3), 219–231.

Beluche, I., Carrière, I., Ritchie, K., & Ancelin, M. L. (2010) A prospective study of diurnal cortisol and cognitive function in community-dwelling elderly people. *Psychological Medicine, 40*(6), 1039–1049.

Beluche, I., Chaudieu, I., Norton, J., Carrière, I., Boulenger, J. P., Ritchie, K., & Ancelin, M. L. (2009) Persistence of abnormal cortisol levels in elderly persons after recovery from major depression. *Journal of Psychiatric Research, 43*(8), 777–783.

Binder, E. B., Salyakina, D., Lichtner, P., Wochnik, G. M., Ising, M., Putz, B., ... Muller-Myhsok, B. (2004). Polymorphisms in FKBP5 are associated with increased recurrence of depressive episodes and rapid response to antidepressant treatment. *Nature Genetics, 36*(12), 1319–1325.

Binneman, B., Feltner, D., Kolluri, S., Shi, Y., Qiu, R., & Stiger, T. (2008) A 6-week randomized, placebo-controlled trial of CP-316,311 (a selective CRH1 antagonist) in the treatment of major depression. *American Journal of Psychiatry,165*(5), 617–20.

Bose, M., Oliván, B., & Laferrère, B. (2009). Stress and obesity: The role of the hypothalamic-pituitary-adrenal axis in metabolic disease. *Current Opinion in Endocrinology, Diabetes, and Obesity, 16*(5), 340–346.

Bremmer, M. A., Deeg, D. J. H., Beekman, A. T. F., Penninx, B. W. J. H., Lips, P., & Hoogendijk, W. J. G. (2007). Major depression in late life is associated with both hypo- and hypercortisolemia. *Biological Psychiatry, 62*(5), 479–486.

Bremner, J. D., Narayan, M., Anderson, E. R., Staib, L. H., Miller, H. L., & Charney, D. S. (2000). Hippocampal volume reduction in major depression. *American Journal of Psychiatry, 157*(1), 115–118.

Brilman, E. I., & Ormel, J. (2001). Life events, difficulties and onset of depressive episodes in later life. *Psychological Medicine, 31*(5), 859–869.

Brown, E. S., Varghese, F. P., & McEwen, B. S. (2004). Association of depression with medical illness:

Does cortisol play a role? *Biological Psychiatry, 55*(1), 1–9.

Buchanan, T. W., & Lovallo, W. R. (2001). Enhanced memory for emotional material following stress-level cortisol treatment in humans. *Psychoneuroendocrinology, Psychoneuroendocrinology, 26*(3), 307–317.

Buckley, T. M., & Schatzberg, A. F. (2005). On the interactions of the hypothalamic-pituitary-adrenal (HPA) axis and sleep: Normal HPA axis activity and circadian rhythm, exemplary sleep disorders. *Journal of Clinical Endocrinology and Metabolism, 90*(5), 3106–3114.

Budziszewska, B. (2002). Effect of antidepressant drugs on the hypothalamic-pituitary-adrenal axis activity and glucocorticoid receptor function. *Polish Journal of Pharmacology, 54*(4), 343–349.

Butters, M. A., Bhalla, R. K., Mulsant, B. H., Mazumdar, S., Houck, P. R., Begley, A. E., Reynolds, C. F., III. (2004). Executive functioning, illness course, and relapse/recurrence in continuation and maintenance treatment of late-life depression: Is there a relationship? *American Journal of Geriatric Psychiatry, 12*(4), 387–394.

Byers, A. L., & Yaffe, K. (2011). Depression and risk of developing dementia. *Nature Reviews Neurology, 7*(6), 323–331.

Carroll, B. J. (1980). Dexamethasone suppression test in depression. *Lancet, 2*(8206), 1249.

Carroll, B. J. (1982). Use of the dexamethasone suppression test in depression. *Journal of Clinical Psychiatry, 43*(11 Pt 2), 44–50.

Carroll, B. J., Curtis, G. C., Davies, B. M., Mendels, J., & Sugerman, A. A. (1976). Urinary free cortisol excretion in depression. *Psychological Medicine, 6*(1), 43–50.

Caspi, A., Sugden, K., Moffitt, T. E., Taylor, A., Craig, I. W., Harrington, H., Poulton, R. (2003) Influence of life stress on depression: Moderation by a polymorphism in the 5-HTT gene. *Science, 301*(5631), 386–389.

Colla, M., Kronenberg, G., Deuschle, M., Meichel, K., Hagen, T., Bohrer, M., & Heuser, I. (2007). Hippocampal volume reduction and HPA-system activity in major depression. *Journal of Psychiatric Research, 41*(7), 553–560.

Davis, K. L., Davis, B. M., Mathé, A. A., Mohs, R. C., Rothpearl, A. B., Levy, M. I., Gorman, L. K., et al. (1984). Age and the dexamethasone suppression test in depression. *American Journal of Psychiatry, 141*(7), 872–874.

De Kloet, E. R., Vreugdenhil, E., Oitzl, M. S., & Joels, M. (1998). Brain corticosteroid receptor balance in health and disease. *Endocrine Reviews, 19*(3), 269–301.

Deuschle, M., Hamann, B., Meichel, C., Krumm, B., Lederbogen, F., Kniest, A., … Heuser, I. (2003). Antidepressive treatment with amitriptyline and paroxetine: Effects on saliva cortisol concentrations. *Journal of Clinical Psychopharmacology, 23*(2), 201–205.

Evans, D. L., Charney, D. S., Lewis, L., Golden, R. N., Gorman, J. M., Krishnan, K. R., … Valvo, W. J. (2005). Mood disorders in the medically ill: Scientific review and recommendations. *Biological Psychiatry, 58*(3), 175–189.

Evanson, N. K., Herman, J. P., Sakai, R. R., & Krause, E. G. (2010). Nongenomic actions of adrenal steroids in the central nervous system. *Journal of Neuroendocrinology, 22*(8), 846–861.

Everson-Rose, S. A., & Lewis, T. T. (2005). Psychosocial factors and cardiovascular diseases. *Annual Review of Public Health, 26*, 469–500.

Fleury, I., Beaulieu, P., Primeau, M., Labuda, D., Sinnett, D., & Krajinovic, M. (2003). Characterization of the BclI polymorphism in the glucocorticoid receptor gene. *Clinical Chemistry, 49*(9), 1528–1531.

Frasure-Smith, N., & Lesperance, F. (2005). Reflections on depression as a cardiac risk factor. *Psychosomatic Medicine, 67*(Suppl 1), 19–25.

Ganne, S., Arora, S., Karam, J., & McFarlane, S. I. (2007). Therapeutic interventions for hypertension in metabolic syndrome: A comprehensive approach. *Expert Reviews in Cardiovascular Therapy, 5*(2), 201–211.

Gordon, I., Ben-Eliyahu, S., Rosenne, E., Sehayek, E., & Michaelson, D. M. (1996). Derangement in stress response of apolipoprotein E-deficient mice. *Neuroscience Letters, 206*(2–3), 212–214

Gotlib, I. H., Joormann, J., Minor, K. L., & Hallmayer, J. (2008). HPA axis reactivity: A mechanism underlying the associations among 5-HTTLPR, stress, and depression. *Biological Psychiatry, 63*(9), 847–851.

Halbreich, U., Asnis, G. M., Shindledecker, R., Zumoff, B., & Nathan, R. S. (1985a). Cortisol secretion in endogenous depression: II. Time-related functions. *Archives of General Psychiatry, 42*(9), 909.

Halbreich, U., Asnis, G. M., Shindledecker, R., Zumoff, B., & Nathan, R. S. (1985b). Cortisol secretion in endogenous depression: I. Basal plasma levels. *Archives of General Psychiatry, 42*(9), 904–908.

Hammen, C., Henry, R., & Daley, S. E. (2000). Depression and sensitization to stressors among young women as a function of childhood adversity.

Journal of Consulting and Clinical Psychology, 68(5), 782–787.

Hartaigh, B. Ó., Loerbroks, A., Thomas, G. N., Engeland, C. G., Hollands, M. A., Fischer, J. E., & Bosch, J. A. (2011). Age-dependent and -independent associations between depression, anxiety, DHEAS, and cortisol: From the MIPH Industrial Cohort Studies (MICS). *Psychoneuroenpdocrinology, 37*(7), 929–936.

Hatzinger, M., Brand, S., Herzig, N., & Holsboer-Trachsler, E. (2011). In healthy young and elderly adults, hypothalamic-pituitary-adrenocortical axis reactivity (HPA AR) varies with increasing pharmacological challenge and with age, but not with gender. *Journal of Psychiatric Research, 45*(10), 1373–1380.

Hatzinger, M., Reul, J. M. H. M., Landgraf, R., Holsboer, F., & Neumann, I. (1996). Combined dexamethasone/CRH test in rats: Hypothalamo-pituitary-adrenocortical system alterations in aging. *Neuroendocrinology, 64*(5), 349–356.

Henckens, M. J. A. G., Pu, Z., Hermans, E. J., van Wingen, G. A., Joels, M., & Fernandez, G. (2011). Dynamically changing effects of corticosteroids on human hippocampal and prefrontal processing. *Human Brain Mapping*, Sep 21. [Epub ahead of print].

Heuser, I. J., Schweiger, U., Gotthardt, U., Schmider, J., Lammers, C. H., Dettling, M., Holsboer, F. (1996). Pituitary-adrenal-system regulation and psychopathology during amitriptyline treatment in elderly depressed patients and normal comparison subjects. *American Journal of Psychiatry, 153*(1), 93–99.

Heuser, I., Yassouridis, A., & Holsboer, F. (1994). The combined dexamethasone/CRH test: A refined laboratory test for psychiatric disorders. *Journal of Psychiatric Research, 28*(4), 341–356.

Hildrum, B., Mykletun, A., Hole, T., Midthjell, K., & Dahl, A. A. (2007). Age-specific prevalence of the metabolic syndrome defined by the International Diabetes Federation and the National Cholesterol Education Program: The Norwegian HUNT 2 study. *BMC Public Health, 7*, 220–220.

Hinkelmann, K., Moritz, S., Botzenhardt, J., Muhtz, C., Wiedemann, K., Kellner, M., & Otte, B. (2012). Changes in cortisol secretion during antidepressive treatment and cognitive improvement in patients with major depression: A longitudinal study. *Psychoneuroendocrinology, 37*(5), 685–692.

Hiroi, N., Wong, M. L., Licinio, J., Park, C., Young, M., Gold, P. W., … Bornstein, S. R. (2001). Expression of corticotropin releasing hormone receptors type I and type II mRNA in suicide victims and controls. *Molecular Psychiatry, 6*(5), 540–546.

Horstmann, S., Dose, T., Lucae, S., Kloiber, S., Menke, A., Hennings, J., ... Ising, M. (2009). Suppressive effect of mirtazapine on the HPA system in acutely depressed women seems to be transient and not related to antidepressant action. *Psychoneuroendocrinology, 34*(2), 238–248.

Ising, M., Depping, A. M., Siebertz, A., Lucae, S., Unschuld, P. G., Kloiber, S., ... Holsboer, F. (2008). Polymorphisms in the FKBP5 gene region modulate recovery from psychosocial stress in healthy controls. *European Journal of Neuroscience, 28*(2), 389–398.

Jokinen, J., & Nordström, P. (2009). HPA axis hyperactivity and attempted suicide in young adult mood disorder inpatients. *Journal of Affective Disorders, 116*(1–2), 117–120.

Karst, H., Nair, S., Velzing, E., Rumpff-van Essen, L., Slagter, E., Shinnick-Gallagher, P., & Joels, M. (2002). Glucocorticoids alter calcium conductances and calcium channel subunit expression in basolateral amygdala neurons. *European Journal of Neuroscience, 16*(6), 1083–1089.

Keitner, G. I., Ryan, C. E., Kohn, R., Miller, I. W., Norman, W. H., & Brown, W. A. (1992). Age and the dexamethasone suppression test: Results from a broad unselected patient population. *Psychiatry Research, 44*(1), 9–20.

Kendler, K. S., Kuhn, J. W., Vittum, J., Prescott, C. A., & Riley, B. (2005). The interaction of stressful life events and a serotonin transporter polymorphism in the prediction of episodes of major depression: a replication. *Archives of General Psychiatry, 62*(5), 529–535.

Köhler, S., Thomas, A. J., Lloyd, A., Barber, R., Almeida, O. P., & O'Brien, J. T. (2010). White matter hyperintensities, cortisol levels, brain atrophy and continuing cognitive deficits in late-life depression. *The British journal of psychiatry : the journal of mental science, 196*(2), 143–149.

Knoops, A. J. G., van der Graaf, Y., Mali, W. P. T. M., & Geerlings, M. I. (2010). Age-related changes in hypothalamic-pituitary-adrenal axis activity in patients with manifest arterial disease. *Endocrine, 37*(1), 231–238.

Kraaij, V., Arensman, E., & Spinhoven, P. (2002). Negative life events and depression in elderly persons: A meta-analysis. *Journal of Gerontology Series B, Psychological sciences Social sciences, 57*(1), P87–P94.

Lange, T., Dimitrov, S., & Born, J. (2010). Effects of sleep and circadian rhythm on the human immune system. *Annals of the New York Academy of Sciences, 1193*, 48–59.

Lenze, E. J., Mantella, R. C., Shi, P., Goate, A. M., Nowotny, P., Butters, M. A., ... Rollman, B. L. (2011). Elevated cortisol in older adults with generalized anxiety disorder is reduced by treatment: A placebo-controlled evaluation of escitalopram. *American Journal of Geriatric Psychiatry, 19*(5), 482–490.

Lovallo, W. R., Robinson, J. L., Glahn, D. C., & Fox, P. T. (2010). Acute effects of hydrocortisone on the human brain: An fMRI study. *Psychoneuroendocrinology, 35*(1), 15–20.

Lowry, C. A. (2002). Functional subsets of serotonergic neurones: Implications for control of the hypothalamic-pituitary-adrenal axis. *Journal of Neuroendocrinology, 14*(11), 911–923.

Lupien, S. J., de Leon, M., de Santi, S., Convit, A., Tarshish, C., Nair, N. P., ... Meaney, M. J. (1998). Cortisol levels during human aging predict hippocampal atrophy and memory deficits. *Nature Neuroscience, 1*(1), 69–73.

MacQueen, G. M., Campbell, S., McEwen, B. S., Macdonald, K., Amano, S., Joffe, R. T., ... Young, L. T. (2003). Course of illness, hippocampal function, and hippocampal volume in major depression. *Proceedings of the National Academy of Sciences USA, 100*(3), 1387.

Maglione, J. E., Ancoli-Israel, S., Peters, K. W., Paudel, M. L., Yaffe, K., Ensrud, K. E., & Stone, K. L. (2012) Depressive symptoms and subjective and objective sleep in community-dwelling older women. *Journal of the American Geriatrics Society, 60*(4), 635–643.

Manthey, L., Leeds, C., Giltay, E. J., van Veen, T., Vreeburg, S. A., Penninx, B. W. J. H., & Zitman, F. G. (2011). Antidepressant use and salivary cortisol in depressive and anxiety disorders. *Eur Neuropsychopharmacol, 21*(9), 691–699.

Mehta, K. M., Yaffe, K., Langa, K. M., Sands, L., Whooley, M. A., & Covinsky, K. E. (2003). Additive effects of cognitive function and depressive symptoms on mortality in elderly community-living adults. *Journal of Gerontology, 58A*, 461–467.

McCaffery, J. M., Niaura, R., Todaro, J. F., Swan, G. E., & Carmelli, D. (2003). Depressive symptoms and metabolic risk in adult male twins enrolled in the National Heart, Lung, and Blood Institute twin study. *Psychosomatic Medicine, 65*(3), 490–497.

McEwen, B. (1998). Stress, adaptation, and disease: Allostasis and allostatic load. *Annals of the New York Academy of Sciences, 840*, 33–44.

McEwen, B. (2007). Physiology and neurobiology of stress and adaptation: Central role of the brain. *Physiological Reviews, 87*(3), 873–904.

Mitra, R., & Sapolsky, R. M. (2008). Acute corticosterone treatment is sufficient to induce anxiety and amygdaloid dendritic hypertrophy. *Proceedings of the National Academy of Sciences USA, 105*(14), 5573–5578.

Nemeroff, C. B., & Musselman, D. L. (2000). Are platelets the link between depression and ischemic heart disease? *American Heart Journal, 140*(4 Suppl), 57–62.

Nikisch, G. (2009). Involvement and role of antidepressant drugs of the hypothalamic-pituitary-adrenal axis and glucocorticoid receptor function. *Neuro-Endocrinology Letters, 30*(1), 11–16.

Nikisch, G., Mathe, A. A., Czernik, A., Thiele, J., Bohner, J., Eap, C. B.,…Baumann, P. (2005). Long-term citalopram administration reduces responsiveness of HPA axis in patients with major depression: Relationship with S-citalopram concentrations in plasma and cerebrospinal fluid (CSF) and clinical response. *Psychopharmacology, 181*(4), 751–760.

O'Brien, J. T., Lloyd, A., McKeith, I., Gholkar, A., & Ferrier, N. (2004). A longitudinal study of hippocampal volume, cortisol levels, and cognition in older depressed subjects. *American Journal of Psychiatry, 161*(11), 2081–2090.

O'Connor, C. M., Gurbel, P. A., & Serebruany, V. L. (2000). Depression and ischemic heart disease. *American Heart Journal, 140*(4 Suppl), 63–69.

O'Hara, R. (1986). Stress, aging, and mental health. *Am J Geriatr Psychiatry, 14*(4), 295–298.

O'Hara, R., Schröder, C. M., Mahadevan, R., Schatzberg, A. F., Lindley, S., Fox, S., Hallmayer, J. F. (2007) Serotonin transporter polymorphism, memory and hippocampal volume in the elderly: Association and interaction with cortisol. *Molecular Psychiatry, 12*(6), 544–555.

O'Hara, R., Coman, E., & Butters, M. (2006). Late life depression. In P. J. Snyder & P. D. Nussbaum (Eds.), *Clinical neuropsychology: A pocket handbook for assessment* (2nd ed., pp. 183–231).

Pariante, C. M., Pearce, B. D., Pisell, T. L., Su, C., & Miller, A. H. (2001). The steroid receptor antagonists RU40555 and RU486 activate glucocorticoid receptor translocation and are not excreted by the steroid hormones transporter in L929 cells. *Journal of Endocrinology, 169*(2), 309–320.

Pariante, C. M., Thomas, S. A., Lovestone, S., Makoff, A., & Kerwin, R. W. (2004). Do antidepressants regulate how cortisol affects the brain? *Psychoneuroendocrinology, 29*(4), 423–447.

Paslakis, G., Krumm, B., Gilles, M., Schweiger, U., Heuser, I., Richter, I., & Deuschle, M. (2011). Discrimination between patients with melancholic depression and healthy controls: Comparison between 24-h cortisol profiles, the DST and the Dex/CRH test. *Psychoneuroendocrinology, 36*(5), 691–698.

Penninx, B. W. J. H., Beekman, A. T. F., Bandinelli, S., Corsi, A. M., Bremmer, M., Hoogendijk, W. J., Ferrucci, L. (2007). Late-life depressive symptoms are associated with both hyperactivity and hypoactivity of the hypothalamo-pituitary-adrenal axis. *American Journal of Geriatric Psychiatry, 15*(6), 522–529.

Raikkonen, K., Matthews, K. A., & Kuller, L. H. (2002). The relationship between psychological risk attributes and the metabolic syndrome in healthy women: Antecedent or consequence? *Metabolism, 51*(12), 1573–1577.

Reuter, M. (2002). Impact of cortisol on emotions under stress and nonstress conditions: A pharmacopsychological approach. *Neuropsychobiology, 46*(1), 41–48.

Rosenbaum, A. H., Schatzberg, A. F., MacLaughlin, R. A., Snyder, K., Jiang, N. S., Ilstrup, D., Kliman, B. (1984). The dexamethasone suppression test in normal control subjects: Comparison of two assays and effect of age. *American Journal of Psychiatry, 141*(12), 1550–1555.

Rosmond, R., & Bjorntorp, P. (2000). Low cortisol production in chronic stress. The connection stress-somatic disease is a challenge for future research. *Läkartidningen, 97*(38), 4120–4124.

Rowe, W., Steverman, A., Walker, M., Sharma, S., Barden, N., Seckl, J. R., & Meaney, M. J. (1997). Antidepressants restore hypothalamic-pituitary-adrenal feedback function in aged, cognitively-impaired rats. *Neurobiology of Aging, 18*(5), 527–533.

Rubin, R. T., Phillips, J. J., Sadow, T. F., & McCracken, J. T. (1995). Adrenal gland volume in major depression. Increase during the depressive episode and decrease with successful treatment. *Archives of General Psychiatry, 52*(3), 213–218.

Sapolsky, R.M. (1986). Glucocorticoid toxicity in the hippocampus: reversal by supplementation with brain fuels. *J Neurosci., 6*(8), 2240–4.

Sapolsky, R. M. (2000). Glucocorticoids and hippocampal atrophy in neuropsychiatric disorders. *Archives of General Psychiatry, 57*(10), 925–935.

Sapolsky, R. M., & Altmann, J. (1991). Incidence of hypercortisolism and dexamethasone resistance increases with age among wild baboons. *Biological Psychiatry, 30*(10), 1008–1016.

Sapolsky, R. M., Krey, L. C., & McEwen, B. S. (1984). Stress down-regulates corticosterone receptors in a site-specific manner in the brain. *Endocrinology, 114*(1), 287–292.

Sapolsky, R. M., Krey, L. C., & McEwen, B. S. (1984). Glucocorticoid-sensitive hippocampal neurons are involved in terminating the adrenocortical stress response. *Proc Natl Acad Sci U S A*, 81(19), 6174–7.

Sapolsky, R. M., Krey, L. C., & McEwen, B. S. (1986). The neuroendocrinology of stress and aging: The glucocorticoid cascade hypothesis. *Endocrine Review*, 7(3), 284–301.

Sarginson, J. E., Lazzeroni, L. C., Ryan, H. S., Schatzberg, A. F., & Murphy, G. M. (2010). FKBP5 polymorphisms and antidepressant response in geriatric depression. *American Journal of Medical Genetics Part B*, 153B(2), 554–560.

Sarrieau, A., Dussaillant, M., Agid, F., Philibert, D., Agid, Y., & Rostene, W. (1986). Autoradiographic localization of glucocorticosteroid and progesterone binding sites in the human post-mortem brain. *Journal of Steroid Biochemistry*, 25(5B), 717–721.

Scharnholz, B., Weber-Hamann, B., Lederbogen, F., Schilling, C., Gilles, M., Onken, V.,...Deuschle, M. (2010). Antidepressant treatment with mirtazapine, but not venlafaxine, lowers cortisol concentrations in saliva: A randomized open trial. *Psychiatry Research*, 177(1–2), 109–113.

Smith, G. S., Lotrich, F. E., Malhotra, A. K., Lee, A. T., Ma, Y., Kramer, E.,...Pollock, B. G. (2004). Effects of serotonin transporter promoter polymorphisms on serotonin function. *Neuropsychopharmacology*, 29(12), 2226–2234.

Spath-Schwalbe, E., Gofferje, M., Kern, W., Born, J., & Fehm, H. L. (1991). Sleep disruption alters nocturnal ACTH and cortisol secretory patterns. *Biological Psychiatry*, 29(6), 575–584.

Steffens, D. C., Byrum, C. E., McQuoid, D. R., Greenberg, D. L., Payne, M. E., Blitchington, T. F.,...Krishnan, K. R. (2000). Hippocampal volume in geriatric depression. *Biological Psychiatry*, 48(4), 301–309.

Steiger, A., & Kimura, M. (2010). Wake and sleep EEG provide biomarkers in depression. *Journal of Psychiatric Research*, 44(4), 242–252.

Stetler, C., & Miller, G. E. (2011). Depression and hypothalamic-pituitary-adrenal activation: A quantitative summary of four decades of research. *Psychosomatic Medicine*, 73(2), 114–126.

Ta, A. T., Huang, S-E., Chiu, M-J., Hua, M-S., Tseng, W-Y. I., Chen, S-H. A., & Qiu, A. (2011). Age-related vulnerabilities along the hippocampal longitudinal axis. *Human Brain Mapping*. 2011 Sep 6, ePub ahead of print. doi: 10.1002/hbm.21364.

Thompson, W. K., Hallmayer, J., O'Hara, R., & Alzheimer's Disease Neuroimaging Initiative. (2011). Design considerations for characterizing psychiatric trajectories across the lifespan: Application to effects of APOE-ε4 on cerebral cortical thickness in Alzheimer's disease. *American Journal of Psychiatry*, 168(9), 894–903.

Traustadottir, T., Bosch, P. R., & Matt, K. S. (2003). Gender differences in cardiovascular and hypothalamic-pituitary-adrenal axis responses to psychological stress in healthy older adult men and women. *Stress*, 6(2), 133–140.

Tsukiura, T., Sekiguchi, A., Yomogida, Y., Nakagawa, S., Shigemune, Y., Kambara, T.,...Kawashima, R. (2011). Effects of aging on hippocampal and anterior temporal activations during successful retrieval of memory for face-name associations. *Journal of Cognitive Neuroscience*, 23(1), 200–213.

Vakili, K., Pillay, S. S., Lafer, B., Fava, M., Renshaw, P. F., Bonello-Cintron, C. M., & Yurgelun-Todd, D. A. (2000). Hippocampal volume in primary unipolar major depression: A magnetic resonance imaging study. *Biological Psychiatry*, 47(12), 1087–1090.

Vance, D. E., Heaton, K., Eaves, Y., & Fazeli, P. L. (2011). Sleep and cognition on everyday functioning in older adults: Implications for nursing practice and research. *Journal of Neuroscience Nursing*, 43(5), 261–271.

Van Cauter, E. (1996). Effects of gender and age on the levels and circadian rhythmicity of plasma cortisol. *Journal of Clinical Endocrinology and Metabolism*, 81(7), 2468–2473.

van Rossum, E. F. C., Koper, J. W., van den Beld, A. W., Uitterlinden, A. G., Arp, P., Ester, W.,...Lamberts, S. W. (2003). Identification of the BclI polymorphism in the glucocorticoid receptor gene: Association with sensitivity to glucocorticoids in vivo and body mass index. *Clinical Endocrinology (Oxford)*, 59(5), 585–592.

Vgontzas, A. N., Bixler, E. O., Lin, H. M., Prolo, P., Mastorakos, G., Vela-Bueno, A.,...Chrousos, G. P. (2001). Chronic insomnia is associated with nyctohemeral activation of the hypothalamic-pituitary-adrenal axis: clinical implications. *Journal of Clinical Endocrinology and Metabolism*, 86(8), 3787–3794.

Vogelzangs, N., & Penninx, B. W. (2007). Cortisol and insulin in depression and metabolic syndrome. *Psychoneuroendocrinology*, 32(7), 856.

Vythilingam, M., Vermetten, E., Anderson, G. M., Luckenbaugh, D., Anderson, E. R., Snow, J.,...Bremner, J. D. (2004). Hippocampal volume, memory, and cortisol status in major depressive disorder: Effects of treatment. *Biological Psychiatry*, 56(2), 101–112.

Watzka, M., Beyenburg, S., Blumcke, I., Elger, C. E., Bidlingmaier, F., & Stoffel-Wagner, B. (2000). Expression of mineralocorticoid and glucocorticoid receptor mRNA in the human hippocampus. *Neuroscience Letters, 290*(2), 121–124.

Watzka, M., Bidlingmaier, F., Beyenburg, S., Henke, R. T., Clusmann, H., Elger, C. E., ... Stoffel-Wagner, B. (2000). Corticosteroid receptor mRNA expression in the brains of patients with epilepsy. *Steroids, 65*(12), 895–901.

Wirth, M. M., Scherer, S. M., Hoks, R. M., & Abercrombie, H. C. (2011). The effect of cortisol on emotional responses depends on order of cortisol and placebo administration in a within-subject design. *Psychoneuroendocrinology, 36*(7), 945–954.

Wirtz, P. H., von Kanel, R., Emini, L., Ruedisueli, K., Groessbauer, S., Maercker, A., & Ehlert, U. (2007). Evidence for altered hypothalamus-pituitary-adrenal axis functioning in systemic hypertension: Blunted cortisol response to awakening and lower negative feedback sensitivity. *Psychoneuroendocrinology, 32*(5), 430–436.

Wolkowitz, O. M., Reus, V. I., & Mellon, S. H. (2011). Of sound mind and body: Depression, disease, and accelerated aging. *Dialogues in Clinical Neuroscience, 13*(1), 25–39.

Woolley, C. S., Gould, E., & McEwen, B. S. (1990). Exposure to excess glucocorticoids alters dendritic morphology of adult hippocampal pyramidal neurons. *Brain Research, 531*(1–2), 225–231.

Wüst, S., van Rossum, E. F. C., Federenko, I. S., Koper, J. W., Kumsta, R., & Hellhammer, D. H. (2004). Common polymorphisms in the glucocorticoid receptor gene are associated with adrenocortical responses to psychosocial stress. *Journal of Clinical Endocrinology and Metabolism, 89*(2), 565–573.

Yau, J. L. W., Noble, J., Hibberd, C., Rowe, W. B., Meaney, M. J., Morris, R. G. M., & Seckl, J. R. (2002). Chronic treatment with the antidepressant amitriptyline prevents impairments in water maze learning in aging rats. *Journal of Neuroscience, 22*(4), 1436–1442.

Yau, J. L., Olsson, T., Morris, R. G., Meaney, M. J., & Seckl, J. R. (1995). Glucocorticoids, hippocampal corticosteroid receptor gene expression and antidepressant treatment: Relationship with spatial learning in young and aged rats. *Neuroscience, 66*(3), 571–581.

Yehuda, R., Teicher, M. H., Trestman, R. L., Levengood, R. A., & Siever, L. J. (1996). Cortisol regulation in posttraumatic stress disorder and major depression: A chronobiological analysis. *Biological Psychiatry, 40*(2), 79–88.

41

CLINICAL PREDICTION MODELS

Wesley K. Thompson, Ji-in Choi, and Stewart Anderson

CLINICAL TRIALS of mood disorders in late life frequently use time to the occurrence of an event as the primary study outcome. Examples include time to remission for an acute episode in a bipolar treatment study or time to onset of major depression in a late-life depression prevention study. In recent years it has become common to collect auxiliary post-randomization variables on subjects, often repeatedly over multiple time points, augmenting the primary time-to-event study outcome. A growing proportion of prospective observational studies of late-life mood disorders also collect repeated measurements of auxiliary variables in addition to clinical assessments of disorder severity, including variables related to physical health and functioning, biological correlates of illness, contextual variables such as negative life events, and cognitive impairments. Aims for collecting auxiliary longitudinal variables in addition to primary clinical outcomes differ across studies but include (1) characterizing the etiology and mechanisms of late-life mood disorders; (2) determining which variables mediate treatment outcomes; and (3) using them as surrogate markers for the primary outcome. These three goals are closely related to each other and to a fourth, less common goal: (4) performing individualized subject predictions of future illness states, perhaps in response to treatment.

Predictive models, in general, use auxiliary information previously incorporated into the model to *predict* a current or future observation. Predictive models are particularly useful in a clinical setting where the interest is to use a set of patient characteristics to project his or her outcome of interest. For example, an elderly patient with poor cognitive ability, poor family support, and previous incidences of major depression may have a high probability of having future episodes of major depression. If a model could accurately predict that the probability of the occurrence of a future episode was high, then a clinician could try to provide an intervention to avoid that occurrence. Hence, based on the elderly patient's previous trajectory of cognitive functioning, comorbidities, and other subsyndromal depressive characteristics, predictive models could potentially enable a clinician to provide an appropriate *personalized intervention*.

More generally, a predictive model that incorporated longitudinal assessments of auxiliary variables might be used to determine whether patterns of *change* in these variables impacted the probability of an episode of major depression. To be effective in this scenario, a predictive model would need to incorporate the ability to update patient predictions as repeated assessments were collected over time.

Example One of the simplest types of predictive models can be demonstrated with a multiple linear regression model:

$$Y_i = \beta_0 + \beta_1 X_1 + \beta_2 X_2 + \beta_{p-1} X_{p-1} + \epsilon_i, \quad i = 1,\ldots, n$$

where Y_i is the outcome of interest for subject i; the X_j, $j = 1, \ldots, p$ are potential *predictors* of Y_j; $\beta_0, \beta_1, \ldots, \beta_{p-1}$ are *parameters* to be estimated from the data, and the errors are independent and normally distributed with constant variance, or $\epsilon_i \sim N(0, \sigma^2)$, $i = 1, \ldots, n$. A convenient way to rewrite this model involves the use of linear algebra, that is,

$$\underbrace{\mathbf{Y}}_{n \times 1} = \underbrace{\mathbf{X}}_{n \times p} \underbrace{\beta}_{p \times 1} + \underbrace{\epsilon}_{n \times 1}$$

where $\mathbf{Y} = \begin{pmatrix} Y_1 \\ Y_2 \\ \vdots \\ Y_n \end{pmatrix}$, $\mathbf{X} = \begin{pmatrix} 1 & X_{11} & \cdots & X_{1,p-1} \\ 1 & X_{21} & \cdots & X_{2,p-1} \\ \vdots & \vdots & \cdots & \vdots \\ 1 & X_{n1} & \cdots & X_{n,p-1} \end{pmatrix}$,

$$\beta = \begin{pmatrix} \beta_0 \\ \beta_1 \\ \vdots \\ \beta_{p-1} \end{pmatrix} \quad \text{and} \quad \epsilon = \begin{pmatrix} \epsilon_1 \\ \epsilon_2 \\ \vdots \\ \epsilon_n \end{pmatrix} \qquad (1.1)$$

Denoting the average, or expectation, of a random variable by $\mathcal{E}(\cdot)$, we have that $\mathcal{E}(\epsilon) = \mathbf{0}$. Thus, we can represent the model in equation (1.1) as $\mathcal{E}(\mathbf{Y}) = \mathbf{X}\beta$, where $\mathbf{Y}$ is an $n \times 1$ vector of observations, $\mathbf{X}$ is an $n \times p$ design matrix, and β is a $p \times 1$ parameter vector. Recall that the least squares (best linear unbiased) estimator of β is given by $\hat{\beta} = (\mathbf{X}'\mathbf{X})^{-1}\mathbf{X}'\mathbf{Y} = \mathbf{A}^{-1}\mathbf{X}'\mathbf{X}$ where "′" denotes the transpose of a matrix, "^" indicates that β is being estimated from the data, and $\mathbf{A} = \mathbf{X}'\mathbf{X}$.

Suppose we obtain a new observation (subject) but only have access to his or her $1 \times p$ row vector of auxiliary variables, $\mathbf{x}_{n+1}$. The *predictive equation* for this subject's outcome is given simply by

$$\hat{Y} = \mathbf{x}_{n+1}\hat{\beta}$$

After obtaining the actual outcome Y_{n+1}, we can assess the *prediction error*, $\hat{e}_{n+1} = Y_{n+1} - \hat{Y}$. Moreover, this subject's data can now be incorporated into future predictions as follows. We add the new observation to each variable, that is, we add Y_{n+1} to $\mathbf{Y}$ and a $1 \times p$ row vector, $\mathbf{x}_{n+1}$, to $\mathbf{X}$. It can be shown that the inverse of $\mathbf{B} = \mathbf{A} + \mathbf{x}'_{n+1}\mathbf{x}_{n+1}$ is

$$\mathbf{B}^{-1} = \mathbf{A}^{-1} - \left(\mathbf{A}^{-1}\mathbf{x}'_{n+1}\mathbf{x}_{n+1}\mathbf{A}^{-1}\right) / \left(1 + \mathbf{x}_{n+1}\mathbf{A}^{-1}\mathbf{x}'_{n+1}\right)$$

From this, one can derive an *updating formula* for observation $n + 1$ using the first n points of the model:

$$\hat{\beta}_{n+1} = \hat{\beta}_n + \mathbf{A}^{-1}\mathbf{x}'_{n+1} (Y_{n+1} - \mathbf{x}_{n+1}\hat{\beta}_n) / (1 + \mathbf{x}_{n+1}\mathbf{A}^{-1}\mathbf{x}'_{n+1})$$

where the subscripts n and $n + 1$ on $\hat{\beta}$ indicate estimates of β with n and $n + 1$ points, respectively (Kendall & Stuart, 1983). From this last equation, it can be seen that updating the prediction model with new observations depends on the accuracy of the prediction (i.e., the prediction error) for the new observation using the data from prior observations. Note that this prediction model is severely limited by the ability to obtain only one observation and to make only one prediction per subject. Moreover, this prediction model does not allow assessment of the predictive implications of longitudinal patterns of change in auxiliary variables $\mathbf{x}$.

The past three decades have seen dramatic developments in the statistical models available for the analysis of longitudinal data (see, e.g., Fitzmaurice & Molenberghs, 2009, for an overview). Far from relying on fairly restrictive models (e.g., multivariate or repeated measures analysis of variance), it is now possible for example to implement analyses of longitudinal data using linear mixed-effects models (LMMs; Diggle, Heagerty, Liang, & Zeger, 2002) for normally distributed data or generalized linear mixed-effects models (GLMMs; McCulloch & Neuhaus, 2009) from the more inclusive exponential family of distributions. LMMs and GLMMs form an extremely flexible class of models allowing for irregular follow-up times and missing data, nonnormal, including discrete, responses, intuitive and flexible parametrization of within-subject correlation, integrated analysis of longitudinal assessments from multiple domains (e.g., Fieuws, Verbeke, Maes, & Vanrenterghem, 2008), and the ability to use individual estimates of random effects to perform subject-level predictions of current and future outcomes (e.g., Rabe-Hasketh & Skrondal, 2009).

The development of sophisticated new multivariate models for the analysis of longitudinal data has been abetted by the concomitant rise in computing power and user-friendly statistical software packages that implement LMMs and GLMMs, such as the software distributed by SAS (2000–2004), SPSS (2006), Stata (2011), Mplus (1998–2007), and the freely available R statistical language (Hornik, 2011). The ability to fit more realistically complex models to multivariate longitudinal data has also been aided by simultaneous developments in modern Bayesian computational methods, especially the development of inferential procedures relying on Markov Chain Monte Carlo (MCMC) simulations (Tanner & Wong, 2010). Bayesian methods have consequently been extensively employed as inferential tools in the analysis of complex hierarchical and longitudinal data (Gelman & Hill, 2007) and are especially germane for purposes of prediction, since Bayes's rule is essentially a formula for sequentially updating probability models as new information becomes available.

While mixed models have appropriately become widely used in the analysis of longitudinal data from studies of late-life mood disorders, many of these more recent theoretical developments have not yet seen widespread use in this area. In particular, models involving nonnormal responses and joint models of multiple auxiliary longitudinal variables and a time-to-event outcome have not been extensively exploited. In this context, joint models promise to provide improved understanding of the mechanisms of late-life mood disorders and how these mechanisms interact to mediate time-to-event treatment outcomes. Moreover, joint models implemented with Bayesian inferential procedures potentially allow for updatable patient-level, individualized prediction of treatment outcomes utilizing all of the information available from a rich stream of repeated patient-level auxiliary variables.

The remainder of the chapter is structured as follows. First, we briefly describe static prediction models, typically involving Cox proportional hazards models. Second, we describe a related class of longitudinal prediction models called *joint models*, wherein auxiliary longitudinal measures are included to obtain improved subject-level predictions of event times. Third, we briefly describe a

Bayesian approach to updating information and performing sequential prediction. We conclude with some remarks on future directions and potential applications to studies of late-life mood disorders. Most technical details are contained in examples and asides distributed throughout the chapter, and they may be glossed over by the reader if desired.

STATIC PREDICTION MODELS

To date, the vast majority of clinical prediction models involve static predictors, in other words, predictions from data collected from a subject at one time point (Steyerberg, 2009). Perhaps the best-known static clinical prediction model is the Framingham risk score, which assesses the probability that an individual will develop cardiovascular disease in the next 10 years given a set of cross-sectional variables (Wilson et al., 1998). Specifically, the risk score was based on a multivariate regression involving age, total cholesterol, presence of diabetes, smoking status, among other variables. The risk of developing coronary heart disease over the next 10 years can be computed by plugging in the responses for a given subject at a specific point in time. In mental health applications, static prediction models have been developed for traumatic brain injury (Maramrou et al., 2007), schizophrenia (Carter, Schulsinger, Parnas, Cannon, & Mednick, 2002), hazardous drinking (King et al., 2002), eating disorders (Fichter, Quadflieg, & Rehm, 2003), and psychosis (Cannon et al., 2008), among others.

Most static prediction models employ methods from the field of survival analysis to predict time to the occurrence of an event. The most commonly used model from survival analysis is the Cox proportional hazards model (Cox, 1972), which evaluates the impact of static or *fixed* predictor variables on the hazard rate. The hazard rate at time t is the probability of experiencing the event of interest in the next instant, given that the event has not yet occurred. The regression coefficients of the predictors scale the baseline hazard rate up or down, depending on whether the coefficients are positive or negative, thus increasing or decreasing the estimated risk for future occurrence of the event. One of the primary advantages of the Cox model is that it allows for right censoring of event times. Right censoring occurs when the event of interest takes place after the end of the measurement period. For right-censored observations, the time of the event is not observed; it is only known that the event time was longer than the length of time on study. A necessary condition is that the censoring times are independent of the event times conditional on the observed independent variables, as is the case if censoring occurs because of study completion.

Technical Note: Denote the primary study outcome (event time) for the ith subject by T_i, for $i = 1,\ldots, n$. In practice, what is observed is $\{T_i^*, \delta_i\}$, where $T_i^* = \min\{T_i, C_i\}$, C_i is a censoring time for subject i, and $\delta_i = 1$ if the event is observed and zero otherwise. The censoring times C are assumed to be independent of the event times T conditional on the observed data; this assumption is generally valid if, for example, censoring times are caused by the (planned) study completion date. Perhaps the most commonly implemented model used for assessing the impact of baseline covariates $\mathbf{x}_i$ on right-censored, time-to-event outcomes is the Cox proportional hazards model (Cox, 1972)

$$\lambda_i(t) = \lim_{dt \to 0} \frac{Pr\left(t \leq T_i < t + dt \mid T_i \geq t, X_i\right)}{dt}$$
$$= \lambda_0(t)\exp\{\mathbf{x}_i^T \alpha\} \qquad (1.2)$$

where $\lambda_i(t)$ is the hazard function at time t for subject i and λ_0 is a baseline hazard rate. Note that, in equation (1.2), by dividing both sides of the equation by $\lambda_0(t)$, one obtains $\lambda_i(t)/\lambda_0(t) = \exp\{\mathbf{x}_i^T\alpha\}$, which is constant as a function of time. Hence, we use the term *proportional* hazards. Based on the first n data points, we can obtain an estimate $\hat{\alpha}$ of α. An estimate $\hat{\lambda}_0$ of the baseline hazard λ_0 can be obtained by assuming either a parametric model for λ_0 or using nonparametric methods (e.g., Anderson & Senthilselvan, 1980). Predictions of event times can then be made from the model (1.2) based on new baseline observation $\mathbf{x}_{n+1}$ and simply plugging in the new observation to obtain the subject-specific hazard function

$$\hat{\lambda}_{n+1}(t) = \hat{\lambda}_{0,n}(t)\exp\{x_{n+1}^T \hat{\alpha}_n\} \qquad (1.3)$$

where $\hat{\lambda}_{0,n}$ and $\hat{\alpha}_n$ denote estimates based on the first n observations. A prediction that the event will occur in a given time interval is then obtained by exponentiating equation (1.3) and integrating over the desired interval.

In practice, clinical prediction models focus on a defined future time interval. The Framingham risk score, for example, estimates the probability of onset of cardiovascular disease in the next 10 years from the time of prediction. This probability can be easily obtained from the estimated hazard rate. A simple yes/no prediction can then be obtained by thresholding the probability. For example, if we threshold the estimated probability at 0.5, we predict the subject will experience the event within the time period if his or her estimated probability of occurrence is greater than 0.5. The predictive utility of the model can then be assessed by computing the *sensitivity* (the proportion of subjects who experience the event who were predicted to) and the *specificity* (the proportion of subjects who did not experience the event who were predicted not to). One can use sensitivity and specificity to assess whether, indeed, 0.5 is the best value to use as a threshold. Overall accuracy of the prediction algorithm is just the proportion of correct predictions. Another commonly used overall assessment of the predictive utility is the *Area Under the Curve* (AUC). The AUC is the probability that for any two randomly chosen subjects, one of whom experiences the event and the other does not, the person who experiences the event is assigned a higher probability of experiencing the event by the prediction model.

Note that predictions from a Cox model and assessment of its predictive utility are *static* quantities. While the survival model is fitted on data measured over time, the predictors in the model are time invariant. Event time predictions do not consider trajectories of predicting variables, nor are predictions dynamically updated as more (longitudinal) assessments of predictors are collected. For example, if the Framingham risk score was computed on a subject at two or more time points, the risk scores would not reflect any information about the *trajectory* of risk factors. Instead, each time of measurement would be considered in isolation, without regard to prior time points. Extensions to model (1.2) that allow for inclusion of time-varying auxiliary variables and dynamic updating are considered next.

JOINT LONGITUDINAL AND TIME-TO-EVENT MODELS

An area of predictive modeling where many recent methodological developments have occurred is that of predicting time-to-event outcomes based on baseline covariates and auxiliary variables that have been measured longitudinally (for a review, see Tsiatis & Davidian, 2004). In this setting, prediction models provide an estimate, either point or interval, for future events based on trajectories of auxiliary variables obtained from previous observations. To obtain predictions of event times that efficiently use the information contained in the trajectories of auxiliary variables, both the event times and trajectories should be modeled simultaneously, that is, *jointly*. This can be accomplished in a number of ways, for example, by letting the survival and trajectories depend on shared parameters or by making the estimation of the survival function conditional on the underlying (noise-free) trajectories. One advantage of joint models is that measurement error in the longitudinal measurements is assessed simultaneously with the uncertainty in event times due to censoring (Rizopoulos, 2011).

Technical Note: Suppose that in addition to baseline covariates and the primary time-to-event outcome, we collect auxiliary longitudinal data $Y_{ij} = Y(t_{ij})$ for subject i at times t_{ij}, $j = 1, \ldots, m_i$. Model (1.2) is incapable of incorporating longitudinal auxiliary variables or assessing the impact of patterns of variation in these auxiliary variables on time-to-event predictions. Note that the number and timing of measurements can vary considerably across subjects, either randomly or by design; we make the assumption that the observation times $\mathbf{t}_i = (t_{i1}, \ldots, t_{im_i})$ are independent of the measured values of Y_{ij} and the time-to-event outcome T_i. A linear mixed effects model is assumed to describe the subject-specific longitudinal evolutions

$$Y_i(t) = \mathbf{f}_i(t)^T \boldsymbol{\beta} + \mathbf{r}_i(t)^T \mathbf{b}_i + \epsilon_i(t)$$
$$= W_i(t) + \epsilon_i(t) \qquad (1.4)$$

where $W_i(t) = \mathbf{f}_i(t)^T \boldsymbol{\beta} + \mathbf{r}_i(t)^T \mathbf{b}_i$ is the underlying noise-free longitudinal process, $\boldsymbol{\beta}$ denotes the vector of the unknown fixed-effects parameters, $\mathbf{b}_i$ the vector of random effects, $\mathbf{f}_i(t)$ and $\mathbf{r}_i(t)$ are the column vectors of time-varying covariates corresponding to fixed and random effects, respectively, and $\epsilon_i(t)$ is the normally distributed measurement error term with variance σ^2. Following Diggle et al. (2009), we call (1.4) the *measurement submodel* of the joint model. We can incorporate the longitudinal submodel into (1.2) via the *hazard submodel*

$$\lambda_i(t) = \lambda_0(t) \exp\{\mathbf{x}_i^T \boldsymbol{\alpha}^* + \gamma W_i(t)\} \qquad (1.5)$$

where γ quantifies the dependence of the time-to-event outcome on the underlying process giving rise to the longitudinal measurement Y_{ij}. Note that more general formulations of model (1.5) have been given in the literature (e.g., see Diggle, Henderson, & Philipson, 2009). In particular, it is possible to specify the dependence of $\lambda_i(t)$ on W_i through a function of the history of the process, defined as $W_i^H(t) = \{W_i(u) \mid 0 \le u \le t\}$ (Tsiatis & Davidian, 2004); the formulation given in equation (1.5) is a function of $W_i^H(t)$ only through the current level $W_i(t)$. Submodels (1.4) and (1.5) together specify a *joint model* for auxiliary longitudinal variables and the time-to-event outcome.

Note that longitudinal measurements up to a time t imply survival up to time t. Consequently, predictions from models (1.4) and (1.5) are often focused on the conditional probability of surviving time $u > t$ given survival up to time t, that is

$$\pi_i(u \mid t) = \Pr\left(T_i \ge u \mid T_i > t, W_i^H(t), \mathcal{D}_n\right)$$

where $\mathcal{D}_n = \{T_i^*, \delta_i, \mathbf{Y}_i; i = 1, \ldots, n\}$ denotes the sample on which the joint model is fitted and on which the prediction model is based. Rizopoulos (2011) derives a first-order estimate of $\pi_i(u \mid t)$ using the empirical Bayes estimate for $\mathbf{b}_i$. To produce valid standard errors for the estimate of $\pi_i(u \mid t)$, a standard asymptotic Bayesian formulation (Cox & Hinkley, 1974) is used.

Joint models are ideal for realizing aims (1)–(3) described earlier. For example, if Z indicates application of a treatment to prevent depression onset, and W is an underlying longitudinal post-treatment biomarker of illness, W mediates the effect of Z on time to depression onset T if (a) Z predicts time to depression onset T; (b) Z predicts W; and (c) the effect of Z on T disappears when W is included in the model (Kraemer, Stice, Kazdin, Offord, & Kupfer, 2001). Note that condition (a) is equivalent to showing that $\boldsymbol{\alpha} \ne \mathbf{0}$ in equation (1.2) and condition (c) is equivalent to showing that $\boldsymbol{\alpha}^* = \mathbf{0}$ in equation (1.5) in which case by necessity $\gamma \ne 0$. Condition (b) is satisfied if we include the treatment indicator Z as a baseline predictor in equation (1.4) and if Z has a nonzero coefficient. The conditions (a)–(c) are also consistent with requirements for consideration of W as a surrogate end point (Prentice, 1989; Tsiatis & Davidian, 2004). Note that all three aims would need to be validated in further studies. Mechanistic and mediational claims involve determining how systems behave under interventions, that is, causal relationships, and would need to be validated from multiple streams of evidence, including data from controlled experiments. Surrogacy arguably involves both prediction and causal claims (Berger, 2003). Joint models could also potentially be used for aim (4), that is, performing individualized assessments of the probability of mental illness onset given a longitudinal trajectory of clinical symptom and other measures, such as cognitive or biomarker trajectories. For example, it might be found that rapid decline in cognition from one time point to another, perhaps in conjunction with onset of disability, predicts higher probability of depression onset in a given time period. Other information, for example, age, gender, previous mental health history, familial risk, may also contribute substantially to such a multivariate, longitudinal risk model.

A number of authors have considered the use of joint models for making individualized predictions in biomedical settings (Garre, Zwinderman, Geskus, & Sijpkens, 2008; Proust-Lima & Taylor, 2009; Yu et al., 2004). For example, Rizopoulos (2011) applied individualized prediction models to AIDS patients, using longitudinal CD4 cell count measurements to predict time to death in a sample of 467 patients using the joint model specified by equations (1.4) and (1.5). In particular, he used this time-dependent covariate to compare the probabilities of survival in two individual patients with similar baseline characteristics but one who had stable CD4 counts over time and one whose CD4 counts deteriorated over time. In a clinical setting, having quantitative information like this could facilitate the initiation of another treatment intervention in the latter patient. In this model, longitudinal measurements on a variable represent an endogenous time-dependent covariate (Kalbfleisch & Prentice, 2002). Hence, longitudinal measurements are directly related to the failure mechanism; longitudinal measurements up to t, in fact, imply survival up to t. Consequently, predictions are focused on the conditional probability of surviving time $u > t$ given survival up to t.

Technical Note: To assess the predictive performance of time-to-event models, estimates of sensitivity and specificity measures can be derived under the joint modeling framework. In particular, we assume the quantity of estimation is the probability a given subject will experience an event in the clinically relevant interval $(t, t + \Delta t]$ given that he or she has not experienced the event up to time t. A prediction rule for event occurrence can be formed based on the prior longitudinal history, $W_i^H(t)$, for some time-dependent risk set A_t. For example, A_t may consist of thresholds for the longitudinal process at times $t_{ij} \leq t$. Let $\mathcal{S}_i(t) = \{W_i^H \in A_t\}$ denote prediction that the event will happen in interval $(t, t + \Delta t]$ and let $\mathcal{F}_i(t)$ denote its complement. Rizopoulos (2011) defines the time-dependent sensitivity of the prediction rule as

$$\Pr\left(\mathcal{S}_i(t) \mid T_i > t, T_i \in (t, t + \Delta t]\right)$$

and the time-dependent specificity measure as

$$\Pr\left(\mathcal{F}_i(t) \mid T_i > t, T_i > t + \Delta t\right)$$

Based on these definitions, Rizopoulos (2011) proposes estimates of dynamic receiving operator characteristic (ROC) curves and area under the curve (AUC) estimates of prediction performance.

Often more than one set of auxiliary variables will be collected. One approach, motivated by predicting renal graft failures in 432 subjects using multiple auxiliary longitudinal variables, was investigated by Fieuws et al. (2008). This approach employs multivariate mixed models (MMMs) to handle prediction from multiple correlated longitudinal markers of graft failure. The goal was to utilize information from four separate longitudinal markers to obtain a probability of the risk that the graft will fail within a 10-year period following transplantation. This probability function was calculated using Bayes's rule (see later). Due to computational complexity, all pairwise mixed models are fit and results averaged across fits, as in Fieuws and Verbeke (2006). The pattern-mixture approach (Little, 1993; Molenberghs & Verbeke, 2005) was used to factorize the joint model for the longitudinal measurement process and the event times. Fieuws et al. (2008) conclude that MMMs of correlated markers significantly outperformed other prediction strategies.

Several authors have performed individual prediction via the use of a longitudinal-survival-cure model (Law, Taylor, & Sandler, 2002; Yu, Law, Taylor, & Sandler, 2004). For example, Yu et al. (2004) divided the patients into "cured" or "susceptible" groups depending on whether the patient has his or her tumor completely killed by the treatment. Since it is not known a priori which patients will fall into which group, this aspect of the study is incorporated into the joint modeling by using mixture cure models (e.g., Farewell, 1982; Kuk & Chen, 1992; Taylor, 1995). The cured fraction is modeled as a logistic function of baseline covariates, measured before the end of the radiation therapy period. The longitudinal data are modeled using nonlinear mixed models with different models for the cured and susceptible groups. The time to event outcomes are modeled using a time-dependent proportional hazards model for those in the susceptible group, where the time-dependent covariates include both the current value and the slope of posttreatment longitudinal measurement profile. This model has the disadvantage that it is highly parameterized, and hence estimation and interpretation of the parameters can be difficult (Farewell, 1986; Li, Taylor, & Sy, 2001).

DYNAMICALLY UPDATING PREDICTIVE MODELS

An advantage of joint models over standard survival models is that longitudinal trajectories are incorporated, utilizing within-subject patterns of variation (e.g., rapid decline of a given biomarker) for event time predictions, potentially leading to large gains in predictive accuracy.

A framework that is well suited to the task of dynamically updating a predictive model involves the use of a *Bayesian* paradigm. In a Bayesian paradigm, the parameters of a probability distribution assumed to be associated with a process or event of interest are considered to be random. In addition, one has some notion of how that parameter or set of parameters is distributed (based on either one's subjective opinion or based on previous scientific evidence) and, hence, a *prior distribution* is constructed. Usually, one wishes to construct a prior distribution with a large variance so that a reasonable amount of uncertainty will ensure that the amount of subjectivity built into a given model is minimized. Once the data are observed, the evidence for parameter(s) of interest is updated (through the use of Bayes's rule; hence, the term "Bayesian" is used). The updated distribution is known as a *posterior distribution*.

Technical Note: Formally, we consider observations $\mathbf{y} = (y_1, y_2, \ldots, y_n)'$ to be *fixed* and are interested in making inference about $\boldsymbol{\theta} = (\theta_1, \theta_2, \ldots, \theta_q)'$, $q < n$. The posterior probability of $\boldsymbol{\theta}$ given the data is represented by $p(\boldsymbol{\theta}|\mathbf{y})$, whereas the prior distribution and the probability of a certain set of data given the parameters in the model are given by $p(y|\boldsymbol{\theta})$ and

$p(\boldsymbol{\theta})$, respectively. The three quantities can be linked via the use of *Bayes's rule*:

$$p(\boldsymbol{\theta}|\mathbf{y}) = \frac{p(\mathbf{y}|\boldsymbol{\theta})p(\boldsymbol{\theta})}{p(\mathbf{y})} \propto p(y|\boldsymbol{\theta})p(\boldsymbol{\theta}) \qquad (1.6)$$

where $p(\mathbf{y}) = \int p(\mathbf{y}|\boldsymbol{\theta})p(\boldsymbol{\theta})d\boldsymbol{\theta}$ and "$\propto$" denotes proportional to the (fixed) quantity $p(\mathbf{y})$. In equation (1.6), we think of $p(\mathbf{y}|\boldsymbol{\theta})$ as a function of $\boldsymbol{\theta}$. When we have n independent observations, we form the *likelihood function*, $L(\boldsymbol{\theta}|\mathbf{y})$ of $\boldsymbol{\theta}$, so that the Bayes's formula can be rewritten as

$$p(\boldsymbol{\theta}|\mathbf{y}) \propto L(\boldsymbol{\theta}|\mathbf{y})p(\boldsymbol{\theta})$$

Good overviews of Bayesian methodology can be found in Box and Tiao (1973), Lee (1997), and Leonard and Hsu (1999). For readers who are more theoretically inclined, overviews by Lindley (1971) and Berger (1985) are recommended.

One reason that Bayesian methods are useful as a predictive tool is because of how easily sequential sets of observations are incorporated into the model. Following Box and Tiao (1973), if $\mathbf{y}_1$ is a sample of observation and $\mathbf{y}_2$ is a second sample independent from the first, we have

$$p(\boldsymbol{\theta}|\mathbf{y}_1, \mathbf{y}_2) \propto L(\boldsymbol{\theta}|\mathbf{y}_1)L(\boldsymbol{\theta}|\mathbf{y}_2)p(\boldsymbol{\theta}) \propto p(\boldsymbol{\theta}|\mathbf{y}_1)L(\boldsymbol{\theta}|\mathbf{y}_2)$$

Thus, the posterior distribution given *both* $\mathbf{y}_1$ and $\mathbf{y}_2$ is proportional to the product of the posterior given $\mathbf{y}_1$ alone times the likelihood of sample 2 (that is, the updated information from sample 2).

For example, the posterior predictive distribution of the event time based on the joint probability model can be calculated as

$$p(t^j|\mathbf{y}, \bar{\mathcal{D}}) \propto p(t^j, \mathbf{y}^*|\bar{\mathcal{D}})$$
$$= \int p(t^j, \mathbf{y}, \boldsymbol{\theta}^j, \boldsymbol{\theta}|\bar{\mathcal{D}})d\boldsymbol{\theta}\, d\boldsymbol{\theta}$$
$$= \int p(t^j|\boldsymbol{\theta}, \boldsymbol{\theta})p(\mathbf{y}^j|\boldsymbol{\theta}^j, \boldsymbol{\theta})\, p(\boldsymbol{\theta}|\boldsymbol{\theta})p(\boldsymbol{\theta}|\bar{\mathcal{D}})d\boldsymbol{\theta}^j d\boldsymbol{\theta}$$

where t^j denotes the time to event for the patient under consideration with an additional (or new) vector of longitudinal measurements $\mathbf{y}^j$, $\bar{\mathcal{D}}$ denotes data from all previous patients for which posterior distributions are available, $\boldsymbol{\theta}$ denotes the patient-specific random effects vector, and $\boldsymbol{\theta}^j$ denotes the new random effects vector for the additional subject (Pauler & Finkelstein, 2002).

A biomedical example of a Bayesian model for the joint modeling of longitudinal and right-censored event-time data was proposed by Pauler and Finkelstein (2002). The motivation was to use longitudinal prostate-specific antigen (PSA) markers to predict recurrence in a sample of 1,011 patients diagnosed and treated for prostate cancer. The joint model is closely related to that described by equations (1.4) and (1.5). In particular, they specified a simple parametric mixed model for the longitudinal measurements, with a subject-specific change point allowing for steeper PSA slopes, indicative of recurrence. The prior distribution on the subject-specific change point was chosen with the consideration that many patients do not have a recurrence within the study period and their longitudinal PSA measurements tend to be flat. For the event time data, a Bayesian version of Cox proportional hazard model was assumed. The posterior predictive distribution of the event time based on the joint probability model was computed, using Bayes's rule to update individual prediction probabilities as new longitudinal observations became available within subjects.

To continue the hypothetical example of the last section, suppose onset of late-life depression is predicted from longitudinal trajectories of cognition and biomarkers, as well as static risk factors. At a given point in time, a patient's risk for depression onset is computed from the a posteriori distribution of the risk parameters (e.g., the hazard rate) given the observed data up to that time. If the subject is assessed again at a future time point, the hazard rate distribution is recomputed using Bayes's rule incorporating the new data, and an updated personalized prediction of depression onset can be made.

DISCUSSION AND FUTURE DIRECTIONS

The last 30 years have witnessed tremendous growth in the ability of researchers in late-life mood disorders to model complex multivariate longitudinal processes. This has resulted from the confluence of many factors, including methodological developments in mixed-effects models, the explosive increase in computing power and availability of user-friendly statistical software, and the development of modern Bayesian computational algorithms based on MCMC methods. In no small degree, this growth has been spurred by the desire of biostatisticians to develop more realistically complex models for use in biomedical research. Many of these statistical methods have been widely utilized for the study of late-life mood disorders; for example, Cox proportional hazards models are de rigueur for time-to-event data and the repeated measures ANOVA has largely, though not entirely, been replaced by more flexible linear mixed-effects models. However, despite their potential utility, joint models encompassing both primary time-to-event outcomes and auxiliary longitudinal markers of illness have been little used, either in clinical trials or in observational studies of late-life mood disorders. The reasons for this are probably two-fold: Most methods do not yet have readily available software implementations, and most researchers in late-life mood disorders are not yet aware of the potential advantages of joint modeling approaches.

One such advantage lies in the potential for improved individualized treatment algorithms. Prognosis, or prediction of future patient outcomes, is crucial for determining course of treatment or prevention. Individualized treatment requires individualized predictions that reflect the temporal changes in course of illness. Joint models have been successfully applied to individualized prediction of event times in AIDS and cancer research.

Though promising, it remains to be demonstrated that similar good results will be obtained in research of late-life mood disorders. For example, while onset of AIDS in HIV-positive patients has a fairly good surrogate marker (CD4 cell count), no such clear surrogate marker exists for late-life mood disorders. More likely a combination of longitudinal markers would need to be incorporated into prediction models for late-life mood disorders, including physical health and functioning, psychosocial and contextual variables, cognitive impairments, and biomarkers of illness. In practical implementations, prediction models would also need to involve ease of implementation and interpretation, as well as the ability to be updated in real time. Bayesian prediction models are promising in this respect, perhaps in combination with simple prediction rules similar to Rizopoulos (2011).

In conclusion, many research studies in late-life mood disorders already collect multiple auxiliary longitudinal variables in addition to a primary time-to-event outcome. Determining whether these auxiliary variables are involved in mechanisms of illness or mediate treatment effects implicitly involves the ability to predict patient outcomes, whether it be future outcomes of currently treated patients or of a new patient yet to be treated. Moreover, prediction of future illness states is crucial in terms of individualized prevention or treatment of mood disorders. Joint models of longitudinal and time-to-event data are a class of statistical methods ideally suited for this task and deserve increased attention from researchers in the field.

DISCLOSURES

The authors have no disclosures to make. All three authors were supported by NIH grant P30MH090333.

REFERENCES

Anderson, J., & Senthilselvan, A. (1980). Smooth estimates for the hazard function. *Journal of the Royal Statistical Society Series B (Methodological)*, 42, 322–327.

Berger, J. O. (1985). *Statistical decision theory and Bayesian analysis*. New York: Springer–Verlag.

Berger, J. O. (2004). Does the Prentice criterion validate surrogate endpoints? *Statistics in Medicine*, 23, 1571–1578.

Box, G. E. P., & Tiao, G. (1973). *Bayesian inference in statistical analysis*. New York: Wiley.

Cannon, T. D., Cadenhead, K., Cornblatt, B., Woods, S. W., Addington, J., Walker, E., Heinssen, R. (2008). Prediction of psychosis in youth at high clinical risk: A multisite longitudinal study in North America. *Archives of General Psychiatry, 65*, 28–37.

Carter, J. W., Schulsinger, F., Parnas, J., Cannon, T., & Mednick, S. A. (2002). A multivariate prediction model of schizophrenia. *Schizophrenia Bulletin, 28*, 649–682.

Cox, D. R. (1972). Regression models and life-tables. *Journal of the Royal Statistical Society Series B (Methodological), 34*, 187–220.

Cox, D., & Hinkley, D. (1974). *Theoretical statistics*. London: Chapman & Hall.

Diggle, P. J., Heagerty, P. J., Liang, K-Y., & Zeger, S. L. (2002). *Longitudinal data analysis*. New York: Oxford University Press.

Diggle, P. J., Henderson, R., & Philipson, P. (2009). Random-effects models for joint analysis of repeated-measurment and time-to-event outcomes. In G. Fitzmaurice, M. Davidian, G. Verbeke, & M. Molenberghs (Eds.), *Longitudinal data analysis* (pp. 349–366). Boca Raton, FL: CRC Press.

Farewell, V. T. (1982). The use of mixture models for the analysis of survival data with long-term survivors. *Biometrics, 38*, 1041–1046.

Farewell, V. T. (1986). Mixture models in survival analysis: Are they worth the risk? *Canadian Journal of Statistics*, 14, 257–262.

Fichter, M. M., Quadflieg, N., & Rehm, J. (2003). Predicting the outcome of eating disorders using structural equation modeling *International Journal of Eating Disorders, 34*, 292–313.

Fieuws, S., & Verbeke, G. (2006). Pairwise fitting of mixed models for the joint modelling of multivariate longitudinal profiles. *Biometrics, 62*, 424–431.

Fieuws, S., Verbeke G., Maes, B., & Vanrenterghem, Y. (2008). Predicting renal graft failure using multivariate longitudinal profiles. *Biostatistics, 9*, 419–431.

Fitzmaurice, G., & Molenberghs, G. (2009). Advances in longitudinal data analysis: An historical persepctive. In G. Fitzmaurice, M. Davidian, G. Verbeke, & M. Molenberghs (Eds.), *Longitudinal data analysis* (pp. 3–30). Boca Raton, FL: CRC Press.

Garre, F. G., Zwinderman, A. H., Geskus, R. B., & Sijpkens, Y. W. J. (2008). A joint latent class change point model to improve the prediction of time to graft failure. *Journal of the Royal Statistical Society Series A, 171*, 299–308.

Gelman, A., & Hill, J. (2007). *Data analysis using regression and multilevel/hierarchical models*. New York: Cambridge University Press.

Hornik, K. (2011). *The R FAQ*. Retrieved October 2012, from http://CRAN.R-project.org/doc/FAQ/R-FAQ.html

Kalbfleisch, J., & Prentice, R. (2002). *The statistical analysis of failure time data* (2nd ed.). New York: Wiley.

Kendall, M. G., & Stuart, A. (1983). *The advanced theory of statistics, Vol. 2. Inference and relationship* (4th ed.). Ann Arbor, MI: MacMillan Press.

King, M., Marston, L., Švab, I., Maaroos, H. I., Geerlings, M. I., Xavier, M., Nazareth, I. (2011). Development and validation of a risk model for prediction of hazardous alcohol consumption in general practice attendees: The predictAL study. *PLoS One, 6*, e22175.

Kraemer, H. C., Stice, E., Kazdin, A., Offord, D., & Kupfer, D. (2001). How do risk factors work together? Mediators, moderators, and independent, overlapping, and proxy risk factors. *American Journal of Psychiatry, 158*, 848–856.

Kuk, A. Y. C., & Chen, C. H. (1992). A mixture model combining logistic regression with proportional hazards regression. *Biometrika, 79*, 531–541.

Law, N. J., Taylor, J. M. G., & Sandler, H. (2002). The joint modeling of a longitudinal disease progression marker and the failure time process in the presence of cure. *Biostatistics, 3*, 547–563.

Lee, P. (1997). *Bayesian statistics: An introduction*. New York: Wiley.

Leonard, T., & Hsu, J. S. J. (1999). *Bayesian methods: An analysis for statisticians and interdisciplinary researchers.* Cambridge, England: Cambridge University Press.

Li, C. S., Taylor, J. M. G., & Sy, J. P. (2001). Identifiability of cure models. *Statistics and Probability Letters, 54*, 389–395.

Lindley, D. V. (1971). *Bayesian statistics: A review.* Philadelphia, PA: Society for Industrial and Applied Mathematics.

Little, R. J. A. (1993). Pattern-mixture models for multivariate incomplete data. *Journal of the American Statistical Association, 88*, 125–134.

Marmarou, A., Lu, J., Butcher, I., McHugh, G. S., Murray, G. D., Steyerberg, E. W., Maas, A. I. (2007). Prognostic value of the Glasgow Coma Scale and pupil reactivity in traumatic brain injury assessed pre-hospital and on enrollment: An IMPACT analysis. *Journal of Neurotrauma, 24*, 270–80.

McCulloch, C. E., & Neuhaus, J. M. (2005). Generalized linear mixed models. In *Encyclopedia of biostatistics* (2nd ed., pp. 1–5). Published Online: 15 JUL 2005. John Wiley & Sons, Ltd.

Molenberghs, G., & Verbeke, G. (2005). *Models for discrete longitudinal data.* New York: Springer.

Muthen, L. K., & Muthen, B. O. (1998–2007). *Mplus users guide* (5th ed.). Los Angeles, CA: Muthen & Muthen.

Pauler, D. K., & Finkelstein, D. M. (2002). Predicting time to prostate cancer recurrence based on joint models for non-linear longitudinal biomarkers and event time outcomes. *Statistics in Medicine, 21*, 3897–3911.

Prentice, R. (1989). Surrogate endpoints in clinical trials: Definition and operation criteria. *Statistics in Medicine, 8*, 431–440.

Proust- Lima, C., & Taylor, J. M. G. (2009). Development and validation of a dynamic prognostic tool for prostate cancer recurrence using repeated measures of posttreatment PSA: A joint modeling approach. *Biostatistics, 10*, 535–549.

Rizopoulos, D. (2011). Dynamic predictions and prospective accuracy in joint models for longitudinal and time-to-event data *Biometrics, 67*(3), 819–829.

SAS 9.1.3 help and documentation. (2000–2004). Cary, NC: SAS Institute.

Skrondal, A., & Rabe-Hesketh, S. (2009). Prediction in multilevel generalized linear models. *Journal of the Royal Statistical Society, 172*(3), 659–687.

SPSS 15.0 command syntax reference. (2006)., Chicago, IL: SPSS Inc.

Stata statistical software: Release 12. (2011). College Station, TX: StataCorp LP.

Steyerberg, E. T. (2009). *Clinical prediction models.* New York: Springer.

Tanner, M. A., & Wong, W. H. (2010). From EM to data augmentation: The emergence of MCMC Bayesian computation in the 1980s. *Statistical Science, 25*(4), 506–516.

Taylor, J. M. G. (1995). Semi-parametric estimation in failure time mixture models. *Biometrics, 51*, 899–907.

Tsiatis, A. A., & Davidian, M. (2004). Joint modelling of longitudinal and time-to-event data: An overview. *Statistica Sinica, 14*, 809–834.

Wilson, P. W. F., D'Agostino, R. B., Levy, D., Belanger, A. M., Silbershatz, H., & Kannel, W. B. (1998). Prediction of coronary heart disease using risk factor categories. *Circulation, 97*, 1837–1847.

Yu, M., Law, N. J., Taylor, J. M. G., & Sandler, H. M. (2004). Joint longitudinal-survival-cure models and their application to prostate cancer. *Statistica Sinica, 14*, 835–862.

Yu, M., Taylor J. M., & Sandler H. M. (2004). *Individual prediction in prostate cancer studies using a joint longitudinal-survival-cure model.* The University of Michigan Department of Biostatistics Working Paper Series 2004. Ann Arbor: University of Michigan.

42

INTEGRATION OF BIOLOGICAL, CLINICAL, AND PSYCHOSOCIAL PREDICTORS OF TREATMENT RESPONSE VARIABILITY IN LATE-LIFE DEPRESSION

Linda Garand, Ellen M. Whyte, Meryl A. Butters, Elizabeth R. Skidmore, Jordan F. Karp, and Mary Amanda Dew

THREE PARAMETERS of key interest to clinicians and researchers in the treatment of depression are the degree of resolution of depression symptoms, the rapidity of treatment response, and the maintenance of symptom remission (Papakostas et al., 2008). Although safe and effective treatments for late-life depression (LLD) are available, their effects may be slow to occur, and remission may be incomplete and unstable (Alexopoulos, Buckwalter, et al., 2002; Mendlewicz, 2008). About half of the older adults who are treated for depression do not reach rapid and full symptom remission (Driscoll et al., 2005; Hybels, Blazer, & Steffens, 2005; Mitchell & Subramaniam, 2005), and they are at increased risk for medical comorbidity, symptom recurrence, increased health care utilization and mortality (Charlson et al., 2002; Frojdh, Hakansson, Karlsson, & Molarius, 2003). Conversely, depressed elderly patients who reach rapid and full symptom remission with treatment have a better level of psychosocial functioning (Hirschfield et al., 2002) than patients who are slow, partial, or nonremitters.

But how can we best predict which older adults are likely to show which pattern of response to depression treatment? Are some individuals likely to show a complete, rapid, and durable response to some types of treatment but not to others? The notion of personalized treatment for depression in late life hinges on answering these questions, and the present chapter reviews the full range of factors that—separately and in combination—may contribute to our ability to provide effective, personalized treatment.

CONCEPTUALIZATION OF FACTORS CONTRIBUTING TO DEPRESSION TREATMENT RESPONSE VARIABILITY

Potential predictors of treatment response variability can be conceptualized as falling into several domains (Fig. 42.1). They include biological, clinical, and psychosocial domains, the latter of which

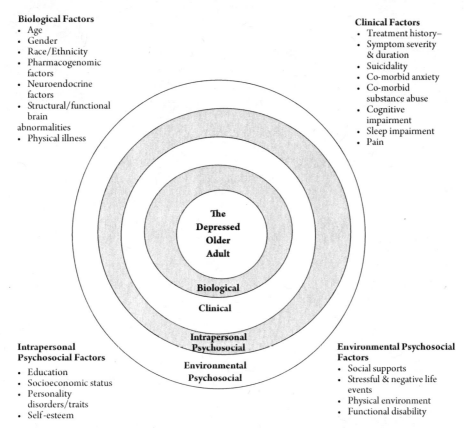

Biological Factors
- Age
- Gender
- Race/Ethnicity
- Pharmacogenomic factors
- Neuroendocrine factors
- Structural/functional brain abnormalities
- Physical illness

Clinical Factors
- Treatment history–
- Symptom severity & duration
- Suicidality
- Co-morbid anxiety
- Co-morbid substance abuse
- Cognitive impairment
- Sleep impairment
- Pain

The Depressed Older Adult

Biological

Clinical

Intrapersonal Psychosocial

Environmental Psychosocial

Intrapersonal Psychosocial Factors
- Education
- Socioeconomic status
- Personality disorders/traits
- Self-esteem

Environmental Psychosocial Factors
- Social supports
- Stressful & negative life events
- Physical environment
- Functional disability

FIGURE 42.1. Nested domains of potential predictors of treatment response variability in late life depression

can be divided into intrapersonal characteristics and environmental characteristics. These domains logically proceed from features most integral to the person (his or her biology) to features of the environment. The figure also illustrates the reality that these factors and their effects are entwined, despite the fact that most studies focus on their individual effects. In this chapter, we explore the relative impact of each of these sets of factors on older adults' response to treatment, and—when possible given available literature—we consider the factors' combined effects as well. We focus on their impact on the three key parameters of treatment response in geriatric depression: degree of depressive symptom resolution, the rapidity of treatment response, and/or the durability of symptom remission. We focus our review primarily on literature published since 2000.

Table 42.1 provides an overview and guide to the current state of knowledge regarding factors' influence on these outcomes. As shown in the table, and discussed further in the sections that follow, evidence for the factors' impact varies greatly.

Some factors are supported by relatively consistent evidence. For others, equivocal findings have been reported. There is even less evidence on the combined (additive or synergistic) effects of multiple factors. As we will discuss, although multivariable models have received the least attention to date in this field, they may be most important for the design of future studies to better understand treatment response variability. The chapter concludes with a summary of issues important for new research in this area as well as what the existing evidence suggests for optimal clinical care of patients.

Biological Factors

Among older adults, key biological attributes have been proposed as predictors or determinants of depression treatment response variability, including demographic characteristics (age, gender, race/ethnicity), genetic vulnerability, neuroendocrine factors, structural and functional brain abnormalities, and the presence of physical illness. Demographic factors are perhaps the most easily identified, yet

Table 42.1 Factors Affecting Response Variability in Late-Life Depression Treatment

	MAGNITUDE		SPEED		DURABILITY	
	EVIDENCE OF EFFECT	WHO IS LESS LIKELY TO RESPOND? ELDERS WITH:	EVIDENCE OF EFFECT	WHO RESPONDS MORE SLOWLY? ELDERS WITH:	EVIDENCE OF EFFECT	WHO HAS A MORE BRITTLE RESPONSE? ELDERS WITH:
Biological Factors						
Age	No	N/A	No	N/A	Yes	older age
Gender	?	?	?	?	NS	N/A
Race/ethnicity	No	N/A	No	N/A	NS	N/A
Pharmacogenomic factors	Yes	Certain genotypes	Yes	Certain genotypes	NS	N/A
Neuroendocrine factors	NS	N/A	NS	N/A	NS	N/A
Brain abnormalities	?	?	?	?	?	?
Physical illness	Yes	CVD	?	?	Yes	High medical burden
Clinical Factors						
Treatment history	Yes	Inadequate/failed or prior treatment for index episode	Yes	Inadequate/failed or prior treatment for index episode	NS	N/A
Severity and/or duration of symptoms	?	?	Yes	Severe and long-lasting symptoms	NS	N/A
Suicidality	?	?	Yes	Persistent ideation	Yes	Persistent ideation
Anxiety	Yes	Comorbid anxiety	Yes	Comorbid anxiety	Yes	Comorbid anxiety
Substance abuse	Yes	Alcohol abuse	NS	N/A	NS	N/A
Cognitive impairment	Yes	Executive dysfunction	?	?	Yes	Executive dysfunction

(Continued)

Table 42.1 (Continued)

	MAGNITUDE		SPEED		DURABILITY	
	EVIDENCE OF EFFECT	WHO IS LESS LIKELY TO RESPOND? ELDERS WITH:	EVIDENCE OF EFFECT	WHO RESPONDS MORE SLOWLY? ELDERS WITH:	EVIDENCE OF EFFECT	WHO HAS A MORE BRITTLE RESPONSE? ELDERS WITH:
Sleep impairment	Yes	Comorbid sleep impairment	No	N/A	Yes	Comorbid sleep impairment
Pain	Yes	Higher pain levels	No	N/A	NS	N/A
Intrapersonal Psychosocial Factors						
Educational level	?	?	No	N/A	NS	N/A
SES	Yes	Low SES	Yes	Low SES	NS	N/A
Personality disorders/traits	Yes	Neurotic traits	Yes	Cluster C personality disorders	NS	N/A
Self-esteem	Yes	Low self-esteem	Yes	Low self-esteem	NS	N/A
Environmental Psychosocial Factors						
Social support	Yes	Lower social support	Yes	Lower social support	Yes	Lower social support
Stressful life events	NS	N/A	NS	N/A	NS	N/A
Physical environment	NS	N/A	No	N/A	NS	N/A
Functional disability	?	?	NS	N/A	NS	N/A

Question marks indicate inconsistent evidence of treatment effects or equivocal findings. CVD, cerebrovascular disease; N/A, not applicable because there is no empirical evidence of an effect; NS, no studies have explored this effect; SES, socioeconomic status.

their impact on the prognosis of LLD has received surprisingly little attention. While comorbidities have long been important areas of investigation in late-life populations, studies focused on genetic or endocrine vulnerability, and structural/functional brain abnormalities are in their infancy and often show mixed results.

AGE

There is a long-standing belief that treatment response in LLD is slower and less complete than that in young and middle-aged adults. However, there is a growing body of evidence suggesting that this view may be inaccurate. For example, with respect to symptom resolution, Ell and colleagues (2010) recently pooled intent-to-treat data from three similarly designed randomized clinical trials of multidisciplinary collaborative care that incorporated problem-solving therapy and antidepressant medications, offered individually or in combination. They found no significant differences in the degree or speed of symptom reduction among patients aged 60 years or greater versus those aged 18 to 59 years. Similarly, a systematic review of the literature comparing older adults to middle-aged adults on prognosis for depression treatment concluded that these age groups showed similar levels of symptom resolution (Mitchell et al., 2005).

Even within elderly cohorts, there appears little evidence that the old-old show any less marked symptom reduction or any slower speed of response than younger-old adults (Dew et al., 2007; Gildengers et al., 2002; Reynolds et al., 1999a). In fact, Gildengers et al. (2002) found that the oldest patients (aged 76 and older) showed a slightly faster symptom reduction than the young-old (aged 59–69) and middle-old patients (aged 70–75). Meta-analytic and systematic reviews of empirical findings support the conclusion that within older cohorts, increasing age does not appear to adversely affect magnitude or speed of response to depression treatment (Pinquart, Duberstein, & Lyness, 2007; Whyte, et al., 2004).

In contrast, increasing age appears to have a negative impact on treatment response durability. For example, Reynolds and colleagues (1999a) found that 60% of patients aged 70 and older experienced a recurrence of symptoms during the first year of maintenance therapy compared to 30% of patients aged 60 to 69. This generally elevated risk for recurrence was also one of the key observations of the systematic review comparing outcomes in older versus middle-aged adults (Mitchell et al., 2005).

GENDER

The influence of gender on the course of LLD treatment remains poorly understood. One clinical trial among adult subjects found no gender differences in response to different classes of antidepressant drugs (Martenyi, Dossenbach, Mraz, & Metcalfe, 2001). In a larger prospective, observational, epidemiological study of 5,454 adults of all ages (mean age 53) receiving outpatient treatment with an selective serotonin reuptake inhibitor (SSRI), gender did not predict the magnitude or speed of recovery (Thiels, Linden, Grieger, & Leonard, 2005). Contrary to these finding, an exploratory analysis of 1,500 outpatients aged 18 to 75 initially treated with an SSRI in the STAR-D trial (Sequenced Treatment Alternatives to Relieve Depression) showed that women had a significantly slower depression treatment response than men when age was controlled (Marcus et al., 2005).

The inconsistencies in gender-specific antidepressant treatment response across studies have led investigators to examine the influence of sex hormones rather than gender per se. Results of several studies suggest that women are less responsive to SSRIs during their peri- and postmenopausal years than during their younger, reproductive years (Grigoriadis, Kennedy, & Bagby, 2003; Kornstein et al., 2000; Martenyi et al., 2001). However, these studies assumed the women's menstrual status based on their age, not the prolonged cessation of the menstrual cycle. When examined in relation to actual menstrual status, Pinto-Meza and associates (2006) found that postmenopausal women (i.e., women with no menstrual cycle for at least 1 year) had slower responses to SSRI treatment than either nonmenopausal women or men. These results suggest that it is menopausal status, rather than gender alone, that affects speed of depressive symptom reduction. Even so, for subgroups of depressed older adults—for example, those who require augmentation pharmacotherapy due to poor initial response to treatment—there is little evidence that gender affects rate or speed of recovery (Dew et al., 2007). Whether gender affects response durability remains unknown.

RACE/ETHNICITY

Racial or ethnic group membership may influence the use of, or access to, mental health treatment for depression, yet we have no evidence that, once in treatment, individuals' race or ethnicity influence treatment outcomes in LLD. Among the general (all ages) population, a review of depression treatment studies suggests no differences in outcomes among persons of various racial or ethnic backgrounds (Schraufnagel, Wagner, Miranda, & Roy-Byrne, 2005). In late life, findings from the Improving Mood-Promoting Access to Collaborative Treatment (IMPACT) study are particularly noteworthy. The IMPACT study evaluated outcomes of treatment (which consisted of stepped care with both medications and problem-solving therapy [PST]) among a large, ethnically diverse, low-income sample of elderly primary care clinics patients across five states. Results indicated comparable levels of symptom improvement and remission rates in European American versus African American and Latino patients (Areán et al., 2005). This study, as well as those reviewed by Schraufnagel et al. (2005), suggests that individualized treatment that is designed to meet patients' specific needs and preferences is equally effective in treating depressed ethnic minorities. No data exist on response durability as a function of race/ethnicity.

PHARMACOGENOMIC FACTORS

The field of pharmacogenomics is in its infancy. To date, the few studies that have examined the influence of genes on treatment outcome in LLD have selected candidate genes based on either the presumed mechanism of action of an antidepressant or on the unique association of LLD with specific medical illnesses.

Serotonin Transporter Gene (SLC6A4) Promoter Region Polymorphism (5-HTTLPR)

The serotonin transporter (5-HT) is the principal site of initial action for several antidepressants, most prominently the SSRIs. The serotonin transporter gene (SLC6A4) contains an insertion/deletion polymorphism within its promoter (5HTTLPR) that influences transcriptional efficiency and activity (Heils et al., 1996; Lesch et al., 1996). Specifically, the "short" repeat polymorphism (e.g., the S allele) is associated with decreased transcription of the transporter protein and decreased serotonin reuptake

compared to the "long" repeat polymorphism (e.g., the L allele; Heils et al., 1996).

In LLD, carriers of the S allele experience a slower initial response to treatment with an SSRI antidepressant but ultimately are as likely to respond to a trial of a SSRI antidepressant as individuals homozygous for the allele (Durham, Webb, Milos, Clary, & Seymour, 2004; Pollock et al., 2000). This polymorphism is not associated with speed of initial response to antidepressants that do not depend on serotonin transporter protein blockade (Pollock et al., 2000). Furthermore, there is evidence that serum drug concentration is influenced by genotype (Lotrich, Pollock, Kirshner, Ferrell, & Reynolds, 2008), suggesting that persons carrying an S allele may require higher medication doses to achieve a response. Unfortunately, S allele carriers appear to be at greater risk of SSRI side effects and early drug discontinuation compared to persons not carrying the S allele (Murphy, Hollander, Rodrigues, Kremer, & Schatzberg (2004). Hence, this polymorphism may also contribute to poor drug response through a negative effect on drug tolerability (Gerretsen et al., 2008).

DAT1 VNTR 10/10 Polymorphism

Adding methylphenidate to standard antidepressant treatment (typically an SSRI) to accelerate treatment response (Lavretsky, Park, Siddarth, Kumar, & Reynolds, 2006) is an attractive idea because methylphenidate blocks dopamine reuptake at the dopamine transporter (Bannon, Michelhaugh, Wang, & Sacchetti, 2001), especially in the mesolimbic dopaminergic projections (Willner, 1997). In a small study comparing an SSRI plus methylphenidate versus SSRI plus placebo in the treatment of LLD, individuals homozygous for the 480-bp allele (VNTR 10/10) in the human dopamine transporter (DAT1) gene demonstrated a faster response to combined SSRI and methylphenidate treatment than persons with other genotypes also exposed to methylphenidate. The DAT1 VNTR 10/10 polymorphism was not associated with time to response in individuals who received SSRI plus placebo (Lavretsky, Siddarth, Kumar, & Reynolds, 2008).

Brain-Derived Neurotrophic Factor Val66Met Polymorphism

Although antidepressants acutely affect the monoamine neurotransmitter(s), the actual antidepressant effect may be due to longer term effects on neurogenesis, plasticity, and modulation of signal transduction and gene expression (Duman et al., 2006; Manji, Drevets, & Charney, 2001). Hence, brain-derived neurotrophic factor (BDNF) has received considerable attention due to its role in synaptic plasticity, repair, and connectivity (Escobar, Figueroa-Guzman, & Gomez-Palacio-Schjetnan, 2003, Nagappan et al., 2005; Poo, 2001).

The Val66Met (rs6265) is a functional polymorphism in the coding region of the BDNF gene that results in a valine (Val) to methionine (Met) substitution in the 5′ prodomain of the human BDNF protein (Neves-Pereira et al., 2002). This polymorphism affects the intracellular distribution, packaging, and release of the BDNF protein in vitro, and in humans, this polymorphism has significant effects on verbal episodic memory and hippocampal activity (Egan et al., 2003).

In late life, carriers of the Met66 allele have increased risk of depression (Taylor et al., 2011). Interestingly, however, the Met66 allele was associated with an increased rate of response in an 8-week antidepressant trial in a Korean population (Choi, Kang, Lim, Oh, & Lee, 2006). Additionally, Met66 allele carriers were more likely to achieve remission after 6 months of treatment compared to Val66 homozygous individuals (Taylor et al., 2011). These findings support a role for BDNF in LLD treatment response, but these preliminary studies must be followed by more in-depth studies to more fully understand the specific nature of the effect of the Met66 allele on treatment response variability.

Angiotensin II Receptor, Vascular Type 1 (AGTR1) A1166C Polymorphism

Unique to late life is the association of cerebrovascular disease (CVD) and late-onset depression (Alexopoulos et al., 2011). Hence, genetic polymorphisms that are associated with CVD may also be associated with late-onset depression. Angiotensin II is an important hormone of the renin-angiotensin system that regulates blood pressure and volume homeostasis. The gene angiotensin II receptor, vascular type 1 (AGTR1) codes for a G protein–coupled cell surface receptor that is believed to mediate the cardiovascular effects of angiotensin II (Murphy, Alexander, Griendling, Runge, & Bernstein, 1991). The A1166C polymorphism is associated with several cardiovascular disorders, including ischemic stroke (Rubattu et al., 2004) and essential hypertension (Bonnardeaux et al., 1994) with the C/C homozygote persons being most severely affected.

Consistent with the hypothesis that CVD can modify the presentation of and treatment responsiveness of LLD, in a large, prospective cohort study in which patients with LLD received individualized treatment using a standardized algorithm, individuals with AGTR1 homozygous C/C status were less likely to respond to treatment than those with other allelic configurations (Kondo et al., 2007). No studies have yet examined the influence of genetic factors on the durability of depression treatment response in older adults. Furthermore, pharmacogenetic study findings have not been translated into clinical practice.

NEUROENDOCRINE FACTORS

Neuroendocrine systems, including those associated with the thyroid gland, the hypothalamic–pituitary–adrenal axis, inflammation, and testosterone production, have been etiologically linked to depression. These associations have led to investigations of novel agents as depression therapies (e.g., testosterone replacement), none of which have firmly established efficacy. No studies have been conducted to examine the effects of neuroendocrine factors in the context of treating LLD. However, studies in mixed-age samples (some of which included older adults) are informative to consider.

HPA Axis

The hypothalamus–pituitary–adrenocortical (HPA) axis has long been implicated in the underlying pathophysiology of major depression across the life span. Acutely depressed persons have been shown to have impaired regulation of the HPA system (e.g., failure to suppress cortisol production during the dexamethasone suppression test) compared to healthy controls across the life span; however, this finding is inconsistent (Stetler & Miller, 2011). Normalization of some aspects of HPA function (specifically the release of adrenal androgen dehydroepiandrosterone [DHEA] together with its sulfated conjugate, DHEA-S) is correlated with response to treatment in LLD (Fabian et al., 2001). Recently, interest has focused on whether this "normalization" of the HPA function predicts long-term outcome of antidepressant treatment. Studies of mixed-aged samples suggest that failure to normalize HPA during successful antidepressant treatment predicts eventual relapse (Appelhof et al., 2004; Zobel et al., 2001).

Inflammation

Several lines of evidence implicate inflammation in the pathophysiology of major depression (Maes, 2011). Recently, it has been hypothesized that inflammation may have a unique contribution to LLD based on several age-related immune changes, including increased peripheral immune responses, impaired peripheral-central nervous system immune communication, and a shift of the brain into a pro-inflammatory state. These age-related changes in inflammation may predispose to geriatric depression (Alexpoulos et al., 2011). This hypothesis would suggest that markers of inflammation may predict treatment response. The role of pro-inflammatory cytokines as markers of treatment response in LLD has not been investigated. However, a few small studies, generally in mixed-aged samples, found that elevated IL-6 levels and increased TNF-alpha levels at baseline were associated with reduced likelihood of responding to treatment with an SSRI antidepressant (Janssen, Caniato, Verster, & Baune, 2010).

Thyroid Hormones

The use of the thyroid hormone triiodothyronine (T3) to accelerate treatment response or to treat refractory depression is a long-standing clinical practice. The use of T3 is based upon its ability to desensitize the serotonin inhibitory 5-hydroxytryptamine1a autoreceptor, leading to increased serotonergic neurotransmission (Bauer, Heinz, & Whybrow, 2002; Moreau, Jeanningros, & Mazzola-Pomietto, 2001). A meta-analysis of studies in mixed-aged samples concluded that T3 augmentation increases speed of response when combined with tricyclic antidepressants (TCAs; Altshuler et al., 2001). However, a study investigating the use of T3 combined with an SSRI antidepressant found no evidence of an accelerated response in a midlife sample (Appelhof et al., 2004).

Testosterone

The age-related decline in testosterone secretion in men (Gray, Feldman, McKinlay, & Longcope, 1991) is of particular interest in geriatric psychiatry because hypogonadism is associated with depression, anxiety, irritability, insomnia, and cognitive impairment (Sternbach, 1998). Hence, testosterone replacement may be beneficial in the treatment of depressive symptoms. One small study supported this hypothesis in older men with hypogonadism with subthreshold depression (Shores, Kivlahan, Sadak, Li, & Matsumoto, 2009). Another small study in midlife indicated that testosterone augmentation was useful in the treatment of treatment refractory depression in men with low/borderline-low testosterone levels (Pope, Cohane, Kanayama, Siegel, & Hudson, 2003). However, these results were not replicated in a larger subsequent study, and no correlation between improvement in depression symptoms and increase (improvement) in serum total testosterone levels was observed (Pope et al., 2010).

STRUCTURAL AND FUNCTIONAL BRAIN ABNORMALITIES

Characterizing structural brain abnormalities associated with LLD has been a growing focus of research over the past decade. However, few studies have examined whether brain abnormalities are related to treatment response among older adults. This is surprising since LLD is associated with reduced volume of regional gray matter and the presence of vascular lesions in the white matter and basal ganglia, each of which may interfere with treatment response.

Results of studies examining relationships between cerebral gray matter volume and pharmacotherapy response depend on the area of the brain examined. An early study found that higher global ventricular-brain ratio on computerized tomography (CT) scan was associated with poorer response to the TCA nortriptyline (Young, Kalayam, Nambudiri, Kakuma, & Alexopoulos, 1999). All subsequent imaging studies have employed magnetic resonance imaging (MRI) to measure brain structure and response to SSRI pharmacotherapy; not all of them have replicated the finding that reduced volume is associated with worse response.

Investigators surveying volumes of large, broadly distributed regions found that lower volume of the frontotemporal lobes was associated with greater treatment resistance (Simpson, Baldwin, Burns, & Jackson, 2001). Hsieh and colleagues (2002) examined hippocampal volume and found that lower right, as well as bilateral volume, was associated with lower remission rate. In a study focusing on anterior cingulate and subgenual cortex volumes, Gunning and colleagues (2009) found that reduced volume of the former, but not the latter, was associated with nonresponse. Another study showed that higher ratings of Virchow-Robin dilatation (a measure of cerebrospinal fluid spaces associated with microangiopathy of small cerebral vessels) in the corona radiat was associated with worse symptom course over 3 years (Baldwin et al., 2004). Lastly, Patankar et al. (2007) found higher ratings of basal ganglia Virchow-Robin dilatation in individuals who did not, compared with those who did, respond to antidepressant pharmacotherapy. In contrast to these studies, a study assessing global gray matter volumes found no difference in any cerebral gray matter structures between individuals who did and did not respond to pharmacotherapy (Janssen et al., 2007). Similarly, Baldwin and colleagues (2004) found no difference in cerebral atrophy in groups of individuals who did or did not respond to antidepressant pharmacotherapy.

Equivocal findings are also evident among studies examining whether the structural integrity of cerebral white matter influences LLD treatment response. In two studies, Alexopoulos and colleagues (Alexopolus, Kiosses, et al., 2002; Alexopoulos et al., 2008) found that reduced fractional anisotropy measured with diffusion tensor imaging (representing microstructural white matter abnormalities) was associated with poorer antidepressant response rates. However, Taylor and colleagues (2008) found just the opposite: Increased fractional anisotropy, or superior integrity of the white matter, was associated with poorer treatment response. They concluded that the discrepant findings may have been due to differences in methods, sample sizes, or pathophysiologic heterogeneity of LLD.

Studies examining whether white matter lesion load or volume influences LLD treatment response also have yielded discrepant findings. Baldwin and colleagues (2004) found that nonresponse to antidepressant treatment was associated with greater volume of periventricular white matter hyperintensities (based on semiquantitative ratings), but not with lesions in other brain regions (including subcortical frontal areas). A study that employed objective quantitative measures of white matter lesions also showed that individuals with more white matter lesion volume were less likely to respond to antidepressant treatment (Gunning-Dixon et al., 2010). Furthermore, Patankar and colleagues (2007) assessed white matter hyperintensities with semiquantitative ratings of severity and found that individuals who failed to respond to pharmacotherapy tended to have more white matter lesion load than those who responded. Baldwin and colleagues (2000) examined the relationship between MRI abnormalities in individuals with LLD and subsequent 3-year symptom course. They found that hyperintense lesions in the pons were associated with worse clinical course. Taylor et al (2008) found that greater increase in white matter hyperintensity volume over their 2-year study period was associated with failure to sustain remission. In contrast, other studies have found no effects on response to antidepressant pharmacotherapy (Janssen et al., 2007; Sneed et al., 2007).

There are very few studies of brain function in LLD and even fewer that have examined associations with treatment response. In an early study, Kalayam and Alexopoulos (1999) found that long P300 latencies (a measure of prefrontal lobe function) assessed with auditory evoked potentials was associated with both delayed and poor response to antidepressant pharmacotherapy. They subsequently assessed event-related potentials in an emotional go/no go task that activates the rostral anterior cingulate. Individuals who remained symptomatic after treatment had larger error-related negativity and smaller error positivity amplitude compared with those who achieved remission (Alexopoulos et al., 2007). These data suggest that two distinct conflict-processing functions of the anterior cingulate are important for antidepressant response in LLD (Alexopoulos et al., 2007).

PHYSICAL ILLNESS

There are several ways to examine the impact of the medical illness on degree, speed, and maintenance of response to treatment in LLD. These include examining the effect of the overall burden of medical illness (e.g., such as a count of comorbid medical diagnoses), as well as considering the possible effects of specific medical illnesses.

In general, the overall burden of comorbid medical illness is not associated with either the likelihood or the speed of response to antidepressant treatment among subjects enrolled in studies of LLD treatment (Nelson et al., 2007; Whyte et al., 2004). However, Dew and colleagues (2007) found that medical illness burden did predict slower treatment response among persons who failed an initial trial of antidepressant therapy and who were subsequently treated using an augmentation strategy. Furthermore, overall medical burden predicted a brittle long-term course of LLD after remission. Specifically, Reynolds and colleagues found in a randomized controlled trial of maintenance pharmacologic and psychotherapy for LLD that older persons with a greater number and severity of medical illness are more likely to experience a relapse of their depressive illness while on

SSRI monotherapy compared to persons with less medical burden (Reynolds et al., 2006).

The patterns of effects of medical illness burden on long-term response to treatment likely arise because medical illness burden may best be considered as a proxy measure of functional disability. Functional disability and depression have a reciprocal and reinforcing relationship (Bruce, 2001). Hence, persons with the greatest burden of medical illness likely have the greatest degree of functional disability; it is this degree of disability, with its associated negative impact of independence, self-image, and social relationships, which make long-term management of depression challenging.

The relationship of specific diseases and treatment response in LLD has also been investigated. Typically, investigators have examined the effects of cerebrovascular risk factors and CVD. CVD, as a proxy for vascular disease in general, has been found associated with a decreased rate of response to open-label antidepressant monotherapy, even after controlling for the presence of impaired executive function (Alexopoulos, Kiosses, Murphy, & Heo, 2004). In contrast, risk factors for CVD have consistently been shown not to be associated with treatment response (Oslin et al., 2002). For example, in a study of older persons with depression, an elevated burden of CVD risk factors was not associated with likelihood of response, time to remission, or risk of recurrence during maintenance treatment (Miller et al., 2002). The association between CVD and acute treatment response is likely explained in large part by the impact of CVD on specific brain regions and circuits thought to be associated with mood regulation (as noted in the section on "Pharmacogenomic Factors"). Hence, the location of the cerebrovascular insult, and not the disease process itself, may be the critical link to depression treatment variability.

SUMMARY

Of the biological factors considered, certain genotypes and physical illness influence the magnitude of treatment response, and there is growing evidence that genotypes play a role in speed of response. There is no evidence that advanced age or the race of older adults negatively impacts the magnitude or speed of treatment response. However, advanced age and higher medical burden negatively impact the durability of treatment response. For the remainder of the biological variables that we considered, either studies show equivocal results or there is as yet

no evidence regarding effects on LLD treatment response. In particular, we have little understanding of the influence of neuroendocrine factors on LLD treatment outcomes. Furthermore, few studies have considered the role of any biologic factors in the context of nonpharmacologic (in contrast to pharmacologic) therapies.

Clinical Factors

A range of clinical factors are associated with treatment outcomes in LLD. Like most biologic factors, clinical factors such as treatment history, symptom severity, and duration are characteristics that cannot be modified. However, although they themselves may not be amenable to intervention, their effects on treatment response must be understood to identify which patients may, for example, require pharmacologic augmentation or more intensive psychosocial interventions and/or support to reach desired therapeutic outcomes. On the other hand, clinical factors such as cognitive or sleep impairment, pain, comorbid anxiety or substance abuse, and suicidality may themselves be targeted for intervention in order to facilitate improvements in treatment outcomes among older adults with depression.

TREATMENT HISTORY

There is consistent evidence that receipt of past treatment for a given episode of depression, and the quality of that treatment, influences both the overall magnitude and speed of response to additional acute treatment for the LLD. For example, Tew and colleagues (2006) retrospectively examined the treatment history of depressed older adults who entered acute treatment before being randomized in a maintenance therapy trial (Reynolds et al., 1999b). Persons who had not received any pharmacological treatment during the index episode of major depression (e.g., "treatment-naïve") were more likely to respond to pharmacologic treatment than those who, during the index episode, either had failed an adequate trial of pharmacotherapy or had received an "inadequate" trial of pharmacotherapy (i.e., the maximum prescribed dose was less than the generally accepted therapeutic range for a specific drug or the duration of pharmacotherapy was less than 4 weeks at a therapeutic dose). Prior treatment experience remained a strong predictor of treatment outcomes even when other putative predictors of treatment outcomes were examined, including duration and severity of index episode, burden of medical illness, and presence of cognitive impairment. Furthermore, those individuals naïve to treatment experienced a faster response than those who had failed a previous adequate trial of pharmacotherapy.

This finding is consistent with that of Dew and colleagues (2007), who examined the subset of the Tew et al. cohort who went on to demonstrate "treatment resistance," that is, they failed to respond during acute treatment with antidepressant monotherapy or relapsed after an early response to treatment. These individuals were subsequently treated using an augmentation strategy. Although a majority recovered, they were less likely to do so than were individuals not requiring augmentation. In addition, individuals who received augmentation because they did not respond to the initial monotherapy trial experienced a slower time to response compared to those persons who received augmentation because of failure to maintain their initial response to monotherapy.

In sum, older adults who have required previous treatment for their major depression, those whose treatment was inadequate, and, in particular, those who have failed to respond to an adequate trial of treatment for depression are at heightened risk for a slow or poor response to additional depression treatment. It should be noted that these effects have been examined primarily in the context of pharmacologic treatment; whether they apply to psychotherapeutic treatment strategies remains unknown. In addition, studies have focused on past treatment for the index episode, and treatment history for previous episodes may also affect response to treatment for the new episode. Finally, among older adults who do respond to treatment, it is not yet known whether treatment history predicts whether recovery will be sustained in the long term.

SYMPTOM SEVERITY AND DURATION OF CURRENT EPISODE

The majority of studies demonstrate that older adults with more severe depressive symptoms at baseline require a longer period of treatment before demonstrating a response, a finding paralleled in the midlife literature (Whyte et al., 2004). Despite the slower speed of response, the severity of symptoms at baseline may not have a strong impact on whether an individual ultimately responds to treatment. A few studies have reported a negative effect

on response rate, but these studies were generally of short duration (e.g., 6 weeks) (Ackerman, Greenland, Bystritsky, & Small, 2000; Saghafi et al., 2007). Given their slower speed of response, those subjects with high baseline symptom burden might have met response criteria if the trial length had been longer. Indeed, this was seen in the Dew et al. (2007) study of treatment-resistant older adults receiving augmentation therapy. They found that symptom severity was not associated with ultimate response.

Episode duration is also an index of depression severity. Duration of a given episode of LLD appears to bear only a small, nonsignificant relationship to acute treatment response (Dew et al., 2007; Saghafi et al., 2007). Duration has not been investigated as a predictor of speed of response, and neither duration nor baseline symptom severity has been examined in relation to the success of maintenance treatment.

SUICIDALITY

Suicidal patients are often excluded from depression treatment studies due to safety concerns. This is unfortunate since suicidality may play a role in variable treatment responses in LLD. The small number of studies conducted to date show mixed results. For example, among depressed older adults followed during standardized open treatment with pharmacotherapy (Reynolds et al., 1999b), suicidal and nonsuicidal patients had almost identical remission rates and similar average times to remission (Szanto et al., 2001). However, the patients with suicidal ideation had higher relapse rates during continuation treatment. In contrast, in older primary care patients enrolled in the PROSPECT study (Prevention of Suicide in Primary Care Elderly; Collaborative Trail, Boa et al., 2011), patients with suicidal ideation had significantly lower rates of remission than nonsuicidal patients (Alexopoulos, Katz, et al., 2005).

The course of suicidal ideation during treatment may account for the inconsistent findings across these two reports. Specifically, Szanto and colleagues (2007) examined treatment outcomes among older adults receiving open treatment with either medications alone or combined pharmacologic and psychotherapy interventions. They found that depressed elderly patients with emergent or persistent suicidal ideation had slower rates of remission and higher relapse rates than either patients with no suicidal ideation or patients whose suicidality had resolved.

COMORBID ANXIETY

Nearly 50% of community-dwelling older adults endorse comorbid depression and anxiety symptoms or the presence of lifetime or current diagnosable anxiety disorder (Beckman et al., 2000). Most recent studies suggest that the presence of comorbid anxiety (either during the depressive episode or earlier in life) reduces the magnitude and speed of treatment response, and it may shorten the durability of treatment effects. Cohen and associates (2009) pooled data from the open-label, nonrandomized phases of two trials of maintenance therapies for LLD and found that preexisting anxiety symptoms levels predicted a lower likelihood of treatment response independent of other factors' effects. Similarly, secondary analysis of the PROSPECT study data showed that patients with high levels of self-reported anxiety symptoms had significantly lower remission rates than remaining patients (Alexopoulos, Katz, et al., 2005).

Several reports have shown that older depressed adults with elevated anxiety symptoms or a comorbid anxiety disorder have a delayed response (from 1 to 5 weeks) to antidepressant medications, compared to individuals without anxiety (Dew et al., 1997, 2007; Flint et al., 1997, Lenze et al., 2002; Mulsant, Reynolds, Shear, Sweet, & Miller, 1996). Steffens and McQuoid (2005a) showed that anxiety disorders predicted a significantly longer time to remission in a naturalistic study of LLD treatment response.

Similar results are found in the few studies that have examined the effects of premorbid anxiety on the outcomes of psychotherapy or combined medication and psychosocial treatment for LLD. Gum and associates (2006) found that depressed older adults with comorbid anxiety symptoms had higher depression scores than nonanxious depressed patients after 6 months of treatment. Pretreatment anxiety was also found to be associated with lower rates and longer time to remission of depression among older adults who partially responded to acute treatment and were subsequently randomized to receive augmentation (Greenlee et al., 2010).

One exception to this pattern of effects is reported in a secondary analysis conducted by Lenze et al. (2003). They failed to find that either anxiety symptom levels or comorbid anxiety disorders were associated with time to response to either paroxetine or nortriptyline in two LLD randomized clinical trials. The results may have been influenced

by the fact that subjects in both trials received antidepressant dose adjustments based on their clinical response and they received lorazepam as needed. This interpretation is supported by a study showing that the co-prescription of a benzodiazepine during treatment for LLD significantly increases a patient's likelihood of response (Buysse et al., 1997). This suggests that aggressive treatment of both the depression and the anxiety may overcome any negative effects of comorbid anxiety.

Two studies have explored the effects of comorbid anxiety symptoms on the durability of LLD treatment response. Secondary analyses of a randomized trial of maintenance therapies showed that both pretreatment and residual anxiety symptoms predict depression recurrence (Andreescu et al., 2007; Dombrovski et al., 2007).

SUBSTANCE ABUSE

Both drug and alcohol abuse in mixed-age populations worsen depression and interfere with response to antidepressant pharmacotherapy (Davis et al., 2006; Rae, Joyce, Luty, & Mulder, 2002; Watkins, Paddock, Zhang, & Wells, 2006). Benzodiazepines and opioids, both central nervous system depressants, are the most commonly abused prescription drugs in older adults (Gallo & Lebowitz, 1999). However, the most commonly abused substance in late life, especially among those with depression, is alcohol (Devanand, 2002). Therefore, in this chapter we focus on the effect of beverage alcohol on antidepressant treatment response.

Up to 20% of older adults regularly drink in excess of recommended guidelines (i.e., no more than three drinks on any given day or seven drinks per week) and can be considered at-risk drinkers (Blow & Barry, 2000; Meier et al., 2008). In a group of mixed-age adults, the degree of alcohol consumption prior to beginning pharmacologic treatment for depression was a significant predictor of weaker treatment response, even after adjusting for severity of depression at baseline (Worthington et al., 1996). Similar findings have been obtained in older adults. For example, Oslin (2005) found that older patients with major depression comorbid with alcohol dependence have lower treatment response rates and higher treatment costs than non-alcohol-dependent patients.

Studies have not yet been designed to explore the influence of alcohol abuse or dependence (or other drug abuse or dependence) on the speed or durability of LLD treatment response. This will be an important area of future investigation. The work of Oslin, Katz, and colleagues (2000) suggests that even a modest reduction in alcohol consumption improves pharmacologic treatment response. This points to the importance of screening for and ongoing attention to a use reduction in the treatment of LLD.

NEUROPSYCHOLOGICAL FACTORS

Cognitive impairment is highly prevalent in LLD (Butters et al., 2004; Sheline et al., 2006) and tends to persist beyond remission (Bhalla et al, 2006; Murphy & Alexopoulos, 2004; Nebes et al., 2003). Whether cognitive impairment that accompanies a depressive episode predicts treatment response is understudied, but the evidence suggests that neuropsychological dysfunction in general, and especially in executive functions, predicts poor treatment response. Recent studies have focused on response to pharmacologic intervention, and the vast majority of these have focused on the magnitude of treatment response rather than either speed of response or relapse/recurrence. Next we consider effects as a function of the breadth and depth of the cognitive domains that have been examined.

Steffens et al. (2006) examined data from a large geriatric depression intervention trial in primary care patients in which cognitive function was measured with a screener designed primarily to detect dementia. Screener scores were not associated with treatment response. However, the measure may have been insensitive to differences that are either relatively small or lie in specific domains of cognition.

Alexopoulos and colleagues have focused a series of studies exclusively on executive function, as assessed by the Initiation/Perseveration subscale of the Dementia Rating Scale (DRS; Mattis, 1988). They report that impaired executive function predicted poor and delayed treatment response among subjects receiving TCAs (Kalayam et al., 1999). They also found that poor Initiation/Perseveration performance was associated with slow (Alexopoulos et al., 2007), incomplete (Alexopoulos et al., 2007; Murphy & Alexopolous, 2004), and nonresponse to antidepressant treatment with either SSRIs or serotonin-norepinephrine reuptake inhibitors (SNRIs).

Impaired executive function is also associated with early relapse and recurrence (Murphy &

Alexopolous, 2004). Sneed et al. (2008) examined performance on the Stroop Color-Word Interference Test (a widely used measure of response inhibition, considered to be an executive function) and found that it predicted antidepressant treatment response. Sneed et al. (2007) found similar results: Deficient response inhibition led to poorer response to antidepressants (compared with placebo). They concluded that there may be a deleterious interaction between deficient response inhibition and antidepressants, and that the mechanism of SSRI and placebo response is different.

Additional studies have examined whether executive function is selectively associated with treatment response or whether performance in other neuropsychological domains, or cognitive function more generally, are also predictors. For example, Alexopoulos et al. (2000) found that over a 2-year postintervention follow-up period, the baseline scores of the DRS Initiation/Perseveration subscale, but not the Memory Subscale, predicted fluctuations of depressive symptoms as well as relapse and recurrence of major depression. Similar findings based on other cognitive assessment measures have been reported elsewhere (Morimoto et al., 2011; Murphy & Alexopolous, 2004).

Other studies have attempted to dissociate executive function from other cognitive domains more broadly, by comparing performance on an executive measure with that on screening measures of other domains. For example, in a study examining subscales of the DRS as well the Stroop Color Word Interference Test, Alexopoulos, Kiosses, et al. (2005) found that poorer performance on both the Initiation/Perseveration subscale and the Stroop, but not performance on other DRS subscales, were associated with poor antidepressant treatment response. However, in a report examining relapse and recurrence in two independent antidepressant pharmacotherapy trials, Butters et al. (2004) found that neither overall performance on the DRS nor performance on the Initiation/Perseveration subscale was associated with either relapse or recurrence.

Four studies have employed broad-based measures of multiple cognitive domains, thus providing a more complete test of whether various domains are particularly sensitive predictors of treatment response. Baldwin et al. (2004) found that measures indicating impaired visuospatial ability, language, and executive function were associated with antidepressant treatment nonresponse. Potter et al. (2004) employed a battery with basic measures of attention, processing speed, and multiple measures of executive function and found that attention and perseverative responding were associated with poorer response. Taylor et al. (2008) found that better processing speed and episodic memory were associated with better treatment response and that mental flexibility did not predict response, while Sneed et al. (2007) found that processing speed was related to speed of response but, otherwise, no task or domain other than response inhibition measured with the Stroop predicted treatment response.

In sum, although there are some studies in which executive functioning was not associated with treatment response, as well as some that suggest that other domains predict treatment response, on the whole, findings generally suggest that poorer executive functioning is associated with poorer antidepressant treatment response and that it may be associated with poorer response durability as well. However, more often than not, studies have employed either measures of executive function exclusively or very limited, insensitive measures of other neuropsychological domains. Future studies should employ sensitive measures of broad-based domains, especially episodic memory and information processing speed, to fully confirm the specificity of the executive function–treatment response relationship.

SLEEP IMPAIRMENT

Depression may lead to disruption of normal sleep patterns as reflected in the inclusion of sleep impairment as a diagnostic feature of major depression across the life span. For older adults, sleep disturbance is also a risk factor for both for incident and recurrent depressive episodes (Buysse, 2004; Cole et al., 2003; Kim et al., 2009; Perlis et al., 2006). While the pathways underlying this reciprocal relationship are complex and unknown, the neurocircuitry responsible for mood and sleep is highly connected, leading to the hypothesis that an underlying neurodegenerative disorder could lead to the presentation of both insomnia and LLD (Naismith et al., 2009).

Studies consistently show that sleep impairment is associated with LLD treatment response. During acute treatment of LLD, the presence of subjectively reported "poor sleep" in the context of little early response to antidepressant treatment by week 4 predicts a low likelihood of antidepressant response by week 12 (Andreescu et al., 2008). Similarly, during maintenance treatment, the presence of subjectively

reported (Dombrovski, 2007) as well as objectively measured (Buysse et al., 1996) sleep impairment predicts recurrence of LLD, independent of ongoing maintenance antidepressant therapy. In the context of other predictors of recurrence during maintenance treatment, the presence of poor subjective sleep, but not residual mood symptoms, predicts recurrence (Dombrovski, 2007).

PAIN

While patients rarely present to mental health professionals for the management of pain, mental health practitioners frequently care for patients with comorbid pain and psychiatric disorders. Due to the common co-occurrence of psychiatric, cognitive, and functional disability associated with persistent pain, in this chapter we focus on the relationship between depression treatment response and pain that is chronic (i.e., of at least a 3- to 6-month duration).

In a secondary analysis of 1,801 depressed older adults enrolled in the IMPACT trial, Thielke et al. (2007) observed that higher pain levels differentially impaired response magnitude. Others have found that high levels of pain severity (Karp et al., 2006) and interference with work activities (Mavandadi et al., 2007) blunted improvements in depressive symptoms. Mavandadi and associates (2007) also showed that pain interference has a greater effect on depression symptom levels than pain severity and it is a moderator of depression levels over time.

Karp and associates (2006) found that individuals receiving acute treatment were less likely to respond if they reported more severe pain at baseline. Yet, after controlling for severity of baseline depression levels, pain had no effect on time to remission, which occurred in approximately 7 weeks. This time to response is consistent with other studies of LLD in older adults without documented comorbid pain, in which time to response occurred within 6–8 weeks (Flint et al., 1997; Reynolds et al., 1996, Sackeim, Roose, Burt, 2005; Whyte et al., 2004). Interestingly, when older adults with both major depression and chronic low back were treated with duloxetine (an antidepressant with analgesic properties), improvement in pain occurred twice as fast as improvement in mood (Karp et al., 2009).

The effect of persistent pain on depression treatment response durability has not been tested. However, the presence of general medical conditions in which pain is common (e.g., arthritis) is routinely listed as a risk factor for depression relapse (Karp & Reynolds, 2004).

SUMMARY

Of the range of factors potentially influencing treatment response, clinical factors have received perhaps the greatest attention to date in studies of LLD treatment. A history of inadequate treatment or failed treatment during an index episode negatively influences both the magnitude and speed of symptom remission during additional treatment. Yet consensus has not been reached regarding the influence of severe and long-lasting symptoms on treatment response variability or how treatment history or severe/long-lasting symptoms affect the durability of LLD treatment response. On the other hand, a consistent body of literature suggests that comorbid anxiety, alcohol abuse, cognitive impairment (particularly in executive function), sleep impairment, and pain negatively influence the magnitude of treatment response. This literature also indicates that executive dysfunction, suicidality, anxiety, and sleep impairment negatively impact the speed of treatment response. With regard to treatment response durability, suicidality, anxiety, and sleep impairment appear to exert important effects. As with biological factors, additional work is required to understand the impact of clinical factors on the maintenance of treatment response. Furthermore, clinical factors' influence on treatment outcomes in the context of nonpharmacologic therapies requires greater examination.

Intrapersonal Psychosocial Factors

Older adults bring a variety of intrapersonal resources and vulnerabilities that may affect their likelihood of responding to depression treatment. These include socioeconomic characteristics, such as educational attainment and economic resources, and dispositional characteristics, such as self-esteem and personality traits or disorder. Personality factors have received the most attention to date; few studies consider the influence of other intrapersonal factors on the magnitude, speed, and/or durability of LLD treatment response.

EDUCATION

An individual's level of education may indicate his or her ability to acquire positive social, psychological, and economic resources, and such assets are beneficial when recovering from illness (Winkelby, Jatulis, Frank, & Formann, 1992). Thus, it is plausible that a patient's level of educational attainment may influence depression treatment outcomes. However, studies do not necessarily support this idea in persons of any age. Among older adults in particular, several studies of pharmacologic treatment of depression have found no reliable association between educational level and either the magnitude or speed of depression treatment response (Cohen, Gilman, Houck, Szanto, & Reynolds, 2009; Cui et al., 2008; Dew et al., 2007). However, the IMPACT trial (which focused on an ethnically diverse, low-income elderly sample) showed that more highly educated patients had fewer depression symptoms after 12 months of psychotherapy and/or clinical case management (Gum, Areán, & Bostrom, 2006). Whether education affects maintenance of symptom remission is unknown.

SOCIOECONOMIC STATUS

Socioeconomic status (SES) is a complex phenomenon often conceptualized as a combination of educational as well as occupational and financial influences. Here, we focus on SES primarily as an economic construct since it may reflect the patient's spending power, housing, diet, and medical care (Winkleby et al., 1992).

Low SES is generally associated with high psychiatric morbidity, more disability, and poorer access to health care (Lorant et al., 2003), and a small literature points to independent associations between SES and treatment outcomes in LLD. In particular, Cohen et al. (2009) found that low SES (as indicated by Census tract median household income) was an independent predictor of both reduced likelihood and speed of response to LLD treatment. There appears to be no research to date, however, evaluating the influence of SES on durability of LLD treatment responses.

PERSONALITY DISORDERS AND TRAITS

Studies examining the effects of personality disorder on the outcomes of LLD treatment show mixed results. Gum and associates (2006) found that IMPACT trial participants with and without comorbid personality disorder had similar levels of symptom improvement. Yet other studies of late-life samples with depression have found that greater personality pathology was associated with a reduced likelihood of, and a longer time, to remission (Lenze, Miller et al., 2001; Morse, Pilkonis, Houck, Frank, & Reynolds, 2005). In particular, persons with Cluster C personality disorders (avoidant, dependent, or obsessive-compulsive) take longer to respond to acute treatment and have less stable remission (Morse et al., 2005).

Conceptually, neuroticism is a personality trait that represents the individual's tendency to experience psychological distress and an underlying difficulty coping with stress (Costa & McCrae, 1985). Studies show that patients with high levels of neuroticism have less favorable LLD treatment responses. In a naturalistic follow-up study of community-residing older adults (The Longitudinal Aging Study Amsterdam, LASA), Steunenberg and associates (2007) found that the presence of high levels of neuroticism at baseline independently decreased the likelihood of LLD recovery. Furthermore, Canuto et al. (2009) and Hayward et al. (2012) found that greater neuroticism at baseline independently predicted a reduced magnitude of depression treatment response among geriatric patients. While no studies have examined whether neuroticism influences in the speed or durability of LLD treatment, greater neuroticism increases the risk for depression recurrence among adults of all ages (Berlanga, Heinze, Torres, Apiquián, & Caballero, 1999).

SELF-ESTEEM

Self-esteem is conceptualized as the overall affective evaluation of one's own worth, and it may impact the experience of distress when confronted with a stressor (Takagishi, Sakata, & Kitamura, 2011). Although it is closely related to depression (Nuns & Loas, 2005), it reflects a relatively stable trait rather than a fluctuating characteristic (state). Studies show that higher self-esteem is associated with an increased likelihood of symptom remission (Saghafi et al., 2007) and a more rapid response (Gildengers et al., 2005) in LLD treatment. No studies have explored the effects of self-esteem on the durability of treatment response.

SUMMARY

In general, the literature on the role of interpersonal psychosocial factors on LLD treatment response is small relative to the biologic and clinical literatures. Low SES, low levels of self-esteem, and certain personality traits/disorder may predict a reduced

magnitude of response and slower time to respond, but the existing evidence is slim. With regard to personality factors, neurotic personality traits may play a role in the magnitude of treatment response and Cluster C personality disorders may play a role in speed of response. Studies provide mixed evidence as to whether an individual's education level affects magnitude of treatment response, but they suggest that it does not affect speed of response. No studies have examined the influence of intrapersonal factors on treatment response durability. Additionally, there are a wide range of intrapersonal factors that have not received scientific attention but may be influential as well, including an individual's sense of mastery or control and the use of particular styles of coping with life stressors.

Environmental Psychosocial Factors

Similar to intrapersonal factors, the effects of only a very limited range of environmental characteristics have been considered to date. These include social support, stressful life events, characteristics of one's physical environment and living arrangements, and physical functional disability. Although one might conceptualize disability as a personal (rather than environmental) characteristic, we have included it in this section of the chapter because the extent to which a characteristic acts as a disability is highly dependent on the circumstances in which an individual lives.

SOCIAL SUPPORT

Social support variables have long been recognized as important predictors of the occurrence of geriatric depression and the persistence of depressive symptoms over time (De Beurs et al., 2001; Steffens et al., 2005b; Taylor et al., 2004). Social support may also play an important role in LLD treatment response variability, as evidenced by findings from one study showing that the likelihood of achieving remission was significantly increased for individuals with higher levels of perceived social support (Hybels et al., 2005).

Social supports may also predict speed of recovery in LLD treatment. Bosworth and colleagues (2002) prospectively followed a sample of 239 initially clinically depressed elderly patients for 4.5 years. They found that two aspects of social support: (1) a lack of instrumental support (for sick care, errands, chores, finances, transportation, etc.)

and (2) a lack of subjective support (feeling useful, listened to, satisfied with relationships, etc.) were both significant predictors of longer time to remission. However, social network size (household size, number of family, friends, and coworkers) and social interaction (family proximity, in-person or telephone contact with friends and family, group affiliation) did not influence the speed of treatment in this study.

In terms of influence on durability of LLD treatment response, Solomon et al. (2004) studied adults age 17 to 76 and reported that overall psychosocial impairment (encompassing not only interpersonal relationships but impairments in work, satisfaction derived from activities in the past week, and level of involvement in recreational activities during the past week) was significantly associated with subsequent recurrence of major depression, with an odds ratio of 1.12 (95% CI 1.06 to 1.19). In other words, for every 1-point increase in the psychosocial impairment score, the risk of recurrence increased by 12%. Similar results were found in a sample of 211 older adults, where Oddone and associates (2011) found that subjective social support was significantly associated with the durability of depression symptom remission.

STRESSFUL LIFE EVENTS

Stressful life events are well documented to predict depression onset across the life span (Kraaij, Arensman, & Spinhoven, 2002). However, little is known about whether such events affect likelihood, speed, or durability of recovery from depression. One report examining adults of all ages found little evidence of any impact of such events on rates of recovery during receipt of cognitive-behavioral therapy (CBT; Spangler, Simons, Monroe, & Thase, 1997). This area deserves more attention because, to the extent that stressful events can provoke depression, they would appear likely to be related to depression recurrence (i.e., predict shorter durability of treatment response).

PHYSICAL ENVIRONMENT

An individual's physical environment, defined by one's living conditions (i.e., living alone or with another person, urban or rural residence, good or poor quality of the residence or neighborhood) has been associated with the onset of LLD (Alexopoulos et al., 1996; Flint et al., 1997; Schulman, Gairola,

Kuder, & McCulloch, 2002). However, the role of the physical environment in treatment response remains unclear. Alexopoulos et al. (1996) assessed depressed older adults' subjective views of their housing and neighborhood (adequate air temperature and circulation year round, enough space, and safe neighborhood at night) and found that these perceptions were not associated with time to response to pharmacologic treatment. Additional studies examining objective or other indicators of living conditions appear warranted.

FUNCTIONAL DISABILITY

Functional disability refers to limitations in the capacity and actual performance of basic activities of daily living (i.e., self-care, functional mobility) and instrumental activities of daily living (i.e., meal preparation, financial management, home maintenance). It is both a risk factor and an outcome of LLD (Alexopoulos, Buckwalter, et al., 2002; Bruce, 2002; Lenze, Rogers et al., 2001). In addition, treatments that reduce disability in older adults have a modest effect on depressive symptoms (Horowitz, Reinhardt, & Boerner, 2005; Lai et al., 2006; Milani & Lavi, 2007), and treatments that reduce or lead to the remission of depressive symptoms are associated with modest reductions in disability (Hirschfeld et al., 2002; Lenze, Miller et al., 2001; Oslin, Streim et al., 2000). Given these reciprocal associations, and the high incidence of comorbid depression and disability in late life, it is difficult to isolate specific causal contribution of disability to LLD treatment response.

Nevertheless, there is some evidence that the severity of physical or cognitive disability attributed to chronic illness in late life predicts the magnitude of LLD treatment response (Lenze, Miller et al., 2001; Oslin et al., 2002). Specifically, Lenze, Miller et al. (2001) found that greater instrumental activities of daily living (IADL) disability predicted failure to achieve depression remission in older adults. Yet, when potential predictors of remission status (age, education, depressive symptom burden, personality, social adjustment, and self-rated health) were controlled, the impact of IADL disability status was attenuated. This could indicate that the mechanisms that give rise to disability and depression do not highly overlap (Rush et al., 2006). To date, no empirical evidence exists to suggest that disability influences either the speed or durability of remission.

SUMMARY

Although the literature on environmental psychosocial factors' role in treatment response variability remains small, studies consistently show that low levels of perceived social support negatively influence the magnitude, speed, and durability of LLD treatment responses. We continue to have a poor understanding of the influence of stressful life events, the patient's living conditions, and functional disability on LLD treatment outcomes. While the aforementioned circumstances may not be amenable to intervention, if we had evidence that these factors were important, it would suggest that interventions to maximize individuals' ability to cope with these factors should be developed.

INTERACTION OF FACTORS AFFECTING TREATMENT RESPONSE

Thus far, we have discussed the individual effects of a variety of factors on depression treatment response. An equally important issue concerns the combined, potentially interactive effects of these factors when modeling treatment response variability in LLD. To date, very few investigators have examined the interaction effects between biologic, clinical, and/or psychosocial factors on LLD treatment response. Instead, it has been more common to examine whether these factors moderate the impact of treatment or interact with type of treatment received in affecting treatment outcomes. Next we offer several examples of studies examining variables' combined effects.

A recent study examined the influence of social support on the association between disability and depressive symptoms. Taylor and Lynch (2004) analyzed four waves of data from an epidemiological study of older adults (N = 3,872) and found that trajectories of perceived, but not received support provide a buffer against the negative effect of disability on depression symptoms levels. Using random coefficient (growth) models, they found that the effect of growth in disability on growth in depressive symptoms was weakened or eliminated by the inclusion of perceived social support.

Some studies have searched for interaction effects but found no evidence for them. For example, Cohen and colleagues (2009) examined the combined influence of SES and anxiety symptoms during open-label pharmacotherapy in LLD and found no evidence of an interaction between these

variables and depression treatment responses. Instead, their findings suggest that income level (based on a respondent's Census tract) and anxiety levels are independent predictors of response to LLD treatment. In another analysis of data from some of the same subjects, Miller and colleagues (2002) examined the effects of age and CVD risk factors on depression treatment outcomes. They found no evidence that these variables had either main effects or interacted in affecting remission, recurrence, or the need for adjunctive medication to achieve remission.

Several reports have considered biological, clinical, and psychosocial moderators of treatment itself on depression outcomes. Analysis of data from a study comparing the effects of pharmacologic and psychosocial maintenance treatments for LLD showed an interaction between the type of treatment and medical burden on long-term depression levels (Reynolds et al., 2006). In this study, maintenance pharmacotherapy (paroxetine) was effective in preventing recurrence if an individual had fewer and less severe medical illnesses; neither medication nor placebo was effective in individuals with higher levels of medical burden. No interactions effects were detected between type of treatment and cognitive status, coexisting anxiety, or sleep impairment on LLD maintenance treatment outcomes (Reynolds et al., 2006).

Taylor and colleagues (1999) examined interactions between depression symptom severity at the start of maintenance therapy and type of maintenance treatment among older adults with a history of recurrent depression. After making full or partial recovery in the acute and continuation phase of depression treatment, subjects with greater symptom severity had a significantly greater risk for recurrence if they went on to receive maintenance psychotherapy (interpersonal therapy). The effect was not observed in patients maintained on placebo, on nortriptyline, or combined nortriptyline and interpersonal therapy. These data suggest that older adults who enter maintenance phase of treatment with higher levels of depression symptoms are at greater risk of recurrence following discontinuation of medication.

To further understand patterns of recurrence, Dew and associates (2001) found that initial response profiles during acute/continuation treatment predicted which persons were most likely to stay well, given the receipt of maintenance combined therapy (nortriptyline plus interpersonal therapy) versus monotherapy (nortriptyline or interpersonal therapy) versus placebo. They found that subjects with rapid and sustained response during open treatment were likely to do well (i.e., not experience a recurrence) as long as they received any active treatment (i.e., either combined therapy or monotherapy). However, individuals who showed a bumpy pattern toward recovery needed combined therapy to stay well; monotherapy was less effective. Lastly, none of the active maintenance treatments were effective in stemming recurrence of depression among individuals who had initially shown prolonged nonresponse to acute/continuation treatment. Thus, initial response profile data are important to consider when making decisions about maintenance therapy for depressed older adults.

SUMMARY OF FINDINGS AND IMPLICATIONS FOR RESEARCH AND CLINICAL CARE

Although considerable progress has been made in delineating a range of factors that contribute to treatment response variability in LLD, large gaps still remain in the literature. We have noted these throughout the chapter and they are summarized in Table 42.1. In general, much of the scientific effort to date has focused on understanding factors' individual rather than combined effects. Within studies of factors' individual effects, the emphasis has been on the impact of biological and clinical factors on the magnitude and speed of late-life treatment response, with considerably less attention to the role of intrapersonal and environmental factors that might affect these outcomes. Although durability of response has less often been the focus of research than magnitude and speed of initial response, the same pattern of emphasis on biological and clinical factors appears, with considerably less information on other types of factors that could influence patient outcomes.

While multivariable models have received the least attention to date in this field, they may be most important for the design of future studies to better understand the combined (additive or synergistic) effects of multiple factors on LLD treatment response variability. The combined impact of predictors of treatment response durability also needs to be investigated to move the field forward. Such studies will require investigators to recruit heterogeneous samples (including very old and ill older adults), collect detailed longitudinal data

(measuring multiple factors), and extend the periods of follow-up in order to fully understand patterns of risk for recurrence.

The literature also suggests that future studies of LLD treatment must include outcomes that go beyond specific measures of depression, including measures of general health, overall medical burden, and aspects of disability (Alexopoulos, Buckwalter, et al., 2002). Targeting interventions not only to depression, but to medical burden and resulting disability (utilizing, for example, physical and occupational therapy), may have considerable promise for reducing levels of depression. In addition, because disability can be both a cause and an outcome of depression, a few research groups have argued that it is critical to explore the efficacy and effectiveness of multimodal approaches to managing both conditions (Alexopoulos, Buckwalter, et al., 2002; Bruce, 2002; Lenze, Rogers et al., 2001). Moving in that direction, investigators at the University of Pittsburgh are preparing to launch a study to determine whether treating pain and disability in older adults with knee osteoarthritis and minor depression prevents conversion to major depression over the course of 2 years. This study, which blends intervention and prevention science, will be the first to determine whether treating pain and associated disability reduces rates of depression.

Viewed together, the literature suggests there are multiple categories of patient characteristics that are identifiable at the time of treatment initiation and provide important prognostic information to clinicians. However, not all prognostic factors are equal. It is quite possible that various patient characteristics that negatively impact treatment outcomes may require different combinations of pharmacotherapy, psychotherapy, and social service interventions to mitigate their effects (Pinquart et al., 2007). For example, a person of low SES who is depressed may require depression treatment that includes or is linked to additional assistance in locating and accessing community-based services, while a depressed individual with comorbid anxiety may benefit from a combination of therapies that address the anxiety explicitly (e.g., CBT plus pharmacotherapy).

LLD treatment studies, to the extent that they clearly identify factors responsible for response variability, have the potential to contribute to personalized medicine, that is, enable mental health care providers to choose pharmacotherapy, psychotherapy, and supportive services based on the patient's biological, clinical, and psychosocial profile. Although personalized care for LLD has not advanced very far to date, one might envision selecting an antidepressant based on an older adult's genetic profile as well as whether there are other clinical or psychosocial factors that may impact treatment response such as suicidality and low levels of social support. For such personalized treatment to become a reality, not only must research fully delineate the biologic and other factors that affect response variability, but both mental health researchers and clinical care providers will need to strengthen ties with colleagues in internal medicine, neurology, nursing, pharmacy, and social work in an effort to share information on assessment and treatment strategies and monitoring needs.

CONCLUSION

Advances in health care increasingly result in successful management of severe chronic illnesses into late life, such that we now have illness burden in our elderly population that has not previously been encountered. LLD is both part of this illness burden and may complicate other coexisting conditions. Thus, being able to select the most effective depression treatment, given a patient's unique biologic, clinical, and psychosocial profile, has great value to patients, their families, and clinicians. We only partially understand the myriad factors that comprise this profile, and how those factors work individually and in combination. The path ahead requires that clinical trials of innovative treatment approaches include a full range of such factors so that efficacy of treatment is always determined within the context of patient characteristics that may influence response.

Disclosures

Dr. Garand has no conflicts to disclose. She was funded by NIMH. Grant Support: No K23 MH070719.

Dr. Whyte Grant Support NIMH U01 MH062565 (PI: Whyte; 06/01/11–03/31/16)

Grant Support NICHD/NCMRR 1R01HD055525 (PI: Whyte; 12/1/2008–11/30/2013)

Grant Support NICHD R01 HD069620 (PI: Kline; 4/1/2012–3/31/2017)

Grant Support DOD W81XWH-10-1-0920 (PI: Raina: 9/2011–9/2013)

Grant Support NINDS 2R44 NS052948 (PI: Debra Fox, FoxLearningSystems; 2008–2010)

Research supplies provided by Pfizer and Lilly for NIMH U01 MH062565 (PI: Whyte; 06/01/11–03/31/16)

Dr. Butters NIMH Grant Support: No R01 MH080240 (MA Butters) and P30 MH090333 (CF Reynolds). Over the past three years Dr. Butters has received honoraria for lectures from the following organizations: the International Neuropsychological Society, Fundació ACE, University of Texas Southwestern Medical Center, and the Southern Illinois University School of Medicine; for grant reviews from the Michael J. Fox Foundation, the Department of Veterans Affairs, and the NIMH; and for mentorship from the NIMH. Dr. Butters also has been a consultant for Fox Learning Systems. She also has received remuneration for providing neuropsychological assessment services for clinical trials conducted by Northstar Neuroscience and Medtronic.

Dr. Skidmore has no conflicts to disclose. She currently receives research support from the NIH through the National Institute for Child and Human Development (K12 HD055931, R01 HD055525, R03 HD073770, and R21 HD071728) and the National Institute of Mental Health (P30 MH090333).

Dr. Karp receives research support in the form of medication supplies from Pfizer and Reckitt Benckiser. He is a stockowner of Corcept. He receives or has received research funding from NIH, RAND, and the Brain and Behavior Research Foundation.

Dr. Dew has no conflicts to disclose.

REFERENCES

Ackerman, D. L., Greenland, S., Bystritsky, A., & Small, G. W. (2000). Side effects and time course of response in a placebo-controlled trial of fluoxetine for the treatment of geriatric depression. *Journal of Clinical Psychopharmacology, 20,* 658–665.

Alexopoulos, G. S., Buckwalter, K. C., Oslin, J., Martinnez, R., Wainscott, C., & Kirshnan, R. R. (2002). Comorbidity of late-life depression: An opportunity for research on mechanisms and treatment. *Biological Psychiatry, 52*(6), 543–558.

Alexopoulos, G. S., Katz, I. R., Bruce, M. L., Heo, M., Ten Have, T., Raue, P., ... Reynolds, C. F., III. (2005). Remission in depressed geriatric primary care patients: A report from the PROSPECT study. *American Journal of Psychiatry, 162*(4), 718–724.

Alexopoulos, G. S., Kiosses, D. N., Choi, S. J., Murphy, C. F., & Lim, K. O. (2002). Frontal white matter microstructure and treatment response of late-life depression: A preliminary study. *American Journal of Psychiatry, 159*(11), 1929–1932.

Alexopoulos, G. S., Kiosses, D. N., Heo, M., Murphy, C. F., Shanmugham, B., & Gunning-Dixon, F. (2005). Executive dysfunction and the course of geriatric depression. *Biological Psychiatry, 58*(3), 204–210.

Alexopoulos, G. S., Kiosses, D. N., Murphy, C., & Heo, M. (2004). Executive dysfunction, heart disease burden, and remission of geriatric depression. *Neuropsychopharmacology, 29*(12), 2278–84.

Alexopoulos, G. S., Meyers, B. S., Young, R. C., Kakuma, T., Feder, M., Einhorn, A., & Rosendahl, E. (1996). Recovery in geriatric depression. *Archives of General Psychiatry, 53*, 305–12.

Alexopoulos, G. S., Meyers, B. S., Young, R. C., Kalayam, B., Kakuma, T., Gabrielle, M., ... Hull, J. (2000). Executive dysfunction and long-term outcomes of geriatric depression. *Archives of General Psychiatry, 57*(3), 285–290.

Alexopoulos, G. S., & Morimoto, S. S. (2011). The inflammation hypothesis in geriatric depression. *International Journal of Geriatric Psychiatry.* 2011 Mar 2,. ePub ahead of print. doi: 10.1002/gps.2672.

Alexopoulos, G. S., Murphy, C. F., Gunning-Dixon, F. M., Kalayam, B., Katz, R., Kanellopoulos, D., ... Foxe, J. J. (2007). Event-related potentials in an emotional go/no-go task and remission of geriatric depression. *NeuroReport, 18*(3), 217–221.

Alexopoulos, G. S., Murphy, C. F., Gunning-Dixon, F. M., Latoussakis, V., Kanellopoulos, D., Klimstra, S., ... Hoptman, M. J. (2008). Microstructural white matter abnormalities and remission of geriatric depression. *American Journal of Psychiatry, 165*(2), 238–244.

Altshuler, L. L., Bauer, M., Frye, M. A., Gitlin, M. J., Mintz, J., Szuba, M. P., ... Whybrow, P. C. (2001). Does thyroid supplementation accelerate tricyclic antidepressant response? A review and meta-analysis of the literature. *American Journal of Psychiatry, 158*, 1617–1622.

Appelhof, B. C., Brouwer, J. P., van Dyck, R., Fliers, E., Hoogendijk, W. J., Huyser, J., ... Wiersinga, W. M. (2004). Triiodothyronine addition to paroxetine in the treatment of major depressive disorder. *Journal of Clinical Endocrinology and Metabolism, 89*(12), 6271–626.

Andreescu, C., Lenz, E. J., Dew, M. A., Begley, A. E., Mulsant, B. H., Dombrovski, A. Y., Reynolds, C. F., III. (2007). Effect of comorbid anxiety on treatment response and relapse risk in late-life depression: Controlled study. *British Journal of Psychiatry, 190*, 344–349.

Andreescu, C., Mulsant, B. H., Bouck, P. R., Whyte, E. M., Mazumday, S., Dombrovski, A., ... Reynolds, C. F., III. (2008). Empirically derived decision trees for the treatment of late-life depression. *American Journal of Psychiatry, 165*, 855–862.

Areán, P. A., Ayalon, L., Hunkeler, E., Lin, H. B., Tang, L., Harpole, L., ... Unützer, J. (2005). Improving depression care for older, minority patients in primary care. *Medical Care, 43*(4), 381–390.

Baldwin, R., Jeffries, S., Jackson, A., Sutcliffe, C., Thacker, N., Scott, M., & Burns, A. (2004). Treatment response in late-onset depression: relationship to neuropsychological, neuroradiological and vascular risk factors. *Psychological Medicine, 34*(1), 125–136.

Baldwin, R. C., Walker, S., Simpson, S. W., Jackson, A., & Burns, A. (2000). The prognostic significance of abnormalities seen on magnetic resonance imaging in late life depression: Clinical outcome, mortality and progression to dementia at three years. *International Journal of Geriatric Psychiatry, 15*(12), 1097–1104.

Bannon, M. J., Michelhaugh, S. K., Wang, J., & Sacchetti, P. (2001). The human dopamine transporter gene: Gene organization, transcriptional regulation, and potential involvement in neuropsychiatric disorders. *European Neuropsychopharmacology, 11*(6), 449–455.

Beckman, A. T., de Beurs, E., van Balkom, A. J., Deeg, D. J., Van Dyck, R., & van Tilburg, W. (2000). Anxiety and depression in late life: Cooccurrence and community of risk factors. *American Journal of Psychiatry, 157*, 89–95.

Berlanga, C., Heinze, G., Torres, M., Apiquián, R., & Caballero, A. (1999). Personality and clinical predictors of recurrence of depression. *Psychiatric Services, 50*(3), 376–380.

Bauer, M., Heinz, A., & Whybrow, P. C. (2002). Thyroid hormones, serotonin and mood: Of synergy and significance in the adult brain. *Molecular Psychiatry, 7*, 140–156.

Bhalla, R. K., Butters, M. A., Mulsant, B. H., Begley, A. E., Zmuda, M. D., Schoderbek, B., ... Becker, J. T. (2006). Persistence of neuropsychologic deficits in the remitted state of late-life depression. *American Journal of Geriatric Psychiatry, 14*(5), 419–427.

Blow, F. C., & Barry, K. L. (2000). Older patients with at-risk and problem drinking patterns: New developments in brief interventions. *Journal of Geriatric Psychiatry and Neurology, 13*, 115–123.

Boa, Y., Alexopoulos, G. S. Casalino, L. P., Ten Have, T. R., Donhue, J. M., Post, E. P., Schackman, B. R., & Bruce, M. L. (2011). Collaborative depression care management and disparities in depression treatment and outcomes. *Archives of General Psychiatry, 68*(6), 627–636.

Bonnardeaux, A., Davies, E., Jeunemaitre, X., Féry, I., Charru, A., Clauser, E., ... Soubier, F. (1994). Angiotensin II type 1 receptor gene polymorphisms in human essential hypertension. *Hypertension*, 24, 63–69.

Bosworth, H. R., McQuoid, D. R., George, L. K., & Steffens, D. C. (2002). Time-to-remission from geriatric depression. Psychosocial and clinical factors. *American Journal of Geriatric Psychiatry*, 10(5), 551–559.

Bruce, M. L., (2001). Depression and disability in late life, directions for future research. *American Journal of Geriatric Psychiatry*, 9, 102–112.

Bruce, M. L. (2002). Psychosocial risk factors for depressive disorders in late life. *Biological Psychiatry*, 52, 175–184.

Butters, M. A., Bhalla, R. K., Mulsant, B. H., Mazumdar, S., Houck, P. R., Begley, A. E., … Reynolds, C. F., III. (2004). Executive functioning, illness course, and relapse/recurrence in continuation and maintenance treatment of late-life depression: Is there a relationship? *American Journal of Geriatric Psychiatry*, 12(4), 387–394.

Butters, M. A., Whyte, E. M., Nebes, R. D., Begley, A. E., Dew, M. A., Mulsant, B. H., … Becker, J. T. (2004). The nature and determinants of neuropsychological functioning in late-life depression. *Archives of General Psychiatry*, 61(6), 587–595.

Buysse, D. J. (2004). Insomnia, depression and aging: Assessing sleep and mood interactions in older adults. *Geriatrics*, 59, 47–51.

Buysse, D. J., Reynolds, C. F., III, Hoch, C. C., Houck, P. R., Kupfer, D. J., Mazumdar, S., & Frank, E. (1996). Longitudinal effects of nortriptyline on EEG sleep and the likelihood of recurrence in elderly depressed patients. *Neuropsychopharmacology*, 14(4), 243–52.

Buysse, D. J., Reynolds, C. F., III, Houck, P. R., Perel, J. M., Frank, E., Begley, A. E., … Kupfer, D. J. (1997). Does lorazepam impair the antidepressant response to nortriptyline and psychotherapy? *Journal of Clinical Psychiatry*, 58, 426—432.

Canuto, A., Giannakopoulos, P., Meiler-Mititelu, C., Delalye, C., Herrmann, F. R., & Weber, K. (2009). Personality traits influence clinical outcome in day hospital-treated elderly depressed patients. *American Journal of Geriatric Psychiatry*, 17(4), 335–340.

Charlson, M., & Peterson, J. C. (2002). Medical comorbidity n late life depression. *Biological Psychiatry*, 52, 226–235.

Choi, M. J., Kang, R. H., Lim, S. W., Oh, K. S., & Lee, M. S. (2006). Brain-derived neurotrophic factor gene polymorphism (Val66Met) and citalopram response in major depressive disorder. *Brain Research*, 1118, 176–182

Cohen, A., Gilman, S. E., Houck, P. R., Szanto, K., & Reynolds, C. F., III. (2009). Socioeconomic status and anxiety as predictors of antidepressant treatment response and suicidal ideation in older adults. *Social Psychiatry and Psychiatric Epidemiology*, 44, 272–277.

Cole, M. G., & Dendukuri, N. (2003). Risk factors for depression among elderly community subjects: A systematic review and meta-analysis. *American Journal of Psychiatry*, 160, 1147–1156.

Costa, P. T., & McCrae, R. R. (1985). *The NEO Personality Inventory Manual*. Odessa, FL : Psychological Assessment Resources.

Cui, X., Jeffrey, M. S., Lyness, J. M., Tang, W., Tu, X., & Conwell, Y. (2008). Outcomes and predictors of late-life depression trajectories in older primary care patients. *American Journal of Geriatric Psychiatry*, 16(5), 406–415.

Davis, L. L., Frazier, E., Husain, M. M., Warden, D., Trivedi, M., Fava, M., … Rush, A. J. (2006). Substance use disorder comorbidity in major depressive disorder: A confirmatory analysis of the STAR*D cohort. *American Journal on Addictions*, 15, 278–285.

De Beurs, E., Beekman, A., Geerlings, S., Deeg, D. Y., Van Dyck, R., & Van Tilburg, W. (2001). On becoming depressed or anxious in late life: Similar vulnerability factors but different effects of stressful life events. *The British Journal of Psychiatry*, 179, 426–431.

Devanand, D. P. (2002). Comorbid psychiatric disorders in late life depression. *Biological Psychiatry*, 52, 236–242.

Dew, M. A., Reynolds, C. F., III, Houck, R. P., Hall, M., Buysse, D. J., Frank, E., & Kupfew, D. F. (1997). Temporal profiles of the course of depression during treatment: Predictors of pathways toward recovery in the elderly. *Archives of Geriatric Psychiatry*, 54, 1016–1024.

Dew, M. A., Reynolds, C. F., III, Mulsant, B., Frank, E., Houck, P. R., Mazumdar, S., … Kupfer, D. J. (2001). Initial recovery patterns may predict which maintenance therapies for depression will keep older adults well. *Journal of Affective Disorders*, 65, 155–166.

Dew, M. A., Whyte, E. M., Lenze, E. J., Houck, P. R., Mulsant, B. H., Pollock, B. G., … Reynolds, C. F., III. (2007). Recovery from major depression in older adults receiving augmentation of antidepressant pharmacotherapy. *American Journal of Psychiatry*, 164(6), 892–899.

Dombrovski, A. Y., Mulsant, B. H., Houck, P. R., Mazumdar, S., Lenze, E. J., Andreescu, C., … Reynolds, C. F., III. (2007). Residual symptoms and recurrence during maintenance treatment of late-life depression. *Journal of Affective Disorders*, 103, 77–82

Driscoll, H. C., Basinski, J., Mulsant, B. H., Butter, M. A., Dew, M. A., & Houck, P. R. (2005). Getting better, getting well: Understanding and managing partial and non-response to pharmacological treatment of non-psychotic major depression in old age. *Drugs and Aging*, 24, 801–814.

Duman, R. S., & Monteggia, L. M. (2006). A neurotrophic model for stress-related mood disorders. *Biological Psychiatry*, 59, 1116–1127.

Durham, L. K., Webb, S. M., Milos, P. M., Clary, C. M., & Seymour, A. B. (2004). The serotonin transporter polymorphism, 5HTTLPR, is associated with a faster response time to sertraline in an elderly population with major depressive disorder. *Psychopharmacology*, 174(4), 525–529.

Egan, M. F., Kojima, M., Callicott, J. H., Goldberg, T. E., Kolachana, B. S., Bertolino, A., ... Weinberger, D. R. (2003). The BDNF val66met polymorphism affects activity-dependent secretion of BDNF and human memory and hippocampal function. *Cell*, 112(2), 257–69.

Ell, K., Aranda, M. P., Xie, B., Lee, P. J., & Chou, C. P. (2010). Collaborative depression treatment in older and younger adults with physical illness: Pooled comparative analysis of three randomized clinical trials. *American Journal of Geriatric Psychiatry*, 18(6), 520–530.

Escobar, M. L., Figueroa-Guzman, Y., & Gomez-Palacio-Schjetnan, A. (2003). In vivo insular cortex LTP induced by brain-derived neurotrophic factor. *Brain Research*, 991, 274–279.

Fabian, T. J., Dew, M. A., Pollock, B. G., Reynolds, C. F., III, Mulsant, B. H., Butters, M. A., ... Kroboth, P. D. (2001). Endogenous concentrations of DHEA and DHEA-S decrease with remission of depression in older adults. *Biological Psychiatry*, 50(10), 767–774.

Flint, A. J., & Rifat, S. L. (1997). Effect of demographic and clinical variables on time to anti-depressant response in geriatric depression. *Depression and Anxiety*, 5, 103–7.

Frojdh, K., Hakansson, A., Karlsson, I., & Molarius, A. (2003). Deceased, disabled, or depressed—a population-based 6-year follow-up study of elderly people with depression. *Social Psychiatry and Psychiatric Epidemiology*, 38(10), 557–562.

Gallo, J. J., & Lebowitz, B. D. (1999). The epidemiology of common late-life mental disorders in the community: Themes for the new century. *Psychiatric Services*, 50, 1158–1166.

Gerretsen, P., & Pollock, B. G. (2008). Pharmacogenetics and the serotonin transporter

in late-life depression. *Expert Opinion in Drug Metabolism and Toxicology*, 4(12), 1465–1478.

Gildengers, A. G., Houck, P. R., Mulsant, B. H., Dew, M. A., Aizenstein, H. J., Jones, B. L., ... Reynolds, C. F., III. (2005). Trajectories of treatment response in late-life depression. Psychosocial correlates. *Journal of Clinical Psychopharmacology*, 25(1), S8-S13.

Gildengers, A. G., Houck, P. R., Mulsant, B. H., Pollock, B. G., Mazumdar, S., Miller, M. D., ... Reynolds, C. F., III. (2002). Course and rated of antidepressant response in the very old. *Journal of Affective Disorders*, 69, 177–184.

Gray, A., Feldman, H. A., McKinlay, J. B., & Longcope, C. (1991). Age, disease and changing sex hormone levels in middle-aged men: Results from the Massachusetts make aging study. *Journal of Clinical Endocrinology and Metabolism*, 73, 1016–25

Greenlee, A., Karp, J. F., Dew, M. A., Houck, P., Andreescu, C., & Reynolds, C. F., III. (2010). Anxiety impairs depression remission in partial responders during extended treatment in late-life. *Depression and Anxiety*, 27, 451–456.

Grigoriadis, S., Kennedy, S. H., & Bagby, R. M. (2003). A comparison of antidepressant response in younger and older women. *Journal of Clinical Psychopharmacology*, 23, 405–407.

Gum, A. M., Areán, P. A., & Bostrom, A. (2006). Low-income depressed older adults with psychiatric comorbidity: Secondary analyses of response to psychotherapy and case management. *International Journal of Geriatric Psychiatry*, 22, 124–130.

Gunning, F. M., Cheng, J., Murphy, C. F., Kanellopoulos, D., Acuna, J., Hoptman, M. J., ... Alexopoulos, G. S. (2009). Anterior cingulate cortical volumes and treatment remission of geriatric depression. *International Journal of Geriatric Psychiatry*, 24(8), 829–836.

Gunning-Dixon, F. M., Walton, M., Cheng, J., Acuna, J., Klimstra, S., Zimmerman, M. E., ... Alexopoulos, G. S. (2010). MRI signal hyperintensities and treatment remission of geriatric depression. *Journal of Affective Disorders*, 126(3), 395–401.

Hayward, R. D., Taylor, W. D., Smoski, M. U. J., Steffens, D. C., & Payne, M. E. (2012). Association of five-factor model personality domains and facets with presence, onset, and treatment outcomes of major depression in older adults. *American Journal of Geriatric Psychiatry*. 2012 March 15, ePub ahead of print.

Heils, A., Teufel, A., Petri, S., Stober, G., Riederer, P., Bengel, D., & Lesch, K. P. (1996) Allelic variation of human serotonin transporter gene expression. *Journal of Neurochemistry*, 66, 2621–2624.

Hirschfeld, R. M. A., Dunner, D. L., Keitner, G., Klein, D. N., Koran, L. M., Kornstein, S. G., ... Keller, M. B. (2002). Does psychosocial functioning improve independent of depressive symptoms? A comparison of nefazdodone, psychotherapy and their combination. *Biological Psychiatry, 51,* 123–33.

Horowitz, H., Reinhardt, J. P., & Boerner, K. (2005). The effect of rehabilitation on depression among visually disabled older adults. *Aging and Mental Health, 9,* 563–70.

Hsieh, M. H., McQuoid, D. R., Levy, R. M., Payne, M. E., MacFall, J. R., & Steffens, D. C. (2002). Hippocampal volume and antidepressant response in geriatric depression. *International Journal of Geriatric Psychiatry, 17*(6), 519–525.

Hybels, C. F., Blazer, D. G., & Steffens, D. C. (2005). Predictors of partial remission in older patients treated for major depression. *American Journal of Geriatric Psychiatry, 13*(8), 713–721.

Janssen, D. G., Caniato, R. N., Verster, J. C., & Baune, B. T. (2010). A psychoneuroimmunological review on cytokines involved in antidepressant treatment response. *Human Psychopharmacology: Clinical and Experimental, 25,* 201–215.

Janssen, J., Hulshoff Pol, H. G., Schnack, H. G., Kok, R. M., Lampe, I. K., de Leeuw, F. E., Kahn, R. S., & Heeren, T. J. (2007). Cerebral volume measurements and subcortical white matter lesions and short-term treatment response in late life depression. *International Journal of Geriatric Psychiatry, 22*(5), 468–474.

Kalayam, B., & Alexopoulos, G. S. (1999). Prefrontal dysfunction and treatment response in geriatric depression. *Archives of General Psychiatry, 56*(8), 713–718.

Karp, J. F., & Reynolds, C. F., III. (2004). Pharmacotherapy of depression in the elderly: Achieving and maintaining optimal outcomes. *Primary Psychiatry, 11,* 37–46.

Karp, J. F., Reynolds, C. F., Butters, M. A., Dew, M. A., Mazumdar, S., Begley, A. E., ... Weiner, D. K. (2006). The relationship between pain and mental flexibility in older adult pain clinic patients. *Pain Medicine, 7*(5), 444–452.

Karp, J. F., Skidmore, E. R., Lotz, M., Lenze, E. J., Dew, M. A., & Reynolds, C. F. (2009). Use of the late-life function and disability instrument to assess disability in major depression. *Journal of the American Geriatrics Society, 57,* 1612–1619.

Kim, J. M., Stewart, R., Kim, S. W., Yang, S. J., Shin, I. S., & Yoon, J. S. (2009). Insomnia, depression, and physical disorders in late life: A 2-year longitudinal community study in Koreans. *Sleep, 32*(9), 1221–1228.

Kondo, D. G., Speer, M. C., Krishnan, K. R., McQuoid, D. R., Slifer, S. H., Pieper, C. F., ... Steffens, D. C. (2007). Association of AGTR1 with 18-month treatment outcome in late-life depression. *American Journal of Geriatric Psychiatry, 15*(7), 564–72.

Kornstein, S. G., Schatzberg, A. F., Thase, M. E., Youngers, K. A., McCullough, J. P., Keitner, G. I., ... Keller, M. B. (2000). Gender differences in treatment response to sertraline versus imipramine in chronic depression. *American Journal of Psychiatry, 157,* 1445–1452.

Kraaij, V., Arensman, R., & Spinhoven, P. (2002). Negative life events and depression in elderly persons: A meta-analysis. *Journal of Gerontology: Psychological Sciences, 57B*(1), P87–94.

Lai, S. M., Studenski, S., Richards, L., Perera, S., Reker, D., Rigler, S., & Duncan, P. W. (2006). Therapeutic exercise and depressive symptoms after stroke. *Journal of the American Geriatrics Society, 54,* 240–7.

Lavretsky, H., Siddarth, P., Kumar, A., & Reynolds, C. F., III. (2008). The effects of the dopamine and serotonin transporter polymorphisms on clinical features and treatment response in geriatric depression: A pilot study. *International Journal of Geriatric Psychiatry, 23,* 55–59.

Lavretsky, H., Park, S., Siddarth, P., Kumar, A., & Reynolds, C. F., III. (2006). Methylphenidate enhanced antidepressant response to citalopram in the elderly: A double-blind, placebo-controlled pilot trial. *American Journal of Geriatric Psychiatry, 14*(2), 181–185.

Lenze, E. J., Miller, M. D., Dew, M. A., Martire, L. M., Mulsant, B. H., Begley, A. E., ... Reynolds, C. F. (2001). Subjective health measures and acute treatment outcomes in geriatric depression. *International Journal of Geriatric Psychiatry, 16,* 1149–55.

Lenze, E. J., Mulsant, B. H., Dew, M. A., Shear, M. K., Houck, P., & Reynolds, C. F., III. (2002). Anxiety symptoms in elderly patients with depression: What is the best approach to treatment? *Drugs and Aging, 19*(10), 753–60.

Lenze, E. J., Mulsant, B. H., Dew, M. A., Shear, M. K., Houck, P., Pollock, B. G., & Reynolds, C. F., III. (2003). Good treatment outcomes in late-life depression with comorbid anxiety. *Journal of Affective Disorders, 77,* 247–254.

Lenze, E. J., Rogers, J. C., Martire, L. M., Mulsant, B. H., Rollman, B. L., Dew, M. A., ... Reynolds, C. F., III. (2001).The association of late-life depression and anxiety with physical disability. *American Journal of Geriatric Psychiatry, 9,* 113–135.

Lesch, K. P., Bengel, D., Heils, A., Sabol, S. Z., Greenbert, B. D., Petri, S., ... Murphy, D. L.

(1996). Association of anxiety-related traits with a polymorphism in the serotonin transporter gene regulatory region. *Science, 274,* 1527–1531.

Lotrich, F. E., Pollock, B. G., Kirshner, M., Ferrell, R. F., & Reynolds, C. F., III. (2008). Serotonin transporter genotype interacts with paroxetine plasma levels to influence depression treatment response in geriatric patients. *Journal of Psychiatry and Neuroscience, 33*(2), 123–130.

Lorant, V., Deliege, D., Eaton, W., Robert, A., Philippot, P., & Ansseau, M. (2003). Socioeconomic inequalities in depression: A meta-analysis. *American Journal of Epidemiology, 157*(2), 98–112.

Maes, M. (2011). Depression is an inflammatory disease, but cell-mediated immune activation is the key component of depression. *Progress in Neuro-Psychopharmacology and Biological Psychiatry, 35,* 664–675.

Manji, H. K., Drevets, W. C., & Charney, D. S. (2001). The cellular neurobiology of depression. *Nature Medicine, 7,* 541–547.

Marcus, S. M., Young, E. A., Kerber, K. B., Kornstein, S., Farabaugh, A. H., Mitchell, J., ... Rush, A. J. (2005). Gender differences in depression: Findings from the STAR-D study. *Journal of Affective Disorders, 87,* 141–150.

Martenyi, F., Dossenbach, M., Mraz, K., & Metcalfe, S. (2001). Gender differences in the efficacy of fluoxetine and maprotiline in depressed patients: A double-blind trial of antidepressants with serotonergic or norepinephrinergic reuptake inhibition profile. *European Neuropsychopharmacology, 11,* 227–232.

Mattis, S. (1988). Dementia Rating Scale (DRS). Odessa, FL : Psychological Assessment Reources.

Mavandadi, S., Ten Have, T. R., Katz, I. R., Durai, U. N., Krahn, D. D., Llorente, M. D., ... Oslin, D. W. (2007). Effect of depression treatment on depressive symptoms in older adulthood: The moderating role of pain. *Journal of the American Geriatrics Society, 55*(2), 202–211.

Meier, P., & Seitz, H. K. (2008). Age, alcohol metabolism and liver disease. *Current Opinion in Clinical Nutrition and Metabolic Care, 11,* 21–26.

Mendlewicz, J. (2008). Towards achieving remission in the treatment of depression. *Dialogues in Clinical Neuroscience, 10*(4), 371–374.

Milani, R., & Lavie, C. (2007). Impact of cardiac rehabilitation on depression and its associated mortality. *American Journal of Medicine, 120,* 799–806.

Mitchell, A. J., & Subramaniam, H. (2005). Prognosis of depression in old age compared to middle age: A systematic review of comparative studies.

American Journal of Psychiatry, 162(9), 1588–1601.

Moreau, X., Jeanningros, R., & Mazzola-Pomietto, P. (2001). Chronic effects of triiodothyronine in combination with imipramine on 5-HT transporter, 5-HT(1A) and 5-HT(2A) receptors in adult rat brain. *Neuropsychopharmacology, 24,* 652–662

Morimoto, S. S., Gunning, F. M., Murphy, C. F., Kanellopoulos, D., Kelly, R. E., & Alexopoulos, G. S. (2011). Executive function and short-term remission of geriatric depression: The role of semantic strategy. *American Journal of Geriatric Psychiatry, 19*(2), 115–122.

Morse, J. Q., Pilkonis, P. A., Houck, P. R., Frank, E., & Reynolds, C. F., III. (2005). Impact of cluster C personality disorders on outcomes of acute maintenance treatment of late-life depression. *American Journal of Geriatric Psychiatry, 13*(9), 808–814.

Mulsant, B. H., Reynolds, C. F., III, Shear, M. K., Sweet, R. A., & Miller, M. (1996). Comorbid anxiety disorders in late-life depression. *Anxiety, 2*(5), 242–247.

Murphy, T. J., Alexander, R. W., Griendling, K. K., Runge, M. S., & Bernstein, K. E. (1991). Isolation of a cDNA encoding the vascular type-1 angiotensin II receptor. *Nature, 351,* 233–236.

Murphy, C. F., & Alexopoulos, G. S. (2004). Longitudinal association of initiation/ perseveration and severity of geriatric depression. *American Journal of Geriatric Psychiatry, 12*(1), 50–56.

Murphy, G. M., Jr., Hollander, S. B., Rodrigues, H. E., Kremer, C., & Schatzberg, A. F. (2004). Effects of the serotonin transporter gene promoter polymorphism on mirtazapine and paroxetine efficacy and adverse events in geriatric major depression. *Archives of General Psychiatry, 61*(11), 1163–1169.

Nagappan, G., & Lu, B. (2005). Activity-dependent modulation of the BDNF receptor TrkB: Mechanisms and implications. *Trends in Neuroscience, 28,* 464–471.

Naismith, S. L., Norrie, L., Lewis, S. J., Rogers, N. L., Scott, E. M., & Hickie, I. B. (2009). Does sleep disturbance mediate neuropsychological functioning in older people with depression? *Journal of Affective Disorders, 116*(1–2), 139–143.

Nebes, R. D., Pollock, B. G., Houck, P. R., Butters, M. A., Mulsant, B. H., Zmuda, M. D., & Reynolds, C. F., III. (2003). Persistence of cognitive impairment in geriatric patients following antidepressant treatment: A randomized, double-blind clinical trial with nortriptyline and paroxetine. *Journal of Psychiatry Research, 37*(2), 99–108.

Nelson, J. C., Holden, K., Roose, S., Salzman, C., Hollander, S. B., & Betzel, J. V. (2007). Are there predictors of outcome in depressed elderly nursing home residents during treatment with mirtazapine orally disintegrating tablets? *International Journal of Geriatric Psychiatry, 22*(10), 999–1003.

Neves-Pereira, M., Mundo, E., Muglia, P., King, N., Macciardi, F., & Kennedy, J. L. (2002). The brain-derived neurotrophic factor gene confers susceptibility to bipolar disorder: Evidence from a family-based association study. *American Journal of Human Genetics, 71,* 651–655.

Nuns, N., & Loas, G. (2005). Interpersonal dependency in suicide attempters. *Psychopathology, 38,* 140–143.

Oddone, C. G., Hybels, C. F., McQuoid, D. R., & Steffens, D. C. (2011). Social support modifies the relationship between personality and depressive symptoms in older adults. *American Journal of Geriatric Psychiatry, 19*(2), 123–131.

Oslin, D. W. (2005).Treatment of late-life depression complicated by alcohol dependence. *American Journal of Geriatric Psychiatry, 13*(6), 491–500.

Oslin, D. W., Datto, C. J., Kallan, M. J., Katz, I. R., Edell, W. S., & Ten Have, T. (2002). Association between medical comorbidity and treatment outcomes in late-life depression. *Journal of the American Geriatrics Society, 50*(5), 823–8.

Oslin, D. W., Katz, I. R., Edell, W. S., & Ten Have, T. R. (2000). Effects of alcohol consumption on the treatment of depression among elderly patients. *American Journal of Geriatric Psychiatry, 8,* 215–220.

Oslin, D. W., Streim, J., Katz, I. R., Edell, W. S., & Ten Have, T. (2000). Change in disability follows inpatient treatment for late life depression. *Journal of the American Geriatrics Society, 48,* 357–362.

Papakostas, G. I., & Fava, M. (2008). Predictors, moderators, and mediators (correlates) of treatment outcome in major depressive disorder. *Dialogues in Clinical Neuroscience, 10*(4), 439–452.

Patankar, T. F., Baldwin, R., Mitra, D., Jeffries, S., Sutcliffe, C., Burns, A., & Jackson, A. (2007). Virchow-Robin space dilatation may predict resistance to antidepressant monotherapy in elderly patients with depression. *Journal of Affective Disorders, 97*(1–3), 265–270.

Perlis, M. L., Smith, L. J., Lyness, J. M., Matterson, S. R., Pigeon, V., & Xin, T. (2006). Insomnia as a risk factor for onset of depression in the elderly. *Behavior and Sleep Medicine, 4,* 104–113.

Pinquart, M., Duberstein, P. R., & Lyness, J. M. (2007). Effects of psychotherapy and other behavioral interventions on clinically depressed older adults: A meta-analysis. *Aging and Mental Health, 11*(6), 645–657.

Pinto-Meza, A., Usall, J., Serrano-Blanco, A., Suarez, D., & Haro, J. M. (2006). Gender differences in response to antidepressant treatment prescribed in primary care. Does menopause make a difference? *Journal of Affective Disorders, 93,* 53–60.

Poo, M. M. (2001). Neurotrophins as synaptic modulators. *Nature Reviews: Neuroscience, 2,* 24–32.

Pollock, B. G., Ferrell, R. E., Mulsant, B. H., Mazumdar, S., Miller, M., Sweet, R. A., … Kupfer, D. J. (2000). Allelic variation in the serotonin transporter promoter affects onset of paroxetine treatment response in late-life depression. *Neuropsychopharmacology, 23*(5), 587–590.

Pope, H. G., Jr., Amiaz, R., Brennan, B. P., Orr, G., Weiser, M., Kelly, J. F., … Seidman, S. N. (2010). Parallel-group placebo-controlled trial of testosterone gel in men with major depressive disorder displaying an incomplete response to standard antidepressant treatment. *Journal of Clinical Psychopharmacology, 30*(2), 126–134.

Pope, H. G., Jr., Cohane, G. H., Kanayama, G., Siegel, A. J., & Hudson, J. I. (2003). Testosterone gel supplementation for men with refractory depression: A randomized, placebo-controlled trial. *American Journal of Psychiatry, 160*(1), 105–11.

Potter, G. G., Kittinger, J. D., Wagner, H. R., Steffens, D. C., & Krishnan, K. R. (2004). Prefrontal neuropsychological predictors of treatment remission in late-life depression. *Neuropsychopharmacology, 29*(12), 2266–2271.

Rae, A. M., Joyce, P. R., Luty, S. E., & Mulder, R. T. (1982). The effect of a history of alcohol dependence in adult major depression. *Journal of Affective Disorders, 70,* 281–290.

Reynolds, C. F., III, Dew, M. A., Pollock, B. G., Mulsant, B. H., Frank, E., Miller, M., … Kupfer, D. J. (2006). Maintenance treatment of depression in old age. *New England Journal of Medicine, 354*(11), 1130–1138.

Reynolds, C. F., III, Frank, E., Kupfer, D. J., Thase, M. E., Perel, J. M., Mazumdar, S., & Houck, P. R. (1996). Treatment outcome in recurrent major depression: A post hoc comparison of elderly ("young old") and midlife patients. *American Journal of Psychiatry, 153*(10), 1288–1292.

Reynolds, C. F., III, Frank, E., Dew, M. A., Houck, P. R., Miller, M., Mazumdar, S., … Kupfer, D. J. (1999a). Treatment of 70 +—year olds with recurrent depression. Excellent Short-term but brittle long-term response. *American Journal of Geriatric Psychiatry, 7*(1), 64–69.

Reynolds, C. F., III, Frank, E., Perel, J. M., Imber, S. D., Cornes, C., Miller, M. D., ... Kupfer, D. J. (1999b). Nortriptyline and interpersonal psychotherapy as maintenance therapies for recurrent major depression: A randomized controlled trial in patients older than 59 years. *Journal of the American Medical Association, 281*, 39–45.

Rubattu, S., Di Angelantonio, E., Stanzione, R., Zanda, B., Evangelista, A., Pirisi, A., ... Volpe, M. (2004). Gene polymorphisms of the renin-angiotensin-aldosterone system and the risk of ischemic stroke: A role of the A1166C/AT1 gene variant. *Journal of Hypertension, 22*, 2129–2134.

Rush, A. J., Kraemer, H. C., Sckeim, H. A., Fava, M., Trivedi, M. H., Frank, E., ... Schatzberg, A. F. (2006). Report by the ACNP Task Force on response and remission in major depressive disorder. *Neurospchophamacology, 31*, 1841–1853.

Sackeim, H. A., Roose, S. P., & Burt, T. (2005). Optimal length of antidepressant trials in late-life depression. *Journal of Clinical Psychopharmacology, 25*(4 Suppl 1):S34–S37.

Saghafi, R., Brown, C., Butters, M. A., Cyranowski, J., Dew, M. A., Frank, E., ... Reynolds, C. F., III. (2007). Predicting 6-week treatment response to escitalopram pharmacotherapy in late-life major depressive disorder. *International Journal of Geriatric Psychiatry, 22*(11), 1141–1146.

Schraufnagel, T. J., Wagner, A. W., Miranda, J., & Roy-Byrne, P. R. (2005). Treating minority patients with depression and anxiety: What does the evidence tell us? *General Hospital Psychiatry, 28*, 27–36.

Schulman, E., Gairola, G., Kuder, L., & McCulloch, J. (2002). Depression and associated characteristics among community-based elderly people. *Journal of Allied Health, 31*, 140–146.

Sheline, Y. I., Barch, D. M., Garcia, K., Gersing, K., Pieper, C., Welsh-Bohmer, K., ... Doraiswamy, P. M. (2006). Cognitive function in late life depression: Relationships to depression severity, cerebrovascular risk factors and processing speed. *Biological Psychiatry, 60*(1), 58–65.

Shores, M. M., Kivlahan, D. R., Sadak, T. I., Li, E. J., & Matsumoto, A. M. (2009). A randomized, double-blind, placebo-controlled study of testosterone treatment in hypogonadal older men with subthreshold depression (dysthymia or minor depression). *Journal of Clinical Psychiatry, 70*(7), 1009–1016.

Simpson, S. W., Baldwin, R. C., Burns, A., & Jackson, A. (2001). Regional cerebral volume measurements in late-life depression: Relationship to clinical correlates, neuropsychological impairment and response to treatment. *International Journal of Geriatric Psychiatry, 16*(5), 469–476.

Sneed, J. R., Keilp, J. G., Brickman, A. M., & Roose, S. P. (2008). The specificity of neuropsychological impairment in predicting antidepressant non-response in the very old depressed. *International Journal of Geriatric Psychiatry, 23*(3), 319–323.

Sneed, J. R., Roose, S. P., Keilp, J. G., Krishnan, K. R., Alexopoulos, G. S., & Sackeim, H. A. (2007). Response inhibition predicts poor antidepressant treatment response in very old depressed patients. *American Journal of Geriatric Psychiatry, 15*(7), 553–563.

Solomon, D. A., Leon, A. D., Endicott, J., Mueller, T. I., Coryell, W., Shea, M. T., & Keller, M. B. (2004). Psychosocial impairment and recurrence of major depression. *Comprehensive Psychiatry, 45*(6), 423–430.

Spangler, D. L., Simons, A. D., Monroe, S. M., & Thase, M. E. (1997). Response to cognitive-behavioral therapy in depression: Effects of pretreatment cognitive dysfunction and life stress. *Journal of Consulting and Clinical Psychology, 65*(4), 568–575.

Steffens, D. C., & McQuoid, D. R. (2005a). Impact of symptoms of generalized anxiety disorder on the course of late-life depression. *American Journal of Geriatric Psychiatry, 13*(1), 40–47.

Steffens, D. C., Pieper, C. F., III, Bosworth, H. B., MacFall, F. J., Provenzale, J. M., Payne, M. E., ... Krishnan K. R. R. (2005b). Biological and social predictors of long-term geriatric depression outcome. *International Psychogeriatrics, 17*(1), 41–56.

Steffens, D. C., Snowden, M., Fan, M. Y., Hendrie, H., Katon, W. J., & Unutzer, J. (2006). Cognitive impairment and depression outcomes in the IMPACT study. *American Journal of Geriatric Psychiatry, 14*(5), 401–409.

Sternbach, H. (1998). Age-associated testosterone decline in men: Clinical issues for psychiatry. *American Journal of Psychiatry, 155*, 1310–8.

Stetler, C., & Miller, G. E. (2011). Depression and hypothalamic-pituitary-adrenal activation: A quantitative summary of four decades of research. *Psychosomatic Medicine, 73*(2), 114–126.

Steunenberg, B., Beckman, A. T. F., Deeg, D. J. H., Bremmer, M. A., & Kerkhof, A. J. F. M. (2007). Mastery and neuroticism predict recovery of depression in late life. *American Journal of Geriatric Psychiatry, 1393*, 234–242.

Szanto, K., Mulsant, B. H., Houck, P. R., Dew, M. A., Dombrovski, A., Pollock, B. G., & Reynolds,

C. F., III. (2007). Emergence, persistence, and resolution of suicidal ideation during treatment of depression in old age. *Journal of Affective Disorders*, *98*, 153–161.

Szanto, K., Mulsant, B. H., Houck, P. R., Miller, M. D., Mazumdar, S., & Reynolds, C. F., III. (2001). Treatment outcomes in suicidal vs. non-suicidal elderly patients. *American Journal of Geriatric Psychiatry*, *9*(3), 261–168.

Takagishi, Y., Sakata, M., & Kitamura, T. (2011). Effects of self-esteem on state and trait components of interpersonal dependency and depression in the workplace. *Journal of Clinical Psychology*. 2011 June 8, ePub ahead of print. doi: 10.1002/jdp.20815.

Taylor, W. D., Kuchibhatla, M., Payne, M. E., Macfall, J. R., Sheline, Y. I., Krishnan, K. R., & Doraiswamy, P. M. (2008). Frontal white matter anisotropy and antidepressant remission in late-life depression. *PLoS One*, *3*(9), e3267.

Taylor, M. G., & Lynch, S. M. (2004). Trajectories of impairment, social support, and depressive symptoms in later life. *Journal of Gerontology: Social Sciences*, *59B*(4), S238-S246.

Taylor, W. D., McQuoid, D. R., Ashley-Koch, A., MacFall, J. R., Bridgers, J., Krishnan, R. R., & Steffens, D. C. (2011). BDNF Val66Met genotype and 6-month remission rates in late-life depression. *Pharmacogenomics Journal*, *11*, 146–154.

Tew, J. D., Jr., Mulsant, B. H., Houck, P. R., Lenze, E. J., Whyte, E. M., Miller, M. D., ... Reynolds, C. F., III. (2006). Impact of prior treatment exposure on response to antidepressant treatment in late life. *American Journal of Geriatric Psychiatry*, *14*(11), 957–965.

Thielke, S., Vannoy, S., & Unutzer, J. (2007). Integrating mental health and primary care. *Primary Care; Clinics in Office Practice*, *34*, 571–592.

Thiels, C., Linden, M., Grieger, F., & Leonard, J. (2005). Gender differences in routine treatment of depressed outpatients with selective serotonin reuptake inhibitor sertraline. *International Clinical Psychopharmacology*, *20*(1), 1–7.

Watkins, K. E., Paddock, S. M., Zhang, L., & Wells, K. B. (2006). Improving care for depression in patients with comorbid substance misuse. *American Journal of Psychiatry*, *163*, 125–132.

Willner, P. (1997). The mesolimbic dopamine system as a target for rapid antidepressant action. *International Clinical Psychopharmacology*, *12*(Suppl 3), S7–S14.

Winkelby, M. A., Jatulis, D. E., Frank, E., & Formann, S. P. (1992). Socioeconomic status and health: How education, income, and occupation contribute to risk factors for cardiovascular disease. *American Journal of Public Health*, *82*(6), 816–820.

Worthington, J., Fava, M., Agustin, C., Alpert, J., Nierenberg, A. A., Pava, J. A., & Rosenbaum, J. F. (1996). Consumption of alcohol, nicotine, and caffeine among depressed outpatients: Relationship with response to treatment. *Psychosomatics*, *37*(6), 518–522.

Whyte, E. M., Dew, M. A., Gildengers, A., Lenze, E. J., Bharucha, A., Mulsant, B. H., & Reynolds, C. F., III. (2004). Time course of response to antidepressants in late-life major depression: Therapeutic implications. *Drugs and Aging*, *21*(8), 531–554.

Young, R. C., Kalayam, B., Nambudiri, D. E., Kakuma, T., & Alexopoulos, G. S. (1999). Brain morphology and response to nortriptyline in geriatric depression. *American Journal of Geriatric Psychiatry*, *7*(2), 147–150.

Zobel, A. W., Nickel, T., Sonntag, A., Uhr, M., Holsboer, F., & Ising, M. (2001). Cortisol response in the combined dexamethasone/CRH test as predictor of relapse in patients with remitted depression. A prospective study. *Journal of Psychiatric Research*, *35*(2), 83–94.

43

CONCLUSION

Helen Lavretsky, Martha Sajatovic, and Charles F. Reynolds III

FOLLOWING THIS comprehensive review of recent advances in research in late-life mood disorders, we can say that we have come a long way in understanding risk factors and pathophysiology in late-life mood disorders. Various psychosocial and neurobiological risk factors for developing mood disorders in later life are relatively well understood. Neuroimaging studies have helped us to gain a better understanding of the anatomy, functional circuitry, and biochemistry of mood disorders in older people. New developments in information technology have helped to improve the assessment and management of late-life mood disorders. However, more needs to be done in developing personalized pharmacological and psychosocial treatments for late-life depression and bipolar disorders. Promoting understanding of genetic and epigenetic contribution to late-life mood disorders can lead to the development of selective and indicated preventive approaches that increase resilience in later life. Integration of biomarkers in the development of interventions remains a challenge. Understanding the contribution of cognitive impairment and biological aging-related physiological changes is still in the early stage. Global mental health initiatives are likely to be more prominently present in prevention research. Next we outline the current state of art in research and clinical care, and the immediate and distant goals for future research.

DIAGNOSIS

Late-life mood disorders continue to be significantly underdiagnosed in primary care, which is the health care setting used most often by elderly persons. Depression is missed in approximately half of all elderly persons with mood disorder. Given the risks for deleterious effects of depression on health, the failure to diagnose late-life mood disorders remains a serious public health problem and suggests that geriatric psychiatrists need to be more proactive in working with primary health care systems.

There are a variety of barriers in primary care to the recognition and diagnosis of late-life depression. Primary care providers may miss the diagnosis of late-life depression because of insufficient training, a focus on medical conditions that mask the presence of depression, or overlapping symptoms of dementia. Time constraints, inadequate reimbursement, and lack of support staff also hinder the recognition of late-life mood disorders in primary care settings. Patient barriers include stigma about a psychiatric diagnosis. Better education and training of primary care providers and general public can improve appropriate and timely diagnosis of mood disorders and aid in suicide prevention.

Diagnosis of late-life mood disorders can be difficult, in part, because patients often present with somatic symptoms, overlapping symptoms of medical illness, or coexisting mild cognitive impairment. Depression should be suspected and investigated in elderly persons with anhedonia, apathy, hopelessness, anxiety, psychomotor retardation, and unexplained fatigue and weight loss. Among older adults, mood and anxiety disorders are associated with physical illness and cognitive impairment, and result in reduced quality of life and increased functional disability and suicide risk. Dimensional diagnosis can be very useful in approaching geriatric depression given significant medical, neurological, and psychiatric comorbidity. Of particular concern, a significant risk associated with late-life depression is that of excess mortality. Depression has been shown to predict less successful outcomes of treatment for other physical conditions, particularly cardiovascular and cerebrovascular disease, and to increase death rates among the elderly. Depression should be considered in the differential diagnosis of hospitalized elderly persons with myocardial infarction, congestive heart failure, stroke, hip fracture, cancer, or alcohol/substance abuse who exhibit delayed recovery, poor compliance with rehabilitation programs, or treatment refusal. Depression should also be investigated in patients who are apathetic, withdrawn, or agitated, or who exhibit increased dependency, functional decline, or delayed rehabilitation, and in patients receiving long-term care.

The *DSM-5/ICD-10* diagnostic criteria for major depression and bipolar disorder are explicit and may improve diagnosis of late-life depression and include such common features as comorbid anxiety (e.g., in the category of mixed Anxiety-Depression) or comorbid mild-cognitive impairment. However, the language used to describe other milder forms of mood disorder remains imprecise and consists of poorly defined terms, including clinical depression, depressive symptoms, subsyndromal or subthreshold depression, minor depression, and depressed mood. This continuous ambiguity about clinical significance of subclinical depression might still interfere with the ability to make substantive changes in clinical practice. Current diagnostic tools do not adequately address an individual's potential for suicide. Clinicians would benefit from the development of assessment tools that assist in identifying patients with acute and chronic suicidal risk. The effect of possible correlates of suicide (e.g., hopelessness and anxiety) and protective factors (e.g., resilience, ethnicity, and religious beliefs) needs further study. However, future research encouraged by the National Institute of Mental Health "R-DoC" research criteria for dimensional diagnosis of depression or anhedonia may improve the nature of diagnosis in research and clinical practice to include subclinical mood symptoms.

Several subtypes of late-life depression have been identified that may benefit from further study and subsequent development of age-specific diagnostic criteria. Vascular depression may be associated with a later age at onset, and patients may exhibit symptoms of motor retardation, anhedonia, apathy, poor insight, functional disability, and impaired executive function. The features, treatment response, and illness course of late-onset depression, which is defined as a first episode of depression occurring after age 60 years, may differ from those of depression in younger adults. Late-onset depression can be characterized by a greater degree of apathy, cognitive dysfunction, and temporal lobe abnormalities that are similar to changes associated with dementia. Understanding brain aging contribution to the pathophysiology of late-life mood disorders will open new opportunities for the development of new treatment approaches.

The diagnosis of late-life bipolar disorder is an especially neglected and understudied area. Patients with late-onset bipolar disorder may be more likely to have medical comorbidity, particularly cerebrovascular illness, and psychotic features. The differential diagnosis of late-life bipolar disorder must include assessment of comorbid conditions or medications that can cause mania. Once these factors are excluded, a detailed cognitive assessment may inform the potential for recovery and long-term outcome. A better understanding of the risk of precipitating mania in depressed elderly individuals treated with antidepressant agents is also needed. Stigma can delay treatment initiation and a favorable outcome in patients who screen positive for depression.

TREATMENT

While a range of effective interventions are available for mood and anxiety disorders, there remains a considerable need for developing innovative approaches that overcome the shortcomings of these interventions when applied to geriatric mental health care. Current psychopharmacological approaches to the treatment of late-life mood disorder have been shown to be effective for alleviating symptoms in about two thirds of those receiving treatment. Medications are effective in treating late-life depression and combination therapies (medications and psychotherapy) are effective as well. However, a large proportion of patients still do not fully recover and can remain disabled and at risk for other negative outcomes. Moreover, older adults' response to treatment often occurs somewhat more slowly and/or proves to be less sustained over time than that of younger adults. Although such treatment shortcomings are not unique to older adults, they may pose more acute problems for geriatric patients.

Advances in delineating the pathophysiology of mood and anxiety disorders have opened pathways for developing novel interventions that, for example, might target different or additional neurotransmitter systems to those addressed by current antidepressant medications, or that might utilize varied techniques (e.g., pharmacological, psychosocial, cognitive, device-driven) to modulate the activity of brain circuits that have been identified as hyper- or hypoactive in depression and anxiety. This proliferation of studies has contributed to increased understanding of the public health impact of late-life mood disorders, including data needed to guide treatment and inform basic research. Treatment is effective across settings, including primary care, rehabilitation, and long-term care. Controlled studies have demonstrated the efficacy of medication therapy, psychotherapy, and electroconvulsive therapy. Compared with younger adults, older persons often exhibit higher and more variable drug concentrations and a greater sensitivity to adverse effects.

The gold standard of treatment remains the achievement of full remission and a return to wellness. It is now known that antidepressant drug therapy, interpersonal psychotherapy, and the combination of medication use and psychotherapeutic intervention are as efficacious in preventing recurrent major depression in elderly patients as in younger adults. Treatment of psychotic depression and bipolar disorder in late life remains especially understudied, although two major collaborative studies have been recently been completed. There is a critical need to both better understand how pharmacotherapies widely used in younger patients with mood disorders should be optimally used in older patients as well as research with novel agents that may be particularly helpful for older adults. Partial response to the first-line treatment is common and occurs in 30%–50%. Some elderly patients with mood disorders do not respond to treatment, and more needs to be known about factors associated with treatment response and nonresponse. Developing biomarkers of response or nonresponse can accelerate development of individualized and biomarker-driven treatment approaches.

Underlying the positive evidence from treatment studies is the need to address nonadherence. Patients who do not follow treatment advice do so for many different reasons, including stigma associated with antidepressants, inadequate education and support from providers, adverse effects or perceived lack of efficacy, drug–drug interactions, complexity of dosing regimens, medication cost, inadequate insurance coverage, and lack of awareness about the sequelae and chronicity of mood disorders. Although medication adherence is associated with favorable outcomes, approximately 40% of patients of all ages with major depression and 50% with bipolar disorder are nonadherent to antidepressant therapy. Compared with nondepressed persons, depressed medical patients are three times more likely to be nonadherent to medication regimens, exercise, diet, other health-related behaviors, vaccinations, and appointments. These observations suggest the need to improve collaboration with families and care providers and develop therapeutic alliances to improve treatment adherence. Treatment studies need to move progressively to primary care and community populations to treat representative older adult populations.

STUDIES OF RISK AND PROTECTIVE FACTORS FOR LATE-LIFE MOOD DISORDERS AS A BASIS FOR SELECTIVE PREVENTION

Depression and bipolar disorder in the elderly are not necessarily associated with the same risk factors as in younger adults. It is necessary to identify temporal relationships, correlates, and causal patterns to develop clinically useful profiles for high-risk patients and to inform prevention and intervention studies and health care policy.

Late-life depression and mania often occur in the context of chronic medical illness and the medications used to treat them. Medical illness, chronic pain and insomnia, inflammatory processes, functional disability, family and personal histories of mood disorders, social isolation, bereavement, caregiving, and other losses frequently co-occur with depression. Temporal and causal relationships between depression and such correlates are not known with precision and are likely to be bidirectional. Risk factors for depression may also be consequences of depression. Social isolation may contribute to depression risk, but depression can also lead to loneliness and isolation. Correlates of risk for late-life bipolar disorder are less well studied but include comorbid neurological illness, cerebrovascular disease, and a family history of affective disorder. Depression and cardiovascular and cerebrovascular diseases are also strongly correlated. Stroke is a risk factor for depression, and, conversely, depression predicts a poor outcome after stroke. Depression occurs in roughly one third to one half of individuals after stroke. A few intervention studies on antidepressant treatment of post-stroke depression are promising and suggest a pathway for larger prevention and intervention studies.

Late-life depression and depressed mood are common correlates of cognitive impairment and may be prodromes for subsequent cognitive dysfunction and dementia. The presence of mild cognitive impairment during an episode of major depression in late life may precede the development of dementia, particularly if the depression is severe, untreated, and associated with psychomotor retardation or psychosis. Depressive symptoms, especially those with a late-life onset, can herald the onset of Alzheimer disease in nondemented patients. Some cognitive abnormalities such as abnormal performance in response inhibition or in initiation and perseveration tasks and structural neuroimaging indices (e.g., white matter hyperintensities and hippocampal atrophy) may predict a treatment-resistant depression. These findings are preliminary and require further study and replication.

Mood disorders in late life are a major correlate of suicidal behavior. In the United States, suicide is more common in elderly White men than in the general population. Although medical illness and

functional disability also are associated with late-life suicide, the risk associated with these factors is mediated by the presence of depression. Other risk factors such as personal or family history of mood and anxiety disorders, family history of suicide, loneliness, hopelessness, access to handguns, and insufficient social support systems are also important. Suicidal intent or behavior often is not recognized by physicians, and many older adults who commit suicide have visited a physician in the month before their suicide. Suicide prevention for elderly persons must be a primary focus of intervention efforts in the community.

CONCLUSION

Despite increased awareness of older age mood disorders in recent decades, there are still a number of questions that remain unanswered. Based on the rapid development of neuroimaging, genomic, and computer technologies, we anticipate a shift in research priorities that will address immediate needs of the field. Better understanding should encompass better methods of assessment, more appropriate treatment options for older people and their families, and public education about these conditions. Future research will also seek to translate findings into clinical practice to improve the well-being of older people. Given increasing economic globalization, international efforts in mental health research will focus on alleviation of the global burden of depression and associated disability, and they are likely to utilize simple algorithm-based approaches to the management and prevention of common mental disorders in primary care settings.

Current and Future Research Priorities

- Longitudinal studies that assess interactions between psychosocial and biological factors and inform the development of clinically useful high-risk profiles for late-life mood disorders, including better delineation of acute versus chronic risk factors for suicide
- Selective and indicated prevention and intervention studies to identify and reduce risk for first-episode and recurrent late-life mood disorders
- Studies of genetic liability to mood disorders with late-life onset with integration of biomarkers of inflammation and biological and cognitive aging

- Studies of depression subtypes, including dimensional diagnosis of depression and anhedonia, vascular depression, depression associated with inflammation, depression of Alzheimer's disease, dysthymia, and late-onset depression, and development of clinically useful diagnostic tools that facilitate recognition and appropriate treatment
- Studies of the mechanisms by which mood disorders predispose to dementing illnesses
- Studies of depression and suicide prevention, screening, and diagnosis in primary care settings and in underserved minorities
- Longitudinal, early-treatment studies (including psychotherapy and combined pharmacotherapy and psychotherapy) that address prevention of treatment resistance, relapse, recurrence, persistence, and chronicity
- Studies to measure the effect of psychotherapeutic and psychoeducational interventions on treatment adherence
- Development of treatment algorithms specifically tailored to the elderly, including guidelines to optimize treatment response in partially or slowly responding and nonresponding patients and to guide long-term treatment planning
- Studies of pharmacogenetic and pharmacodynamic sources of treatment response variability
- Development of new classes of therapeutic agents for late-life depression (including vascular depression, inflammatory mechanisms, biological aging, and cognitive impairment) and bipolar disorder
- Development of a public health model for mental health care that encompasses case finding, facilitation of access to and delivery of care, and evaluation of reimbursement for service innovations to improve outcome
- Development of partnerships among the research community, health care providers (including agencies that provide home-based nursing care), and health care payers such as the Centers for Medicare and Medicaid Services to design economically sustainable models of mood disorder care in the general medical sector and to further effectiveness and cost-effectiveness studies of evidence-based, clinical disease management models
- Development of partnerships between researchers and religious and other community agencies for outreach to underserved elderly people and for overcoming mistrust of research and mental health care among minorities
- Development of international collaborations for global mental health initiatives

INDEX

Page numbers followed by *t* and *f* indicate tables and figures

Acceptance and commitment therapy (ACT), 154–155, 155*f*
Activities of daily living (ADL). *See also* Instrumental activities
    of daily living
  Alzheimer patient needs, 178
  caregiver/care recipient trajectory and health, 238*f*
  cognitive impairments and, 119
  community need surveys, 36
  depression's influence on, 270
  examples of, 47
  functional disability and, 730
  geriatric BP patient study, 117
  informal caregiver provision of, 237
  men in hospice care needs, 517
  needs when in nursing home, 478
  neuropsychiatric illness and, 135
  number of medical conditions and, 440
  pain's influence on, 330
  post-stroke depression risk factors, 256, 257
  subsyndromal depression and, 134
  suicide association, 212
Acupuncture, 432, 433*t*, 435*t*, 441–442
Acute coronary syndrome, 274, 677
AD. See Alzheimer's disease
Adherence to medication treatment, 279, 457–468
  African Americans data, 464–465
  case study, 457
  conceptual model, 458–459

CRN (cost-related nonadherence), 462
Health Behavior Model, 458
IMPACT study findings, 465
modifiable factors, 460–461
nonmodifiable factors, 464–465
potentially modifiable factors, 461–464
in primary care settings, 508
promising interventions, 465–468
PROSPECT trial findings, 464
provider-/system-level factors, 458
suggested approaches, 467*t*
Theory of Reasoned Action, 458–459
Transtheoretical Model, 458
Treatment Initiation and Participation Program, 466–467
Adjustment disorder
  complicated grief comparison, 228
  with depressed mood, 80, 83, 84b, 85*f*
Administration of Aging (AoA), 533–534
Adult life expectancy data (U.S.), 32
Advancing DSM: Dilemmas in Psychiatric Diagnosing (Hyman),
  69–70
Affective disorders
  BP-type, 106
  comorbid pain and, 334
  treatment referral for, 452
African Americans
  access to information issues, 239

African Americans (*Cont.*)
    alleles frequency data, 644
    Black women diabetes mortality, 272
    complicated grief in, 229
    depression diagnosis gap, 34–35
    depression epidemiology, 35
    depression level data, 167
    grief practices, 222–223
    hopelessness, suicidal thoughts and, 276–277
    income-depression relation, 172
    late-late depression remission data, 719
    psychotherapy adaptions for, 396
    risk variant meta-analysis data, 5
    spiritual/religious practices integration, 442, 460, 504
    SSD risk factors, 132
    treatment adherence data, 464–465
    treatment response, 172
Age and Gender Considerations (Narrow, First, Sorpvatka, Regier), 70–71
Agoraphobia, 145, 148
AGS Panel on Persistent Pain in Older Persons, 329
Aizenstein, H. J., 589, 590
Alcohol dependency. *See* Substance abuse comorbidity
Alcohol Use Disorders Test (AUDIT), 321, 322*f*
Alexopoulos, G. S., 10–11, 82, 259, 261, 368*t*, 369
Almeida, O. P., 85–86, 592
Alpha-2 delta ligands, possible neuropsychiatric side effects, 340*t*
Altered cognition biomarkers
    state biomarkers, 607–608, 610–611, 615–616
    trait biomarkers, 607–608, 611, 614–615
Alzheimer's disease (AD)
    antidepressant first-line treatment, 21
    caregiver burden and, 49
    clinical course, 178
    coding of depression in, 81
    comorbidities
        depression, 36
        MinD, 133
        NMD, 135
        SSD, 133, 135
    differential diagnosis, 84
    DSM coding discussions, 81
    epidemiology, 177–178
    fMRI study, 332
    hippocampal neurodegeneration in, 25
    informal caregiving in, 238
    lithium's prevention association, 24
    in long-term care residents, 491–492
    manic phenomenology association, 109
    medical pain system influenced by, 332
    neuronal pathology, 632
    neuropsychiatric symptoms, 178–179
    in nursing home residents, 478
    patient anxiety, 25
    psychiatric disorders and risks of, 627
    U.S. prevalence data, 177–178
American Geriatrics Society (AGS), 329, 330
American Psychiatric Association
    consensus on ECT, 412
    diagnostic systems development, 68
    Practice Guidelines for Depressive Disorders, 63, 71
    Task Force for ECT, 416
American Telemedicine Association, 547
Amitriptyline
    anticholinergic properties, 194
    for depression in dementia, 189*t*
    HPA axis and, 693

influence on sleep, 353
    non-use recommendation, 487
    open-trial for MDD, 137
    for pain conditions, 339
    pharmacokinetics, 659*t*
    receptor affinity data, 299*t*
    relapse prevention study, 366
    SAMe comparison, 437
Andreescu, C., 591
Anesthetic choice, in ECT, 415–416
Angst, J., 81, 106–107
Anhedonia
    absence in SSD, 130
    as depression symptom, 33, 72, 150
    mortality influence, 274
Anosognosia, 75, 255, 256
Anticholinergic medications
    cautious use recommendations, 194, 299–300, 487
    cognitive toxicity of, 182
    mimicking of depression in dementia, 183*t*
    possible side effects, 340*t*
    use for pre-ECT treatment, 416
Antidepressant medications. *See also* Antidepressant-resistant depression, adjunctive therapy; Monoaminergic antidepressants; Selective serotonin reuptake inhibitors; Serotonin-norepinephrine reuptake inhibitors; Tricyclic antidepressants
    affective network associated with response to, 597*t*
    for anhedonia, 298
    for anxious depression, 152, 154
    as augmentation therapy component, 21
    bipolar disorder and, 107
    cerebral metabolic effects of, 597*t*
    for cerebrovascular disease, 297
    cognitive network associated with response to, 597*t*
    for depression in dementia, 188*t*–190*t*, 196
    for depression in hospice care settings, 524–525
    for depression in long-term care, 480–481, 482*t*–485*t*
    differing response rates to, 83
    efficacy/effectiveness of treatment, 90–92, 90*t*
    interpersonal psychotherapy with, 377, 591, 744
    for late-life depression, 20
    male mortality and, 43
    pharmacokinetics of, 658, 659*t*–662*t*
    placebo comparison, 9, 95
    for post-stroke depression, 256, 257–258, 297
    preventative for depression, 20, 213–214
    relapse possibility, 89
    for sleep-depression disorders, 353
    social determinants for receiving, 171
    in structural brain abnormalities, 87
    tolerability issues, 22
Antidepressant-resistant depression, adjunctive therapy
    acceleration trials, 364
    adjunctive agents
        antipsychotics, 368*t*
        atypical agents, 369–370
        cognitive enhancing agents, 373–374
        donepezil, 374
        hormone therapy, 372–373
        lithium, 365–366, 367*t*
        memantine, 374
        modafinil, 371–372
        nutritional supplements, 374–375
        pindolol and buspirone, 372
        stimulants, 370–371

testosterone, 373
thyroid, 366, 369
algorithm for treatments, 377–381
initial minimal responders, 381
partial responders, 378–380, 379t
specific residual symptoms, 380–381
combination treatments, 365
novel treatments, 375–376
sequential use of treatments, 376–377
Antiepileptic drugs (AEDs), 303, 304t. See also Felbamate;
Levetiracetam; Tiagabine; Vigabatrin; Zonisamide
Antihistamines, 183t
Antipsychotic medications. See also Aripiprazole; Quetiapine
adherence in BP patients, 119
adjunctive trials, for LLD, 368t
adjunctive uses, 9, 91, 154, 379t, 666
atypical antipsychotics, 301, 368t, 369–370, 418, 493
differing response rates to, 83, 94
health/mortality-related risks, 9, 45
for late-life anxious depression, 154
new formulations, 664
new formulations of, 664
non-use recommendations, 194–195
pharmacokinetics of, 658, 663
for psychotic depression, 487, 525
regulatory considerations, 487
side effects, 45, 667
tardive dyskinesia from, 370
Anxiety disorders. See also Generalized anxiety disorder
adverse consequences, 24
cardiovascular disease and, 24, 148
comorbidity data, 4
in depression in hospice care setting, 519
future research directions, 26
neurobiology of, 147
neurotransmitter modulation of, 331
in nursing home residents, 478
problem-solving therapy, 148
psychotropic medications for, 9
research priorities
anxiety-cognitive decline association, 25
diagnostic criteria, 25
prevention, detection, treatment, 25–26
thought suppression association, 149–150, 153f
Anxious depression, 144–157
behavioral avoidance, 150–151
cognitive avoidance and, 150
co-occurrence explanations, 146–148
as emotion regulation, 148–151
in ICD-10, 64
as maladaptive, emotional experience, 148–151
MDD comorbidity, 145
pharmacological treatment, 152, 154
prevalence, negative outcomes, 144–146
psychotherapy, unified models, 154–157
safety signals in, 150–151
tripartite model, 148
unified models, 151–152
Arean, P., 154, 230
Aripiprazole
adjunctive use, 91, 154, 368t, 381
for antidepressant-resistant depression, 369, 370, 379t
for anxious/non-anxious, mixed-depression, 380
controlled trials data, 369–370
for late-life anxious depression, 154
pharmacokinetic studies of, 663
Armitage, R., 353

Asian Americans
health care access issues, 171
information access issues, 239
Assisted living facilities (ALFs), 477, 492–493
Atomoxetine, 301
Atypical antipsychotics, 301, 368t, 369–370, 418, 493. See also
Clozapine; Quetiapine
AUDIT (Alcohol Use Disorders Test), 321, 322f
Autonomic arousal (AA), 148, 150
Avery, D. H., 419
Ayurveda, 433t, 435t, 439, 442

Baglioni, C., 351
Bakshi, N., 107, 114
Baltimore Epidemiologic Catchment Area (ECA) study, 270
Barbiturates, 303, 415, 657
Barlow, D. H., 148
Bartels, S. J., 277
Bauer, M., 366
Beach, S.R.H., 70
Beekman, A.T.F., 88
Behavioral avoidance, 150–151
Behavioral mechanisms, of medical burdens, 45–46
Behavioral pathways, linking medical illness
and depression, 278–279
Behavioral Risk Factor Surveillance System (BRFSS), 34, 237
Benton Visual Retention Test, 261
Benzodiazepines
adjunctive uses, 9
for anxiety disorders, 24
for late-life anxious depression, 154
mimicking of depression in dementia, 183t
new formulation, 664
pharmacokinetics of, 664
substance abuse comorbidity and, 317–318, 320, 324
Benztropine, 183t
Bereavement, 220–232. See also Complicated grief syndrome;
Grief; Mourning among older adults
antidepressants for, 91
of caregivers, 224–225
CLOC study findings, 221–222
defined, 221–222
differential diagnosis, 84
friends/family influenced by, 220
grief therapy for, 89
influences on depression, 168–169
meta-analysis, longitudinal studies, 222–223
posttraumatic stress disorder and, 229
social determinants, 169–170
subsyndromal depression and, 133
by suicide, 209
suicide risk factors, 221
from widowhood, spousal loss, 167, 169, 221, 223–224
Bereavement in older adults
strengths and resources, 225–227
Berkman, L. F., 169
Berrios, G. E., 107, 114
Berry, D.T.R., 350
Beta-amyloid deposition, 593, 596, 599
Beta-amyloid imaging, 599
Beta-blockers, 89
Bibliotherapy
efficacy/effectiveness of, 90t
Biochemical changes, in depression, 86–87
Biological mechanisms, of medical burdens, 45
Biological pathways, linking medical illness and depression,
279–281

Biomarkers. *See also* Altered cognition biomarkers; Cognitive biomarkers in depression; Neuropathological markers, in late-life depression
  of aging, 6–7
  application in clinical practice, 19
  in ECT and antidepressants, 407
  fMRI and
    bipolar disorder, 591–592
    late-life depression, 588–591
  future depression research, 22
  metabolites and respective markers, 578*t*
  neurocognitive biomarkers, 607, 609, 614, 617
  "Use of Biomarkers in the Elderly," 71
Biopsychosocial model of depression, 89
Bipolar depression, 37, 111
  ECT treatment for, 408–409
  learning/memory issues, 35%5
  pharmacotherapy response, 118–119
  sleep, 20%6
Bipolar disorder (BPD), 104–120. *See also* Bipolar depression; Mania/manic syndromes
  affective course factors, 113–114
  alterations in fMRI BOLD signal change, 594*t*
  brain cell pathological changes, 632
  comorbidities
    medical/neurological, 115
    psychiatric, 106, 115
  differential diagnosis, 106
    chronic psychoses, 106
    manic states, 105
    organic mental disorders, 105–106
    substance abuse, 106
    type I, II BPDs, 105
  disability and, 47, 113, 115
  DSM-V proposals, 72–73
  economic costs, 48–49
  epidemiology of, 37, 106–107
  episodes: affective features
    bipolar depression, 111
    mania, 110–111
    mixed states, 111
    psychotic features, 111
  episodes: cognitive impairments, 111–113
  familial factors, 110
  family burdens from, 49–50
  global prevalence data, 23
  hospitalization rates, 49
  in *ICD-9-CM,* 62
  in *ICD-10-CM,* 65*t*–66*t*
  late-life admissions data, 627–628
  late-life bipolar disorder studies, 560
  life events, daily routine, 110
  medical burdens, 45
  medical comorbidity, 109–110
  mortality and, 43–44
  MRS studies, 578, 580–582
  nonaffective outcomes
    cognitive impairment, 116
    emergent dementia, 116
    functional, behavioral disability, 117
    nonsuicide mortality, 115–116
  pathophysiology and etiology
    age/age at onset, 107
    age-associated factors, 107
    brain lesions and mania, 107–108
    functional neuroimaging, 109
    neurological disorders, treatments, 109

    structural imaging abnormalities, 108–109
    vascular risk factors, 107
  quality of life issues, 47
  relapse/recurrence, 114–115
  research challenges, directions, 23–24, 120
  social support issues, 115
  standardized mortality ratios, 43–44
  treatment outcomes, modifiers
    adherence issues, 119–120
    bipolar depression, pharmacotherapy response, 15–16
    relapse recurrence in maintenance, 119
    slowed, attenuated antimanic response, 117–118
  treatment strategies
    lithium, 23
    types of, 37
    unipolar depression vs., 105
Bipolar disorder (BPD) schizoaffective disorders, 106
Black, D. W., 109
Blazer, D. G., 81, 317
Boerner, K., 225
BOLD functional MRI, 586–587
Borbély, A. A., 350
Borderline personality disorder
  sleep disorders and, 348
Bowlby, John, 227, 228
Brain. *See also* Cerebrovascular disease; Functional magnetic resonance imaging; Hypothalamic-pituitary-adrenal (HPA) axis; Neurotransmitters; Prefrontal cortex; Structural magnetic resonance studies; White matter; White matter hyperintensities
  age-associated changes, 332
  amygdala/prefrontal cortex patterns, 147
  biological changes, in chronic illness, 46*f*
  bipolar disorder
    age-related changes, 107
    OFC dysfunction, 108
    PFC research, 632
    prefrontal cortex, limbic regions, 591–592
    structural neuroimaging, 108–109
  cerebral neoplasms, 305
  circuitry modulation methods, 9
  deep brain stimulation treatment, 94
  disorders (examples), 85*f*
  estrogen effects on, 8
  frontal lobe studies, 560
  hippocampal neurodegeneration, Alzheimer's disease, 25
  lesions, 84
  LLD: frontostriatal, frontolimbic circuitry, 588–590
  molecular aging research, 5
  neuroimaging methods, 19
  organic cerebral impairment, in mania, 109
  positron emission tomography studies, 572–573
  postmortem studies with relevant MDD findings, 628*t*–631*t*
  structural abnormalities in depression, 87
  subcortical structure studies, 561–562
  suicide and brain volume, 210
  task-specific regions, functional processes, 587*t*
  temporal lobe studies, 560–561
  in vascular depression, 260–262
Brain lesions
  mania and, 105, 107–108
  in post-stroke depression, 256
  role in depression, 84
  white matter lesions, 87, 561–562
Brain-derived neurotrophic factor (BDNF), 5, 187, 280
  Val66Met polymorphism, 577, 648, 719–720
Brandy Handgun Violence Prevention Act (1994), 215

Brassen, S., 590
Brief recurrent depression, 129
Broadhead, J., 107, 110–111, 114
Brofaromine, 353
Bromocriptine, 300–301
Brown, G. W., 168
Brown, T. A., 148
Bruce, M. L., 10–11
Bunney, W. E., 353
Buprenorphine, 376
Bupropion, 91, 301
    for antidepressant-resistant depression, 365, 379t
    for depression in hospice care, 525
    for late-life anxious depression, 154
    pharmacokinetics, 659t
Burden of illness
    defined, 42
Burdens of late-life mood disorders
    disability, 47
    on formal care, 48–49
    increased mortality
        bipolar disorder, 43–44
        increased morbidity, 44
        late-life depression, 43
        suicide, 44
    loss of productivity, 48
    medical burdens
        of bipolar disorder, 45
        of depression, 44–45
    medical burdens, mechanisms
        behavioral, 45–46
        biological, 45
        psychological/cognitive, 46–47
        social, 47
    quality-of-life issues, 47
    socioeconomic status factors, 50
    strategies for addressing
        prevention, early detection, 50–51
        treatment, 51
Burns, A., 180t
Burrows, A. B., 482t
Burton, A. M., 225
Buspirone
    adjunctive uses, 372, 380
    for antidepressant-resistant depression, 372
    bupropion comparison, 365
Bustin, J., 410

Cache County Study on Memory, Health and Aging, 167, 179, 180t, 182
Caine, E. D., 81
Cairney, J., 165
Calcium channel blockers, 262, 376. See also Nimodipine
California Verbal Learning Test (CVLT), 596
Callahan, C. M., 43, 277
Cancer
    depression in hospice care and, 517–518
    MDD as risk factor, 273
    mimicking of depression in dementia, 183t
    in nursing home residents, 478
Carbamazepine
    mimicking of depression in dementia, 183t
Cardiac disease/coronary heart disease
    NMD association, 133
Cardiovascular disease
    anxiety and, 24, 148
    brain changes in, 19
    caregivers' depression and, 242
    clinical trial needs, 22
    ECT pretreatment assessment, 412–413
    emotional stress and, 280
    MDD as risk factor, 9, 44, 87, 88f, 270, 273–274
    white matter hyperintensities and, 82
Cardiovascular Health Study, 179, 180t
Care deliver systems. See Home-based services and interventions; Hospice care settings, late-life depression in; Internet-based interventions and telepsychiatry; Long-term care, depression and dementia in; Long-term care, depression in; Primary care settings, late-life depression in
Care management models, home-based services
    aging services network, 540
    home health care, 538–540
    mental health care, 540
    telephone, telehealth care, 540
Caregiver burden
    Alzheimer's disease and, 49
    benefits from caregiving and, 246
    bipolar disorder and, 117
    causes of, 249
    CBT intervention for, 391
    in families of depressed adults, 49, 391, 531
    health issues of caregivers, 178
    patient nursing home placement from, 478
    positive/negative effect reconciliation, 246–247
    psychiatric services use and, 115
    U.S. national survey findings, 49–50
Caregivers/informal caregivers
    anxiety disorder risk factors, 24
    bereavement of, 224–225
    challenges faced by, 239, 247
    characteristics of, 237–238
    complicated grief syndrome and, 225
    decreased mortality of, 243–244
    health risks of, 178
    indeterminate prevalence of, 236–237
    interventions for, 247–248
    minor depression in, 49–50
    physical health measures, 240t
    prevalence of, 236–237
    productivity issues, 50
    psychological health measures, 241t
    recipient characteristics, 238
    roles and responsibilities of, 238–239
    skills trainings for, 195
    as societal resource, 236
    U.S. prevalence data, 237–238
Caregiving
    beneficial effects, 243–247
    complicated grief and, 225, 229
    in depression in dementia, 195t–196t, 197–198
    detrimental effects, 239–243
    impact on caregivers, 49–50
    informal caregiving, 236–238
    by older adults, 224–225
    prevalence of, 236–237
    reciprocal-altruism theory, 245
    social support aspect of, 277–278
    societal prevalence of, 249
    U.S. national survey findings, 49
Caregiving Satisfaction Scale, 246
Carr, D., 224
CBT. See cognitive behavioral therapy
Celecoxib
    for antidepressant-resistant depression, 376

Census Bureau (U.S.)
  aging demographic data, 329
  BP nonsuicide mortality data, 115–116
  Hispanic population projections, 271
  home-based care needs data, 532
  nursing home data, 36
  SES/LLD data, 728
  2010 age data, 4
Center for Epidemiological Studies Depression Scale (CES-D), 130
Centers for Disease Control and Prevention (CDC), 11, 477
Centers for Medicare and Medicaid Services (CMS), 478. *See also* Medicare
Cerebral neoplasms, 305
Cerebrovascular disease. *See also* Vascular depression
  comorbidities
    bipolar disorder, 23
    depression, 45, 254, 258
  DED syndrome and, 259
  mortality rates, 116
  neuroimaging evaluation, 258–259
  risk factors, 107
  therapeutic outcomes, 118
  treatment considerations, 297
  white matter hyperintensities and, 261
CES-D (Center for Epidemiological Studies Depression Scale), 37
Changing Lives of Older Couples (CLOC) study, 221–222
Charlton, R., 224
Chemotherapeutic agents
  mimicking of depression in dementia, 183t
Chepenik, L. G., 592
China, complicated grief rates, 229
Chlorpromazine, 183t
Cholinergic-aminergic hypothesis, 348–349. *See also* Sleep-depression relationship
Chorpita, B. F., 148
Chronic obstructive pulmonary disease (COPD)
  depression comorbidity, 87
  ECT risks, 414
  medical comorbidities, 134
  mimicking of depression in dementia, 183t
  suicide risks, 211
Chronobiological models, of sleep regulation, 349–350
Chu, D., 109
Ciapparelli, A., 409
CIDI. See Composite International Diagnostic Interview
Ciechanowski, P., 540
Circadian hypotheses of depression, 350
Citalopram, 91
  for depression in dementia, 188t
  for depression in hospice care, 525
  for late-life anxious depression, 152
  pharmacokinetics, 659t
  for post-stroke depression, 258
Clements, P. T., 223
Clements-Cortes, A., 523
Clinical prediction models
  Area Under the Curve (AUC), 707
  Cox proportional hazards model, 706–707, 711
  dynamically updating of, 710–711
  future research directions, 711–712
  general linear mixed models, 705–706
  hazard submodel, 708
  information used by, 704–705
  joint models, 706–712
  linear mixed-effects models, 705–706, 708, 711

longitudinal submodel, 708
  Markov Chain Monte Carlo simulation, 706
  measurement submodel, 708
  multiple linear regression model, 705
  nonlinear mixed-effects models, 658, 710
  static prediction models, 706–707
  time-to-event models, 704, 706–712
Clinical trials. *See also* Improving Mood-Promoting Access to Collaborative Treatment (IMPACT) study; STAR*D study
  aging service clients, 540
  antidepressants, nursing home trials, 481, 482t–485t, 486–487
  citalopram vs. perphenazine, 195
  depression prevention trials, 452
  escitalopram effectiveness, 137
  future research directions, 22
  monoaminergic antidepressants, 187
  multidisciplinary collaborative care, 718
  neuroimaging trials' importance, 19
  NIMH intramural research program, 3
  non-major depression, 137
  olanzapine plus sertraline, double-blind, 21
  omega-3 fatty acids, depression, 436
  paroxetine vs. mirtazapine, double-blind, 647
  population pharmacokinetic studies, 658, 668
  relapse recurrence rates, 37
  SAMe, 436
  St. John's wort, 437–438
  stepped-care approach effectiveness, 51
  substance use, depression, 320–321
  symptom outcomes assessment, 89
  transcranial magnetic stimulation, 419
  vagal nerve stimulation, 420
Clomipramine
  for depression in dementia, 188t
  pharmacokinetics, 659t
Clozapine, 301, 657
Cochrane Database review
  antidepressant efficacy study, 91
  of psychopharmacological approaches, 9
Cognitive avoidance, 150
Cognitive behavioral therapy (CBT)
  advantages of, 92
  for anxiety, 148
  comparative studies, 92–93, 134
  comparison with other therapies, 395t
  for depression, 20, 26, 148
  efficacy/effectiveness of, 90t
  evidence base, 391
  for insomnia in depression, 354–355
  intervention theory, overview, 391
  for NMD, 137
  for pain management, 341t
  for post-stroke depression, 258
  pros and cons, 391–392
  research studies, 11
  for sleep problems, 352
Cognitive biomarkers in depression, 606–617
  altered cognition, underlying causes, 607
  altered cognition biomarkers
    state biomarkers, 607–608, 610–611, 615–616
    trait biomarkers, 607–608, 610–611, 614–615, 615–616
  "cold" cognition in depression
    at-risk populations, 611
    executive function, 610–611
    learning and memory, 610
  described, 606–607
  functional imaging

at-risk individuals, 614
  cold cognition, 612–613
  hot cognition, 613–614
genetic links, 615
"hot" cognition in depression, 611–612
modeling in health individuals, 607
  monamine manipulation, 614–615
  mood manipulation, 615
neurocognitive biomarkers, 607, 609, 614, 617
specific effects in LLD
  chronic relapsing depression, 608–609
  comparative research, 609
  late-onset depression, 608
treatment impact on markers
  state biomarkers, 615–616
  trait biomarkers, 616
uses of
  better identification, 616–617
  improved treatment outcomes, 617
  promoting resilience, 617
Cognitive decline
  comorbidities
    anxiety, 24–25, 146
    bipolar disorder, 23, 24
    depression, 19
  lithium treatment for, 23
Cognitive enhancing agents
  for antidepressant-resistant depression, 373–374
Cognitive impairment
  bereavement and, 224
  cognitive biomarkers, effects of, 608
  comorbidities
    anxiety disorders, 26
    bipolar disorder, 23
    depression, 19, 21
    mania, 104–105
  mania with, 104–105
  in nursing home residents, 478
  in post-stroke depression, 257
  psychotherapy adaptations, 397
Cognitive mechanisms, of medical burdens, 46–47
Cohen, A., 172
Cohen, L. M., 483t, 484t
Cold cognition, in depression, 609–611, 612–613
Collaborative care programs, 51
  for depression management, 93–94
Collaborative depression care model, 21, 214, 538
Community interventions, 11
Community service settings
  bipolar disorder epidemiology, 37
  depression epidemiology, 36–37
Community-based studies
  major depression, 131–132, 270
  non-major depression, 130–131
Comorbid neurological illness, 295–305
  cerebral neoplasms, 305
  cerebrovascular disease
    bipolar disorder association, 23
    treatment considerations, 297
    vascular depression, 296–297
  degenerative dementias
    Alzheimer's disease, 298
    apathy in dementia, 297–298
    frontotemporal dementias, 106, 108, 298
    treatment considerations, 298–299
  disorders of movement
    Huntington's disease, 301–302

Parkinson's disease, 299–300
    treatment considerations, 300–301
  epilepsy, 303
  mood symptoms (defined), 295–296
Comorbid pain disorders, 329–341. See also Pain (in older adults)
  fibromyalgia, Pope and Hudson criteria, 338t
  mental health care for, 727
  psychiatric conditions and, 332–335
    affective disorders, 106, 334, 452
    disordered sleep, 334–335, 681
    somatoform disorders, 65t, 71, 333–334, 339
    substance use, 334
  treatment modalities
    nonpharmacologic, 339–340
    pharmacologic, 338–339
    psychiatric evaluation, 337–338
Complementary and alternative medicine (CAM), 432–443
  acupuncture, 432, 433t, 435t, 441–442
  aromatherapy massage, 523
  ayurveda, 433t, 435t, 439, 442
  conventional physical exercise, 439–441
  definitions and domains, 433
  exercise, 436t
  expressive therapies, 436t
  folate and B12, 435t
  gingko biloba, 435t
  late-life mood disorder studies, 433–434
  mindful physical exercise, 438
  mindfulness meditation, 441
  omega-3 fatty acids, 434, 435t, 436–437
  religion and spirituality, 436t, 442
  SAMe, 374–375, 379t, 437
  St. John's Wort, 434t, 437–438, 657
  tai-chi, 433t, 438–439, 680–681
  US usage data, 432–433
  yoga, 432, 433t, 436t, 438–439, 442
Complicated grief syndrome, 223, 227–228
  assessment, 224
  caregiving and, 225, 229
  diagnostic criteria proposals, 228
  epidemiology, risk, protective factors, 229–230
  population-based studies, 229
  smoking risks, 229
  suffering from, 228
  treatment, 230–231
Complicated mania, 105
Composite International Diagnostic Interview (CIDI), 33
Computed tomography (CT)
  bipolar patient scanning, 108
  brain ventricular enlargement observations, 559
  depression-multiple sclerosis study, 302
  single photon emission CT, 354
The Conceptual Evolution of DSM-V (Regier, Narrow, Kuhl), 71
Congestive heart failure
  differential diagnosis, 743
  etomidate success in, 415
  HPA axis hyperactivity and, 45
  inpatient recovery study data, 133
  mimicking of depression in dementia, 183t
  nonmajor depression association, 134
  psychomotor retardation symptoms in, 182
  suicide association, 277
Conradsson, M., 193t
Consent process, in ECT, 416
Continuing-care retirement communities, 477
Controlled Oral Word Association Test (COWAT), 596
Conversion disorder, 333

Cook, J. M., 148
Cooper, L. A., 458
Cornelius, J. R., 321
Cornell Scale for Depression in Dementia (CSDD), 183–184, 525
Corticosteroids
  grief association, 228
  HPA axis and, 690
  manic state association, 109
  mimicking of depression in dementia, 183t
  possible neuropsychiatric side effects, 340t
  use in multiple sclerosis, 302
Cost-related nonadherence (CRN), to medication, 462
Cotter, D., 628t
Cox proportional hazards model, 706–707, 711
C-reactive protein (CRP), 86–87, 278–279, 281, 677–678
Crum, R. M., 135
CYP2D6, 304t, 643–646, 656–657
Dahabra, S., 560

DAT1 VNTR 10/10 polymorphism, 719
DED syndrome. See Depression-executive dysfunction (DED) syndrome
Deep brain stimulation (DBS)
  for depression, 94
  mania occurrence from, 300
  for treatment-resistant depression, 420
Deep white matter hyperintensities, 562–563
Degenerative dementias. See also Alzheimer's disease (AD)
  apathy in dementia, 297–298
  frontotemporal dementias, 106, 108, 298
  treatment considerations, 298–299
Delaloye, C., 561
DeLeo, D., 214
Delirium
  from alcohol withdrawal, 323
  clinical trial results and, 482t, 486
  depression comparison, 518
  diminished concentration in, 182
  ECT-induced delirium, 409
  manic features of, 104–105
  mimicking of depression in dementia, 183t
  as neurotoxicity side effect, 366
  as possible medication side-effect, 340t
  postictal delirium, 194
  suicide association studies, 210
Dementia. See also Alzheimer's disease; Depression in dementia
  anxiety disorder risk factors, 24
  comorbidities
    BPD, 115
    depression, 492, 525–526, 627
    mania, 105–106
    NMD, 134
  frontotemporal dementia, 106, 108
  in long-term care residents, 491–492
  neuropsychiatric symptoms, 178–179
  in nursing home residents, 478
  pain assessment, 336
  positron emission tomography studies, 572–573
Depression care management (DCM), 11
Depression CAREPATH (CARE for PATients at Home)
    Intervention, 539–540
Depression in dementia, 87, 177–198
  assessment
    apathy vs. depression, 182
    caregiver input, caregiver bias, 181
    instruments for, 183–184, 184t–185t
    neuroimaging, 187

symptom clusters, diagnostic dilemmas, 179–181
  caregiver intervention
    sample intervention, 195t–196t
    supportive care checklist: caregiver, 197
    supportive care checklist: patient, 198
  causes
    genetic factors, 187
    neurochemical factors, 186–187
    psychosocial factors, 186
  diagnostic workup, 183t
  epidemiology of, 179
  mimicking conditions and medications, 183t
  premorbid depression, 178
  prevalence studies, 180t
  treatment
    choosing a medication, 194–195
    medications, 187, 188t–190t, 191
    nonpharmacologic, 191, 192t–193t, 194
Depression without sadness, 150, 479
Depression-executive dysfunction (DED) syndrome, 259
Depression-pain syndrome, 330–331
Depressive disorders. See also Bipolar disorder; Depression in
    dementia; Dysthymic disorder; Early onset depression;
    Late-life depression; Major depressive disorder; Post-
    stroke depression; Social determinants of depression;
    Subsyndromal depression; Subthreshold depression;
    Vascular depression
  Alexopoulos/Bruce intervention schema, 10–11
  biological mechanisms, 45
  burden of, 272
  collaborative depression care model, 21, 214, 538
  current knowledge, summary, 19
  depression-pain syndrome, 330–331
  disabilities and, 47
  economic costs (2000), 48
  endogenous depression, 10, 67t, 255, 347
  epidemiological factors
    community service settings, 36–37
    medical settings, 35–36
    population representative samples, 34–35
  ethnic diversity data, 271–272
  family burdens from, 49–50
  future research directions, 22–23
  home-based services and interventions, 536–538
  issues/gaps in knowledge
    detection/diagnosis, 21
    prevalence, 21
    prevention, 21
    treatment, interventions, 22
  melancholic depression, 83, 90, 94–95, 96t, 680, 691
  mortality and, 43, 271
  prevalence, 42, 271
  productivity losses and, 48
  psychoneuroimmunology of, 675–683
  research priorities, 18–23
    detection, diagnosis, 19
    interventions, 21
    prevalence, 19–20
    prevention, 20, 21–22
    treatment, 20–21
  thought suppression association, 149–150, 153f
Desai, M. M., 48
Desvenlafaxine, 152
Devanand, D. P., 135
Developmental trajectories of late-life mood disorders
  earlier exposures, experiences, 8
  mechanisms of excess mortality, 8–9

menopause, 8
study methodologies, 7–8
Dew, M. A., 172
Dextroamphetamine
adjunctive use, 370, 379t
for antidepressant-resistant depression, 371, 379t
as Category 3 agent, 380
initial testing, 364
placebo-controlled trials, 371
Diabetes
Ayurvedic treatment, 442
comorbidities
bipolar disorder, 23
depression, 9, 44–46, 270–271, 463
HPA axis reactions, 695
non-major depression, 135
day-to-day management, 270
depression mortality comparison, 271
geriatric psychiatrist management role, 337
late-life cognition influenced by, 113
life course projections, 283
MDD as risk factor, 273–274
medical burden of, 44, 48–49, 272
mini-depression and, 2135
muti-ethnic study, 274
need for clinical trials, 22
non-Hispanic White women mortality, 272
nonmajor depression association, 134
nurse-led intervention study, 453
in nursing home residents, 478
patient hopelessness issues, 276–277
in primary care settings, 501
quality of life issues, 47
race/ethnicity risks, 282
renal decline exacerbation, 657
as risk factor for LLD, 88f
subcortical nuclei Glu, Gln levels, 581
vascular depression and, 82
white matter hyperintensities and, 82
Diabetic peripheral neuropathic pain, 338
Diagnosis. See also Differential diagnosis
African Americans, diagnosis gap, 34–35
of Alzheimer's disease, 178, 182, 572
barriers in hospice care, 517, 518–519
barriers in hospice care settings, 518–519
of bipolar disorders, 80, 105–106
of cancer-related depression, 453
challenges, in late-life depression, 743
Chinese medicine and, 441–442
of chronic illness-related depression, 274, 282
comorbidity issues, 318
of dementia, 210
of depression in Alzheimer's disease, 184t, 188t
of depression in homebound adults, 534
depressive disorders, gaps, 21
of generalized anxiety disorder, 145
geriatric research focus, 19
Hispanic adults, gaps, 34–35
intrapersonal therapy strategy, 393
of late-life depression, 79–83, 171, 241t, 450
linking treatment with, 95
of non-major depression, 132–133
post-diagnosis treatment gaps, 458
of prolonged grief disorder, 170
regulatory treatment considerations, 487
of secondary depression, 318
staff observations in nursing homes, 480

of stroke-related mood disorder, 255
uncertainty issues, 502, 504–505
underdiagnosis issues, 300, 335, 675, 742–743
Diagnostic and Statistical Manual of Mental Disorders (DSM), 5,
68–71, 68t, 74
Diagnostic and Statistical Manual of Mental Disorders-III (DSM-
III), 68, 69, 270
Diagnostic and Statistical Manual of Mental Disorders-III-R (DSM-
III-R), 68, 69
Diagnostic and Statistical Manual of Mental Disorders-IV
(DSM-IV)
altered cognition in depression, 607
anxiety disorders criteria, 25
dysthymic disorder description, 33–34
major depression
anxiety disorders symptom overlap, 146
diagnostic criteria, 181
subtype classifications, 83
minor depression diagnostic criteria, 181
mood disorder divisions, presentation, 69, 79–80
post-bereavement depression, 84
post-stroke depression, diagnostic criteria, 255
shortcomings of, 80–81
SSD adult prevalence, 130
Structured Clinical Interview for depression, 228, 517
Diagnostic and Statistical Manual of Mental Disorders-IV-TR
(DSM-IV-TR)
anxiety disorders criteria, 24, 25
bipolar disorder, 105
Diagnostic Criteria sets, 69
Global Assessment of Relational Functioning Scale, 70
"late onset" definition, 74
minor depression description, 34
sleep disorder listing, 356
stroke/post-stroke depression listing, 254
subsyndromal depression description, 34
Diagnostic and Statistical Manual of
Mental Disorders-V (DSM-V)
bipolar disorder proposals, 72–73
ICD-11 organization and, 68
"late onset" inclusion discussion, 74–75
mixed anxiety/depression proposal, 72–73
Mood Disorders Work Group, 72
presentations/proposals for, 69–71
Sleep-Wake Disorders Work Group, 72
Task Force, 71–73
Differential diagnosis
of Alzheimer's disease, 84
of bipolar disorder, 105, 106
of congestive heart failure, 743
of dysthymic disorder, 83, 84b
of late-life depression, 83–84, 84b, 612
of old age depression vs. AD dementia, 352
of substance abuse, 106
of vascular dementia, 84
Diffusion tensor imaging (DTI) studies
benefits of, 6
description, 565–566
late-life bipolar disorder, 566
late-life depression, 566, 576–577, 591
in vascular depression, 260–262
Digoxin toxicity, 183t
Dimensional Approaches in Diagnostic Classification (Helzer,
Kraemer, Krueger, Wittchen), 71
Dimensional Models of Personality Disorders (Widiger, Simonsen,
Sirovatka, Regier), 70
Dimsdale, J. E., 71

Disability
  bipolar disorder and, 47, 113, 115
  prevalence data, 47
  suicide risks, 212
  WHO definition, 42, 47
Discomfort Scale—Dementia of Alzheimer Type (DS-DAT), 336
Djernes, J. K., 167
Dombrovski, A. Y., 210
Donepezil, 374
Dopamine agonists, 300–301. *See also* Bromocriptine;
    Pramipexole; Ropinirole
Dopamine system, 596, 598–599
Doshi, J. A., 48
Driscoll, H. C., 91–92
DSM-5 Working Group on Mood Disorders, 71
DSM-V Task Force, 71–73
Duloxetine
  for antidepressant-resistant depression, 369
  for diabetic peripheral neuropathy, 338
  for fibromyalgia, 338
  for late-life anxious depression, 152
Dyslipidemia
  depression association, 86
  vascular depression and, 82
Dysphoric mania, 111
Dysthymic disorder
  comorbidities, 145
  differential diagnosis, 83, 84b
  DSM-IV, DSM-IV-TR description, 33–34, 80, 83
  in *ICD-9-CM, ICD-10-CM*, 62, 67t
  prevalence rates, 34, 131

Eagles, J. M., 106
Early-onset depression (EOD)
  antidepressant efficacy, effectiveness, 91
  differential diagnosis, 82
  EAAT 1 levels, 635
  genetic factors, 281
  late onset depression vs., 82, 91, 111
  neurological trajectory considerations, 7
  neuronal pathophysiology, 632
  pathophysiology, 107
  patient self-esteem in, 91
  phenomenology of, 82
  white matter hyperintensities and, 259, 564
Eastman, George, 206, 211
Eating disorders, 67t, 348–349, 706
Edell, W. S., 458
Edland, S. D., 180t
Eisenbach, Z., 224
Electroconvulsive therapy (ECT)
  availability factors, 406–407
  complication risks, 413t
  consent process, 416
  continuation, maintenance of, 418–419
  for depression, 94
  for depression in dementia, 194
  for depression in hospice care, 524
  for depression in hospice care settings, 524–525
  for depression with Parkinson's disease, 301
  future research directions, 421
  for late-life bipolar disorder, 408–409
  for late-life depression, 407–408
  mechanism of antidepressant action, 407
  methodology
    algorithmic approach, 411t
    anesthetic agents, 415–416

  electrode placement, 410–412
  neuromodulation of, 419–420
  in neuropsychiatric disorders, 409–410
  for post-stroke depression, 258
  pretreatment medical assessment, 412–415
  relapse rates, prevention, 418–419
  side effects, 416–418
  stigma related to, 406, 410
EMBLEM (European Mania in Bipolar Longitudinal Evaluation
    of Medication) study, 110–111
Endogenous depression, 10, 67t, 255, 347
End-stage renal disease, 133
Enhancing Recovery in Coronary Heart Disease (ENRICH-D)
    Trial, 282
Epidemiologic Catchment Area (ECA) study, 106, 130, 135, 318, 533
Epidemiology of late-life mood disorders, 32–38
  depression assessments, 33
  future research directions, 20
  unipolar depression
    community service settings, 36–37
    medical settings, 35–36
    population representative samples, 34–35
    types of, 33–34
  U.S. life expectancy data, 32
Epilepsy
  carbamazepine and, 663
  depression in, 303, 304t
  mood stabilizers and, 666
  suicide risks, 211
Escitalopram
  for antidepressant-resistant depression, 369
  for depression in hospice care, 525
  for late-life anxious depression, 152
  MDD open-label trial, 145
  pharmacokinetics, 660t
Estradiol, and depression, 86
Estrogen
  adjunctive replacement therapy, 372–373, 657
  effects on aging brain findings, 8
Ethnicity. *See also* African Americans; Asian Americans;
    Hispanic adults; Non-Hispanic Whites
  atherosclerosis study, 274
  depressive disorders data, 271–272
  diabetes risk factors, 274, 282
  epidemiological depression studies, 167–168
  grief variations, 222–223
  Medicare antidepressant data, 171
  population data, 271–272
  social determinants of depression and, 167–168
  treatment response variability, in LLD, 716t, 719
Evidence-based practice (IOM definition), 11
Exercise. *See* Physical activity

Faces Pain Scale (FPS), 335
Facial Action Coding System (FACS), 335
Family therapy, 93
Fawcett, J., 371
Fedoroff, P., 255
Felbamate, 303
Figuel, G. S., 563–564
Finch, E.J.L., 367t
Fink, M., 81
First, Michael, 63
First, Michael B., 68t, 69
First-episode mania, 104
5-HT systems, 147
5HT2a serotonin receptor, 647

5-HTTLPR (serotonin transporter promoter gene) studies, 85–86, 146, 151, 165, 524, 615, 668, 682, 719
Flint, A. J., 367t
Fluoxetine
    for depression in dementia, 189t
    for depression in hospice care, 525
    for depression in nursing homes, 483t, 484t
    for late-life anxious depression, 152
    for pain conditions, 339
    pharmacokinetics, 660t
    for post-stroke depression, 258
    for sleep-depression disorders, 353
Fluvoxamine
    CYP1A2 metabolizing enzyme of, 657
    for late-life anxious depression, 152
    pharmacokinetics, 660t
Folate supplementation, 20, 22, 86, 90t, 375, 435t
Ford, D. E., 351
Formal care
    burdens of mood disorders on, 48–49
Framingham Heart Study, 169
Frances, Allen, 68t
Frasure-Smith, N., 274
Fredman, L., 242
Freud, Sigmund, 228, 230
From Discovery to Cure report (National Advisory Mental Health Council Workgroup), 9–10
Frontotemporal dementias, 106, 108, 298
Functional magnetic resonance imaging (fMRI)
    Alzheimer's disease study, 332
    and biomarkers
        bipolar disorder, 591–592
        late-life depression, 588–591
    BOLD functional MRI, 586–587
    BPD alterations in BOLD signal change, 594t
    future directions of, 592–593
    historical background, 586
    late-life anxious depression study, 589
Functional neuroimaging, 586–600

Galantamine, 373–374
Garre-Olmo, J., 180t
Gatekeeper models, of homebound depression delivery services, 536–537
General Health Questionnaire, 275
General linear mixed models (GLMMs), 705–706
General neurotic syndrome, 146
Generalized anxiety disorder (GAD)
    behavioral avoidance in, 150–151
    diagnostic hierarchy rule, 145
    MDD comorbidity, 146
    negative affect and, 148
    prevalence rates, 4
Genetic vulnerability, to late-life unipolar depression, 84–86
Genome-wide association (GWAS) methods, 5
Genomic research, 5–6
Geriatric Depression Scale (GDS), 185t, 375, 523, 533–534
Germain, A., 350
"Geropsychiatric" nursing, 492
Glasser, M., 114
Glial cell pathology, 633–635
Global Assessment of Relational Functioning Scale (GARF) (DSM-IV-TR), 70
Graff, M. J., 192t
Grief. See also Complicated grief syndrome
    of caregivers, 196
    chronic problematic grief, 221–222

cultural variations, 222
defined, 222
experience of C.S. Lewis, 220
gender variations, 223
from loss of loved ones, 221, 225
prolonged grief disorder, 170, 228
therapy intervention, 89
Gruenberg, Ernest M., 68t
Gum, A. M., 34, 230
Gustafson, Y., 193t
Guze, S. B., 228

Haggerty, R. J., 448
Haley, W. E., 242
Halgin, R. P., 458
Hamilton Depression Rating Scale (HAM-D), 130, 131, 184t, 259, 369, 524
Hannestad, J., 561
Harris, T. O., 168
Harwood, D., 210
Health and Retirement study (HR), 35, 272, 273f
Health Behavior Model, 458
Health Care Financing Administration (U.S.), 478
Healthcare for Communities (HCC)
    unipolar depression telephone survey, 34
Healthy IDEAS (Identifying Depression, Empowering Activities for Seniors) program, 540
Heart disease. See also Cardiovascular disease; Hypertension
    Baltimore DCA study, 273
    care recipient profile, 238
    collaborative care strategy, 51
    depression comorbidity, 35, 45, 87, 132, 274
        CBT therapy for, 391
        C-reactive protein risks, 678
        ECT treatment for, 413
        PST therapy for, 413
    depression mortality comparison, 42
    development predictions, 706
    ENRICH-D Trial, 282
    global mortality data, 4
    omega-3 fatty acids for, 434
    quality of life issues, 47
    smoking cessation recommendation, 323
    as SSD risk factor, 133
    suicide risks, 211
Helzer, J. E., 71
Hendricksen, M., 630t
Herr, K., 335
Herrmann, J. H., 259
Himmelhoch, J. M., 114
Hindi, F., 95
Hindu culture, grief practices, 222–223
Hippocrates, 347
Hirono, N., 187
Hispanic adults
    access to health care issues, 171
    depression diagnosis gap, 34–35
    depression epidemiology, 35
    grief practices, 222–223
    income-depression relation, 172
    levels of depression data, 167
    psychotherapy adaptions for, 396
    treatment response, 172
Hitchings, S. E., 224
HIV/AIDS
    suicide risks, 211
Holley, C., 261

Holtzheimer, P. E., III, 373
Home-based services and interventions, 532–541
  Administration of Aging services, 533–534
  barriers to detection in, 532
  care management models
    aging services network, 540
    home health care, 538–540
    mental health care, 540
    telephone, telehealth care, 540
  depression service delivery models
    gatekeeper model, 536–537
    integrated screening into routine care, 537–538
  depression treatments
    psychotherapy, 534–535
    telephone, telehealth psychotherapy, 535–536
  mobility restrictions of patients, 532–533
Hormone therapy, 372–373, 657
Horowitz, M. J., 228
Hospice care settings, late-life depression in, 516–526
  antidepressants, 524–525
  assessment scales, 521
  barriers to diagnosis, 518–519
  clinical manifestations, 519–520
  depression and advanced dementia, 525–526
  electroconvulsive therapy, 524–525
  future research directions, 526
  management of depression, 522–524
  non-major depression, 131
  patient wish to hasten death, 520–521
  prevalence of depression data, 517
  psychosocial interventions research, 522–524
  reasons for depressions treatment, 517–518
  spiritual pain of patients, 519–520
  Terminally Ill Grief for Depression Scale, 521t
Hot cognition, in depression, 611–612, 613–614
Household Telephone Survey of unipolar depression rates, 34
HPA axis. See hypothalamic-pituitary-adrenal (HPA) axis
Huang, X., 580
Huntington's disease (HD), 301–302
Hyman, Steve, 69–70
Hypericum perforatum (St. John's Wort), 434t, 437–438, 657
Hypertension
  A1166C polymorphism in, 720
  comorbidity factors, 338
  depression and
    Ayurvedic treatment for, 442
    cortisol levels, 280
    ECT treatment for, 413
    post-stroke depression model, 257f
    risk factors, 88f
  in nursing home residents, 478
  PET studies, 573
  quality of life issues, 47
  renal decline and, 657
  as risk factor for widowed people, 229
  vascular depression and, 82
  white matter hyperintensities and, 82
Hypochondriasis, 82, 210, 333, 443
Hypothalamic-pituitary-adrenal (HPA) axis
  cigarette smoking and, 278
  cognitive biomarkers and, 608–609
  description, 689–691
    overview, 689–691
  high-fat/high-sugar foods and, 278–279
  immune response and, 281, 676–677
  late-life depression and
    cognitive function, 694

  genetic factors, 696–697
  HPA dysregulation, 281, 676–677, 691–693
  mediators and moderators, 694–697
  medical comorbidities, 695–696
  pharmacotherapy, 693–694
  types of abnormalities, 691–692
  mood disorder implication, 146
  role in stress response mediation, 280
  SSRIs influences, 693–694
Hypothyroidism, 183t

Imipramine, 188t
Immune system
  alterations in depression
    assays of in vivo responses, 679
    dissociation between declines of innate immunity and
      inflammatory markers, 678
    inflammation, 677–678
    neuroimmune changes, 636–637
    nonspecific functional measures, 676
    stimulated cytokine production, 676–677
    viral specific measures, 678
  ayurveda influences on, 442
  caregiving and, 49, 240t, 243
  clinical moderating factors, 679–681
    activity and exercise, 680–681
    alcohol dependence, 680
    depression treatment, 679–680
    disordered sleep, 681
    smoking, 680
  complicated grief and, 228–229
  HPA dysregulation and, 281, 676–677, 691–693
  ICD-10 and, 63t
  inflammatory regulation of depressive symptoms, 681–682
  influences on central nervous system, 675
  positive emotions and, 226
  substance abuse and, 315
Improving Mood-Promoting Access to Collaborative Treatment
    (IMPACT) study, 11, 51, 171–172, 214, 465, 505, 508,
    538–539
Inflammation. See also Inflammatory markers
  biomarker research, 745–746
  enzymatic pathway alterations, 681
  gene polymorphisms, 682
  ICAM-1 mediator, 637
  increased IL-6 levels, 679
  links to depression, 275, 600, 681–682, 721
  measurement of, 593
  neuroendocrine factors, 720
  neuroinflammation markers, 600
  omega-3 fatty acids and, 434
  pathways studies, 6
  risk factors associated with, 675, 681
  systemic inflammatory responses, 6, 677
Inflammatory markers
  biological domains, pathways, 281, 450
  circulating levels of, 677
  in depression, 86–87, 261, 682
  dietary associations, 278–279
  HPA axis and, 677
  innate immunity and, 678
  in smoking, 680
Insomnia. See also Sleep disorders
  anxiety and, 25
  bereavement and, 229
  depression and
    depression predictability, 350–352

emotional relationships, 350
 major depression episode, 80
in depression in dementia, 177, 179
in *DSM-5*, 74
in pain disorders, 338*t*, 339
in Parkinson's disease, 300
as a psychiatric tridiagnostic factor, 356
psychotherapy treatment
 IBT/CBT, 354–355
 outcome on depression, 355
 prevention of depression, 355–356
as TCA side effect, 340*t*
Institute of Medicine (IOM)
 evidence-based practice definition, 11
 suicide prevention interventions, 213–215
Instrumental activities of daily living (IADL). *See also* Activities
 of daily living
 caregiver/care recipient trajectory and health, 238*f*
 cognitive IADLs, 666
 deficits and suicide, 212
 examples of, 47
 functional disability and, 730
 informal caregiver provision of, 237
Interleukin 6, 86–87
International Advisory Group for the Revision of *ICD-10* Mental
 and Behavioral Disorders, 61
International Classification of Diseases
 Clinical Modifications by nations, 61–62
 DSMs relationship to, 74
 focus of earlier editions, 61, 68
 non-major depression studies, 131
 variations 1–11 approval dates, 62*t*
International Classification of Diseases (ICD-9-CM), 62, 75
International Classification of Diseases (ICD-10)
 chapter listings, 64*t*
 chapter V, mental, behavior disorders outline, 65*t*
 dimensional model of depression, 81
 shortcomings of, 80–81
 U.S. implementation issues, 63
International Classification of Diseases (ICD-10-CM), 65*t*–67*t*
International Classification of Diseases (ICD-11), 63, 81
Internet-based interventions and telepsychiatry, 546–553
 advantages, disadvantages, dangers, 548–549
 common components, 540*t*, 549–550
 described, 547
 effects on mood disorders, 550–551
 future directions, 552
 for home-based services, 534–536, 540
 Internet effects on mood disorders, 550–551
 self-help without professional support, 547
 telepsychiatry effects on mood disorders, 551–552
Interpersonal psychotherapy (IPT)
 antidepressants with, 377, 591, 744
 for bereavement-associated depression, 230
 cognitive benefits in older adults, 609
 for complicated grief, 228
 depression care management vs., 145
 depression care management with, 90*t*, 93
 paroxetine combination trial, 376
Inventory of Complicated Grief, 228
Iowa Pain Thermometer (IPT), 335
IPT. See interpersonal therapy (IPT)

Jacoby, R., 107, 110–111, 114, 180t
Japan, suicide intervention studies, 215
Jarvis, E., 164
Jewish culture, grief practices, 222–223

Jones, G. T., 330
Jorge, R., 180t, 420
Judd, L. L., 129–130
Jururlink, D. N., 211, 277

Kamerow, D. B., 351
Kaplan, G. A., 165
Katon, W., 43, 48, 51
Katona, C.L.E., 367*t*
Katz, I. I., 482*t*
Kay, D.W.K., 109
Kellner, C. H., 408, 412
Kendler, K. S., 168, 274
Kendrick neuropsychological battery, 112
Kenney, B. A., 320
Khundakar, A. A., 629*t*–630*t*
Kleinman, A., 71, 276
Klerman, G., 109
Kohler, S., 563
Kohli, M. A., 5–6, 86
Kok, R. M., 367*t*
Kraemer, H. C., 71
Kraepelin, E., 104, 347
Krause, N., 165
Krauthammer, C., 109
Krishnan, K. R., 82, 107, 258–259, 561, 564
Kroenke, K., 540
Krueger, R. F., 71
Kuhl, E. A., 71
Kumar, A., 560, 580
Kunovac, J. L., 130
Kunz, M., 335–336
Kupfer, David J., 68*t*, 69, 347, 350

Lafferman, J., 367*t*
Late-life anxious depression (LLAD), 152, 154, 589
 HPA axis and, 689–697
Late-life bipolar disorder (LLBD) studies, 560–562, 566
Late-life depression (LLD). *See also* Depressive disorders;
 Hospice care settings, late-life depression in; Late-life
 depression (LLD), prevention strategies; Long-term care,
 depression and dementia in; Long-term care, depression in;
 Major depressive disorder; Post-stroke depression; Primary
 care settings, late-life depression in; Vascular depression
 adjunctive antipsychotic trials, 368*t*
 alterations in cerebral glucose metabolism, 597*t*
 associated factors, 85*f*
 biochemical changes, 86–87
 genetic vulnerability, 84–86
 medical comorbidity, 87–88
 psychosocial factors, lifestyle, 88
 structural brain abnormalities, 87
 bipolar disorder vs., 105
 cell death/cell proliferation markers, 635–636
 classifications, 81–82
 shortcomings of, 80–81
 cognitive biomarkers, specific effects
 chronic relapsing depression, 608–609
 comparative research, 609
 cognitive impairment, types and subtypes, 609
 complexities of, 18
 developmental stages, 449*f*
 differential diagnosis, 83–84, 84*b*
 diffusion tensor imaging studies, 566, 576–577
 disability risks, 36, 45, 47
 early detection, 50–51
 early-onset depression vs., 6, 79

Late-life depression (LLD) (*Cont.*)
  ECT for, 407–408
  factors in development of, 85*f*
  fMRI/biomarker studies
    default network mode, 590–591
    frontostriatal, frontolimbic circuitry, 588–590
  functional neuroanatomy of, using PET, 593–599
  HPA axis and, 689–697
    cognitive function, 694
    genetic factors, 696–697
    HPA dysregulation, 281, 676–677, 691–693
    mediators and moderators, 694–697
    medical comorbidities, 695–696
    pharmacotherapy, 693–694
    types of abnormalities, 691–692
  implications of psychoneuroimmunology on, 675–683
  male vs. female prevalence, 43
  management of, 88–94
    antidepressant medications, 20, 90–92, 90t
    assessment of reasons for, 88–89
    collaborative care programs, 51, 93–94
    combination therapy, 9
    intervention schema studies, 10–11
    physical treatments, 94
    psychotherapy, 92–93
    therapeutic interventions, 20, 51
    treatment strategies (summary), 96t
  medical burden of, 44–45
  molecular imaging in l, 572–582
  mortality and, 4, 43
  neuropathological markers in, 627–638
  neurovascular, neuroimmune changes, 636–637
  pharmacogenetics of, 643–650
  phenomenology of, 82
  recurrence rate data, 37
  research needs for, 23
  SES considerations, 50
  suicide risk factors, 44
  suicide risks, 210
  TMS potential use in, 419
  treatment response variability in, 714–733
Late-life depression (LLD), prevention strategies
  aims of, 448–449
  developmental stages of LLD, 449*f*
  effectiveness of
    indicated prevention, 453–454
    selective prevention, 453
    universal prevention, 453
  MDD cohort data summary, 450*f*
  preventative intervention
    indicated prevention, 452
    relapse prevention, 452
    selective prevention, 451–452
    universal prevention, 451
  staging and profiling LLD, 95, 448–454, 449–450
Latino culture, grief practices, 222–223
Lee, M., 224
Leventhal, H., 276
Levetiracetam, 303
Levin, F. R., 321
Levine, P. M., 106
Levy, R., 180t
Lewis, C.S., 220
Life course perspective
  Baltimore ECA study, 270–271
  on late-life depression, 164–165
    gender differences, 167

    patterns of social, environmental patterns, 166*f*
    social determinants of depression, 170–171
    socioeconomic status and, 168
  neurocognitive impairments, 609
  resilience promotion influences, 617
  stressful life events, 694
  suicide, 207, 213, 216
Lind, K., 187
Lindelof, N., 193t
Lindemann, E., 227, 228
Linear mixed-effects models (LMMs), 705–706, 708, 711
Lipsey, J. R., 255
Lithium
  age-related outcomes, 119
  for antidepressant-resistant depression,
    365–366, 367t, 379t
  with antidepressants, 91
  augmentation usage, 21, 91–92, 94, 154, 367t, 418
  BP MRS studies, 581
  for BPD treatment, 23–24, 105, 117
  contraindications of, 301
  declining renal clearance and, 655–656
  for dementia, 24
  efficacy research needs, 24
  interactions with other drugs, 23
  negative outcomes, 114, 118, 301
  older adult dosage adjustments, 663
  placebo-controlled trials, 365–366
  postictal agitation side effect, 417
  side effects, 24
  STAR*D open-label comparison, 369
  tolerability issues, 380
  toxicity of, 183t
Littbrand, H., 193t
Little, J. D., 409
LLD. See late-life depression
Longitudinal Aging Study Amsterdam (LASA),
    132–133, 145
Long-term care, depression and dementia in, 491–492
Long-term care, depression in, 477–493. *See also*
    Assisted living facilities; Nursing homes
  advanced dementia and, 525
  for borderline personality disorder, 23
  caregiver assistance in, 237–238, 242
  community-based studies, 130, 215
  facility presentation variations, 35
  minor to major depression conversion, 36
  National Long Term Care survey, 237
  nonpharmacological treatment, 488t–489t, 490–491
  pharmacological treatment
    antidepressant clinical trials, 482t
    antidepressant comparison trials, 484t
    clinical approach, 487
    clinical trials findings-adverse effects, 486–487
    clinical trials findings-efficacy, 481, 486
    open-label antidepressant trials, 483t
    regulatory considerations, 487, 490
  placement considerations, 238
  types of facilities, 477
Long-term care, suicide and, 491
Loranger, A. W., 106
Lund, D., 230
Lundquist, G., 114
Lung disease. *See* Chronic obstructive pulmonary disease
Luszczynska, H., 180t
Lyketsos, C. G., 180t
Lyness, J. M., 131–132

MacDonald, J. B., 114
MacFarlane, G. J., 330
Magai, C., 482*t*
Magee, J. C., 149
Magnetic resonance imaging (MRI). *See also* Functional
    magnetic resonance imaging
  fundamentals
    affective tasks, 587–588
    BOLD functional MRI, 586–587
    cognitive tasks, 587, 587*t*
    resting state, default mode network, 588
  historical background, 586
  human gene expression studies, 5
  vascular depression studies, 259–260
Magnetic resonance spectroscopy (MRS)
  for bipolar disorder, 578, 580–582
  clinical studies findings summary, 579*t*–580*t*
  geriatric/bipolar disorder studies, 578, 580–582
  for late-life depression, 577–578, 580–582
  neuroimaging studies, 5–6
  for neuropsychiatric disorders, 578
Magnetic seizure therapy (MST), 420
Major depressive disorder (MDD), 33–37. *See also*
    Antidepressant-resistant depression; Depressive disorders;
    Late-life depression
  addictive substance comorbidity, 318
  anxiety disorder comorbidity, 145
  burden of, 272
  as cardiovascular disease risk factor, 9, 44, 87, 88*f*, 270,
    273–274
  CIDI interview used for, 33
  classification, 81–82
    shortcomings of, 80–81
  cognitive biomarkers in, 606–617
  community-based studies, 270
  conceptual model of interactions, 46*f*
  criterion, 80b
  depression-pain syndrome, 330–331
  diabetes risk factors, 273–274
  diagnostic indications, 450
  epidemiology
    community service settings, 36–37
    medical settings, 35–36
    population representative samples, 34–35
    types of, 33–34
  escitalopram open-label trial, 145
  excess morbidity, mortality association, 273–274
  in *ICD-10-CM*, 67*t*
  lifetime prevalence, 273*f*
  and medical comorbidity (diagram), 282*f*
  minor depression conversion risks, 131–132, 132*t*
  mortality and, 273–274
  pathways linking medical illness, 275–281
    behavioral pathways, 278–279
    biological pathways, 279–281
    life course framework, 275
    psychological pathways, 276–277
    social pathways, 277–278
    stressors/psychological distress, 275–276
  PHQ-9 depression scale assessment, 36, 478
  in primary care settings, 501
  relapse/recurrence of, 37
  risk factors, 273
  SCID criteria, 228
  stress, resources, behavior and, 281–283
  symptom manifestations, 4, 129
  treatment adherence issues, 279

WHO 2020 projections, 273
Malhi, G. S., 89, 90
Mania Rating Scale, 114
Mania/manic syndromes. *See also* Bipolar disorder
  characteristics, 104
  cognitive impairments with, 104–105, 112
  "disinhibition syndrome" and, 108
  dysphoric mania, 111
  EMBLEM study, 110–111
  first-episode mania, 104
  in Huntington's disease, 301
  manic depressive reactions, 68
  medical conditions, drug treatment associations, 105
  Modified Mania Scale, 110–111
  in multiple sclerosis, 302
  prevalence rates, 106
  psychopathology of, 105–106
Manic depressive reactions (defined), 68
Mann, J. J., 210
Manor, O., 224
MAO inhibitors, 353. *See also* Brofaromine; Phenelzine;
    Tranylcypromine
Marital therapy, 93
Markov Chain Monte Carlo (MCMC) simulation, 706
Martire, L. M., 51
Marty, M. A., 211
Mathias, J. L., 224
Mattis Dementia Rating Scale, 259
McCaffery, M., 335
McCrae, C. S., 350
McDonald, W. M., 560, 563
McInnes, E., 317
MDD. *See* Major depressive disorder
Meals on Wheels program, 239
Medical burdens
  of bipolar disorder, 45
  of depression, 44–45
  mechanisms
    behavioral, 45–46
    biological, 45
    psychological/cognitive, 46–47
    social, 47
  in nursing home residents, 478
Medical comorbidity. *See also* Substance abuse comorbidity
  adherence to treatment and, 459*t*
  with bipolar disorder, 24, 38, 109–110, 118
  caregiving burden and, 49
  in depression in primary care settings, 501–503
  depression-pain syndrome, 330–331
  description, 270
  electroconvulsive therapy and, 406
  in hospice care patients with depression, 517–518
  HPA axis, late-life depression, 695–696
  late-life depression links, 87–88, 272–276, 280–283, 479,
    501–503, 714
  in late-onset bipolar disorder, 743
  with non-major depressions, 134–135
  polypharmacy and, 463
  with stroke, 297
  in subsyndromal depression, 134–135
Medicare
  depression in beneficiaries, 35, 48
  description/coverage data, 34
  device payment limitations, 420
  eligibility criteria expansion, 537
  ethnic antidepressant data, 171
  health care costs data, 48

Medicare (*Cont.*)
  home health care study, 533–534
  homebound patient "care plan," 539
  homebound patient definition, 533
  hospice care definition, 516
  nursing home reimbursement issues, 487, 493
  Outcome and Assessment Information Set, 537–538
  Part D enrollment, 239
  patient spending data, 48
  prescription drug plan addition, 462
  standardized OASIS, 537
  U.S. certified home health care agencies, 539
Medicare Current Beneficiary Survey (MCBS), 34
Meeks, T. W., 130–131
Melancholia, 83
  antidepressants for, 90–91
  cerebrovascular disease and, 296
  cholesterol connection, 86
  as *DSM-IV* subclassification, 83
  DSM V establishment recommendation, 81
  as late-life depression factor, 85*f*
  sleep disorders and, 347
  sleep issues with, 347
Melancholic depression, 83, 90, 94–95, 96*t*, 676–677, 680, 691
Mellon, S., 7
Memantine, 374
Menopause, 8
Methylphenidate
  acceleration trials, 364
  adjunctive uses, 91, 370, 379*t*, 380, 599, 648, 719
  for antidepressant-resistant depression, 371, 379*t*
  for depression in hospice care, 524
  hospice-care controlled-study, 524
  placebo-controlled study, 370–371
  specific recommendation for, 195
Meyers, B. S., 370
Mianserin, 353, 660*t*–661*t*
Miech, R. A., 165
Migliorelli, R., 180t
Migneco, O., 187
Migraine headache, 273, 416–417, 551
Miguel-Hidalgo, J. J., 628*t*
Milnacipran, 152, 338
Mindfulness-based approaches, 156, 441
Mini Mental Status Examination (MMSE), 409, 563
Minimum Data Set (MDS), 478
Minor depression (MinD). *See also* Dysthymic disorder
  characteristics of, 88
  CIDI interview used for, 33
  community-based study, 130
  conversion to major depression, 36, 96
  diagnostic criteria, 83
  DSM-IV definition, 130
  DSM-IV-TR definition, 34
  hospital-based prevalence, 35
  medical comorbidities, 134
  need for research, studies, 22
  prevalence rates, 131
  in primary care settings, 501
  relapse/recurrence of, 37
Mirtazapine
  for antidepressant-resistant depression, 365, 379*t*
  for depression in nursing homes, 483*t*
  pharmacokinetics, 661*t*
Mixed states, in bipolar disorder, 111
Mixed states (dysphoric mania), in bipolar disorder, 111
Mizrahi, R., 180t

Mock, P., 92
Moclobemide
  for depression in dementia, 188*t*
  pharmacokinetics, 661*t*
Modafinil, 371–372
Modified Mania Scale, 110–111
Moellentine, C., 410
Molecular imaging, 572–582. *See also* Positron emission
    tomography
  diffusion tensor imaging studies, 565–566
    benefits of, 6
    description, 565–566
    late-life bipolar disorder, 566
    late-life depression, 566, 576–577
    in vascular depression, 260–262
  magnetic resonance spectroscopy
    for bipolar disorder, 578, 580–582
    clinical studies findings summary, 579*t*–580*t*
    description, 577–578
    geriatric/bipolar disorder studies, 578, 580–582
    for late-life depression, 577–578, 580–582
    neuroimaging studies, 5–6
    for neuropsychiatric disorders, 578
  quantitative PET data analysis, 574–576
Monamine manipulation, 614–615
Monk, T. H., 352
Monoaminergic antidepressants, 187
Montgomery-Asberg Depression Rating Scale (MADRS), 185*t*,
    366, 419
Mood Disorders Work Group (for *DSM-V*), 72
Mood stabilizers. *See also* Lithium
  in borderline personality disorder, 105
  cognitive enhancement and, 112–113
  co-prescriptions of, 649
  interactions with other drugs, 23
  neuroprotective effects of, 118
  pharmacokinetics of, 663–664
  SAMe interactions with, 437
  in suicide prevention, 24
Morbidity
  bipolar patients, 119
  BPD research directions, 24
  caregiving and, 246
  depression factors, 84, 271, 273–274, 275, 502, 675
  diagnostic challenges, 25
  drug selection association, 299, 353
  ECT and, 407–408
  generalized anxiety disorder, 4
  hormone replacement risks, 86
  ICDs and, 61, 64*t*
  medical burdens associated with, 44–45, 49
  mood disorders research, 9–12
  nursing homes and, 243
  SES and, 728
  suicide-related, 215
  tobacco and, 317
Morris, J. C., 256
Mortality
  anhedonia influence, 274
  antipsychotic medication risks, 9, 45
  Black women and diabetes, 272
  burdens associated with, 43–44
  of caregivers, 243–244
  Census Bureau BP nonsuicide data, 115–116
  cerebrovascular disease, 116
  global heart disease data, 4
  grief practices, cultural variations, 222–223

MDD association, 273–274
men/antidepressant medications, 43
non-major depression and, 134
Motenko, A. K., 245, 246
Mourning among older adults, 222–224
Mrazek, P. J., 448
MRS. *See* magnetic resonance spectroscopy
Mueller, S. G., 187, 414
Mukherjee, S., 408
Mulsant, B., 254, 258
Multi-Ethnic Study of Atherosclerosis, 274
Multiple sclerosis
depression in, 302–303
mimicking of depression in dementia, 183t
Myocardial infarction (MI)
C-reactive protein links, 678
depression mortality comparison, 271
ECT and, 413
post-MI depression, 35, 44, 132–133, 274
donepezil treatment, 380
SSRIs treatment, 667
SSD association, 134
stroke patient comparisons, 255

Narrow, W. E., 70
National Advisory Mental Health Council Workgroup, 9–10
National Center for Complementary and Alternative Medicine (NCCAM)
National Center for Health Statistics (NCHS), 62–63
National Comorbidity Study, 318
National Comorbidity Study-Replication (NCS-R), 34, 145, 167
National Comorbidity Survey, 165, 272, 273f
National Consensus Development Conference on Caregiver Assessment, 249
National Institute of Mental Health (NIMH)
Alzheimer's disease, consensus conference, 180
drug development research support, 9
mission of, 3
project group study decisions, 5
Provisional Diagnostic Criteria for Depression of AD, 181t
RDoC project, 4–5
research/intervention support, 10–12
National Institutes of Health (NIH), 3
Navajos, grief practices, 222–223
Nefazodone
antidepressant receptor affinity, 299t
CYP3A4 activity inhibition by, 657
pharmacokinetics, 661t
sleep treatments, 353
Negative affect (NA), 148, 151, 350, 489t, 608, 611, 615–616
Negative affect syndrome, 146
Nelson, J. C., 91, 369, 483t
Nemeroff, C. B., 147
NEO-Personality Inventory, 210–211
Neurobiology/neuroscience, integration of studies with, 5–7
Neurochemical hypotheses, of sleep-depression relationship, 354
Neurocognitive biomarkers, 607, 609, 614, 617
Neuroimaging. *See* Computed tomography; Functional neuroimaging; Positron emission tomography; Structural magnetic resonance studies; Structural neuroimaging
Neuronal pathology, 632–633, 638
Neuropathic pain, 331, 334, 337–339
Neuropathological markers, in late-life depression, 627–638
brain postmortem studies, MDD findings, 628t–631t
cell death and cell proliferation, 635–636

glial cell pathology, 633–635
neuronal pathology, 632–633, 638
neurovascular, neuroimmune changes, 636–637
Neuropsychiatric disorders
dementia symptoms, 178–179
ECT treatment for, 409–410
genomic research, 5
magnetic resonance spectroscopy for, 578
in nursing home residents, 478
omega-3 fatty acids for, 436
Neurosyphilis, 183t
Neurotransmitters
age-related changes, 85f
functional neuroimaging studies, 632
pain-related, 331–332
Nicotine dependency, 278
NIMH Strategic Plan, 4
Nimodipine
adjunctive uses, 91–92, 262, 376
for antidepressant-resistant depression, 376
for vascular depression, 96t
NMD. *See* non-major depression
Nociceptive pain, 331, 339
Non-Hispanic Whites, 271–272, 490
Nonlinear mixed-effects models, 658
Non-major depression (NMD), 129–138. *See also* Minor depression
clinical trials, 137
comorbidity, 134–136
distinctive categories of, 129–130
epidemiology, community-based studies, 130–131
health outcomes, 133–134
illness course, 131–133, 132t
neurobiology research, 136
prevention, 137
in primary care settings, 501
successful aging and, 136
treatment strategies, 136–137
Non-REM sleep, 348–350, 354. *See also* Sleep disorders
Nonsteroidal antiinflammatory drugs (NSAIDs), 340t, 657, 682
Non-tricyclic antidepressants, 90t
Noradrenergic (excitatory) system, 146, 152, 157
Norepinephrine (NE) pathways, 146–147
Norton, M. C., 167
Nortriptyline
for antidepressant-resistant depression, 379t
for depression in dementia, 194
for depression in nursing homes, 482t, 484t, 485t
for late-life depression, 92–94
for pain conditions, 339
pharmacokinetics, 661t
for post-stroke depression, 257–258
for recurrent major depression, 21
Numeric Rating Scale (NRS), 335
Nunes, E. V., 321
Nursing homes (NHs), late-life depression in
assessment/detection, 479–480, 481t
delivery of mental health services, 492–493
federal legislation for, 478, 493
prevalence, risk, consequences, 479
psychiatric disorders, 478, 491–492
resident profile, 477–478
treatment, nonpharmacological, 488t–489t, 490–491
treatment, pharmacological
antidepressant clinical trials, 482t
antidepressant comparison trials, 484t

Nursing homes (*Cont.*)
   clinical approach, 487
   clinical trials findings-adverse effects, 486–487
   clinical trials findings-efficacy, 481, 486
   dose/duration clinical trials, 485t
   open-label antidepressant trials, 483t
   regulatory considerations, 487, 490
Nutrition, Aging, and Memory in Elders (NAME) Study, 37

O'Brien, J., 187
Obsessive-compulsive disorder
   behavioral therapies, 156
   brain changes in, 147
   negative affect and, 148
   PET use in, 593
   psychological vulnerabilities in, 152
   TMS use in, 419
O'Connor, D. W., 408
Oksuzyan, A., 224
Olanzapine
   adjunctive uses, 21, 369, 418, 525
   age and clearance data, 658
   for antidepressant-resistant depression, 369, 370
   CYP1A2 metabolizing enzyme of, 657
   for depression in hospice care, 525
Oldehinkel, A. J., 261
Olin, J. T., 89
Omega-3 fatty acids, 374, 379t, 434, 435t, 436–437
Omnibus Budget Reconciliation Act (OBRA-87), 478
Openness to Experience (OTE) factor (NEO-Personality
   Inventory), 210–211
Opioid analgesics
   abuse potential, 323, 334–335, 725
   cognitive toxicity risks, 182
   historical use background, 376
   mechanisms of action, 725
   mimicking of depression in dementia, 183t
   palatable food consumption and, 279
   pharmacist's use input, 525
   possible neuropsychiatric side effects, 340t
O'Reardon, J. P., 419
Ostroff, R. B., 369
Outcome and Assessment Information Set (OASIS, Medicare),
   537–538
Oyama, H., 215

PACE (Program for All-Inclusive Care for the Elderly), 239
Pain (in older adults). *See also* Comorbid pain disorders
   age-associated brain changes, 331–332
   assessment of, 335–337, 336t
   chronic malignant pain, 331
   depression-pain syndrome, 330–331
   effect of age on perception of, 331
   epidemiological measurement considerations, 330
   idiopathic pain, 337
   neuropathic pain, 331, 334, 337–339
   nociceptive pain, 331, 339
   significant neurotransmitters, 331–332
   treatment modalities
     nonpharmacologic, 339–340
     pharmacologic, 338–339
     psychiatric evaluation, 337–338
Pain Assessment in Advanced Dementia (PAINAD), 336–337
Panel on Persistent Pain in Older Persons (American Geriatrics
   Society), 329, 330
Panic disorder, 33, 145–148, 152, 156, 551
Paranoid schizophrenia, 106

Parker, G. B., 81, 83, 90
Parkinson's disease
   comorbid with depression, 299–301
   ECT and, 409
   mimicking of depression in dementia, 183t
   neuropsychiatric illness and, 135
   NMD association, 133
   TMS use in, 419
Paroxetine
   for depression in dementia, 189t
   for depression in hospice care, 525
   for depression in nursing homes, 482t, 484t
   for pain conditions, 339
   pharmacokinetics, 661t–662t
Patel, V., 71
Patient Protection and Affordable Care Act, 510
Patten, C. A., 320
PEARLS (Program to Encourage Active and
   Rewarding Lives for Seniors), 11–12, 540
Peptic ulcer, suicide risks, 211
Periventricular hyperintensities, 259–260, 562–563
Personalizing interventions, 9–10
PET. See positron emission tomography
Petkus, A. J., 154
Petrides, G., 408
Pharmacodynamics
   alterations in older adults, 89
   brain-related changes, 656
   drug interactions, 667
   markers, 643
     additional markers, 648
     5HT2A, 647
     5HTTLPR, 647–648
   side effects in older adults, 666–667
   SSRIs, 665–666
Pharmacogenetics of late-life depression, 643–650
   issues in, 649–650
   other markers, 648–649
   pharmacodynamic markers, 647–648
     additional markers, 648
     5HT2A, 647
     5HTTLPR, 647–648
   pharmacokinetic markers
     CYP2D6, 304t, 643–646, 656–657
     P-glycoprotein (ABCB1, MDR1), 646–647
Pharmacokinetics
   age-associated physiological changes and
     absorption, 656
     distribution, 656
     excretion, 657
     metabolism, 656–657
   antidepressants, 658, 659t–662t
   antipsychotics, 658, 663
   benzodiazepines, 664
   described, 657–658
   markers
     CYP2D6, 304t, 643–646, 656–657
     P-glycoprotein (ABCB1, MDR1), 646–647
   metabolism, 656–657
   mood stabilizers, 663–664
   new drug formulations, 664–665
Phase shift hypothesis, of sleep-depression relationship, 350
Phenelzine, 353, 377
Phenytoin toxicity, 183t
PHQ-2 (Patient Health Questionnaire-2), 538
PHQ-8 (Patient Health Questionnaire-8)
   depression scale, 34

PHQ-9 (Patient Health Questionnaire-9) depression scale, 36, 478, 538
Physical activity
  antibody response promotion, 680–681
  antidepressant comparison, 90t
  cross-sectional study findings, 439–441
  depression prevention study, 454
  efficacy/effectiveness of, 90t
  outcomes in depression, 21, 46, 95
  patient education programs, 340
  quality of life and, 270, 282
  randomized trials findings, 137
Physician-assisted suicide, 518
Pincus, Harold Alan, 68t
Pindolol, for antidepressant-resistant depression, 372
Plato, 347
Polsky, D., 274
Polysomnographic research, 347, 348f. See also Sleep disorders;
  Sleep-depression relationship
Porter, F. L., 332
Positive affect (PA), 148, 151, 180, 181t, 350, 489t, 617
Positron emission tomography (PET)
  brain regions/cerebral glucose metabolism measures, 597t
  functional neuroanatomy of LLD
    midlife depression comparison, 595
    mood/cognitive networks of treatment response, 596
    neural circuitry of depression, 593, 595
  functional neuroanatomy of LLD, treatment response
    midlife depression comparison, 595
    neural circuitry of depression, 593, 595
  historical background, 593
  in late-life depression, 572–573
    mood/cognitive networks of treatment response, 595
  molecular imaging
    beta-amyloid imaging, 599
    dopamine system, 598–599
    serotonin system, 596–598
  quantitative PET data analysis, 574–576
  sleep studies, 349, 353–354
Post, F., 104, 109, 114
Postherpetic neuralgia, 331
Postictal agitation (PIA), from electroconvulsive therapy, 417–418
Post-stroke depression (PSD)
  definition/clinical features, 254–255
  diagnostic criteria issues, 254–255
  mechanism (cause), 256
  model, 257f
  prevalence, 255
  prognosis and course, 256–257
  risk factors, 255–256
  treatment, 257–258
Poststroke mania, 296
Posttraumatic stress disorder (PTSD), 228, 229, 419
Powell, J., 317
Pramipexole, 300–301
Preadmission Screening and Resident Review (PASRR), 478
Prefrontal cortex (PFC)
  affect regulation role, 588
  age-associated brain changes, 332
  bipolar disorder and, 591–592, 594t
  cold cognition and, 612
  in depression with anxiety, 146–147
  diffusion tensor imaging studies, 260, 577
  fMRI studies of, 589, 594t
  functional processes of, 587t
  hot cognition and, 607

HPA and, 280, 691
  inflammatory regulation and, 682
  major depression and, 581
  MRS studies, 579t
  neuropathological studies focus, 632
  suicidal behavior and, 210
  white matter hyperintensities and, 260–261
Premorbid depression, 178
Present State Examination, 255
Prevention of late-life depression (LLD)
  aims of, 448–449
  developmental stages of LLD, 449f
  effectiveness of
    indicated prevention, 453–454
    selective prevention, 453
    universal prevention, 453
  MDD cohort data summary, 450f
  preventative intervention
    indicated prevention, 452
    relapse prevention, 452
    selective prevention, 451–452
    universal prevention, 451
  staging and profiling LLD, 95, 448–454, 449–450
Prevention Research Centers' Health Aging Network (PRC-
  HAN), 11
Prigerson, H. G., 228
Primary care settings, late-life depression in, 500–510
  IMPACT study findings, 505, 508
  importance of primary care settings, 500–501
  interventions for depression, 505–506
  medical comorbidities, social strains, 501–503
  patient expectations, values, beliefs, priorities, 503–504
  patient-centered future directions, 509–510
  patient-centered mental health care, 508–509
    collaborative care approaches, 502, 505–506
    treatment-centered vs., 507t
  physician perspectives, 504–505
  PRISM-E study findings, 505
  PROSPECT study findings, 505
  RESPECT-D study findings, 505
  simple, complicated, complex problems, 502, 503t
  spectrum of depression in, 501
Prince, M. J., 88
Problem adaptation therapy (PATH), 534–535
Problem-solving therapy (PST), 148
  comparison with other therapies, 395t
  efficacy/effectiveness of, 90t
  evidence base, 393
  for homebound patients, 534–535, 538
  intervention overview, 392
  for late-life anxious depression, 154
  pros and cons, 393
  steps of, 155f
Program for All-Inclusive Care for the Elderly (PACE), 239
Prolonged grief disorder, 170, 228
PROSPECT (Prevention of Suicide in Primary Care Elderly:
  Collaborative Trial), 51, 94, 214, 464
Protective ("resilience") factors research, 7, 8
Prudic, J., 408
PSD. See post-stroke depression
Pseudopsychopathic syndrome, 105
Psychogeriatric Assessment and Treatment in City Housing
  (PATCH) (Maryland), 536–537
Psychological autopsy (PA) study, of suicide, 207, 209–210
Psychological mechanisms, of medical burdens, 46–47
Psychological pathways, linking medical illness and depression,
  276–277

Psychoneuroimmunology, of depressive disorders, 675–683
  alterations in depression
    assays of in vivo responses, 679
    clinically relevant alterations, 675
    dissociation between declines of innate immunity and
      inflammatory markers, 678
    inflammation, 677–678
    neuroimmune changes, 636–637
    nonspecific functional measures, 676
    stimulated cytokine production, 676–677
    viral specific measures, 678
  clinical moderating factors, 679–681
    activity and exercise, 680–681
    alcohol dependence, 680
    depression treatment, 679–680
    disordered sleep, 681
    smoking, 680
  immunological alterations, 676–679
  inflammatory regulation of symptoms, 681–682
Psychotherapy treatment, 390–399. See also
    Cognitive behavioral therapy; Problem-solving therapy
  adaptations for late-life populations
    cognitive impairment, 397
    cultural considerations, 396
    disabilities, 396–397
  for antidepressant-resistant depression, 365
  for anxious depression, 154–157
  based on unified models, 154–157
  in collaborative care settings, 51
  in combination therapy, 9, 89, 95, 171
  group treatment, 11, 321
  for insomnia, 354–356
  interpersonal psychotherapy, 228, 230,
    376–377, 393–394
  in late-life depression
    comparison chart, 395t
    efficacy, effectiveness of, 90t, 92–93
    family therapy, 394
    management strategies, 92–93
    maximizing treatment fidelity, 397
    as preferred treatment, 390–391
    reminiscence therapy, 394
    supportive therapy, 394
  for non-major depression, 136–137
  pharmacotherapy vs., 94
  psychodynamic psychotherapy, 230
  for sleep-related depression, 354–355
  transdiagnostic treatments, 144
Psychotic depression, 83
Psychotropic medications
  adverse effect potential, 194, 655
  age-related difficulties with, 23, 656–657
  cognitive enhancement with, 112–113, 113f
  gait disturbance issues, 380, 666
  lithium difficulties, 366
  menopause and, 8
  mortality-related risks, 9
  nursing home abuse, 478
  pharmacokinetics of, 657
Pyne, J. M., 47

Quality adjusted life years (QALYs), 47
Quality of life (QOL)
  bipolar disorder issues, 23, 113
  burden of mood disorders on, 47
  GAD/MDD influences on, 4
Quantitative PET data analysis, 574–576

Quetiapine
  for antidepressant-resistant depression, 369
  for depression in hospice care, 525
  for late-life anxious depression, 154

Rabins, P., 114, 560
Rabkin, J. G., 371
Raines, George, 68t
Rajkowska, G., 628t–630t, 629t
RDoC project. See Research Domain Criteria (RDoC) project
Recipients of care, characteristics, 238
Reciprocal-altruism theory, 245
Regenold, W. T., 45
Regier, Darrel A., 68t, 69, 70
Reifler, B. V., 80
Relational Processes and DSM-V: Neuroscience, Assessment,
    Prevention, and Treatment (Beach), 70
REM sleep, 347–350, 352–355. See also Sleep disorders
Reminiscence therapy, 394
Renal ulcer, suicide risks, 211
Repetitive transcranial magnetic stimulation (rTMS), 262
A Research Agenda for DSM-V (Kupfer, First, Regier), 69
Research Domain Criteria (RDoC) project (NIMH), 4–5
Research priorities, in late-life mood disorders, 17–27
Ressler, K. J., 147
Reynolds, C. F., III, 72, 93, 352–353
Rifat, S. L., 367t
Risperidone
  adjunctive use, 418
  adverse effects, 666
  age-related metabolism issues, 656, 658–659
  for antidepressant-resistant depression, 369–370
  metabolism study, 646
  renal clearance issues, 655–656, 663
Robins, E., 228
Robinson, R. G., 180t, 258
Roose, S. P., 483t
Ropinirole, 300–301
Rosendahl, E., 193t
Rosenquist, J. N., 169
Roshanaei-Moghaddam, B., 43
Roth, M., 104, 114
Roy-Byrne, P. P., 321
Rutherford, B., 368t, 369
Ryan, J., 43

Sackeim, H. A., 408
Safety signals, 150–151
SAMe (S-adenosyl-L-methionine)
  for antidepressant-resistant depression, 374–375, 379t
  description, 437
  vs. placebo, 435t
Satlin, A., 109
Scheltens, P., 562
Schizoaffective disorder, 84b, 106
Schizophrenia
  hospitalization rates, 49
  neuropsychiatric illness and, 135
  in nursing home residents, 478
  paranoid schizophrenia, 106
  TMS use in, 419
Schizophrenic reactions (defined), 68
Schneider, L. S., 89
Schulz, R., 43
Secondary mania, 105
Selective Optimization and Compensation model
    (of successful aging), 154–155

Selective serotonin reuptake inhibitors (SSRIs). *See also* Citalopram; Escitalopram; Sertraline
adjunctive uses, 339, 364–366, 369, 372, 379
adult cancer patient study, 524–525
for alcohol withdrawal, 322
for antidepressant-resistant depression, 365
for anxiety disorders, 148–149, 380
brain region activity findings, 595
cross-sectional observational studies, 679
for dementia, 299
for depression in hospice care, 524
for depression in long-term care, 480
double-blind trial findings, 369–370
drug interactions, 667
efficacy/effectiveness of, 90–91, 90t
gait issues, 191
HPA axis influences of, 693–694
intolerability risks, 154
for late-life anxious depression, 152–153
for late-life MDD, 148
new formulation, 664
for nursing home patients, 486
for pain conditions, 339
pharmacodynamics of, 665–666
pharmacokinetic differences among, 658
for post-stroke depression, 258, 297
response rate comparisons, 258
SAMe comparison, 435t
side effects, 486–487, 666–667
St. John's wort comparison, 438
STAR*D outpatient study findings, 718
trait markers, 616
tricyclic antidepressants comparisons, 94, 300
UK population-based study, 191
usage data, 480
Self-esteem
causative/contributory factors, 97
in depressed patients, 79, 83, 85f
in EOD patients, 91
interventions for, 92–93, 96t
Selye, Hans, 280
Sequenced Treatment Alternatives to Relieve Depression (STAR*D) study, 172, 365, 369, 375, 377–379, 649–650, 718
Serotonin system, 146–147, 157, 356, 596–598, 697. *See also* 5-HT systems; 5HT2a serotonin receptor
Serotonin transporter promoter gene (5-HTTLPR) studies, 85–86, 146, 165, 524
Serotonin-norepinephrine reuptake inhibitors (SNRIs). *See also* Atomoxetine; Desvenlafaxine; Duloxetine; Milnacipran; Venlafaxine XR
adjunctive uses, 364
brain interactions, 682
criteria for choosing, 194
for late-life anxious depression, 152
for persistent pain, 331, 338, 524
pharmacodynamic markers, 648
for post-stroke depression, 297
tolerability issues, 486
Sertraline
for depression in dementia, 189t, 190t
for depression in hospice care, 525
for depression in nursing homes, 482t, 483t, 484t, 485t
for late-life anxious depression, 152
for pain conditions, 339
pharmacokinetics, 662t
for post-stroke depression, 258, 297

Shanahan, M. J., 165
Sheeran, T., 540
Sheffrin, M., 368t, 369
Shulman, K., 109
Si, X. H., 628t
Siedlecki, K. L., 149
Signal hyperintensities (SHs), in BPD, 108–109
Simonsen, E., 70
Sirovatka, P. J., 70
Slater, E., 104
Sleep disorders. *See also* Insomnia; Sleep-depression relationship
from alcohol withdrawal, 323
in Alzheimer's disease, 180, 181t
circadian rhythms (process C) and, 349
complicated grief and, 228, 229
cytokine involvement, 87
dangers of, 116
DSM-5 and, 74
ICD-10-CM coding, 67t
late-life depression and, 79
in MDD/GAD, 146
NA/5-HT system deregulation and, 147
non-REM sleep, 348–350, 354
pain and, 334–335, 336t, 337–340
polysomnographic research, 347, 348f
REM sleep, 347–350, 352–355
slow-wave activity and, 349–350
Sleep-depression relationship
insomnia and depression
depression predictability, 350–352
emotions, 350
psychotherapy treatment, 354–355
sleep continuity, architecture
age/gender influences, 352–353
shortened REM latency, 352
sleep regulation theories
cholinergic-aminergic hypothesis, 348–349
chronobiological models, 349–350
neurochemical hypotheses, 354
treatments
antidepressants, 353
sleep-wake manipulations, 353–354
Sleep-Wake Disorders Work Group (for *DSM-V*), 72
Smetana, G. W., 413
Smith, M. E., 225
Smoking prevalence, in older adults, 317
Snowdon, J., 107
SNRIS. See serotonin-norepinephrine reuptake inhibitors
Social determinants of depression, 164–172
social integration: unifying framework, 168–171
across the life course, 170–171
bereavement, depression nosology, 169–170
disruptions in social connections, 169
social networks and support, 169
socioeconomic, demographic factors
gender, 167
race/ethnicity, 167–168
socioeconomic status, 168
theoretical models, 164–165, 166f
treatments, 171–172
Social pathways, linking medical illness and depression, 277–278
Social phobia
behavior therapy for, 156
cognitive avoidance strategies, 150
comorbidities, 145
development of, 152
diagnostic criteria, 25

Social phobia (*Cont.*)
    Internet-based therapies, 551
    MDD study findings, 145
    negative affect association, 148
Social rhythm model, of sleep-depression relationship, 350
Socioeconomic status (SES)
    associated risk factors, 229
    burden of depression and, 50
    cross-sectional associations, 133
    depression behavioral pathways and, 278
    depression management and, 522
    hormone therapy outcomes, 372
    importance of assessment of, 168
    Medicare variability and, 171
    physical health association, 165, 240t
    psychological health measures, 241t
    risks of depression and, 88
    treatment predictors, 715f
Somatic Presentations of Mental Disorders (Dimsdale, Xin,
        Kleinman, Patel), 71
Somatization disorder, 333
Somatoform disorder not otherwise specified, 333
Somatoform disorders, 65t, 71, 333–334, 339
Sorpvatka, P. J., 70
Spencer, P. G., 458
Spicer, C. C., 106
Spinal cord injury, suicide risks, 211
Spitzer, Robert L., 68t
Spousal loss and bereavement, 167, 169, 221
SSD. See subsyndromal depression
SSRIs. See selective serotonin reuptake inhibitors
St. John's Wort (*Hypericum perforatum*), 434t, 437–438, 657
Standardized mortality ratios (SMRs), 43–44
Stanford Self-Management Program (for chronic pain), 340
STAR*D study. See Sequenced Treatment Alternatives to Relieve
        Depression (STAR*D) study
Starkstein, S. E., 180t, 187
State biomarkers, 607–608, 610–611, 615–616
Steffens, D. C., 35, 107, 258, 591
Stein, D. J., 228
Stimulants, for antidepressant-resistant depression, 370–371
Stirling County study, 167
Stone, K., 109, 112, 114
Stroke. *See also* Post-stroke depression
    B12/B6 supplement studies, 86
    comorbidities, 45, 87, 145
    NMD association, 133
    in nursing home residents, 478
    risk factors
        with BP, 107
        cerebrovascular disease, 296
        with depression, 44
        spousal caregiving, 242
        with SSD, 133
        suicide, 277
    "silent strokes" in BP patients, 108
    vascular depression and, 19
Stroop Color-Word Interference, 261
Structural magnetic resonance studies
    cortical structures
        frontal lob, 560
        generalized atrophy, 560
        other regions, 561
        temporal lobe, 560–561
    subcortical structures, 561–562
Structural neuroimaging, 559–567. *See also* Computed
        tomography; Structural magnetic resonance studies

bipolar disorder abnormalities, 108–109
diffusion tensor imaging studies, 565–566
    benefits of, 6
    description, 565–566
    late-life bipolar disorder, 566
    late-life depression, 566, 576–577
    in vascular depression, 260–262
Hoptman's argument in favor of, 19
white matter hyperintensities, 260, 261t
    deep intensities, 562–563
    periventricular hyperintensities, 562–563
    subcortical gray matter hyperintensities, 563–564
Structured Clinical Interview for DSM-IV (SCID), 228, 517,
        533–534
Structured Clinical Interview for *DSM-IV* for depression, 517
Subcortical ischaemic depression, 82
Substance Abuse and Mental Health Services Administration
        (SAMHSA) report, 11
Substance abuse comorbidity, 315–324
    alcohol addictions, later life, 316–317, 318
    benzodiazepines, 317–318
    bipolar disorder, mania, 115, 118
    complicated grief, 228
    consequences, 319–320
    late-life depression co-occurrence, 318, 319f
    MDD, PTSD, anxiety, insomnia, 316
    misuse, abuse, dependence (defined), 228
    pain association, 334
    psychiatric disorders, 106
    sedatives/hypnotics, 317
    sleep disorders, 348
    tobacco use, 317, 318
    treatment considerations, 320–324
Substance-induced mood disorder, 84
Subsyndromal depression (SSD), 5, 33, 129
    African American risk factors, 132
    CIDI interview used for, 33
    community-based study, 130
    conversion to major depression, 36
    DSM-IV-TR description, 34
    medical comorbidities, 134–135
    meta-analysis of interventions, 51
    neuropsychiatric illness and, 135
    prevalence rates, 131
    in primary care setting, 35
    in primary care settings, 501
    prognosis success, 132–133
    relapse/recurrence of, 37
    research needs, 22
    suicide ideation and, 134
Subthreshold depression (SubD), 129
    community-based study, 130
    neuropsychiatric illness and, 135
    in primary care settings, 501
Suicide, physician-assisted, 518
Suicide/suicide ideation, in older adults
    antiepileptic drugs and, 303
    bereavement risk factors, 221
    BPD and, 115
    coping strategies (with ideation), 211
    in depression in hospice care setting, 519
    ECT treatment for, 408
    epidemiology of, 207
    hopelessness and, 276–277
    long-term care and, 491
    morbidity factors, 215
    mortality and, 44

neuropsychiatric illness and, 135–136
prevention strategies, 212–215
  barriers to prevention, 213
  indicated approaches, 213–214
  selective approaches, 214–215
  universal approaches, 215
psychological autopsy studies, 207, 209–210
rates, by age and gender
  global rates, 207*f*
  U.S. rates, 208*f*
risk factors associated with, 207–208
  Axis I: psychopathology, 208–209, 209*f*
  Axis II: personality, coping style, 209–210, 209*f*
  Axis III: physical health, illness, 209*f*, 210
  Axis IV: social context, 209*f*, 211–212
  Axis V: functioning, disability, 209*f*, 212
subsyndromal depression and, 134
thought suppression and, 149
Sultzer, D. L., 187
Survey on Income and Program Participation (NFCA & FCA), 237
Symptomatic mania, 105
Systemic lupus erythematosus, 211

Tai-chi, 433*t*, 438–439, 680–681
Tappen, R. M., 193*t*
Taylor, M. A., 81
Taylor, W. D., 577
TCAs. See tricyclic antidepressants
Teachman, B. A., 148–149
TEAM care programs, 51
Telephone and telehealth psychotherapy, 535–536, 540. *See also*
  Internet-based interventions and telepsychiatry
Telepsychiatry. *See* Internet-based interventions and
  telepsychiatry
Temporal lobe epilepsy, suicide risks, 211
Ten Have, T. R., 484*t*
Teri, L., 192*t*
Terminally Ill Grief for Depression Scale, 521*t*
Terminally ill patients. *See* Hospice care settings, late-life
  depression in
Tess, J. D., Jr., 413
Testosterone
  age-related declining levels, 372, 721
  low levels and depression, 86, 720
  replacement therapy findings, 372–373
Tetrabenazine, 301
Theory of Reasoned Action, 458–459
Thioridazine, 183*t*, 666
Thomas, A. J., 629*t*
Thought suppression, 149–150, 153*f*
Three-City study, 167
Thyroid (triiodothyronine), for antidepressant-resistant
  depression, 366, 368
Tiagabine, 303
Tohen, M., 109
Trait biomarkers, 607–608, 610–611, 614–615, 615–616
Transcranial magnetic stimulation (TMS). *See also* Repetitive
  transcranial magnetic stimulation
  in ECT, 419–420
  FDA approval for, 420
  for late-life depression, 94, 419
Transdiagnostic treatment, 154, 157
Transtheoretical Model, 458
Tranylcypromine, 353
Trappler, B., 483*t*, 484*t*
Treatment development research, 9

Treatment Initiation and Participation Program (TIP), 466–467
Treatment response variability, in late-life depression, 714–733
  biological factors
    age, 716*t*, 718
    gender, 716*t*, 718
    race/ethnicity, 716*t*, 719
  clinical factors, 716*t*–717*t*, 723
    comorbid anxiety, 725
    neuropsychological factors, 726–727
    pain, 727–728
    sleep impairment, 727
    substance abuse, 725–726
    suicidality, 724
    symptom severity, current episode duration, 724
    treatment history, 723–724
  environmental psychosocial factors, 717*t*, 728
  findings, research implications, 732–733
  functional disability, 730
  interactions of factors, 731–732
  intrapersonal psychosocial factors, 717*t*, 728–729
    education, 728
    personality disorders, traits, 728–729
    self-esteem, 729
    socioeconomic status, 728
  neuroendocrine factors, 720–721
    HPA axis, 720
    inflammation, 721
    testosterone, 721
    thyroid hormones, 721
  neuropsychological factors, 726–727
  pain, 727–728
  pharmacogenomic factors, 719–720
    angiotensin II receptor, vascular Type 11 A1166C
      polymorphism, 720
    brain-derived neurotrophic factor Val66Met polymorphism,
      577, 648, 719–720
    DAT1 VNTR 10/10 polymorphism, 719
    serotonin transporter gene promoter region polymorphism,
      719
  physical environment, 730
  physical illness, 722–723
  social support, 729–730
  stressful life events, 730
  structural, functional brain abnormalities, 721–722
Treatment-resistant depression, 371, 374, 379, 420, 458. *See also*
  Antidepressant-resistant depression
TRIAD (Training in the Assessment of Depression)
  intervention, 537–539
Tricyclic antidepressants (TCAs)
  for dementia-related depression, 191, 299
  for depression in hospice care, 524
  efficacy/effectiveness summary, 90–91, 90*t*
  for late-life anxious depression, 154
  mimicking of depression in dementia, 183*t*
  for pain conditions, 339
  for persistent pain relief, 331
  possible neuropsychiatric side effects, 340*t*
  for post-stroke depression, 297
  for sleep-depression disorders, 353
  social determinants for receiving, 171
  SSRI comparison, 258
  SSRIs, discontinuation comparison, 94
Trimipramine, 662*t*
Tsoh, J., 212
Tsopelas, C., 629*t*
Tumor necrosis factor alpha, 86–87
Type I bipolar disorders, 105

Type II bipolar disorders, 105

Uncinate fasciculus (UF) white matter tract, 591
Undifferentiated somatoform disorder, 333
Unipolar depression. *See* Major depressive disorder (MDD)
United States (U.S.)
  adult life expectancy data, 32
  aging population data, 271
  Alzheimer's prevalence data, 177–178
  baby boomer cohort data, 206
  benzodiazepine use, 317
  Brandy Handgun Violence Prevention Act, 215
  CAM usage data, 432
  complicated grief rates, 229
  depression, economic costs, 48
  disability prevalence data, 47
  epidemiological depression studies, 167–168
  ethnic diversity data, 271
  home-based care data, 532
  ICD Clinical Modification, 62–63
  increasing pain complaints, 329
  informal caregiving data, 237–238
  Medicare certified home health care agencies, 539
  2010 age data, 4
  widowed adults data, 221
Unützer, J., 12, 47, 48
U.S. Department of Health and Human Services, 62

Vagal nerve stimulation (VNS), 94, 420
Vahia, I. V., 136
Van der Velde, C. D., 114
Van Marwijk, H. W., 367*t*
Van Praag, H. M., 81
Vascular dementia
  antidepressant comparison trial, 484*t*
  causative for dementia, 177
  comorbidities, 135, 608
  depressed mood in, 84b, 187
  differential diagnosis, 84
  frontal white matter lesions in, 187
  MMSE evaluation, 481
  MRI evaluation, 480
  open-label antidepressant trial, 483*t*
Vascular depression, 81
  definition/clinical features, 258–259, 296–297
  description, 81–82
  mechanism (causes), 259–261
  prognosis and treatment, 262
  relapse prevention, 91
  risk assessment, treatment, 19
  TMS treatment benefits, 94
  treatment
    antidepressants, 96*t*
    TMS, rTMS, 94, 262
Vascular depression hypothesis of late-life depression, 6, 19,
  81–82, 178, 187
Venkatraman, T. N., 578, 580
Venlafaxine
  for antidepressant-resistant depression, 365
  for depression in dementia, 189*t*
  for depression in hospice care, 525
  for depression in nursing homes, 484*t*
  for pain conditions, 338–339
  pharmacokinetics, 662*t*
  for sleep-depression disorders, 353

Venlafaxine XR, 152
Verbal Descriptor Scale (VDS), 335
Vietnam Twin Study of Aging, 147–148
Vigabatrin, 303
Vink, D., 167
Visual impairment, NMD association, 133
Vitamin B6 supplementation, 86
Vitamin B12 supplementation, 86, 90*t*
Vogel, G. W., 354
Vuorilehto, H., 132

Waern, R., 212
Wagner, G. J., 371
Wagner Chronic Care Model, 540
Wallace, R. B., 370–371
Wang, L., 589–590
Ward, L., 224
Weaver, D. D., 458
Webb, W. B., 350
Weiner, M. F., 180t, 337
Wells, K. B., 129
Wertham, F. L., 106, 114
Wetherell, J. L., 154
Whalley, L. J., 106
White matter
  of cortical/subcortical regions, in LLD, 627
  diffusion tensor imaging study, 591
  disease of, 8
  electroconvulsive therapy and, 411*f*
  frontal, in vascular depression, 261*f*
  neuropathological study findings, 87
  of the prefrontal cortex (PFC), 635
  uncinate fasciculus tract, 591
White matter hyperintensities, 260, 261*t*
  deep intensities, 562–563
  periventricular hyperintensities, 259–260, 562–563
  subcortical gray matter hyperintensities, 563–564
White matter lesions (WML), 87, 561–562
Whyte, E. M., 254, 258
Widiger, T. A., 70
Wilamoska, Z., 156
Wilkinson, D., 366
Williams, C. L., 193*t*
Williams, Janet B., 68*t*
Wirz-Justice, A., 350
Wittchen, H-U., 71
Wittig, R. M., 334
Wolkowitz, O. M., 7
Women's Health Across the Nation Study, 8
World Health Organization (WHO), 42
  disability definition, 42, 47
  major depression 2020 projection, 273
  suicide rates, patterns, 207
Wu, J. C., 353, 591

Xin, Y., 71

Yoga, 432, 433*t*, 436*t*, 438–439, 442
Young, R. C., 560
Yuan, Y., 576
Yurgelun-Todd, D. A., 592

Zisook, S., 81, 136
Zonisamide, 303
Zung Depression Rating Scale, 185*t*